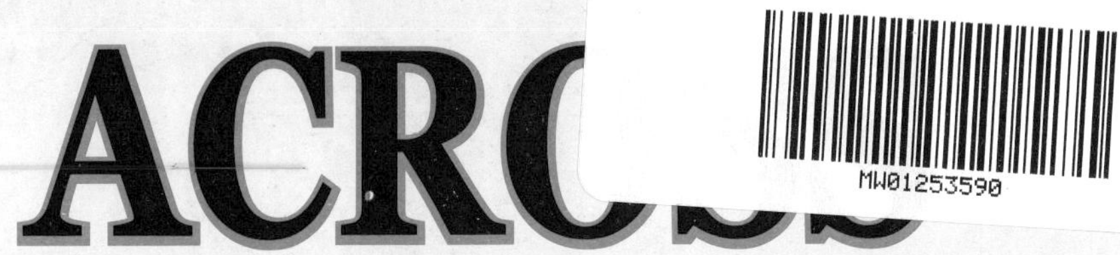

ACROSS

A complete Review of Short Subjects

Volume

Part A

- Skin
- Radiotherapy
- Radiodiagnosis
- Anaesthesia
- Nuclear Medicine

Eighth Edition

Authored by

Saumya Shukla DNB Radiodiagnosis
Assistant Professor
Nizam's Institute of Medical Sciences
Hyderabad, India

Anurag Shukla MS MCh (Orth), UK

Edited and Procfread by

Monika Shukla
Vibha Shukla

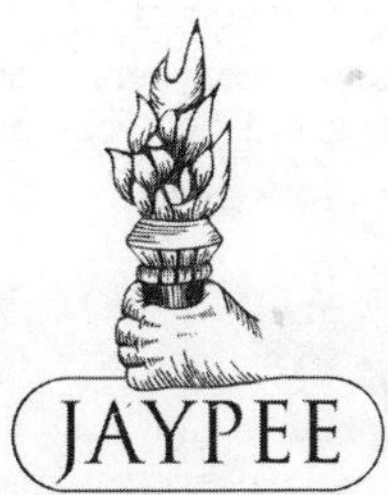

JAYPEE BROTHERS MEDICAL PUBLISHERS (P) LTD

New Delhi • London • Philadelphia • Panama

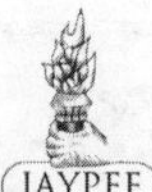

Jaypee Brothers Medical Publishers (P) Ltd

Headquarters
Jaypee Brothers Medical Publishers (P) Ltd
4838/24, Ansari Road, Daryaganj
New Delhi 110 002, India
Phone: +91-11-43574357
Fax: +91-11-43574314
Email: jaypee@jaypeebrothers.com

Overseas Offices

J.P. Medical Ltd
83, Victoria Street, London
SW1H 0HW (UK)
Phone: +44-2031708910
Fax: +44 (0)20 3008 6180
Email: info@jpmedpub.com

Jaypee Medical Inc
The Bourse
111, South Independence Mall East
Suite 835, Philadelphia, PA 19106, USA
Phone: +1 267-519-9789
Email: joe.rusko@jaypeebrothers.com

Jaypee Brothers Medical Publishers (P) Ltd
Bhotahity, Kathmandu, Nepal
Phone: +977-9741283608
Email: Kathmandu@jaypeebrothers.com

Jaypee-Highlights Medical Publishers Inc
City of Knowledge, Bld. 237, Clayton
Panama City, Panama
Phone: +1 507-301-0496
Fax: +1 507-301-0499
Email: cservice@jphmedical.com

Jaypee Brothers Medical Publishers (P) Ltd
17/1-B, Babar Road, Block-B, Shaymali
Mohammadpur, Dhaka-1207
Bangladesh
Mobile: +08801912003485
Email: jaypeedhaka@gmail.com

Website: www.jaypeebrothers.com
Website: www.jaypeedigital.com

A Complete Review of Short Subjects (Vol-1)

Eighth Edition: 2014

ISBN : 978-93-5152-345-1

Printed at Sanat Printers, Kundli

Not only this book, my whole life is dedicated to

"Bhagwan Ratneshwar, my Mother and Father"

Preface to the Eighth Edition

We are thankful for your reviews that has given us a fresh impetus to completely change this book in a more systematic way.

In this edition, the entire book has been revised, with a view to eliminating errors, incorporating suggestion of readers, updating concepts and discarding material that is no longer relevant. Our aim was to update all subjects according to recent available text. For convenient reading *subject has been divided into theory and MCQ portion and further subdivided into chapters and sub-chapters; according to their topics.* In this way the book has been kept concise while remaining as up to date and accurate as possible. Our major goal was to make this book *more interesting and user-friendly, with a substantial reduction in overall size of the subject.* To achieve this goal the book has been rigorously edited involving their amalgamation, division, or deletion. This has been put to effect without loss of crucial information but with gain in conciseness and clarity. We have kept the book succinct and to the point. The job that was no mean feat has become possible only because of the best endeavours of our team.

Many MBBS students do not have a good background in these subjects. This examination-oriented book is written with these students in mind. The *language is simple, explanations clear and presentation very systematic.* Our commitment to simplicity is total! This book will help you overcome the fear of these subjects. Topics, which usually confuse the students, are explained in greater detail. This text will help you learn faster and enjoy it more! Stress is on understanding as well as memorization. It is intended that every topic should be approached in a pragmatic and flexible manner.

This book is an important text for Postgraduate Entrance Exams. Your choice of a book can mean success or failure. Because today you need a book, that can help you streak ahead of competition and succeed. No one knows more about your needs than us. It is a tall claim, but it is true!

Phenomenon of Contradiction (POC)

I think the time has come to make you realize the importance of the **phenomenon of contradiction (POC)** in medical preparatory exams. You all must understand, that medical science is a dynamic (ever changing) and relative science which is made-up of innumerable number of research papers from different part of world (some of them contradicting each other and with their own most common, most preferred and best, etc). And each topic has been explained in books of various specialties (like a topic about kidney is explained in books of nephrology, urology, radiodiagnosis, genitourinary imaging, nuclear medicine, oncology, radiotherapy, medicine, surgery, anatomy, physiology and so on) giving their own shades to the topic focusing more on their aspect of that topic; and not to mention about numerous authors of each subject.

So when a book by an author (many times even Harrison) says anything, it is not always an absolute truth, if it is against the basic broad concept of that topic. So be very cautious before blatantly remarking any answer wrong on the basis of single line written in one book. And try to avoid amending answers on the basis, of one British/American/French research paper until and unless it is a ground breaking/Nobel prized research paper because most of the times you even do not know the statistical significance of that paper.

Your standard reference/textbooks tell you the extract of statistically significant research papers (most of which are paid review papers comparing the contradictory papers about that topic and few new statistically significant research papers). So leave this cumbersome responsibility of which paper to include/believe or exclude/not to believe on reference books.

In nut shell, **never try to believe an answer on the basis of journals (freely available on internet) when you are getting a logical answer in your reference textbooks.** Because most of the PGMEE questions are concept (not research) based.

We have elaborately explained this phenomenon in few selected answers, which were controversial/wrong according to some reviews. In last 12 years (initial 6 years in CROSS) we have explained few of these questions at least 6 times but the answer always remained same. It is not always possible to elaborate all answers to such a huge extent but believe us research done to find a perfect fitting answer is always far more extensive and exhaustive and many times include reading hundreds of pages and spending weeks of time for getting one perfect line.

Knowledge with Purpose: Why, How, What Algorithm

Knowledge without purpose is only a useless collection of words. So before attempting any question, always follow the algorithm of why, how, and what, i.e. why this question has been asked?, how it is going to make me a better clinician? and what have I learnt while finding the correct answer? After following this approach you would realize that most questions are based on very basic concepts of medical science used to differentiate various diseases. And this process of giving **purpose to your learning** would never allow you to forget the concept, making your remembering easy.

Never restrict your imagination by thinking that only purpose of reading is to pass PGMEE. Instead, always think that how this information makes me a better, safer clinician. Believe me, a student who approaches the exams in this way always gets success, whatever the pattern of examination maybe because purpose of all examinations is only and only this.

This book has helped students to secure good ranks in various patterns of entrance exams including **AI, AIIMS, PGI, DNB, JIPMER, CMC, AFMC, AMU and various state PGME exams for last 14 years.** So, do not worry about the pattern of NEET and its conducting body (presently DNB) because this book incorporates the latest text and 20 year questions about most important topics in a sequential manner.

May 21, 2014

Dr Anurag Shukla
Dr Saumya Shukla
Dr Siddharth Dixit
Dr Khushi Shukla

Preface to the First Edition

"Try to achieve what you like, otherwise you have to like what you achieved".

Friends, have you ever given your few valuable minutes to think about the reasons of being successful (or unsuccessful) in PGMEE.

What I feel, that this success is an art which not only requires a lot of grey matter but also needs – **an intense will to succeed, a lot of devotion, a positive attitude and above all a firm determined constant effort in right direction with proper strategy.**

Now question arises that what is the proper strategy?

And in most simple words – **"The only part of your knowledge, which is retained between your two ears, is going to help you in your exams."**

- So do not waste your very precious time in reading worthless incomprehensible unretainable guides or books.
- Be to the point in remembering things.
- Let your confusions clear by repeated revisions, before exams.
- Reading how many times is more important than reading how much?
- Knowing few things about every topic and everything about few topics is important aspect of your preparation.

I have kept all these things in my mind while writing this book. **This book provides at least three to four times revision of almost each and every important topic in a single reading. And with every repetition the topic gets more concise and more lucid.**

I have worked a lot, to make this book **easily retainable**, which you will realize as you proceed further with the book.

In this book there is collection of **21 years solved papers of AI, AIIMS and PGI PGMEE.** All answers have been referenced from the most recent and standard textbooks available. Relevant questions of JIPMER, AMU, Kerala, UP, Tamil Nadu, Karnataka, MP, West Bengal, Rohtak, CMC Vellore, Delhi, Rajasthan, Bihar, Jharkhand, MAHE are also solved.

Kindly let me know your opinion and send me your invaluable suggestions to further improve this book and make it more readable and enjoyable.

I know you are going to fight in the toughest of battleground!

Best of luck.

Saumya Shukla

Acknowledgments

"To Bhagvan Ratneshwar"

At the very outset, I fail to find adequate words, with limited vocabulary at my command, to express my emotions to 'Dear God', whose eternal blessings, divine presence, and masterly guidance helps us to fulfill all our goals.

It is very difficult to find a true Guru in this materialistic world. But I am lucky and I fail to find words to express my emotions to "Swami Swayambodhanand Sarawasati" (Swami Ji) for his colossal and beatific spiritual cosseting, without which I would never have been like this.

I will always remain obliged and grateful to my teachers Prof OP Singh, MS, FICS, MAMS; Prof VD Sharma, MS, FICS, Prof Vineet Sharma, MS, FICS, Dr Ashish Mahendra, MS, MCh, FRCS, Orthopaedics Department, KGMC, Lucknow, Prof KD Khare Retd HOD, AFMC, Pune and Dr RK Singh, MS, D Orth for their inspiration and encouragement, which gave succour and strength to my thoughts and mapped my way to find a modus operandi for myself.

Sometimes it is not easy to express your emotions in words especially when you have to say thanks to your parents for their constant undemanding love, dedication, sacrifice, inspiring guidance, affectionate encouragement and never ending enthusiasm; without which this book would not have seen the light of the day.

An ostentatious use of word will not be sufficient to express my heartiest thanks to Dr SK Dikshit, Mr LN Dikshit, Dr (Mrs) Arti Shukla (MD, Obs and Gynae), Dr Smita (RIMS) and Dr Sneha Dikshit (AMU), Dr Harish Dikshit, Dr VN Shukla, Dr Shraddha Shukla, Smt Kamla Devi, Mr PS Shukla and Mr Dev S Shukla, Mr Sujit Kumar Mishra, Aditi and Kriti Tripathi for their meticulous efforts during the making of this book. Their valuable and critical suggestions, constant inspiration and encouragement, instinctive corrective measures, tireless efforts, unstinted cooperation and sentimental support throughout have made this marathan task a smooth journey.

It is hard to envisage how it could have happened without the assiduously deligent and ingenious editing effort and proof reading of Dr Monika, Mrs Vibha Shukla, Mr VS Shukla. And infact this book would never have been like this without the expert technical consultations and dexterous work of Mr Sayeed and Mr Saleem and their team at Compsphere.

It would be a sacrilege if I do not mention the names of my friends, whom I always find with me in every filed of life.

- Dr Sunil Kumar Paltan (Asst Prof Ortho, Safai)
- Dr Sachin Awasthi, MS Ortho, KGMC
- Dr Saurabh Agarwal, MS Ortho, KGMC
- Dr Mukul Singh, MD Ortho, KGMC
- Dr Harish Ghoota, MS Orthopaedics, KGMC
- Dr Ankur Das, MS Orthopaedics, KGMC
- Dr Nitin Joshi, MS ENT, KGMC
- Dr Sandeep Tripathi, MD Pediatrics, LHMC, New Delhi
- Dr Suneel Chamoli, MD Psychiatry, KGMC
- Dr Sharad Chandra, DM Cardiology, AIIMS
- Dr Anil Kumar Singh, MD, Medicine MAMC, New Delhi
- Dr Jai Jag Tambe, SR, Pediatrics, LHMC, New Delhi
- Dr Chitwan Dubey, MS Obs and Gyne, Grants, Mumbai
- Dr Ambuj, MS General Surgery (Pune)
- Dr Chander Shekher Kumar, MS, Ophtha, AIIMS
- Dr Parul Kakkar, Dr Gaurav Mittal
- Dr Rohit Jain, MD Patho, Ahmedabad
- Dr Vineet Kumar, MD Psychiatry, PGI Chandigarh
- Dr Prajna Latika
- Dr Anurag Yadav, MD Pediatrics
- Dr Gopal Singh, MS Ortho, KGMC
- Dr Pradeep Pandey, MS Ortho, KGMC
- Dr Rudra Pratap Singh, SR Orthopaedics, GTB, Delhi
- Dr Atul Jain, MS Orthopaedics, KGMC
- Dr Shaleen Verma, MS Orthopaedics, KGMC
- Dr Abhishek Manu
- Dr Sandeep Buratodi, MD Radiology, KGMC
- Dr Sandeep Rai, MS Gen Surgery, GSVM
- Dr Ashish Gupta, MD Radiology, KGMC
- Dr Vipin Gupta, MS Gen. Surgery
- Dr Nasir Ahmed, BRDMC, Gorakhpur
- Dr Gunjan Das Agarwal, MD Radiology, KGMC
- Dr Anubhav Pandey, MD Microbiology, AIIMS
- Dr Sandhya Mishra, DNB, Obs and Gynae, Mumbai
- Dr Vikas Mathur, NRSMC
- Dr Arijit Mitra, NRSMC
- Dr Gunjan Raghuvanshi, MD Patho, Agra
- Dr Nilanjana Gosh
- Dr Avneet, KGMC, Dr Gopal Singh, GSVM
- Dr Athar Mohammad, KGMC

- Dr Shobhna Singh, KGMC, Lucknow
- Mr Rajpal Singh
- Mr Inder Mohan, Mr Sumit Solanki
- Mr Ananad Singh
- Mr Rajan Singh
- Mr Pranav, Mr Ravi

When it comes to expressing the emotions, I feel hopelessly inarticulate to Dr Abu Hatim A. Rashid, MS, SKIMS, MCh Pediatrics Surgery KGMC, Dr Sheeba Sarvat, Dr Shafat MD, Pediatrics, SKIMS, Srinagar (JandK) and Dr Mozzam Jah, Dr O. P. Gupta, MS Ortho, Dr Arif Kamal MS Ortho, Dr Arvind Kumar, KGMC, for their excellent constructive evaluation, humour at the time of depression and assistance at each and every step of our work.

We are greatly indebted to many individuals who helped with the preparation of this book. And we would like to express our gratitude to those who were especially helpful- Dr Mudit Khanna, MS Ortho, Dr Sandeep Buratodi, SR Radiodiagnosis Sri Chitra Institute, Dr Athar SR Oncology KGMC, Dr Javed MS Optha., Dr Parthiv Desai, DM Neurology, KGMC, Dr Devangi Desai, Dr Mohit Dhingra MS Ortho, Dr Vandana Dhingra MD, Nuclear Medicine, Dr Atul Dhawan MS Ophtha, Dr Gaurav Anand Mishra, MS Ophtha., Dr Pallavai Chaudhary MS Ophtha. and Dr Deepak Chaudhary (ELMC).

It gives me great pleasure to thank Dr Farzana Mahdi (Director Academics), Prof Jayant Bajpai, Prof RP Agarwal, Dr Shakeel A Quidwai and Dr MP Singh (Associate Professor), Dr AN Mishra, Dr Sohail Ahmad and Dr Farid Mohammad (Assistant Professor), Dr Sanjeev Kumar, Dr Amir Khan, Dr Firoz Ahmad, Dr Rakshit, Dr Yasir Ali Khan, Dr Fahad-ul-Islam, Dr Mayank Chauhan, Dr Sudheer Rajauria and Dr Deepak Chaudhary (Orthopaedic Resident, EMLC and Hospital, Lucknow), without whose support and constructive suggestions this edition could hardly have been undertaken.

We thank Shri Jitendar P Vij (Group Chairman) and Mr Bhupesh Arora (Associate Director Sales and Marketing M/s Jaypee Brothers Medical Publishers (P) Ltd, New Delhi, India for their thoroughly professional approach. Their constant interest and input have had a significant impact on the final structure of this book. It has been a pleasure to work with an individual who constantly offered wise and superb skilled suggestions. And at last but not the least, I am thankful to Mr. Inder Mohan, Mr Sumit Solanki, Mr Pranav, Mr Rajkumar, Mr Shadab, Mr Manish and Mr Ravi Sharma for their extremely diligent efforts.

We are grateful to the readers of the previous edition. Suggestions from students around the country have been most helpful in the formulation of this edition. We look forward to receiving similar input in the future. We hope that anyone with an idea, suggestion, or criticism regarding this book will feel free to contact us.

Such comments are always welcome and I solicit additional corrections and criticism, which maybe addressed to us at- dr_anurag_ortho@yahoo.co.in, dr_saumyadikshit@yahoo.com, siddharth_dikshit@yahoo.com.

From the Publisher's Desk

We request all the readers to provide us their valuable suggestions/errors (if any)

at: ***jaypeemcqproduction@gmail.com***

so as to help us in further improvement of this book in the subsequent edition.

Contents

PART A

VIII. Orthopaedics OR.1161 - OR.1488

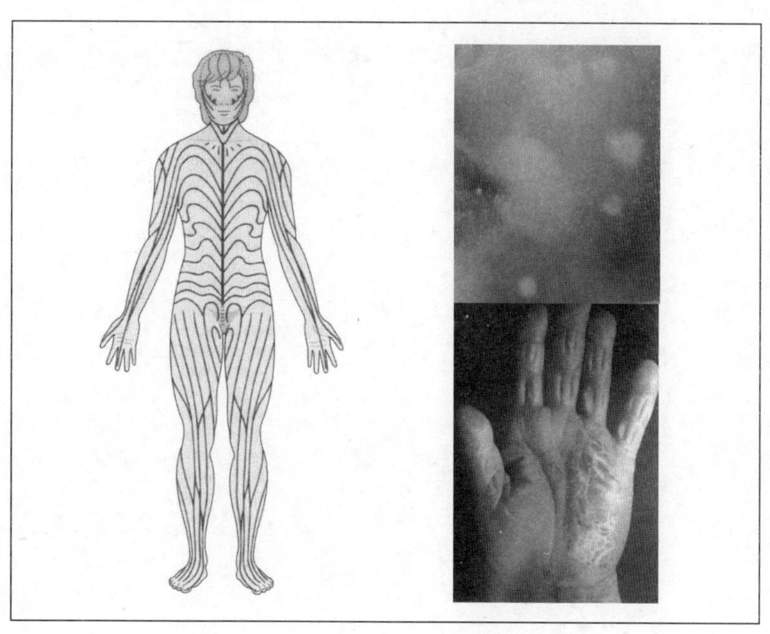

Dermatology
(Skin & Venereal Diseases)

1 GENERAL ANATOMY & APPENDAGEAL DISORDERS

Structural Morphology of Skin Epidermis

- The epidermis is a continually renewing, ***stratified squamous epithelium***Q that keratinizes and gives rise to derivative structures (pilosebaceous units, nails & sweat glands) called appendages.
- Intercalated among the **keratinocytes** in epidermis are the ***immigrant cells- melanocytes and Langerhans cells – and Merkel cells***Q. The melanocytes & langerhans cells migrate into the epidermis during embryonic development while merkel cells probably differentiate in situ.

Epidermal Cells

I. **Keratinocytes :** The **keratinocyte** is an ectodermally derived cell that ***constitutes 95% of the epidermal cells. Keratin filaments are a hallmark of keratinocytes & other epithelial cells***Q. The filamentous cytoskeleton of all mammalian cells comprises: *actin, tubulin and intermediate filaments*. There are 6 types of intermediate filaments: **Keratins** in epithelial cells (keratinocytes); **neurofilaments** in neurones; **desmin** in muscle cells; **peripherin** in peripheral cells; **vimentin** in mesenchymal cells; and **glial filament acidic protein (GFAP)** in glial cells. Keratonocytes move from basement membrane to skin surface forming 4 layers during transit.

II. **Melanocytes: Pigment producing cells** (melanocytes) develop from precursor cells k/a **melanoblasts**, which emerge from ***neural crest cells***Q and migrate to skin, developing hairfollicle, choroid & iris.

- ***Melanocytes are located in the epidermial basal layer (stratum basale or germinativum)***Q, and project their dendrites into epidermis where they transfer **melanosmes** (melanin packed in membrane bound orgenellae) to keratinocytes, which, in turn contain the majority of cutaneous pigment. *36 keratinocytes per melanocytes* giving rise to ***epidermal melanin unit***.
- Melanocytes account for 5-10% of cells in stratum basale and produce two forms of melanin: brown/black **eumelanin** and yellow/red **pheo-melanin** from aa tyrosine with help of copper containing tyrosinase, which protect from UV radiation.
- Number of melanocytes in skin is same regardless of the degree of racial pigmentation. It is the type of melanin pigment, rate of pigmentation and their distribution that differs.
- Unlike keratinocytes, melanocytes do not have desmosomes, but have long branding dendritic projections that transport melanin to the surrounding cells.

III. **Merkel (Tastzellen) cells**: Originate from epidermal keratinocytes in situ or from stem cells of neural crest origin and are located amongst basal keratinocytes mainly in tactile areas of glabrous/hairy skin, anal canal, labial epithelium, sweat glands & taste buds.

- Merkel cells are clustered near unmyelinated sensory nerve endings to form **touch spots (domes/corrpuscles)** or **hair discs** or **Iggo discs** at the bottom of rete ridges.

IV. **Langerhan's cells:** Are also *dendritic cells* like melanocytes but *free from pigment* and are *dopa negative* & *found within the Malphigian layer* rather than in basal layer.

- Langerhan's cells are derived from reticuloendothelial system and exhibit a unique motion k/a *dendrite surveillance extension and retraction cycling habitude **(d SEARCH)*** characterized by rhythmic extension & retraction of dendritic process between intercellular space among keratinocytes. *Topical dinitrofluorobenzene* l/t greater d SEARCH motion and a more efficient antigen sampling through scanning of wider area. L_H cells then leave the epidermis & migrate via lymphatics to regional lymph node. In paracortical region of lymph node these are k/a **interdigitating reticulum cell**.
- L_H cells, like melanocytes, have a lobulated nucleus, clear cytoplasm, and well developed ER, GC and lysosome. But they differ in lacking premelanosomes or melanosomes and in possessing a characteristic **rod- or racquet shaped Birbeck granules** representing subdomains of endosomal recycling compartment & form at sites where protein Langerin accumulates.

- **Four (4) Layers (From Deep to Superficial) of Epidermis**

I. **Basal layer or stratum germinativum (stratum basale)** is attached to basement membrane and it contains ***mitotically active keratinocytes (containing house keeping organelle***Q – *RER, golgi complex, mitochondria, lysosomes & ribosomes*) and gives rise to superficial layer.

II. **Spinous layer** or **Stratum spinosum** are named for the spine like appearance of the cell margins in histological sections. These ***spines are abundant desmosomes, calcium dependant cell surface modification***Q that promote adhesion of epidermal cells and resistance to mechanical stresses. Upper spinous layer cells (and granular cells) contain organelles called **lamellar granules/membrane coating granules or Odland bodies.**

* The term **Malpighian layer** includes both *basal & spinous layer*.

III. **Granular layer** or **stratum granulosum** is characterized by buildup of components necessary for the process of programmed cell death & formation of a superficial water impermeable barrier. The most apparent structures with in these cells are ***– basophilic keratino hyline granules***Q (composed of *profilaggrin, keratin intermediate filament & loricrin)*. Conversion of profilaggrin to filaggrin (filament aggregation protein) occurs during transition of granular cell to cornified cells.

IV. **Corny or Horny layer** or **Stratum corneum (Corneocytes)** is formed of *cornified or horny cells* which *is the largest cell of the epidermis* and have highest concentration of free aminoacids (esp in mid layers). The St. corneum cells retain some metabolic function and thus is *not the inert covering* it has been previously considered. **Filaggrin**, the protein component of keratinohyaline granule (found in granular layer) is responsible for keratin filament aggregation of corneocytes. Whereas highly insoluble cornified envelope is formed by cross linking of soluble protein precursor, **involucrin**.

- In *palmo-plantar skin*, there is an additional *electron-lucent* zone, the **stratum (corneum) lucidum,** ***between the st.granulosum and st.corneum***Q. These cells are still nucleated, and may be referred to as **transitional cells** (Rooks). The **cells degenerates** as they

Keratinization

Keratinization is a genetically programmed, carefully regulated, complex series of morphological changes & metabolic events that occur progressively *in postmitotic keratinocytes,* and involve

- increase in cell size & flattening of cell shape
- appearance of new cellular organelles & structural reorganization of those present
- change from generalized cellular metabolism to a moore focused metabolism associated with the synthesis of molecules (structural proteins & lipids) related to keratinization.
- alteration in properties of plasma membrane, cell surface antigen & recceptors.
- eventual degradation of cellular organelles including internucleosomal chromatin fragmentation characteristic of apoptosis ***dehydration***Q

move into the st. lucidum an ill defined layer in which the cells loose their identity & the nuclei fades. The cytoplasm contains eosinophilic keratohylin (Behl).

- Normally the cellular progression (ascend of new cells) from basal layer to skin surface takes about ***28-30 days (4 weeks)***Q. And the normal average thickness of epidermis is about *3-4 cells.* Skin turnover is accelerated in ***psoriasis*** so that turnover time decreases to ***4 days*** and epidermal thickness increases to *12-15 cells.*

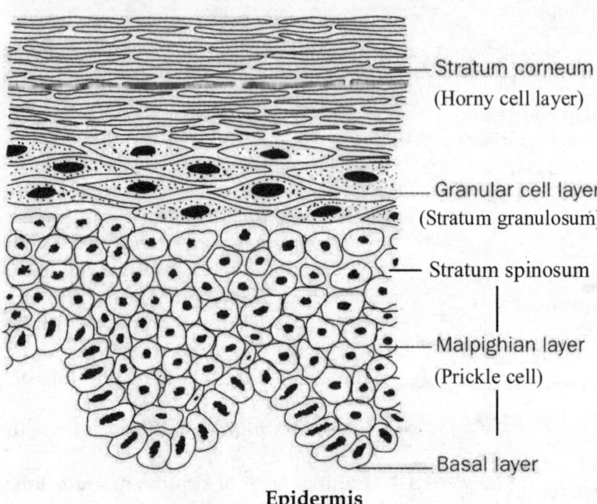

Epidermis

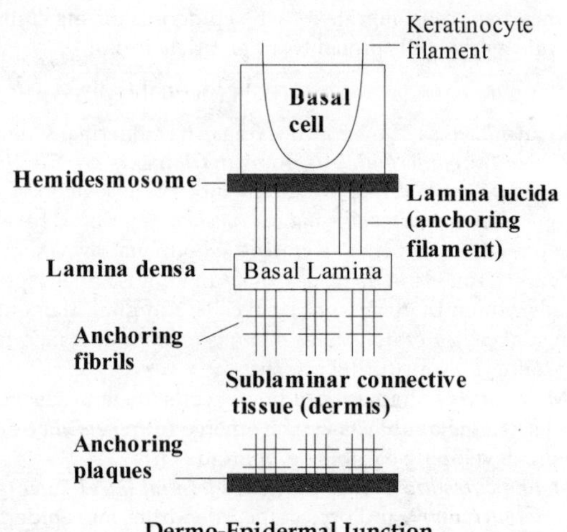

Dermo-Epidermal Junction

Development

Blaschko's Lines

- Lines of Blaschko ***represent the developmental growth pattern of skin and do not correspond to any known nervous, vascular or lymphatic structures***Q. These *nonvisible , non random lines* of development of skin fundamentally ***differ from the system of dermatomes***Q.
- Blaschko's lines are characteristic of **mosaicism** and **lyonization** (ie an individual with ≥2 cell lines of different genotype derived from same zygote and an inactivation of one in early stage of development like one x chrmosomes in female) of epidermis and propbably represent the **routes of ectodermal cell migration from the neural crest.**
- First described by Blaschko in 1901 in his article as a *system of lines on the surface of human body (skin) which the linear naevi and dermatoses follow.*
- As a result of lyonization, the heterozygous state of various *X-linked gene defects* may give rise to a mosaic pattern of cutaneous lesions which conform to Blaschko's line. The shape and distribution of epidermal naevi *reflect both the paths of cell migration and timing of mosaicism and cell type.* Abnormal clones arising at very *early blastocyst stage* will be *widely distributed* along the paths of mirgating cells & appear *linear,* whereas those *arising* late in fully formed fetus are more likely to be *single, small,* oval or round lesions. *Keratinocytes,* which migrate by directional proliferation, produce *linear* lesions, while melanocytes which migrate singly usually form *block like or leaf shaped (phylloid) lesions.* All naevi reflect genetic mosaicism and word naevoid is applied to mosaic forms of inherited skin conditions following lines of Blaschko, eg naevoid psoriasis.
- On *trunk* these lines form *transverse bands* (differing from dermatomes in being more numerous and in their S shaped wave form on lateral trunk) and form *V shape in middle of back.* They never cross the anterior truncal midline, but run along it. Posteriorly the Blaschko's midline is often shifted from anatomical midline. On *extremities,* lines roughly parallel with the *axis of limb.* The lines *spiral on scalp,* are *vertical in mid face* and extend *laterally from the angles of mouth.*

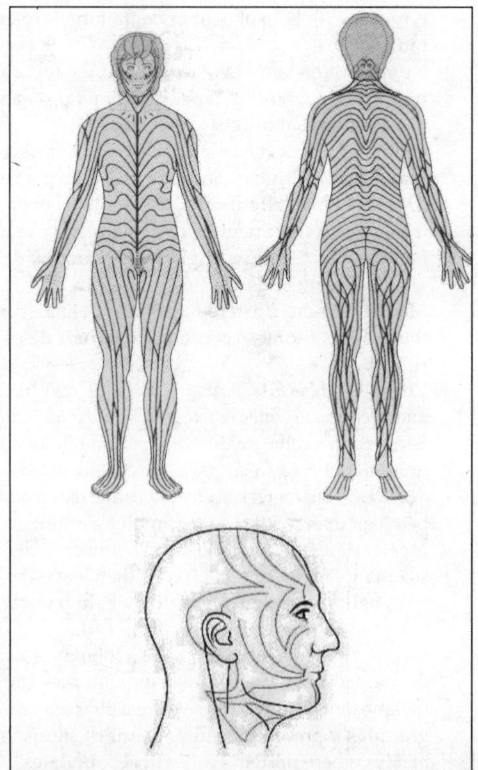

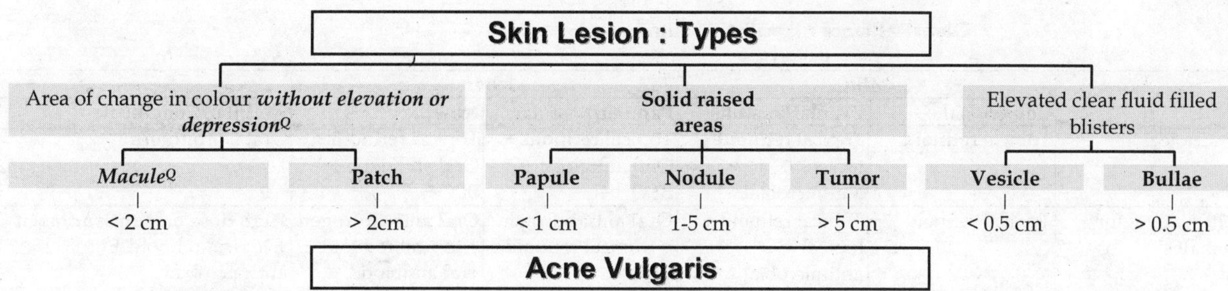

Acne Vulgaris

It is a chronic inflammatory disease of ***pilosebaceous units***[Q] characterized by **seborrhoea**, open & closed **comedones**, **erythematous papules & pustules** and in more severe cases **nodules, deep pustules**, pseudo cysts & even scarring.

Etiology

Four key element (all of these interrelated and under hormonal & immune influence) include

1. **Follicular epidermal lyperproliferation** ie epithelium of infundibulum (upper hair follicle becomes hyperkeratotic with increased cohesion of keratinocytes, resulting in a plug in the follicular ostium l/t concentration of keratin, sebum & bacteria. Small cyst called **micro comedo** form in hair follicle d/t blockage. **Stimulus for keratinocyte hyperproliferation** include **androgen stimulation** (because of increased 17β hydroxysteroid dehydrogenase & 5α reductase enzyme activity of follicular keratinocytes causing enhanced conversion of DHEA-S to dihydrotestosterone = DHT), **decreased linoleic acid, increased interleukin (IL) 1 α activity** (so IL1 receptor antagonist inhibit microcomedone formation), **fibroblast growth factor receptor (FGFR)2 signaling** (association between Apert syndrome & acne) and effects of P. acnes.
2. **Excessive (increased) sebum production by** sebaceous gland under the influence of androgen, CRH. There is ***obstruction of pilosebaceous duct***[Q] due to retention of ***sebum and keratinous material***[Q] (**hypercornification/ hyperkeratosis of pilo sebaceous duct**). Comdones continue to expand and rupture increasing the already existed dermal inflammation.
3. ***Abnormal microbial flora e.g. proprionobacterium acnes (gram positive, anaerobic, and microaerobic bacterium)***[Q] ***and pityrosporum orbiculare (yeast)***[Q] infects comedones.
4. **Inflammation** is caused by pro inflammatory cytokines eg IL 1α/2/8 and TNF-α and antimicrobial peptides eg histone H_4 & cathelicidin etc.
5. Impact of **diet** (particularly relating to **glycemic index & dairy consumption**) on acne is an imerging area of interest. Both increase **insulin like growth factor (IGF)-1** & androgen activity and have proacne effects.

Aggravating Factors

- *Androgens*[Q]
- Glucocorticosteroids (topical & systemic) in high doses
- Cosmetics, hair preparations, industrial compounds, lubricating & cutting oil.
- Friction & trauma
- Drugs – *lithium, isoniazid, halogens, phenytoin, and phenobarbitone*
- Chloronated napthalenic compounds & dioxin (**chlor acne**), pomades (**pomade acne**), topical steroid & other drugs (**drug induced acne**)

Clinical Feature

- Self limiting disorder primarily of *teen agers* and *young adults.* Earliest feature in **greasy skin (seborrhoea).**
- Lesions consist of ***papules, nodules, pustules and comedones***[Q].
- ***The clinical hallmark of acne vulgaris is comedones***[Q], which may be ***closed (white head) or open (black head)***
- *Closed comedones* appear as 1-2 mm white papules (accentuated when skin is stretched). They are precursors of *inflammatory* lesions and their *contents are not easily expressed.*
- *Open comedones rarely* result in *inflammatory* acne, have a large dialated follicular orifice & are filled with *easily expressible* oxidized, darkned oily debris.
- **Sand paper comedones** (multiple, very small white heads, frequently on fore head), **macrocomedones** (> 1mm mostly white heads), **submarine** comedones (>0.5 cm in diameter & deeply situated) and **secondary comedones** (like **chlor acne** and **pomade acne**) are other subtypes.
- The *earliest lesions* are generally mildly inflammed or non inflammaroty *comedones on the forehead.* Most common location is face (*cheeks, chin, forehead & sides of nose*) but *shoulder, upper chest & back* involvement is not uncommon
- Most cases does not develop scarring.

Treatment (Drugs)

Antimicrobial agents reduce bacterial population; **comedolytic** agents encourage shedding of follicular horny plugs and remove obstruction; sebum production is decreased **by sebotrophic agents** (directly) and **antiandrogens** (indirectly); whereas **anti-inflammatory** agents reduce damaging effects of acne inflammation on skin.

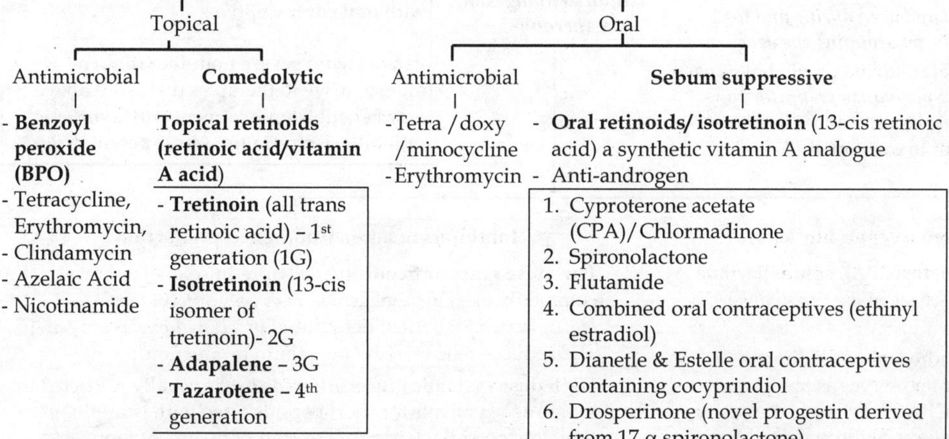

★ Topical salicylic acid, dapsone, sulphur, resorcin, even weak steroids, **UV radiation**, N lite laser therapy, and **cryotherapy** are also less common modes of treatment.

Global Alliance Algorithm (Gollinick et al)

Acne / Drug	Mild		Moderate		Severe
	Comedonal	Papular/Pustular	Papular/Pustular	Nodular	Nodular/Conglobate
1st Choice	Topical **retinoid**	Topical **retinoid** + topical antimicrobial	Topical **retinoid** + Oral antibiotic ± BPO	Topical **retinoid** + Oral antibiotic ± BPO	Oral **isotretinoin**
Alternatives for **Females**	Topical retinoid	Topical retinoid + topical antimicrobial	**Oral antiandrogen** + tropical retinoid ± **topical** antimicrobial	**Oral anti-androgen** + topical retinoid ± **oral** antibiotic	**High dose oral antiandrogen** + topical retinoid ± topical antimicrobial

Treatment of Moderate & Severe Acne Vulgaris

Systemic antibiotics

- Tetracyclines (tetracycline, doxycycline minocycline etc.) are *the sheet anchor of treatment*
- Tetracyclines must *not be given to pregnant* women as they are teratogenic, and must not be given to infants, as they cause bone & tooth dystrophy
- ***Minocycline can cause dark brown pigmentation of skin or acne scars or acral areas on exposed skin***[Q]
- **Erythromycin:** its efficacy is similar to that of tetracycline
- Clindamycin, Quinolines & sulfonamides are less effective drugs, and used when both of first line antibiotics can't be given

Isotretinoin (13-cis-retinoic acid)

- It is ***drug of choice for multiple nodulocystic lesions with pustules and comedones (severe cases)***[Q] unresponsive to therapies discussed
- It reduces sebum secretion by shrinking the sebaceous gland, may also alter keratinization of mouth of hair follicle and have a anti-inflammatory action
- Toxic side effects are frequent, ranging from the trivial, of which most common is drying and cracking of lips, to the very serious which include teratogenicity, hepatotoxicity, bone toxicity (hyperostosis & osteoporosis) & a blood lipid elevating effect (↑ TG, cholesterol, and ratio of VLDL/HDL) and depression (±).
- **Teratogenic effects** are worrisome, as the acne age group is almost identical to the reproductive age group. The effect on fetus include facial, cardiac, renal and neural defects. Because of this it is strongly recommended that if it is planned to prescribe isotretinoin for women who can conceive, ***effective contraceptive measures must also be planned and used during and for 2 months after stopping the drug.***
- All female patients should have ***two negative pregnancy test prior to initiating* therapy and a negative test prior to each refill.**

Hormonal Therapy

- The goal is to counteract the effects of androgen on sebaceous glands with *antiandrogens*, or agents that *decrease the endogenous production of androgens by ovary or adrenal glands including oral contraceptives, glucocorticoids or gonadotropin releasing hormone (Gn RH) agonists.*
- **Systemic hormones for acne in female patients** may be indicated when 1) Standard antibiotics have failed; 2) Oral isotretinoin is inappropriate or not available; 3) ***Menstrual control and/or contraception are required alongside acne therapy***[Q]

Treatment Plan of Acne Vulgeris

Microcomedo is the precursor to inflammatory & non-inflammatory lesions, so even in patients even with predominantly inflammatory acne a **topical retinoid** should be prescribed as a part of regimen. And it should be applied to **all areas** (even clinically normal looking skin) within the active site- as a concept of acne prevention. Topical retinoids have anti-inflammatory and comedolytic activity which makes them suitable for treatment of comedonal and mild to moderate inflammatory disease and they should therefore be used at the onset of treatment combined with topical or oral antimicrobials.

Minimal to moderate, pauci – inflammatory acne may respond adequately to *local therapy alone*

↓

Removal of surface oil has positive, and vigorous scrubbing has a negative role in treatment

↓

Patient with moderate to severe acne with **prominent inflammation** will benefit from addition of ***systemic therapy, such as tetracycline or erythromycin***[Q]

↓

Female patient not responding to oral antibiotics may respond to **hormonal therapy with oral contraceptives**

↓

Patients with **severe nodulocystic acne** unresponsive to therapies discussed above may benefit from treatment with **synthetic retinoids, isotretinoin, (most potent drug)**

Antiandrogens (Androgen receptor blockers)

- These include **cyproterone acetate (CPA), spironolactone and flutamide,** which *supress sebum production* in dose /drug dependent manner.
- **CPA** is a progestational antiandrogen which directly inhibits the androgen receptor and serves as progestogen in oral contraceptives (OCP). CPA 25 mg has been used with success in males but it reduces libido and produces *gynaecomastia & azoospermia.* **Co-cyprindiol (Dianette and Estelle 35)**, a mixture of antiandrogen CPA (2 mg) & an

Inhibitors of adrenal androgen production

- **Low dose glucocorticoids** (usually prednisolone) are most commonly used to manage *late onset congenital adrenal hyperplasia*, an inherited defect in *11 or 21- hydroxylas enzyme.* It also reduces acne by reducing sebum production.
- **High dose systemic glucocorticoids** use is usually restricted to severe acne patients for short periods often with isotretinoin to limit any potential flaring at the start of treatment (anti inflammetory action)

oestrogen ethinyl oestradiol (35µg) is an OCP that a metiorates acne. *It is a central antiandrogen, blocking the pituitary drive to androgen secretion. It also suppress ovulation and acts as an oral contraceptive. It is not suitable for men because of its feminizing properties.* It has greater risk of *deep venous thrombosis embolism* (VTE) than conventional OCP b/o higher oestrogen content.

- **Spironolactone** is an *aldosterone inhibitor used to treat fluid retention or hypertension,* which also functions as a *weak androgen receptor blocker and a weak inhibitor of testosterone synthesis (5α reductase).* It improves acne, hirsutism and side effects include *menstrual irregularity* (combining with OCP alleviate this symptom), *breast tenderness,* headache, fatigue, occasional fluid retention, rarely, melasma and risk of *fiminization of male fetus* (in pregnants).
- **Flutamide, Bicalutamide,** & **Nilutamide** are potent androgen receptor antagonist and used in treatment of metastatic prostatic cancers. In combination with OCP it is used for treatment of acne or hirsutism in women. *Fetal hepatotoxicity* cautions its use for cosmetic purpose. Pregnancy should be avoided.

Inhibitors of ovarian androgen production

- **Gonadotropin-Releasing Hormone (Gn RH) agonists such as leuprolide, nafarelin & buserelin,** block ovulation by disrupting cyclic release of gonadotropins (LH & FSH) from pituitary gland. The net effect is suppression of ovarian steroidogenesis (both androgen & oestrogen), potentially l/t *reduced bone mass & menopausal symptoms.* These are used in treatment of ovarian hyper androgenism, acne & hirsutism in females. However, S/E limit their use.
- **Oral contraceptives (OCP)** contain oestrogen (mostly ethinyl oestradiol) & a progestin. Oestrogen act on liver to *increase synthesis of sex hormone binding globulin (SHBG)* which binds testosterone and *reduces free circulating testosterone.* Hence all OCP will improve acne. In addition, OCP *suppress ovulation* by inhibiting-production of ovarian androgens. Progestins (estranes & gonanes) in combined OCP are derivatives of *19-nortestosterone, cyproterone acetate & drosperinone.* Drosperinone is a new progestin derived from 17 α-spironolactone and has antimineralocorticoid and antiandrogenic activity making it useful in acne like parent compound.

Fordyce's Spot (Disease)

- **Fordyce's spot** (and **Montgomery's tubercle**) represent ***occurrence of ectopic sebaceous glands on lips & buccal mucosa***[Q], (and on breast areola, respectively)
- Despite the ectopic locations both conditions have *normal histopathological sebaceous glands,* but are not associated with hair follicles and are therefore best regarded as *hamartomas.*
- Fordyce's spot are extremely common probably ***80% of normal population have them***[Q]**. It is totally *benign condition***[Q].
- Clinically present as *asymptomatic tiny white* / yellowish focally grouped *papules in buccal mucosa on the lips vermilion portion,* particularly near commisures, & sometimes in retromolar region & upper lip.
- Are ***confused with Koplik's spot (Pathognomic sign of measels). These are differentiated by presence of erythematous halo around Koplic's spot***[Q].
- Fordyces spots are often not noticeable in children until after puberty (although present histologically), increase in some rheumatic disorders.
- *No treatment* is indicated other than reassurance. The large disfiguring spots become less prominent with *oral isotretinoin.*

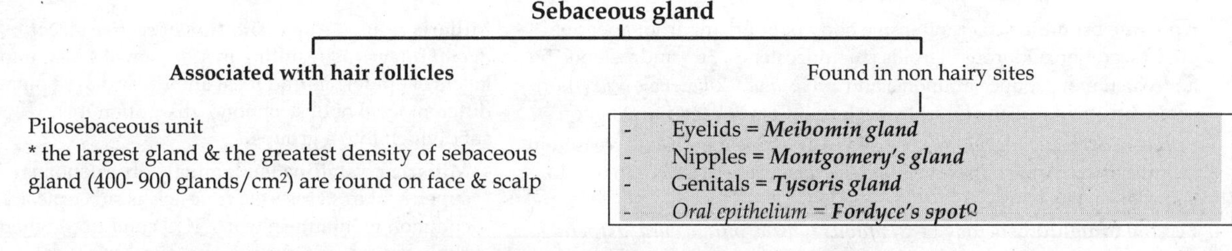

Rosacea (Acne rosacea)

- It is characterized by ***erythema of central face persisting for months or more***[Q]. *Convex areas of nose, cheeks, chin & forehead* are characteristically involved, whereas perioral and periorbital areas are spared.
- *Intermittent flushing* followed by more permanent *telangiectasia, papules, pustules* (rarely nodules but never comedones) are primary features.
- Secondary features include *facial burning or stinging, edema, plaques,* a dry appearance, *phyma,* peripheral flushing, and ocular manifestations.
- The primary **differentiating feature** b/w acne vulgaris & rosacea ***is presence of open & closed comedones in acne***[Q]. Both conditions may coexist, although rosacea most often begins & reaches its peak incidence in the decades after acne declines. However **rosacea fulminans (pyoderma faciale / rosacea conglobata)** occurs mainly in women in their 20's and characterized by sudden onset of confluent papules, pustules, nodules, and draining sinuses on chin, cheeks, forehead with in background of diffuse facial erythema. Rosea is of 5 types. Rosacea is of 5 types

1. **Erythemato – telangiectatic rosace (ETR)**
2. **Papulo – pustular rosace (PPR)**
3. **Ocular rosacea**

4. Phymatous rosacea

- Characterized by patulous follicular orifices, thickened skin, nodularities & irregular surface contours in convex areas
- ***Mostly occurs on nose (rhinophyma)***Q f/b chin (gnathophyma), forehead (metophyma), eyelids (blepharophyma), & ears (otophyma).
- It is ***d/t hyperplasia of sebaceous glands***Q. Women d/t hormonal resons do not develop phyma

5. Granulomatous rosacea

- Yellow brown (or red) monomorphic papules or nodules on cheeks & periorificial facial skin.
- Diascopy reveal *apple jelly like colour change* (similar to sarcoid or lupus vulgaris)
- Biopsy show *granuloma formation.*

3 Types of Sweat Glands

Eccrine

- Humans have 2 to 4 million eccrine sweat glands, ***most numerous on sole of foot***Q (620/cm²) and ***least abundant on the back***Q (64/cm²)
- Glands ***first appear on volar surface of hands & feet***Q in 3.5 month old fetus > (followed by) axilla (early 5th month) > rest of body (late 5th month)
- **Preoptic hypothalamic area** plays a *key role in regulating body temperature.* Sweating, vasodilation & rapid breathing occurs if it's heated, whereas local cooling causes generalized ***vasoconstriction & shivering***Q
- **Hypothalmic temperature** (reflected by tympanic membrane temperature) is the ***strongest stimulus for sweating***Q
- **Emotional sweating** is usually confined ***to palms, soles and axilla***Q & in some instances the forehead or even whole skin
- ***Ductal reabsorption conserves NaCl***Q; (& make it hypotonic from isotonic). In cystic fibrosis mutated chloride channels increase NaCl loss.

Apo-eccrine (AEG)

- Develop *during puberty from eccrine like* precursor glands & is consistently present in *axilla*
- It's frequency varies and in *axillary hyperhydrosis*, it accounts for 50% of all axillary glands
- Like eccrine it has long duct which opens directly on to skin surface (*unlike apocrine which opens into hair follicles*).
- Like eccrine gland, AEG is *both cholinergic & adrenergic*, but its secretory rate is 10 times more.

Apocrine

- Develop from upper bulge of hair follicle in 4th month of gestation and *remain quiescent until puberty*
- Present in *axilla, anogenital (perineal) region,* periumblical area, nipples, external auditory meatus (**ceruminous glands**) and eyelids (**Moll's glands**). Breast (mammary gland) is also modified apocrine gland.
- Their ***development not the functional activity is dependent on sex hormone. So gonadectomy in adults does not affect function***Q.
- ***Apocrine glands are adrenergic***Q; stimulated by epinephrine > nor epinephrine given locally or systemically (in marked contrast to **eccrine glands** which are ***under cholinergic control***Q)

Disorders of Sweat Gland

Bromhidrosis

- **Apocrine bromhidrosis** is offensive body odor arising from apocrine gland secretion. Odorous steroids (16-androstenes, 5α - androstenol, 5α-androstenone) produce ammonia and *ε-3 methyl – 2-hexenoic acid* (short chain fatty acid causing odor) by bacterial (Corynebacterium) action.
- Levels of *5α reductase type I* expressed in apocrine glands is increased in bromhidrosis. And so the levels of *dihydrotestosterone* (as compared to testosterone) in skins.
- **Eccrine bromhidrosis** may be d/t ***foods (garlic, onion, cury, asfoetida, alcohol)***Q, drugs (bromides), toxins or metabolic disorders such as hypermethioninemia, isovaleric acedmia, phenylketonuria, trimethylaminuria (fish odor syndrome), Cat-odor syndrome and sweaty feet syndrome.

Fox Fordyce Disease (Apocrine Miliaria)

Fox Fordyce disease is characterized by *pruritic (itchy) follicular papules* localized to anatomical regions that bear *apocrine sweat glands (i.e., axillae & genito femoral area)*, due to apocrine duct obstruction, rupture or inflamation. 90% of patients are *female* and onset tends to be after puberty.

Miliria

Miliaria results from ***disruption of eccrine sweat ductal integrity***Q resulting in secretion of sweat into layers of epidermis and focal anhidross. Based on different level of obstruction / disruption it is subdivided into 4 groups.

- **Miliaria crystallina (sudamina)** : obstruction is superficial in *st. corneum* & vesicle is subcorneal. It is common in infants in warm ICU conditions where cholinergic & adrenergic agents are employed.
- **Miliaria rubra (prickly heat)**: include keratinization of intraepidermal part of sweat duct with leakage of sweat into epidermis & upper dermis causing pruritic papules around sweat pores.
- **Miliaria pustulosa** : miliaria rubra becoming pustular
- **Miliaria profunda** : rupture of duct at or below dermal – epidermal junction with sweat leaking into deeper dermis.

Summary of Disorders of Sweat Gland

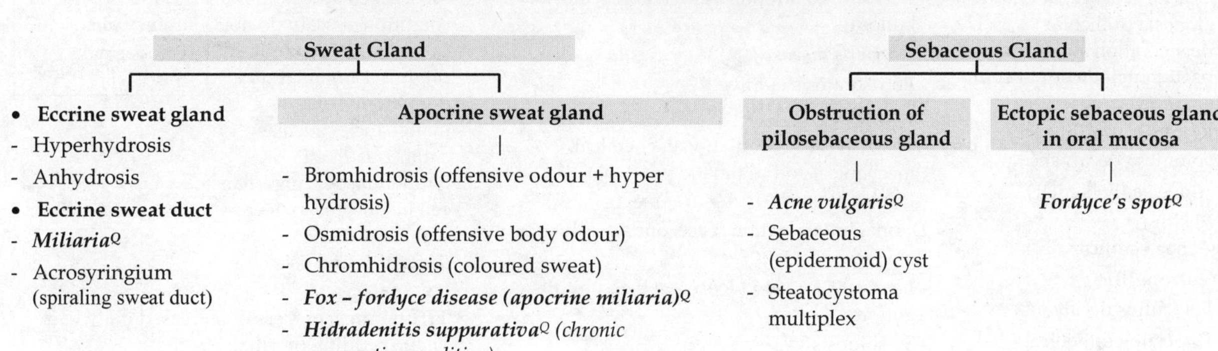

Sweat Gland
Sebaceous Gland
• Eccrine sweat gland
- Hyperhydrosis
- Anhydrosis
• Eccrine sweat duct
- Miliaria[Q]
- Acrosyringium (spiraling sweat duct)
Apocrine sweat gland
- Bromhidrosis (offensive odour + hyper hydrosis)
- Osmidrosis (offensive body odour)
- Chromhidrosis (coloured sweat)
- Fox – fordyce disease (apocrine miliaria)[Q]
- Hidradenitis suppurativa[Q] (chronic suppurative condition)
Obstruction of pilosebaceous gland
- Acne vulgaris[Q]
- Sebaceous (epidermoid) cyst
- Steatocystoma multiplex
Ectopic sebaceous gland in oral mucosa
Fordyce's spot[Q]

Stages of Hair Growth

- A normal human being has ~ 1 million hair follicles on his body, of which 1 lac are on the scalp (10%). A hair normally grows at the rate of 1 cm/month (~10 cm / year). Normal individual *lose about 100 hair from the scalp every day.*
- The hair during its life passes through three different phases of growth & shedding. This cycle is independent of cycle of neighbouring follicles i.e. the neighbouring cycle are not synchronised in growth. The proportion of hair in each phase can be estimated by looking at the plucked hair – this is called **trichogram**. Stages of hair cycle are

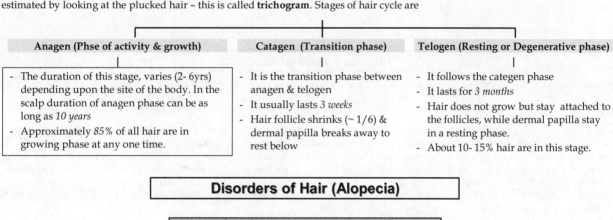

Anagen (Phse of activity & growth)
- The duration of this stage, varies (2- 6yrs) depending upon the site of the body. In the scalp duration of anagen phase can be as long as *10 years*
- Approximately *85%* of all hair are in growing phase at any one time.

Catagen (Transition phase)
- It is the transition phase between anagen & telogen
- It usually lasts *3 weeks*
- Hair follicle shrinks (~ 1/6) & dermal papilla breaks away to rest below

Telogen (Resting or Degenerative phase)
- It follows the categen phase
- It lasts for *3 months*
- Hair does not grow but stay attached to the follicles, while dermal papilla stay in a resting phase.
- About 10- 15% hair are in this stage.

Disorders of Hair (Alopecia)

Etiology of Alopecia

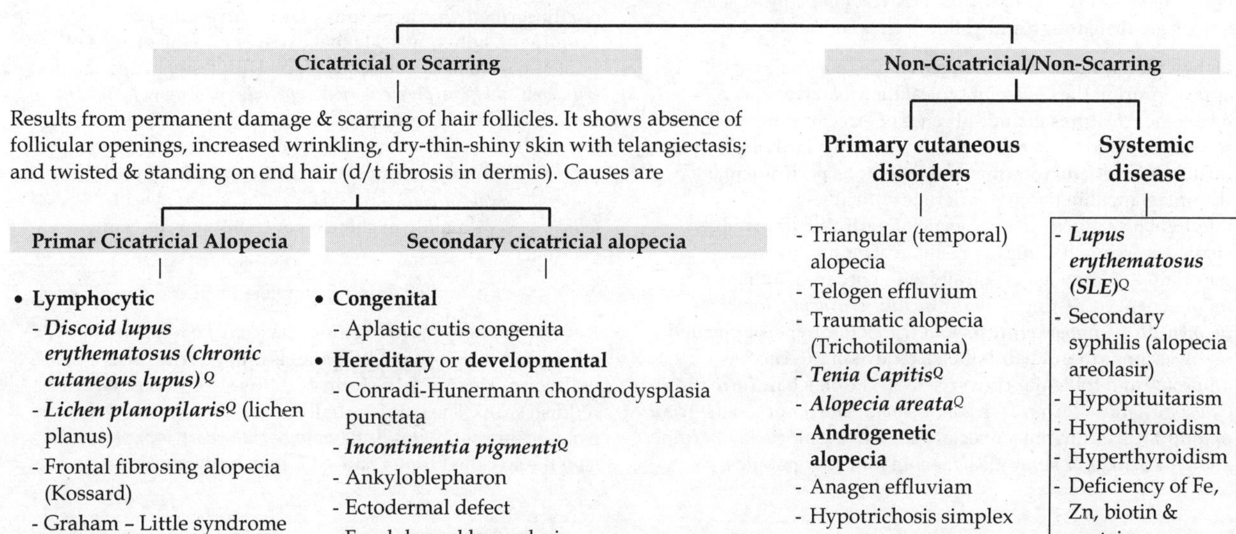

- ***Pseudopelade of Brocq***[Q]
- Central centrifugal cicatrical alopecia (follicular degeneration syndrome or **pseudo pelade** or hot comb alopecia)
- Keratosis follicularis spinulosa decalvans
- Alopecia (Follicular) mucinosa
- Acne necrotica

• **Neutrophillic**
- Folliculitis decalvans
- Dissecting folliculitis (perifolliculitis capitis abscedens et suffodiens)

• **Mixed**
- Acne keloidalis (nuchae)
- Erosive pustular dermatosis

• **Systemic** – sarcoid, ***SLE***[Q] & secondaries involving skin

- Hallerman Streiff Syndrome
- Generalized atrophic benign epidermolysis bullosa
- ***Darrier's disease***[Q]
- Porokeratosis of mibelli

• **Traumatic**
- Thermal (burn), radiational, chemical, mechanical and traumatic tractional (trichotillomania)

• Dermal inflammation l/t secondary follicular damage
- ***Leprosy***[Q], ***Lupus Vulgaris***[Q], TB, Syphillitic gumma
- Sarcoidosis
- ***Linear scleroderma (morphea)***[Q]
- Cicatrical pemphigoid

• **Follicular inflammation**
- Tenia capitis with favus & kerion
- Infections e.g. bacterial folliculitis, impetigo, herpes zoster
- Lichen sclerosis et atrophicus

• **Neoplastic**
- Basal & squamous cell Ca, Lymphoma, Secondaries (cutaneous)

- Pattern hair loss
- Most eczematous condition of scalp do not cause hair loss except pityriasis amiantacea, dermatomyositis, malignancies such as cutaneous T cell lymphoma or Langerhans cell histiocytosis severe scalp seborrheic dermatitis and psoriasis (very rarely).

- Drugs - Alopecia universalis - Ectodermal dysplasia

★ **Effluvium** is process of increased daily hair shaft shedding (normal: 25- 100)

★ **Pattern hair loss (male androgenetic alopecia or male balding)** is the most common type of hair loss in both sexes.

★ *Most common* congenital cicatrial alopecia is aplasia cute's congenita (i.e. focal absence of epidermis with or with or with out other layers)

Various Types of Alopecia

Cicatrising alopecia in Lichen planus

- Hyperpigmented spiny lesions around hair follicles (i.e. ***perifollicular erythema, hyperpigmentation, hyperkeratosis and scale) with cicatrising alopecia***[Q] are characteristic features of **follicular lichen planus** of scalp (**lichen planopilaris**). So it may be a/w other features of lichen planus like *shiny, flat topped, polygonal, purple, pruritic (violaccons) papules which retain the skin lines* most often of volar aspect of wrists, the lumbar region and around the ankles. ***White line (Wickham's striae) transversing surface of papules and white streaks, forming a lace work, on buccal mucosa are highly characteristic***[Q]. On palms & soles lesions are firm, rough and yellow.
- **Lichen planopilaris** affects females more than males and appears during the course of typical LP. Characteristic histological features include absence of errector pili muscles & sebaceous glands, a perivascular & **perifollicular lymphocytic infiltrate in reticular dermis and mucinous perifollicular fibroplasia** within the upper dermis with abscence of interfollicular mucin, and **superficial perifollicular wedge shaped scarring**. It clinically result in **atrophic**, scarred, porcelain – colored area centrally with bordering follicular involvement consisting of ***perifollicular erythema, hyper pigmentation, hyperkeratosis and scale***[Q] (i.e. hyperpigmented scally lesions around hair follicle), **cicatrising** / ***scarring alopecia***[Q] and follicular convergence (l/t **doll's hair formation**). *Graham – Little – Piccardi – Lassueur syndrome* comprises the triad of multifocal cicatricial alopecia, non-scarring alopecia of groin and / or axillae, & keratotic lichenoid follicular papules.

Cicatrising alopecia in DLE

- ***Cicatrising alopecia with follicular accentuation &keratotic plugging***[Q] (i.e. horny / keratotic plugs occupying **dilated follicles / pilosebaceous canals**) and producing **carpet tack or tin tack sign** (i.e. when adherent scale is lifted from advanced lesions, keratotic spikes similar in appearance to carpet tacks are seen to project from under surface of scale) is seen in **DLE**.
- DLE begins as red-purple macule / papule / or plaque and rapidly develop a hyper keratotic (scaly) surface. Classical lesion is sharply demarcated, **coin – shaped (i.e. discoid or circumscribed) erythematous plaque covered by a prominent, adherent scale** that extends into the orifices of dilated hair follicles, mostly on face. DLE lesions *expand with erythema and hyperpigmentation at periphery, leaving hallmark central scarring, telangiectasia, and hypopigmentation.* Resolving *perioral lesions* characteristically show **acneiform / cribriform pattern of pitted scarring. Wide follicular pits**, sometimes *containing scale or blackcheads (i.e. dilated, hyperpigmented follicles)* occur mainly in choncha or triangular fossa of external ear.

Non cicatrising alopecia in SLE

- **Reversible, non – scarring alopecia** (may be telogen effluvium) develops in SLE patients often during active phase of disease. This takes the form of diffuse loss of hair with a reddish scalp. The hair is usually *coarse, dry, and fragile* esp on frontal margin l/t *unruly appearance with short, broken – off – hair*, the so called **lupus hair**. SLE may be a/w *arthritis*.

Telogen and Anagen Effluvium

Telogen Effluvium

Pathogenesis & Clinical Feature

- Every hair passes through 3 phases (anagen, catagen, & telogen) but adjoining hair follicles are not synchronous in their cycle.
- However, sometimes ***growing anagen phase of several adjoining hair follicles is aborted and these hair follicles enter catagen phase at the same time (i.e. the hair cycle becomes synchronous)***Q, which is then followed by telogen phase.
- So several hair are shed simultaneously, after completion of telogen phase.
- Therefore it ***starts ~ 3 months after the onset of causative factor***Q, and when the new hairs have actually already started growing in these places.
- Since in most cases the causative influence disappears by this time, the patient tends to attribute the hair loss to unrelated factors.
- The diagnosis is confirmed by examination of falling hairs, which contain *club like swelling at the root end* and therefore called **club hairs** and are *shorter than the maximal hair length of that area* (d/t premature stoppage of growing anagen phase).

Etiological Factors

1. ***Fever of any cause, especially if it is high, prolonged or recurrent.***Q
2. ***Child birth***Q (esp. prolonged & difficult)
3. Abortion, cessation of oral contraceptives or treatment with hormones.
4. Surgical operations, accidents or severe blood loss
5. Psychiatric disturbances or acute mental stress.
6. Nutritional dificiencies, crash dieting or anemia
7. Hypothyroidism, hyperthyroidism or treatment with antithyroid drugs
8. Severe general illness.
9. Treatment with anticoagulants, antihypertensive drugs, lithium or oral retinoids.

* Loss of all hair from scalp is called **alopecia totalis**
* Loss of hair from *whole body* is called **alopecia universalis**
* **Ophiasis** is *band like* pattern of hair loss at *periphery of skull.*

Anagen Effluvium

- It is alway abnormal to shed anagen hair. The **onset is rapid within 2-4 weeks of cause**Q
- Causes include
  - *Radiotherapy to head*
  - *Systemic chemotherpy* esp. with alkylating agents (eg. *cyclophosphamides*) disrupt anagen cycle & cause hair follicle dystrophy. Replacement with normal pelage usually occur rapidly after discontinuation of chemotherapy although *high dose busulfan may l/t permanent alopecia* d/t irreversible damage to hair follicle stem cell. Lower dose cytostatic regimen or less cytotoxic agents (eg. methotrexate, decarbazine) induce premature catagen & more often l/t telogen effluvium.
  - *Mercury / Boric acid / Thalium intoxication*
  - *Colchicine poisoning*, Vit A poisoning
  - Severe protein malnutrition, iron deficiency anemia

Androgenetic Alopecia (Male Balding) or Pattern Hair Loss

Aetiology

Androgen dependent traitQ
- Male *castrated before puberty* do not develop balding unless treated withtestosterone
- No balding in XY individuals with *complete androgen insensitivity syndrome* who fail to express androgen receptor (despite having normal circulating testosterone)
- Although testosterone is the major circulating androgen n men the ***balding process is driven by its metabolite dihydrotestosterone which has greater affinity & avidity for androgen receptor***Q.

Clinical Presentation

Essential clinical feature in both sexes is *patterned hair loss over the crown.* Pigmented terminal hairs are progressively replaced by finer, short & virtually nonpigmented hair. *A female pattern of hair loss may be seen in males, & vice versa*Q.

Male Pattern (Hamilton – Norwood scale)

Two major features are
- *recession of frontal hair line &*
- *balding of scalp vertex*, eventually leaving a rim of normal hair at the sides & back of scalp

Male pattern

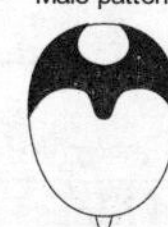

Female Pattern

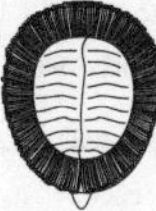

Female pattern (Ludwig scale)

- **More *diffuse process.* Typically *there is diffuse reduction in hair density involving the crown & frontal scalp with maintenance of frontal hair line*Q.**
- *Parietal region* may also be involved
- There may be miniaturized hairs in fronto temporal region but deep recession of hair line is uncommon
- Presence of high proportion of miniaturized follicles on biopsy differentiates it from telogen effluvium.

Treatment

In males

- **Topical minoxidil**
  Show maximum benefit in first 6 months of use. On taking orally it is a potent vasodilator & antihypertensive
- **5 α-reductase inhibitors**
  - *Finasteride*Q a non competitive irreversible highly selective antagonist of 5 α reductase type 2 that inhibits conversion of testosterone to DHT. It causes a *50% reduction in serum prostate specifc antigen (PSA) levels, thus resulting in underestimation of prostatic cancer risk (so the value should be doubled* to correct finasteride effect.
  - **Dutasteride**
    Combined type 1 & 2 - 5α-reductase inhibitor.

In Females

- **Topical minoxidil**
- Oral anti-androgen therapy with
  - **Cyproterone acetate**
    It is androgen receptor blocker, a potent progestin & has antigonadotrophic effect
  - **Spironolactone**
    A diuertic – antihypertensive synthetic steroid, which structurally resemble aldosterone & acts by competitively blocking cytoplasmic receptors for dihydrotestosterone. It also weakly inhibits androgen biosynthesis.
  - **Flutamide**
    Non steroidal anti androgen which acts by inhibiting androgen uptake & by inhibiting nuclear binding of androgen with its target tissue. Potentially *fatal hepatotoxicity* limits its use.

* Cyproterone acetate & ethinylestranol is **dianette**.

Alopecia Areata

Aetiology

- **Genetic factors**
  - *10-20% patients give a* family history *& inheritance is polygenic*
  - Strong association between alopecia areata & *major histo compatibility complex (MHC) class II antigens HLA- DR4, DR II (DR 5) & DQ3*
  - DQB1* 0301 allele
  - *DR4, DR5, DQ3* are associated with *severe alopecia & DQ3 and DR11* (allele DRB1* 1104) with *alopecia totalis & universalis.*
  - Severity of alopecia areata is associated with polymorphisms in antiinflammatory *IL-1 receptor antagonist (IL-1 RN) & its homologue IL1F5 cytokine genes*
  - AR autoimmune polyglandular syndrome type 1 (APS-1, *antoimmune polyendocrinopathy – candidiasis – ectodermal dystrophy syndrome) and Down's syndrome* (both involving chromosome 21) have high incidence of alopecia areata.
- **Autoimmunity**[Q]
  - It's a chronic organ specific *autoimmune disease,* mediated by CD8+ T-cells ***affecting hair follicles (bullb)***[Q] & sometimes nail.
  - Associated with other autoimmune diseases eg, myxoedema, pernicious anemia etc.
  - Frequency of type 1 DM is increased in relatives of patients with alopecia areata but not in patient themselves (i.e., protects against DM type 1)

Clinical Presentation

- Onset may be at any age peaking b/w 2-4th decade. Sex incidence is equal
- Characteristic ***initial lesion is a circumscribed, totally bald, smooth patch***[Q], often noticed by chance. The skin within the bald patch appears normal or slightly reddened.
- Short easily extractable broken hairs' k/a **exclamation mark hairs** are seen at margins of bald patch.
- ***Scalp is the first affected site in most cases***[Q], but any hair bearing skin eg. beard, eyebrows, or eyelashes can be affected.
- **Alopecia totalis** is total or almost total loss of scalp hair, and **alopecia universalis** is loss of all body hair. **Ophiasis** is alopecia along scalp margin.
- Classical feature is ***sparing of gray /white hairs***[Q]. and preferentially affecting pigmented (black) hairs. This results in a dramatic change in hair colour if alopecia progress rapidly & k/a "**going white overnight phenomenon**"
- In 10-15% cases ***nail show fine stippled pitting***[Q], trachyonychia (roughening of nail plate), onychomadesis, modesis, mottled lunula.

Differential Diagnosis

Feature	**Alopecia areata**	**Tinea capitis**
Age group	***Adults***[Q]	***Children***[Q]
Inflamation, Itching & Scales	Absent	***Present***[Q]
Exclamation (!) mark sign	Stumps are scanty & ***form exclamation mark (!)***[Q]	Stumps of broken hair are *numerous* but *do not form exclamation mark*
Pattern of hair loss	Complete in center	Incomplete in centre

Exclamation mark hair, is the hair which is broken off about *4 mm* from the scalp, due to constriction in the shaft. The broken hair is *paler and narrower* than normal with broader distal end.

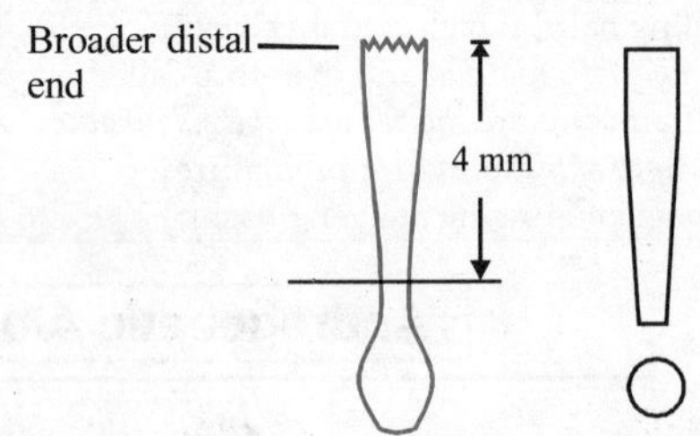

Disorders of Nail

Koilonychia (Spoon nail)	The nail is concave with raised edges	- ***Fe deficiency anemia***[Q] associated with Plummer – Vinson's syndrome - Sideropenic anemia
Racquet Nail	Width of nail bed & nail plate is greater than their length	- Premature obliteration of epiphyseal line
Anonychia	Absence of all or part of one or several nails	- ***Lichen panus***[Q] - With cong. bone anomalies
Beau's Line	Poor nutrition to matrix l/t a defective band of nail formation resulting in *transverse groove of thin nail plate.* By measuring the position of this groove, it is possible to date previous illness.	- High fever, **Viral illness (hand-foot-mouth disease, measles)** - Peripheral nerve injury (ischemia) - Surgery, Kawasaki syndrome - Drug.

Longitudinal ridges with **beaded** & /or **Fir tree appearance**		- Median canaliform dystrophy of Heller
Trachyonychia (Rough Sand paper nail)		- 20 nail dystrophy (alopecia areata) - External chemical treatment
Leuconychia	White discolouration of nail	- Nail matrix dysfunction
Apparent leuconychia	White appearance d/t changes in underlying tissue	- Tery's nail, half & half nail & muchrke's paired narrow white band
Onychogryphosis (Ram's horn or Oyster – Nail)	Nail is severly distorted, thickened, opaque, brownish, sparaled & with out attachment to nail bed	- Pressure from foot wear in elderly
Hook Nail		- Lack of support from short bony phalynx
Pterygium	Gradual shortening of proximal nail groove l/t proximal thinning of nail plate & secondary fissuring caused by *fusion of proximal nail fold to matrix & subsequently to nail bed*. The portion of divided nail plate progressively decrease in size (as pterygium widens) ultimately resulting in total loss of nail with permanent atrophy & scarring (sometimes)	- ***Dorsal pterygium in lichen planus***[Q] - Ventral pterygium in scleroderma with Raynaud's phenomenon, causalgia of median nerve, trauma, formaldehyde containing nail cosmetics.
Onychomadesis	Seperation of nail from matrix	- Same as Beau's line
Onycholysis	Detachment of nail plate from its bed starting at its distal & /or lateral attachment	- ***Psoriasis***[Q] - ***Reiter's syndrome***
Onychorrhexis	Splitting & roughness of nail plate	Lichen planus
Onychoptosis defluvium (Alopecia Unguim)	Component of alopecia	***Alopecia areata***[Q]
Koenen's Periungal Fibroma		- ***Tuberous sclerosis***[Q] (50% cases)
Mee's Line		- ***Arsenic Poisoining***[Q].
Pitting		- ***Deep & irregular pits in psoriasis & atopic dermatitis***[Q] - ***Superficial & geometric pits in alopecia areata***[Q].
Melanonychia	Presence of melanin in nail plate presenting as single /multiple longitudinal brown- black band.	- Single band: nail matric nevus or melanoma (deserve biopsy), trauma (usually in 4/5th toe nail) - Multiple band: dark race, pregnancy, inflmatory nail disorder, Lauiger-Huntziker syndrome (with pigmented macules on lip & genitals), AIDS, Addison syndrome
Muehreke's lines		Hypoalbuminemia

Questions

GENERAL ANATOMY

1. **True about corneum lucidum:** *(PGI June 09)*
   A. Sadwitched b/w s.spinosum & s. granulosum ☐
   B. Sandwitched b/w s. corneum & s. granulosum ☐
   C. Contain hair follicle ☐
   D. Also k/a prickle cell layer ☐
   E. Contain degenerated cells ☐
2. **All statements are true regarding skin except** *(PGI –96)*
   A. Skin is stratified squamous epithelium ☐
   B. Melanocyte & merkel cells are immigrant cells ☐
   C. Keratin filaments are a hall mark of epidermal cells ☐
   D. Keratinization process cause hydration of cells. ☐
   E. Spines of spinous cells are formed from house keeping organelle. ☐
3. **Which layer of epidermis is underdeveloped in the VLBW infants in the initial 7 days:** *(AIIMS Nov 02)*
   A. Stratum germinativum ☐
   B. Stratum granulosum ☐
   C. Stratum lucidum ☐
   D. Stratum corneum ☐
4. **Normal turnover time of epidermis (skin doubling time) is** *(AIIMS 91)*
   A. 2 weeks ☐
   B. 4 weeks ☐
   C. 6 weeks ☐
   D. 8 weeks ☐
5. **Melanocytes are present in:** *(PGI 99)*
   A. Stratum corneum ☐
   B. Stratum basale ☐
   C. Stratum granulosum ☐
   D. Dermis ☐
6. **The correct sequence of cell cycle is:** *(AI 03)*
   A. G0-G1-S-G2-M ☐
   B. G0-G1-G2-S-M ☐
   C. G0-M-G2-S-G1 ☐
   D. G0-G1-S-M-G2 ☐

DEVELOPMENT

7. **Lines of Blaschko represent:** *(AI 2011)*
   A. Lines along lymphatics ☐
   B. Lines along blood vessels ☐
   C. Lines along nerves ☐
   D. Lines of development ☐

SKIN LESION

8. **Neither raised nor depressed is** *(PGI 97)*
   A. Macule ☐
   B. Plaque ☐
   C. Nodule ☐
   D. Papule ☐
9. **A flat discolouration on skin as 1 cm is called :**
   A. Macule *(Rohatak 97)* ☐
   B. Plague ☐
   C. Boil ☐
   D. Papule ☐
   E. Wheal ☐
10. **Which among is not a primary skin lesion of:**
    A. Plaque *(Bihar – 2006)* ☐
    B. Macule ☐
    C. Abscess ☐
    D. None ☐

ACNE VULGARIS

11. **Causative factor of acne include(s)** *(PGI May 13)*
    A. Hypersecretion of sebum ☐
    B. ↑IgE level ☐
    C. Follicular duct hypercornification ☐
    D. ↑ Colonisation of propionibacterium acnes ☐
    E. IGF-1 ☐
12. **Acne vulgaris is caused by-** *(JIPMER 91)*
    F. Staph aureus ☐
    G. Diphtheroids ☐
    H. Sweat gland hyperplasia ☐
    I. Obstruction to pilosebaceous duct ☐
13. **Causative factor for acne are all *except*:**
    A. Androgen *(PGI 2000)* ☐
    B. Only food ☐
    C. Bacterial contamination ☐
    D. Hypercornification of duct ☐
    E. Lipophilic yeast ☐
14. **Causative factor for acne are following except**
    A. Androgen *(SGPGI – 2000)* ☐
    B. Only food ☐
    C. Keratin ☐
    D. Cell nucleus ☐
15. **Comedones are characteristics of -** *(AIIMS 95, Kerala 94)*
    A. Acne vulgaris ☐
    B. Acne rosasea ☐
    C. SLE ☐
    D. Adenoma sebaeceum ☐
16. **19 years old girl has multiple papulo pustular erythematous lesions on face and neck, the likely diagnosis is**
    A. Acne rosacae *(AIIMS 94)* ☐
    B. Acne Vulgaris ☐
    C. Pityriasis Versicolour ☐
    D. Lupus Vulgaris ☐
17. **Treatment of acne-** *(PGI June 2005)*
    A. 13 cis retionol ☐
    B. Minocycline/Tetracycline ☐
    C. Erytromycin ☐
    D. Dapsone ☐
    E. Rifampicin ☐
18. **Treatment of acne vulgaris may include all except-**
    A. Cryotherapy *(PGI 96, AIIMS 03)* ☐
    B. Oestrogens ☐
    C. UV light ☐
    D. Androgens ☐
19. **A patient presented with multiple nodulocystic lesions on the face. The drug of choice is :** *(AIIMS May 02)*
    A. Retinoids ☐
    B. Antibiotics ☐
    C. Steroids ☐
    D. UV light ☐
20. **Treatment of nodulocystic acne is** *(AIIMS 95, AI 95)*
    A. Erythromycin ☐
    B. Tertacycline ☐
    C. Isoretinonine (Retinoic acid) ☐
    D. Steroids ☐
21. **Recalcitrant Pustular Acne is treated by**
    A. Oral Erythromycin *(AIIMS 92)* ☐
    B. Oral tetracycline ☐
    C. Steriod ☐
    D. Retinoid ☐

22. **Treatment of choice for Acne vulgaris** *(PGI Dec 05)*
A. Minocycline for inflammatory acne ☐
B. Retinoids for comedonal acne ☐
C. Etretinate ☐
D. Rifampicin ☐
E. Dapsone ☐

23. **A 24-year-old unmarried women has multiple nodular, cystic, pustular and comadonic lesions on face, upper back and shoulders for 2 years. The drug of choice for her treatment would be:** *(AI 2006)*
A. Acitretin ☐
B. Isotretinoin ☐
C. Doxycycline ☐
D. Azithromycin ☐

24. **Most common side effects of retinoids is**
A. Headache *(AIIMS 94)* ☐
B. Skin rashes ☐
C. Photosensitivity ☐
D. Diarrhoea ☐

25. **A teenager girl with moderate acne is also complaining of irregular menses. Drug of choice will be:**
A. Oral isotretinon *(AIIMS Nov 2010)* ☐
B. Oral acitretin ☐
C. Oral minocycline ☐
D. Cyproterone acetate ☐

26. **A 17 year old girl with Acne has been taking a drug for the last two years. Show now presents with blue black pigmentation of nails. The likely medication causing the above pigmentation is** *(AI 2010)*
A. Tetracycline ☐
B. Minocycline ☐
C. Doxycycline ☐
D. Azithromycin ☐

27. **Acne vulgaris is due to involvement of:**
A. Sebaceous glands *(PGI June 06, AIIMS 01)* ☐
B. Eccrine glands ☐
C. Pilosebaceous glands ☐
D. Apocrine glands ☐
E. Sweat glands ☐

FORDYCE SPOTS

28. **Regarding Fordyce spots :** *(PGI 02)*
A. Represent internal maliganancy ☐
B. Ectopic sebaceous glands ☐
C. Present in axillae ☐
D. Found in healthy people ☐
E. Are erythematous ☐

29. **Fordyce's disease mainly involves :** *(PGI 97, AIIMS 2K)*
A. Lips ☐
B. Buccal mucosa ☐
C. Neck ☐
D. Trunk ☐

ROSACEA

30. **Rhinophyma is (a complication of) -** *(AI 97, UP 04, AP 98)*
A. Glandular form of acne rosacea *(PGI 96)* ☐
B. Form of acne vulgaris ☐
C. Affects the scalp ☐
D. A form of dermatofibroma ☐

31. **Rhinopyma is (Potate nose) -** *(AP 96)*
A. Septal deviation of nose ☐
B. Sweat gland hypertrophy ☐
C. Mucous gland hypertrophy ☐
D. Sebaceous gland hypertrophy ☐

32. **A 40 year old woman presents with a 2 year old h/o erythematous papulo pustular lesions on convexities of the face. There in a background of erytherma & telengiec-tasia. The most likely diagnosis is:**
A. Acne valgaris *(AI 2005)* ☐
B. Rosacea ☐
C. SLE ☐
D. Polymorphic light eruption ☐

33. **Morphological features of rosacea includes:** *(PGI May 12)*
A. Papules ☐
B. Pustules ☐
C. Vesicles ☐
D. Telangiectasia ☐
E. Comedones ☐

TYPES & DISORDERS OF SWEAT GLANDS

34. **Sweat glands of palm can be defferentiated from others by the following :** *(Jipmer 91, Delhi 93)*
A. Apocrine glands ☐
B. High chloride content ☐
C. Secretion stimulated by emotional stimuli ☐
D. Chemical mediators mediators control control the secetion. ☐

35. **All are false except** *(PGI June 08)*
A. Sweat glands are most numerous on back & least on sole ☐
B. Palm & sole sweat glands are last to appear ☐
C. Sweat duct produce isotonic sweat ☐
D. Hypothalmic preoptic nucleus has key role in sweating ☐
E. Gonadectomy of adults impair apocrine sweat secretion ☐
F. Apocrine glands are under cholinergic control ☐

36. **True about apocrine gland is A/E** *(PGI June 09)*
A. Modified sweat gland ☐
B. Modified sebaceous gland ☐
C. Present in groin & axilla ☐
D. Infection is k/a hydradenitis suppurativa ☐

37. **Bromhidrosis may be produced by intake of the following except :** *(Jipmer 93, Rohtak 96)*
A. Asafoetida ☐
B. Ginger ☐
C. Onions ☐
D. Garlic ☐

38. **Crystaline miliaria is due to obstruction to-** *(JIPMER 93)*
A. Sebaceous glands ☐
B. Sweat glands ☐
C. Hair roots ☐
D. Accessory sweat glands ☐

39. **Miliaria is a disorder of:** *(PGI Dec 07)*
A. Sebaceous glands ☐
B. Apocrine glands ☐
C. Merocrine- glands ☐
D. Holocrine. Glands ☐
E. Eccrine Glands ☐

40. **In Fox Fordyce disease, true is/are:** *(PGI 2002)*
A. Common in adult woman ☐
B. Bullous lesions are common ☐
C. Common in areola & axilla ☐
D. Associated with other malignancies ☐

DISORDERS OF HAIR (ALOPECIA)

41. **Anagen phase of the hair indicates:**
A. The phase of activity and growth ☐
B. The phase of transition ☐
C. The phase of resting *(AIIMS May 06)* ☐
D. The phase of degeneration ☐

42. Growth phase of hair is *(PGI 97, 99, AI 98)*
A. Anagen ☐
B. Metagen ☐
C. Telogen ☐
D. None ☐

43. The time period that elapses between the physic emotional stress and the hair loss is about- *(Jipmer 99, DNB 01)*
A. 21 days ☐
B. 30 days ☐
C. 3 months ☐
D. 6 months ☐

44. A female patient presents with diffuse alopecia to you. She had suffered from typhoid fever 4 months back. Most probable diagnosis is: *(AIIMS Nov 07)*
B. Androgenetic alopecia ☐
C. Telogen effluvium ☐
D. Anagen effluvium ☐
E. Alopecia areata ☐

45. A 30 year old female developed diffuse hair loss 3 months after delivery of her first child. The probable diagnosis is *(PGI01,SGPGI 03)*
A. Androgenic alopecia ☐
B. Endocrinal alopecia ☐
C. Telogen effluvium ☐
D. SLE ☐

46. Cicatrising alopecia with perifollicular blue-gray patches hyperpigmentation is most commonly associated with:
A. Pitting of nails *(AI 2011)* ☐
B. Whitish lesions in the buccal mucosa ☐
C. Arthritis ☐
D. Discoid plaques in the face ☐

47. Cicatrisial alopecia is seen in: *(PGI Dec 07)*
A. DLE ☐
B. Psoriasis ☐
C. Alopecia areata ☐
D. Lichen planus ☐
E. SLE ☐

48. Cicatrial Alopecia is seen in: *(AI 99)*
A. Tenia Capitis ☐
B. Psoriasis ☐
C. DLE ☐
D. Alopecia Aereta ☐

49. Pseudo pelade is synonym of - *(AIIMS 91, PGI 94)*
A. Alopeciasteatoides ☐
B. Premature alopecia ☐
C. Traction ☐
D. Cicatricial alopecia ☐

50. Cicatricial alopecia is seen in: *(PGI Dec 04)*
A. DLE ☐
B. SLE ☐
C. Secondary syphilis ☐
D. Psoriasis ☐
E. Lichen planus ☐

51. Scarring alopecia is seen in: *(AI 2009)*
A. T. capitis ☐
B. Androgenic alopecia ☐
C. Alopecia areata ☐
D. Lichen planus ☐

52. Non cicatrical alopecia is present in- *(AIIMS 98)*
A. Scleroderma ☐
B. Lichen planus ☐
C. Psoriasis ☐
D. Parva virus ☐

53. All of the following are causes of cicatrizing alopecia except: *(AIIMs Nov 07)*
A. Lichen planus ☐
B. Discoid lupus erythematosus ☐
C. Alopecia areata ☐
D. Lupus vulgaris ☐

54. Alopecia aerata is: *(SGPGI – 2004)*
A. Cicatricial scar ☐
B. Non cicatricial scar ☐
C. Fungal infection ☐
D. None ☐

55. Non-circatrical alopecia is seen in *(PGI May 11)*
A. Alopecia aerate ☐
B. Androgenetic alopecia ☐
C. Pseudopalade ☐
D. DLE ☐
E. SLE ☐

56. Alopecia aerate is presumed to be:
A. Androgenic in nature *(AIIMS 92)* ☐
B. Autoimmune in etiology ☐
C. Infective in etiology ☐
D. Part of lichenoid in spectrum ☐

57. Exclamation mark hairs is seen in :
A. Alopecia areata *(Bihar 06, Kerala 01)* ☐
B. Traumatic alopecia ☐
C. Lichen planus ☐
D. All ☐

58. In alopecia areata, seen is: *(PGI 97)*
A. Exclamatory mark hair ☐
B. Scaring ☐
C. Fungal infection ☐
D. Traumatic ☐

59. Exclamation mark alopecia is a feature of:
A. Telogen effluvium *(AIIMS Nov 05)* ☐
B. Androgenic alopecia ☐
C. Alopecia aerata ☐
D. Alopecia mucinosa ☐

60. Male with patchy loss of scalp hair and grey hair in the eyebrows and beard diagnosis is
A. Anagen effluvium *(AI 08)* ☐
B. Alopecia areata ☐
C. Telogen effluvium ☐
D. Androgenic alopecia ☐

61. Alopecia areata is treated by- *(Jipmer 92, DNB 07)*
A. Minoxidil ☐
B. Tranquilizers ☐
C. Whitfields oinment ☐
D. Parenternal penicillin ☐

62. Diagnosis of a man with diffuse hair loss involving crown & frontal scalp with maintenance of frontal hair line *(Jipmer 98, DNB 01)*
A. Alopecia areata ☐
B. Anagen effluvium ☐
C. Male pattern baldness ☐
D. Female pattern baldness ☐

63. Contraindicated in Androgenic Alopecia:
A. Testosterone *(AI 2K, DNB 10)* ☐
B. Minoxidil ☐
C. Cyproterone ☐
D. Finasteride ☐

DISORDERS OF NAIL

64. Nail are involved in *(AIIMS 94)*
A. Pemphigus ☐
B. Pemphgoid ☐
C. Psoriasis ☐
D. Dermatitis Herpetiformis ☐

65. Nail is involved in: *(PGI Dec 07)*
A. Psoriasis ☐

B. Lichen planus ☐
C. Fungal infection ☐
D. Alopecia ☐
E. Viral infection ☐

66. Nail involvement is not a feature of
A. Psoriasis *(SGPGI 05, AIIMS 94)* ☐
B. Lichenplanus ☐
C. Dermatophytosis ☐
D. DLE ☐

67. Nail involvement is not a feature of :
A. Psoriasis *(AIIMS 92)* ☐
B. Drug induced lupus erythematous ☐
C. Dermatophytosis/Tenia ☐
D. Lichen Planus ☐

68. Pterygium of nail is characteristically seen in
A. Lichen planus *(AI 06, DNB 03)* ☐
B. Psoriasis ☐
C. Tinea unguium ☐
D. Alopecia areata ☐

69. Wrong statement is: *(AI 2000)*
A. Mees line in Arsenic poisoning ☐
B. Pterygium of nails in Lichen Planus ☐
C. Oncholysis in Psoriasis ☐
D. Koilonychia in Megaloblastic Anemia (B_{12} def.) ☐

70. Pitting of nails is seen in : *(AIIMS 01, UPSC 04, Jipmer 98, DNB 99)*
A. Lichen planus ☐
B. Psoriasis ☐
C. Phemphigus ☐
D. Arsenic poisoning ☐
E. Leprosy ☐

71. Pitting nail dystrophy seen in: *(PGI June 08, DNB 09)*
A. Dermatophytic infection ☐
B. Psoriasis ☐
C. Lichen planus ☐
D. Seborrhic dermatitis ☐

72. Oil drop is seen in : *(AP 96)*
A. Psoriasis of nails ☐
B. Lichen planus of nails ☐
C. Clubbing ☐
D. T. Unguim ☐

73. Which of the following is wrong statements: *(AI 00)*
A. Koilonychia in Vit B_{12} deficiency ☐
B. Oncholysis in Psoriasis ☐
C. Mees lines in Arsenic poisoning ☐
D. Pterygium of nailis in Lichen Planus ☐

74. Koenen's periungal fibroma is seen in *(PGI 96, Jipmer 02)*
A. Tuberous sclerosis ☐
B. Neurofibromatosis ☐
C. Psoriasis ☐
D. Alopecia aerata ☐

75. Tinea ungum effects *(AI 95)*
A. Nail fold ☐
B. Nail plate ☐
C. Joints ☐
D. Inter digital space ☐

76. A Patient presented with yellowish discoloration and thickening of nails. He also has tunneling of 2 toe and 1 Finger nails. Diagnosis can be done by *(PGI Nov 11)*
A. Wood's Lamp ☐
B. KOH. Mount ☐
C. Biopsy ☐
D. Trank Smear ☐

ANSWERS AND EXPLANATIONS

General Anatomy

1. **B, E i.e. Sandwitched b/w s. corneum & s. granulosum; Contain degenerated cells**
2. **D i.e. Keratinization process cause hydration of cells; E i.e. Spines of spinous cells are formed from house keeping organelle**
3. **D i.e. Stratum corneum**
4. **B i.e. 4 weeks**
5. **B i.e. Stratum basale**
6. **A ie $G_0 - G_1 - S - G_2 - M$**

[Rook's 8/e p. 3.1-3.2; Roxburgh's 18/e p. 4-7, 146; Thomas Hubif 4/e p. 549; Fitzpatric's 7/e p. 57-69, 130]

- *"Stratum corneum is permeable in preterm infants and becomes similar to the adult and full term infant after 2-3 weeks, postnatal maturation."*
- **Normal** turnover time of epidermis = *28 days (4 weeks)*[Q] but turnover time in psoriasis = *4 days*[Q]
- **Cell cycle sequence is -** $G_0 - G_1 - S - G_2 - M$
- **Acantholytic cells** are derived from ***stratum basale***[Q] ***in pemphigus vulgaris.***
- **Melanocytes** are present in ***stratum basale***[Q]
- ***Stratum corneum***[Q] is under developed in **VLBW infants in initial 7 days**
- **Dermatophytes (Ring worm)** live in ***stratum corneum***[Q]

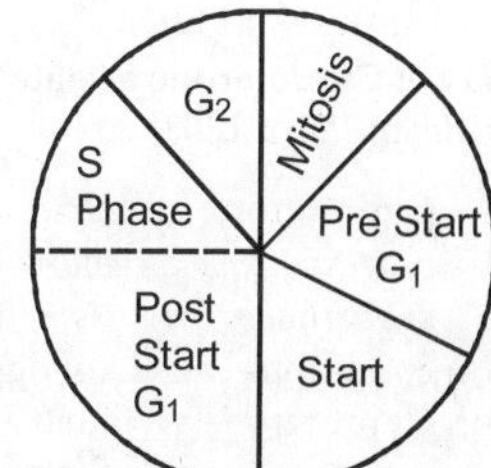

Development

7. **D i.e. Lines of development** *[Ref: Rook's 8/e p. 15.6 - 15.7, 18.2/4; Millington & Wilkinson 1/e p 18-19; Neurocuteneous disorders- Ruggieri (Springer 2008)- 364]*

Lines of Blaschko ***represent the developmental growth pattern of skin and do not correspond to any known nervous, vascular or lymphatic structures***[Q]. These *nonvisible* , *non random lines* of development of skin fundamentally ***differ from the system of dermatomes***[Q].

Skin Lesion

8. A i.e. Macule 9. A. i.e. Macule 10. C. i.e. Abscess *[Ref: Behl 8/e P-24]*

Acne Vulgaris

11. **A,C,D,E i.e. Hypersecretion of sebum; Follicular duct hypercornification; ↑Colonisation of propionibacterium acnes; IGF1**
12. **D i.e. Obstruction to pilosebaceous duct**
13. **B i.e. Only food**
14. **B. i.e. Only food**
15. **A. i.e. Acne Vulgaris**
16. **B i.e. Acne Vulgaris**
17. **A i.e. 13 cis retionol; B i.e. Minocycline; C i.e. Erytromycin**
18. **D. i.e. Androgen**
19. **A i.e. Retinoids**
20. **C i.e. Isoretinonine**
21. **D i.e. Retonoid**
22. **A, B i.e Minocycline for inflammatory acne , Retinoids for comedonal acne**
23. **B i.e. Isotretinoin**
24. **B i.e. Skin Rash**

[Roxburgh's 18/e p. 159-172; Rook's 8/e vol 2 p. 42.17-70; Fitzpatrick's 8/e p 897-907; Harrison's 18/e p. 403-409]

- **Acne vulgaris** is characterized by ***seborrhea (greasy skin), comedones (hallmark)***Q, *erythematous papules, pustules, nodules & psedo cysts.* It is caused by multiple factors like **follicular epidermal hyperproliferation, excessive sebum production, obstruction of pilosebaceous duct** (d/t hyperkeratosis/hypercornification)Q. **P. acnes bacteria, inflammation, androgen, insulin like growth factor (IGF)2, increased IL 1α activity, FGFR2 signaling, decreased linoleic acid and diet (but not only food)**Q. Treatment of acne vulgaris depends on type of severity of lesion but the **mainstay of treatment** or **drug of choice** remains ***synthetic retinoids*** Q (topical in most and oral **isotretinoin** in severe cases).
- Synthetic retinoids are drug of choice in acne vulgaris with
  1. ***Comedones*** Q
  2. ***Severe nodulocystic (conglobate)*** Q
  3. Mild to moderate **papulopustular** (with antibiotics)
  4. **Moderate nodular (with anti-biotics).**

Feature \ Type	Comedones	Inflammatory lesions
Seen in	Pre-teens	Teen-agers
Most effective drug (of choice)	**Topical retinoids** Q eg tretinoin	**Antibiotics**Q like ***oral tetracycline & doxycycline*** Q. **Minocycline** is reversed for resistant cases

Side effects of **isotretinoin (oral retinoid)** are

1. **Muco-cutaneous problems** like **skin rash** Q, Cheilitis, conjunctivitis, blepharitis, desquamation etc are **most common** (also occur with topical retinoids)
2. **Teratogenicity** Q (is most serious; so contraindicated in pregnancy)
3. **Hyper-triglyceridemia** (↑ TG, cholesterol), hepatotoxicity, bone toxicity (disseminated interstitial skeletal hyperostosis, & osteoporosis) on prolonged use especially in older.
4. Depression, achillis tendonitis, high toned deafness etc.

Agent	Sebum suppressive	**Comedolytic**	**Antimicrobial**	**Anti-inflammatory**
Retinoids eg. Adapalene, tretinoin	No except isotretinoin	High	No	Mild-moderate
Antimicrobial eg. BPO, Clindamycin, erythromycin, tetracycline, nicotinamide (NM)	No	Mild	High except BPO & NM (both have mild)	

25. **D i.e. Cyproterone acetate** *[Ref: Novak's 14/e p 1085; Fitzpatrick's 7/e p. 698; Shaw's 14/e p 287; Rook's 8/e p. 42.52; Goodman & Gilman 12/e p 1205]*

- **Cyproterone acetate** is a **progestin and a weak anti androgen** by virtue of binding to the androgen receptor (*i.e. progestational antiandrogen that blocks androgen receptor*). Because of antiandrogen action, it is efective in conditions like ***acne seborrhoea, hirsutism, female pattern hair loss (androgenetic hair loss in females), hidreadinitis suppurativa***Q –i.e. conditions caused or aggravated by androgenic hormones.
- Cyproterone acetate (CPA) is *effective in treatment of acne as it reduces sebum production (dose dependent) & comedogenesis.* In **premenopausal women** it is usually combined with ethinyloestradiol (Dianette & estelle 35) or other oral contraceptive agents to ***regulate menstrual cycle irregularities***Q (caused by high dose cyproterone) and *prevent pregnancy* (d/t concerns of feminising effects of cyproterone on male fetus). Whereas, in **postmenopausal women,** it is not necessary to combine ethinyl oestradiol (EOD) with CPA.
- **Reverse sequential regimen (CPA** 100 mg / day on days 5 to 15, **and EOD** 30-50 mg /day on cycle days 5to 26) ***regulates menstrual bleeding, provides excellent contraception and is effective in treatment of even severe hirsutism and acne***Q. Acne usually improves 40-50% by 3rd and 80-90% by 9th cycle.

Other Disorders of Sebaceous Glands

26. **B i.e. Minocycline** *[Ref: Harrison 17/e p. 328, Horn dermatology (2003) 1/e p-67; Atlas of disease of nail (2003) p-35-36]*

- **Amongst tetracyclines** (tetracycline/ minocycline/ doxycycline) ***pigmentation is most commonly associated with minocycline***Q. A diffuse ***blue-black/blue- gray/ muddy hyper pigmentation***Q is an uncommon but troublesome side effect of **prolonged minocycline therapy**. Sites of involvement include sun exposed ***skin, mucus membranes (eg conjunctiva), nails, teeth, sclera, thyroid & bones***Q.
- Two side effects unique to minocycline are *drug induced lupus & blue black pigmentation*. Tetracycline induced nail discolouration is *yellow*.

27. **C i.e. Pilosebaceous glands**

28. **B i.e. Ectopic Sebaceous gland; D i.e. Found in healthy people**

Acne vulgaris is due to obstruction of ***pilosebaceous glands***Q l/t formation of ***comedones***Q, papules, pustules & cyst. Also remember obstruction of following structures lead to

Pilo-Sebaceous gland	**Sweat gland**	**Apocrine gland**	**Hair-root**
- *Acne vulgaris*Q - *Fordyce spot*Q	*Crystalline miliaria*Q	Fox Fordyce's disease	Boil

29. **A. i.e. Lips > B i.e. Buccal mucosa**

30. **A i.e. Glandular form of acne rosacea**

31. **D i.e. Sebaceous gland hypertrophy**

32. **B i.e. Rosacea**

33. **A i.e. Papules; B i.e. Pustule; C i.e. Talangiectasia**

[Ref: Rook's 8/e p. 43.1-43.10; Fitzpatric's 7/e, p-704-08; Neena Khanna 3/e, p-104-105; Roxburgh's 18/e p. 172-78; Harrison 18/e p 444, 404]

Rosacea (Acne Rosacea)

- Definition – Rosacea is a chronic inflammatory disorder of the skin of the *facial convexities, characterized by persistent erythema and telangiectasia punctuated by acute episodes of swelling, papules & pustules*Q.
- Clinical features
  - Seen almost exclusively in adults, only ***rarely affecting patients under 30 years***Q of age
  - Seen ***more often in women***, but those most severly affected are men
  - Central face (cheeks, forehead, nose & chin) is most frequently affected, making typical *cruciate pattern of skin involvement.*

    The flexures & periocular areas are conspicuously spared. Chest & back involvement is also rare.
  - It is characterized by ***erythemato-telangiectatic state.*** Superimposed on this are episodes of *swelling & papules.* The papules are dull red, dome shaped & non tender, in contrast to acne, in which they tend to be irregular & tender. *Pustules* also occur, but are less frequent than in acne; *comedones, blackheads, cysts and scars do not.*
  - Pronounced flushing in response to heat, emotional stimuli, alcohol, hot drink, or spicy food may be the initial feature
  - Long standing rosacea may lead to connective tissue overgrowth, particularly of nose (***rhinophyma***) Q
- **Treatment**
  - Topical corticosteroid are contraindicated
  - Mild case respond to topical metronidazole or sodium sulfacitamide
  - Acute (severe) episodes treated by systemic tetracycline, erythromycin or metronidazole.
- **Differential diagnosis**

I. Acne vulgaris

- Occurs in *younger* age grup
- **Distinguished by the *greasy* skin, *comedones and scars* as wells as lesions on sites other than face (ie *back & chest*)**

II. SLE

- *No symptoms of systemic disease* (eg. Arthropathy, positive antinuclear antibody etc) in rosacea

III. Polymorphic Light Eruption (PLE)

- Mostly present with ***often intensely pruritic erythematous papules that may coalesce into plaques in a patchy distribution on sun exposed areas of trunk & forearms***Q.
- Morphological **skin findings remain similar for each patient with** subsequent recurrences, **significant individual variations** in skin findings are characteristic (**hence** term **polymorphous**).

Sweat Gland and Disorders

34. **C i.e. Secretion stimulated by emotional stimuli**

35. **D i.e. Hypothalmic preoptic nucleus has key role in sweating**

[Ref: Rooks Textbook of Dermatology 8/e p. – 44.15-44.16]

36. **B i.e. Modified sebaceous gland**

37. **B i.e. Ginger**

38. **B. i.e. Sweat glands**

39. **E i.e. Eccrine gland**

40. **A i.e. Common in adult women, C i.e. Common in axilla & areola**

Hair Growth and Disorders of Hair (Alopecia)

41. **A i.e. The phase of activity & growth**

42. **A i.e. Anagen** *[Ref: Roxburgh's 18/e p. 280-88; Rooks 8/e vol 4 p. 66.7, 66.16 – 66.60; Fitzpatrick's 7/e p 761-62; Neena Khanna 4/e p. 129-136; Behl 10/eP 418; Harrison's 18/e p. 407-408]*

Anagen is *anabolic stage* of hair cycle, *causing* ***activity and growth of hair***[Q].

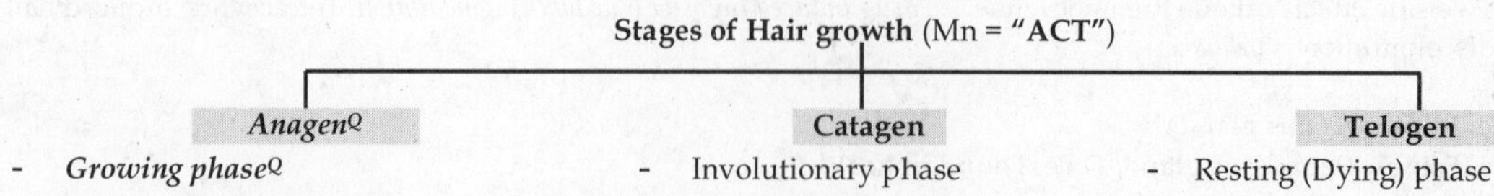

43. **C. i.e. 3 months** **44.** **B i.e.Telogen effluvium** **45.** **C i.e. Telogen effluvium**

Diffuse hair loss after 3 months of prolonged, high grade, recurrent fever of any cause (eg typhoid) or difficult & prolonged child birth[Q] indicates diagnosis – **telogen effluvium.** The onset of hair loss is rapid within 2-4 weeks of causes (like radio/chemotherapy, poisoning/intoxication and malnutrition) in anagen effluvium.

46. **B i.e. Whitish lesions in the buccal mucosa** *[Ref: Rook's 8/e p. 41.7/11, 51.4/22; Fitzpatrick's 7/e p. 248, 1524]*

Cicatrising alopecia with perifollicular erythema / hyperpigmentation / hyperkeratosis & scale[Q] are seen in **lichen planus** (lichen planopilaris or spinosus et folliculitis decalvans). Whereas, ***Ciratrising alopecia with follicular accentuation / widening / dilation and keratotic plugging (i.e dilated hyperpigmented follicular orifices)***[Q]. are seen in **DLE.**

47. **A i.e. DLE; D i.e. Lichen planus; E i.e. SLE**
48. **C. i.e. DLE**
49. **D. i.e. Cicatrical alopecia**
50. **A i.e. DLE; B i.e. SLE; E i.e. Lichen planus**
51. **D i.e. Lichen planus**
52. **C. i.e. Psoriasis**
53. **C i.e. Alopacia aerate**
54. **B. i.e. Non Cicatrial**
55. **A i.e. Alopecia aerata ; B i.e. Androgenetic alopecia; E i.e. SLE**

- **Scarring Alopecia** is seen in "5L, 4F, 3S" i.e. Lichen planus[Q], Leprosy, Lupus vulgars, Linear scleroderma (morphea), *Lupus eryrhematosus (DLE & SLE)*, Folliculitis decalvans, ***Follicular degeneration syndrome (pseudo pelade of Broq), Frontal fibrosing alopecia of Kossard, Favus & Kerion; Sarcoid, Syphilitic gumma & Secondaries.***
- In **DLE** (a form of SLE) there is **cicatrial alopecia** & in **SLE** there is **non cicatrial alopecia**; thus SLE has both forms of alopecia.
- In **psoriasis** there is no alopecia inspite of very common scalp involvement.
- ***Lichen planus, lupus vulgaris, DLE, pseudopelade & tenia capititis with kerion***[Q] leads to **scarring alopecia**; whereas ***Alopecia areate, androgenetic alopecia, tenia capitis (without kerion) and psoriasis***[Q] (alopecia is very rare) leads to **non-scarring alopecia.**

56. **B. i.e. Autoimmune in etiology** **57.** **A. i.e. Alopecia areata** **58.** **A i.e. Exclamatory mark**

Stumps in alopecia areata form exclamation mark[Q] (constriction) just above the skin surface. ***Exclamation mark hair is pathognomic of alopecia areata***[Q].

59. **C i.e. Alopecia aerate** **60.** **B i.e. Alopecia areata**

Single or multiple circumscribed smooth patchy hair loss, most obviously on scalp but frequently involving any hair bearing skin eg beard, eyebrows, eye lashes, with pathognomic "exclamation mark" & "going gray overnigth" phenomenon (i.e., white or gray hairs are frequently spared)[Q] indicate the diagnosis of **alopecia areata.** Scanty stumps form ***'Exclamation mark (!) in alopecia areata***

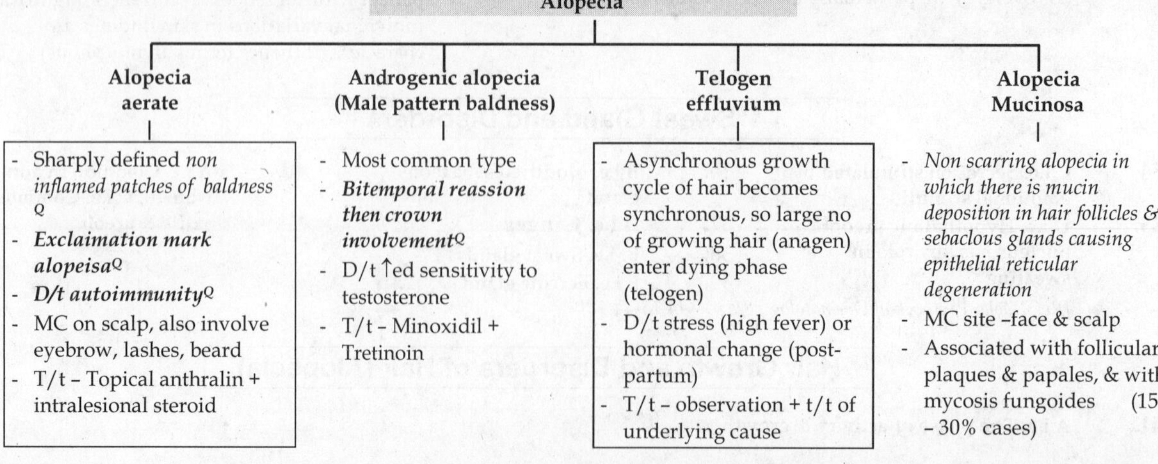

Alopecia
Alopecia aerate
- Sharply defined non inflamed patches of baldness Q
- Exclaimation mark alopeisa Q
- D/t autoimmunity Q
- MC on scalp, also involve eyebrow, lashes, beard
- T/t – Topical anthralin + intralesional steroid
Androgenic alopecia (Male pattern baldness)
- Most common type
- Bitemporal reassion then crown involvement Q
- D/t ↑ed sensitivity to testosterone
- T/t – Minoxidil + Tretinoin
Telogen effluvium
- Asynchronous growth cycle of hair becomes synchronous, so large no of growing hair (anagen) enter dying phase (telogen)
- D/t stress (high fever) or hormonal change (post-partum)
- T/t – observation + t/t of underlying cause
Alopecia Mucinosa
- Non scarring alopecia in which there is mucin deposition in hair follicles & sebaclous glands causing epithelial reticular degeneration
- MC site –face & scalp
- Associated with follicular plaques & papales, & with mycosis fungoides (15 – 30% cases)

61. **A. i.e. Minoxidil** **62.** **D i.e. Female pattern baldness** **63.** **A i.e. Testosterone**

[Ref: Fitzpatric's dermatology in general medicine 7/e p- 762-67]

***Testosterone is an etiological agent so it is contraindicated*[Q] *& antiandrogens are used in t/t of androgenic alopecia*[Q].**

Disorders of Nail

64. **C i.e. Psoriasis**
65. **A i.e., Psoriasis B Lichen planus C i.e., Fungal infection D i.e., Alopecia E i.e., Viral infection**
66. **D i.e. DLE**
67. **B i.e. DLE**
68. **A i.e. Lichen planus**
69. **D i.e. Koilonychia in megaloblastic anemia (B12 def)**
70. **B. i.e. Psoriasis**
71. **B. i.e. Psoriasis**
72. **A. i.e. Psoriasis of nails**
73. **A. i.e. Koilonychia in vit B12 deficiency**
74. **A i.e. Tuberous sclerosis**
75. **B i.e. Nail plate**

[Ref: Roxburgh's 18/e p. 288-292; Rooks 8/e vol 4 p. 65.1-65.50, 51.12; Fitzpatrick's 7/e p 778-98; Neena Khanna 4/e p. 139-144; Harrison's 18/e p. 398-401; API 6/e p. 1179]

- ***Pterygium of nail is characteristically seen in lichen planus & Koilonychia is found in Iron deficiency anemia*[Q]** (not megaloblastic anemia).
- In 10-15% of cases, **alopecia areata** causes ***fine stippled pitting of nails*[Q]** or less commonly well defined roughening of nail plate (trachyonychia) or a non specific atrophic dystrophy.

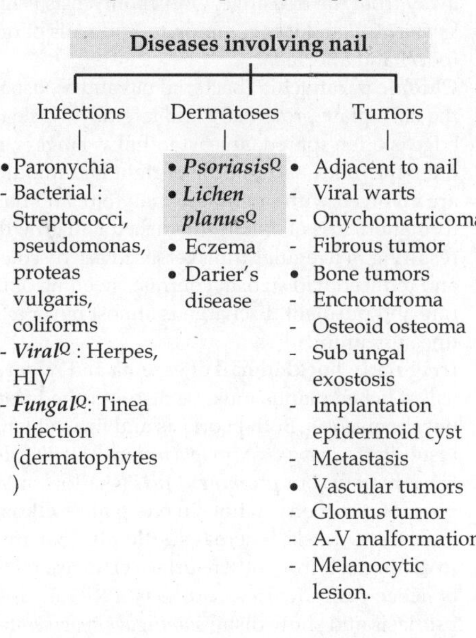

Diseases involving nail
Infections
Dermatoses
Tumors
• Paronychia
- Bacterial : Streptococci, pseudomonas, proteas vulgaris, coliforms
- Viral[Q] : Herpes, HIV
- Fungal[Q]: Tinea infection (dermatophytes)
• Psoriasis[Q]
• Lichen planus[Q]
• Eczema
• Darier's disease
• Adjacent to nail
- Viral warts
- Onychomatricoma
- Fibrous tumor
• Bone tumors
- Enchondroma
- Osteoid osteoma
- Sub ungal exostosis
- Implantation epidermoid cyst
- Metastasis
• Vascular tumors
- Glomus tumor
- A-V malformation
- Melanocytic lesion.

Pattern of nail involvement

- **DLE**
  - ***No nail involvement*** (relatively). However chloroquin responsive subungal hyperkeratosis, red-blue nail plate with stria may be seen.
  - Usually in females, Butterfly malar rash with carpet track appearence found.
  - Chloroquin is used in patients not responding to steroids
- **Fe deficiency Anemia**
  - *Koilonychia*[Q]
- **As poisoning**
  - *Mee's Line*[Q]
- **Lichen Planus**
  - *Pterygium*[Q]
  - Anychia
  - Onychorrhexia
  - Pitting
- **Psoriasis**
  - ***Pitting of nail*[Q]** (thimble nail)
  - Oil (spot) drop nails
  - ***Onycholysis (detachment of nail plate)*[Q]**
  - ***Discolouration of nail plate***
  - ***Subungal hyperkeratosis (i.e. keratin debris under nail plate)***

Disease	Nail involvement
Dermatophytosis (Tinea ungum)	***Nail plate*[Q] > Nail bed**
Psoriasis	Nail plate > Nail bed
Lichen planus	Nail plate > Nail matrix

76. **B i.e. KOH mounting** *[Ref: Rook's 8/e p. 36.24, 65.23/27]*

Asymmetric involvement of toe>finger nail, yellow discoloration, nail thickening and tunneling indicate the diagnosis of **tinea unguium**, which can be confirmed by **KOH mounting.**

Tinea unguium (Ringworm of nails or Onychomycosis caused by Dermatophytes)

Etiopathogenesis

- **Onychomycosis** means any infection of nail caused by drmatophyte or nondermatophyte fungi and yeast. Whereas, **tinea unguium** refers strictly to ***dermatophyte infection of nail plate*[Q]**
- **T. rubrum** (71%) is the most common cause, f/b T. mentagrophyte (20%), of tinea unguium involving finger and toe nails.
- Invasion of nail plate usually occurs either from lateral nail fold or from the free edge. It begins with *invasion of stratum corneum of hyponychium and distal nail bed forming a **white to brownish yellow opacification** at the distal edge of nail.* The infection then spreads proximally up the nail bed

Clinical Features (5 patterns)

1. **Distal & lateral subungual onychomycosis** is most common pattern & usually presents as **patch or streak of yellow or white to brown or black discoloration** at the free edge of nail plate often near the lateral nail fold. ***Nail plate thicking and cracking*[Q]** f/b TDO are late features.
2. **Proximal subungual onychomycosis**- is particular a/w **AIDS.** Rapid invasion of nail plate from posterior nail fold may develop to produce a **white to beige opacity on proximal** nail plate that gradually enlarges to affect *entire nail,* leukonychia, proximal onychomycosis with only marginal increase in thickness

1

DERMATOLOGY

to the ventral nail plate.

- In response to infection, there is ***nail bed hyperproliferation*** creating ***subungual hyperkeratosis***. The *nail plate becomes thickened* and may *crack* as it is lifted up by accumulation of soft subungual hyperkeratosis. Nail plate thickening & subungual hyperkeratosis contribute to ***nail discoloration (yellow appearance)*** particularly common in toes. Green color is usually caused by candida and pseudomonas infection & destruction
- In late stage, progressive invasion of nail plate leads to an *increasingly dystrophic nail*.

3. **Superficial white onychomycosis** is direct invasion of *dorsal nail plate* resulting in ***white to dull yellow sharply circumscribed (bordered)*** powdery patches anywhere on the surface of toe nail (often away from free edge). *Easily scrappable powdery nature* distinguishes it from other causes of leukonykia. **Striate banding** may also occur.
4. **Endonyx onychomycosis** is caused by dermatophytes that cause end-thrix scalp infection mainly T. soudanense. Nail plate is scarred with **pits and lamellar splits**.
5. **Totally dystrophic nail (TDO)**

Differential Diagnosis

	Fungal infections	Psoriasis	Chronic Paronychia	Dermatitis
Color	*Yellow or brown* (often); part or whole of nail	***Maybe normal or yellow or brown***Q	Edge of nail often discolored brown or black	May be normal
Onycholysis	Common (frequent)	Common	Usually absent	Confined to tips or absent
Pitting	Infrequent	***Frequent &Fine***Q	Uncommon	Coarse pits frequent
Cross ridging	Absent	Uncommon	***Frequent; irregular transverse ridges***Q	Frequent; transverse ridges and furrows (Similar to psoriatic nail)
Filaments or spores in **KOH mount**	Filaments, usually abundant	Absent	Spores in edge of nail; spores and filament in scraping from nail folds may be seen	Absent
Other Association	Fungal infection elsewhere	F/H or personal h/o psoriasis elsewhere	Mostly women; wet work and cold hands thumb sucking	Recent h/o hand dermatitis

- In **onychomycosis, toes** are more commonly affected, whereas **finger nails** are more commonly affected in **psoriasis**. If there is fingernail involvement in **onychomycosis**, it is usually of ***only one or a few of digits***Q, whereas in *psoriasis*, there are usually *several digits* affected. The changes are often on the *nail surface in psoriasis*, whereas in onychomycosis features are usually *with in or beneath the nail plate*. Fine pitting of dorsal nail plate is never produced by fungal infections and strongly suggests psoriasis, as does the oil drop sign away from the free edge. Onlychomycosis is *rarely symmetrical* and it is common to find nails of one foot/hand affected.
- **Chronic paronychia** (bacterial or candia), usually affects the nails plate proximally and laterally, while the free edge is often spared, at least initially. Fingers, most often the index and middle of right and middle of left are involved with swelling of nail fold, and pus formation, loss of cuticle, disturbed nail growth resulting in irregular transverse ridges, discoloration and reduced nail size. In contrast, swelling of nail fold is rare and purulent discharge is almost never a feature of tinea unguium.
- **Irregularly buckled nail** of eczema and *ridged dysplastic nail* of lichen planus must be distinguished from onychomycosis. Both psoriasis and lichen planus may result in *trachyonychia (roughened nails) with subungal hyper keratosis* but **prominent pits** (shallow or large to the point of punched out hole in nail plate = **elkonyxis**) indicate psoriasis, whereas **subtle pits** that are difficult to distinguish from other surface changes, may be part of lichen plans. *Reiter's disease and PRP* can also mimic psoriasis and show distal *subungual hyperkeratosis and splinter hemorrhage*.
- Nail signs of psoriasis in reducing order of freacuency are pits, onycholysis, subungual hyperkeratosis, nail plate discoloration, uneven nail surface, splinter hemorrhages, acute and chronic paronychia and transverse midline depression in thumbnails. It can also be classified into.

Nail plate changes	Diseased area	Disease duration
Pits	Proximal matrix	Short; episodic
Transverse furrows	Proximal matrix	1-2 weeks
Leukonychia with rough surface	Proximal (± distal) matrix	Variable
Crumbling nail plate	Entire matrix	Prolonged

Nail bed and hyponychium change	Diseased area	Duration
Splinter hemorrhage	Nail bed	Short
Oily spot/onycholysis	Nail bed	Prolonged
False nail following onychomadesis.		
Subungual hyperkeratosis		
Yellow-green discoloration of nail bed	2° inf. by yeast or pseudomonas	Prolonged

2 DISORDERS OF PIGMENTATION

Causes of Hypopigmentation/Hypomelanosis

Primary Cutaneous Disorder

- Localized
  1. ***Vitiligo (Halo/ Sutton's nevus)***Q
  2. Tinea (pityriasis) versicolour
  3. ***Nevus anaemicus***Q
  4. ***Nevus depigmentosus***Q
  5. ***Piebaldism***Q
- Diffuse
  - Generalized vitiligo (absence of melanocytes)

Systemic Disease

- Localized
  1. ***Tuberous sclerosis***Q
  2. ***Tuberculoid & indeterminate leprosy***Q
  3. Cutaneous T- cell lymphoma
  4. Hypomelanosis of Ito /mosaicism
  5. Melanoma associated leukoderma
  6. ***Scleroderma***Q
  7. Sarcoidosis
  8. ***Incontinentia pigmenti (stage IV)***Q
  9. Vogt koyanagi Harada syndrome
- Diffuse
  1. ***Occulocutaneous albinism***Q (normal no. of melanocytes)
     - Hermansky –pudlak syndrome
     - Chediak – Higashi syndrome
  2. *Phenylketonuria*
  3. *Homocystinuria*

Genetic & Naevoid Disorders

- Oculocutaneous albinism (OCA)
  - Tyrosine positive/negative
  - Hermansky-Pudlak syndrome
  - Chediak-Higashi syndrome
- Ocular albinism
- Albinoidism
- Cross syndrome
- Piebaldism
- Phenylketonuria
- Waardenburg syndrome
- ***Vitiligo***Q
- Tuberous sclerosis
- Achromic naevus
- In continentia pigmenti achromians

Acquired Hypomelanosis

- Endocrine disorders
  - Diffuse loss of pigment d/t lack of MSH- **Hypopituitarism**
  - Circumscribed vitiligo like areas eg **Addison's disease, thyroid disease**
- Chemical factors
  - **Monobenzylether** and **monomethyl ether** (eg P-tertiary butyl or amyl phenol) cause circumscribed vitiligo like areas
  - **Chloroquin & hydroxychloroquine**
  - **Arsenic** (partial loss of pigment in circumscribed area = PLC)
- Nutritional factors eg chronic protein deficiency & pernicious anemia (l/t loss of pigment in hair).
- Post inflammatory & infections (all cause PLC).
  - ***Eczema (pityriasis alba)***Q
  - ***Pityriasis versicolar***Q
  - ***Psoriasis***Q
  - ***Pinta, syphilis, yaws***Q
  - Lupus erythematosus
  - ***Lichen planus***Q
  - Sarcoidosis
- Neoplasm eg *Halo naevus & malignent melanoma* (both circumscribed vitiligo like area).
- Miscellaneous eg *Vogt-koyanagi-Harada syndrome & idiopathic guttate hypomelanosis* (both PLC).

Vitiligo

Aetiology

- **Genetic** *factor is undoubtly* ***involved***Q, since 30-40% of patients have positive family history. Inheritance may be *polygenic or AD*.
- **Autoimmune hypothesis**
  - Associated with autoimmune disorders eg. thyroid ds, diabetes mellitus etc.
  - Autoantibodies to *thyroid, gastric parietal cells & adrenal tissue.*
  - *Antibodies to melanocyte* in vitiligo patients who also had alopecia areata, mucocutaneous candidiasis & multiple endocrinal insufficiencies.
  - ***Pathology shows marked absence of melanocytes & melanin in epidermis with infiltration of Langerhans cells, lymphocytes & histiocytes.***Q
- **Neurogenic hypothesis**
  - *Dermatomal distribution of segmental vitiligo* & abnormalities of terminal portions of peripheral nerve

Associated disorders

- **Endocrine disorders**
  - Addison's disease
  - ***Diabetes mellitus***Q
  - Thyroid disease (hypo & hyper)
  - Hypoparathyrodism
- Appendageal disorder
  - Alopecia areata
  - *Halo naevus (often antedate the onset of vitiligo)*
  - Morphea
  - Lichen sclerosis
  - Malignant melanoma
  - Mysthenia gravis
- Pernicious anemia
- 4 systemic disease – ***Vogt-Koyanagi Harada Syndrome, Scleroderma, Onchocerciasis and melanoma associated leukoderma*** should be considered in vitiligo.

Epidemiology

Affects 1% of world population with same frequency *in both sexes*

Types

- **Vitiligo vulgaris**

Commonest progressive variety

- **Segmental vitiligo**
  - Dermatomal/quasidermatomal distribution,
  - Stable/static course
  - Leucotrichia
  - Not associated with autoimmune disease
- **Generalized vitiligo**
  - **Lip-tip vitiligo** involves lips & tips of penis, vulva & nipples.
  - **Acrofacial vitiligo**
  - **Vitiligo universalis** widespread disease oftenly associated with multiple autoimmune endocrinopathies

Treatment

- **Topical corticosteroids** are the *1st line of t/t for children.* It is indicated for ***localized new lesions.*** **Lesions on *face have best response***Q (d/t high permeability) and lesions on neck & extremities (except finger & toes) also have favourable response. Recurrence after cessation, & *side effects eg. skin atrophy, telengiectases, striae & contact*

suggest that a toxin released from endings could destroy melanocytes & inhibit melanogenesis
- *Neuropeptide Y* may have a role
- **Self destruct theory of Lerner**
- Melanocytes destroy themselves d/t defect in natural protective mechanism to remove toxic melanin precursor
- Defective keratinocyte metabolism, low catalase levels in epidermis, defective tetra hydrobiopterin & catecholamine biosynthsesis play a role.

Poor prognostic factors

- Long standing vitiligo
- ***Leucotrichia (depigmented hair)***[Q]
- *Acrofacial lesion* i.e.,
  - *acral = palms, soles & periungal area*
  - facial = periorificially around eyes & lips
- *Lesions on resistant areas* .i.e.,
  - bony prominences = elbow, wrist, ankle
  - nipples, areolae, genitals
  - non hairy, non fleshy & mucosal areas.

Treatment algorithm

<20% skin surface involved	≥ 20% skin surface involved
↓	↓
Topical steroids, tacrolimus or calcipotriol or a combination	**Phototherapy** i.e., NB-UVB / **PUVA**/ PUVASOL
↓ No response	↓
Topical PUVA or phototherapy	no response & >50% skin involved
↓ No response	↓
Grafting / melanocyte transplant	Depigmentation

PUVASOL = Psoralen, UV A, & solar light

dermatitis are limiting factors.

- **Topical immunomodulators** i.e., **tacrolimus** (0.03 –0.1%) is considered *safer for children than topical steroids particularly on face & neck.* Its more effective when combined with *ultraviolet B (UVB) or excimer (308 nm) laser*
- Topical calcineurin inhibitor & calcipotriol
- Pseudocatalase
- Systemic steroids
- **Narrow band ultraviolet B (NBUB-311nm) radiation** is first choice for extensive generalized vitiligo
- **Topical or oral psoralen (8 methoxy psoralen) with UV-A (320 – 400nm) radiation (PUVA)**
  - topical PUVA is used for old lesion involving <20% of body surface area
  - oral psoralen is used in extensive disease or in patients not responding to topical PUVA
- **Excimer (308 nm) laser**
- Depigmentation of residual normal skin by *monobenzyl ether of hydroquinone (monobenzone)*
- Systemic corticosteroid (pulse therapy)
- Autologous thin thiersch split thickness /mini punch/ suction blister grafting
- Transplantation of autologous cultured melanocytes

Causes of Hyperpigmentation/Hypermelanosis

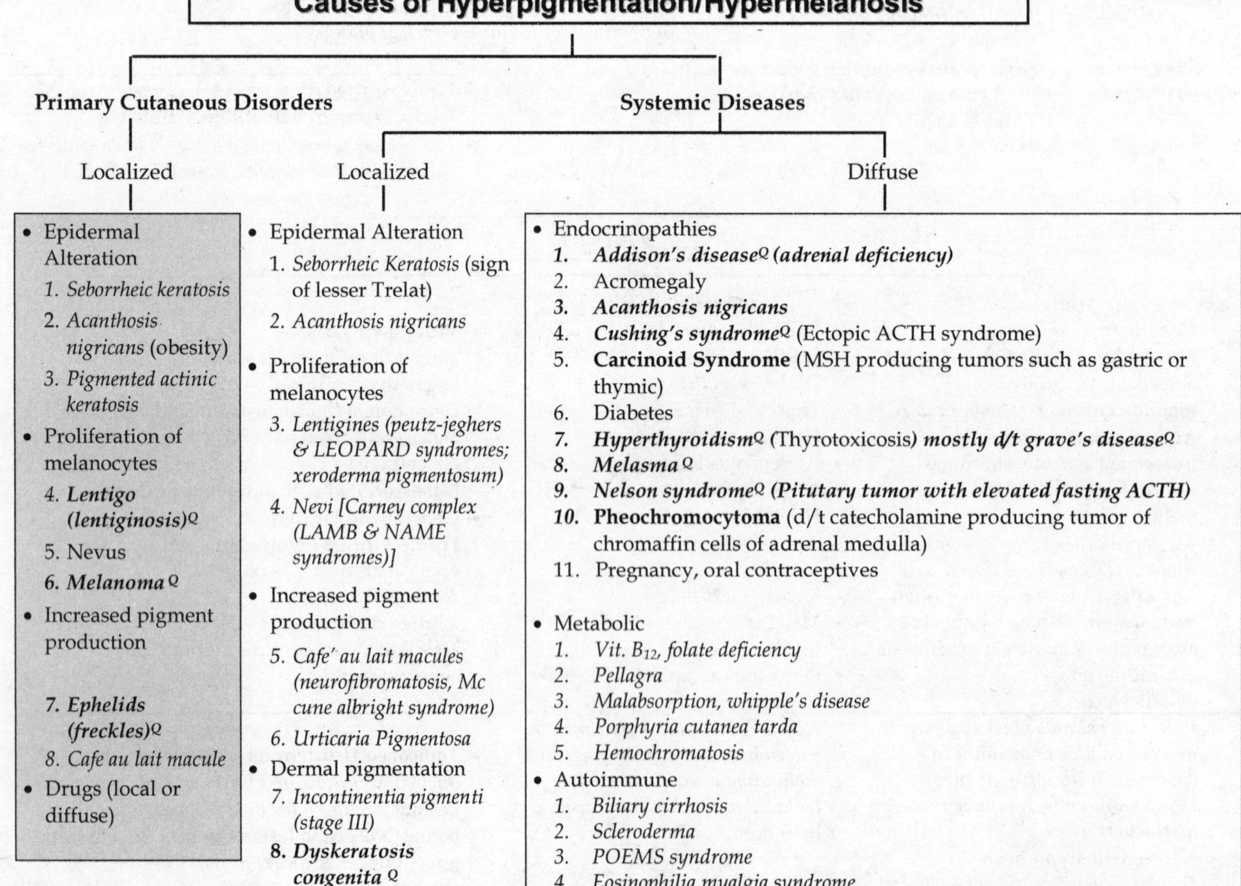

Primary Cutaneous Disorders
Systemic Diseases
Localized
Localized
Diffuse
• Epidermal Alteration
1. Seborrheic keratosis
2. Acanthosis nigricans (obesity)
3. Pigmented actinic keratosis
• Proliferation of melanocytes
4. Lentigo (lentiginosis)[Q]
5. Nevus
6. Melanoma [Q]
• Increased pigment production
7. Ephelids (freckles)[Q]
8. Cafe au lait macule
• Drugs (local or diffuse)
• Epidermal Alteration
1. Seborrheic Keratosis (sign of lesser Trelat)
2. Acanthosis nigricans
• Proliferation of melanocytes
3. Lentigines (peutz-jeghers & LEOPARD syndromes; xeroderma pigmentosum)
4. Nevi [Carney complex (LAMB & NAME syndromes)]
• Increased pigment production
5. Cafe' au lait macules (neurofibromatosis, Mc cune albright syndrome)
6. Urticaria Pigmentosa
• Dermal pigmentation
7. Incontinentia pigmenti (stage III)
8. Dyskeratosis congenita [Q]
• Endocrinopathies
1. Addison's disease[Q] (adrenal deficiency)
2. Acromegaly
3. Acanthosis nigricans
4. Cushing's syndrome[Q] (Ectopic ACTH syndrome)
5. Carcinoid Syndrome (MSH producing tumors such as gastric or thymic)
6. Diabetes
7. Hyperthyroidism[Q] (Thyrotoxicosis) mostly d/t grave's disease[Q]
8. Melasma [Q]
9. Nelson syndrome[Q] (Pitutary tumor with elevated fasting ACTH)
10. Pheochromocytoma (d/t catecholamine producing tumor of chromaffin cells of adrenal medulla)
11. Pregnancy, oral contraceptives
• Metabolic
1. Vit. B12, folate deficiency
2. Pellagra
3. Malabsorption, whipple's disease
4. Porphyria cutanea tarda
5. Hemochromatosis
• Autoimmune
1. Biliary cirrhosis
2. Scleroderma
3. POEMS syndrome
4. Eosinophilia myalgia syndrome

* Seborrheic keratosis is a sign of systemic disease when it occurs as *sudden appearance* of multiple lesions, with *inflammatory base* and in association with *acrochordons (skin tags) and acanthosis nigricans*. This is termed as **sign of leser Trelat** and *signifies internal malignancy*

* **Acanthosis nigricans** can also be a reflection of *internal malignancy*, most commonly of *gastrointestinal tract* & it appears as velvety hyperpigmentation, primarily in flexural areas. In majority of patients, it is associated with *obesity* and *insulin resistance*, but may be reflection of endocrinopathy such as *acromegaly, Cushing's syndrome, Stein – leventhal syndrome* or *insulin resistant diabetes mellitus* (type A, B, & lipoatrophic form).

- Melanosis secondary to metastatic melanoma
- Drugs & metals (**arsenic=** ***rain drop pigmentation***Q, chlorpromazine/phenothiazines = blue grey; chloroquine/ hydroxychloroquine= blue-grey to blue black)
  - Busulfan (diffuse brown), bleomycin, cyclophosphamide, daunorubicin, adriamycin, fluorouracil, hydroxyuria, methotrexate, mithramycin, mitomycin, thiotepa, adriamycin produce hyperpigmentation.
  - Topical cytostatic drugs carmustine,fluorouracil & mechlorethamine produce localized hyperpigmentation
  - Busulfan & doxorubicin cause mucous membrane pigmentation.
  - Bleomycin, cyclophosphamide, dauno & doxo-rubicin and fluorouracil l/t banded or diffuse nail pigmentation. Methotrexate cause hair & cyclophosphamide cause teeth pigmentation
- **Post inflammatory hpermelanosis**
  - Slate brown hypermelanosis d/t disruption of basal epidermal layer in ***lichen planus***Q or lupus erythematosus, fixed drug erruptions.
  - Chronic graft-verses-host reaction (late stage), nostalgia paraesthetica, erythema ab igne, prurigo pigmentosa, late secondary syphilis.

Ptyriasis Rosea (PR)

- PR is an acute, exanthematous papulo-squamous eruption of ***unknown etiology probably infective in origin***Q often with a ***characteristic self limiting course***Q.
- PR most commonly affect ***children and young adults (b/w 10 to 35 years of age)***Q with a slight predominance in females. It is a viral exanthema associated with ***reactivation of human herpes virus 7 (HHV - 7) and sometimes HHV-6***Q.
- Classicial clinical picture: ***First feature is development of larger single annular plaque lesion (k/a herald or primary or mother patch) usually on trunk***Q followed 2 hours to 2 months (usually 2 weeks) later by the onset of numerous smaller secondary lesions in ***Christmas or fir tree appearance*** distributed along the lines of cleavage. Mostly the patients are asymptomatic as the prodromal ***(constitutional) symptoms are usually absent or minimal***Q.

Cutaneous Lesions

- **Primary plaque** or **Herald/Mother patch** is *sharply (well) demarcated, larger* (2-6 cm in diameter), *oval or round*, erythematous, salmon colored or **hyperpigmented** (red to brown) plaque that is *usually located on trunk* in areas covered by clothes. Sometimes it is on neck or proximal extremities and very rarely on face, penis, vulva and palms. Lesions demonstrate ***fine (cigarette paper) collarette of scale just inside the periphery of plaques***Q.
- **Secondary eruption (similar appearing but smaller lesions)** occurs in **crops** at intervals of 2 hours to 2 months (usually **2 weeks**) distributed along the skin tension lines of cleavage on the trunk in **Christmas or Fir tree pattern**. The long axis of oval lesions follow the skin fold lines of cleavage.
- Lesions may be slightly- moderately pruritic and commonl fade after 3-9 weeks (i.e. **self limiting course**)

Diagnosis and Treatment

- Diagnosis is clinical and histopathologic findings are non specific.
- Usually no treatment is required. But in cases of troublesome itch & distressing appearance treatment consists of antihistaminics, topical glucocorticoids & in few cases, UVB-phototherapy.

Differential Diagnosis

- **Secondary syphilis:** lesion typically involving palms & soles, history of primary chancre, condylomalata, systemic symptoms, lymphadenopathy, absence of herald patch and presence of plasma cells on histology suggest this diagnosis.
- **Pityriasis lichenoides chronica:** has smaller lesions with thick scales more commonly on extremities and disease has longer course.
- **Nummular dermatitis:** has circular (not oral) plaques commonly with tiny vesicles but without collarettes of scale.
- **Drug eruption:** acute onset, progressive, irritable (pruritic), atypical pityriasis form eruption in patient taking drug are suggestive features.

Mnemonic	Characterstic features
Her	***Herald patch***Q***, HHV-6 & 7***Q
Young	*Young adults (females)* and children are mostly affected
Mother	***Mother (herald) patch***Q***, minimal constitutional & symptoms (asymptomatic)***
Smokes	***Secondary syphilis like lesion except for palm & sole involvement***Q
Fir-tree	***Fir-tree or Christmas-tree appearance***Q due to distribution of lesion along the line of clevage on trunk
Ciggarette	*Ciggarette paper (fine) collarette of scales*Q

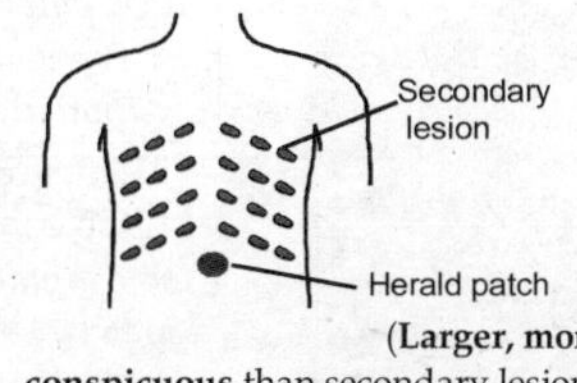

(Larger, more conspicuous than secondary lesions usually on upper thigh, arm, trunk or neck)

Christmas (Fir)-Tree Pattern

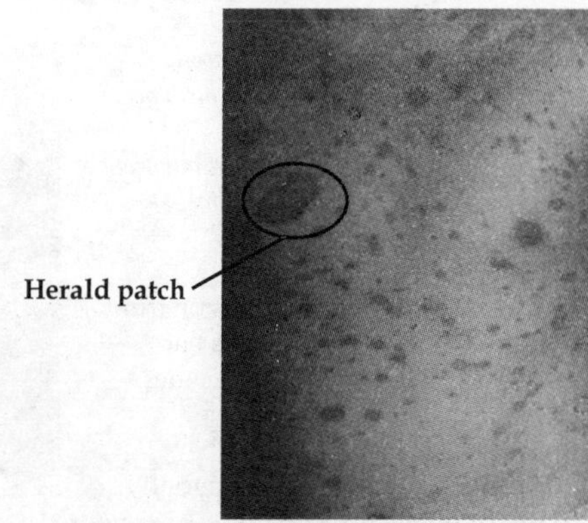

1

DERMATOLOGY

Ptyriasis (Tinea) Versicolor

Etiology

- This *superficial mycosis* (also k/a *tinea flavea, dermatomycosis furfuracea, liver spots or chromophytosis*) is caused by polymorphic **yeast Malassezia sp.** of which **M. globosa, M. sympodialis** and **M. furfur** (old name **Pityrosporum ovale** & P. orbiculare) are most frequently associated.
- P. versicolor develops when round yeast phase (saprophyte of skin) changes to a parasitical mycelial phase d/t genetic, endogenous (like intake of oral anticoagulants or systemic steroids & malnutrition) and environmental factors (hot humid climates).

Clinical Features

- Presents with ***multiple, small, scaly macules of varying skin color (hypopigmented***[Q], pink, salmon colored or ***hyperpigmented***) that develop insidiously over the ***trunk, chest, back and shoulders in young adult***[Q].
- The characteristic scale is **dust like** or **furfuraceous (fine, branny scaling)**.
- Macules start around the hair follicles and then merge with each other to form large confluent areas with scalloped border.
- The name versicolor is appropriate as the color of scales may vary from pale ochre to medium brown and the affected area look *darker* (hyperpigmented) than normal *in untanned* white skin; whereas the affected skin is paler in suntanned and black people. So the presenting complaint is usually cosmetic, because ***hypopigmented lesions often fail to tan with sun exposure***[Q].

Laboratory Diagnosis

- **Microscopic scale examination** mounted in **10-20% KOH** and *Parker ink (calcofluor white)* demonstrate short *hyphae/mycelium (diagnostic of condition) and blastospores* in typical **sphagetti and meat-balls** or **bananas and grapes appearance**.
- Skin patches often fluoresce an **apple (yellow) green** in long wave ultra violet radiation (**Wood's light examination**).
- **Skin surface biopsy** using a **cyanoacrylate adhesive (crazy or super glue)** to remove superficial layer of stratum corneum on glass slide and staining with PAS reagent.

Treatment

- ***Griesofulvin is not effective***[Q]
- Systemic Keto/Itraconazole
- Topical Mi/E/Keto/Itra- conazole; Clotrimazole, ***Whitfield's ointment (3% salicylic acid + 6% Benzoic acid)***[Q], ***Selenium disulphide, Sodium thiosulphate***[Q]
- Antidendruff shampoo containing *ketoconazole, zinc pyrithione or selenium disulphide.*

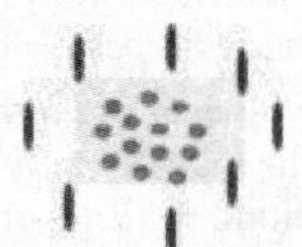

Grapes & Bananas or Meatball & Sphagetti appearance in KOH scale slide

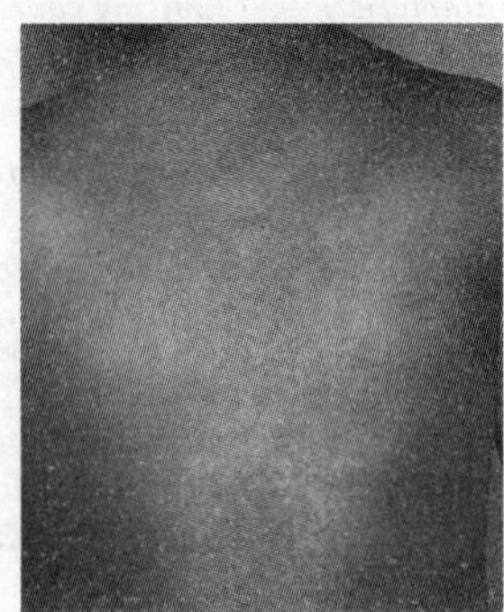

Ptyriasis alba (simplex)/PA

Etiology

- Commonly characterized as a mild manifestation of **atopic dermatitis** but PA is not only confined to atopic individuals.
- *Excessive & unprotected sun* exposure or hygienic habits (like frequent bathing and **hot baths**)
- Lack of sebaceous secretion before puberty
- Pigmented PA is associated with superficial *dermatophyte infection.*

Differential Diagnosis

- **Naevus depigmentosus** most commonly presents as *single, well marginated* lesions on *trunk* at *birth or before 3 years of age.*
- **Discoid eczema** presents with *intensely pruritic, larger & more oedematous* lesions in atiopic child.
- In adults & older children early erythematous phase of lesions on trunk may be mistaken for **psoriasis** but *distribution and mild scaling* excludes this diagnosis.
- Mycosis fungoides may even be difficult to distinguish histologically, so repeat follow ups & biopsies are required.

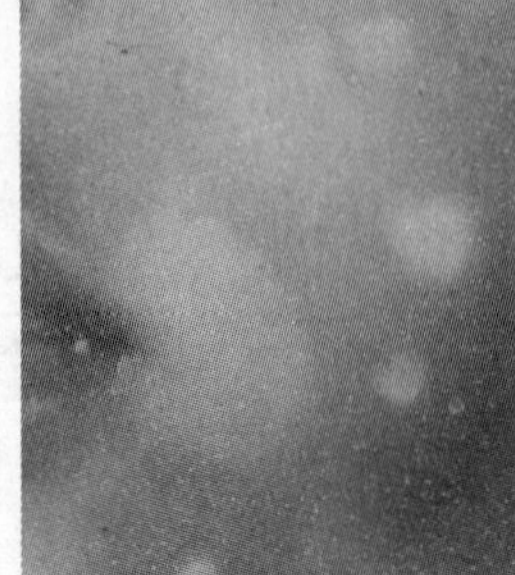

Clinical Presentation

- Common benign condition predominantly affecting the ***head and neck regions of preadolescent children between the ages of 3 & 16 years***[Q].
- Classical PA has 3 stages which may occur simultaneously

I. Slightly ***erythematous pink patch with an elevated border & fine scaling,*** fading after several weeks into
II. A ***paler spot covered with powdery white fine scale***
III. The lesion progress to ***non scaly hypopigmented macules*** persisting for months or years.

- There are usually several patches of *0.5 to 2 cm* diameter often confined *to face,* and are most common on *cheeks and around the mouth and chin.* The individual patch/lesion is *ill defined (marginated) round, oval or irregular* macule.
- The disease is ***self limiting (disappear spontaneously) with frequent recurrences***[Q].

Treatment

- ***Assurance***[Q] is the main stay as treatment (like topical steroids, emollients, tretinoin, UV therapy & antifungals) is often not completely successful.

Ptyriasis rubra pilaris (PRP)

Clinical Presentation
(Griffith & Gonzales-Lopez classification)

- Commonest type (I, classic adult type) occurs in *late middle aged or elderly (40-60 yrs)* and is often of *sudden onset without* obvious precipitating factor.
- Characteristically the disease *begins on face and scalp* (head, neck or upper trunk) as an ***erythematous (pink), slightly scaly macule and spreads*** in ***cephalocaudal direction***Q within a few days or weeks to involve the rest of the body.
- Then patients show an eruption of **erythematous perfollicular hyperkeratotic** (i.e. with central keratotic acuminate plug) **papules** that spread in **cephalo-caudal direction**.
- With further evolution of disease, an **erythematous scaling dermatitis with a characteristic reddish orange hue** appears which often progresses to a generalized **erythroderma** over a period of 2-3 months.
- **A** diagnostic hallmark **is sharply demarcated** islands of normal (unaffected) skin, **1 cm in diameter (k/a** island of sparing or nappes claires **or skip areas) in a random distribuition.**
- Palms & soles become **waxy, thickened, hyperkeratotic and yellow (PRP sandal). Scalp shows diffuse bran like scaling.**
- **Follicular accentuation** d/t presence of hyperkeratotic spines.
- Nail show distal yellow brown discoloration, nail plate thickening, splinter haemorrhage, subungal hyperkeratosis, but unlike psoriases pitting is minimal and there is no *dystrophy of nail plate.* Mucous membranes may be affected but hair & teeth are normal.
- 2nd most common type IV (circumscribed juvenile type) presents in pre pubertal children as well demarcated scaly, erythematous plaque on elbow & knees resembling localized psoriasis.
- Type III (classical juvenile) is similar to type I but begins in year 1 or 2 of life.
- Type II (atypical adult), type V (atypical juvenile) show follicular hyperkeratosis, icthyosiform like lesions or scleroderma and type VI is a/w HIV.

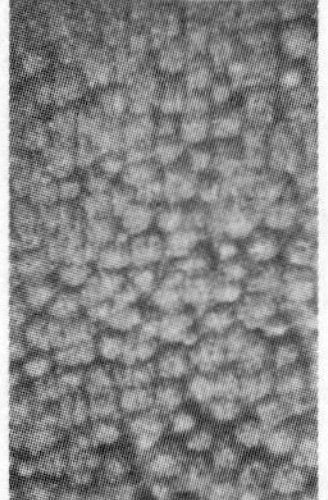
Acuminate follicular papules of Ptyriasis rubra pilaris. Confluent lesion

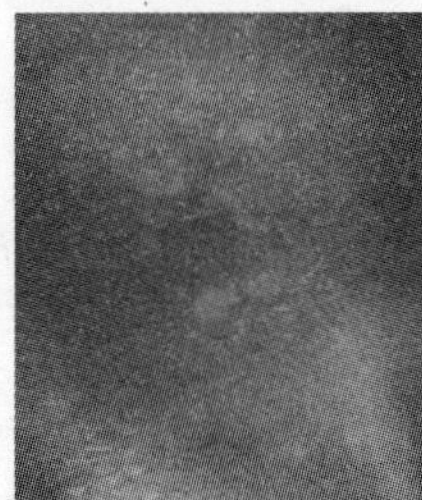
Ptyriasis rubra pilaris with islands of normal skin (napppes claires)

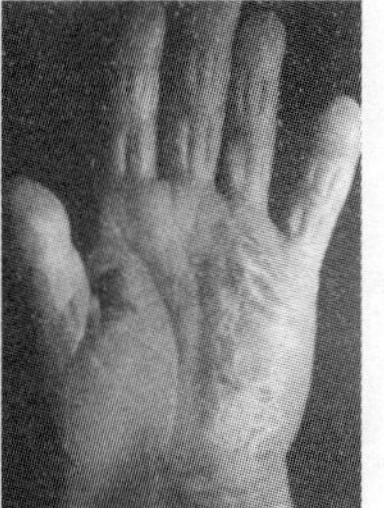
Keratoderma in Ptyriasis rubra pilaris. Palmar

Differential Diagnosis

Feature	PRP	Psoriasis
Age at onset	Biomodal (1st & 5th decade)	2nd decade
Scalp scaling	**Furfuraceous (fine bran)**	Adherent (thick)
Keratoderma	Constant	Rare
Island of pale (normal) skin = Nappes Claires	*Constant (diagnostic)*Q	Rare
Seronegative arthropathy	Rare	Common
Munromicro abscess	Absent	Common
Salmon patches in nail	Absent	Present
Nail growth rate & epidermal kinetics	Moderate increase	Marked increase
Response to UVB, corticosteroid or methotrexate	Poor (Variable)	Good (positive)

Histopathology

Biopsy is diagnostic aid and findings include

- *Dense (horny) follicular plugging,* acanthosis with exaggerated follicular shoulders (broad short rete ridges) and *alternating spotty parakeratosis* (in perifollicular shoulder and interfollicular epidermis) and *orthokeratosis* in both horizontal & vertical directions.
- *Basket-weave hyperkeratosis* overlying a prominent granular layer and *perivascular lympho-histiocytic infiltrate.*
- **Prominent granular layer** and **dilated but not tortuous, capillaries differentiate** PRP from psoriasis. Unlike psoriasis, the acanthotic epidermis is not thinned above the dermal papillae & there is no neutrophilic infiltration.

Treatment

- **Oral retonoids** are the first line of therapy. **Acitretin** more effective than **isotretinoin** in erythroderma phase. However, in children isotretinoin has best response.
- **Systemic Methotrexate**, triple antiretro viral therapy (in HIV), **topical** emollients, keratolytics (salicylic acid, urea) and vitamin D_3 (calcipotriol); and physical options like **photochemotherapy** (oral or systemic psoralen + UVA), **extracorporeal photopheresis** are other first line treatments.
- 2nd line treatment (with unpredictable effect) includes **systemic cyclosporine**, azathioprine, TNF α antagonists, fumaric acid esters; topical steroids & vitamic A analogue; and physical UV A_1 or UV B phototherapy.

Woods Lamp Examination

It is a source of ultra violet light (mainly long wave UV-A), from which virtually all variable rays have been excluded by ***filter (made of nickel oxide i.e.*** NiO_2 ***and Si***Q*)*. It is used in:

1. Fungal infections like:
   - **Tinea capitis** = *yellow green fluorescence*
   - **Pityriasis versicolor**Q = *golden yellow/ apple green*
2. Bacterial infections like:
   - **Erythrasma**Q **& Acne** = Coral red / pink
   - **Pseudomonas pyocyanea** = yellow-green
3. Infestations like - Scabies
4. Pigmentary disorder
   - **Vitiligo** = total white
   - Ash-**leaf** macules in tuberous sclerosis = blue white
5. Urine examination in ***porphyria***Q (red/pink urine)
6. Detection of tetracycline/mepacrine in tissues and photosensitizers/fluorescent contact in skin.
7. **Squamous cell carcinoma** of skin = *red fluorescence*
8. Detection of *lipofuschins in sweat* from patients with *chromhidrosis.*

Questions

HYPERPIGMENTATION & HYPOPIGMENTATION

1. Hyperpigmentation is not seen in: *(DNB 98, AI 93)*
A. Addison's disease
B. Cushing's Disease
C. Graves Disease
D. Hypothyroidism (Myxedema)

2. Hyperpigmented lesions are *(PGI Nov 11)*
A. Pityriasisalba
B. Melanoma
C. Naevus anaemicus
D. Dyskeratosis congenital
E. Lentigines lichen planus

3. Which of the following is/are not the cause of hypopigmentation: *(PGI May 10)*
A. Leprosy
B. Pinta
C. Syphilis
D. Pityriasis alba
E. Pityriasis versicolor

4. Hypopigmentation is/are seen in: *(PGI May 11)*
A. Vitiligo
B. Pityriasis versicolor
C. Lichen planus
D. Melasma
E. Scleroderma

5. Hypopigmented patches can be seen in : *(PGI Dec 05, 02)*
A. Becker naevus
B. Freckles
C. Nevus Ito
D. Nevus Ota
E. Nevus anemicus

6. Hypo-depigmented lesion seen in : *(PGI 04)*
A. Naevas Ito
B. Naevus depigmentosa
C. Naevas Ota
D. Naevas anaemicus
E. Freckles

7. A newborn child presents with solitary white well defined hypopigmented patch on his right thigh. Diagnosis is : *(AIIMS 2K)*
A. Piebaldism
B. Albinism
C. Nevus achromicus
D. Acral vitiligo

VITILIGO

8. True about vitiligo are all except *(Jipmer 04, WB 05)*
A. Genetic predisposition is known
B. Leucotrichia is associated with good prognosis
C. PUVA-B is used for treatment
D. Topical steroids give good results.

9. An increased incidence of vitiligo is found in:
A. Psoriasis *(Karnatak 98, AIIMS 94)*
B. Nutritional deficiency
C. Old age
D. Diabetes mellitus

10. In a patch of vitiligo - *(AIIMS 04, PGI 94)*
A. Melanin synthesis is inhibited
B. Melanosomes are absent
C. Melanocytes are absent
D. Melanocytes are reduced

11. Psoralen - A is used in the treatment of : *(Jipmer 91)*
A. Pemphigus
B. Vitiligo
C. Pityriasis alba
D. Icthyosis

12. Vitiligo vulvaris, best treatment is : *(Bihar 03, DNB 01)*
A. PUVA
B. Steroids
C. Coaltar
D. All

13. Vitiligo vulvaris, treatment is :
A. PUVA *(Jharkhand 06, DNB 04)*
B. Steroids
C. Coaltar
D. All

PITYRIASIS ROSEA

14. Pityriasis rosea true *(AI 07, AIIMS Nov 06)*
A. Self limiting
B. Chronic relapsing
C. Life threatening infection (autoimmune disease)
D. Caused by dermatophytes

15. 'Fir-tree' type of distribution is seen in-
A. Pityriasis Rosea *(PGI 92, Jipmer 98)*
B. Psoriasis
C. Measles
D. Secondary syhilis

16. Which viral association is found in pityriasis rosea :
A. HHV 7 *(Jharkhand 2004)*
B. CMV
C. Vericella Zoster
D. E B V

17. Annular herald (mother) patch is seen in *(PGI 03, 96)*
A. Psoriasis *(TN,Kerala 98, AIIMS 97, 91, 90)*
B. P. alba
C. P. rosea
D. Nocardiasis

18. A 16 year old boy presented with asymptomatic, multiple erythamatous annular lesions with a collarette of scales at periph-ery of the lesions present on the trunk. The most likely diagnosis is: *(AI 12, 05)*
A. Pityriasis versicolor
B. Pityriasis alba
C. Pityriasis rosacea
D. Pityriasis rubra pilaris

19. Photosensitive lichenoid drug eruption is seen in ...... therapy: *(Kerala 90, DNB 99)*
A. Rifampicin
B. Tetracycline (old)
C. Gold
D. Streptomycin

20. A patient of hypertension on ACE inhibitors developed rosea skin erruptions. True statement regarding this situation is *(SGPGI 2003)*
A. Drug may be the cause and discontinuation may improve the skin condition
B. High dose steroids are needed initially

C. ACE inhibitors are safe and cannot lead to skin errruptions. ☐
D. Drug may be the cause discontinuation is not required ☐

21. **Tinea Versicolour is caused by:** *(AI 05, 02, PGI 98)*
A. E. Flaccosum ☐
B. Malassezia Furfur ☐
C. T. rubrum ☐
D. T. Schonleini ☐

22. **An adult presents with oval scaly hypopigmented macules over chest and back. The diagnosis is**
A. Leprosy *(AIIMS 2001, AI 12)* ☐
B. Lupus Vulgaris ☐
C. Pityriasis Versicolour ☐
D. Lichen Planus ☐

23. **A 24 year old man had multiple, small hypopigmented macules on the upper chest and back for the last three months. The macules were circular, arranged around follicles and many had coalesced to form large sheets. The surface of the macules showed fine scaling. He had similar lesions one year ago which subsided with treatment. The most appropriate investigation to confirm the diagnosis is;**
A. Potassium hydroxide preparation of scales ☐
B. Slit skin smear from discrete macules ☐
C. Tzanck test *(AIIMS May 12, Nov 03)* ☐
D. Skin biopsy of coalesced macules ☐

24. **All of the following is given for the treatment for Pityriasis versicoler Except:** *(AI 05, 02)*
A. Ketoconazole ☐
B. Griseofulvin ☐
C. Clotrimazole ☐
D. Selenium sulphate ☐

25. **Griseofulvin is not useful in one of the following-**
A. Tinea capitis *(AI 02)* ☐
B. Tinea cruris ☐
C. Tinea versicolor ☐
D. Tinea pedis ☐

26. **Treatment of tinea versicolor -** *(Kerala 97)*
A. Clotrimazole ☐
B. Sod. thiosulphate ☐
C. Selenium Sulphide ☐
D. Micanazole ☐
E. All of the above ☐

27. **The following drug is indicated in the treatment of pityriasis versicolar :** *(AIIMS May 03)*
A. Ketoconazole ☐
B. Metronidazole ☐
C. Griseofulvin ☐
D. Chloroquine ☐

28. **Babloo around 5 to 10 year boy presents with multiple small hypopigmented scaly macule patch on cheek. Some of his classmates also have similar lesions. The most probable diagnosis is**
A. Pityriasis rosea *(AIIMS 01, 2K, 99, 98, 95)* ☐
B. Pityriasis versicolour ☐
C. Indeterminate leprosy ☐
D. Pityriasis alba ☐

29. **A 5 year boy has recurrent multiple asymptomatic oval and circular faintly hypopigmented macules with fine scaling on his face. The most probable clinical diagnosis is:** *(AI 03, AIIMS 96)*
A. Ptyriasis versicolor ☐
B. Indeterminate leprosy ☐
C. Ptyriasis alba ☐
D. Acrofacial vitiligo ☐

30. **True about pitryiasis alba :** *(PGI 01)*
A. No active treatment required ☐
B. Common in elderly ☐
C. Variant of vitiligo ☐
D. Common over the face ☐
E. Presents as scaly, whitish macules ☐

31. **Which of the following statements is true regarding Pityriasis Rubra Pilaris:** *(PGI 01)*
A. Isolated patches of normal skin are found ☐
B. Cephalocaudal distribution ☐
C. I.V. cyclosporine is effective and 1st line drug ☐
D. More common in females ☐
E. Methotrexate is effective ☐

32. **A boy comes from Bihar with non-anesthetic hypopigmented atropic patch over face, diagonosis is**
A. P. alba *(AIIMS 99)* ☐
B. P. versicolour ☐
C. Indeterminate leprosy ☐
D. Borderline leprosy ☐

33. **Woods lamp used in diagnosis of :** *(PGI Dec 06)*
A. P. versicolor ☐
B. Vitiligo ☐
C. Porphyria ☐
D. Psoriasis ☐
E. Lichen Planus ☐

34. **Skin pigmentation is caused by:** *(AIIMS 93)*
A. Methotrexate ☐
B. Dactinomycin ☐
C. Cyclophosphamide ☐
D. Busulphan ☐

35. **Rain drop pigmentation is seen in** *(AP 96)*
A. Chronic lead poisoing ☐
B. Chronic Arsenic poisoning ☐
C. Chronic Mercury poisoning ☐
D. All of the above ☐

36. **Slate like discoloration of the skin is caused by all these drugs except-**
A. Chlorpromazine *(PGI 98, AIIMS 99)* ☐
B. Minocycline ☐
C. Amiodarone ☐
D. Thiacetazone ☐

ANSWERS AND EXPLANATIONS

HYPERPIGMENTATION

1. **D i.e. Hypothyroidism**
2. **B i.e. Melanoma; D i.e. Dyskeratosis congenital; E i.e. Lentigines lichen planus** *[Ref: Rooks 8/e p. 58.10-58.39; 18.18; Roxburgh's 18/e p. 311-14; Fitzpatrick's 7/e p 727-40; Neena Khanna 4/e p. 156; Harrison's 18/e p. 412]*

- **Hyperpigmentation (hyper melanosis)** of skin is seen in endocrine disorders like ***Addison's disease***[Q], acromegaly, Nelson's syndrome, ***Cushing's (ectopic ACTH) syndrome***[Q], carcinoid syndrome, pheochromocytoma, and ***hyperthyroidism (Grave's disease) but not in hypothyroidism or myxedema***[Q].
- ***Melanoma, dyskeratosis congenita & lentigines lichen planus***[Q] cause hyperpigmentation.

3. **None** *[Ref: Rook's 8/e p. 30.63, 58.39, 58.51, 34.10]*
4. **D i.e. Melasma**

- ***Pityriasis alba, pityriasis versicolor, pinta, yaws, syphilis (secondary syphilis – leukoderma syphiliticum), tuberculoid and indeterminate leprosy***[Q] – all can cause **hypopigmentation (hypomelanosis)**.
- A few papules or erythematosquamous plaques develop in primary stage of pinta which become more extensive in secondary stage (pintids) after an interval of months or years. Initial red color of pintids changes to brown, slate blue, black or grey, and eventually there is **depigmentation intermixed with hyperpigmentation**. Primary & secondary stages are infectious. In tertiary (late) stage, which takes several years to develop, there is irregular pigmentation, **vitiligo like achromia (hypopigmentation)**, areas of hyperkeratosis and eventually atrophy.
- Nonscaly, non itchy, transient (evanescent) **macular syphilide (roseolar rash)** of secondary syphilis is generalized, symmetrical, coppery red oval or round spots. Fading roseolar rash may sometimes, leave a pattern of **depigmented spots** on a hyperpigmented background (**k/a leukoderma syphiliticum**) most commonly located on the back or sides of neck (**k/a necklace of venus**).
- ***Melasma (mask of pregnancy) l/t hyperpigmentation***[Q]***. Lichen planus usually l/t hyperpigmentation***[Q]***. Lichen planus usually l/t hyperpigmentation but hypopigmentation may also occur***[Q].

5. **E i.e. Naevus anemicus** *[Ref: Rooks 8/e p. 58.10-58.51; 18.17-18.18]*
6. **B & D i.e. Naevus depigmentosa & Naevus anaemicus**

- **Freckles (or ephelides), Melasma (chloasma or mask of pregnancy),** *Mongolian* **spots, Café au lait, Becker's nevus** or melanosis (pigmented hairy epidermal nevus), **nevus of Ota** and **nevus of Ito** cause **hyperpigmented patches** (Mn: **"Free Meal & Mongolian Café BOY = BOI** arer hyperpigmented"). Whereas, **Nevus depigmentosus (or achromicus), nevus anaemicus, Sutton's (Halo) nevus** (leukoderma acquisitum centrifugum), hypomelanosis of Ito and **Piebaldism** leads to **hypopigmentation.** (Mn- **"Pie DASH nevus** are hypopigmented").
- **Becker's nevus** is sporadically acquired disorder (may be of familial occurance), 5 times more commonly affecting *males*. It is usually first noticed during *adolescence*, initially pale in colour which becomes more prominent during sun exposure. It follows Blaschko's lines, but with lack of conformity (d/t late occurance). It starts as an area of **irregular macular (hyper) pigmentation** with **geographical outline** usually on shoulder, anterior chest or scapular region. Once present it remains *indefinitely* and shows predisposition to *androgen sensitivity* (since it is prone to *acne & hypertrichosis*). Lesion may show central thickening and increased terminal hairs on & around the lesion. **Becker's nevus syndrome** is Becker's nevus with ipsilateral non cutaneous developmental abnormalities like breast hypoplasia, supernumerary nipples, spina bifida etc.
- **Nevus of Ota** (oculo-dermal melanocytosis/nevus fuscocaeruleus ophthalmo-maxillaris) is usually congenital & unilateral slate brown or blue hyperpigmentation in the areas of skin, sclera, cornea, iris, retina, ocular muscles, orbit & hard palate supplied by ophthalmic and maxillary division of trigeminal nerve, more prevalentally in Japanese. **Nevus of Ito** is hyperpigmentation in area supplied by posterior supraclavicular and lateral brachial cutaneous nerves, commonly in Japanese.

HYPOPIGMENTATION

7. **C i.e. Nevus achromicus** *[Ref: Rooks 8/e p. 58.39-58.51; 18.17-18.18; Roxburgh's 18/e p. 307-310; Fitzpatrick's 7/e p 624-25; Neena Khanna 4/e p. 147-56; Harrison's 18/e p. 409-412]*

Hypopigmented Patch

Unilateral

Nevus achromicus (depigmentosus)

- Mostly presents with *unilateral, stable single, well circumscribed oval or rectangular localized area of hypomelanosis (depigmented skin) with feathered margins.*
- It is ***congenital (i.e. present at birth)***Q but sometimes may not be apparent at birth.
- It ***remains stable in size and color over time and typically has no associated findings***Q.
- Lesions occur most commonly on trunk. *Hairs within the lesiosn are usually depigmented.* Histology shows normal or reduced number of melanocytes. 3 variants of lesion are single (mc), segmental and systematized (very rare).
- Erythema appears on massage
- Pressure with glass slide does not make the lesion disappear.

Nevus anaemicus

- Developmental, solitary (unilateral) white (pale) round flat patch, usually on trunk and present at birth. It is stable (i.e. does not increase in size). Thought to have vascular filling defect.
- ***Massage fails to develop erythema in lesion***Q. Pressure with glass slide makes the lesion disappear & indistinct from surrounding skin.

Hypomelanosis of Ito (Linear nevoid hypopigmentation/ Pigmentary Mosacism / Incontinentia pigmenti achromians of Ito)

- This neurocutaneous disorder results from migration of 2 clones of melanocytes, each with a different pigment potential.
- It may present with *widespread bilateral (symmetrical) or unilateral areas of hypopigmentation in form of whorls (swirls) and streaks occurring along Blaschko's lines.*
- One third cases are associated with abnormalities involving musculoskeletal system (asymmetry), CNS (convulsions & mental retardation), teeth, and eyes (hypertelorism & strabismus).

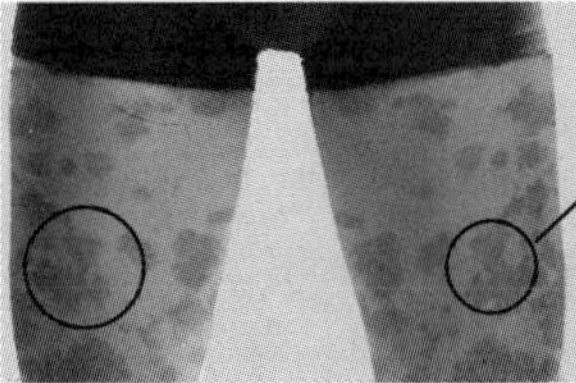

Island of normal or hypermelanotic skin in white depigmented area

Piebaldism

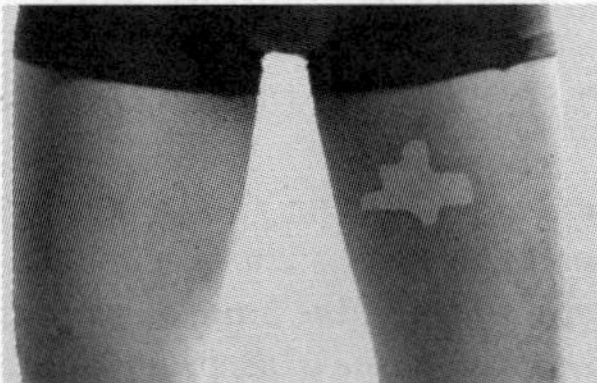

Nevus achromicus (depigmentosus)

Bilateral

Piebaldism

- It is AD condition characterized by congenital stable areas of vitiligo like amelanotic skin with white forelock.
- Amelanotic patches of skin totally devoid of pigment are ***present at birth (congenital) and remain unchanged throughout life (stable)***Q.
- Frontal median or paramedian **patch with** a mesh of white hair (**white foelock**) is most common lesion; rest of scalp hair are pigmented.
- Often, white patches occur **bilaterally mostly** but not necessarily (always) **symmetrically on ventral trunk** (chest & abdomen) **and limbs** (upper & lower extremities). Occasionally they are found on face esp. chin
- Back as well as **hands and feet (acral area)** remain normally pigmented **(acral sparing).**
- ***Islands of normal or hypermelanotic skin occur in white depigmented areas***Q.
- Piebaldism can be distinguished from vitiligo (where the lesions are acquired later in life) ***by almost invariable presence of white forelock and islands of normal pigmented skin in hypomelanotic areas***Q as well as configuration & distribution of lesions.
- Piebaldism may be associated with 2 systemic neurocristopathies d/t abnormal embryonic migration or survival of 2 neural crest derived elements, one being **melanocytes** and other **myenteric ganglion cells** (l/t Hirschprung disease in *Shah-Waardenburg syndrome*) or **auditory nerve cells** (l/t sensorineural deafness in Waardenburg's syndrome). *Waardenburg's syndrome* is characterized by dystopia canthorum (lateral displacement of inner canthi but normal interpupillary distance), hetero chromic irises, broad nasal root, sensorineural hearing loss and piebaldism.

Vitiligo

- Usually *not present at birth*, oftenly starts in childhood (before 20 years age)
- *Hypomelanotic (milky white) macule with scalloped hyper pigmented border* usually first noted at *sun exposed area* of face & dorsa of hands.
- Affect particularly areas that are *hyper pigmented* (i.e., face, axilla, groin, areola & genitalia) or *subjected to repeated trauma* (i.e., dora of hand, feet, elbow, knee & ankles).
- Usually symmetrical but may be segmental (i.e. U/L dermatomal involving trigeminal distribution) or generalized (complete).
- ***Increase in size***, older lesions show ***amelanotic hair (leucotrichia)***Q and damage to normal skin results in depigmentation i.e., **Koebner / isomorphic phenomenon**
- May be associated with ***diabetes mellitus***Q, pernicious anemia, mysthenia gravis, alopecia areata, Addison's ds, thyroid ds, hypoparathyroidism, morphea, lichen sclerosus, halo nevus & malignant melanoma
- Eyes are not involved
- Show partial / near complete response to treatment

Albinism (Oculo-cutaneous)

- *Present at birth* (autosomal recessive)
- ***Diffuse hypopigmentation of skin, & hair throughout the body***Q.
- Absence of pigment in iris & retina (eye) with visual defects in form of nystagmus, poot eye sight, photophobia, transulent iridis & red reflex.
- *Frecklies, non- pigmented melanocytic nevi, & amelanotic melanomas* may develop on sun exposed area
- No response to treatment

VITILIGO

8. **B i.e., Leucotrichia is assiciated with good prognosis**
9. **D i.e. Diabetes mellitus**
10. **C. i.e. Melanocytes are absent**
11. **B. i.e. Vitiligo**
12. **A. ie. PUVA**
13. **D. i.e. All**

[Ref: Rooks 8/e p. 58.46-58.49; Roxburgh's 18/e p. 309-11; Fitzpatrick's 7/e p 616-21; Neena Khanna 4/e p. 149-153; Harrison's 18/e p. 411-10]

- **Vitiligo** is a focal failure of pigmentation d/t ***genetically predisposed destruction of melanocytes***[Q] by immunological mechanism. So a patch of vitiligo shows ***marked absence of melanocytes & melanin in epidermis***[Q].
- Vitiligo is more common in (or a/w) ***diabetes mellitus***[Q], alopecia areata, Addison's disease and thyroid diseases.
- ***Long standing vitiligo with leucotrichia (depigmented hair), acrofacial lesions (acral i.e, periungal, palm, sole & facial around eyes & lips) and lesion on resistant area are indicators of poor prognosis for therapy***[Q].
- Treatment includes ***topical steroids***[Q] (for localized, <20% skin surface involved), tacrolimus (topical immunomodulators, considered safer for children) and ***PUVA (= psoralen + UV - A)***[Q] etc.

PITYRIASIS ROSEA

14. **A i.e. Self resolving**
15. **A. i.e. Pityriasis rosea**
16. **A. i.e. HHV-7**
17. **C i.e. P. rosea**
18. **C i.e. Pityriasis rosea**

[Ref: Rooks 8/e p. 33.78-33.81; Fitzpatrick's 7/e p 362-366; Neena Khanna 4/e p. 53; Harrison's 18/e p. 400]

Pityriasis rosea is a ***self limiting disorder***[Q] of unknown etiology, with a suspected association with ***Herpes virus 7 and 6***[Q]. It presents with development of usually **asymptomatic** (i.e. no prodromal or constitutional system), **sharply (well) demarcated, larger** (2-6 cm), **annular** (oval-round), ***erythematous***[Q] (red to brown) lesion k/a **primary/herald/mother patch** mostly located on **trunk** ***in children and young adults (10-35 yrs)***[Q]. Similar but **smaller secondary eruptions** appear in crops at interval of usually 2 weeks distributed along lines of cleavage in ***christmas (fir) tree appearance***[Q]. Lesions demonstrate ***fine (cigarette paper) collarette of scale***[Q] just inside the peripheray of plaque.

19. **C i.e. Gold** *[Ref: Harrison 16/e p. 296]*
20. **A i.e. Drug may be the cause and discontinuation may improve the skin condition**

When ever the diagnosis of **pityriasis rosea or lichen planus** is made, it is important to review the patients medication because the ***eruption can be treated by simply discontinuing the offending agent***[Q].

Pityriasis rosea like drug eruptions

- ACE inhibitors
- β blockers
- Metronidazole
- **Gold**

Mn – "**Aβ Metro Gold**"

Lichenoid drug eruptions

1. ACE inhibitors
2. **Anti**malarials
3. **Gold**
4. **Thi**azides
5. Pheno**thi**azines
6. **Quini**dine
- Sulfonyl ureas
- Chronic graft –versus- host disease

Mn **"A Anti Gold Thai Queen"**

PITYRIASIS (TINEA) VERSICOLOR

21. **B i.e. Malazzezia furfur**
22. **C i.e. Pityriasis versicolor**
23. **A i.e. KOH preparation of scale**
24. **B i.e. Griseofulvin**
25. **C i.e. Tinea versicolor**
26. **E i.e. All**
27. **A i.e. Ketoconazole** *[Ref: Roxburgh's 18/e 38-40; Rook's 8/e p. 36.10-36.12; Fitzpatrick's 7/e p. 623,626, 1828-30; Neena Khanna 4/e p. 290]*

- **Pityriasis versicolor** is superficial mycosis caused by **mycelial phase of yeast** ***Malassezia (furfur, globosa, sympodialis)***[Q]. It presents with *multiple, small,* **hypopigmented (usually or pink-salmon or hyperpigmented)** *scaly macules* that develop insidiously over the ***trunk, chest, back and shoulders in young adults***[Q]. ***Macules start around the hair follicle and then merge with each other to form large areas***[Q]. The characteristic scale is ***furfuraceous or dust like (fine, branny scaling)***[Q]. **Microscopic examination (in 10% KOH) show bananas and grapes** (or **spaghetti and meat balls) appearance** and Wood's lamp examination show **apple (yellow) green fluoresce.**
- **Griseofulvin** is used systemically for dermatophytosis (tinea infections) but it is ***ineffective topically***[Q] and ***has no role in treatment of tinea versicolor and candida***[Q].

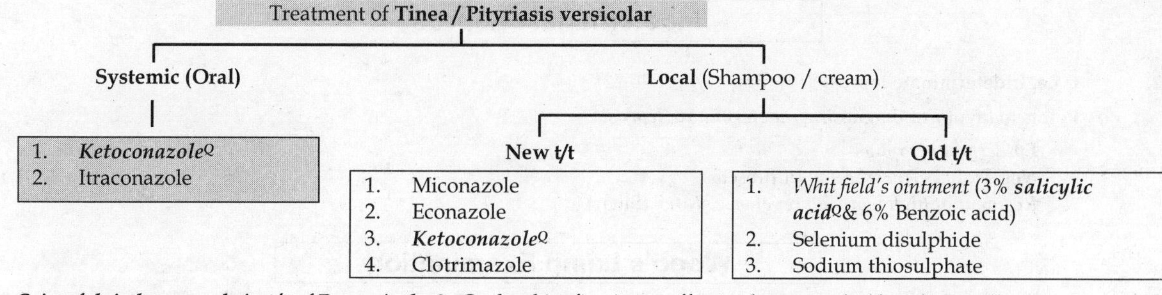

Griesofulvin has no role in t/t of P. versicolar[Q]. Oral terbinafine is not effective but topical terbinafine is effective.

Capsofungin, an echinocandin, is a *cell wall* antagonist that *blocks glucan synthetase.* It's an *intravenous drug* used in treatment of *aspergillosis or candidosis (resistant species)*

PITYRIASIS ALBA

28. **D i.e. Pityriasis alba** **29.** **C i.e. Ptyriasis alba**

30. **A i.e. No active treatment required; D i.e. Common over face; E i.e. presents with scaly, whitish macules**
[Ref: Rook's 8/e p. 23.27; Neena Khanna 4/e p. 267; Fitzpatrick's 7/e p-623-626]

Pityriasis alba characteristically presents with recurrent scaly hypopigmented macules on cheeks and face of young children[Q]***. It requires no active treatment (i.e. assurance only).***

PITYRIASIS RUBRA PILARIS (PRP)

31. **A i.e. Isolated patches of normal skin are found; B i.e. Cephalo caudal distribution; E i.e. Methotrexate is effective**
[Ref: Rook's 8/e p. 19.76-19.84; Fitzpatrick's 7/e p. 232-36; Neena Khanna 4/e p. 62; Roxburgh's 18/e p. 152-54]

PRP presents with erythematous slightly scaly macules (or dermatitis) and perifollicular hyperkeratotic papules, erythroderma with ***characteristic orange hue, diagnostic islands of normal - unaffected skin (nappes claires)***[Q]; waxy-hyperkeratotic – thickened and yellow palm & soles (**PRP sandal**) and ***follicular accentuation***[Q].

Nonscaly Hypopigmented macule

- **Indeterminate leprosy**
  - More common in children
  - More frequent in patients belonging to ***high leprosy prevalence (endemic) state as Tamil Nadu, Bihar, Orrisa etc.***
  - Anaesthetic/Non anaesthetic lesion
  - ***Epidermal atrophy***[Q]
- **Tuberous sclerosis**
  - ***Ash leaf macule***[Q]
  - ***Shagreen patch***[Q]
  - ***Adenoma sebacium***[Q]
  - ***Seizure, mental retardation***[Q]
- **Vitiligo**
  - Sharply defined
  - Non pigmented patches
  - Anywhere

Recurrent Scaly Nonanesthetic Hypopigmented macule

- **Pityriasis alba** (Predominant **face** involvement)
  - Self limiting benign condition mostly affecting **head & neck** regions (**most common on cheeks, around the mouth & chin**) of ***preadolescent children***[Q] b/w the ages of 3 & 16 years (before puberty).
  - More frequent in children of *hill station exposed to excessive & unprotected sun,* and hot baths.
  - Presents with ***multiple ill defined, irregular, round or oval, erythematous or hypopigmented macule without or with fine powdery white scale***[Q].
- **Pityriasis versicolor** (Predominant **trunk** involvement)
  - Common in ***young adults (rare in children)***[Q]. Cushing's syndrome steroids, oral anticoagulants, hot & humid climate aggrevate lesions.
  - ***Multiple small scaly hypopigmented (pale, non erythematous) macules***[Q] (may also be hyperpigmented/brown, pink or salmon colored) develop ***insidiously over trunk, chest, back and shoulders***[Q]. Macules start around the hair follicle. Face involvement is rare. Hands & lower limbs are usually not involved.
  - ***Scales are dust like (fine, branny) or furfaceous***[Q].

Erythematous Scaly Lesions

- **Pityriasis rubra pilaris** (starts from face)
  - Sudden onset without precipitating factor in ***late middle aged or elderly (40-60 yr)***[Q]
  - Begins on face and scalp & spreads in ***cephalo caudal direction***[Q] to involve rest of body within weeks.
  - Patient shows **erythematous slightly scaly macules and perifollicular hyperkeratotic papules.** Gradually *erythematous scaling dermatitis* with ***characteristic orange hue***[Q] appears which often progresses to generalized **erythroderma.**
  - **Diagnostic hallmark** is sharply demarcated ***islands of sparing or normal/unaffected skin (k/a nappes claires)***[Q].
  - Waxy, thickened, hyperkeratitic & yellow palms & soles (**PRP sandal**), ***follicular accentuation***[Q] and diffuse bran scaling are other features.
- **Pityriasis rosea** (predominant trunk involvement)
  - ***Self limiting disorder***[Q] of sudden onset mostly affecting *children & young adults (10-35 years).* May be a/w reactivation of HHV 7 and 6.
  - **Ist feature** is development of ***larger, single, sharply (well) demarcated, annular, erythematous or hyperpigmented, asymptomatic, scaly patch usually on trunk***[Q] (k/a **herald/ primary / mother patch**).
  - Lesions ***show fine cigarette paper collarette of scale just inside the periphery of plaque***[Q].
  - Similar but smaller secondary eruptions appear in crops in ***christmas or fir tree pattern***[Q].

Indeterminate Leprosy

32. **C i.e. Indeterminate leprosy** *[Ref: Behl's 9/e p. 220-22]*

Points in favour of diagnosing ***indeterminate leprosy:***

- ***Epidermal atrophy***Q
- ***Non scaly & Anesthesia***Q (if present)
- ***Resident of high leprosy prevelence state***Q (Bihar)

Wood's Lamp Examination

33. **A i.e. P. Versicolor; B i.e Vitiligo; C i.e. Porphyria** *[Ref: Rook's 8/e p. 5.19; Harrison 18/e p. 394]*

Skin Discoloration (Pigmentation)

34. **D i.e. Busulphan** **35.** **B. i.e. Chronic Arsenic poisoning** **36.** **D. i.e. Thiacetazone**

[Ref. Rook's 8/e p. 58.38, 58.56; Neena Khanna 4/e p. 159; IADVL 2/e p. 1289; Harrison 18/e p. 413]

- **Blue, grey or slate like discoloration** of skin is caused by argyria (silver), **chrysiasis (gold), bismuth, *amiodarone***Q (phototoxic eruption = exaggerated sunburn slate gray to violaceous discoloration of sun exposed skin, & yellow brown granules in dermal macrophage), **minocycline**Q (diffuse blue-gray, muddy pigmentation skin, mucous, teeth, nails, bones and thyroid), **chlorpromazine**Q, phenothiazine and fixed drug eruptions (barbiturates, phenolphthalein), hemo chromatosis and pinta.
- **Brown discoloration of skin** is caused by ***arsenic (rain drop pigmentation)*** Q, ACTH therapy, adriamycin, busulfan, bleomycin, cyclophosphamide, contraceptive pills, oestrogens, and psoralens. (Berloque & phytophoto dermatitis).
- Mepacrine, picric acid, di/tri-nitrophenol, santonin and acriflavine stain skin yellow (like jaundice).
- **Busulfan** is used in CML and it l/t ***busulfan lung (pulmonary fibrosis) and hyperpigmentation*** Q of skin. Busulfan causes mucous membrane & zidovudine l/t nail pigmentation.
- **Cyclophosphamide** l/t ***haemorragic cystitis***Q *due to metabolite acrolein.*
- **Methotrexate** ***blocks DHFR-ase***Q & prevents conversion of DHFA to THFA. It's toxicity can be overcomed by ***folinic acid (citrovorum factor)***Q ***& thymidine***Q ***but not by folic acid.***Q In **low** doses l/t ***megaloblastic anemia***Q. In **high** doses l/t ***pancytopenia***Q

Complications (features) and causing Drugs

Skin pigmentation Mn-"ABCD of PM"

A. **Arsenic** = ***rain drop pigmentation***Q; ***Amiodarone = purple coloration, Argyria (silver)***
B. ***Busulfan***Q, ***Bleomycin=generalized hyperpigmentation, Bismuth***
C. ***Clofazamine***Q ***(orange pigmentation),*** chloroquin, ***Chlorpromazine***Q, Contraceptive (cause melasma), ***Cancer drugs eg. Bleomycin, busulfan, cyclophosphamide, daunorubicin, hydroxyl urea, 5FU & methotrexate.***
D. ***Dapsone***Q
P. **Psoralens** = brown pigmentation; phenothiazines = gray-brown pigmentation
M. ***Minocycline/pefloxacin (blue black/blue-gray) pigmentation of mucosa, shins and healing acne) Mercury***

Pulmonary Fibrosis Mn = "BBC – MAN"

Busulfan, Bleomycin
Cyclophosphamide
Methotrexate, Methysergide
Amiodarone
Nitrofurantion

No Pulmonary fibrosis

Doxorubin & Methyl-dopa

Minimum Bone marrow toxicity & Maximum Nausea & Vomitting

Cisplatin

Maximum immunosuppression

Methotrexate

Maximum alopecia

Cyclophosphamide
Dactinomycin

3 ALLERGIC DISORDERS AND DERMATITIS (ECZEMA)

ATOPIC DERMATITIS (AD)

AD is a cutaneous expression of the atopic state, characterized by a ***family history of asthma, hay fever or dermatitis***Q in ~ 70% of patients.

Etio-Pathology

- Etiology is only partially defined but there is a clear *genetic predisposition.* When both parents are affected, over 80% and when only one parent is affected ~50% of their children manifest the disease
- *Increased IgE synthesis*; increased *serum IgE;* increased *specific IgE* to food, aeroallergins, bacteria & bacterial products.
- *Increased expression of CD23* (low affinity IgE receptor) on monocyte & B- cells
- *Impaired delayed type hypersensitivity* reactions.

Histology

SpongiosisQ of epidermis is the hallmark of eczema. In chronic stage, lesions show *hyperkeratosis* (thickening of stratum corneum) & *acanthosis* (thickening of viable epidermis)

Diagnostic criteria

- ***Hanifin and Rajka*** *defined major and minor criteria for diagnostic accuracy of atopic dermatitis.* Three major and three minor criteria should be present.

Major criteria

- ***Pruritis***Q
- ***Involvement of face and convexities (extensor surface) in infants (< 2 years)***Q and distribution over ***flexures (popliteal and anticubital fossa) in older children*** & adultQ.
- Tendency to chronicity or chronically relapsing
- ***Personal or family history of atopy such as hay fever, asthma, allergic rhinitis or atopic dermatitis***Q.

Minor criteria

- Facial pallor/Suborbital shadowing
- ***Infra-orbital folds (Dennie's line/Denny Morgan fold***Q***)***
- ***Xerosis (dry skin)*** Q
- Icthyosis vulgaris with accentuation over palmar crease (palmar hyperlinearity)
- Recurrent skin infections
- Tendency to non specific dermatosis of hand
- Immediate (type I) skin reactivity
- Delayed blanching to cholinergics
- Raised serum total IgE
- Anterior subcapsular cataract
- Keratoconus, conjunctivitis (recurrent)
- Cheilitis, food intolerance, keratosis pilaris, nipple dermatitis, perifollicular accentuation, ***pityriasis alba, white dermographism***Q, wool intolerance.

Clinical Presentation

- The clinical presentation often varies with age. Half of the patients present within the first year of life, & 80% present by 5 years of age
- The ***infantile pattern*** is characterized by ***weeping inflammatory patches and crusted plaques, that occur on face, neck and extensor surfaces***Q. **(Infantile eczema)**
- **The childhood and adolescent pattern** is marked by dermatitis of ***flexural skin particularly in antecubital & popliteal fossa***Q
- Clinical course lasting longer than **6 weeks**Q
- About 80% ultimately *co express allergic rhinitis or asthma.*
- AD may resolve spontaneously, but over half of affected children will have dermatitis in adult life, i.e. ***coure is marked by exacerbations and remissions***Q. However, adults frequently have localized disease, manifesting as *hand eczema* or *lichen simplex chronicus.*
- Clinical features can be remembered in an easy way by understanding the cause.

Pruritis (Itching) & ScratchingQ

- ***Severely itchy, erythematous papular or papulo-vesicular lesions***Q, mostly involve ***face, popliteal fossae, antecubital fossae, wrist***Q. Itchiness is made worse by:
  - Minor environmental alteration
  - ***Sundry (in rainy seasons)***Q
  - ***Changes in temperature***Q
  - Rough clothings (woolen)
- Perpetual rubbing & scratching l/t
  - ***Excoriation***Q (simple, linear scratch marks)
  - ***Lichenification***Q (exaggeration of skin markings)
  - Dryness / Xeroderma
  - *Hyperlinear palms* (prominent skin markings on palm)
  - **Denny Morgan fold**Q *extrafold of skin beneath lower eyelid.*

Increased tendency for vasoconstriction

- *Pallor* on skin especially cheeks (i.e. perioral pallor)
- ***White dermatographism***Q (running a blunt object as key on affected skin produces a white line)

Personal or Family History of atophy

- ***Asthma***Q
- Hay fever
- Rhinitis (allergic)
- ***Chronic urticaria***Q
- Food allergies
- Eczema

Associated with

- Alopecia areata
- ***Susceptibility to skin infections***Q particularly to staphylococcus aureus, warts & molluscus contagiosum
- **Antena sign** - Follicular openings are filled with horny plugs
- **Head light sign** – cheilitis i.e. inflammation of skin on & around lips (perioral pallor)
- **Hertoghe's sign** – thinning of lateral half of eyebrows

Clinical Phase of Atopic Dermatitis

Infantile phase (Infantile eczematous dermatitis)

- Rarely starts before 4-6 weeks of age & *usually* ***begins between 2-3 months***Q of age (Roxburgh); but in Neena Khanna after 3 months).
- *First begin on face*Q & may quickly spread to other areas. Although, oftenly then *napkin area is relatively*

Childhood phase

- *From 1½ – 2years* ***onwards***Q
- Most characteristically involve ***elbow & knee flexures***Q, wrist & ankle.
- Sides of neck show a

Adult phase

- Lichenification, esp of *flexures & hands* (similar to that in later childhood)
- Involvement of *vermition of lip (like dermatitis)*
- **Nipple**

DERMATOLOGY

UK refinement of Hanifin & Rajka's diagnostic criteria of atopic dermatitis-

Major- *Itchy skin condition*[Q] (or parental reporting of scratching or rubbing)

Minor- 1. Onset below 2 years of age (not used if child is under 4 years)

2. History of skin crease involvement (including cheeks in child < 10 years age)
3. History of *dry skin*[Q]
4. ***Visible flexural dermatitits (or cheeks, forehead & other limb dermatitis in children < 4 years)***[Q]
5. ***Personal or family (in 1st degree relative) h/o other atopic disease.***[Q]

spared[Q], as a result of the area being kept moist.

- *Excoriation & lichenification* appear at about 6 months of age, when the ability to scratch develops
- *Initialy* the disorder involves flexural distribution. But when the *child starts to crawl,* the exposed *extensor aspect of knees, are most involved*[Q].

reticulate pigmentation k/a **atopic dirty neck.**

- *Uncommon extensor distribution & inability to lichenify*[Q] (even after prolonged rubbing) are very difficult to treat and take longer time to remit.

involvement in young / adolescent women

- Photosenstivity with ultraviolet & infrared radiation.

KAPOSI VERICELLIFORM ERUPTIONS / ECZEMA HERPETICUM

Most serious complication of atopic dermatitis is widespread herpes simplex virus infection resulting in kaposi's varicelliform eruption. KVE is wide spread cutaneous infection with a virus which normally causes localized or mild vesicular eruption occurring in patients with pre-existing skin disease.

Etiopathogenesis

It is **wide spread (disseminated cutaneous) herpes simplex virus 1 (HSV1) infection** in patients of damaged skin.

Infectious agent	Predisposing factor (damaged skin)
- ***Herpes simplex virus (HSV1) is most common cause (Eczema herpaticum)***[Q] - Coxsackie A 16 - Vaccinia - ***Small pox vaccination (Eczema vaccinatum)***[Q]	- ***Atopic dermatitis or eczema***[Q] (most common predisposing factor), Allergic contact dermatosis, ***Darrier's disease (keratosis follicularis)***[Q] - Various bullous diseases (particularly if receiving immunosuppressive therapy). Pemphigus foliaceous, benign familial pemphigus - Icthysosis vulgaris, congenital icthyosiform erythroderma - Mycosis fungoides, Sezary syndrome, SSSS - Burns (2nd and 3rd degree) - Contact dermatitis, Hailey-Hailey disease, Grover disease, Psoriasis, PRP etc.

Treatment

- In infants early treatment with acyclovir is life saving
- **Acyclovir** or **valacyclovir** in adults.

Clinical features

- ***History of herpes labialis in a parent in previous week***[Q] (in 1/3rd cases)
- After **incubation period of 5-12 days, *multiple itchy, vesiculo-pustular lesions erupt in a disseminated pattern***[Q].
- Vesicular lesions are ***markedly umblicated***[Q], tend to crop & often become ***hemorrhagic & crusted***[Q]. Punched out & extremely painful erosions result that may coalesce to large, denuded & bleeding areas.
- Most common in areas of active or recently healed atopic dermatitis, *particularly the face*, but nomal skin may be involved.
- ***High fever & adenopathy***[Q] occurs 2-3 days after onset of vesication.
- *10% mortality* without treatment is d/t bacterial super infection & bacteremia caused by staph. aureus, streptococcus & pseudomonas.
- It is usually d/t *primary HSV1 infection* in a child with atopic dermatitis (cathelicidins control susceptibility).
- *Recurrences are uncommon & usually far milder.*
- Should be *always considered in children with infected eczema, particularly if child is more ill systemically* than one might anticipate with impetigo (D/D).

★ **Eczema vaccinatum** is severe wide spread eruption (similar to eczema herpeticum) in **atopic dermatitis** patients who are *vaccinated for **small pox*** or even exposed to vaccinated individuals. So in AD patients small pox vaccination is contraindicated unless there is a clear risk of small pox. Even decision to vaccinate family members is cautiously taken.

CONTACT DERMATITIS

It is an inflammatory process in skin caused by an exogenous agent that directly or indirectly injure skin.

Irritant Contact Dermatitis (ICD)	Allergic Contact Dermatitis (ACD)
- Caused by inherent characteristic of a compound eg acid or base - Strictly demarcated & often localized to areas of thin skin (eyelides inter trigenous areas) or to areas, where irritant is applied. - *Chronic low grade irritant dermatitis* is the most common type of ICD, and most common area of involvement is the hands. - The most common irritants encountered are ***chronic wet work, soaps and detergents***[Q]	- Agent causing ACD induce an antigen specific immune response. (delayed type hypersensitivity mediated by memory T lymphocytes) - The ***most common cause is exposure to plants especially members of family Anacardiaceal including the genus Toxicodendrun***[Q], poison ivy, poison oak, poison sumac are members of this genus. The sensitizing antigen common to these plants is *urushiol*, an oleoresin containing the active ingredient *pentadecylcatechol*.

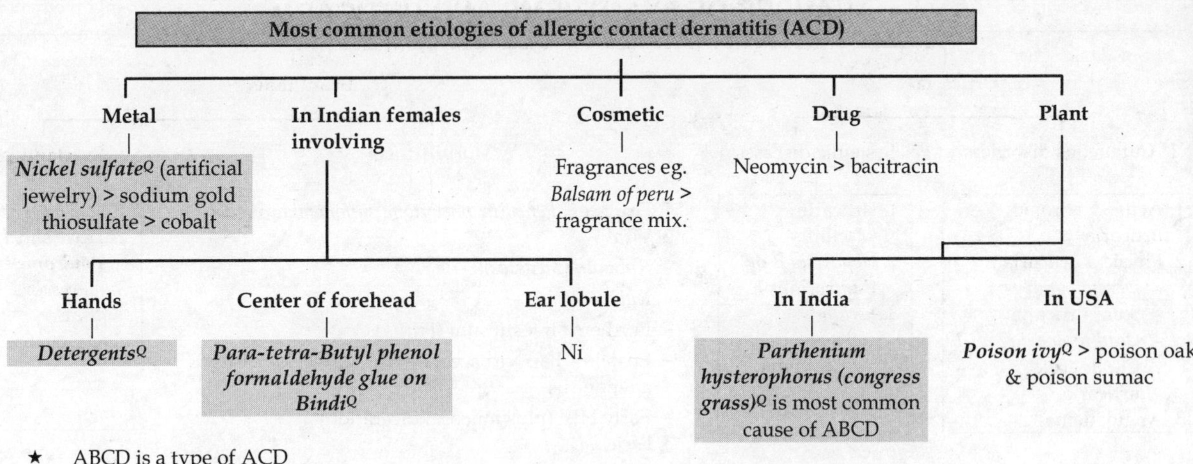

★ ABCD is a type of ACD

PATCH TEST

- The **gold standard method** for the diagnosis of ***allergic dermatitis resulting from type IV delayed hypersenstivity***[Q]. Such as ***allergic contact dermatitis (ACD) & air borne contact dermatitis (ABCD)***[Q] remains the patch test. It is ***read after 48 hours (2 days)***[Q]
- In this a battery of suspected allergen is applied to *patient's back under occlusive dressing* (**closed patch test**) and allowed to remain in contact with the skin. The adhesive bandage is removed in ***48 hours***[Q] (2days) for initial interpretation. Second reading is taken at 96 hours (4 days) or at 3-7 days. Second reading (b/w 4- 7 days) is important for ***elderly***[Q], who mount an allergic reaction more slowly tha younger patients and also in ***neomycin allergy***[Q] (as > 50% cases are not evident until 96 hours). In **open patch test** allergen is applied on outer arm skin & *left uncovered*. In **use test** suspected cosmetic is used on a site distant from original eruption twice daily for 7 days.
- Thin – layered **R**apid **U**se **E**picutaneous **(T.R.U.E) test** is a ready to use patch test containing 23 allergens & 1 allergen mix. TROLAB herbal and American cotact dermatitis group tay (containing 50 antigens) are also ready to use patch test.
- **Photopatch test** is necessary when the allergen requires photo activation, as in *photoallergic contact dermatitis* caused by *sunscreen oxybenzone*. Everything remains same except at 24 hours, one set of patches are irradiated with UV – A.

Interpretation

Grade	Reaction	Feature
O	No reaction	Normal skin
±	Doubtful	Minimal macular erythema only
1 +	Weak **(Non vesicular)**	Erythema, infiltration & papule (±)
2+	Strong	Erythema & edema or vesicles
3+	Extreme	Spreading erythema & bulous or ulceration

Avoided in

- Active flaring dermatitis involving > 25% body surface
- ***Excited skin (angry back) syndrome, a major cause of false positive patch test***[Q].

Defered in

Treatments interfering delayed hypersensitivity reactions such as:

- Systemic steroids (delayd for at least 2 weeks)
- Topical steroids on back (delayed for 3 days)
- Immunosuppressants (cyclophosphamide, azathioprine etc)
- **PUVA or ultraviolet B** phototherapy.

Alergic versus irritant test

Strong irritant reaction exhibits a deep erythema, resembling a burn. Whereas, strong allergic reactions are vesicular & spread beyond the test site.

Test	Read after
Patch Test **Early Fernadez reaction**	*2 days*[Q] *2 days*[Q]
In T.B., induration is seen after	3 days
Skin doubling time in psoriasis	4 days
Kveim's test	***2 weeks***[Q]
Late Mistuda reaction	***3 weeks***[Q]
Normal skin doubling time	4 weeks

CAUSES OF EXANTHEMS AND URTICARIA

Urticaria

1° Cutaneous disorders

1. Acute & chronic urticaria
2. Physical urticaria
   - *Dermatographism*
   - Solar urticaria
   - ***Cold urticaria***Q
   - Cholinergic urticaria
3. Angioedema

Systemic diseases

1. Urticaria vasculitis
2. ***Hepatitis B or C infections***Q
3. ***Serum sickness***Q
4. Angioedema

Exanthems*

Morbilliform

1. Drugs eg. *Pencillin, phenytoin, sulfonamide or gold*
2. Viral
   - ***Rubeola (measles)***Q
   - ***Rubella***Q
   - Erythema infectiosum (Fifth ds.)
   - Epstein – Barr virus, echo virus, coxsackie virus & adenovirus
   - Early HIV (plus mucosal ulceration)
3. *Bacterial*
   - ***Typhoid fever***Q
   - *Early secondary syphilis*
   - *Early Rickettsia*
   - *Early* meningococcemia
4. *Acute graft versus host reaction*
5. *Kawasaki's disease*

Scarlantiform

1. ***Scarlet fever***Q
2. ***Toxic shock syndrome***Q
3. *Kawasaki's disease*

* **Exanthems** are characterized by an *acute generalized eruption.* The most common presentations are *erythematous macules & papules (morbilliform) and confluent blanching erythema (scarlantiform).*

URTICARIA AND ANGIOEDEMA (QUINCKE'S DISEASE)

May appear seperately or together as ***localized nonpitting edema of skin*** and ***mucosal surface of respiratory or gastrointestinal tract***Q. **Urticaria** involves only the *superficial* portion of the *dermis*, presenting as *well circumscribed* wheals with erythematous raised serpiginous borders with blanched centres (characteristic central clearing). **Angioedema** is a well-demarcated localized edema, involving the deeper layers of the skin including *subcutaneous tissue.* It is a *self limiting* disease & episodes of < *6 weeks* are considered acute.

Predisposing Factors, Etiology

- Ingestion of ***fresh fruits, shell fish, fish, milk products, chocolate, legumes including peanuts & drugs***Q.
- Inhalation or physical contact with ***pollens, animal dander, mold spores***Q.
- *Physical stimuli* such as *cold, heat, solar rays, exercise, and mechanical irritation.*
- *Most cases of chronic urticaria* are *idiopathic.*

Classification

1. **IgE dependent**
   a. Specific antigen sensitivity (pollens, foods, drugs, fungi, molds, Hymenoptera venom, helminths)
   b. Physical: dermographism, cold, solar, cholinergic, vibratory, exercise-related.
   c. Autoimmune
2. **Bradykinin mediated**
   a. Hereditary angiodema: ***C1 inhibitor deficiency***Q: null (type 1) and dysfunctional (type 2)
   b. Acquired angioedema: C1 inhibitor deficiency.
   c. ***Angiotensin-converting enzyme inhibitors***Q
3. **Complement mediated**
   a. Necrotizing vasculitis
   b. Serum sickness
   c. Reactions to blood products
4. **Nonimmunologic**
   a. Direct mast cell- releasing agents (opiates, antibiotics, curare, D-tubocurarine, radiocontrast media)
   b. Agents that alter arachidonic acid metabolism (asprin and nonsteroidal anti-inflammatory agents, azo dyes, and benzoates)
5. **Idiopathic**

Clinical Features and Types

- Rapid onset and self limited nature of eruptions are distinguishing feature
- Additional characteristics are occurence of urticarial crops in various stages of evolution & asymmetrical distribution of the angioedema.
- ***Urticarial eruptions are pruritic***Q, ***involve any area of the body from scalp to soles of feet***Q, & appear in ***crops of 24- to 72 hours***Q duration. The most common site for *urticaria* are *extremities & face*, with *angioedema* often being ***periorbital and in the lips***Q.
- Although *self limited* in duration, angioedema of upper respiratory tract may be life threatening d/t laryngeal obstruction, while gastrointestinal involvement may present with abdominal colic, with or without nausea & vomit, and may precipitate unnecessary surgical intervention.
- The diagnosis of **hereditary angioedema** is suggested not only by *family history* but also by the ***lack of pruritus and of urticarial lesions***Q, the prominence of ***recurrent gastrointestinal attacks of colic & episodes of laryngeal edema. (causing hoarseness of voice & stridor)***Q
- Physical urticarias can be distinguished by precipitating events

1. ***Cholinergic urticaria*** : is **distinctive in that the pruritic wheals are of small size (1 – 2 mm)**Q and *are surrounded by large area of erythema; attacks are precipitated by fever, a* **hot bath or shower, or exercise**Q *and are presumptively attributed to a* rise in core body temperature.
2. **Solar Urticaria**Q : *Patients react* only to sunlight & not to heat from other sources. *Lesions are limited to* sun exposed areas *only. It may be a manifestation of porphyria.*
3. **Excercise related anaphylaxis**: Can be precipitated by

Pathophysiology

- Patients with chronic urticaria may have *autoantibodies to IgE/ α chain of Fc ∈ RI*, which leads to *basophilic degranulation* & enhancement of *anaphylatoxic fragment* C_{5a}.
- ***C1 esterase inhibitor (C1INH) deficiency*** causes ***angioedema without urticaria***[Q] d/t generation of bradykinin.
- ***ACE inhibitors***[Q] in hypertensive can provoke *angioedema without urticaria* d/t decreased degradation of bradykinin.
- Urticaria & angioedema associated with serum sickness, hypo complementemic cutaneous necrotizing angiitis are **Immune complex mediated**[Q].
- **Herieditary angioedema** is an ***autosomal dominant***[Q] disease due to ***deficiency (type I, 85%) or dysfunction (type II, 15%) of C1INH***[Q].
- **Acquired angioedema** is d/t excessive consumption of C1INH due either to immune complexes formed between *anti-idiotypic antibody* and monoclonal IgG presented by *B cell lymphomas* or to an auto antibody directed to C1INH,
- C1 inhibitor is a serine protease inhibitor whose target enzyme are ***C1r and C1s of complement cascde, Factor XII (Hageman factor)***[Q] *of* coagulation pathway and *kallikrein system.*
- In patients with heriditary angioedema (HA), activation of C1 by immune complex (i.e. first step of classical complement pathway, which is blocked by C1INH is not properly controlled and increased break down of C_4 & C_2 occurs). During clinical attack there is:
  - *Decline* in complement substrate, C_4 *&* C_2 reflect the action of activated C1
  - Elevated levels of bradykinin, and reduced level of prekallikrein & high *molecular weight kinnogen*, from which bradykinin is cleaved.
  - C1 levels are normal.
- So in **HA**, while levels of C1 are normal, its substrate C4 & C2, are chronically depleted and fall further during attacks.
- **Acquired angioedema** exhibits a reduction of C1 function and C1q protein as well as C1INH, C4 & C2.
- Hereditary, acquired and ACE inhibitor – elicited angioedema are associated with elevated levels of bradykinin.

exertion alone or can be dependent on prior food ingestion. It causes erythema & pruritic urticaria which may progress to angioedema of face, oropharynx, larynx, or intestine; or to vascular collapse. It is distinguished from cholinergic urticaria by presenting with ***wheals of conventional size***[Q] and by ***not occuring with fever or hot bath***[Q].

4. **Cold urticaria** is of two types:
   - **Familial Cold Urticaria -** Huge urticaria with fever & leucocytosis on exposure to cold. **It** occurs in families
   - ***Idiopathic Acquired Cold Urticaria***[Q] - precipitated by exposure to cold water/wind drinks, visit to hill stations, entering A.C. rooms, intake of ice-cream, *exposure to wind, after getting drenched in rains or sitting under fan while sweating.*
5. **Dermographism** : This is *exaggerated 'triple response'* of lewis. In some patients of urticaria, mark easily when their skin is scratched or rubbed with blunt object (key). It is not influenced by an atopic diathesis and has a duration generally of less than 5 years.
6. **Pressure urticaria** : Urticarial lesions develop sometime (upto several hours) after pressure on the skin, for example – *tight belts,* strap of brassiere, elastic of socks, watch strap, swelling of feet after *prolonged walking* & of *hands* after *clapping,* shoulder swelling after carrying heavy weight.
7. **Aquagenic urticaria** : from contact with water of any temperature (may be associated with polycythemia vera)
8. **Urticaria pigmentosa (Mastocytosis) :** there is excess of mast cells in many tissues, but it mainly manifests in the skin as numerous red-brown/pink papules over trunk & limbs. Some patients may have itching & experience erythema when bathing. *Alcohol, Opioids* or other drugs may precipitate attacks. *Juvenile* variety remits in adolescence but *adult* variety persists.
9. **Vasculitic urticaria:** typically persists longer than 72 hours, where as conventional urticaria, often has a duration of less than 24 –48h. Confirmatory biopsy reveals cellular infiltration, nuclear debris & fibrinoid necrosis of venules

✶ *Chronic recurrent urticaria,* generally in *females*, with *arthalgias, elevated ESR*, & normo – or hypo comlementemia suggest **cutaneous necrotizing angiitis.**

✶ Urticaria d/t serum sickness or drugs also includes pyrexia, lymphadenopathy, myalgia, and arthralgia or arthritis.

✶ Note: **Mastocytoma (mast cell naevus):** Is localized collection (one or many) of mast cells presenting as red/pink nodules in *infants & young children* but *disappears later in childhood.* Rubbing/heating results in swelling & red halo- ***Darier's sign***[Q].

URTICARIA (Types and Treatment)

Manifests as sudden eruption of ***itchy wheals***[Q] in any size, shape & location. Types include

Cholinergic Urticaria	Heat Urticaria	Solar Urticaria	Pressure Urticaria	Idiopathic Familial Cold U.	Acquired 2° cold U.
- *Urticaria develops due to ACh liberated from post ganglionic cholinergic enervated sweat glands* ***under the influence of any stimuli which induces sweating by increasing core body temperature***[Q] - Characteristic feature is ***small size pruritic wheals surrounded by large erythema***[Q]. - Precipitating factors are: 1. ***Exercise***[Q] ***/ Physical exertion*** [Q] 2. ***Emotion upset***[Q] 3. ***Exposure to sun / heat***[Q] 4. ***Hot bath / food***[Q]	Urticaria seen after application of *local heat* only	- Urticaria seen after exposure to *sunlight (UV lamp)* - May be seen in: 1. *SLE* 2. *Porphyria cutanea tarda* 3. *Erythropoietic protoporphyria*	Urticaria seen after pressure example belt prolonged clapping/ walking	- A.D. - *Appears soon after birth* - *Urticaria* seen after *drop in body temp precipitated by generalized environmental rather than local cooling*	- More common in *adults* - Precipated by cold contact, be it *cold water/ drink/ food/ air.* **Urticarial vasculitis** **Urticaria pigmentosa**

✶ Exercised related urticaria is precipitated by exertion alone (not by fever, hot bath) or on prior food ingestion

Treatment of Urticaria

Drug of choice	- Acute severe urticaria - Angioedema	Life threatening condition
Antihistamines of H_1 ***recceptor blocker type***[Q]	Oral Corticosteriod	Intravenous hydrocortisone ± tracheostomy

ANGIODERMA (TYPES AND DD)

HEREDITARY ANGIONEUROTIC EDEMA (HAE)

Etiopathogenesis

C1 esterase inhibitor (C_1INH) enzyme is an inhibitor of serine proteases including ***factor XII (Hageman – factor), Kallikrein and activated protein C1***Q (C1r & C1s) of complement cascade. So ***C1 INH deficiency***Q (type 1, ~ 85%) or dysfunction (type 2) l/t

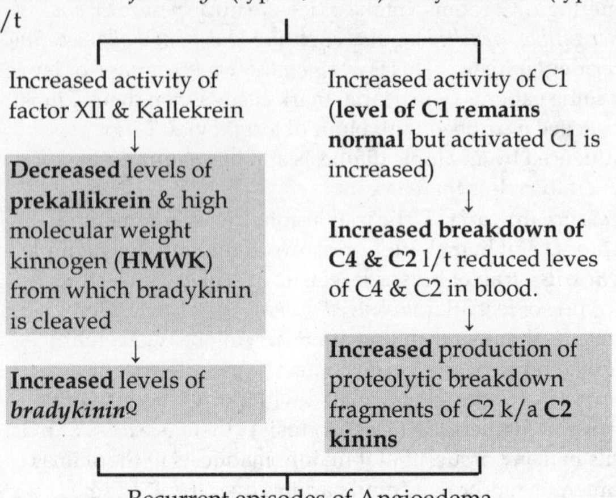

Increased activity of factor XII & Kallekrein
↓
Decreased levels of **prekallikrein** & high molecular weight kinnogen **(HMWK)** from which bradykinin is cleaved
↓
Increased levels of ***bradykinin***Q
Increased activity of C1 **(level of C1 remains normal** but activated C1 is increased)
↓
Increased breakdown of C4 & C2 l/t reduced leves of C4 & C2 in blood.
↓
Increased production of proteolytic breakdown fragments of C2 k/a **C2 kinins**
Recurrent episodes of Angioedema

Differential Diagnosis

Feature	Angioneurotic Edema	Anaphylaxis
Onset	Sudden	Sudden
Association with food allergy	Present	Present
Angioedema (swelling of lips, face, tongue, eyelids etc)	Present	Present
Upper respiratory tract obstruction (d/t laryngeal edema	Present	Present
Abdominal cramps (d/t intestinal edema)	Present	**Present**
Progression	**Slow**	**Rapid**
Pruiritis	**Not** a prominent manifestation (often non- pruiritic)	**Present**
Vascular collapse (hypotension)	**Not** a prominent manifestation (often absent)	**Present**
Family history	**Present** (no. f/h in acquired form)	Often absent

ACQUIRED ANGIOEDEMA

Acquired angioedema (acquired C1 inhibitor deficiency) onsets in *middle age* and occurs in two forms

1. Acquired angioedema **(AAE)** I is associated with malignancies (such as B- cell lymphoprolifeative disorder, breast cancer etc), connective tissue diseases, infections
2. **AAE type II** is an autoimmune form in which auto antibody directed against C1 INH is found.

LABORATORY EVALUATION OF HEREDITARY & ACQUIRED ANGIOEDEMA

Type	C4	C1 INH (functional)	C1 INH (Quantitative)	C1q
HAE Type I	↓	↓	↓	**Normal**
HAE Type II	↓	↓	**Normal**	**Normal**
AAE Type I	↓	↓	↓	↓
AAE Type II	↓	↓	Normal to midly ↓	↓

Questions

1. **'Itch is disease' is true for -** *(UPSC 2K)*
   A. Atopic dermatitis
   B. Insect bites
   C. Seborrheic dermatitis
   D. Tinea cruris
2. **Characteristic feature of atopic drmatitis is**
   A. Pruritus *(MP 05, DNB 08)*
   B. Dennie's Lines
   C. Scalling skin (Lichenification)
   D. Rash
3. **Minor clinical feature in diagnosis of atopic dermatitis A/E-** *(PGI Dec 04)*
   A. Dry skin
   B. Pruritus
   C. Morgagnian fold
   D. Pitriasis alba
   E. Dermographism
4. **Dennie Morgan fold is seen in-**
   A. Mastocytosis *(Karnatak 96, Bihar 06)*
   B. Seborrhoic dermatitis
   C. Sarcoidosis
   D. Atopic dermatitis
5. **Commonest site of Atopic dermatitis is-**
   A. Scalp *(Jipmer 93, DNB 06)*
   B. Elbow
   C. Trunk
   D. Ante cubital fossa
6. **Spongiosis is seen in :** *(Karnataka 03, AI 01)*
   A. Acute eczema
   B. Lichen Planus
   C. Psoriasis
   D. Pemphigus
7. **Atopic Dermatitis is diagnosed by:** *(AI 99)*
   A. Patch test
   B. Wood Lamp
   C. Clinical Examination
   D. -IgE
8. **A 3 yr old child has eczematous dermatitis on extensor surfaces. His mother has a history of bronchial asthma. Diagnosis could be** *(AIIMS Nov 06, May 07, Nov 11)*
   A. Atopic dermatitis
   B. Contact dermatitis
   C. Seborrhic dermatitis
   D. Infantile eczematous dermatitis
9. **An infant presented with erythematous lesions on cheek, extensor aspect of limbs, mother has history of bronchial asthma, the probable diagnosis is** *(AI 2007)*
   A. Air borne contact dermatitis
   B. Atopic dermatitis
   C. Seborraehic dermatitis
   D. Infectious eczematoid dermatitis
10. **Rakesh, a 7-year-old boy had itchy, excoriated papules on the forehead and the exposed parts of the arms and legs for 3 years. The disease was most severe in the rainy season and improved completely in winter. Most likely diagnosis is:** *(AIIMS 04)*
    A. Insect bite hypersensitivity
    B. Scabies
    C. Urticaria
    D. Atopic dermatitis
11. **A 25 year old man presents with recurrent episodes of flexural exzema contact urticaria, recurrent skin infections and severe abdominal cramps and diarrhoea upon taking sea foods. He is suffering from :**
    A. Seborrheic dermatitis *(AI 04)*
    B. Atopic dermatitis
    C. Airborne contact dermatitis
    D. Nummular dermatitis
12. **Coin shaped eczema is :** *(Jharkhand 05)*
    A. Nummular eczema
    B. Atopic ecema
    C. Infantile eczema
    D. Endogenous eczema
13. **Eczema herpeticum seen with**
    A. HSV *(PGI June 07, 2K)*
    B. EBV
    C. CMV
    D. VZV
    E. HPV
14. **Kaposi's varicelliform eruption seen in :**
    A. Darrier disease *(PGI 05, 04)*
    B. Varicella zoster
    C. Pityriasis rosea
    D. Atopic dermatitis
    E. Mumps
15. **After hepatitis B vaccination child with allergic family history and pruritis involving face & convexities developed numerous umblicated vesicles; which became pustular & haemorhagic & crusted. After 2 days child developed high fever and lymphadenopathy. The diagnosis is** *(AIIMS 07)*
    A. Secondary infected atopic dermatitis
    B. Molluscum contagiosum
    C. Eczema herpaticum
    D. Eczema vaccinatum
16. **Most common precipitant of contact dermatitis is**
    A. Gold *(AI 93)*
    B. Nickle
    C. Silver
    D. Iron
17. **Commonest metal causing skin hypersensitivity-**
    A. Nickle *(AIIMS 98, 96, AI 93)*
    B. Cu
    C. Iron
    D. Brass
18. **Most common cause of allergic contact dermatitis in Indian female is** *(AIIMS 2000)*
    A. Vegetables
    B. Nail polish
    C. Detergents
    D. Dyes
19. **Commonest cause of air borne contact dermatitis in India is:** *(AI 99, AIIMS 94)*
    A. Parthenium
    B. Garden grass
    C. Calotropis/Crysophillus
    D. Yellow oleander
    E. Dust
20. **In India, the plant which causes dermatitis most commonly is:** *(AIIMS May 08)*
    A. Parthenium grass

DERMATOLOGY 1

B. Cotton fibers ☐
C. Poison Ivy ☐
D. Ragweed ☐

21. A female has hypopigmented lesion on centre of forehead drug, responsible is: *(AIIMS Nov 2008)*
A. Hydroquinone ☐
B. Mono benzene metabolite of hydroquinone ☐
C. Para tetra butyl catechol ☐
D. Para tetra butyl phenol ☐

22. Berloque dermatitis is due to contact with -
A. Metals *(Jipmer 99, DNB 98)* ☐
B. Cosmetics ☐
C. Food ☐
D. Plants ☐

23. A 55-year-old male, with uncontrolled diabetes mellitus and hypertension, developed severe air-borne contact dermatitis. The most appropriate drug for his treatment would be: *(AIIMS 04)*
A. Systemic corticosteroids ☐
B. Thalidomide ☐
C. Azathioprine ☐
D. Cyclosporine ☐

24. A 27 year old male has itchy, excoriated papules on forehead and exposed parts of arms and legs for 3 years. The disease was most severe in rainy season and improved completely in winters. Most likely diagnosis is:
A. Scabies *(AIIMS May 12)* ☐
B. Urticaria ☐
C. Atopic dermatitis ☐
D. Insect bite hypersensitivity ☐

25. Air-borne contact dermatitis can be diagnosed by:
A. Skin biopsy *(AIIMS May 06, DNB 10)* ☐
B. Patch test ☐
C. Prick test ☐
D. Estimation of serum IgE levels ☐

26. Diagnostic meathod of choice in contact dermatitis
A. Clinical examination *(AI 92)* ☐
B. Skin Biopsy ☐
C. Tzank Smear ☐
D. Patch Test ☐

27. Patch testing is done for : *(PGI Dec 08)*
A. Atopic dermatitis ☐
B. Irritant contact dermatitis ☐
C. Allergic contact dermatitis ☐
D. Discoid eczema ☐
E. Seborrhoeic dermatitis ☐

28. Patch test is a type of: *(AIIMS May 2009)*
A. Immediate hypersensitivity ☐
B. Antibody mediated hypersensitivity ☐
C. Immune complex mediate hypersensitivity ☐
D. Delayed type hypersensitivity ☐

29. Skin test can be done for which hypersensitivity reactions : *(PGI 01)*
A. I ☐
B. II ☐
C. III ☐
D. IV ☐

30. Patch test is read after: *(AI 99)*
A. 2 hours ☐
B. 2 days ☐
C. 2 weeks ☐
D. 2 months ☐

31. All are true/ except regarding patch test *(PGI 08)*
A. Diagnose ABCD ☐
B. Read after 48 hours ☐
C. Angry back l/t false negative test ☐
D. Reading is delayed in neomycin ☐
E. T.R.U.E test ☐

32. Morbilliform eruptions is seen in: *(PGI 01)*
A. Scarlet fever ☐
B. Rubella ☐
C. Toxic shock syndrome ☐
D. Measle s ☐
E. Mumps ☐

33. All may lead to hives and wheels except
A. Cold *(PGI 97)* ☐
B. Hepatitis C ☐
C. Serum Sickness ☐
D. Typhoid Fever ☐

34. A 22 year old woman developed small itchy wheals after physical exertion, walking in the sun, eating hot spicy food and when she was angry. The most likely diagnosis is: *(AIIMSNov 03)*
A. Chronic idiopathic utricaria ☐
B. Heat urticaria ☐
C. Solar urticaria ☐
D. Cholinergic urticaria ☐

35. A patient gets reccurent urticaria while doing exercise and on exposure to sunligh. Which of the following is most like cause: *(AIIMS Nov 12, 2K)*
A. Chronic Idiopathic Utricaria ☐
B. Universal dermographism ☐
C. Cholinergic Utricaria ☐
D. Photdermatitis ☐

36. A 9 year-old has multiple itchy erythematous wheals all over the body for 2 days. There is no respiratory difficulty. Which is the best treatment? *(AIIMS 04)*
A. Antihelminthics ☐
B. Systemic corticosteroids ☐
C. Antihistamines ☐
D. Adrenaline ☐

37. Darriers sign is seen in : *(Jipmer 98, PGI 99)*
A. Xenoderma pigmentosa ☐
B. Urticaria pigmentosa ☐
C. Herpes zoster ☐
D. Glucogonoma ☐

38. A 5 year old male child has multiple hyperprigmented macules over the trunk. On rubbing the lesion with the rounded end of a pen, he developed urticarial wheal, confined to the border of the lesion. The most likely diagnosis is : *(AI 04)*
A. Fixed drug eruption ☐
B. Lichen planus ☐
C. Urticaria pigmentosa ☐
D. Urticarial vasculitis ☐

39. All are true regarding hereditary angioedema, except?
A. Dysfunction of enzyme is most common cause ☐
B. Enzyme involved in C1 INH *(PGI 98)* ☐
C. C1 inhibitor targets Hageman factor ☐
D. Complement C4 & C2 decrease ☐
E. Bradykinin level decrease during attack ☐

40. A person present with recurrent swelling on face and lips due to emotional stress, cause is *(AIIMS May 2009)*
A. C1 esterase inhibitor deficiency ☐
B. Allergy ☐
C. Anaphylaxis ☐
D. None of the above ☐

41. A patient presents with history of episodic painful edema of face and larynx and abdominal pain associated with stress. Which of the following is likely to be deficient
A. Complement C3 *(AI 2009, May 10)* ☐

B. Complement C5 ☐
C. C1 Esterase Inhibitor ☐
D. Properidin ☐

42. Immediately after eating, a man develops swelling of face and lips, respiratory distress, intense pruiritis, hypotension and feeling of impending doom. The most likely diagnosis is *(AI 2009)*
A. Angioneurotic Edema ☐
B. Anaphylaxis ☐
C. Myocardial Infarction ☐
D. Food stuck in throat ☐

43. Laboratory evaluation of a patient with recurrent lip edema shows decreased C4 and C1INH (quantity & function) with normal C1q. Diagnosis is
A. Hereditary angioedema type II ☐
B. Hereditary angioedema type I ☐
C. Acquired AE type II ☐
D. Acquired AE type I ☐

44. Not true about angioneurotic edema? *(AI 2009)*
A. Pitting edema of face, lips and mucous membrane ☐
B. C1 Esterase inhibitor deficiency can cause it ☐
C. Extreme temperature exposure can provoke it. ☐
D. Known with ACE inhibitors. ☐

45. A man takes peanut and develops, tongue swelling, neck swelling, stridor, hoarseness of voice. What is the probable diagnosis. *(AIIMS Nov 06)*
B. Angioneurotic edema ☐
C. FB bronchus ☐
D. Parapharyngeal abscess ☐
E. FB in larynx ☐

46. Quincke's disease is popularly known as - *(PGI 95, AIIMS 98)*
A. Norweigian scabies ☐
B. Angioneurotic oedema ☐
C. Seborrohea olesa ☐
D. Saddle nose ☐

ANSWERS AND EXPLANATIONS

ATOPIC DERMATITIS

1. **A i.e. Atopic dermatitis**
2. **A i.e. Pruritis**
3. **B i.e. Pruritis**
4. **D i.e. Atopic dermatitis**
5. **D i.e. Antecubital fossa**
6. **A i.e. Acute eczema**
7. **C i.e. Clinical Examination** *[Ref: Rooks 8/e p.24.1-24.30; 23.15-23.20; Harrison 18/e p. 395-97; Neena Khanna 4/e p.91-95; Fitzpatrick's 7/e p. 146-58; Roxburgh's 18/e p. 114-22]*

- *Itch (or pruritis)*Q is a **major** diagnostic criteria whereas, **Denny Morgan infra orbital fold** is a **minor** criteria for diagnosis of atopic dermatitis.
- Atopic dermatitis **most commonly involves** *flexural surfaces like antecubital and popliteal fossa* Q. However, in infantile phase, face and extensor surface (convexities) are more commonly involved.
- *Spongiosis of epidermis* Q is the **histological hallmark** of dermatitis (eczema).

Contact dermatitis *is diagnosed by patch test*Q & **Atopic dermatitis** *is diagnosed by clinical examination*Q. **Clinical criteria** for diagnosis of atopic dermatitis

1. **Family h/o allergy/atophy**
2. Personal history of allergy/atophy i.e. presence of *other atopic condition as*Q – *rhinitis, hay fever, asthma, food allergy or eczema*Q.
3. *Extremily pruritic lesions commonly on antecubital or popliteal fossa*Q
4. *Dienny morgan fold*Q, white dermographism
5. Exacerbation & remissions.
6. *Pruritis and scratching made worse by environmental alteration, changes in temperature, sundry (in rainy season) & rough (woolen) clothing*Q *and leading to excoriation, lichenification*Q, dryness & Dennie's line.
7. *Clinical course lasting longer than 6 weeks*Q.
8. Lesions typical of eczematous dermatitis i.e. *papules, erythematous macules and vesicles, which can coalesce to form patches and plaques.*

Disease	Diagnosis made by
Atopic Dermatitis	*Clinical Examination*Q
Contact Dermatitis	*Patch Test*Q
Donovanosis	*Microscopy*Q (demonstration of *Donovan bodies or safety pin appearance*)Q
Syphilis	*Dark field microscopy*Q, FTA-ABS, VDRL, MHA-TP, TPI
Chancroid	*Gram staining*Q *(gram –ve cocco-bacilli, school of fish or rail road appearance)*Q
LGV	- Microscopic examination of giemsa stained scrapings for inclusion or elementary bodies - Culture, ELISA
Tinea (Dermatophytes)	*KOH Smear*Q
Lupus vulgaris	*Biopsy*Q

8. **A i.e. Atopic Dermatitis**
9. **B i.e. Atopic Dermatitis**
10. **D i.e. Atopic dermatitis**
11. **B i.e. Atopic dermatitis**

*History of atophy (asthma) in family, with erythematous lesions on face (cheek and extensor surface of limbs*Q in infant is diagnostic of **atopic dermatitis (infantile eczematous dermatitis)**

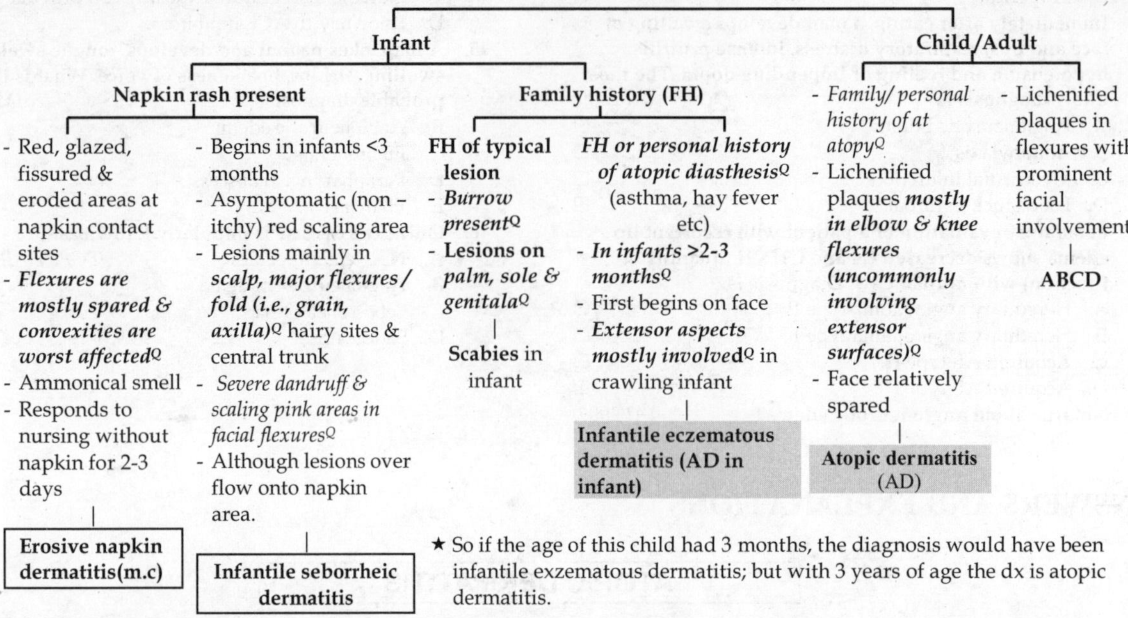
Infant
Child/Adult
Napkin rash present
Family history (FH)
- Red, glazed, fissured & eroded areas at napkin contact sites
- Flexures are mostly spared & convexities are worst affectedQ
- Ammonical smell
- Responds to nursing without napkin for 2-3 days
Erosive napkin dermatitis(m.c)
- Begins in infants <3 months
- Asymptomatic (non – itchy) red scaling area
- Lesions mainly in scalp, major flexures/ fold (i.e., grain, axilla)Q hairy sites & central trunk
- Severe dandruff & scaling pink areas in facial flexuresQ
- Although lesions over flow onto napkin area.
Infantile seborrheic dermatitis
FH of typical lesion
- Burrow presentQ
- Lesions on palm, sole & genitalaQ
Scabies in infant
FH or personal history of atopic diasthesisQ (asthma, hay fever etc)
- In infants >2-3 monthsQ
- First begins on face
- Extensor aspects mostly involvedQ in crawling infant
Infantile eczematous dermatitis (AD in infant)
- Family/ personal history of at atopyQ
- Lichenified plaques mostly in elbow & knee flexures (uncommonly involving extensor surfaces)Q
- Face relatively spared
Atopic dermatitis (AD)
- Lichenified plaques in flexures with prominent facial involvement
ABCD
★ So if the age of this child had 3 months, the diagnosis would have been infantile exzematous dermatitis; but with 3 years of age the dx is atopic dermatitis.

12. **A. i.e. Nummalar eczema**
[Ref: Rooks 8/e p.23.9-23.11; Harrison 18/e p. 397; Fitzpatrick's 7/e p. 158-59; Roxburgh's 18/e p. 126-127]

Circular or oval ***coin shaped lesions***Q are seen in **nummular (discoid) eczema.**

Dermatitis / Eczema

Nummular (Discoid) Eczema

- More frequently a disease of *middle aged adult (50-65 years) men.* However a second peak around 15-25 years in women and rarely childhood onset (at 5 years age) is also seen. *Dry skin* in elderly is a contributory factor.
- **Diagnostic lesions** is a ***well demarcated, coin shaped eryrhematous plaque***Q arising, quite rapidly, from the *confluence of tiny, closely set, thin walled papules and papulovesicles.*
- *Pin point oozing, crusting and scaling* eventuate. *Pruritis* varies from severe (in acute phase) to minimal. Later *central clearing* (resolution) and peripheral extension leads to *annular or ring shaped lesions.*
- Secondary lesions in a **mirror-image configuration** on opposite side of body and **reactivation of apparently dominant lesions** (particularly on premature discontinuation of treatment) is very characteristic.
- Common locations are *trunk or extensor surfaces of extremities,* particularly on the *pretibial areas (in men) or dorsal aspects of hands (in women).*
- **Differential Diagnosis: Contact dermatitis** should be suspected in *chronic recalcitrant and unusually severe* case where patches are *few, asymmetrical and of unusual configuration.* **Psoriasis** has usually more well defined, thickened, scaly and more number of plaques. **Bowen's disease** usually has 1 or 2 red, scaly patches mostly restricted to light exposed areas.
- Treatment is similar to that of atopic dermatitis.

Contact Dermatitis

I. *Air borne C.D.*Q
- Is due to ***parthenium (congress grass)***Q

II. Primary irritant C.D
- Due to ***direct contact with toxic irritating material***Q
- ***Palmar surface of hands***Q are m.c. involved

III. Allergic C.D.
- Due to contact with an agent to which delayed hypersensitivity has developed.
- ***Ex-Nickel (m.c.)***Q dye, cosmetics, local anesthetic.

Seborrheic Dermatitis

Occurs on hairy sites, flexures or on central trunk. It is chracterized by:
- Itching or burning
- ***Severe dandruff***Q
- ***Greasy yellow scales***Q over erythematous patch **(stuck on appearance)**
- ***Cradle cap***Q is seen in pityriasis capitis complicated by seborrheic dermatitis.

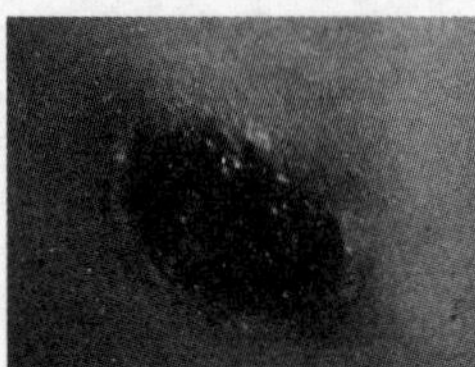

Coin shaped – Numular Eczema

Kaposi's Varicelliform Eruption

13. **A i.e. HSV**

14. **D i.e Atopic eczema > A i.e. Darrier disease**

15. **C. i.e. Eczema herpaticumx** *[Ref: Thomas Habif 4/e p. 388; Neena Khanna 3rd/p-81; Fitzpatrick 7/e p. 1877, 152, 153, 156, 1883; Dermatology by Jean & Joseph 1/e p. 1237; Rook's 8/e p. 24.24, 33.35-33.37]*

- **Eczema herpeticum** or **Kaposi's varicelliform eruption** results from wide spread (usually) ***primary HSV- 1 (herpes simplex1) infection in skin damaged by atopic dermatitis (eczema)***Q.
- Patients with *atopic eczema* may develop severe ***orofacial herpes simplex virus (HSV) infection***Q ***(eczema herpaticum),*** which may rapidly involve extensive areas of skin & occasionally disseminate to visceral organs. *Systemic acyclovir or valaciclovir* is treatment of choice.
- *In atopic dermatitis* patients, *small pox vaccination or even exposure to vaccinated individual,* may cause severe wide spread erruption (**k/a eczema vaccinatum**) that resembles to eczema herpaticum.
- Kaposis varicelliform eruptions manifest either as – eczema herpeticum or eczema vaccinatum.

Disease	Causative Virus
Eczema herpeticum	***HSV-1 (Herpes simplex honimis virus)***Q
Eczema vaccinatum	Vaccinia virus due to inadvertent vaccination of small pox with live virus vaccine
Milker's node	Paravaccinia / Pseudocowpox

CONTACT DERMATITIS

16. **B i.e. Nickle**

17. **A. i.e. Nickle**

18. **C i.e. Detergents**

19. **A i.e. Parthenium**

20. **A i.e., Parthenium grass**

21. **D i.e. Para tetra butyl phenol**

[Ref: Thomas Habif 4/e p. 101-84; API 17/e P-1313; Harrison 17/e p. 101; Neena Khanna 3/e p. 86-89; Pasricha-Illustrated Dermatology 3/e p. 92; Fitzpatrick's 7/e p-135-145; Rooks 7/e p.17.7-17.37; Roxburgh's 17/e p- 105-109]

- Most common cause of **air borne contact dermatitis (ABCD)** in India is ***parthenium hysterophorus (congress grass) plant***Q
- **Metal** most commonly l/t allergic contact dermatitis (ACD) is ***nickel (Ni)***Q and drug is neomycin. Whereas ***detergent***Q are most common cause of **ACD in Indian females.**
- ***Para-tetra (p-test)-Butyl phenol formaldehyde glue (resin) on Bindi***Q is most common cause of ACD or hypopigmentation on centre of forehead in Indian females.

22. **B i.e. Cosmetics** *[Ref: Thomas Habif clinical dermatology 4/e p-682-83; Fitzpatric's 7/e p-2361]*

Berlock dermatitis is a phototoxic reaction due to ***bergamot fragrance oil (5 methoxy psoralen) present in some perfumes & cosmetics***Q. It causes erythema followed by prolonged hyperpigmentation after exposure to sun light.

23. **C i.e. Azathioprine** *[Ref:Pasricha 4/e p 154; Roxburgh's 17/e p. 313; KDT 5/e p. 265; Fitzpatrick's 6/e p1181-1203; Rooks 7/e p.19.1-19.20]*

In contact dermatitis, the allergic reaction is mediated by *delayed hypersensitivity (cell mediated immunity).* It is treated by:
- Antihistamincis
- Steroids (topical/systemic)
- Agents depressing cell mediated immunity as cyclosporine, tacrolimus, azathioprine

Now let's concentrate on individual drug

Contraindication of ***Gluco-corticosteroid***Q:
1. ***Diabetes mellitus***Q
2. ***Hypertension***Q, Herpes simplex Keratitis
3. Pregnancy, Peptic ulcer, Psychosis
4. Epilepsy, CHF, Renal failure
5. Osteoporosis, Tuberculosis

S/E of **Cyclosporin**
1. Nephrotoxic
2. ***Hypertension***Q, & hirsutism, hyperkalemia
3. Precipitates diabetes

- Thalidomide causes – Phocomalia (is banned in 1960)
- S/E of **Azathioprine**
  1. ***Myelosuppression***Q

So I think azathioprine is the most appropiate answer as it may be given in diabetes & hypertension.

24. **D i.e. Insect bite hypersensitivity** *[Ref: Rook's 8/e p. 35.19; Neena Khanna 4/e p. 336-37]*

	Scabies	Insect Bite Hypersensitivity	Atopic Prurigo
Age	Any	***Children: if adults rule out underlying malignancy or HIV***Q	***Adults***Q (usually)
Morphology	***Burrow (Pathognomic)***Q **Papulo-vesicles** (itchy)	**Papules** surmounted with **vesicles** or **hemorrhagic crust** (itchy)	*Papulonodules (pruritic)*
Distribution	Webs of fingers, wrist, periumbilical area, genitals and thighs	***Exposed parts***Q (mostly on legs)	Flexures (mainly); face relatively spared
Family history	Present (similar lesions)	Absent	F/H of atophy, dry skin etc. present
Worsening		Summer>rainy	***Rainy season (sundry)***Q, change in temperature, ***woolen clothing***Q

DERMATOLOGY

PATCH TEST

25. B i.e. Patch Test
26. D i.e. Patch Test
27. C. Allergic contact dermatitis
28. D i.e. Delayed type hypersensitivity
29. A i.e. I; D i.e. IV (1st choice if only one answer)
30. B i.e. 2 days
31. C. i.e. Angry back l/t false negative test

[Ref: Thomas Habif 4/e p. 98 – 103; Fitzpatrick 7/e p.142-143; Harrisons 17/e p-312; Neena Khanna 3rd/e p- 89; Roxburgh's 17/e p21-24; Rooks 7/e p. 19.1- 19.20; API- 6/e p-1189, www.truetest.com]

- The **gold standard method** for the diagnosis of ***allergic dermatitis resulting from type IV delayed hypersenstivity***Q. Such as ***allergic contact dermatitis (ACD) & air borne contact dermatitis (ABCD)***Q remains the patch test. It is ***read after 48 hours (2 days)***Q
- **Type 1 hypersensitivity (eg atopic dermatitis) is detected by prick test (of debatable significance). And type IV delayed hypersensitivity (eg contact dermatitis) is diagnosd by patch skin test (gold standard). So skin test** can be done for **Type I (atophy) & type IV (contact dermatitis).**

Type of hypersensitive reaction	Clinical Syndrome
Type I : IgE type	***Anaphylaxis***Q ***Atopy***Q ***(prick test)***
Type II : Cytolytic & Cytotoxic	Antibody mediated damage– Thrombocytopenia– agranulocytosis, hemolytic anemia etc.
Type III : Immune complex	Arthrus reaction Serum sickness
Type IV : Delayed Hypersensitivity	Tuberculosis *Contact dermatitis (patch test)*Q

URTICARIA

32. B i.e. Rubella & D i.e. Measles
33. D i.e. Typhoid fever

[Ref: Rooks 8/e p.22.1-22.35]

Typhoid, rubella and **rubeola (measles)** leads to ***morbilliform - exanthems (not to urticaria or hives)***Q

34. D i.e. Cholinergic Urticaria
35. C i.e. Cholinergic Urticaria
36. C i.e. Antihistamines

- Patients developing **urticaria (itchy wheals surrounded by erythema)** under the influence of any stimulus which includes **sweating by increasing core body temperature** ***like physical exertion, emotional upset, and exposure to sun, heat, hot bath or spicy food***Q favours the diagnosis of **cholinergic urticaria.**
- ***Antihistaminics of H_1 receptor blocker***Q are **drug of choice** for treatment of urticaria.

URTICARIA PIGMENTOSA

37. B. i.e. Urticaria pigmentosa
38. C i.e. Urticaria pigmentosa

[Ref: Rook's 8/e p. 22.31-22.32; Fitzpatrick's 7/e p. 2247, 1438-40, 2255; Roxburgh's 18/e p. 214-15]

Darrier sign is ***development of urticaria and erythema around the pale-yellow to reddish-brown macules after mild trauma, including scratching or rubbing of the lesion***Q. It is seen mostly (but not always) in **urticaria pigmentosa**. However, it is not 100% specific for **mastocytosis** as it is also rarely seen in *juvenile Xanthogranuloma* and *acute lymphoblastic leukaemia* of *neonates*.

Urticaria Pigmentosa (UP)/Mastocytosis

- Mastocytosis is mast cell hyperplasia in ≥ 1 organs: *bone marrow, liver, spleen, lymph nodes, gastrointestinal tract and skin.* So mast cell activation may produce symptoms like, *pruritis, flushing, urtication, abdominal pain, nausea, vomiting, diarrhea, musculo skeletal pain, vascular instability, headache and neuropsychiatric difficulties.*
- UP (a type of cutaneous mastocytosis) is the *most common manifestation* of mastocytosis, both in adults & children.

Urticarial Vasculitis

- An important characteristic of urticaria is its transience but rarerly it may *stay for days rather than* hours & leave a brownish stain
- It is due to involvement of small vessels
- Vasculitis urticari typically persist *longer than 72 hours,* where as conventional urticaria often has a duration of less than 24 –48 hours.

Fixed drug Erruption

- Inflamatory patches appear within hours ***at the same sites on every occasion***Q the drug is administered

- Numerous ***pale yellow tan to reddish brown monomorphic macules or slightly raised papules develop in a symmetrical distribution***Q anywhere on the body with generally less involvement of the sun exposed areas, with the ***highest concentration usually being on the trunk and thighs***Q. Also generally spared (or less involved) are face, scalp, head, palms & soles.
- The edges of lesion are *not completely sharp*. It is not uncommon for lesion to become *pigmented*, hence name urticaria pigmentosa.
- ***Development of urticaria, erythema & itching around the lesion after mild trauma, including scratching or rubbing of lesion***Q is called **Darier Sign**. It is seen in UP.
- Climatic temperature, skin friction, ingestion of hot beverages, spicy foods, alcohol, opioids or other drugs may cause histamine release from mast cells and exacerbate mastocytosis
- 3 types/ forms of UP are

1. Juvenile type develop mostly in 1st year of life and usually remits spontaneously during adolescence
2. Adult papular type persists.
3. Adult telangiectasia macularis eruptive perstans of Parker & Weber: in which telangiectatic macules start to appear, persist and increase in number over the years.

- Leave pigmentation
- Common drugs are dapsone, tetracycline, sulfonamides, mefenimic acid.

Lichen Planus

- ***'6-P' lesion***Q
- ***Plain (flat topped)***Q
- ***Polygonal***Q
- ***Purple (mauve)***Q
- ***Pruritic***Q
- ***Papule***Q with
- ***Pterygium of nail***Q
- ***Whickham striae***Q i.e. whitis lacework pattern on surface
- ***Mucosal involvement***Q
- Kobner's phenomenon
- Associated with
- ***Hepatitis - C***Q
- Hyperpigmentation
- Biopsy
- Band like infiltration of lymphocyte, histiocytes & melanophage in dermis ***(lichenoidband)***Q
- ***Civatte bodies***Q
- May l/t ***Squamous cell C_A***Q

ANGIOEDEMA/QUINCKE'S DISEASE

39. **A i.e. Dysfunction of enzyme is most common case E i.e. Bradykinin level decreases during attack.**
40. **A. i.e. C1 esterase deficiency** 41. **C i.e. C1 esterase deficiency** 42. **B. i.e. Anaphylaxis**
43. **B. i.e. Hereditary angioedema type I**
44. **A i.e. Pitting edema of face, lips and mucous membrane**
45. **A i.e. Angioneurotic edema** 46. **B. i.e. Angioneurotic edema**

[Ref: Trevino & Dixon – Food & allergy 1997/19; Harrison 17/e p.2065-66; Merck Manual of diagnosis and therapy 17/e P. 148; Robbin's pathological Basis of disease 7/e P – 245 66, 67; Fitzpatrick's 6/e p-1181-1203; Rooks 7/e p.47.1-47.29; Ananthanrayan 7/e p. 115-116; Thomas Habif 4/e p. 127-151]

- Recurrent episodes of ***non pitting edema of face,larynx (l/t respiratory distress), intestine (l/t colic pain), skin & extremities***Q provoked by emotional stress (neurotic), food, or inhalational agents, with a positive ***family history (autosomal dominant)***Q, is diagnostic of **hereditary angioneurotic edema**.
- ***Angioneurotic edema (swelling of face & lips) in presence of intense pruritis and evidence of vascular collapse (hypotension)***Q, suggest a diagnosis of **Anaphylaxis.**
- **Hereditary Angioneurotic edema** is a *deficiency / non functioning of C1 inhibitors*, a condition characterized by ***episodic not pitting angioedema of the subcutaneous tissue or the mucosa of respiratory &/or alimentrary tracts***Q elicted by ***ingestion of fresh fruits, shell fish, fish, milk products, chocolate, legumes including peanuts***Q & drugs. Uncommonly it may occur secondary to inhalation or physical contact with pollens, animal dander and mold spores and emotional stress. The diagnossi is suggested not only by family history but also by *lack of pruritiies & of urticarial lesions*, the prominence of ***recurrent gastrointestinal attacks of colic and episodes of laryngeal edema (hoarseness of voice & stridor)***Q.

DERMATOLOGY

4 PAPULOSQUAMOUS DISORDERS

When eruptions are characterized by *elevated lesions, papules* (<1 cm / <0.5 cm in some books), *or plaques / nodules* (>1cm) *in association with scales*, it is referred to as papulosquamous lesion. It can be classified according to causes or course:

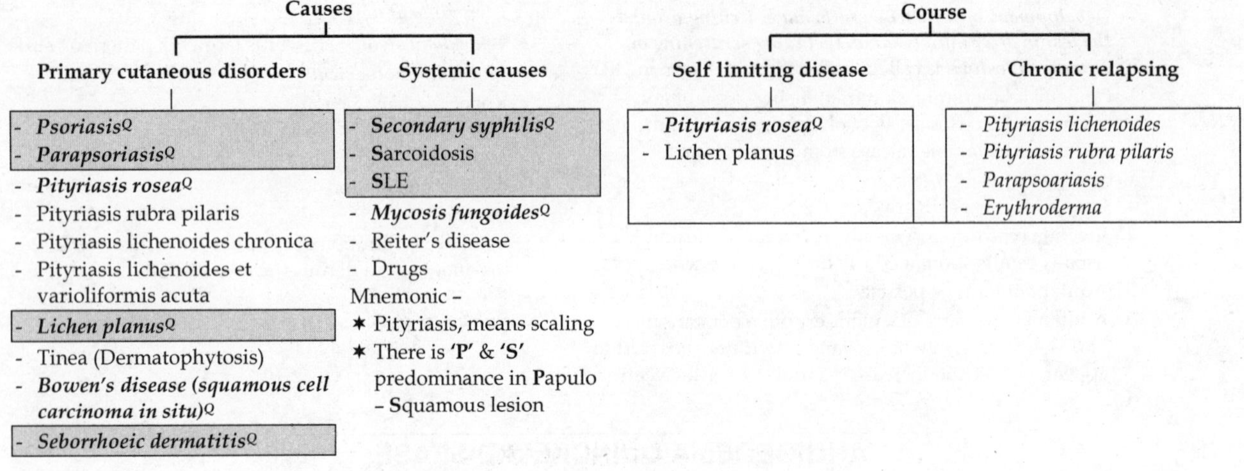

Causes
Primary cutaneous disorders
- Psoriasis[Q]
- Parapsoriasis[Q]
- Pityriasis rosea[Q]
- Pityriasis rubra pilaris
- Pityriasis lichenoides chronica
- Pityriasis lichenoides et varioliformis acuta
- Lichen planus[Q]
- Tinea (Dermatophytosis)
- Bowen's disease (squamous cell carcinoma in situ)[Q]
- Seborrhoeic dermatitis[Q]
Systemic causes
- Secondary syphilis[Q]
- Sarcoidosis
- SLE
- Mycosis fungoides[Q]
- Reiter's disease
- Drugs
Mnemonic –
✶ Pityriasis, means scaling
✶ There is 'P' & 'S' predominance in Papulo – Squamous lesion
Course
Self limiting disease
- Pityriasis rosea[Q]
- Lichen planus
Chronic relapsing
- Pityriasis lichenoides
- Pityriasis rubra pilaris
- Parapsoariasis
- Erythroderma

Types of Scales and Auspitz Sign

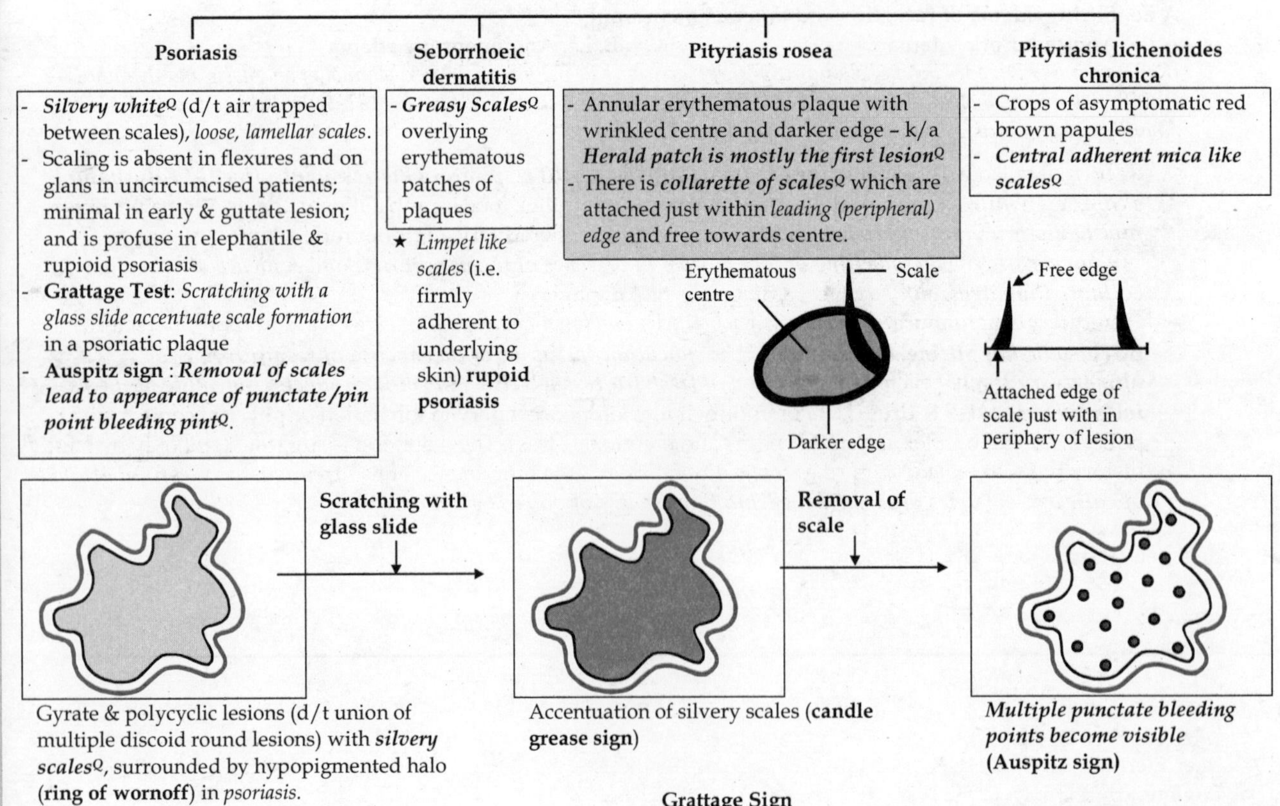

Psoriasis
- Silvery white[Q] (d/t air trapped between scales), loose, lamellar scales.
- Scaling is absent in flexures and on glans in uncircumcised patients; minimal in early & guttate lesion; and is profuse in elephantile & rupioid psoriasis
- Grattage Test: Scratching with a glass slide accentuate scale formation in a psoriatic plaque
- Auspitz sign : Removal of scales lead to appearance of punctate /pin point bleeding pint[Q].
Seborrhoeic dermatitis
- Greasy Scales[Q] overlying erythematous patches of plaques
★ Limpet like scales (i.e. firmly adherent to underlying skin) rupoid psoriasis
Pityriasis rosea
- Annular erythematous plaque with wrinkled centre and darker edge – k/a Herald patch is mostly the first lesion[Q]
- There is collarette of scales[Q] which are attached just within leading (peripheral) edge and free towards centre.
Erythematous centre
Scale
Darker edge
Free edge
Attached edge of scale just with in periphery of lesion
Pityriasis lichenoides chronica
- Crops of asymptomatic red brown papules
- Central adherent mica like scales[Q]
Scratching with glass slide
Removal of scale
Gyrate & polycyclic lesions (d/t union of multiple discoid round lesions) with silvery scales[Q], surrounded by hypopigmented halo (ring of wornoff) in psoriasis.
Accentuation of silvery scales (candle grease sign)
Multiple punctate bleeding points become visible (Auspitz sign)

Grattage Sign

Exfoliative Dermatitis (Erythroderma)

1. **Primary cutaneous disorders**
- ***Dermatitis***[Q] of various types is most common cause (atopic, contact >> stasis, seborrheic)
- ***Psoriasis***[Q] (2nd mc)
- Hereditary disorders like icthyosiform erythroderma & ***pityriasis rubra pilaris***[Q]
- Pemphigus foliaceous, ***Lichen planus***[Q], Crusted scabies, Dermatomyositis, Dermatophytosis
2. **Systemic Diseases** (3rd mc)
- ***Cutaneous T cell lymphoma (Sezary syndrome)***[Q]
- Lymphoma and leukemias
3. **Drugs** (4th mc)
- ***Especially organic arsenic, Gold & Mercury***[Q]
- Penicillins, Phenytoin, Barbiturates
- Carbamazepine, captopril, chloroquin Cimetidine, Calcium channel blockers
- Sulfonamides, Allopurinol, Lithium, Quinidine
4. Idiopathic (2° to solid tumors of lung, liver, prostate, thyroid, & colon)

Clinical Features

- This term is used to any **inflammatory skin disease that affects >90% of body surface** i.e. when the *majority of skin surface is erythematous (red in colour)*. There may be associated *scale, erosions or pustules* as well as *shedding of hair and nails*.
- Systemic features may include fever, chills, hypothermia, reactive lymphadenopathy, peripheral edema, hypoalbuminemia & high output cardiac failure.

★ *Red scaly plaques on elbow & knees* would point to *psoriasis*. Migratory waves of erythema studded with superficial pustules are seen in pustular psoriasis

★ Drug induced erythroderma **(exfoliative dermatitis)** may begin as morbilliform eruption or diffuse erythema. Fever, *peripheral eosinophilia, facial swelling, hepatitis, myocarditis & allergic interstitial nephritis* may accompany and is referred to as **drug reaction with eosinophilia and systemic symptoms.**

★ *Anticonvulsants* can l/t *pseudolymphoma syndrome* (adenopathy, hepatitis, & circulating atypical lymphocytes) and *allopurinol* may cause hepatitis, GI bleed & nephropathy.

★ In the **Sezary Syndrome,** erythroderma is present through out the course with pruritis, lymphadenopathy & circulating atypical T- lymphocytes.

Treatment

Corticosteroids[Q]

Pustules and Abscess

These are cavities within the epidermis or dermis formed by collections of *neutrophil or eosinophil* cells (or rarely other leukocytes).

Subcorneal pustules	Munro microabscess	Kogoj's spongiform pustule	Papillary tip microabscess	Pautrie microabscess
Large, subcorneal collections of neutrophil usually represent either *impetigo or subcorneal pustular dermatosis.*	These are small collections of **neutrophil** usually found within **stratum corneum**[Q] of chronic established ***psoriatic lesions***[Q].	These are multilocular micropustules formed in superficial epidermis (similar to Munro micro abscess but more extensive) in pustular psoriasis.	Small focal collections of *neutrophil* or occasionally *eosinophils* in tips of *dermal papilla.* Although they are characteristic of **dermatitis herpetiformis**, but may also occur in bullous eruptions eg *epidermolysis bullosa aquisita & bullous SLE.*	Small intraepidermal **lymphoid cells** collection (or more commonly single cell colonization) in the absence of marked spongiosis is characteristic of **mycosis fungoides.**

✶ **Grenz zone** refers to a narrow zone of normal dermis between the epidermis and pathological underlying dermis. It is found in ***granuloma faciale (vasculitic skin disease)***[Q].

✶ **Kamino bodies (eosinophilic globules)** are seen in *epidermis or dermal epidermal junction* region in *spindle and epithelioid cell (Spitz) naevi* (almost always) or rarely in melanoma.

✶ *Epidermal degenerations* include *ballooning, hydropic & reticular* degenerations. Ballooning degeneration along with reticular degeneration is characteristic of *acute virus infections of herpes virus & pox virus groups*. Reticular degeneration may also sometimes be seen in acute bullous reaction of contact dermatitis. Hydropic (liquefaction) degeneration (commonly a/w *pigmentary incontinence* & when marked may l/t *subepidermal blister formation*) occurs typically in whole range of lichenoid tissue reactions, including lupus erythematosus, lichen planus, dermatomyositis, poikiloderma atrophicans vasculare & lichen sclerosus.

✶ Whereas **colloid** (typically seen in *colloid milium* & sometimes in epithelial tumors), **elastotic** (develops with increasing age in sun exposed skin), **fibrinoid** (typically in necrotizing vasculitis & also in SLE & collagen diseases), **hyaline** (in tumor cells of *cylindroma*) and **myxoid degeneration** (seen in localized myxoedema, papular mucinosis, scleroderma, & dermatomyosits as well as in various neural, epithelial & adnexal neoplasms) are **dermal degenerations**.

Psoriasis

It is common **(~2.5%), *genetically determined*[Q], *T-cell mediated chronic inflammatory*[Q]** skin disorder of ***unknown cause*[Q].**

Genetics

- Chance of developing psoriasis is 30% when one parent affected, 60% when both parents affected, 20% in non identical twin, 70% in identical twin and 6.4% when relatives affected.
- Associated with CW6 (strongly), HLAB – 13/17/37 as well as with class II antigen DR 7

Histo-Pathology

- Increased epidermal cell turn over results in ***marked epidermal thickening (acanthosis)*[Q],*with regular downward elongation of rete ridges*** (i.e. exaggeration of rete pattern & elongation of epidermal down growths with bulbous club like enlargement of their ends).
- Mitotic figures are easily identified well above the basal cell layer
- *Stratum granulosa is thinned or absent.*
- Epidermal *nuclei* are retained *in the horny layer* **(Parakeratosis)**
- Typical ***thinning of epidermal layer that overlies tips of dermal papillae (supra papillary plates)*[Q]** & dilated tortuous, blood vessels with in these papillae, resulting in *abnormal proximilty of dermal vessel* within dermal papillae *to overlying parakeratotic scale* and it accounts for Auspitz sign
- ***Neutrophils** exit from tips of a subset of dermal capillaries **(the squirting papillae)** leading to their accumulation in the overlying **parakeratotic stratum corneum (Munro's microabscss)** and less frequently in **spinous layer (spongiform pustules of Kogoj). Neutrophils*** form small aggregates within slightly spongiotic foci of the *superficial epidermis* **(spongiform pustules)** & within ***parakeratotic stratum corneum*[Q] *(Munro Microabscess)***
- Superficial *dermis* has *lymphocytic* infiltration.

Clinical Features

1. More common in men & show two peaks of incidence – 2nd half of second decade & 7th decade.
2. It's a life long disorder subject to unpredictable remissions & relapse. There is h/o repeated attacks & *seasonal variations.*
3. *External factors as infection, stress, medications (lithium, β blockers, antimalarials) may exacerbate psoriasis.*
4. Typical lesions are ***well demarcated*[Q], *erythematous, raised papules & plaques, covered by silvery micaceous scale*[Q].**
5. Psoriasis preferentially affects the ***extensor aspects of the trunk (back & lumbosacral area) & limb (elbow, knee)*[Q]**. Scalp is ***frequently affected*[Q].** And *scalp margin, paranasal folds* and *retra-auricular folds* are quite often involved due to *spillage* **(corona psoriatica).**
6. ***Face involvement is uncommon & mucosa seem to be spared*[Q].**
7. **Geographic tongue** (benign migratory glossitis or **glossitis areata migrans**) is oral form of psoriasis resulting in local loss of filiform papillae.
8. The smaller plaques are discoid but merge to form gyrate & polycyclic lesions; *central clearing results in annular lesion*
9. ***Traumatized area often develop psoriatic lesion*[Q]. (Isomorphic or Koebner's phenomenon).**
10. ***Auspitz sign*** [Q], *candle grease sign & grattage test are positive.*
11. Lesions are ***variably pruritic (mildly or no itching)*[Q]** and surrounded by hypopigmented halo **(Wornoff ring)**.
12. **Nail involvement** is common (10 –50%) and may show:
    (i) Small regularly placed ***thimble pitting*[Q]**
    (ii) *Nail plate thickening & tunneling*
    (iii) Accumulation of ***subungal friable debris l/t subungal hyperkeratosis*[Q].**
    (iv) Onycholysis – ***seperation of nail plate from nail bed*[Q].**
    (v) Brownish -black discolouration of nail plate
    (vi) **Oil spots** or staining of nail bed especially of distal part.
13. ***Joint involvement occurs in 10%.*[Q]** cases in form of – polyarticular / monoarticular / axial / rheumatoid arthritis like variety.

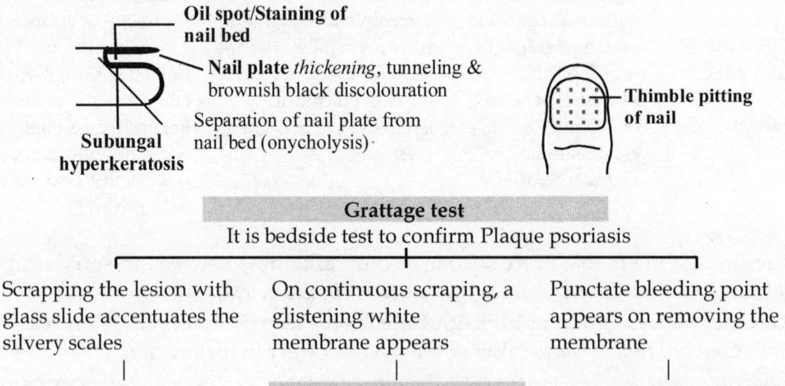

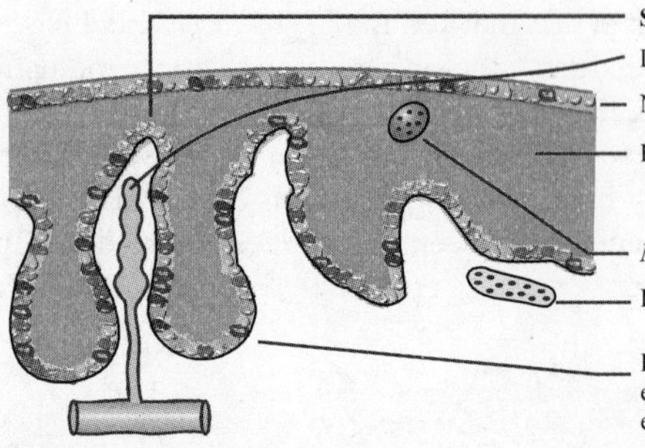

Australian &	**Aus**pitz *sign*Q
Islamic	**I**somorphic/Koebner's *phenomenon*Q
Great &	**G**rattage test
Bulky	**Burkley's** membrane
War	**Warn**off ring
Stories	**S**ilvery - Mica Scales
Can	**Can**dle grease sign
Provoke	**P**itting of nail *plate*Q
Man	**M**unro – micro abscess
On	***On**ycholysis*Q
Exhaustion	**E**xtensor surface of trunk & *limb*Q is preferentially involved, ex-knee, elbow, scalp.

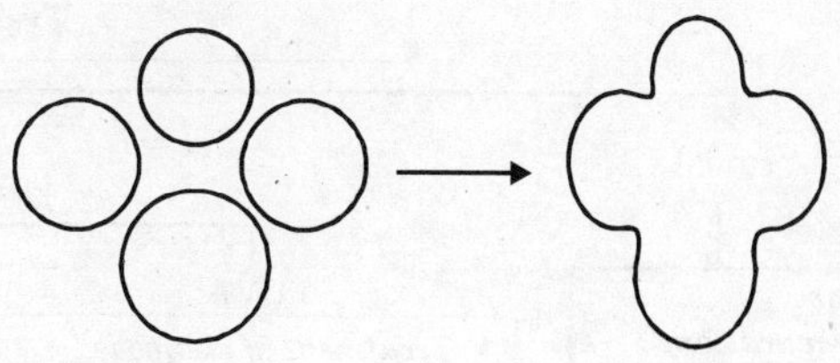

Discoid lesions join to form gyrate & polycyclic lesions

Clinical Variants of Psoriasis

Plaque Type

- *Most common type* with classical presentation ***(well defined, erythematous, dry, scaly plaque on extensor aspect of limbs & trunk.)***Q
- Slow & indolent course

Arthropathic Psoriasis / Arthritis mutilans

- ***Joint involvement*** (~5%)Q
- Characteristically involve *DIP joint*Q.

Type modification by site

1. Flexural (Inverse) Psoriasis

- Occurs when moist flexures like *groin, axillae & body folds like abdominal & inframammary regions* are involved
- Lesion loose their dryness in this area, hence *scaling is reduced.*
- Red, moist, glazed, *nonscaly*Q appearance.
- Some degree of itching is present

2. Scalp Psoriasis –

- Well defined plaques with massive asbestos like scaling, being firmly adherent to scalp (**pityriasis amiantacea**)
- Scalp psoriasis may *spill on to the forehead & nape of neck* (difference from seborrhoeic dermatitis)

3. Penile Psoriasis

- In uncircumcised, scaling is absent on glans, but in circumcised, lesions are similar to classic type

4. Palmo – plantar psoriasis

- Involves palms & soles

5. 5. Napkin Psoriasis

- Occurs in infants

Morphological Variants

1. Erruptive (Guttate) Psoriasis

- Most common in ***children & young adults***Q (7-14 years age), 2-4 weeks after an episode of ***tonsilitis or pharyngitis due to β hemolytic streptococci***Q.
- It develops *acutely* in individuals without psoriasis or in those with chronic plaque psoriasis
- It behaves as exanthema as ***drop size lesions (small erythematous scaly papules)***Q develop *suddenly & at the same time.*
- Lesions usually do not last longer than *8-10 weeks.*

2. Rupioid Psoriasis

- *Healed up scales* so the lesion appears conical. *Scales are firmly adherent to under lying skin* **(limpet like)**
- Classically present in *Reiter's syndrome* (i.e. HLA B 27, preceeding chalmydial genital tract infection or salmonella/ shigella dysentry, acute, asymmetrical, ascending, additive, inflammatory arthritis including severe sacroilitis, iridocyclitis, circinate balanitis & keratoderma blennorhagicum)

Complicated Variants

- **Erythrodermic Psoriasis**
  - Commonest complication, ***precipitated by use of irritant agents like tar & diathranol or by withdrawl of topical or systemic steroids in patients with preexisting psoriasis***Q
  - ***Plaques lose their*** *defined margins & merge; progressing to generalized skin involvement.* The ***skin is universally red & scaly***Q.
  - Hypo / Hyper – thermia, hypo proteinemia, water & electrolyte imbalance may develop in elderly (esp.)
- **Pustular Psoriasis**
  - ***May develop after strong topical or systemic steroid have been used & then abruptly withdrawn***Q or by irritant effect of topical agents as tar.
  - Of 4 types:
    - i) **Palmo – plantar pustulosis** : yellowish white, sterile pustule on *centre parts of palms & soles.*
    - ii) **Acrodermatitis continua** : recalcifrant pustular erosive disorder on *fingers & toes around nails.*
    - iii) **Pustular bacterids** : sterile pustules suddenly develop on the *palms, soles and distal part of limb after infection* .
    - iv) **Generalized Pustular psoriasis / Von Zumbusch disease**: *Suddenly* developing *most serious* disorder characterized by *severe systemic upset, swinging pyrexia, arthralgia & high polymorphonuclear leucocytosis.* ***The skin first becomes erythrodermic & then develops sheets of sterile pustules over trunk & limbs***Q. Pustules may become confluent to form **'lakes of pus'**. Other areas may show superficial peeling without pustule formation.
- **Pustular psoriasis of pregnancy** is k/a *impetigo herpetiformis*Q.

Treatment of Psoriasis

Local

1. *Tar preparations*Q
2. **Vitamin D3 angalogue as** ***calcipotriol***Q ***with*** or ***with***out steroid
3. ***Anthralin (Dithranol)***Q
4. Topical steroid (limited role)
5. Topical retinoid (Tazarotene)

✶ Note: Other drugs are cyclosporin, tacrolimus, polythiouracil, fumaric acid.

Systemic

PUVA

- ***Treatment of choice is PUVA***Q ***-photosensitizing psoralen*** (usually 8-methoxy, sometimes 3-methoxy or 5-methoxy deravitivess) **+ *UV-A (320-400 nm) radiation***Q
- UV-B (290-320 nm) can also be used
- Total dose should be <1500 J/cm²
- Side effects are:
  - ***Skin cancers***Q
  - ***Cataract***Q
  - ***Premature aging***
- Narrow band UVR (311 nm) is claimed to be less hazardous

Retinoids^Q

- Vitamin A analoguses – acitretin (active metabolite of **etretinate**)
- Takes 3-4 weeks to act
- Combination with UV – treatment provides maximum benefit
- S/E
  - **Teratogenic**Q are so fertile women has to use contraception for atleast 2 to 3 years of stopping treatment
  - Hyperlipidaemia
  - Hyperostosis & extraosseous calcification
- Drug of choice in
  - ***Psoriatic erythroderma***Q
  - ***Pustular psoriasis***Q
  - ***Psoriasis with AIDS***Q (b/o no immune supression)

Methotrexate^Q

- **DOC** for ***psoriatic arthropathy***Q
- Very effective in long term management of severe chronic ***pustular psoriasis, psoriatic erythroderma***Q, extensive chronic plaque type psoriasis
- S/E are:
  - ***Hepatotoxicity***Q
  - Bone marrow suppression
  - ***Teratogenic***Q
- Mainly suitable for those who would otherwise be disabled by disease & for elderly patients with severe psoriasis.

Treatment Plan of Pustular Psoriasis

Localized Pustular Psoriasis

- Palmoplantar psoriasis (PPP)
- Acrodermatitis continua

- It is usual to start with topical therapy, but alone it is ineffective. Superpotent topical steroids may be beneficial in short term.
- *Systemic therapy* offers best opportunity for remission.
- ***Oral retinoids either alone or in combination with PUVA*** **are best of the 2nd line therapy (DOC)**

Treatment of Psoriatic Arthritis

*Oral Methotrexate is drug of choice*Q.

✶ ***Etretinate/Retinoid/Vitamin A analogue*** *is used successfully* in children with generalized pustular psoriasis or psoriatic erythroderma *in short intermittent courses (to lessen skeletal toxicity)* as treatment of choice *if the only alternatives are methotrexate & systemic steroids.*

✶ ***Topical corticosteroids*** *are* treatment of choice for psoriasis (chronic palque type) on the face, neck flexures and genitalia, *where neither dithranol nor tar are well tolerated, even in low concentrations.*

✶ *In psoriatic erythroderma & pustular psoriasis, where gross edema is common, diuretics should not be used. As psoriatic inflammation is controlled spontaneous diuresis will follow.*

✶ *In* ***psoriasis with AIDS***, acitretin (retinoid) *is drug of choice.*

✶ ***Methotrexate*** *is most commonly used in –*
- Severe or refractory plaque type psoriasis *that requires systemic treatment (esp. of hands and feet).*
- *Chronic erythrodermic & generalized pustular forms, where it may be life saving and off weaning such patients off systemic steroids.*
- *It is contraindicated in pregnancy & children.*

✶ **Systemic glucocorticosteroids** are double edged weapons. As rebound may take the form of erythrodermic or

Generalized Pustular Psoriasis (Von Zumbush's)

- If there is no immediate metabolic threat in acute/subacute GPP, (particularly in infancy & childhood), initial treatment should be **conservative** (i.e. bed rest in hospital, mild sedation, bland local application with fluid & protein replacement, maintaining adequate ambient temprature). This may promote spontaneous reversion to quieter erythrodermic psoriasis or even psoriasis vulgaris.
- Most cases require systemic therapy. ***Retinoids (oral acitretin) are probably the treatment of choice***Q. Combination of etretinate with PUVA is beneficial. PUVA therapy is effective in acute & subacute GPP. Very ill patient have to be treated in horizontal position with initial small doses of UVA.
- **Methotrexate (Mtx)** is probably as effective as acitretnin (**drug of 2nd choice**). In fulminating GPP, intravenous (preferred) /intramuscular routes are used. Oral therapy is less predictable because of variable absorption. Sudden unexpected toxicity may occur from repeated Mtx doses, b/o improved absorption of drug as GPP subsides.
- *Razoxane, Colchicine, & 6-Thioguanine* have been effective in acute GPP. Hydroxyurea is less effective. In subacute & chronic GPP, dapsone may be used particularly in atypical variants & children.
- **Oral/parenteral corticosteroid** should be used only when urgent control of metabolic complications is needed. The short term effects of prednisolone are excellent, but serious relapses are liable to occur as dosage is reduced unless another form of therapy (eg Mtx or acitretin) is given simultaneously
- Cytotoxic drugs (Methotrexate), retinoids (acitretin), and

generalized pustular psoriasis, so **systemic steroids should not be used in routine care**. They do have a role in management of persistent otherwise uncontrollable erythroderma i.e. causing metabolic complications & in Fulminating generalized pustular psoriasis of von zumbush type if other drugs are C/I or ineffective

✱ Treatment plan of Stable Discoid Ps
- Topical - Tar & Vit D analogees
↓
± Corticosteroids for localized psoriasis
↓
Dithranol / sunlight or UVB

PUVA cannot be used in GPP of pregnancy unless termination has become inevitable. *Fulminating disease in pregnancy is best treated with prednisolone, the drug that carries the least hazard for fetus, but cyclosporin has been used safely for the treatment of impetigo herpetiformis[Q].* Oral retinoids, Mtx or PUVA are needed after delivery to allow weaning off the **steroid or cyclosporin**.

- **TNF-antagonists** & **basiliximab**, an antibody directed at IL-2 receptor, have been reported to rapidly control acute GPP. It is *likely that TNF- antagonists will become the treatment of choice in cases of fulminant disease*, however there are cases of paradonical exacerbation of PPP by these agents.

Role of Corticosteroid in Psoriasis

- *Oral corticosteroids should not be used for treatment of psoriasis due to potential for developing life threatening pustular psoriasis when therapy is discontinued[Q].* (Harrison)
- There is only very limited role for topical corticosteroids in the treatment of psoriasis. They are useful for patients with *fluxaral lesion* for which other irritant preparations are not suitable. For the same reason, weak topical corticosteroids are also suitable for lesions on *genitalia and the face*. Potent topical steroids should not be used, because eventual withdrawl may lead to severe rebound and even the appearance of pustular lesions. Potent topical steroids (eg flucinolone & betamethasone) may be suitable for use on the *scalp and palms & soles* (Roxburg)
- Systemic steroids should be used only when *urgent control of metabolic complications* is needed. The short term effects are excellent but serious relapses are likely to occur as doses are reduced unless another form of therapy is given (eg. Methotrexate or acitretin) simultaneously - *Rook's*.
- Systemic steroids should be restricted to few selected patients with *refractory psoriasis* – Fitzpatrick's
- Clinical guidelines of British Dermatologist association for use of **steroids** are:
 - *Persistent, otherwise uncontrollable erythrodermic psoriasis with metabolic complications[Q]* (not in pregnancy).
 - *Fulminant Generalized pustular psoriasis (von Zumbusch type), if other drugs are contraindicated or ineffective[Q].*
 - *Severe psoriatic polyarthritis threatening severe irreversible joint damage[Q]* (not moderate arthritis).
 - Pustular psoriasis in pregnancy is called **impetigo herpatiformis**. *In pregnancy, safest drug for treatment of pustular psoriasis is prednisolone[Q]*

Photochemotherapy (PUVA)

Method & Mechanism

- *Photosensitizing drug Psoralens mostly 8 – MOP (i.e. methoxsalen or Xanthotoxin) or some times 5 MOP or TMP (4, 5¹, 8 – Trimethyl psotulen) is administered orally* **1-3 hours before exposure to UVA[Q].**
- *In bath PUVA body is immersed for 15-20 min in solution of 0.5-5 mg 8 MOP/ lit of water. Irradiation needs to be performed immediately*
- *Dose of oral 8 MOP is 0.6 – 0.8 mg/kg leads to formation of 3, 4 or 41, 51 cyclobutane addition products with*

Responsive Diseases

For Therapy
- Psoriasis[Q]
- *Palmoplantar pustulosis*
- **Mycosis fungoides or cutaneous T cell lymphoma (stages IA,IB), and sezary syndrome[Q]**
- **Vitiligo[Q]**
- *Atopic dermatitis*
- *Generalized lichen planus*
- Urticaria pigmentosa
- *Generalized granuloma annulare*
- Cutaneous graft versus host

Mn "My pigmented Generalized Granular

For prevention
Tolerance to sunlight can be induced in several photodermatoses eg.
- *Polymorphou s light eruption*
- Solar urticaria
- Hydroa vacciniforme*
- Erythopoietic protoporphyria*
- Chronic actinic dermatitis&

* = Less common

Important Side Effects

- Acute s/e include nausea, vomiting (d/t drug intolerance), erythema/blisters, fever, malaise (d/t UVA overdose) and *pruritis[Q]*.
- Erythema is at present the only available parameter that allows an assessment of the magnitude of the PUVA reaction with psoralens; thus it represents an important criterian for *UVA dose adjustment*. PUVA erythema differs from sunburn or UVB erythema that appears after 4-6 h and peak 12-24 h after exposure. PUVA erythema does not appear before 24-36 hours. and it peaks at 72 to

Contraindications

- Renal disease, hepatic disease, severe cardiovascular disease
- Preexisting light aggrevated disease – SLE, porphyria, multiple melanocytic naevi (particularly in family with h/o malignant melanoma). Previous summer exacerbation is not contraindication.
- H/O previous exposure to arsenic, radiotherapy or h/o cutaneous malignancy are relative contraindications.
- Is of no value for psoriasis in areas where UVA access is impossible eg. in *scalp (except in bald) & certain body flexures*.
- Should not be given in pregnancy or <18 years age except in most compelling

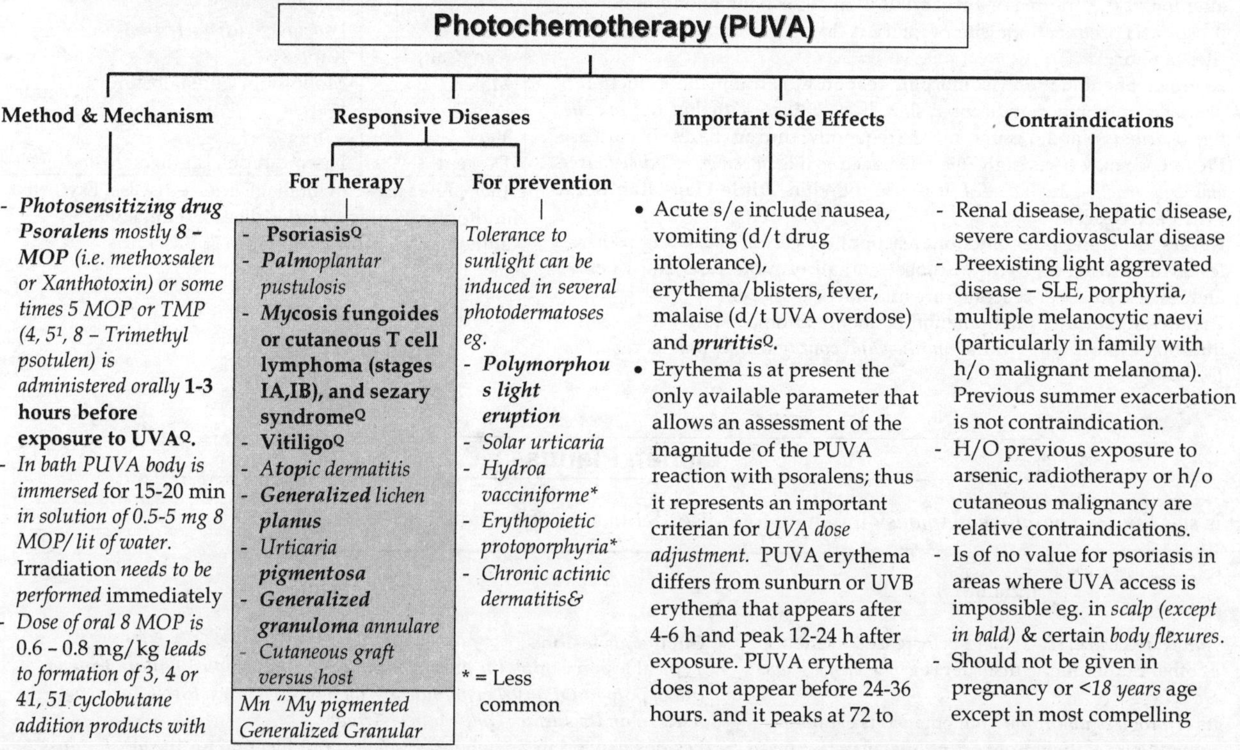

pyrimidine base of native DNA and 5, 6 double bond of pyrimidine base of opposite strandQ. *This l/t suppression of both DNA synthesis & cell division.*
- ***UV-A** doses are given in* **350- 360 nm** range. *(Although action spectrum of antipsoriatic activity & phototoxic erythema peaks at 335nm)*

plans Vil Top Palmar Psoriasis"

- *Pityriasis lichenoides**
- *Pityriasis rubra pilaris**
- ***Pigmented purpuric dermatosis of Gougerot & Blum (lichenoid)***Q *and Schamberg's (progressive)*
- Pompholyx
- *Localized scleroderma**
- *Lymphomatoid papulosis**

96 h or even later.
- **Pigmentation** is the 2nd important effect & is particularly *important in the treatment of vitiligo* and for prevention therapy of photo dermatoses.
- ***Skin cancer (squamous cell carcinoma & melanoma but not of basal cell Ca), premature aging & cataract***Q

★ **Balenophototherapy** is highly concentrated salt water >20%) bath together with UVB. exposure.

conditons.
- Should be considered as primary treatment in patients *over 55 years* of age where psoriasis covers *at least 20%* of body surface and who cannot be controlled by conventional topical therapy.
- UV light therapy is contraindicated in patients taking cyclosporine & used very carefully in immunocompromized d/t increased risk of skin cancers.

UV - Radiation

There are 3 segments of UVR

UV-C /short wave UV-radiation
- 250-280 nm
- **Filtered by ozone layer** & would only become biologically important if the ozone layer becomes seriously depleted
- ***Circulating lymphocytes are most sensitive to UV-C***Q

UV-B / medium wave UV-radiation
- **280-320 nm**
- ***mainly responsible for sunburn, suntan, skin cancers***Q (mainly 290 nm)
- **medically most important UV Rays**

UV-A /long wave UV-radiation
- **320-400 nm**
- ***Wood's lamp***Q produce long wave UVR (360 nm)
- **Used in photo-chemotherapy (PUVA)**Q

Koebner's (Isomorphic) Phenomenon or reaction

- It is appearance of lesion at site of minor trauma usually **7 to 14 days** after injury (i.e. trauma or surgery). It is an **all or none phenomenon** (i.e. if psoriasis occurs at one site of injury it does so means will occur at all sites of injury).
- **Koebner phenomenon** (**isomorphic response**) is traumatic induction of psoriasis on nomal non-lesional skin. It is ***characteristic but not specific for psoriasis***Q and occurs more frequently during flares of disease. Prevalence may be as high 76% when factors like *infection, emotional stress and drug reaction are included.* It is also found in **"Little Plans Kan Make Win Very Descent"**
- **Reverse Koebner phenomenon** (reaction) is clearing of existing psoriasis lesions following injury. It also obeys an **all or none rule**, and Koebner and reverse Koebner reactions are mutually exclusive.
- **Pseudo-isomorphic phenomenon** is due to autoinoculation & is seen in infections like **plane warts, *molluscum contagiosum, and eczematous lesions***Q.

Mnemonic		Causes
Little	-	***Lichen planus***Q
Plans	-	***Psoriasis***Q *(characterstic)*
Kan (Can)	-	Kaposi SA
Make	-	Molluscum Contagiosum] Pseudo
Win	-	*Warts*Q] Pseudo
Very	-	Vitiligo
Descent	-	Discoid lupus Erythematosus

Other causes are- carcinoma, Darier's disease, Erythema multiforme, Hailey – Hailey disease, Leukemia, Xanthoma, Necrobiosis lipoidica & Vasculitis.

Lichen Planus

It is ***self limiting papulo squamous***Q inflammatory disorder of skin of ***unknown origin***Q.

Etiology
- *Autoimmune disease,* so there is increased incidence of other autoimmune disorders eg. *mysthenia gravis & vitiligo.*
- Its ***etiology is unknown***Q but cutaneous eruptions resembling LP (**lichenoid eruptions**) may be caused

Clinical Feature
- **Cutaneous lesions**
- Typical lesion is ***pink (or purple or mauve or violaceous***Q***), plain topped (flat), polygonal, pruritic papule***Q, which often has a ***whitish lacework pattern on its surface (wickham's striae)***Q
- Lesions may occur anywhere but have a predilection for the *wrist, shins,*

by:
1. Drugs eg *gold, antimalarials (chloroquin), thiazide diuretics, penicillamine, phenothiazines* & rarely NSAIDs (eg brufen)
2. Contact sensitiser eg colour photograph sensitizer
3. ***Hepatitis C infection***Q
4. Graft vs host reaction (chronic)

Pathology

- The basic process is thought of as an immunological attack on the basal layer of epidermis causing ***dense continuous infiltration of lymphocytes & histiocytes along dermoepidermal junction***Q **(sub epidermally lichenoid band)**
- This results in ***vacuolar degeneration and necrosis of basal keratinocytes (basal epidermal cell)***Q, and their *resemblance* in size & contour to more mature cells of the *stratum spinosum (squamatization)*
- As a consequence of this lymphocytic infiltration & basal cell degeneration

1. Epithelial connective tissue interface weakenes resulting in formation of **histological cleft** known as ***Max. Joseph space***Q.
2. Redefinition of normal smoothy undulating configuration of *dermo – epidermal interface* to a more ***angulated zig zag contour (saw toothing)***Q
3. Anucleate, necrotic basal cells may become incorporated into inflammed papillary dermis and form eosinophilic – **cytoid / colloid / Civatte bodies**. Although characteristic of LP, these bodies may be detected in any chronic dermatitis where basal keratinocytes are injured & destroyed.

- Show changes of chronicity, namely **epidermal hyperplasia** (or rarely atrophy) and *thickening of granular cell layer* (**hyper granulosis**) and *stratum corneum* (**hyper keratosis**), which differentiate it from erythema multiforme.

Characteristic Histopathology

- ***Basal epidermal cell degeneration***Q causing *saw tooth profile* & eosinophilic ***cytoid bodies (civatte body)***Q
- **Epidermal thickening** esp. of granular cell layer
- ***Subepidermal-Lichenoid Band***Q due deposition of lymphocytes & histiocytes
- ***Max Joseph histological cleft***Q

lower back and genitalia, Face is generally not involved.
- Lesions may appear at sites of trauma **(*isomorphic or koebner's phenomenon*)**
- In dark (black coloured people, lesion may acquire dark brown colour d/t. loss of melanin pigment into dermis as basal cell layer is destroyed.

- **Mucosal lesions** (30%)
- ***Commonly involves mucous membranes***Q, particularly the *buccal mucosa* (30%)
- ***A white lacework pattern in buccal mucosa is most common***Q type of lesion – But the tongue & else where in the mouth may also be involved with - ***white lace work, whitis macule or punctate type of lesions***Q.
- May be *asymptomatic or* patient may *complain of intolerence to spicy food.*
- **Genital** mucosal lesions (25%) are annular shaped
- **Scalp involvement** leads to ***cicatricial (scarring) alopecia***Q.

- **Nail changes** (15%)
- **Pterygium formation (diagnostic)**: There is ***wing shaped projection (prolongation) of proximal nail fold onto nail bed, splitting and destroying naiplate***Q.
- **Onychorrhexia** - Slight roughness of nail plate with longitudinal ridges and brittleness.
- ***Thinning***Q, tenting & distal splitting of nail plates
- **Anychia** - Complete loss (absence) of nail plate.

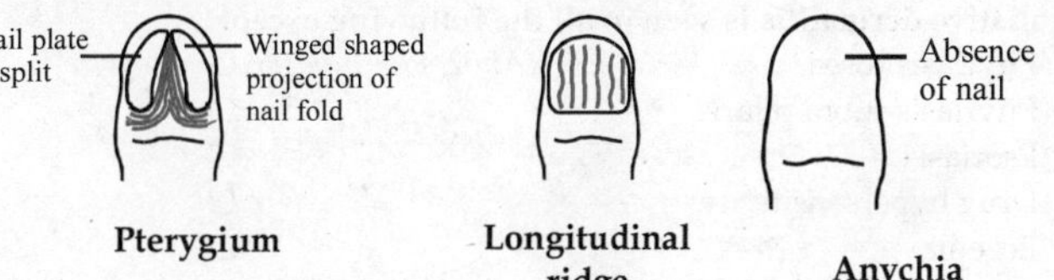

- **Course & Complications**
- A *chronic but self limiting* disease mostly showing *spontaneous remissions* in 6 months – 2 years duration.
- ***As lesions heal, they flatten and often leave hyperpigmented patch***Q.
- Nail & hair loss is irreversible
- *Very rarely* chronic ulcerative lesions may develop malignant changes ***(squamous cell Ca)***Q.

- **Treatment**

In Lichen planus, Steroids are main stay of treatment initally given topically f/b systemic.

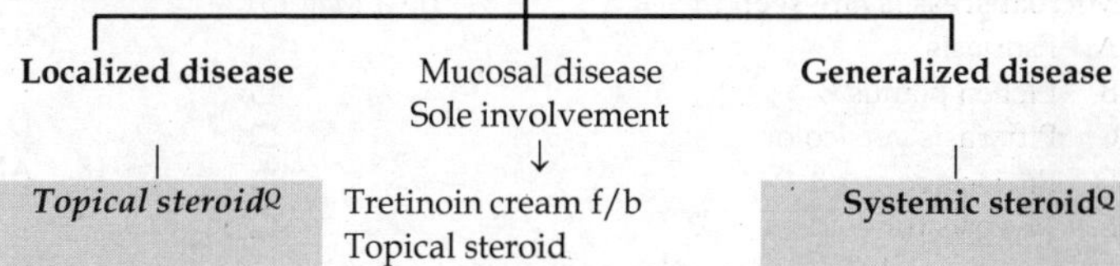

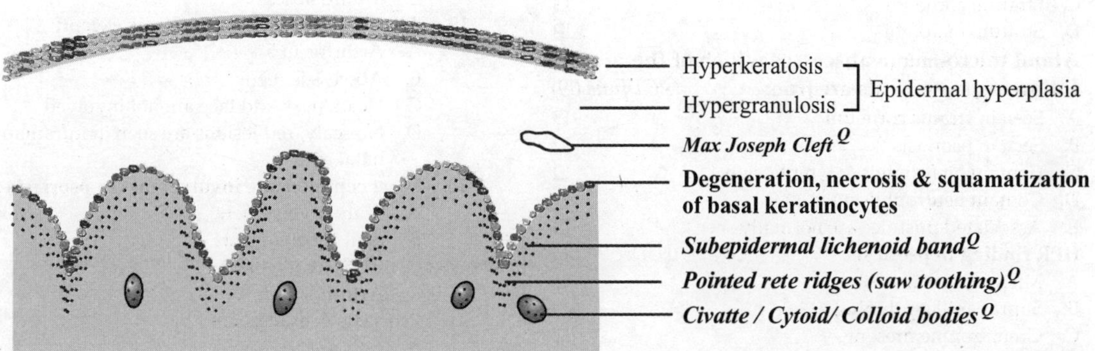

DERMATOLOGY

1

Questions

1. **Which is/are papulosquamous disorder:** *(PGI Nov 12)*
   A. Psoriasis
   B. Dermatitis herpetiformis
   C. Lichen planus
   D. Pityriasis rosea
   E. Morphea
2. **All are causes of papulo squamous lesions except**
   A. Psoriasis *(PGI 02, 2K)*
   B. Para psoriasis
   C. Squamous cell carcinoma
   D. Mycosis fungoides
   E. Congenital syphilis
3. **All of the following may lead to plaque formation except**
   A. Psoriasis *(PGI 99, SGPGI 2003)*
   B. Lichen planus
   C. Pityriasis rosea
   D. Pemphigus
4. **Exfoliative dermatitis is seen in all the following except**
   A. Pityriasis rosea *(AI 02, PGI June 06)*
   B. Pityriasis rubra pilaris
   C. Psoriasis
   D. Drug hypersensitivity
   E. Eczema
5. **Causes of erythroderma-** *(PGI June 05, 11)*
   A. Pityriasis alba
   B. Pityriasis versicolor
   C. Psoriasis
   D. Lichen planus
   E. Eczema
6. **Gold poisioning leading to exfoliative dermatitis is treated by :** *(AIIMS 95)*
   A. Chloroquin
   B. Steroid
   C. Antibiotics
   D. Antihistaminics
7. **Microabscess is /are seen in :** *(PGI May 13)*
   A. Psoriasis
   B. Lichen planus
   C. Pitryiasis versicolor
   D. Pitriasls roseas
   E. Mycosis fungoides
8. **Munro micro abscess is seen in:**
   A. Dermal tissue *(PGI 99)*
   B. Stratum basale
   C. Stratum corneum
   D. Stratum malpighi
9. **About micro-munro abscesses which of the following statements are true:** *(PGI June 09)*
   A. Seen in stratus corneum
   B. Seen in psoriasis
   C. Contain neutrophils & lymphocyte
   D. Contain neutrophils only
   E. Associated pustules are normally seen
10. **HPR finding in psoriasis:** *(PGI June 09, Dec 07, 06)*
    A. Micromunro abscess
    B. Suprapapillary thining
    C. Grenz zonme present
    D. Pautrier's abscess
    E. Hyperkeratosis
11. **Bleeding spots seen on removal of scales in psoriasis is called as:** *(PGI June 2008)*
    A. Auspitz sign
    B. Punctuate hemorrhage
    C. Nikolyski's sign
    D. Darrier sign
12. **"Auspitz" sign is characteristically seen in:**
    A. Plaque Psoriasis *(Bihar 05, AIIMS May 08)*
    B. Pustular Psoriasis
    C. Lichen Planus
    D. Inverse Psoriasis
13. **A patient presents with erythematous scaly lesions on extensor aspect of elbows and knee. The clinical diagnosis is got by :** *(AIIMS May 02)*
    A. Auspitz sign
    B. KOH smear
    C. Tzanck smear
    D. Skin biopsy
14. **A 30 years old male presented with silvery scales on elbow and knee, that bleed on removal. The probable diagnosis is:** *(AI 08)*
    A. Pityriasis
    B. Seborrhoeic dermatitis
    C. Psoriasis
    D. Secondary syphilis
15. **Bulkeley membrane is seen in :** *(DNB 99, PGI 02)*
    A. Psoriasis
    B. Pemphigus
    C. Tinea
    D. Pityriasis
16. **The important feature of psoriasis is -** *(Bihar 04, AMC 99)*
    A. Crusting
    B. Scaling
    C. Oozing
    D. Erythema
17. **All of the following are seen in psoriasis except:**
    A. Auspitz sign present *(SGPGI – 2003)*
    B. 10% associated with arthritis
    C. It is premalignant disease
    D. Worsening of disease during winter
18. **All are true about psoriasis except** *(PGI 2000)*
    A. Very pruritic
    B. Pitting of nails
    C. Joint involvement in 5-10%
    D. Parakeratosis & acanthosis
    E. Munro abscess
19. **All are true regarding Psoriasis except:** *(AI 2000)*
    A. Arthritis in 5%
    B. Abscess is seen
    C. Head, neck and face are not involved
    D. No scaly, red lesions are seen in inframammary and natal area.
20. **Least common site involvemnet in psoriasis is**
    A. Scalp involvement *(AI 98, PGI 02)*
    B. Nail Involvement
    C. CNS involvement
    D. Arthritis
21. **Psoriasis is exacerbated by-** *(All India 98)*
    A. Lithium
    B. B- blockers

C. Antimalarials ☐
D. All of the above ☐

22. Chloroquine cause exacerbation of : *(AI 91)*
A. Malaria ☐
B. Psorisasis ☐
C. DLE ☐
D. Photosensitivity ☐

23. Vitamin D analogue calcitriol is useful in the treatment of
A. Lichen Planus *(AI 94, UP 04, Jhar 05)* ☐
B. Psoriasis ☐
C. Phemphigus ☐
D. Leprosy ☐

24. Treatment of psoriasis- *(PGI June 05)*
A. PUVA ☐
B. Methotrexate ☐
C. Systemic steroids ☐
D. Femicycline ☐
E. Terbinafine ☐

25. In psoritic arthropathy TOC is *(AIIMS 93)*
A. Mtx ☐
B. 5FU ☐
C. PUVA ☐
D. Steroid ☐

26. The treatment of choice for erythrodermic psoriasis is:
A. Corticosteriods *(SGPGI 04)* ☐
B. Methotrexate ☐
C. Coaltar topically ☐
D. Topical corticosteroids ☐

27. The treatment of psoriatic erythroderma is - *(PGI 96)*
A. Methotrexate ☐
B. Retinols ☐
C. Diethrenol ☐
D. Corticosteroid ☐

28. Treatment of pustular psoriasis is :
A. Thalidomide *(AIIMS May 02, PGI 03)* ☐
B. Retinoids ☐
C. Hydroxyurea ☐
D. Metholtrexate
E. Steroid ☐

29. DOC of pustular psoriasis *(AIIMS 91)*
A. PUVA ☐
B. Methotrexate ☐
C. Steroid ☐
D. Cyclophosphamide ☐

30. Treatment of choice in Pustuar psoriasis
A. Psorialin + UV therapy *(AI 94)* ☐
B. Systemic steroid ☐
C. Methotrexate ☐
D. Estrogen ☐

31. A patient with psoriasis was started on systemic steroids. After stoping the treatment, patient developed universally red scaly skin with plaques losing their margins all over his body. The most likely cause is *(AIIMS 01)*
A. Drug induced reaction ☐
B. Pustular psoriasis ☐
C. Bacterial infection ☐
D. Erythrodermic Psoriasis ☐

32. A patient with psoriasis was started on systemic steroids. After stopping treatment, the patient developed generalized pustules all over the body. The cause is most likely to be: *(AI 02)*
A. Drug induced reaction ☐
B. Pustular psoriasis ☐
C. Bacterial infections ☐
D. Septicemia ☐

33. Treatment of erythematous skin rash with multiple pus lakes in a pregnant woman is: *(AI 2010)*
A. Corticosteroids ☐
B. Retinoids ☐
C. Methotrexate ☐
D. Psoralen with PUVA ☐

34. The only indication of giving corticosteroids in pustular psoriasis is *(AI 2005)*
A. Psoriatic erythroderma with pregnancy ☐
B. Psoriasis in a pt. With alchoholic cirrhosis ☐
C. Moderate arthritis ☐
D. Extensive lesions ☐

35. DOC for a pregnant woman in 2nd trimester with pustular psoriasis is
A. Prednisolone *(AI 08)* ☐
B. Dapsone ☐
C. Acitretin ☐
D. Methotrexate ☐

36. Only definitive indication of systemic steroids in psoriasis is *(AIIMS Nov 11)*
A. Pustular psoriasis ☐
B. Erythroderma ☐
C. Psoriatic arthropathy ☐
D. Impetigo herpetiformis ☐

37. Koebner's phenomenon is characteristic of
A. Psoriasis *(PGI 99, 97, AI 02)* ☐
B. Pemphigus vulgaris ☐
C. Pityriasis rosea ☐
D. Lupus vulgaris ☐

38. Koebners phenomenon is seen in- *(Delhi 98, AI 92)*
A. Lichen Planus ☐
B. Psoriasis ☐
C. Icthyosis ☐
D. Pitriasis rubra ☐
E. Phemphigus ☐

39. Koebner's phenomenon is seen in-
A. Lichen planus *(PGI Dec 04)* ☐
B. Warts ☐
C. Bechet syndrome ☐
D. Psoriasis ☐
E. Vitiligo ☐

40. Pseudo koebner's phenomenon is/are seen in:
A. Warts *(PGI Nov 10, AI 11)* ☐
B. Molluscum contagiosum ☐
C. Lichen planus ☐
D. Psoriasis ☐
E. Vitiligo ☐

41. The mechanism of action of psoralen is:
A. Binding to DNA *(Jipmer 98, PGI 96)* ☐
B. Inhibiting protein synthesis ☐
C. Inhibiting angiogenesis ☐
D. Inhibiting keratinization ☐

42. Which is not a complication of PUVA therapy:
A. Premature aging of skin *(AIIMS 97, PGI 2K)* ☐
B. Cataracts ☐
C. Skin cancers ☐
D. Exfoliative ☐

43. Photochemotherapy (Psoralent + UVV) is used in
A. Pityriasis rosea *(SGPGI 03, AIIMS 95, AI 92, 91)* ☐
B. Erythroderma ☐
C. Scabies ☐
D. Psoriasis ☐

44. Photo therapy (PUVA therapy) is used in: *(PGI Nov 12, 02)*
A. Psoriasis ☐
B. Lichen planus ☐
C. Freckles, Melasma ☐

D. Dermatitis herpetiformis
E. Vitiligo

45. **Psoralen - A is used in the treatment of :** *(Jipmer 96)*
A. Pemphigus
B. Vitiligo
C. Pityriasis alba
D. Icthyosis

46. **Psoralen + ultraviolet light (PUVA) therapy is useful in the treatment of:** *(KARN 94)*
A. Psoriasis
B. Vitiligo
C. Mycosis fungoides
D. All of the above

47. **Uses of PUVA-** *(PGI Dec 04)*
A. Pigmentd purpuric lesion
B. Herpes zoster
C. Mycosis fungoides
D. Lupus panniculitis
E. Lichenoid dermatitits of Gougerot & Blum

48. **Circulating lymphocytes are most sensitive to :** *(UP 02, AIIMS 94)*
A. UV-A
B. UV-B
C. UV-C
D. 760-800 mm

49. **The most effective treatment of pruritus in uremia is :**
A. Ultraviolet light *(AIIMS 95, PGI 02)*
B. Cholestyramine
C. Eskazine
D. Topical benzocaine

50. **Mouth Lesion are seen in:** *(AI 94,99)*
A. Psoriasis
B. Lichen Planus
C. Basal Cell CA
D. Icthyosis Vulgaris

51. **Mucosa is involved in:** *(PGI Dec 07)*
A. Psoriasis
B. Lichen planus
C. Alopecia
D. Scabies
E. Porphyria

52. **Features of lichen planus are** *(PGI May 11)*
A. Pruritis
B. Purple color
C. Papule
D. Purpura
E. Petechiae

53. **Oral examination is done in case of:** *(PGI 97)*
A. Peutz jegher syndrome
B. Psoriasis
C. Beri-beri
D. Plummer vinson syndrome

54. **Necrotic Keratinocyts occur in** *(PGI Nov 11)*
A. DLE
B. Graft versus host disease
C. Erythema multiformal
D. Lichen planus
E. Psoriasis

55. **Max. Joseph's space is a histopatho-logical feature of:**
A. Psoriasis vulgaris *(AIIMS May 06, DNB 11)*
B. Lichen planus
C. Pityriasis rosea
D. Parapsoriasis

56. **Civatte bodies are found in :** *(Kerala 98)*
A. Lichen Planus
B. Psoriasis
C. Dermatophytosis
D. Vitiligo

57. **True about lichen planus-** *(PGI Dec 04)*
A. Basal cell degeneration
B. Colloid bodies seen
C. Epidermal hyperplasia in chronic cases
D. Wickham's striae seen
E. Autoimmune disease

58. **Basal cell degeneration characteristically seen in:**
A. Lichen planus *(Jipmer 02, 98, PGI 02)*
B. Psoriasis
C. Pemphigus
D. DLE

59. **A young lady presents with lacy lesions in oral cavity and genitals, and her proximal nail fold has extended onto the nail bed. What is the likely diagnosis** *(AI 12, 10)*
A. Psoriasis
B. Geographic tongue
C. Lichen planus
D. Candidiasis

60. **A 30 year old male present with pruritic flat-topped polygonal, shiny violaceous papules with flexural distribution. the most likely diagnosis is-**
A. Psoriasis *(Bihar 05, J&K 06)*
B. Pityriasis
C. Lichen planus
D. Lichenoid dermatitis

61. **Which of the following is pruritic:** *(PGI 93, Kerala 98)*
A. Lichen planus
B. Psoriasis
C. Icthyosis
D. Secondary syphilis

62. **Lacy white lesion in mouth with pterygium is seen in :**
A. Psoriasis *(SGPGI 2001)*
B. Ptirysis alba
C. Lichen planus
D. Leprosy

63. **Regarding Lichen Planus all are true, except :** *(AI 00)*
A. Hypopigmentation in most residual disease
B. Lymphatic infiltration in supradermal layer
C. Itchy polygonal, purple papule
D. Skin, hair and oral mucosa commonly involved

64. **All of the following regarding Lichen planus are true except:** *(MP 2005)*
A. Does not involve mucous membrane
B. Associated with Hepatitis 'C'
C. Topical steroid are the mainstay of therapy
D. Spontaneous remissions 6mo to 2 years

65. **A patient presented with scarring alopecia, thinned nails, hypopigmented macular lesions over the trunk and oral mucosa. The diagnosis is** *(AIIMS 01)*
A. Psoriasis
B. Leprosy
C. Lichenplanus
D. Pemphigus

66. **Characterstic nail finding in lichen planus**
A. Pitting *(AIIMS 01)*
B. Pterygium
C. Beau's Lines
D. Hyperpigmentation of nails

67. **10 year old chld has violaceous papule and pterygium of nails. The diagnosis is**
A. Psoriasis *(AIIMS 99)*
B. Pemphigus
C. Pemphigoid
D. Lichen Planus

68. Wickehm's stria seen in - *(SGPGI 02, Bihar 03, AI 02)*
A. Lichen niditus ☐
B. Lichenoid eruption ☐
C. Lichen striates ☐
D. Lichen planus ☐

69. Itchy polygonal violaceous (itchy/prusitic) palpules seen in *(AI 98, PGI 2K)*
A. Psoriasis ☐
B. Pemphigus ☐
C. Lichen planus ☐
D. Pitriasios rosea ☐

70. Features of lichen planus are *(PGI May 11)*
A. Pruritis ☐
B. Purple ☐
C. Papule ☐
D. Purpura ☐
E. Petechiae ☐

71. Most characteristic Feature oF lichen planus is: *(PGI 98)*
A. Thinning of nail plate is most common ☐
B. Non scarring alopecia ☐
C. Violaceous lesions on skin and mucous membrane ☐
D. Wickham striae ☐

72. The most characteristic finding In lichen planus is:
A. Civatte bodies *(PGI 99)* ☐
B. Basal cell degeneration ☐
C. Thinning of nail plate ☐
D. Violaceous lesions ☐

73. In Lichen planus TOC is: *(AIIMS 93)*
A. Topical Salicyclic acid ☐
B. UV ray ☐
C. Systemic steroids ☐
D. Erythromycin ☐

74. Which of the following are pruritic lesions
A. Lichen planus *(PGI 2000)* ☐
B. Sun burns ☐
C. Pemphigoid ☐
D. Psoriasis ☐
E. SLE ☐

ANSWERS AND EXPLANATIONS

Papulo squamous Disorders

1. **A i.e Psoriasis; C i.e. Lichen Planus; D i.e. Pityriasis rosea**
2. **E i.e. Congenital syphilis** 3. **D i.e. Pemphigus** *[Ref: Neena Khanna 4/e p. 39-66; Roxburgh's18/e p. 98-104]*

***Congenital syphilis & pemphigus are vesico bullous disorders*[Q]** whereas **psoriasis, para psoriasis, pityriasis rosea, lichen planus, mycosis fungoides & Bowen's disease are papulo-squamous disorders (l/t plaque formation).**

Erythroderma

4. **A i.e. Pityriasis rosea** 5. **C i.e. Psoriasis; D i.e. Lichen planus; E i.e. Eczema** 6. **B i.e. Steroid**
[Ref: Fitzpatrick's 7/e p-30-31; Harrison 18/e p. 405; Rook's 8/e p. 23.46-23.51]

Exfoliative dermatitis or **erythroderma** is caused by ***dermatitis (eczema), psoriasis, lichen planus, pityriasis rubra pilaris and drugs like gold but not by pityriasis rosea and versicolor. It is treated by steroids*[Q].**

Psoriasis

7. **A i.e. psoriasis; E i.e. Mycosis fungoides**
8. **C i.e. Stratum corneum**
9. **A, B, D i.e. Seen in stratus corneum, Seen in psoriasis, Contain neutrophils only**
10. **A i.e. Micromunro abscess; B i.e. Suprapapillary thining; E i.e. Hyperkeratosis**
[Ref: Fitzpatrick 8/e p. 200-261; Robbin's 8/e p. 1185; Rook's 8/e p. 10.41, 65.25, 23.30]

- **Microabscess** are seen in **mycosis fungoides (Pautrie microabscess) and psoriasis (Munro-microabscess).** The histology of **seborrhoeic dermatitis** (SD) is not diagnostic but shows features of both psoriasis (like squirting papilla, Munro's microabscess) and chronic dermatitis. However, spongiosis distinguishes SD from psoriasis.
- **Histopathological features of psoriasis** include – compact *hyperkeratosis*[Q], orthokeratotic stratum corneum ***suprapapillary thinning*[Q], *Munromicro abscess*[Q]** in stratum corneum , *Kogoj's spongiform pustule,* exaggeration of rette pattern and ***parakeratotic stratum corneum (i.e. nuclei are retained)*[Q]** with marked epidermal thickening (but absent or thinned stratum granulosa).

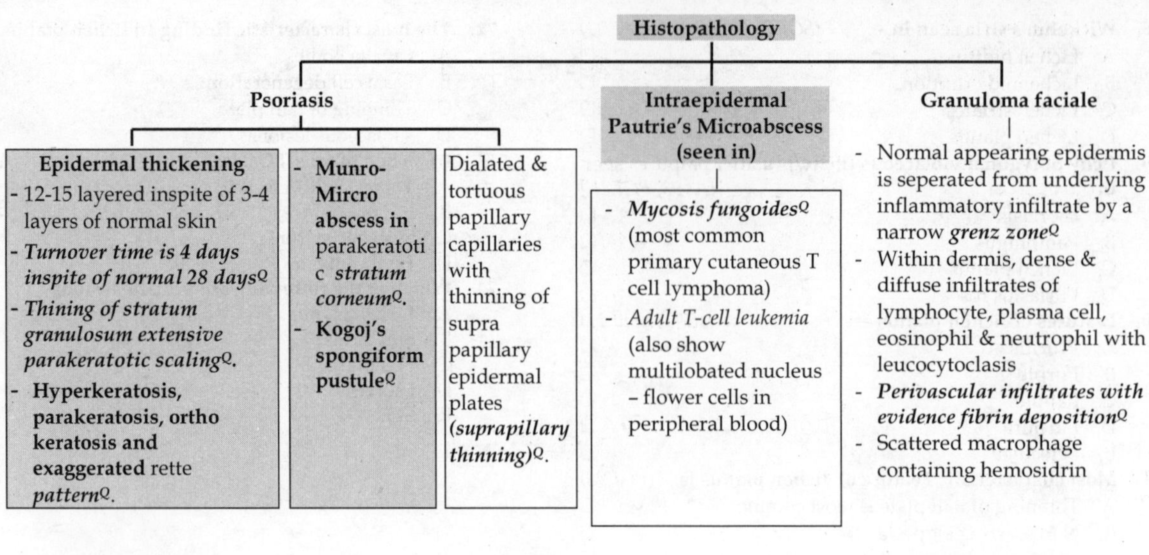

Histopathology
Psoriasis
Epidermal thickening
- 12-15 layered inspite of 3-4 layers of normal skin
- Turnover time is 4 days inspite of normal 28 daysQ
- Thining of stratum granulosum extensive parakeratotic scalingQ.
- Hyperkeratosis, parakeratosis, ortho keratosis and exaggerated rette patternQ.
- Munro-Mircro abscess in parakeratotic stratum corneumQ.
- Kogoj's spongiform pustuleQ
Dialated & tortuous papillary capillaries with thinning of supra papillary epidermal plates (suprapillary thinning)Q.
Intraepidermal Pautrie's Microabscess (seen in)
- Mycosis fungoidesQ (most common primary cutaneous T cell lymphoma)
- Adult T-cell leukemia (also show multilobated nucleus – flower cells in peripheral blood)
Granuloma faciale
- Normal appearing epidermis is seperated from underlying inflammatory infiltrate by a narrow grenz zoneQ
- Within dermis, dense & diffuse infiltrates of lymphocyte, plasma cell, eosinophil & neutrophil with leucocytoclasis
- Perivascular infiltrates with evidence fibrin depositionQ
- Scattered macrophage containing hemosidrin

11. **A i.e. Auspitz sign**
12. **A i.e. Plaque psoriasis**
13. **A i.e. Auspitz sign**
14. **C i.e. Psoriasis**
15. **A. i.e. Psoriasis**
16. **B. i.e. Scaling**
17. **C. i.e. Its premalignant disease**
18. **A i.e. Very Pruritic**
19. **C i.e. Head, neck & face are not involved**
20. **C. i.e. CNS involvement**

[Ref: Harrison 18/e p. 398-99; Robbin's 7/e p. 1256-57; Roxburgh's 18/e p. 138-50; Pasricha 3/e p. 142- 149; Neena Khanna 4/e p 40-60; Behl 10/e p. 253-57; Fitzpatrick's 7/e p 169-93; Rooks 8/e p. 20.1-20.6]

- Psoriasis is ***best diagnosed by clinical presentation***Q. It characteristically presents with **full rich red** (often referred to as **salmon pink, magenta pink**) ***erythematous plaque lesions with well defined sharply demarcated (delineated) edge***Q. These **red, raised, scaly and (usually) symmetrically** distributed plaques are characteristically located on ***extensor aspects of trunk and limbs particularly elbows, knees, scalp***Q, lower lumbosacral, buttocks & genital regions. *Umbilicus & intergluteal clefts* are other sites.
- ***Auspitz sign, Burkley's membrane, candle grease sign, Wornoff ring and Grattage test***Q are characteristically seen in **plaque psoriasis.**
- ***Constant production of large amounts of scale***Q with little alteration in shape or distribution of individual plaques is important feature of plaque type psoriasis. Characteristically scales are ***silvery (mica/asbestos) white***Q with variable thickness.
- When **scaling** is not evident, it can be **induced by light scratchig (Grattage test)**, a useful sign of diagnosis in uncertain lesions.
- **Removal of psoriatic scale** usually reveals underlying glossy red, smooth membranous surface with ***small bleeding points***Q where thin suprapupillary epithelium is torn off traumatizing the dilated capillaries below **(Auspitz sign).**
- **Pityriasis (tinea) amiantacea** is non specific reaction pattern most commonly presenting in children & young adults as *plaques of asbestos like scaling, firmly adherent to the scalp* with sometimes *cicatrical hair loss*. Otherwise scalp psoriasis is a very uncommon cause of alopecia.
- **Ring or halo of Woronoff** is a clear white (hypopigmented) ring of vasoconstriction encircling (peripherally surrounding) the active psoriatic plaque. It is usually a/w UV radiation or topical steroid treatment.
- **Kobner's (isomorphic) phenomenon** i.e. appearance of disease (psoriasis) in previously uninvolved skin at the site of minor injury such as scratch or graze. It is ***characteristic of psoriasis***Q but can also be seen in ***lichen planus and discoid lupus erythematosus***Q.
- **Nail involvement** is ***common***Q and seen in 40% of psoriatic patients. It involves & includes.

Nail matrix & plate	Nail bed & Hyponychium
• ***Thimble pitting (most common)***Q, onychorrhexix, Baeu's lines (ridging). • **Deformity of nail plate (onychodystrophy)** including leukonychia, crumbling nail, thinned nail plate, and ***salmon red/erythematous spots of lunula***Q. Onychodystrophy has strongest association with psoriatic arthritis. • Focal onycholysis.	• **Subungal hyperkeratosis** (d/t accumulation of friable debris) • **Onycholysis** i.e. separation of nail plate from nail bed. • Splinter haemorrhage • **Oil drop spotling sign** or **salmon patches** are yellow red discoloration considered nearly specific for psoriasis.

- Historically, **psoriatic arthritis** is ***uncommon*** (~ ***2.5-7%)***Q but recent literature indicate much higher (40%) prevalence. Presence of **enthesitis (tendonitis), dactylitis and distal interphalangeal (DIP) joint involvement** are hall marks of psoriatic arthritis, which differentiate it from rheumatoid arthritis (RA).

Psoriatic arthritis	Rheumatoid Arthritis
MHC class I susceptibility alleles, **CD8** class of lymphocytes driving inflammation	**MHC class II** susceptibility alleles, **CD-4** class of lymphocyte driving inflammation
Fibroblastic response, sacroilitis, enthesitis, dactyilitis and juxta articular newborn formation present.	Absent (although rarely fibroblastic response may be seen)
Absent	**Small vessel vasculitis, immune complexes, autoantibodies (rheumatoid factor), juxta articular osteopenia** (on X-ray) and amelioration with progressive HIV infection is present.

- **Micro Munro abscess** is collection of polymorphs (neutrophils) in ***stratum corneum in psoriasis***Q.

★ **KOH smear** is used for diagnosis of ***fungal infections***Q such as ringworm infection. **Tzanck test** is used for clinical diagnosis of ***pemphigus***Q. **Tzanck smear** is used in diagnosis of *herpes-virus infection.* **Tzanck** cell is ***Keratinocyte***Q.

Most commonly involved
- *Extensor aspect of knee and elbow*Q
- *Scalp*Q *(head)*

Uncommon
- *Arthritis or Joint involvement (only 5%)*Q
- *Itching*Q
- Alopecia

Not found
- *CNS involvement*Q
- *Mucosal involvement*Q

21. **D. i.e. All**
22. **B i.e. Psoriasis**
23. **B. i.e. Psoriasis**
24. **A i.e. PUVA; B i.e. Mtx**
25. **A i.e. Mtx**
26. **B. i.e. Methotrexate**
27. **B. i.e. Retinoids, A i.e. Methotrexate**
28. **B i.e. Retinoids**
29. **B i.e. Methotrexate**
30. **C i.e. Methotrexate**

Drugs in Psoriasis

Exacerbation (deterioration) of Psoriasis is caused by
- *Antimalarials (eg chloroquine)*Q
- *β-blockers* Q
- NSAIDS
- *Lithium (Li)* Q

- Normaly **drug of choice** in most common type *widespread plaque psoriasis* is **PUVA** (psoralen + UV A i.e. 300-400 nm)
- *Topical vitamin D analogue (calcipotriol), anthralin (dithranol), steroids*Q, and systemic retinoids, methotrexate are also used.

Systemic oral retinoids alone or with **PUVA** are drug of choice in
- *Localized & generalized pustular psoriasis*Q
- *Psoriatic erythroderma*Q
- AIDS with psoriasis (UV B is given)

Methotrexate is DOC in
*Psoriatic arthropathy*Q
- Mtx is very effective in *long term management of severe form of psoriasis, psoriatic erythroderma, pustular psoriasis and chronic plaque type*Q **(drug of 2nd choice)**

31. **D i.e. Erythrodermic psoriasis**
32. **B i.e. Pustular psoriasis**
33. **A i.e. Corticosteroids**
34. **A i.e. Psoriatic erythroderma with pregnancy**
35. **A i.e. Prednisolone**
36. **D i.e. Impetigo herpetiformis**

[Ref: Roxburgh's 18/e p. 148-50; Harrison 18/e p – 399; IADVL – Dermatology 2/e p 827; Rook's dermatology 7/e p –0 35 – 61; Fitzpatrick's 7/e, 192; http://www.bad.org.uk/healthcare/guide/nes/psorcorttcos.asp]

- **Systemic steroids *should be avoided in routine care of psoriasis*** Q because the disease usually breaks through, *requiring progressively higher doses to control symptoms* and withdrawl of drug is usually associated with frequent relapse in form of ***life threatening erythrodermic psoriasis (with exfoliative dermatitis) and pustular psoriasis (with pus lakes)***Q.
- However, systemic steroids may have a role in management of

1. ***Persistent, otherwise uncontrollable (e.g. with metabolic complications), psoriatic erythroderma and in fulminant generalized pustular psoriasis (von Zumbusch type) if other drugs are ineffective or contraindicated***Q.
2. Pustular psoriasis in pregnancy is called **impetigo herpatiformis.** ***In pregnancy, safest drug for treatment of pustular psoriasis is prednisolone***Q.
3. ***Severe psoriatic polyarthritis threatening severe irreversible joint damage***Q.
4. **Pustular psoriasis** ***may develop after strong topical or systemic steroids have been used and then abruptly withdrawn***Q. It ***presents with development of generalized pustules all over the body***Q. Erythematous skin rash with multiple pus lakes suggests a diagnosis of **generalized pustular psoriasis**. As retinoids, methotrexate & PUVA cannot be used (or contraindicated) in pregnancy. ***Corticosteroids form the mainstay of treatment for generalized pustular psoriasis in pregnancy***Q. *Localized disease* is best treated with *topical steroid & fulminiating generalized disease* is best treated with *systemic prednisolone (oral).*

37. **A i.e. Psoriasis**

38. **B > A i.e. Psoriasis > Lichen planus**

39. **A i.e. Lichen Planus; B i.e. Warts; D i.e. Psoriasis; E i.e. Vitiligo**
[Ref: Rooks 8/e p. 20.8; Fitzpatrick's 7/e p. 17; Roxbrough 18/e p. 139]

Kobner's (isomorphic) phenomenon is *characteristic of psoriasis*Q but also found in ***lichen planus, vitiligo & warts***Q.

40. **A i.e. Warts; B i.e. Molluscum contagiosum**

- **Koebner's (isomorphic) phenomenon** is seen in ***psoriasis (characteristic), lichen planus, vitiligo***Q, DLE & Kaposi sarcoma.
- **Pseudo Koebner's (pseudo-isomorphic) phenomenon** is due to auto-inoculation and is seen in ***infections like plane warts, molluscum contagiosum***Q and eczematous lesions.

Photochemotherapy (PUVA)

41. **A. i.e. Binding to DNA**
42. **D. i.e. Exfoliation**
43. **D i.e. Psoriasis**
44. **A i.e. Psoriasis; E i.e. Vitiligo**
45. **B. i.e. Vitiligo**
46. **D. i.e. All**
47. **A i.e. Pigmented purpuric lesin; C i.e. Mycosis fungoides; E i.e. Lichenoid dermatitis of Gougerot & Blum**
48. **C. i.e. UV-C**
49. **A. i.e. Ultraviolet light**

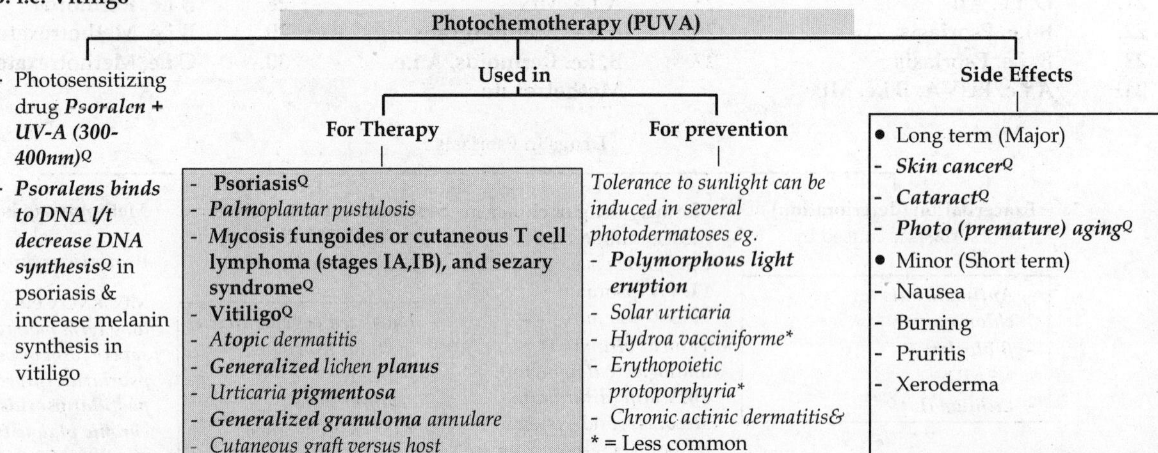

Also Know: *UV-A (300-400 nm) is used in PUVA. UV-B is medically most important as it may l/t skin cancers. UV-C circulating lymphocytes are most sensitive to this light. Best treatment of* ***pruritis in uremia*** *is* **UV light**Q

Lichen Planus

50. **B i.e. Lichen planus**

51. **B i.e., Lichen planus** *[Ref: Roxburgh's 17/e p. 144-45, 292, 301; Fitzpatrick's 6/e p-463-476]*

52. **A i.e. Pruritus, B i.e. Purple, C i.e. Papule**

53. **A i.e. Peutz jegher syndrome**

Mucosal involvement is seen in:
(requiring oral examination)
1. ***Lichen planus***Q***, Leprosy***
2. ***Pemphigus vulgaris (not pemphigoid)***Q
3. ***Peutz Jegher Syndrome***Q
4. ***Erythema multiformae***
5. Syphilis (congenital & secondary)
6. ***Measles (Koplik Spot)***Q
7. Fordyce's spot & disease

Peutz jegher syndrome consists of:
1. ***Melanosis (Brown macules) on oral mucosa, perioral region, lips & fingers***Q
2. ***Familial hamartomatous polyposis***Q affecting the jejunum which leads to haemorrhage & intussusception.

54. **A i.e. DLE; B i.e. Graft versus host disease; C i.e. Erythema multiformal; D i.e. Lichen planus**
[Ref: Fitzpatrick's 57/e p-242/44/51/63; Rooks 8/e p.41/47; www.demussen.net]

- **Lichenoid dermatoses (eruptions)** is used to describe a flat topped, shiny, papular eruption resembling lichen planus (by clincians) or tissue reaction consisting principally of **basal cell liquefaction and a band like inflammatory cell infiltrate in papillary dermis** (by histopathologist).

- Prototype of all lichenoid eruptions is lichen planus. Histologically lichenoid eruption (showing **basal cell liquefaction or necrotic keratinocytes**) are ***dermatomyositis, DLE, drug eruptions (fixed), erythema multiforme, graft versus host disease***Q, ***lichen planus***Q, lichen nitidus, lichen purpuricus (aureus), lichen striatus, lichenoid keratosis, lichenoid drug eruptions, lichen planus-lupus erythematosus overlap syndrome, lichen planus, pemphigoides, keratosis lichenoides chronica (Nekam's disease), pityriasis lichenoides, poikolodermas and viral exanthems.

55. **B i.e. Lichen planus**
56. **A. i.e. Lichen planus**
57. **A i.e. Basal cell degeneration; B i.e. Colloid bodies seen; C i.e. Epidermal hyperplasia in chronic cases; D i.e. Wickham's striae seen; E i.e. Autoimmune disease**
58. **A i.e. Lichen planus**
59. **C i.e. Lichen planus**
60. **C. i.e. Lichen planus**
61. **A. i.e. Lichen planus**
62. **C. Lichen planus**
63. **A. i.e. Hypopigmentation in residual disease**
64. **A. i.e. Does not involve mucous membrane**
65. **C i.e. Lichen Planus**
66. **B i.e. Pterygium**
67. **D i.e. Lichen planus**
68. **D i.e. Lichen Planus**
69. **C. i.e. Lichen planus**
70. **A i.e. Pruritis; B i.e. Purple; C i.e. Papule**
71. **D i.e. Wickham Striae**
72. **B i.e. Basal cell degeneration**
73. **C i.e. Systemic Steroids**

[Ref: Roxburgh's 18/e p. 154-58; Fitzpatrick's 7/e p-244-255; Rooks 8/e p.41.1-41.20; Harrison 18/e p. 399-400]

- ***Max Joseph's space is seen in lichen planus***Q. It is separation of epidermis in small clefts.
- ***Presence of white lacy lesions in the oral cavity together with characteristic nail changes of 'Pterygium' (proximal nail fold prolonged on to nail bed) suggests the diagnosis of Lichen planus.***
- The **hallmark** – ***plain topped, polygonal, purple, pruritic (violaceous) papule***Q are seen on skin (not mucosa)
- In LP, nail plate thinning is seen (but is not most common) and alopecia is of scarring type.
- All are the features of L. planus but violaceous lesions may be seen in many other conditions like lymphoma cutis etc.; thinning of nail plate may be of traumatic origin also – so these are ruled out
- **Characterstic histological** changes of **L. planus** are:

1. ***Basal epidermal cell degeneration***Q causing *saw tooth profile* & eosinophilic ***cytoid bodies (civatte body)***Q
2. **Epidermal thickening** esp. of granular cell layer
3. ***Subepidermal-Lichenoid Band***Q due deposition of lymphocytes & histiocytes

- **Note: As the basal epidermal cell degeneration l/t formation of civatte bodies, it is the 1st choice for answer.**
- **Scarring alopecia** is found in *lichen planus & leprosy both;* but ***oral mucosa involvement and thinning of nails (pterygium)***Q favour the diagnosis of lichen planus.
- The sequela of healing (late waning, resolving) is often slightly **atrophic, hyperpigmented skin.**
- ***Lichen planus usually heals with hyperpigmentation***Q which is more prominent in patients with darker skin color. Hypopigmentation uncommonly (rarely) develop in residual disease.

Lichen Planus (LP)

- LP is a *papulosquamous* disorder in which the primary lesions are ***pruritic, polygonal, plain (flat) topped, purple (mauve/violaceous) papules***Q. But there is no purpura or petechiae.
- The surface of these papules reveals a ***network of gray lines (Wickham's striae)***Q.
- There is predilection for *wrist, shins, lower back and genitals.* Scalp involvement leads to ***scarring alopecia***Q (hair loss), and nail involvement causes ***pterygium (thinning of nail)***Q.
- It commonly involves ***mucous membranes, particularly buccal mucosa***Q, where it can present as a *white net like eruption.* **(lacey pattern).**
- Etiology is unknown, but similar lesions are associated with many drugs eg. *thiazide diuretics, gold, antimalarials, penicillamine, and phenothiazines;* and in patients of ***chronic graft versus host disease and hepatitis – C***Q infections.
- Course is variable but most have ***spontaneous remissions in 6 month to 2 years***Q. As lesions heal, they flaten & often ***leave a hyperpigmented patch***Q.
- **Lichen planus** characteristically shows ***Whickham's striae, mucosal involvement, & scarring alopecia***Q; and may be associated with ***hepatitis C, hyper pigmentation & civatte bodies***Q (d/t liquifactive degeneration of basal cell → Shedding of melanin into dermis, → melanin engulfed by macrophage form civatte bodies), *band like infiltration* and may l/t ***squamous cell carcinoma***Q.
- In **Lichen planus,** the lesions have *whitsh criss cross streaks on their surface* k/a ***Wickham's striae***Q
- ***Topical glucocorticoids are the main stay of therapy***Q.

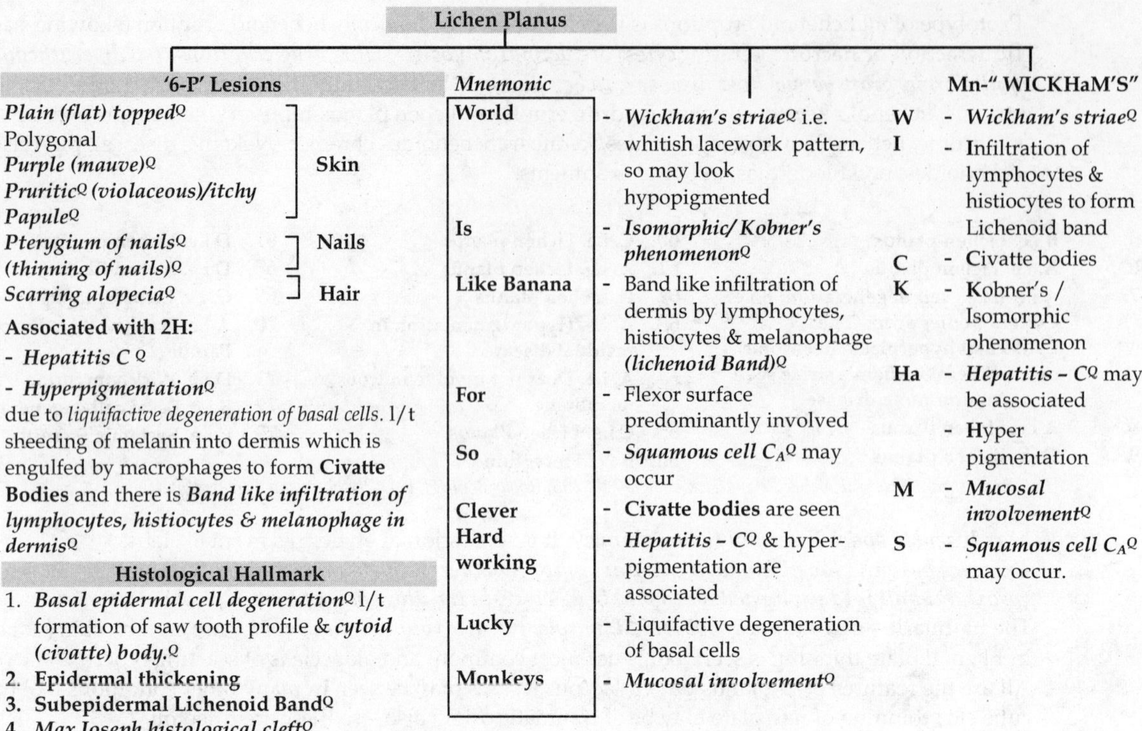

Lichen Planus

'6-P' Lesions

Skin:
- *Plain (flat) topped*Q
- Polygonal
- *Purple (mauve)*Q
- *Pruritic*Q *(violaceous)/itchy*
- *Papule*Q

Nails:
- *Pterygium of nails*Q
- *(thinning of nails)*Q

Hair:
- *Scarring alopecia*Q

Associated with 2H:
- *Hepatitis C* Q
- *Hyperpigmentation*Q due to *liquifactive degeneration of basal cells.* l/t sheeding of melanin into dermis which is engulfed by macrophages to form **Civatte Bodies** and there is ***Band like infiltration of lymphocytes, histiocytes & melanophage in dermis***Q

Histological Hallmark
1. *Basal epidermal cell degeneration*Q l/t formation of saw tooth profile & *cytoid (civatte) body.*Q
2. **Epidermal thickening**
3. **Subepidermal Lichenoid Band**Q
4. ***Max Joseph histological cleft***Q

Mnemonic

World	- *Wickham's striae*Q i.e. whitish lacework pattern, so may look hypopigmented
Is	- *Isomorphic/ Kobner's phenomenon*Q
Like Banana	- Band like infiltration of dermis by lymphocytes, histiocytes & melanophage *(lichenoid Band)*Q
For	- Flexor surface predominantly involved
So	- *Squamous cell C_A*Q may occur
Clever	- **Civatte bodies** are seen
Hard working	- *Hepatitis – C*Q & hyper-pigmentation are associated
Lucky	- Liquifactive degeneration of basal cells
Monkeys	- *Mucosal involvement*Q

Mn-" WICKHaM'S"

- **W** - *Wickham's striae*Q
- **I** - Infiltration of lymphocytes & histiocytes to form Lichenoid band
- **C** - Civatte bodies
- **K** - Kobner's / Isomorphic phenomenon
- **Ha** - *Hepatitis – C*Q may be associated - Hyper pigmentation
- **M** - *Mucosal involvement*Q
- **S** - *Squamous cell C_A*Q may occur.

74. A i.e. Lichen planus; B i.e. Sun burns; C i.e. Pemphigoid; D i.e. Psoriasis

[Ref: Behl 8/e P-385, 109; Fitzpatrick's 6/e p-463-476; Rooks 7/e p.42.1-42.14]

In **SLE** skin lesions are ***neither itchy nor painful***Q

Lesion	Itching
SLE	*Not itchy*Q
Psoriasis	*Very uncommon*Q
Pemphigus	Mild
Pemphigoid	Common
Sun burn	Common
DLE	Very common
Lichen planus	*Voilaceous (extremely itchy)*Q

5 PAPULOVESICULAR / VESICOBULLOUS DISORDERS & IMMUNOLOGICALLY MEDIATED DISEASES

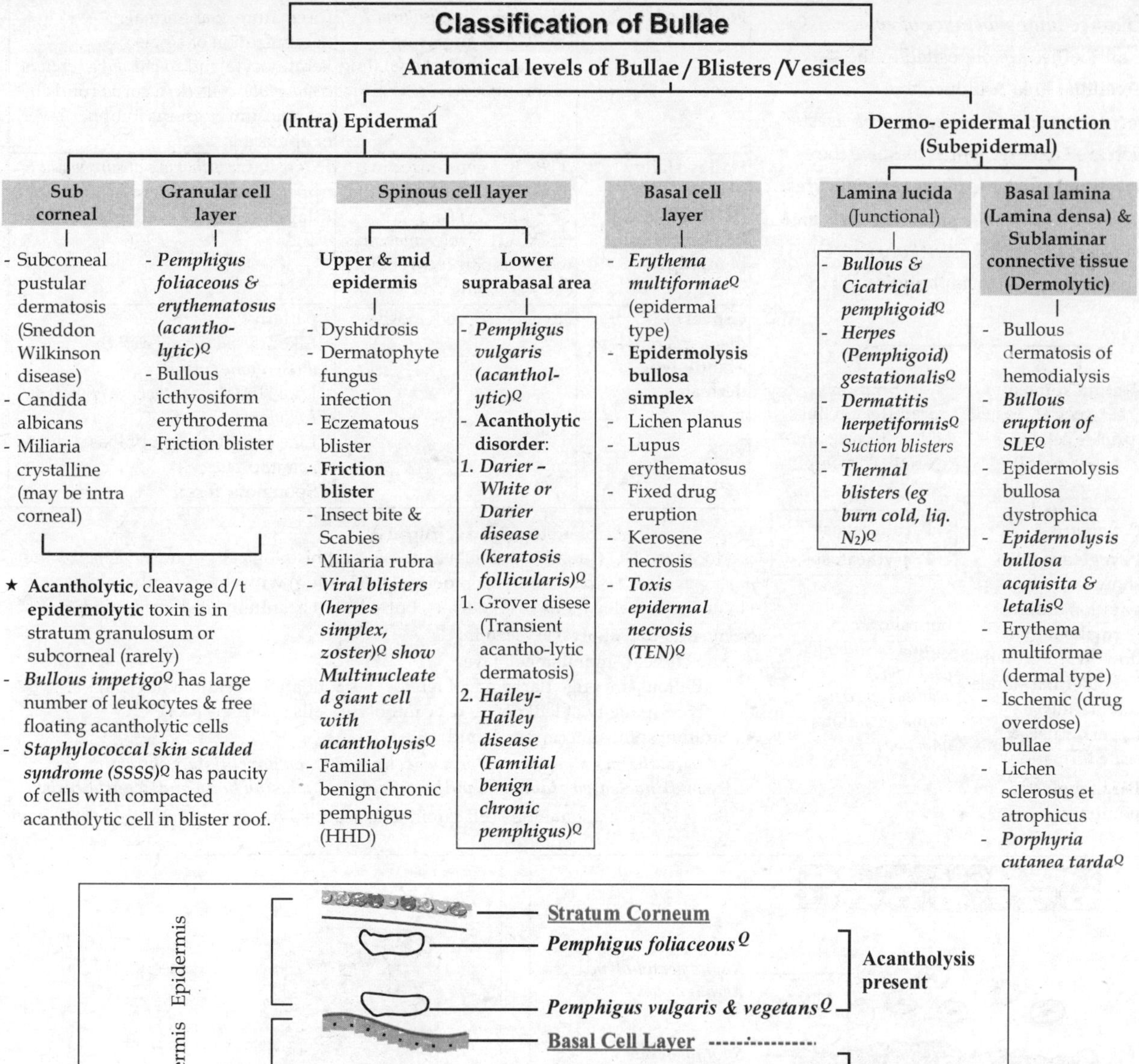

Classification of Bullae
Anatomical levels of Bullae / Blisters /Vesicles
(Intra) Epidermal
Dermo- epidermal Junction (Subepidermal)
Sub corneal
Granular cell layer
Spinous cell layer
Basal cell layer
Lamina lucida (Junctional)
Basal lamina (Lamina densa) & Sublaminar connective tissue (Dermolytic)
- Subcorneal pustular dermatosis (Sneddon Wilkinson disease)
- Candida albicans
- Miliaria crystalline (may be intra corneal)
- Pemphigus foliaceous & erythematosus (acantholytic)Q
- Bullous icthyosiform erythroderma
- Friction blister
★ Acantholytic, cleavage d/t epidermolytic toxin is in stratum granulosum or subcorneal (rarely)
- Bullous impetigoQ has large number of leukocytes & free floating acantholytic cells
- Staphylococcal skin scalded syndrome (SSSS)Q has paucity of cells with compacted acantholytic cell in blister roof.
Upper & mid epidermis
- Dyshidrosis
- Dermatophyte fungus infection
- Eczematous blister
- Friction blister
- Insect bite & Scabies
- Miliaria rubra
- Viral blisters (herpes simplex, zoster)Q show Multinucleated giant cell with acantholysisQ
- Familial benign chronic pemphigus (HHD)
Lower suprabasal area
- Pemphigus vulgaris (acantholytic)Q
- Acantholytic disorder:
1. Darier – White or Darier disease (keratosis follicularis)Q
1. Grover disese (Transient acantho-lytic dermatosis)
2. Hailey-Hailey disease (Familial benign chronic pemphigus)Q
- Erythema multiformaeQ (epidermal type)
- Epidermolysis bullosa simplex
- Lichen planus
- Lupus erythematosus
- Fixed drug eruption
- Kerosene necrosis
- Toxis epidermal necrosis (TEN)Q
- Bullous & Cicatricial pemphigoidQ
- Herpes (Pemphigoid) gestationalisQ
- Dermatitis herpetiformisQ
- Suction blisters
- Thermal blisters (eg burn cold, liq. N2)Q
- Bullous dermatosis of hemodialysis
- Bullous eruption of SLEQ
- Epidermolysis bullosa dystrophica
- Epidermolysis bullosa acquisita & letalisQ
- Erythema multiformae (dermal type)
- Ischemic (drug overdose) bullae
- Lichen sclerosus et atrophicus
- Porphyria cutanea tardaQ
Dermis Epidermis
Stratum Corneum
Pemphigus foliaceous Q
Pemphigus vulgaris & vegetans Q
Acantholysis present
Basal Cell Layer
Bullous pemphigoidQ
Dermatitis herpetiformisQ
Acantholysis absent

Acantholysis, Tzank Test & Nikolsky Sign

Acantholysis

- Acanthosis is a primary ***loss of cohesion between epidermal cells (in epidermis)***Q due to desolution or ***lysis of intercellular adhesion sites (or intercellular substance)***Q. It is characterized by:
  - Seperation of interdesmosomal regions of cell membrane of **keratinocytes**, followed by splitting & disappearance of desmosomes.
  - **Keratinocyte cells** are *intact but no longer attached* to other epidermal cells; loose their polyhedral shape and ***characteristically acquire smallest possible surface and round up. These rounded keratinocytes with hyperchromatic nuclei and perinuclear halo***Q (d/t condensing of cytoplasm in periphery) are k/a **acantholytic cells.**
  - Inter cellular slits & gaps result, and influx of fluid from dermis l/t cavity formation

- Acantholytic cells can be demonstrated in ***bed side Tzanck test***Q. Primary acantholysis is seen in:

Pemphigus

There is production of IgG auto antibodies against polypeptide complexes present in the ***intercellular substance of epidermis***Q. The antibodies are deposited in the intercellular area & induce the ***keratinocyte to release serine proteases***Q which are enzymes which dissolve the intercellular substance. The ***keratinocytes then seperate from the adjoining cells and this process is called acantholysis***Q. On the basis of level of acantholytic split in

Stratum spinosum (i.e. between st. basale & prickle cell layer = **supra basal**)	**Stratum granulosum** (just below st. corneum = Sub- corneal)
- ***P. vulgaris***Q - **P. vegetans** (also show papillomatosis of dermal papillae, downward growth of epidermal stands into dermis, hyperkeratsis & scale formation) - **Paraneoplastic pemphigus**	- **P. foliaceous** - **P. erytheatosus** Both show *sub corneal pustules with neutrophils & acantholytic cells* (same as bullous *impetigo*)

Acantholytic disorders of skin	Defect	Histology
Darier disease (DD)/Keratosis Follicularis	*ATP – 2A2* gene encoding *sarco/endoplasmic reticulum calcium ATP ase isoform 2 (SERCA-2)*, imparing intercellular Ca^{++} signaling of keratinocyte	Suprabasal acantholytic clefts, with *hyperkeratosis, focal dyskeratosis* (premature & abnormal keratinization of single keratinocyte)and *rounded dyskeratotic eosinophilic* cells (k/a **corps ronds** in st spinosum & **grains** in upper layer of epidermis
Hailey Hailey disease (HHD)/Familial benign chronic pemphigus	*ATP- 2C1* gene encoding human secretory pathway *Ca^{++}/Mn^{++} ATPase (hSPCA1) of golgi apparatus,* which impair intra cellular Ca^{++} signaling	Extensive *acantholysis of suprabasal* & upper layers of epidermis l/t **dilapidated brick wall appearance.**
Grover disease/Transient acantholytic dermatosis	No genetic predisposition	4 patterns - Like DD *suprabasal cleft & dyskeratotic* cells - Like HHD, *acanntholysis of most st. Malpighii* - Like pemphigus, suprabasal cell & acantholytic cells - Spongiotic form

Hopf disease (Acrokeratosis verruciformis)
is a localized DD (usually on dorsal hands & feet) histologically showing *hyperkeratosis, hypergranulosis & acanthosis* (i.e. epidermal thickening) with **church spike** circumscribed elevations of epidermis, but **without acantholysis & dyskeratosis.**

Secondary acantholysis is seen in:
- Sub-corneal –granular cell layer
  - Bullous impetigo (large no. of leukocytes & floating acantholytic cells) .
  - SSSS (paucity of leukocytes & acantholytic cells in blister- roof)
- Stratum spinosum (upper & mid)
  - Viral (***herpes simplex, zoster, varicella = chicken pox) blisters show multinucleated giant cells with acidophilic inclusion body and acantholysis***Q.
- Solar Keratosis, squamous cell carcinoma, acantholytic dyskeratotic epidermal nevi.

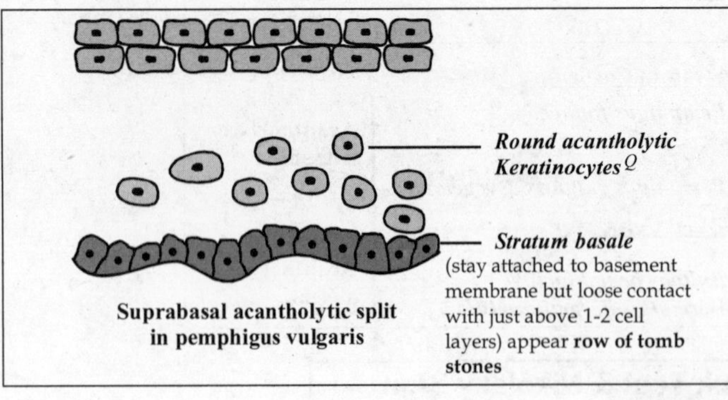

Suprabasal acantholytic split in pemphigus vulgaris

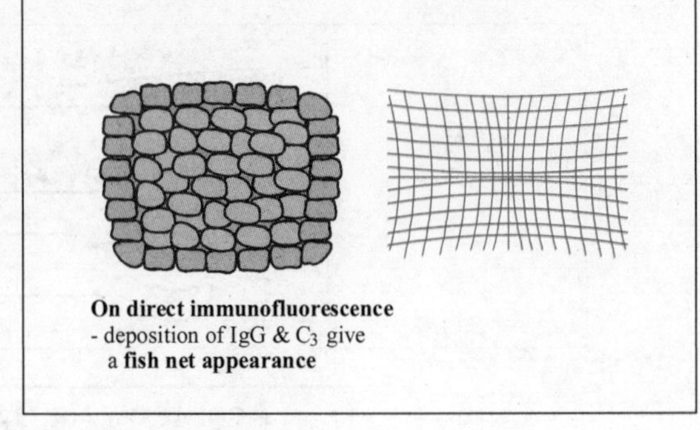
On direct immunofluorescence - deposition of IgG & C_3 give a **fish net appearance**

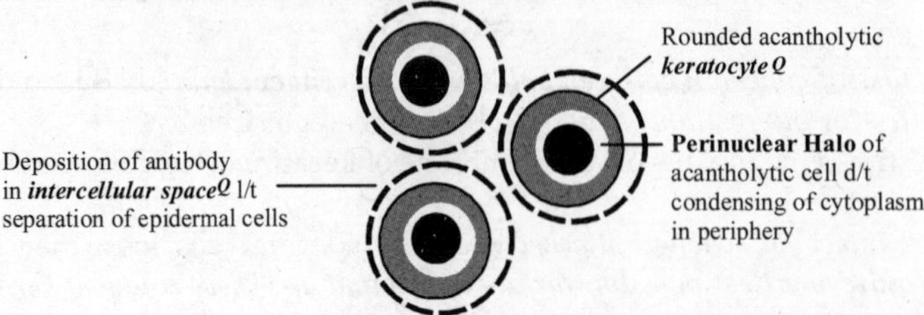

Bed Side Tzanck (Cytodiagnosis smear) Test

- It is an ***easy bed side, rapid cytodiagnosis smear test***[Q] most valuable in bullous disorders, vesicular virus eruptions and basal cell epithelioma.
- An early, small, uninfected lesion (i.e. vesicle not pustule) is unroofed, its base scraped and stained with hematoxylin eosin, giemsa wright's stain or any Romanowsky's (or Papanicolaous) staining for microscopic examination. Microscopic appearances may be.

Acantholysis with numerous acantholytic Keratinocytes

- ***Pemphigus vulgaris & vegetans and Hailey- Hailey disease***[Q] (rounded Keratinocytes of uniform size with pale perinuclear halo and large nuclear cytoplasmic ratio)
- In more superficial forms of pemphigus like **pemphigus foliaceous** and **Senear-Usher pemphigus (syndrome)**, keratinocytes are more cuboidal with prominent cytoplasm and small nucleus.
- **Darier's disease** ***(dyskeratosis with occasional acantholytic cells)***[Q]
- **Bullous impetigo** (numerous neutrophil polymorphs and bacteria in addition to acantholytic cells)

Diagnostic Multinucleated (often ≥ 8 nuclei) giant cells and typical ballooning degeneration of nucleus (i.e. blurring of chromatin pattern & loss of staining)

- ***Herpes simplex & Herpes zoster***[Q] (eosinophilic cowdry Type A intra nuclear inclusion bodies are occasionally identified)
- ***Varicella zoster (chicken pox) virus***[Q].

Vaccinia or Cow pox	Typical ballooning degeneration & multinucleated giant cell formation does not normally occur but occasionally slightly enlarged acantholytic cells and **eosinophilic (acidophilic) intracytoplasmic inclusion bodies** may be detected.
Molluscum contagiosum	Characteristic large, rounded, eosinophilic molluscum bodies are easily identified without H & E stain in a KOH preparation.
Basal cell carcinoma	Closely set, oval or round, deeply basophilic cells with very scantly cytoplasm, finely granular nuclei with poorly defined nucleoli.

Its usefulness in subepidermal bullous eruption is limited as the smear in most cases contain only inflammatory cells.

Toxic epidermal necrolysis	Necrotic cells
Bullous Pemphigoid	Eosinophilic (predominantly)
Chronic bullous disease of childhood	Polymorphs (predominantly

Nikolsky Sign

- **Nikolsky sign** is shearing away (separation/dislodgement or sheet like removal) of normal looking epidermis from dermis producing an erosion by applying firm sliding (lateral or tangenital) pressure on normal skin. It results in *formation of new bullae on stroking normal skin* or if applied to pre existing bullae, results in spread of bullae **(bullae spread sign)**.
- In this, superficial layers slide over deeper layers, which is seen over bony prominences when pressure applied with pulp of thumb. It is positive in pemphigus (differentiating it from other blistering diseases) and more rarely in TEN.
- It is noted in **blistering disorder in which pathology is above the basement membrane zone** such as
  - ***Pemphigus all types (but not in pemphigoid)***[Q]
  - **Epidermal necrolysis** – ***Stevens Johnson syndrome***[Q] (involving <10% body surface area i.e. BSA)
    - **Toxic epidermal necrolysis** (**TEN or Lyell syndrome** involving >30% BSA)
  - ***Staphylococcal scalded skin syndrome (SSSS)***[Q]
  - Epidermolysis bullosa simplex & dystrophic
  - ***Herpes, Leukemia***[Q] etc.

Epidermolysis Bullosa (EB)

It consists of a group of disorders in which the **skin and related epithelial tissue break and blister as a result of minor trauma**[Q]

Congenital (Inherited) Epidermolysis Bullosa

Classification & Molecular Defects

Classification	Level of separation or blistering	Mulated gene	Defective product	**Types**
EB **Simplex**	**Epidermis**	KRT (keratin) 5/14	Major keratin of basal epithelial cells	- Koebner (Generalized EB), - Dawling – Meara (Herpetiformis EB), - Weber- Cockayne (Localized)

Epidermolysis- Bullosa Acquisita

- It is a ***sporadic autoimmune***[Q] bullous (blistering) disease associated with *immunoglobulin G (IgG) autoantibodies* against ***non collagenous 1 (NC-1) amino terminal of α chain of collagen VII (7)***[Q] within anchoring fibrils that fortify the attachment of dermis to epidermis.
  There is ***no family history of bullous disorders***[Q]. It may be associated with *HLADR2+* and have varying presentation.

1. **Classical presentation** is of **non inflammatory tense bullous disease with acral distribution that heals with scarring, scaling, curst formation or erosions and pearl like milia cyst formation**[Q].

				- Ogna, Superficialis & mottled pigmentation (only KRT5)
EB **Hemidesmosomal**	Fissures between *keratinocytes & basal lamina*	PLEC -1	Plectin 1	EB with mild blistering at birth & *late onset muscular dystrophy*
		ITG-A6 ITG – B4	α-6 Integrin β-4 Integrin	EB with ***pyloric atresia and intestinal*** abnormalities
Both hemidesmosomal & Junctional		COL 17A1 LAMB 3	Collagen type 17 α 1 Laminin β 3	Generalized atrophic benign
EB **Junctional**	*Dermal – epidermal junction*	COL 17A1	Collagen type 17α 1	Localized
		LAMB3/ LAMA 3/ LAMG 2	Laminin β 3 Laminin α3 Laminin γ2	Gravis / Herlitz and miltis
EB **Dystrophic** (most severe)	Dermis	**COL 7A1**	***Collagen type 7 α1***[Q]	Pasini , Cockayne – Touraine, localized recessive dystrophic EB (RDEB), Hallopeau – Siemens
EB **Desmosomal**		**PKP1**	Plakophilin 1	Ectodermal dysplasia – skin fragility
EB Variable		KIND 1	Kindilin 1	Kindler syndrome

★ **Epidermolytic icthyosis** is d/t mutation in *keratin 1 and keratin 10*

Presentation & Diagnosis

- It is ***inherited genodermatoses (genetic disorder***[Q]***)*** *characterized by* ***skin that readily breaks and form blisters***[Q].
- As with ***most heritable disorders of connective tissues***[Q], the manifestations range from ***mild to lethal***[Q].
- EB simplex & EB hemidesmosomal are generally milder than EB junctional or EB dystrophica.
- EB dystrophica form large & prominent scars.
- Although milder EB subtypes have normal life span and little or no internal involvement, the most severe recessive types are mutilating multiorgan disorders that threaten both quality & length of life. Nikolsky sign l/t *mitten like* deformity with digits encased in *epidermal coccon.*

  Diagnostic gold standard for grouping EB is ***electron microscopy.*** *Indirect immunofluorescence (IDIF)* is also useful in distinguishing subtypes. *DNA mutation analysis* is also of *prognostic importance.* For example RDEB & severe dominant type may have equivalent blistering but risk of SCC is higher in RDEB.

- It presents with skin fragility, spontaneous or trauma induced blisters within non inflamed skin, scars, & milia *over trauma prone surfaces* such as backs of hands, knuckles, ***elbows, knees, sacral area***[Q], palm, soles & toes in adults & children. It may show *scarring alopecia* and dystrophy of nails.
- It resembles reminiscent of *porphyria cutanea tarda (PCT)* when mild and *recessive dystrophic (EB inherited)* when severe. But unlike PCT hirsutism, photodistribution of eruption, scleroderma like changes are absent and urinary porphyrins are normal.

2. **Bullous pemphigoid** (BP) like presentation with *inflammed, pruritic, widespread* vesico- bullous eruption also *involving trunk, central body, flexural areas & skin folds.*
3. **Cicatricial pemphigoid** like presentation with *predominant mucosal involvement* i.e. erosion & scar in mouth , oesophagus, conjunctiva, vagina or anus ± skin.
4. **Bursting – Perry pemphigoid** like lesions with residual *scarring & predominant head and neck distribution* with no (or minimal) mucosal involvement.
5. Linear IgA bullous dermatosis (LABD) or chronic bullous disease of childhood like presentation.

- Histology show ***subepidermal blister***[Q]
- **Direct immuno fluorescence (DIF)** of perilesional skin shows ***intense, linear, homogenous fluorescent band of IgG & C3 at DEJ***[Q] (dermoepidermal junction). PCT & BP show same picture; however **PCT** also demonstrate. ***immune deposits around blood vessels***[Q].
- Patients with EBA may have autoantibodies in blood ,directed against DEJ. So EBA & BP can be distinguished by:

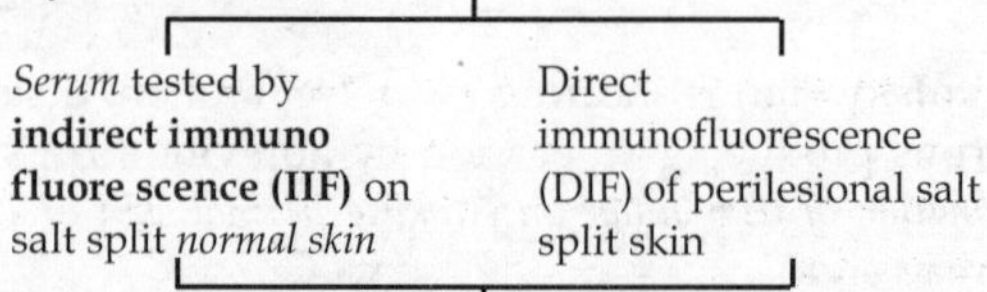

1M NaCl fractures DEJ cleanly through lamina lucida, Deposition of Ig and staining is on

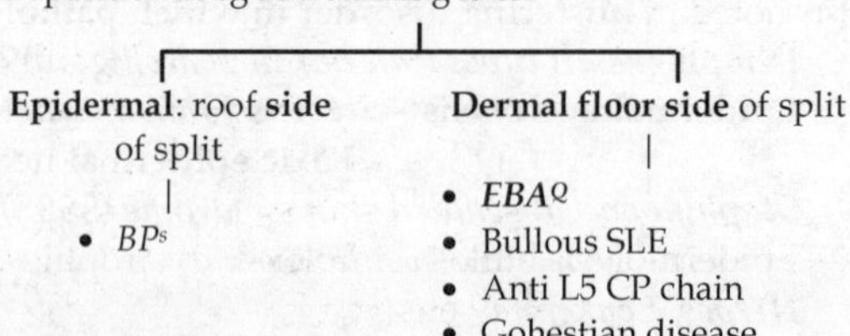

- **Direct Immuno – Electron microscopy** is *gold standard* for diagnosis and show immunoglobin G (IgG) & C_3 *deposits localized to lower lamina densa & / or sub- lamina densa* of dermo-epidermal basement membranes. Whereas these deposits are high up in hemidesmosome area *or lamina lucida* area of BMZ in BP; and confined to *lamina lucida in cicatricial pemphigoid (CP).*

Pemphigus

Pemphigus is an ***autoimmune blistering disorder***[Q] resulting from the loss of integrity of normal intercellular attachments with in the epidermis. Most individuals are in *fourth to sixth decades of life,* and men & women are affected equally. There are five variants : 1) ***pemphigus vulgaris (most common)***[Q], 2) **pemphigus foliaceous** (superficial pemphigus), 3) **pemphigus vegetans** (least common & a type of p. vulgaris that is large & localized to flexural areas), 4) **pemphigus erythematous** (Senear-Usher syndrome is localized pemphigus foliaceous & SLE), 5) **Fogo Selvagem (wild fire)** is an endemic form of pemphigus foliacious.

Comparison of Pemphigus and Pemphigoid

Features	Pemphigus Foliaceous	Pemphigus Vulgaris	(Bullous) Pemphigoid
Level of Blisters	**Superficial intraepidermal, high in granular layer or immediately below stratum corneum (sub corneal)**Q	**Intra- epidermal, in lower suprabasal area in spinous cell layer**Q	**Deep subepidermal** with intact & often viable epidermis forming the roof.
Skin Lesions	- Because the cleavage is superficial and the primary lesions of **small flaccid blisters rupture easily, blistering maynot be found (obvious)** typically. - The onset is usually insidious with **scaly lesions scattered in a seborrheic distribution ie scalp, face, and upper trunk (chest & back)**. Scales separate leaving **well demarcated crusted erosions surrounded by erythema** or rarely small vesicles - **So the characteristic clinical lesions are scaly, crusted erosions often on a erythematous base.** Lesions are **painful burning & offensive.** Term **fogo selvagem** (or **wild fire**) takes into account many of the clinical aspects of PF: the burning feeling, exacerbation of disease by sun, and the crusted lesions that make the patient appear as if they had been burned. Eventually patient becomes erythrodermic with crusted, oozing, red skin. - **Summary:** ***Rarely demonstrate intact blisters***Q ***but rather exihibit shallow erosions associated with erythema, scale & crust formation***Q. Mild cases of PF resemble severe ***seborrheic dermatitis***; severe PF may cause extensive exfoliation.	- Primary lesion is **fragile, flaccid blister,** which may occur anywhere on the skin surface (with a predilection for scalp, face, axilla, trunk and groin preferably upper half of body) but typically *not the palms and soles.* In most patients, **lesions typically begin in the mouth (oral mucosa)**Q, preceeding by months. - Usually the blilsters arise **on normal appearing skin,** but it may develop on erythemathous skin as well. Because **bullae are fragile (rupture easily) the most common skin lesions are erosisons** resulting from broken blisters. - **Pruritic, painful erosions** are often quite **large**, as they have a tendency to **spread peripherally.** A characteristic finding in PV is that **erosions can be extended into visibly normal skin** by pulling the blister wall or rubbing at the periphery of active lesions - Erosions can be induced in normal appearing skin distant from active lesions by manual pressure of mechanical shear force separating the epidermis **(Nikolsky sign).** This finding while **characteristic of PV** is not specific as it can also be seen in *SSSS, Stevens Johnson syndrome & TEN.* - **Pruritis** may be seen in early lesions and **severe pain** is a/w extensive denudation. **Healing is slow** and occurs **without scarring** (except in secondary infection & mechanical denudation) but **pigmentary changes (hyperpigmentation)** & **acanthomas** may occur in resolving lesions for sometime.	- Typically occurs in **elderly patients over 60 years** of age. The lesions are most commonly **found on flexural surfaces, lower (central) abdomen, trunk & thighs (ie lower half of body),** although they may occur anywhere. Although rarely involved *infants* have *acral distribution of lesion* and older *children have genital involvement.* - Prodrome includes **itching pruritis, eczematous rash** (preceding months), **urticaria**, or faint **dusky erytheme in figurate pattern** closely resembling erythema multiforme or dermatitis herpetiformis preceding the blister by weeks. - **Classically blisters are large** (many cm diameter), **tense, dome shaped** arising on *normal skin, or on an erythematous base* and may be a/w *dermal swelling.* - Blisters are **tough** & may remain intact for several days with clear serous or jelly like coagulated or rarely hemorrhagic fluid content. - The **Nikolsky and Asboe-Hansen signs are negative.** - Erosions d/t ruptured blisters heal **rapidly without scaring,** although erythema, **milia** and **hyperpigmentation** may last for several months.
Mucous membrane involvement	- **Almost always spared**Q (very rarely, if ever, involved, even with wide spread disease)	- **Nearly all patients have mucoscal lesion**Q**; oral-pharyngeal mucosa** being earliest & most commonly rinvolved. As with skin inlact blisters are rare and **illdefined, irregularly shaped slowly healing painful erosions** which make drinking & eating difficult are most common presentation. - Involvement of other mucosal surfaces (eg pharyngeal, laryngeal, esophageal, conjunctival, vulval, urethral or retal) can occur in severe cases.	- **Less frequent** (but not uncommon with 10% patient involvement) and **less severe,** and are almost always **limited to oral (buccal) mucosa**. Oral lesions consist of small blisters that may remain intact or more commonly **erode and heal rapidly without scarring.** Unlike erythema mutiformae, the **vermillion border** of lip is **rarely involved**. Scarring suggest cicatricial pemphigoid
Variants	- **Pemphigus erythematosus (Senear-Usher syndrome)** is localized form of PF with **better prognosis** and features of a **pemphigus-lupus erythematosus overlap.** Clinical presentation includes **crusted erosions in a seborrheic distribution**, at times concurrent with more lupus like **discoid lesions with carpet tract scale.** Immunological	- **Pemphigus vegetans** is a rare type of PV which is characterized by a tendency to develop **excessive granulation tissue & crusting** (referred to as **vegetating erosions**), primarily in **flexures (intertriginous areas),** scalp or face. Clinical spectrum of it may rary from *mild Hallopeau to sereve Neumann subtype.*	-

	features of both LE & PF include granular IgG & C_3 at BMZ, intercellular IgG & C_3 in the epidermis and circulating antinuclear antibody. Some patients may progress to generalized PF but **progression to SLE is rare**; i.e. most patients do not develop systemic signs & symptoms of SLE. - Blistering disease endemic to brazil k/a **wild fire** or **fogo selvagem** or **Brazilian pemphigus** is clinically, histologically & immunopathologically indistinguishable from PF that is thought to develop as a result of environmental stimuli (eg insect bite). - **Pemphigus herpetiformis** is PF resembling dermatitis herpetiformis.		
Associated with	- *Thymoma* & or ***myasthenia gravis***[Q] (autoimmune disorders) usually associated with PF. - **Drug** induced pemphigus usually resemble PF rather than PV. Offending drugs include ***penicillamine***[Q] ***(most common), penicillin***[Q], piroxicam, phenobarbitone, rifampin, (captopril (Mn - "**P**" dominant).	- Increased incidence of *HLA-DR4* and *HLA – DRW6* serological halotype - Drugs (penicillamine, rifampicin), neoplasm (thymoma & lymphoma), and mysthenia gravis are rarely associated. - Exposure to UV radiation (sun) exacerbate the disease.	- **Neurological diseases** (most common), hemophilia due to acquired factor VIII inhibitor, and malignancy with gastric carcinoma being the commonest (controversial).
Histology (Tzank test)	- Acantholytic blisters are located **high** within the epidermis ***usually just beneath the stratum corneum***[Q]. So in contrast to PV, PF is a **more superficial** blistering disease that ***almost always spare mucous membranes***[Q]. - ***Acantholytic blister formed either in granular or in sub corneal (superficial) layer of epidermis***[Q].	- ***Acantholytic blister formed in suprabasal (deep) layer of epidermis***[Q] - The single layer of intact basal cells (attached to basement membrane) that form blister base has been likened to a ***row of tombstone***[Q]	**Subepidermal** blister with ***eosinophil rich infiltrate***[Q] in perivascular & vesicular sites.
Immuno pathology	- DIM of perilesional skin demonstrates *IgG on surface keratinocytes.* - IIM (using *guinea pig oesophagus*) demonstrate circulating IgG autoantibodies against keratinocyte cell surface antigen	- Direct immunofluorescence microscopy (DIM) of *lesion or intact* patient skin shows ***deposits of IgG on the surface of keratinocytes in a fish net like pattern***[Q]; in contrast complement components are typically found in lesional (but not uninvolved) skin. - Indirect immuno fluorescence microscopy (using *monkey oesophagus*) demonstrate circulating autoantibodies against keratinocyte cell surface antigen.	**On direct immunofluorescence microscopy:** Linear band of IgG and/or C3 in epidermal BMZ
Autoantigen	- Autoantibodies are directed against **Dsg 1**[Q] and distribution of this antigen account for distribution of lesion (low expression in oral mucosa)	- ***Auto antibodies (IgG) are directed against Dsgs (desmogleins)***[Q], transmembrane desmosomal glycoprotein that belong to cadherin supergene family of calcium dependent adhesion molecules • *Early PV (i.e. mucosal involvement only)* have only anti – ***Dsg3 autoantibodies***[Q] • *Advanced PV* (i.e. *mucosal & skin involvement both*) have both anti *Dsg3* and Dsg – 1 autoantibodies.	*Bullous pemphigoid antigen (BPAG) 1 and 2* (i.e. 230 & 180 K-Da hemidesmosome – associated proteins in basal keratinocytes respectively)
Prognosis	- Less severe & carries better prognosis.	- Can be *life threatening* with mortality of ~5%. Infection & complication of steroid treatment are most common causes of morbidity & mortality.	Less severe, better prognosis usually 3-6 years duration. Waxing-Waning course
Treatment	- Topical or intralesional glucocorticoids for localized disease and systemic glucocorticoids for severe disease	- *Systemic glucocorticoid* is mainstay of treatment.	- Steroid, dapsone, immunosuppressives

Paraneoplastic Pemphigus (PNP)

- Is an *autoimmune acantholytic* mucocutaneous disease associated with an occult or confirmed neoplasm. The predominant causative neoplasms are ***NHL, CLL, castle man's disease, thymoma & spindle cell tumors***[Q].
- Typically show painful mucosal erosions with *papulosquamous* eruptions progressing to blisters. *Palm & sole involvement* is common.
- Biopsy shows acantholysis, keratinocyte necrosis, vacuolar interface dermatitis. And direct immuno fluorescence microscopy show deposits of *IgG & compliment on the surface of keratinocytes & epidermal basement membrane zone.*
- Have IgG auto antibodies against cytoplasmic proteins that are members of plakin family (eg. desmoplakins I & II, bullous pemphigoid antigen 1, envoplakin, periplakin & plectin) and cell surface proteins that are members of cadherin family *(eg Dsg3 = key role).*
- Resistant to convential therapies of (of PV); but may improve following resection of underlying neoplasm.

Direct Immunofluorescence Microscopy

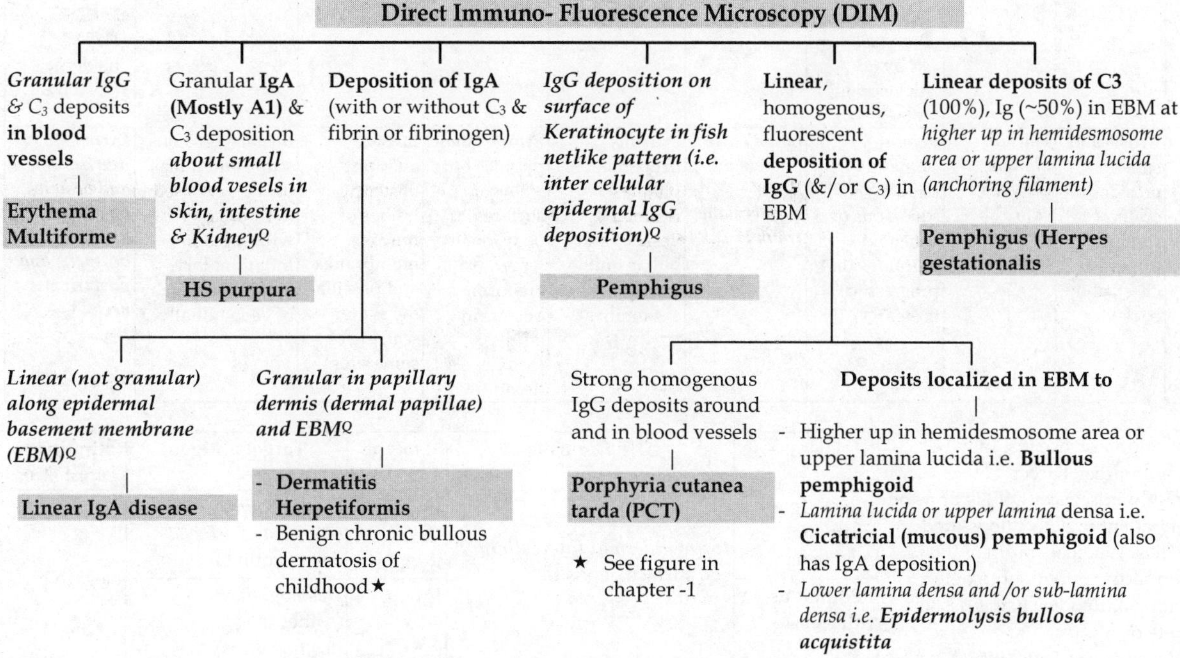

Immunologically Mediated Blistering Disease

Disease	Pemphigus folliaceous	Pemphigus vulgaris	Paraneoplastic pemphigus	Bullous pemphigoid	Pemphigoid gestationis	Linear IgA disease	Ciatricial Pemphigoid	Epidermolysis bullosa acquisita	Dermatitis herpatifosis
Auto antigen	***Desmoglein (Dsg) 1***[Q]	*Dsg3 (plus Dsg1* in patient with skin involvement)	**Plakin** protein family (eg. Desmoplakins I & II, BPAG1, envoplakin, periplakin, & plectin) & cell surface **cadherin** family proteins (eg. Dsg 3 and Dsg 1)	*Bullous pemphigoid antigen (BPAG) 1 and* 2 (i.e. 230 & 180 K-Da hemidesmosome – associated proteins in basal keratinocytes respectively)	BPAG 2 (+ BPAG 1 in some patients)	BPAG 2 (neoepitopes in extracellular domain) = LAD antigen)	BPAG 2, Laminin 5, type VII collagen etc.	***Type VII collagen(anchoring fibrils)***[Q]. This is also involved in bullous SLE	Epidermal transglutaminase 3 & tissue transglutaminase
Histology	**Epidermal acantholytic** blister in *superficial granular cell layer*	**Epidermal acantholytic** blister in *suprabasal spinous cell layer*	**Acantholysis** *keratinocyte necrosis & vacuolar interface dermatitis*	**Subepidermal** blister with ***eosinophil rich infiltrate***[Q] in perivascular & vesicular sites.	Teardrop-shaped, **subepidermal blisters** in dermal papillae with eosinophil-rich infiltrate	**Subepidermal** blister with ***neutrophils in dermal papillae***[Q]	**Subepidermal** blister that may or may not include a leukocytic infiltrate	**Subepidermal blister** that may or may not include a leukocytic infiltrate	***Subepidermal blister with neutrophils in dermal papillae***[Q]

Direct immunofluorescence Microscopy	Cell surface deposits of IgG on keratinocytes	Cells surface **deposits of IgG on keratinocytes in fishnet pattern**	Deposition of IgG & C3 on Keratinocytes cell surface and (+) in epidermal basement membrane zone (BMZ)	Linear band of IgG and/or C3 in epidermal BMZ	Linear band of C3 in epidermal BMZ	Linear band of IgA, in epidermal BMZ	Linear band of IgG, and/or C3 in epidermal BMZ	Linear band of IgG and /or C3 in epidermal BMZ	***Granular deposits of IgA in dermal papillae***[Q]
Associations	Drugs, *thymoma & myasthenia gravis*[Q]	***HLA- DR4 & DRW6***[Q]	- ***NHL, CLL, Castle man's disease***[Q], spindle cell tumors, thymoma, Walden strom macro globulinemia - *Bronchiolitis obliterans* (develop in some PNP)	HLA-DQ β1 * 0301	- Pregnancy & puerperium - HLA – DR3 & DR4	- HLA-B8 (+) - TNF2 allele	HLA-DQB1* 0301 (amino acid at 55 & 71-77)	*HLA – DR2*	- Sub clinical gluten sensitive entero pathy (100%) - *HLA – B8 (60%) / DRw3 (95%) & HLA – DQW2* halotype (95-100%)
Clinical feature	Crusts and shallow erosions on scalp, central face, upper chest, and back	***Flaccid blisters, denuded skin, oromucosal lesions***[Q]	Painful stomatitis with papulo squamous or lichenoid eruptions that progress to blister	***Large tense blisters on flexor surfaces and trunk***[Q]	Pruritic, urticarial plaques, rimmed by vesicles and bullae on the trunk and extremities	Pruritc small papules on extensor surfaces occasionally larger, arciform blisters in adults (usually 4th decade)	Erosive and/or blistering lesions of **mucous membranes** and possibly the skin; scarring of some sites	Blisters, erosions, scars, and milia on sites exposed to trauma; widespread, Inflammatory, tense blisters may be seen initially	***Extremely pruritic small and vesicles on elbows, knees, buttocks and posterior neck***[Q]

- Immunofluorescence test may be direct or indirect. Direct immunofluorescence (DIF) is done on skin of patient to detect deposited antibodies. Whereas, indirect IF is done on serum of patient to detect circulating antibodies using tissue substrate or ELISA.
- *Type of immunoreactants* (IgG/M/A, C3 etc) deposited, *location* of deposits (intraepiderm or BMZ) *and pattern of deposit* (linear, granular, homo/hetro-genous, fishnet etc) are noted.
- **Direct immunofluorescence (DIF)** is useful in diagnosis of ***pemphigus (vulgaris/foliaceus/vegetans & paraneoplastic pemphigus), pemphigoid (bullous/mucous membrane/gestationis), linear IgA disease, chronic bullous disease of childhood, epidermolysis bullosa acquisita, bullous SLE, dermatitis herpetiformis, erythema multiforme, HS purpura and porphyria cutanea tarda***[Q].
- **Darier white disease (keratosis follicularis), Hailey-Hailey disease (familial benign chronic pemphigus)** and **Grover's disease** are acantholytic disorders of skin diagnosed on the basis of histology (**not showing DIF**)

Disease	DIF Deposits	Isotype	Target antigen	Binding to split skin
Pemphigus vulgaris /vegetans	***Intraepidermal intercellular***[Q] cell surface deposits	**IgG** (& few IgM, IgA)	***Desmoglein 3***[Q] (sometimes 1 & desmocollins)	Negative
Pemphigus foliaceus		**IgG**	***Desmoglein 1***[Q] (sometimes desmocollins)	
Paraneoplastic pemphigus	**Intraepidermal intercellular & subepidermal**	**IgG**	**Plakins** (desmoplakin, envoplakin BP 230, periplekin)	
Bullous pemphigoid	Subepidermal, **linear, homogenous BMZ**	IgG (few IgA)	BP1 & 2 (i.e. 230 & 180)	Epidermal (few dermal)
Mucous membrane (cicatrical pemphigoid)		IgG, IgA	BP2 (>>1), α6 β4 integrin	Epidermal
Pemphigoid gestationis		IgG	BP2 & 1	Epidermal
Linear IgA disease (CBDC)		IgA	BP2, LAD 285, BP1, Collagen VII (dermal few)	Epidermal (most)
Epidermolysis bullosa aquisita		IgG	Collagen VII (anchoring fibril)	Dermal
Bullous SLE	Sabepidermal, **linear,** homogenous or non homogenous **BMZ**	IgG, IgA	Collagen VII (anchoring fibril)	Dermal
Dermatitis herpetiformis	Subepidermal, focal granular deposits in dermal papillae (papillary tips)	IgA	Epidermal tissue transglutaminase	Negative

Pemphigoid (Herpes) Gestationalis

- Acute onset *intensely pruritis* urticarial/vescio-bullous disease of pregnancy or immediate postapartum period. 90% patients express class II antigens *(HLA-DR3 & DR-4)* and class III antigen (C4). It is mediated by *IgG1 specific for 180 kd component of hemidesmosome (BPAG2).*
- It typically presents during *late pregnancy* (2nd or 3rd trimester) with ***abrupt onset intensly pruritic urticarial lesions mostly (50%) on the abdomen, often within or immediately adjacent to umbilicus (peri-umbilical)***Q. Others develop typical lesion in atypical distribution i.e. extremities, palms, or soles. *Rapid progression to pemphigoid like eruption, sparing only face, mucous membranes, palms & soles* is the rule (although any site may be involved). *Flare occurs with delivery* (in 75%). It disappears 1-2 months after delivery and ***reccurs with subsequent pregnancies***Q. Newborns are affected in *10%* cases, but the disease is typically *mild & self limiting*. It may be associated with premature & small for gestational age births.
- Histopathology shows *dermal – epidermal split* & DIF shows *linear deposition of C3 (± IgG) along BMZ* on epidermal side of salt split skin.
- Bullous pemphigoid & PG have several differences:
  - BP is a disease of *elderly with no gender* bias; PG is exclusively associated with *pregnancy.*
  - PG has strong a/w *HLA – DR3, - DR4, and C4 null allele.* BP does not.
  - Indirect IF in BP yields *positive results in most* and *titer of anti-BMZ antibody is mostly high.* The titer of anti-BMZ antibody in PG is usually *so low* that antibody cannot be detected without the use of complement added or ELISA technique.
  - Most of BP sera react to 230- 240 kd component of hemidesmosome (BPAG1); whereas, most PG react to 180 kd transmembrane protein with collagen domain (BPAG 2).

Dermatitis Herpetiformis (DH) / Duhring Disease

Associated With

- ***Subclinical gluten sensitive enteropathy***Q (in ~ all)
- ***HLA – B8*** *(60%) / DRw3 (95%) &* *HLA – DQW2* halotype (95-100%)
- Increased incidence of autoimmune disorders eg. *thyroid abnormalities (mostly hypothyroid), achlorhydria, atrophic gastritis, and antigastric parietal cell antibodies,* insulin dependent DM, SLE, Sjogren syndrome, vitiligo, RA, UC, myasthenia and gastrointestinal *non Hodgkins Lymphoma.*
- As in patients with celiac ds., dietary gluten sensitivity in DH is associated with *IgA endo mysial autoantibodies* that target tissue transglutaminase
- ***On direct immunofluorescence, IgA autoantibodies against epidermal trans glutaminase***Q ***& granular deposits of IgA in papillary dermis (dermal papillae)***Q.

Clinical Feature

- ***Intensly (itchy) pruritic***Q*, papulovesicular / urticarial* skin ds characterized by lesions symmetircally distributed over ***extensor surfaces (i.e. elbows, knees, buttocks, back, scalp & posterior neck)***Q
- Primary lesion is a *papule, papulovesicle or urticarial plaque.* Because pruritis is prominent, patients may present with ***excroation & crusted papules with no observable primary lesion***Q.
- Pruritis may have a distinctive *burning* or *stinging* component.
- May present at any age including childhood; but **2nd – 4th decades** are most commonly involved.

Diagnosis & Treatment

- Lesion biopsy reveal *subepidermal blister with neutrophils in dermal papillae i.e.* ***subepidermal bullae with papillary tip abscess***Q.
- ***Diagnosis is confirmed by direct immuno fluorescence microscopy of normal appearing or faintly erythematous perilesional skin (adjacent to active lesion)***Q, by demonstration of ***granular deposits of IgA (with or without complements) in papillary dermis***Q and along the epidermal basement membrane zone (EBMZ)
- IgA deposits in skin are unaffected by control of disease with *medication* dapsone; but decrease or disappear in patients maintained on long periods on a ***strict gluten – free diet***Q ***(treatment of choice).***
- ***Dapsone (diamino diphenyl sulfone = drug of choice), sulfoxone (diasone) & sulfapyridine control but do not cure disease.***
- ***Elemental diet (composed of free amino acids, short chain polysaccharides, & small amount of triglycerides) without full proteins can alleviate skin disease within few weeks.***
- ***Atkins diet with high protein, unlimited fat & low carbohydrate also l/t complete resolution of skin disease.***

Linear IgA Disease

- Once considered a variant form of dermatitis herpetiformis, is actually a ***seperate & distinct entity***[Q]. Clinically, these patients may resemble patients with case of DH, bullous pemphigoid or other ***subepidermal blistering disease***[Q].
- Lesions consist of papulovesicles, bullae, and / or urticarial plaques predominantly on extensor (as in DH), central or flexural sites. ***Severe pruritis***[Q] resembles that in patients with DH. Oral mucosal involvement occurs in some cases.
- Do not have an increased frequency of HLA – B8 / DRW3 halotype or an associated enteropathy & are hence are ***not candidates for gluten free diet***[Q].
- Histology may be indistinguishable from those in DH. However direct immunofluorescence microscopy of normal appearing perilesional skin reveal ***linear (not granular) deposits of IgA***[Q] (and often C_3) in the epidermal basement membrane zone.
- Demonstrate circulating *IgA anti-basement membrane autoantibodies against extracellular domain of BPAG2, a* transmembrane protein found in ***hemidesmosomes of basal keratinocytes.*** Respond to dapsone.

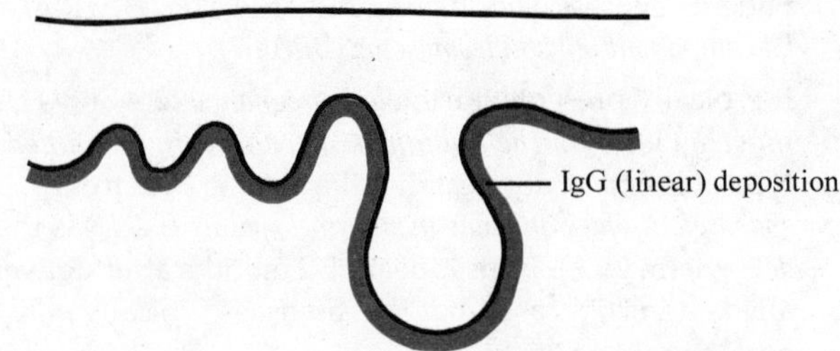

Direct immuno fluorescence of **bullous pemphigoid** showing linear basement membrane zone deposition of IgG

Erythema Multiformae (EM)

It is an *acute self limited, usually mild and often relapsing* mucocutaneous syndrome

Etiology

- **Infection** (*most common cause*)
- ***Herpes simplex virus***[Q] is definitely the **most common** cause; even more common in recurrent cases. **HSV1** is usually the cause but HSV-2 can also induce EM.
- *Mycoplasma pneumonial* is 2nd major cause of EM & may *even be major cause in pediatric cases.*
- ***Orf virus***[Q], varicella – zoster virus, parvo virus B19, hepatitis B & C viruses and infectious mononucleosis and a variety of other infections like histoplasmosis, coccidiomycosis, typhoid, leprosy etc.
- **Drugs** are a *rare* cause of EM
- ***Sulfonamides (most common drug)***[Q]
- Salicylates, penicillin, barbiturates, hydantoins and anti malariaals etc.
- *Malignancies* (such as lymphoma & carcinoma), *collagen vascular diseases* (eg. SLE, PAN, dermatomyosits), ultra violet & x-ray radiation, Crohn's ds & ulcerative colitis etc may be other rare causes.
- It is *type III hypersensitivity*
- May be associated with ***HLA – DQB1* 0301***[Q]

EM Subtypes

- **EM minor**: Skin lesions *without* involvement of mucous membrane
- **EM major**: skin lesions *with involvement of mucous membrane*
- **Mucosal EM (Fuchs syndrome, ectodermosis pluriorificialis):** mucous membrane lesions without cutaneous involvement
- **Herpes associated EM**

Clinic Presentation

- Occurs in all ages but mostly in *adolescents & young adults*, with a slight *male* preponderance' (3:2), *30% cases are recurrent.* Prodromal symptoms are mostly absent; and if present are usually mild, suggesting URTI eg cough, rhinitis, low grade fever.
- **Characteristic Target / Iris / Bull's eye /Annular lesion**
- *Abrupt onset, rapidly spreading* (usually all lesions appear in <3 days) ***symmetrical lesions***[Q] often *first appear acrally, and then spread in a centripetal manner.*
- Most occur in **symmetric acral distribution** on extensor surface of extremities (hand, feet, elbow & knees), face & neck and appear less frequently on thigh, buttocks & trunk.
- Influenced by mechanical factors (Koebner's phenomenon) & actinic factors (predilection of sun exposed sites).
- Usually asymptomatic but occasionally may be burning or itching.
- Typical lesion is highly regular, circular, wheal like erythematous papule or plaque, measuring from few mm-3cm and may expand slightly over 24-48 hours and persisting <2 weeks.
- It consists of atleast 3 concentric components l/t pink raised periphery & a necrotic dark blue violaceous (purpuric) centre **like the iris of eye or target of shooting range**:
  1. **Dusky central disk** or **blister**
  2. **Infiltrated pale edematous ring**
  3. **Peripheral erythematous halo**
- Not all lesions are typical; some display two rings only (raised atypical targets). However, ***all are papular in contrast with macules, which are the typical lesions in SJS-TEN***[Q]. However in contrast to SJS, EM patients are *younger, more often male, have higher recurrence* rates (10 times), & **less frequently** have high fever than 101.3°F (38.5°C) and involvement of **≥2 mucous membrane.**

Treatment

- Frequent recurrences can be prevented by *long term use of* anti-HSV medications (*acyclovir, valacyclovir & famciclovir*). However, it is of no use if HSV recurrence or herpes associated EM has occurred.
- Mild cases are not treated. Severe cases may require prednisone, dapsone, azathioprine, anti malarial or thalidomide.

- Larger lesions may have a central bullae and a concentric marginal ring of vesicles (**herpes iris of Bateman**). It is more frequent in *M. pneumoniae* related EM.
- Residual pigmentation may remain for months but there is no scarring.

- **Mucosal lesions** occur in ~70% patients and ***mostly involve lips, non attached gingivae & ventral side of tongue***[Q] (i.e. oral cavity). Hard palate & attached gingival are usually spared. Eye, nasal, **urethral & anal** mucosae may be involved.

Epidermal Necrolysis

Epidermal necrolysis (EN): Steven Johnson Syndrome (SJS) & Toxic Epidermal Necrolysis (TEN)

- It is *acute life threatening mucocutaneous reactions* characterized by extensive necrosis & detachment of epidermis. SJS & TEN are traditionally considered most severe form of EM. To differentiate both, **EM** is ***mostly post- infectious (HSV1 > M. pneumoniae)***[Q] disorder, often recurrent but with low morbidity and is characterized by **typical papular target lesions**. Whereas EN is usually a severe ***drug induced reaction***[Q] with high morbidity (*more frequent high grade fever & ≥ 2 mucous membrane involvement*) and poor prognosis.
- EN can occur at any age, with the *risk increasing with age after 4th decade*, and more frequently affects female (sex ratio 0 : 6).
- It characteristically presents as *initially symmetrical but irregularly shaped confluent purpuric & erythematous macules mainly localized on trunk & proximal limbs which evolve progressively to form confluent flaccid blisters* l/t epidermal detachment. Distal portions of arms & legs are relatively spared but rash can extend to rest of body with in hours - days.
- **Mucous membrane involvement** (nearly always on at least 2 sites) is present in ~ 90% case. *Oral cavity & vermilian border of lips* are almost invariably affected & show painful hemorrhagic erosions coated by greyish white pseudo membranes & crusts of lips. Approximately *85%* have *conjuctival lesions.*

Classification

- *According to total area in which epidermis is detached or detachable (positive Nikolsky)
  - SJS is < 10% body surface area
  - SJS /TEN over lap between 10-30%
  - TEN is > 30%
- Surface of one hand (palm & fingers) represent a little < 1% BSA.

SCORTEN: Prognostic scoring

Prognostic factor	Points
Body surface area involved > 10%	1
Serum urea >10mM	1
Serum glucose level >14mM	1
Serum bicarbonate <20 mM	1
Age > 40 years	1
Heart rate > 120/min	1
Cancer or hematological malignancy	1

Scorten	Mortality rate (%)
0 - 1	3.2
2	12.1
3	35.8
4	58.3
>5	90

Etiology

- ***Drugs are the most common etiological factor***[Q]. The risk seems confined to first 8 weeks (usually 4 – 30 days) of treatment.

High Risk	No risk
- **Sulfa**- drugs eg. **Sulfa**methoxazole, **Sulfa**diazine, **Sulfa**pyridine, ***Sulfa**doxine, **Sulfa**salazine, **Sulfo**namide (m.c.)*[Q] - **Phen**-drugs i.e. ***Pheno**barbital, **pheny**toin*[Q] (aromatic anticonvulsants), phenyl butazone - Mn: "**NOT ACL**" i.e **N**evirapine, ***O**xicam NSAIDs*[Q], **T**hiacetazone, **A**llopurinol (*HLA – B 5801* association in Han Chinese), **C**arbamazepine (HLA – B 1502), **L**amotrigine	*Sulfonyl urea*[Q] *Aspirin*[Q], Aldactone ACE inhibitor, angiotensin II receptor antagonist *Furosemide, thiazide diuretic*[Q] β blocker, calcium channel blocker Stains, hormones, vitamins.

Low risk	Doubtful risk
Acetic acid NSAIDs eg diclofenac, ***aminopenicillins***[Q], cephalosporins, quinolones, macrolides	*Paracetamol (acetaminophen), pyrazolone analgesic*, other NSAIDs (except aspirin), corticosterioid, sertaline

★ Infections, bone marrow transplantation, graft versus host disease, radiotherapy etc are other rare causes.

1

DERMATOLOGY

Molluscum Contagiosum

Etiology

- **Molluscum contagiosum virus (MCV)** is classified in **poxvirus family** & **molluscipox genus**.
- MCV is a large brick shaped pox virus that replicates within the cytoplasm of epithelial cells and infected cells replicate at twice the baseline rate. *It cannot be grown in tissue culture or eggs* and is not readily transmissible to laboratory animals.
- It infects humans and 98% of cases are caused by **MCV genotype 1**.

Histopathology

- Cup shaped (pear shaped with apex upwards) **epidermal thickening (hypertrophy & hyperplasia both)** with a characteristic generative change in granular cell layer.
- Basal layer remains intact. Above the basal layer, cells enlarge distort and ultimately destroyed and appear as large globular, **intracytoplasmic** eosinophillic inclusions **(hyaline bodies/molluscum bodies/Henderson-Paterson bodies).** These increase in size as the cells reach horny layer.

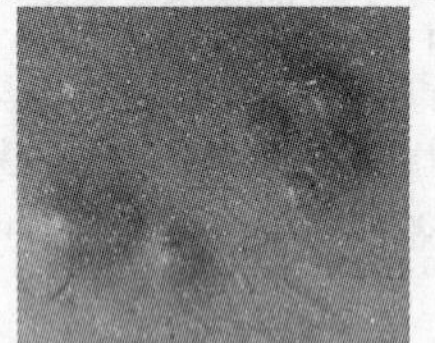

Transmission

- Via *direct skin, or mucous membrane contact or via fomites*. So both towels, swimming pools, Turkish bath, close contact sports (eg wrestling), ***sexual contact***[Q], autoinoculation & Koebnerization play a role in spread.
- In hot countries where children are lightly dressed, close contact within household is common mode.

Clinical Features

- **Characteristic lesions** are ***extremely small, pink, shiny pearly white or flesh/skin colored, dome shaped hemispherical papules***[Q] with a **central dell or umblication** containing a grayish central plug (pore) and white curd like substance.
- **It is commonly seen in school children with a peak b/w 2 to 5 years**[Q]. A later peak incidence in *young adults* with more common *genital lesions* is attributed to *sexual transmission*.
- Most patients develop ***multiple papules***[Q] commonly in *intertriginous regions* (such as axillae, popliteal fossae and groin), *face and genitals*.
- Distribution of lesion is affected by mode of infection, type of clothing (& hence climate). In cold temperate zones, neck or trunk (esp around axillae) and in hot tropics limbs are commonly involved, except in sexual transmission when anogenital region is usually involved. However, perianal & genital lesions in children are only rarely associated with sexual transmission.
- Most cases are self limiting within 6-9 months but some lesions may persist upto 5 years.

Treatment

- Watchful waiting, curettage, cautery, liquid N2 cryotherapy or simply squeezing (but avoid scratching).
- **Topical cantharidin**, cidofovir, podophyllin, imiquimod, silver nitrate, retinoids, trichloroacetic acid.
- Systemic cidofovir, cimetidine and subcutaneous interferon-α.

Lichen Nitidus

Feature	Lichen Nitidus	Molluscum contagiosum	Lichen planus
Symptoms	Asymptomatic	Asymptomatic	Itchy (marked)
Cutaneous lesion Lichen Nitidus	**Multiple, discrete** (or closely grouped**), minute, pinpoint to pinhead sized (1-2mm)**, flat/ round or dome shaped **papule** with a **glistening (shiny surface).** Papules are flesh colored or pink or shiny hypopigmented (in blacks)	**Extremely small, pink/shiny pearly white/or flesh-skin colored**, dome shaped hemispherical papules with a characteristic **central dell** or **umblication** containing a grayish central plug (pore) & **white curd like substance that** can be expressed with pressure. It may **enlarge slowly** to reach a diameter of 5-10 mm in 6-12 weeks (and occasionally, upto 3 cm giant molluscum)	**Larger,** plain (flat) topped, polygonal, pruritic, pink/purple (violaceous) papule
Wickham's striae	Absent	Absent	Present
Grouping	Present	Present	Usually not
Mucous membrane involvement	Uncommon	Not common	**Common** (Variably present)
Site	Anywhere; however most frequently on **flexural surfaces of upper extremities ie arm, forearm, wrist and dorsal surface of hands,** lower abdomen, breast, the **glans & shaft of penis** and other areas of **genital region**	**Intertriginous sites such as axillae, popliteal fossa and groin. Genital & perianal lesions** can develop in children & mostly are non-STD	Flexures (wrist), extremities (shin), lower back & genitals

Histology	- Dense, **circumscribed** & distinctive **infiltrate** of **histio-lymphocytic cells** situated directly beneath **thinned epidermis** results in widening of papillary dermis with **elongation & the appearance of embracement by neighboring rete ridges** (**Ball in clutch appearance**). Dermal infiltrate has histiocytes >> lymphocytes > foreign body / Touton type giant cells. Immunologically most of cells are T lymphocytes (**CD4+**>>> CD8+) intermixed with few to many **histiocyte macrophages (CD 68+)** > epidermal Langerhans cells and indeterminate (S 100+) cells - Thinned epidermis demonstrates **central parakeratosis**, variable / focal hyper keratosis **without hypergranulosis**, minimal hydropic degeneration & few dyskeratotic cells.	**Hypertrophied, hyperplastic epidermis** with intact basal cell layer. Above the basal layer, enlarged cells containing large intracytoplasmic inclusions (**Handerson - Paterson bodies)** are seen.	Hyperkeratotic hypergranulosis dyskeratotic epidermal hyperplasia, sub epidermal band like infiltrate extends through many rete ridges **(lichenoid band); Max Joseph histological cleft; Civatte colloid/ Cystoids bodies**; basal epidermal cell degeneration; CD4+ lymphocytes >>> CD68+ histiocytes > giant cell (none)
		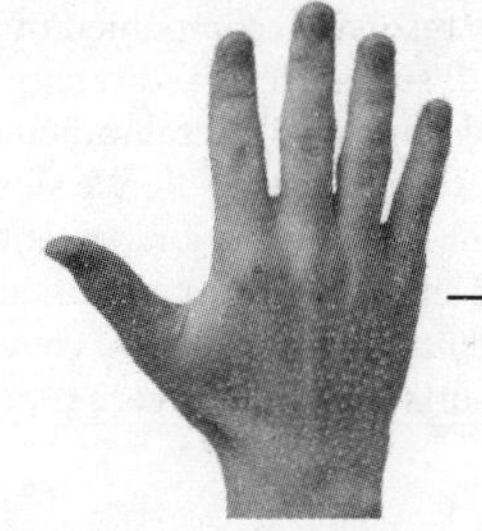	**Lichen Nitidus: Multiple, small, pin point, shiny, papular lesion on dorsal aspect of hand, forearms and penis**

Herpes

Herpes virus	Sub group	Other name
Human (Herpes) **simplex** virus, type 1 (**HSV1**)	α	Herpes virus hominis 1 (**HHV 1**)
Human (Herpes) **simplex** virus, type 2 (**HSV2**)	α	Herpes hominis virus 2 (**HHV2**)
Varicella **zoster virus** (VZV)	α	Herpesvirus varicellae (**HHV3**)
Cytomegalo virus (CMV)	β	HHV 4
Human herpes virus type 6 & 7	β	HHV 6 and 7
Human herpes virus type 8 (HHV 8)	γ	**Kaposi sarcoma associated herpes virus** (KSHV)
Epstein Barr virus (EBV)	γ	

Herpes virus group

Are relatively large, enveloped *DNA viruses* which replicate within the nucleus to produce ***typical eosinophilic intra nuclear inclusion bodies***[Q]. Virus *persists throughout the person's life as a latent infection* even following clinical recovery and may become ***reactivated***[Q].

Herpes Simplex (hominis) virus

- It is one of the commonest human infection throughout the world (HSV1 > HSV2). **HSV1** is mostly (& classically) a/w ***orofacial disease***[Q], whereas **HSV2** mostly causes ***genital infection***[Q]; although both can infect oral & genital areas and cause acute & recurrent infections.
- Both HSV1 & 2 are acquired by direct contact with infected secretion (or droplet) entering via skin or mucous membrane.
- Establishment of latent infection is common with virus persisting in **ganglia of sensory nerve innervating** the primary infection site. Latent virus produce no viral protein & therefore remain undetected by host defence mechanism. Virus may travel peripherally along nerve fiber, ***reactivate, replicate and cause recurrent disease***[Q]. Clinical variants include-

OroFacial (Gingivo-Stomatitis)	Herpes genitalis
- Most commonly a/w ***HSV-1 infection***[Q] and seen in childhood - Primary HSV-1 infections occur mainly in infants & young children (< 5 yr) and are usually	- Genital herpes is ***most prevalent STD worldwide***[Q] & is most common cause of ***ulcerative genital disease***[Q]. - ***Mostly caused by HSV-2***[Q] and rarely by HSV-1 (following oral-genital contact). - HSV-1 infection in a person with prior HSV-2 infection is unusual but HSV-2 acquisition in presence of previous HSV-1 is common. - Rate of **recurrence & reactivation** for genital

Herpes (Varicella) zoster virus

- **Vricella (chicken pox) & herpes zoster (shingles)** are two different clinical entities caused by varicella zoster virus
- *Chicken pox is highly contagious, acute exanthem* that occur mostly in childhood d/t primary infection of a susceptible individual. The rash usually begins on face & scalp and rapidly spreads to the trunk.
- *Lesions are scattered rather than clustered* and progress from *rose-colored macules to papules, vesicles, pustules & crusts* – all stages usually present at the sane time.
- **Herpes zoster** is characterized by ***unilateral dermatomal pain (in course of nerve) preceding rash***[Q] as a result of reactivation of endogenous VZV that had persisted in latent form within sensory ganglia after an earlier attack of varicella. It is *most common in older & immunosuppressed* individuals. *Thoracic*[Q] (53%) > cervical (usually $C_{2,3,4}$, 20%) > trigeminal including ophthalmic (15%) & lumbosacral (11%) dermatomes are most commonly involved. The erythematous, maculopapular and vesicular lesions of *herpes*

minimal, often **subclinical** and rarely produce painful vesicular stomatitis. - Rarely HSV-2 causes a primary orofacial infection, indistinguishable from HSV-1, except that it is seen in *adolescent & young adults* and *following genital-oral contact.* And it is 120 times less likely to reactivate than HSV-1 orolaabial disease.	**HSV-2** is 16 times **more frequent** than HSV-1 henital infection. - Primary HSV-2 infections are more commonly **symptomatic** & occur mainly **after puberty**. - Post HSV-1 infection may decrease the severity of primary HSV-2 infection, shortening the clinical course and reducing systemic symptoms. - Primary **infection** (both 2 & 1) presents with ***extensive genital lesions***Q in different stages of evolution (i.e. vesicles, pustules & erythematous ulcers) that may require 2-3 weeks to resolve, accompanied by pain, itching, dysuria, urethral discharge, ***tender lymphadenopathy***Q, sacral radiculomyelitis, neuralgia and systemic sign & symptoms. Recurrent HSV-2 infection presents with multiple small but grouped vesicular lesions in the genital area (anywhere covered by boxer shorts) with less severe prodrome.

zoster are clustered rather than scattered because virus reaches the skin via sensory nerve. Most important clinical manifestation is pain and similarly most common complication is *chronic pain or postherpetic neuralgia.* Clinical variants include

1. **Zoster sine herpete:** acute segmental neuralgia without ever developing a cutaneous eruption.
2. **Ramsay Hunt Syndrome (Herpes zoster oticus):** d/t involvement of ***facial & auditory nerves***Q, there is facial palsy with herpes zoster of external ear or tympanic membrane, with or without tinnitus, vertigo and deafness.
3. **Zoster ophthalmicus:** d/t involvement of ophthalmic (trigeminal) nerve. Eye is mostly affected in cases with vesicles on the side of nose indicating involvement of **nasociliary nerve (Hutchinson's sign)**.

Questions

Classification of Bullae

1. **All are vesiculo bullous lesions except-***(Kerala 96, PGI 03)*
   A, Dermatitis Herpetiformis ☐
   B. Scabies / Atopic dermatitis ☐
   C. Pemphigus ☐
   D. Pemphigoid ☐
2. **Subepidermal** lesion are *(PGI June 09)*
   A. Bullous pemphigoid ☐
   B. Pemphigus vulgaris ☐
   C. Hailey-Hailey disease ☐
   D. Darier's disease ☐
   E. Acanthosis nigricans ☐
3. **Subepithelial** Bullae are seen in: *(AIIMS 91)*
   A. Dermatitis herpatiforms ☐
   B. Molluscum contagiosum ☐
   C. Pemphigus ☐
   D. Pemphigoid ☐
4. **Subepidermal bulla are seen in -** *(AIIMS 91)*
   A. Pemphigoid ☐
   B. Pemphigus ☐
   C. Pityriasis rosea ☐
   D. Psoriasis ☐
5. **Blister formation in burn case is in :**
   A. Intraepidermal *(AI 2006)* ☐
   B. Subepidermal ☐
   C. Subdermal ☐
   D. Subfascial ☐
6. **Sub-epidermal splitting is not found in:**
   A. Bullous pemphigoid *(PGI 99)* ☐
   B. Pemphigus foliaceus ☐
   C. Dermatitis herpetiformis ☐
   D. Burns ☐
7. **Subepidermal bistreing is seen in all except -**
   A. Pemphigus vulgaris *(JIPMER 91, AMU 96)* ☐
   B. Dermatitis herpetiformis ☐
   C. Toxic epidermal necrolysis ☐
   D. Bullous pemphigoid ☐
   E. Hailey : Hailey disease ☐
8. **Which does not have subepidermal bullous:** *(PGI Nov 12)*
   A. Bullous pemphigoid ☐
   B. Dermatitis herpetiformis ☐
   C. Pemphigus vulgaris ☐
   D. Pemphigus follaceous ☐
   E. Cicatrical pemphigoid ☐
9. **Intra epidermal blisters are seen in:** *(PGI Nov 13, 12, 09)*
   A. Bullous pemphigoid ☐
   B. Pemphigus folliaceous ☐
   C. Dermatitis herpeteformis ☐
   D. Bullous SLE ☐
   E. Bullous impetigo, Hailey-Hailey disease ☐
   F. Pemphigus vulgaris ☐
   G. Trauma (thermal) ☐
10. Intra-**epidermal** acantholytic (blisters) vesicles are seen in
   A. Pemphigus vulgaris *(AIIMS 95, AI 91,PGI 08, 06, 04)* ☐
   B. Carcinomatous (paraneoplastic) pemphigus ☐
   C. Dermatitis herpetiformis ☐
   D. Congenital epidermolysis bullosa ☐
   E. Bullous pemphigoid ☐
11. **Acantholytic cell in pemphigus is derived from :**
   A. Stratum granulosum *(AIIMS 93)* ☐
   B. Stratum basale ☐
   C. Stratum spinosum ☐
   D. Langerhan's cell ☐

Acantholysis, Tzank Test & Nikolsky Sign

12. **Acantholysis is seen in:** *(PGI May 10, June 09)*
   A. Bullous pemphigoid/SSS ☐
   B. Dermatitis herpetiformis/Impetigo ☐
   C. Hailey- Hailey disease ☐
   D. Darrier's disease ☐
   E. Pemphigus vulgaris ☐
13. **Acantholysis is characteristic of:** *(AI 03, AIIMS 91)*
   A. Pemphigus vulgaris ☐
   B. Pemphigoid ☐
   C. Erythema multoforme ☐
   D. Dermatitis herpetiformis ☐
14. **Acantholysis is seen in all of the following except:**
   A. Pemphigus vulgaris & foliaceous*(PGI Nov 13, MP 06)* ☐
   B. Bullous pemphigoid ☐
   C. Grover's disease ☐
   D. Steven- Johnson syndrome, TEN ☐
   E. Darrier's disease, Hailey-Hailey disease ☐
15. **Acantholysis is due to destruction of**
   A. Epidermis *(AIIMS 97)* ☐
   B. Subepidermis ☐
   C. Basement memberane ☐
   D. Intercelluar substance ☐
16. **In pemphigus vulgaris, antibodies are present against:**
   A. Basement member *(SGPGI – 2000)* ☐
   B. Intercellular substance ☐
   C. Keratin ☐
   D. Cell nucleus ☐
17. **Acantholysis involves (is seen in):** *(PGI Dec 08, AI 95)*
   A. Epidermis ☐
   B. Dermis ☐
   C. Epidermis-Dermis junction ☐
   D. Subcutaneous tissue ☐
   E. Adipose tissue ☐
   F. All layers ☐
18. **Acantholytic cells are :** *(SGPGI – 2001)*
   A. Epidermal cells ☐
   B. Plasma cells ☐
   C. Keratinocytes ☐
   D. Giant cells ☐
19. **Acantolytic cells in pemphigus is-** *(PGI 96)*
   A. Cell with hyperchromatic nuclei and perinuclear halo ☐
   B. Cell with hypochromatic nuclei and perinuclear halo ☐
   C. Multinucleated cells ☐
   D. None of the above ☐
20. **A 40 year old male reported with recurrent episodes of oral ulcers, large areas of denuded skin and flacid vesiculo-bullous eruptions. Which is the most important bed-side investigation helpful in establishing the diagnosis -** *(Karn. 94)*
   A. Gram staining of the blister fluid ☐
   B. Culture and sensitivity ☐
   C. Skin biopsy and immunoflurescence ☐

D. Tzanck smear from the floor of bulla ☐

21. A 50 years old man has a 2 year history of facial bullae & oral ulcers. Microscpic smear from skin lesions is most likely to disclose - *(AI 96)*
A. Tzanck cells ☐
B. Acantholytic cells ☐
C. Necrosis ☐
D. Koilogytosis ☐

22. Tzank cell is a - *(AI 98)*
A. Lymphocyte ☐
B. Monocyte ☐
C. Neutrophil ☐
D. Keratinocyte ☐
E. Eosinophil ☐

23. A patient has Bullous Lesion; on Tzank smear *(AI 96)*
A. Langerhans cells are seen ☐
B. AconthＯlysis ☐
C. Leucocytosis ☐
D. Absence of melanin pigment ☐

24. Tzank smear helps in the diagnosis of :
A. Herpes viral infection *(MP 05)* ☐
B. Bullous pemphigoids ☐
C. Carcinoma of cervix ☐
D. None ☐

25. In Tzank smear multinucleated cells are seen in:*(PGI 97)*
A. Chicken pox ☐
B. Psoriasis ☐
C. Molluscum contagiosum ☐
D. Pemphigus vulgaris ☐

26. Nikolsky sign is positive in all of the following except:
A. Staphylococcal scalded skin syndrome ☐
B. Toxic epidermonecrolysis *(MP 06, DNB 08,* ☐
C. Bullous pemphigoid *AIIMS 2K)* ☐
D. Pemphigus ☐

27. Nikolsky sign is seen in - *(PGI 86)*
A. Pemphigus vulgaris ☐
B. Herpes zoster ☐
C. Herpes simlex ☐
D. Leukemia ☐
E. All of the above ☐

28. Nikolsky sign not present in: *(Bihar 06, DNB 09)*
A. Pemphigus ☐
B. Pemphigoid ☐
C. Vitiligo ☐
D. Staphylococcal scalded syndrome ☐

Etiology

29. An auto immune disease is: *(AI 2000)*
A. Pemphigus Vulgaris ☐
B. Psoriasis ☐
C. Lichen Planus ☐
D. Acne Vulgaris ☐

30. Genetic predisposition is seen in which disease: *(PGI 97)*
A. Lichen planus ☐
B. Bullous pemphigoid ☐
C. Pemphigus vulgaris ☐
D. Epidermolysis Bullosa ☐

Dyskeratosis

31. Hailey – hailey disease is: *(Jharkhand 03)*
A. Benign familial chronic pemphigus ☐
B. Pemphigus acutus ☐
C. Pemphigus ☐
D. Lyell's syndrome ☐

32. Dyskeratosis is characteristic feature of : *(PGI 2000)*
A. Darrier's ds ☐
B. Pemphigus vulgaris ☐
C. Psoriasis ☐
D. Boweli's disease ☐
E. Haikey-Hailey ds ☐

Epidermolysis Bullosa

33. Etiology of Epidermolysis bullosa is -
A. Genetic *(Rohtak 97)* ☐
B. Infections ☐
C. Senile ☐
D. Malignant ☐
E. Metabolic ☐

34. In congenital dystrophic epidermolysis bullosa defect is seen in: *(AIIMS Nov 2008)*
A. Laminin 4 ☐
B. Collagen type 7 ☐
C. Collagen 4 ☐
D. Collagen 3 ☐

35. In a 8 day old child with no history of consanguinity in the parents. The mother reports blisters and peeling off of skin at the site of handling and pressure. There was a similar history in previous child which proved to be fatal. The diagnosis:
A. Bullous pemphigod *(AIIMS 01)* ☐
B. Conegntial Syphillis ☐
C. Congential Epidermolysis bullosa ☐
D. Letterrer siwe disease ☐

36. A 2 day old newborn girl born out of non-consanguinous marriage was evaluated for tense blister and areas of denuded skin that had been present since birth. The child develops while mother handles for bathing and feeding. The sibling of child also had h/o developing similar lesions. *(AI 12)*
A. Congenital syphilis ☐
B. Congenital epidermolysis bullosa ☐
C. LCH ☐
D. Congenital bullous icthyosiform erythroderma ☐

37. A patient developed bullae without erythema on elbows, knee & sacral area f/b crust formation, scarring & milia. He had no photo sensitivity and negative family history for bullous diseases. On DIF IgG deposition at DEJ with no blood vessel involvement is seen probable diagnosis is
A. EB dystrophic *(AIIMS Feb 07)* ☐
B. EB acquisita ☐
C. Porphyria CT ☐
D. Pemphigoid bullous ☐

Pemphigus

38. Commonest/rarest veriety of Pemphigus-
A. Pemphigus vulgaris/vegetans *(Kerala 98)* ☐
B. Pemphigus vegetans/vulgaris ☐
C. Pemphigus fliaceus/erythematosis ☐
D. Pemphigus erythematosia/foliaceous ☐

39. 'Row of tombstones' appearance is seen in :
A. Irritant dermatitis *(Jipmer 98, PGI 02)* ☐
B. Pemphigus ☐
C. Pemphigoid ☐
D. Harpes zoster ☐

40. In pemphigus vulgaris, antibodies are present against :
A. Basement membrane *(PGI 2000)* ☐
B. Intercellular substance ☐
C. Cell nucleus ☐

D. Keratin ☐
E. Cell membrane ☐

41. True about pemphigus vulgaris A/E: *(PGI June 09)*
A. Subepidermal ☐
B. Autoimmune disease ☐
C. Tzanck smear shows acanthoyltic cells ☐
D. Antibody are formed against desmogleins ☐
E. Blister on skin & mucosa ☐

42. A patient with Bullous eruption on lower limb and trunk, biopsy show epidermal bullae. The correct diagnosis is: *(AI 2000)*
A. Pemphigoid ☐
B. Pemphigus Vulgaris ☐
C. Impetigo ☐
D. Internal Malignany ☐

43. A 24 years old (middle aged) female has flaccid bullae in the skin and persistent painful oral erosions (palatal & vestibular lesions in buccal mucosa). Histopathology shows intraepidermal acantholytic blister. The most likely diagnosis is
A. Bullous Pemphigoid. *(PGI Dec 05, AI 08, 97)* ☐
B. Erythema multiforme. *(AIIMS May03)* ☐
C. Pemphigus vulgaris. ☐
D. Dermatitis herpetiformis. ☐
E. Epidermolysis bullosa acquista ☐

44. A 40 year old male developed persistant oral ulcers followed by multiple flaccid bullae on trunk and extremities. Direct examination of a skin biopsy immunoflurescence showed intercellular IgG deposits in the epidermis. The most probable diagnosis is: *(AI 03)*
A. Pemphigus vulgaris ☐
B. Bullous Pemphigoid ☐
C. Bullous Lupus erythematosus ☐
D. Epidermolysis bullosa acquisita ☐

45. A 50 year old male known case of myasthe-nia with erythemated shallow erosions with few blisters and scales. Oral mucosa is not involved. Immunopathology demonstrates IgG deposition on keratinocytes and auto antibodies against Dsg – 1. The diagnosis is
A. Pemphigus vulgaris *(PGI – 98)* ☐
B. Bullous pemphigoid ☐
C. Pemphigus foliaceus ☐
D. Dermatitis herpetiformis ☐

46. Drug induced pemphigus is seen in all except *(AI 94)*
A. Penicillin ☐
B. Phenopthelein ☐
C. Iodine ☐
D. Frusemide ☐

47. All are asociated with pemphigus except:
A. Thymoma *(PGI 98, 02)* ☐
B. CLL ☐
C. Myasthenia gravis ☐
D. Non- Hodgkins lymphoma ☐
E. Atrophic gastritis ☐

48. Mucous lesions are seen in : *(PGI 02, AIIMS 92)*
A. Sec. syphilis ☐
B. Dermatitis herpetiformis ☐
C. Psoriasis ☐
D. Pemphigus ☐
E. Porphyria ☐

49. A patient has oral ulcer and skin bullae & large erosions which are slow to heal. The lesion is: *(AIIMS Nov 12)*
A. Intradermal ☐
B. Suprabasal ☐
C. Epidermal ☐
D. Sub corneal ☐

50. A 56 year old male lallu presents with painful bullous lesion in lower extrimity, the most likely diagnosis is
A. Pemphigus Vulgaris *(AIIMS 97)* ☐
B. Bullous pemphigoid ☐
C. Necrotic Pemphigus ☐
D. Contact eczema ☐

51. A 85 year old woman with Nikolsky sign-ve, blisters on thigh & trunk, lesions come on & off. What is the cause :
A. Pemphigus vulgaris *(PGI 2000)* ☐
B. Pemphigoid ☐
C. Lichen planus ☐
D. Dermatitis herpetiformis ☐
E. Leprosy ☐

Direct Immunofluorescence Microscopy

52. 60 years old man presented with itchy tense blisters on normal looking skin and urticarial rash, Investigation done for the diagnosis: *(AIIMS May 13)*
A. Direct immunofluorescence (DIF) ☐
B. Indirect immunofluorescent ☐
C. Histopathology ☐
D. Cytopathology ☐

53. A young boy with multiple flaccid bullous lesions over trunk with oral mucosal lesions. Most likely finding on biopsy would be: *(AIIMS Nov 09)*
A. 'Fishnet' IgG deposits in epidermis ☐
B. Linear IgG in Deposits ☐
C. Linear IgA in dermal papillae ☐
D. Granular IgA in reticular dermis ☐

54. Inter cellular IgG deposition in epidermis is seen in:
A. Pemphigus *(AIIMS May 09, Nov 11)* ☐
B. Sub corneal pustular dermatosis ☐
C. Bullus pemphigoid ☐
D. Dermatitis Herpetiformis ☐

55. Direct immunofluorescence is positive in
A. Atopic dermatitis *(PGI 02)* ☐
B. SLE ☐
C. Pemphigus ☐
D. Secondary syphilis ☐

56. A 40 year old male had multiple blisters over the trunk & Extremities. Direct Immuno fluoresce studies showed linear IgG deposits along the Basement membrane, which of the following is the most likely diagnosis.
A. Pemphigus vulgaris *(AIIMS Nov 2004)* ☐
B. Bullous pemphigoid ☐
C. Pemphigus foliaceous ☐
D. Dermatitis herpetiformis ☐

57. Granular IgA deposit at dermal papilla are found in:
A. Dermatitis Herpetiformis *(AIIMS May 09, Nov 11)* ☐
B. IgA disease of childhood ☐
C. Herpetic gestation ☐
D. Bullous pemphigoid ☐

58. Skin disease not showing DIF (Direct immunofluorescence): *(PGI Nov2010)*
A. Darrier's disease ☐
B. Hailey-Hailey disease ☐
C. Cicatricial pemphigoid ☐
D. Dermatitis herpatiformis ☐
E. Pemphigus ☐

Pemphigoid Gestationalis

59. Spontaneous remission is most frequent with
A. Herpes labialis *(SGPGI 04, DNB 05)* ☐
B. Herpes genitalis ☐
C. Herpetic chancroid ☐
D. Herpes gestationis ☐

60. Commonest site of herpes Gestationis is-
A. Periumbilical region *(AIIMS 93, Delhi 02)* ☐
B. Flanks of abdomen ☐
C. Vulva ☐
D. Infraorbital ☐

Dermatitis Herpetiformis

61. HLA associated with dermatitis Herpetiformis- *(AI 98)*
A. HLA A5 ☐
B. HLB B8 ☐
C. HLA B27 ☐
D. HLA A28 ☐

62. All are true about dermatitis herpetformis except
A. More common in young adult ☐
B. Intense pruritus *(JHARKHAND 05)* ☐
C. Deposist of IgG at the epidermodermal lesion ☐
D. None ☐

63. A 30 year old male had severely itchy papula-vesicular lesions on both knees, elbows, upper back and buttocks for one year. Direct immunofluorescence staining of the lesions showed IgA deposition at dermoepidermal junction and dermal papilla. The most probable diagnosis is : *(AI 12, 04, AIIMS Nov 02)*
A. Pemphigus vulagris ☐
B. Bullous pemphigoid ☐
C. Dermatitis herpetiforms ☐
D. Nummular eczema ☐

64. Extermely pruritic excoriation & papules on buttocks with autoantibodies against epidermal transglutaminase and IgA deposition in dermis on immuno-histological examination of normal perilesional skin. Diagnosis is:
A. Pemphigus vulgaris *(SGPGI 01)* ☐
B. Pemphigoid ☐
C. Linear IgA disease ☐
D. Dermatitis herpetiformis ☐

65. DOC for dermatitis herpetiformis is:
A. Steroids *(AIIMS 97, 92, 91, May 05)* ☐
B. Dapsone ☐
C. PUVA ☐
D. Antihistaminic ☐

66. The treatment of Dermatitis herpetiformis is -
A. Gluten free diet with minerals and vitamins ☐
B. Carbamazepine *(AI 02, Kerala 96)* ☐
C. Acyclovir ☐
D. Corticosteroids ☐

67. What can patient with gluten sensitive hypersensitivity consume as food:
A. Rice *(PGI June 2006)* ☐
B. Barley ☐
C. Oat ☐
D. Corn ☐
E. Rye ☐

Linear IgA Disease

68. All are true about linear IgA disease except
A. Subepidermal involvement *(PGI 2001)* ☐
B. Severe itching ☐
C. Granular deposition of IgA ☐
D. Are candidates for gluten free diet ☐
E. A variant of dermatitis herpetiformis. ☐

Erythema Multiformae

69. Commonest etiology of erythema multiforme is -
A. Viral *(AI 95, DNB 99, UP 02)* ☐
B. Bacterial ☐
C. Food ☐
D. Drugs ☐

70. All are true about erythema multiformis except:
A. Due to herpes simplex *(Jharkhand 05)* ☐
B. Due to sulphonamide ☐
C. Lesion are symmetrical ☐
D. Mucous membrane is involved in all ☐

71. Target or Iris lesion seen in *(AI 97, 98)*
A. Urticaria ☐
B. Erythema mutiformae ☐
C. Scabies ☐
D. Lichen Planus ☐

72. Regarding Erythema multiforme all are true except:
A. No vesicles *(AI 2K)* ☐
B. Target lesions are seen ☐
C. Involves face and neck regions ☐
D. Sign of internal malignancy ☐

Epidermal Necrolysis, SJS, TEN and SSS

73. A 60- year – old patient presented with several bullous lesions for the last 3 days; each bulla was surrounded by an erythematous halo. There were multiple target lesions. Patient also had oral erosions. The most likely diagnosis is: *(SGPGI – 2004)*
A. Chicken pox ☐
B. Herpes simplex ☐
C. Herpes zoster ☐
D. Steven- Johnson syndrome ☐

74. Toxic epidermonercrolysis is caused by: *(PGI 04)*
A. Phenytoin ☐
B. Penicillin ☐
C. Erythromycin ☐
D. Gold ☐

75. All are considered to be high risk agents for TEN except
A. Sulfonamide *(PGI- 07)* ☐
B. Sulfonyl urea ☐
C. Aspirin ☐
D. Oxicam ☐
E. Phenytoin ☐

76. A 3 months old male infant developed otitis media for which he was given a course of Co-trimoxazole. A few days later, he developed extensive peeling of the skin; there were no mucosal lesions and the baby was not toxic. The most likely diagnosis is: *(AIIMS 04)*
A. Toxic epidermal necrolysis ☐
B. Staphylococcal scalded skin syndrome ☐
C. Steven Johnsom syndrome ☐
D. Infantile pemphigus ☐

BURN

77. Which layer of skin causes vesicular chamge in case of burn: *(AIIMS 97)*
A. Basal layer ☐
B. Papillary layer ☐
C. Epidermis ☐
D. Dermis ☐

Molluscum Contagiosum

78. Causative organism of molluscum contagiosum is-
A. Papova virus *(AIIMS 99)* ☐
B. Pox virus ☐
C. Orthomyxo virus ☐
D. Parvo virus ☐

79. An eight year old boy presents with multiple umbilicated pearly white papules on trunk & face following a trivial infection. Diagnosis is : *(AIIMS 98, 96)*
A. Molluscum Contagiosum ☐
B. Chicken Pox ☐

C. Herpes zoster ☐
D. Dermatophytosis ☐

80. **Which of the following is true of molluscum contagiosum-** *(Kerala 97)*
A. Treatment is extirption ☐
B. Is an STD ☐
C. Virall infection ☐
D. Central umbilication ☐
E. All are correct ☐

Lichen Nitidus

81. **A young 8 years old boy with multiple, small, pin point, shiny, papular lesion on dorsal aspect of hand, forearms and his penis also, Diagnosis at:**
A. Molluscum contagiosum *(AIIMS May 13)* ☐
B. Scabies ☐
C. Lichen planus ☐
D. Lichen nitidus ☐

Herpes

82. **Herpes zoster is commonly seen in a :** *(AI 99)* ☐
A. Cervical region ☐
B. Thoracic region ☐
C. Lumbar region ☐
D. Geniculate ganglion ☐

83. **Ballooning is characteristic of :** *(Jipmer 92)*
A. Harpes zoster ☐
B. Pemphigus ☐
C. Pemphigoid ☐
D. Insect bite ☐

84. **A 45 year old male has multiple grouped vesicular lesions present on the T10 segment dermatome associated with pain. The most likely diagnosis is**
A. Herpes zoster *(AIIMS Nov 02)* ☐
B. Dermatitis herpetiformis ☐
C. Herpes simplex ☐
D. Scabies ☐

85. **An old patient presents with painful red vesicular eruption confined to T3 dermatome. Diagnosis:**
A. Varicella zoster *(AIIMS May 13)* ☐
B. Herpes simplex ☐
C. HIV ☐
D. HPV ☐

86. **Most common site of affection of herpes simplex-**
A. Thorax *(UP 96)* ☐
B. Abdomen ☐
C. Face ☐
D. Extremities ☐

87. **The most frequent cause of recurrent genital ulceration in a sexually active male is** *(AI 03)*
A. Herpes genitalis ☐
B. Aphthous ulcer ☐
C. Syphilis ☐
D. Chancroid ☐

88. **Drug of choice in Herpes zoster** *(AIIMS 99, 98, 96)*
A. Acyclovir ☐
B. Vidarabine ☐
C. Idoxuridine ☐
D. Actinomycin ☐

89. **Herpes resistant to acyclovir is treated by** *(Jipmer 02)*
A. Foscarnet ☐
B. Lamivudine ☐
C. Ganciclovir ☐
D. Valocyclovir ☐

ANSWERS AND EXPLANATIONS:

Classification of Bullae

1. **B. i.e. Scabies**
2. **A i.e. Bullous pemphigoid**
3. **D i.e. Pemphigoid; A i.e. Dermatitis herpetiformis**
4. **A. i.e. Pemphigoid**
5. **B. i.e. Sub epidermal**
6. **B i.e. Pemphigus foliaceous**
7. **A. i.e. Pemphigus vulgaris C. i.e. Toxic epidermal necrolysis E. i.e. Hailey- Hailey disease**
8. **C i.e. Pemphigus vulgaris; D i.e. Pemphigus foliaceous**
9. **B, E, F i.e. Pemphigus folliaceous; Bullous impetigo, hailey-Hailey disease; Pemphigus vulgaris**
10. **A & B i.e. (Pemphigus vulgaris) & (Carcinomatous pemphigus)**
11. **C i.e. Stratum spinosum**

[Ref: Harrison's 17/e p-336; Thomas Habif Clinical Dermatology 4/e p. 549; Fitzpatrick 7/e p. 45-47, 349, 459- 84, 1714, 1878, 1892; Rooks Textbook of Dermatology 8/e p.40.3-40.64; Roxburough 17/e p. 89-92]

Pemphigus (vulgaris[Q]*,* vegetans, foliaceus, erythematous, endemic, ***paraneoplastic***[Q]) ***causes intra epidermal***[Q] and ***Pemphigoid***[Q] (bullous, cicatricial, gestations, linear IgA disease) causes ***sub epidermal bullae formation***[Q]. **Blisters (vesicles, bullae or split) are *intra epidermal in pemphigus and subepidermal in pemphigoid and dermatitis herpetiformis***[Q]

Histological site of Bullae (Blister) Formation (Lever Classification)

Intra-Epidermal

- **Acantholytic**
  - *Darier (white) disease*Q
  - *Hailey-Hailey disease*Q
  - Grover disease
  - **Pemphigus** family i.e.
    1. **P.vulgaris** or **vegetans**
    2. **P. foliaceus** or **herpetiformis** or **erythematosus**
    3. Paraneoplastic & induced (eg drug) pemphigus
    4. Intercellular IgA dermatosis or IgA herpetiform vesicopustular dermatosis (pemphigus) or intraepidermal neutrophilic IgA dermatosis
- Viral (Herpes simplex, H. zoster, variola, varicella)
- **Friction blister**, insect bite, scabies, miliaria rubra
- Spongiotic pompholyx & eczema

Sub-Epidermal

The entire epidermis separates from the dermis as in

The	Thermal (*burn*Q, cold, liquid N_2) blisters
Linear	**Linear** IgA disease / chronic bullous disease of childhood / Juvenile (linear) pemphigoid or dermatitis herpetiformis
Erythematous	**Erythema** multiformae
Dermal	***Dermatitis herpetiformis***Q (Duhring Brocq disease)
Epidermal	**Epidermolysis bullosa** acquisita (acquired)/Dermolytic pemphigoid
Bullous	**Bullous** *SLE*Q
	Bullous ***pemphigoid***Q (pemphigoid nodularis or vegetans) — Pemphigoid
	Pemphigoid (Herpes) gestationalisQ — Pemphigoid
Lesions in	**Bullous lichen** planus (lichen planus pemphigoides) — Pemphigoid
Mucous membrane	**Mucous membrane** ***(oral/Cicatrical/scarring/Brunsting Perry) pemphigoid***Q or ocular pemphigus — Pemphigoid

Sub corneal (Superficial)

- Acantholytic blister formed in superficial layer of epidermis at the level of *stratum granulosum*
- *Stratum corneum* forms the roof of bullae
- As in ***bullous impetigo or pemphigus foliaceous***Q

Suprabasal (Deep)

- ***In pemphigus vulgaris***Q and *pemphigus vegetans*, acantholysis selectively involves the layer of cells *immediately above the basal cell layer*
- The single layer of intact basal cells that forms the blister base has been likened to a row of tomb stones.
- The pemphigus vegetans has considerable overlying *epidermal hyperplasia*. The ***suprabasal acantholytic blister is characteristic of pemphigus vulgaris***Q (in which acantholytic cells are derived from ***stratum spinosum***Q).

Acantholysis, Tzank Test & Nikolsky Sign

12. **C, D, E i.e. Hailey- Hailey disease; Darrier's disease; Pemphigus vulgaris**
13. **A i.e. Pemphigus Vulgaris**
14. **B. i.e. Bullous pemphigoid**
15. **D i.e. Intercellular substance**
16. **B. i.e. Intercellular substance**
17. **A. i.e. Epidermis**
18. **C. i.e. Keratinocytes**
19. **A. i.e. Cells with hyper chromatic nuclei & perinuclear halo**

[Ref: Fitzpatrick 7/e p. 46- 47, 60, 432- 41, 1850, 1877-78, 1892, 43; 46, 57-99; Neena Khanna 3rd/e p-63, 15, 61, 66; Roxburgh's 17/e p- 92-91; Harrison's 17/e p- 336; Robbins 6/e p- 1260- 61; Rook's 8/e p- 10.36-10.37; Pasricha 10/e p- 281-83]

- **Acantholysis** is ***seen in epidermis as loss of cohesion between epidermal cells d/t lysis of intercellular substance (intercellular adhesion sites***Q***)***. Acantholytic cells are ***rounded keratinocytes with hyperchromatic nuclei & perinuclear halo***Q. Acantholysis is seen in ***pemphigus, Darier's disease, Grover's disease and Hailey-Hailey disease (but not in pemphigoid)*** Q.
- **Primary acantholysis** (i.e. acantholysis is primary pathological change) is seen in **pemphigus** variants (vulgaris, vegetans, paraneoplastic, foliaceous, erythematosus), **Hailey-Hailey disease** (familial benign chronic pemphigus), **Darrier's disease** (Keratosis follicularis), **Grover's disease** (transient acantholytic dermatosis), persistent acantholytic dermatosis, warty dyskeratoma, and eosinophilic spongiosis. Acantholysis (i.e. loss of cohesion b/w keratinocytes d/t breakdown of intercellular bridges) result in formation of intraepidermal clefts, vesicles & bullae.
- **Secondary acantholysis** (i.e. secondary to some other pathological change like damage in epidermal cells) occurs in *bullous impetigo, SSSS, viral disorders, solar keratosis & squamous cell carcinoma.*

20. **D. i.e. Tzank smear** 21. **B. i.e. Acantholytic cell** 22. **D. i.e. Keratinocyte**
23. **B i.e. Acantholysis** 24. **A. i.e. Herpes** 25. **A i.e. Chicken pox**
[Rooks 8/e p. 5.21, 10.28-10.29, 35.28, 40.8]

- In patients with *vesico-bullous lesions and oral ulcer (mucosal involvement)*, the diagnosis is pemphigus vulgaris and the bed side **diagnostic Tzank test from floor of bullae** shows ***acantholysis with numerous acantholytic keratinocyte cells***Q.
- In Tzank smear **diagnostic multinucleated giant cells with ballooning degeneration** is seen in ***herpes simplex, herpes zoster and varicella zoster (chicken pox) virus***Q.

26. **C. i.e. Bullous pemphigoid** 27. **E. i.e. All** 28. **C. i.e. Vitiligo > B Pemphigoid**

Nikolsky sign is seen in pemphigus (all types), SSS, SJS, TEN, herpes and leukemia but ***not in bullous pemphigoid and vitiligo***Q.

ETIOLOGY

29. **A i.e. Pemphigus vulgaris** 30. **D i.e. Epidermolysis bullosa**
[Ref: Roxburgh's 17/e p. 90; Fitzpatrick's 6/e p-609-615; Rooks Textbook of Dermatology 7/e p.40.7-40.29]

Disease	Etiology
Pemphigus Pemphigoid, Epidermolysis bullosa acquisita	***Autoimmune***Q
Lichen planus	Inflamatory disorder of unknown origin
Acne vulgaris	***Obstruction of pilo-sebaceous gland.***Q
Epidermolysis bullosa congenita Psoriasis	***Genetic disease***Q of unknown origin *Genetic ds*Q unknown (inflamatory) origin

Dyskeratosis

31. **A. i.e. Benign Familial Chronic Pemphigus** *[Ref: Roxburgh's-Common Skin disease 17/e p.*
32. **A i.e. Darrier's ds; D i.e. Bowen's ds; E i.e. Hailey-Hailey ds** *136, 211, 212, 255, 254; Behl's 8/e P-21]*

Dyskeratosis means imperfect & premature keratinization taking on various shapes. It may be:

Benign
- ***Darrier's ds***Q
- ***Hailey-Hailey ds.***Q
  *(chronic benign familial pemphigus)*Q

Mnemonic - **"DH–BSP"**

Malignant

In epithelioma as:
- ***Bowen's ds***Q
- Squamous cell CA
- Pagets ds.

✶ In **Psoriasis** – *parakeratosis* (ie epidermal nuclei are retained in the inefficient horny layer) is seen.

Epidermolysis Bullosa

33. **A. i.e. Genetic** 34. **B. i.e. Collagen 7**
35. **C i.e. Congenital Epidermolysis bullosa** 36. **B i.e. Congenital Epidermolysis bullosa**
37. **B i.e. EB acquisita** *Ref: Fitapatrick 7/e p. 494- 99, 458; Harrison's 17/e p- 2469; Thomas Habif Clinical Dermatology 4/e p. 574- 76; Roxburgh's 17/e p- 90-91; Pasricha 4/e p- 51, 505-12; Rooks 8/e p. 40.51-40.56]*

- **Epidermolysis bullosa congenita** is ***inherited genodermatoses (genetic disorder)***Q, whereas epidermolysis bullosa **acquisita** a *sporadic autoimmune* bullous (blistering) disease, in which the ***skin and related epithelial tissue break and blister as a result of minor trauma***Q. It presents with skin fragility, spontaneous or trauma induced ***non inflammatory (non erythematous) tense bullae (l/t peeling of skin) over trauma prone surfaces such as sacral area, elbow, knee***Q, back of hands, knuckles, palm, soles & toes in adults & children. These lesions ***heal with scarring, scaling, crust formation or erosions and pearl like milia cyst formation***Q.
- **Direct immune-electron microscopy (gold standard) and ditrect immune-fluorescence (DIF)** of perilesional skin shows intense, ***linear, homogenous fluorescent band of IgG & C3 at dermoepidermal junction (DEJ)***Q.
- **α chain of collagen 7** is defective in EB aquisita and congenital (dystrophic type) both. Whereas, in EB congenital – collagen 17 (α1 chain), pelctin 1, laminin α3/β3/γ2, integrin α-6/β-4 and keratin may be defective also.

Pemphigus

38. **A. i.e. Pemphigus vulgaris/vegetans**
39. **B. i.e. Pemphigus**
40. **B i.e. Intercellular substance**
41. **A i.e. Subepidermal**
42. **B i.e. Pemphigus vulgaris**
43. **C i.e. Pemphigus vulgaris**
44. **A i.e. Pemphigus Vulgaris** *[Ref: Rooks 8/e p. 40.1-40.20; Roxburgh's 18/e p. 102-104; Fitzpatrick's 7/e p 459-74; Harrison's 18/e p. 424-26]*

- **Pemphigus vulgaris** is the **commonest** and pemphigus **vegetans** is the **rarest** variety.
- In **pemphigus vulgaris (an auto immune disease)**, *autoantibodies (IgG) are directed against intercellular substance desmogleins (Dsgs)*Q, a transmembrane desmosomal glycoprotein that belong to cadherin supergene family of calcium dependent adhesion molecules causing *loss of cohesion (acantholysis)*Q between epidermal cells of *deep stratum basal layer*Q. That is why, *histology (tzanck smear) show (intra) epidermal acantholytic bullae (blister) in deep supra basal layer of epidermis*Q along with single layer of intact stratum basale cells attached to basement membrane **(row of tomb stone appearance)** that form the base of blister. Indirect immuno fluorescence microscopy demonstrate circulating *autoantibodies against keratinocyte cell surface antigen whereas diagnostic (gold standard) direct immunofluorescence microscopy (DIM) show deposits of IgG on the surface keratinocyte in fishnet like pattern*Q and in intercellular space (causing it to widen).
- Pemphigus vulgaris presents as **muco-cutaneous lesions (blister or erosions)** *predominantly in middle aged patients (> 40 year age). It typically begins on mucosal surface and nearly all patients have mucosal involvement (oral in 70%* Q >> ocular, nasal, pharyngeal, larynx, oesophagus, urethra, vulva, cervix). PV often progresses to **widespread skin involvement** with a predilection for *scalp, face, neck, axillae, groin, trunk* Q and pressure points.
- PV is characterized by *painful, mostly non pruritic, fragile flaccid blisters*Q filled with clear fluid **on a normal or erythematous base** that ruptures to produce extensive denudation of mucous membranes and skin resulting in ill defined irregular shaped erosions. Healing occurs **without scarring but with temporary hyperpigmentation.**

45. **C i.e. Pemphigus foliaceus**

Pemphigus foliaceous (PF) is distinguished from PV by following features-

- Distribution of lesion in both is much the same (i.e. **seborrheic distribution** including face, scalp and upper trunk) except that *in PF the mucous membranes are almost always spared*Q.
- Characteristic clinical lesions of PF are *well demarcated, shallow erosions on an erythematous base with scales, crust formation, erythema*Q and sometimes surrounded with small vesicles along the borders. Patients often complain of both pain & **burning** in the leions. Eventually patient becomes *erythrodermic with crusted, oozing & red skin.*
- Sun exposure (UV rays), environmental stimuli (insect bites), *auto immune diseases particularly thymoma &/or myasthenia gravis*Q, and **drug exposure** (eg drug containing thiol group like penicillamine, captopril, enalapril and non thiol drugs like penicillins, cephalosporins and piroxicams) may be associated and aggrevating factor.
- PF is generally less severe and carries better prognosis than PV.
- Histology (tzank smear) shows **superficial acantholytic blisters** just below stratum corneum and in granular layer. And **DIM** demonstrates *autoantibodies against Dsg1*Q. Because of lack of mucosal involvement *autoantibodies against Dsg3 are not found*Q. Because of superifical cleavage, the small flaccid blisters rupture easily and PF rarely demonstrate intact blisters.

46. **D i.e. Frusemide** *[Ref: Fitzpatrick's 7/e p-359, 350, 465; Rooks 8/e p.40.18-40.19]*

- **Induced pemphigus** is induced by radiotherapy (PV & PF), thermal burns and electrical injury (PV), vegetables of Allium group, Human herpes virus 8 DNA and drugs.
- **Drug induced pemphigus** usually resembles PF (>PV) and is caused by **thiol (sulphydryl)** and **non thiol** containing drugs via biochemical and *immunological mechanisms* respectively. The sulfhydryl group in desmoglein 1,3 becomes more antigenic because of interference of sulfhydryl group of thiol drugs. So the prognosis is better upon drug withdrawl of thiol group drugs.
- Drugs containing **thiol (sulphydryl) group** such as *penicillamine, captopril, enalapril*Q are most commonly associated with drug induced pemphigus (Harrison). Non thiol drugs linked to pemphigus include – *penicillins*Q, cephalosporins, piroxicam, pyrazolam derivatives (eg. phenylbutazone), propranolol, chloroquine, hydroxy chloroquine, rifampicin, montelukast, interferon, other ACE inhibitors eg enalapril, ramapril, fosinopril and angiotension II receptor blockers condesartan and telmisartan (Rook's). *Iodine (radioactive & non radioactive) and phenopthalein*Q may also l/t pemphigus.

47. **E i.e. Atropine gastritis**

Paraneoplastic pemphigus may be associated with ***non Hodgkin's lymphoma***Q (NHL), ***Chronic lymphocytic leukemia***Q (CLL), ***Castleman's disease, thymoma***Q and spindle cell tumors. And pemphigus folliaceus is associated with thymoma & / or ***mysthenia gravis***Q.

48. **D i.e. Pemphigus** *[Ref. Rook's 8/e p. 40.35; Harrison 18/e p. 423]*

- ***Mucosa involvement*** is seen in ***Behcet's syndrome, reactive arthritis (Reiter's syndrome), Peutz Jegher syndrome***Q, erythema multiforme major, Steven Johnson syndrome, TEN, ***lichen planus***Q, lupus erythematousus, leprosy, ***measles (Koplik spots)*** Q, Fordyce spot & disease, syphilis (congenital and secondary), inflammatory bowel disease, acute HIV infection and ***pemphigus vulgaris***Q.
- ***Pemphigus folicaeus and bullous pemphigoid do not involve mucous membrane***Q. However, ocular/oral/scarring/cicatrical/benign mucosal/ or mucous membrane – pemphigoid or bursting perry pemphigoid involve mucosa.

49. **B i.e. Suprabasal**
50. **B i.e. Bullous pemphigoid**
51. **B i.e. Pemphigoid**
52. **A i.e. DIF**

[Ref: Harrison 18/e p 424-26; Rook's 8/e p. 40.30; Fitzpatrick 8/e p 590-93]

Bullous (Blistering) Disorder

Pemphigus Vulgaris

- **Middle aged (30-60yrs) adult presenting with flaccid, fragile (easily ruptured), pruritic, painful, peripherally spreading, blister (or more commonly large erosions which are slow to heal) on upper half of body (scalp, face, axilla, trunk > groin and limbs)** on normal appearing or erythematous skin.
- Nearly all patients have **Mucosal involvement**Q, Acantholysis, Nikolsky sign and Row of tomb stone appearance. And the blisters are Intra Epidermal more specificially **lower suprabasal**Q in spinous cell layer, Mn-"**MAN-R** or **Read NIEMA**"

On direct immune fluorescence microsocopy (DI FM) deposition of IgG on Keratinocyte surface in fishnet pattern and intercellular space (causing it to widen) is **diagnostic (Gold Standard)**

Bullous Pemphigoid

- **Elderly (> 60 to 80 yrs) patient presenting with pruritic eczematous rash/urticaria**/or figurate erytheme resembling erytheme multiforme or dermatitis herpetiformis **prodrome** preceding characteristic large (many cms), **tense, tough (may remain intact), dome shaped blister** on normal or erythematous skin
- **Erosions** formed d/t blister rupture **heal rapidly with out scarring but with milia and** hyperpigmentation
- Lesions (bullae & erosions) predominantly involve **lower half of body** ie **central/lower abdomen or trunk > limb/thigh flexures.**
- **Mucosol involvement is less frequent** (10% cases) **limited** (to buccal mucosa) and **less severe** (vermilion border spared and **heal rapidly without scarring**).
- There is no **"MAN-R"** ie no mucosa involvement (relative & in most cases), Acantholysis, Nikolsky sign and Row of tombstone appearance. The **blisters are deep subepidermal**Q.

- On **direct immune fluorescence microscopy** of normal appearing perilesional skin (within 2cm of lesion but not on blister as immunoreactants are often lost from the roof of blister), there is **linear deposition of IgG** (usually G1 & G4), IgE and/or **C3** in the **epidermal basement membrane zone, (Gold standard diagnostic criteria).**
- Sera of ~70% of these patients contain circulating IgG antibodies that bind the epidermal BMZ of normal human skin (or monkey esophagus) by **indirect immuofluorescence microscopy (IIFM).** IgG from even more (>70%) patients shows reactivity to the epidermal side of **salt (1 mol/liter NaCl) split skin,** (an alternate immune fluorescence microscopy test substrate used to distinguish circulating IgG anti BMZ autoantibodies in patients with BP, from other subepidermal blistering diseases likes epidermolysis bullosa acquisita (EBA) & cicatricial pemphigoid. *In contrast to pemphigus, in BP the indirect IF antibody titer does not usually correlate with disease activity or extent.*
- The use of **salt split skin**, separates epidermis from dermis at the lamina lucida. It *increases the sensitivity* of autoantibody detection and differentiates BP from EBA as circulating autoantibodies in BP react with epidermal side of split skin. Finding of circulating autoantibodies is diagnostic.

Direct Immunofluorescence Microscopy

53. **A i.e. 'Fishnet' IgG deposits in epidermis**
54. **A. i.e. Pemphigus**
55. **C. i.e. Pemphigus > B. i.e. SLE**
56. **B i.e. Bullous pemphigoid**
57. **A.i.e. Dermatitis herpetiformis** *[Ref: Fitzpatrick 7/e p. 459-84; Thoms Habif 4/e p. 550-75; Harrison 17/e p-336-40]*

- **IgG** deposits on ***Keratinocyte surface (i.e in intercellular spaces of epidermis) in fish net pattern***Q is seen in **pemphigus.**

- *Linear IgG deposits along epidermal basement membrane (at dermo-epidermal junction)* Q is seen in **bullous pemphigoid**.
- *Granular IgA deposits in dermal papillae & EBM*Q is seen in **dermatitis herpetiformis** and around small blood vessels in skin, intensive & kidney is seen in **HS purpura**. Whereas linear (not granular) IgA deposits along EBM is seen in **linear IgA disease**.

58. **A i.e. Darrier's disease; B i.e. Hailey-Hailey disease** *[Ref: Rook's 8/e p. 40.27, 13.19, 10.12-10.28, 40.4, Neena Khanna 4/e p. 69-71; Fitzpatrick's 7/e p. 432-41; Harrison 18/e p. 422]*

Darier white disease (keratosis follicularis), Hailey-Hailey disease (familial benign chronic pemphigus) and **Grover's disease** are acantholytic disorders of skin diagnosed on the basis of histology (**not showing DIF**)

Pemphigoid Gestationalis

59. **D. i.e. Herpes gestationis**
60. **A. i.e. Periumblical region**

[Ref: Fitzpatrick 7/e p. 490- 93; Thomas Habif 4/e p. 573; Neena Khanna 3rd/p- 72]

Spontaneous remissions & recurrences are very common in **herpes gestationis** which typically presents with *abrupt onset, intensily pruritic urticarial lesions mostly on abdomen, often periumblical during late pregnancy*Q.

Dermatitis Herpetiformis

61. **C i.e. HLA B8**
62. **C. i.e. Deposition of IgG at the epidermodermal lesion**
63. **C i.e. Dermatitis herpetiformis**
64. **D i.e. Dermatitis herpetiformis**
65. **B i.e. Dapsone**
66. **A. i.e. Gluten free diet with minerals and vitamins**

[Ref: Robbins 7/e p. 1259-63; Thomas Habif Clinical Dermatology 4/e p. 550-59; Harrison 17/e p. 337; Roxburgh's 17/e p. 88, 91-92; Fitzpatrick's 7/e p-500-04; Rooks 7/e p.41.54-41.57]

- **Dermatitis herpetiformis** is associated with *subclinical gluten sensitive enteropathy and HLA B8 halotype*Q. It presents with *severely pruritic (itchy) papulovesicular/urticarial lesions and crusted papules & excoriation symmetrically distributed over extensor surfaces (i.e. elbows, knees, buttocks, back, scalp & posterior neck)* Q.
- On DIM, there is *granular deposition of IgA autoantibodies (directed against epidermal transglutaminase) in papillary dermis (dermal papilla) and epidermal basement membrane (dermo-epidermal junction).*
- *Strick gluten free diet, Atkins diet and elemental diet is treatment of choice and dapsone is drug of choice*Q.

Feature \ Disease	Dermatitis herpetiformis	Pemphigus vulgaris	Bullous pemphigoid	Numular (Discoid) Eczema
Age (mainly)	Adults (20-40 yr)	*Adults (30-60 yr)*Q	*Elderly (>60 to 80 yr)* Q	Middle age & elderly
Area of predeliction (distribution)	***Symmetrically over extensor surfaces (i.e. elbows, knees, buttocks, back, scalp & posterior neck)*** Q	- Asymmetrical on **upper half of body (trunk > limbs)** i.e. scalf, face, neck, axilla & trunk - ***Oral mucosa commonly involved***Q	- Symmetrical on lower half of body (limbs > trunk) i.e. ***flexural aspects of limbs & central abdomens*** Q - ***Mucosa not involved***Q	Lower extremities (mc), upper extremities and trunk
Itching (pruritis)	**Intensely pruritic** (itchy) with a burning/stinging component	Mild in early cases	Itching is common & may persist for months	Intense itching
Lesion	Severely pruritic ***papulovesicular/ urticarial lesions and crusted papules & excoriation*** Q	***Painful, mostly nonpruritic, fragile, flaccid (thin wall delicate) bullae*** Q on a normal or erythematous base that rupture to produce extensive denudation.	- **Urticarial/eczematous prodrome** (preceding 3 weeks to months) f/b faint, dusky **erythema** in a **figurative** pattern. - *Large (many cm), tense, tough, dome shaped* blisters that may remain intact for several days and the contents often becoming jelly like coagulated fibrin or occasionally blood stained	Minute vesicle & papules enlarge to form ***characteristic erythematous scaling coin shaped area*** Q.

Associated with	- ***Gluten sensitive enteropathy (absorptive defect) HLA-B8/DRW3/DQW2 halotype*** Q - Thyroid abnormalities (mostly hypothyroid), achlorhydria, **atrophic gastritis**, SLE, RA, UC, myasthenia gravis and gastrointestinal NHL	Mn: "**Row MAN**" i.e. row of tombstone appearance, mucosal involvement acantholysis & Nikolysky sign present	Row MAN absent	
General health	Fair	Deteriorates	Fair	Fair
Histopathology (of lesion)	- Subepidermal bullae - IgA & neutrophills in papillary tip (**papillary tip absecss**) - **Partial villous atrophy** (on small intestine biopsy)	- ***Intra epidermal bullae with acantholysis*** Q - **IgG** & C3 deposition between epidermal cells in **fishnet pattern**	- ***Subepidermal bullae without acantholysis*** Q - Subepidermal collection of IgG, C3, eosinophils & polymorphs	
Management	***Gluten free diet, (TOC) and dapsone (DOC)*** Q	Systemic steroid, immunosuppressant and Mx of burn	Systemic steroid, immunosuppressant and Mx of burn	Topical steriod

67. **A i.e. Rice > D i.e. Corn** *[Ref: Harrison 16/e p. 1771]*

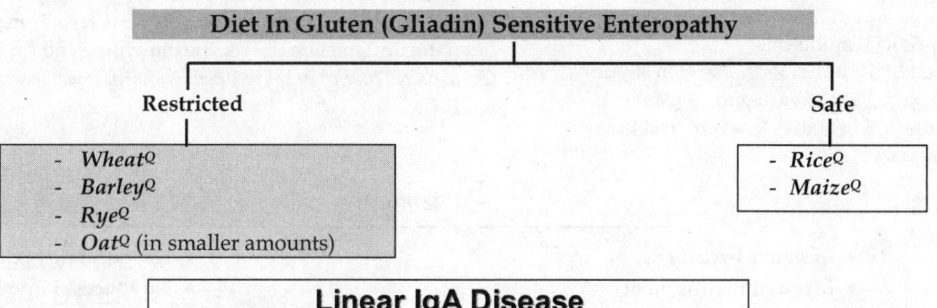

Diet In Gluten (Gliadin) Sensitive Enteropathy
Restricted
Safe
- WheatQ
- BarleyQ
- RyeQ
- OatQ (in smaller amounts)
- RiceQ
- MaizeQ

Linear IgA Disease

68. **C i.e. Granular deposition of IgA; D ie. Are candidates for gluten free diet; E i.e. A variant of dermatitis herpetiformis** *[Ref: Harrison 17/e p. 339; Fitzpatrick's Dermatology in General Medicine 6/e p-587-91; Rooks Textbook of Dermatology 7/e p.41.43-41.47]*

Linear IgA disease presents with *severely pruritic, subepidermal blisters*Q. On DIM, *linear (not granular) deposits of IgA*Q is seen along EBM. It is a ***separate & distinct entity different from dermatitis herpetiformis and so gluten free diet is not required***Q.

Erythema Multiformae

69. **A. i.e. Viral** **70.** **D. i.e. Mucous membrane is usually involved**
71. **B. i.e. Erythema multiformae** **72.** **A i.e. No vesicle**
[Ref: Robbins 7th/e P-1255-56; Roxburgh's 17/e p. 75; Pasricha 4/e p. 161; Neena Khanna 3/e p. 149-50; Fitzpatric's 7/e p-343-54; Thomas Habif Clinical Dermatology 4/e p.626-29; Harrison 17th/311]

Erythema multiforme is caused ***mostly because of virus (herpes simplex virus 1***Q***)*** or rarely d/t ***drugs (sulfonamides mc) and internal malignancies*** Q. **Characteristic target (iris/bull's eye/annular) lesions** is ***purpuric, erythematous-papulo-vesicular lesion resembling target of shooting range*** Q. It first appears acrally & then spread in a centripetal manner to symmetrically involve ***extensor surface of extremities (hand, feet, elbow, knee), face & neck*** Q. Mucosa is involved in 70% cases.

Epidermal Necrolysis

73. **D. i.e. Steven Johnson syndrome** **74.** **A. i.e. Phenytoin B. i.e. Penicillin**
75. **B. i.e. Sulfonyl urea C. i.e. Aspirin**
76. **B i.e. Staphyloccocal Scalded Skin Syndrome** *[Ref: Rudolph Pediatrics 21/e P-1196,1225; Roxburgh's-Common Skin disease 17/e p. 92, 232-3, 75; Fitzpatrick's Dermatology 6/e p-1876-88; Rooks Textbook of Dermatology 7/e p.27.8-40]*

- **SJS** and TEN are most severe form of EM and so may show **atypical target lesions.**
- TEN is caused by ***phenytoin, penicillin & sulfa drugs***[Q] but there is no risk with ***aspirin & sulfonyl urea***[Q].

Staphylococcal scalded skin syndrome (SSSS)

- Caused by ***ET* (Exfollative / erythematogenic toxin) *producing staphylococcus – aureus (phage group II)***[Q]
- 1st site of infection is ***extracutaneous (ex conjunctivitis, pharyngitis, tonsillitis, otitis media, rhinorrhea***[Q]***)***
- There is wide spread *erythematous blisterous eruption* with striking ***desquamation of large areas of skin (Nikolsky sign positive)***[Q] as in scald or burn
- ***Mucosa is not involved***[Q]
- There may be slight fever & some systemic disturbance, but usually the ***children are not severely ill***[Q].
- Initial findings are redness & tenderness of central face, neck, trunk & interiginous zone followed by short lived flaccid bullae & slough or exfoliation or peeling of superficial epidermis.
- Treated by IV antibiotics. The skin should be managed as for burn and concern over dehydration heat loss & severe infection is necessary.

Steven Johnson Syndrome

- It is cutaneous *drug reaction.*
- Presents with ***systemic symptoms***[Q] (fever, malaise, sore throat) followed by ***erosions of multiple mucous membranes***[Q] & blisters developing on *dusky or purpuric macules or* ***atypical target lesions***
- Total % of body surface area blistering & eventual detachment is **<10%.**

Toxic Epidermal Necrolysis (TEN)/Lyell's Syndrome

- It is the *most serious* cutaneous drug reaction
- *Drug* are the primary cause & m.c. offenders are

Punjab	**- Phenytoin, Penicillins**
National	**- NSAID'S**
Bank'	**- Barbiturate**
S	**- Sulfonamides**

- Presents with ***systemic symptoms***[Q] (fever > 102.2° F. malaise),
- Blisters or ulcers on m***ultiple mucous membrane***[Q]***,*** blisters developing on wide spread areas of erythema & then slough.
- **> 30%** of body surface show blistering & epidermal necrosis.

★ Also know

- Most severe form of **SSSS** is termed **Ritter's disease** in *new borns* & **toxic epidermal necrolysis** (TEN) in older (usually <5 years) in dividuals.
- Milder & more common forms of SSSS is K/a **Pemphigus neonatorum** (in neonates) & **Bullous impetigo** (in children & adults)
- Co-trimoxozole may l/t *erythemia multiforme, stevens Johnson syndrome & TEN*

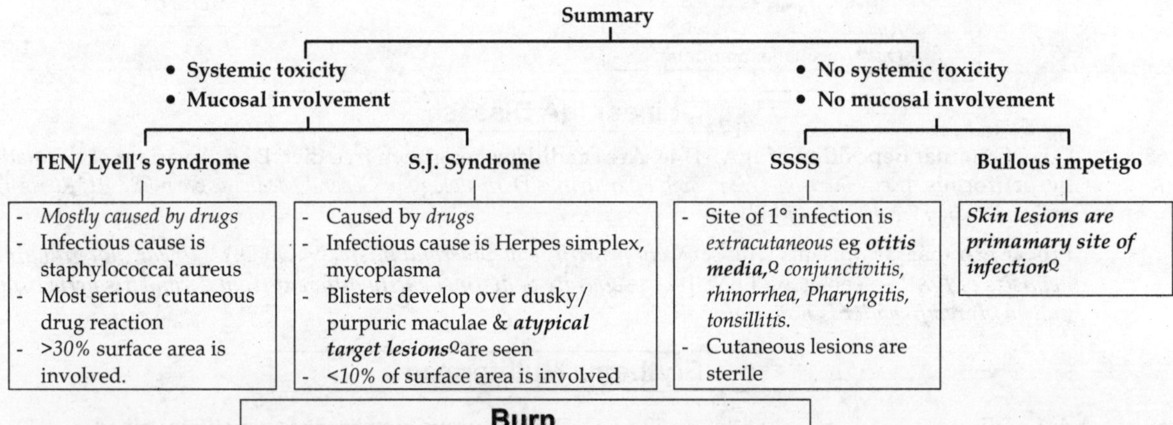

Summary
• Systemic toxicity
• Mucosal involvement
• No systemic toxicity
• No mucosal involvement
TEN/ Lyell's syndrome
- Mostly caused by drugs
- Infectious cause is staphylococcal aureus
- Most serious cutaneous drug reaction
- >30% surface area is involved.
S.J. Syndrome
- Caused by drugs
- Infectious cause is Herpes simplex, mycoplasma
- Blisters develop over dusky/ purpuric maculae & atypical target lesionsQare seen
- <10% of surface area is involved
SSSS
- Site of 1° infection is extracutaneous eg otitis media,Q conjunctivitis, rhinorrhea, Pharyngitis, tonsillitis.
- Cutaneous lesions are sterile
Bullous impetigo
Skin lesions are primamary site of infectionQ

Burn

77. **D i.e. Dermis** *[Ref: Roxburgh's-Common Skin disease 17/e p. 89-92]*

First degree burns involve only the *epidermis* and is characterized by *erythema.* Where as **second degree** or **partial thickness burns** are deeper involving all the epidermis and some of the corium or ***dermis***[Q]**.** The systemic severity of the burn and the quality of subsequent healing are directly related to the amount of undamaged dermis. Superficial burns are characterized by blister formation while deeper partial thickness burns have a reddish appearance or a layer of whitish non viable dermis.

Molluscum Contagiosum

78. **B i.e Pox Virus** **79.** **A i.e. Molluscum Contagiosum** **80.** **E i.e. All**

[Ref. Fitzpatrick 7/e p. 1911-13, 1847-48; Roxborough 18/e p. 55-57; Rooks 8/e p. 33.11-33.14]

Molluscum contagiosum is caused by ***poxvirus family (genus molluscipox) virus***[Q]. Transmission may occur via ***direct skin or mucous membrane contact (eg. touching & sexual contact)*** [Q] or via fomites. Characteristic lesion is ***extremely small, pink, shiny pearly white or skin (flesh) colored, umblicated papule containing a grayish central plug (pore) on face & genitals in children***[Q]. Treatment includes ***watchful waiting, curettage and cryotherapy***[Q].

Lichen Nitidus

81. **D i.e. Lichen nitidus**
[Ref: Rook's 8/e p. 33.11/13, 41.21/23; Fitzpatricks 8/e p. 2418, 312-16; Neena Khanna 4/e p. 5161; Mark 2/e p. 344]

Multiple, discrete (or may be closely grouped), minute, pinpoint to pin head sized small (1-2 mm), smooth, flat/round/dome shaped papules with **a glistening (shiny) surface** on **dorsal hands, forearm and penis** in a young 8 year old boy indicates diagnosis of **lichen nitidus**.

Herpes

82. **B i.e. Thoracic**
83. **A i.e. Herpes zoster**
84. **A i.e. Herpes zoster**
85. **A i.e. Varicella zoster**
86. **C i.e. Face**
87. **A i.e. Herpes genitalis**

[Ref: Harrison 18/e p 270; Fitzpatrick 8/e p. 2383-93; Thomas Habif 4/e p. 381, 394; Roxborough 18/e p. 52-54; Rook's 8/e p. 33.14-33.22]

Herpes	62%
Chancroid	12-20%
Syphilis	13%
LGV & GI	-

- **Varicella zoster (VZ) virus causes chicken pox in childhood and persists in latent from within sensory ganglion. In elderly and immunocopromized individuals,** VZ virusus reactivaties and causes **herpes zoster (HZ).** HZ presents with **localized, unilateral, segmental (dermatomal) painful vesicular eruption** (pain preceding rash) limited to the area of skin innervated by a single sensory ganglion, **trunk from T3 To L2 are most grequently affected.**
- **Herpes zoster** commonly presents with ***painful, closely grouped red papules rapidly becoming vesicular***Q, in area of 1, occasionally 2 or rarely more contiguous **dermatomes**. ***Thoracic dermatome is most commony involved***Q. Histopathology shows ***characteristic ballooning of cytoplasm of Malpighian layer***Q, multinucleated giant cells containing acidophilic intranuclear inclusion bodies (**Cowdry type A inclusions**).
- **Herpes simplex virus (HSV-1)** is mostly associated with *orofacial disease*Q, whereas **HSV-2** mostly causes *genital infections*Q. Most of the HSV infections are caused by HSV-1
- **Genital herpes** is the ***most prevalent sexually transmitted disease (STD) world wide and is the most common cause of ulcerative genital disease***Q.

88. **A. i.e. Acyclovir**
89. **A. i.e. Foscarnet** *Ref: Fitzpatrick's 7/e p- 1895, 2203-08]*

Acyclovir is ***drug of primary choice***Q for herpes infection and **foscarnet** is drug of ***choice for acyclovir resistance HSV, herpes zoster & varicella zoster infection***Q.

Use of Antiviral drugs

Acyclovir
- *Supression* of recurrent & /or *treatment* of symptomatic primary or recurrent mucocutaneous *HSV-1 or HSV-2* infections in normal & immuno compromised patients
- Prevention of perinatal *HSV-1 & HSV-2* infection & treatment of *neonatal HSV infection*
- Treatment of *HSV-1 encephalitis*
- Treatment of primary VZV infection in adults & immuno compromised children
- Treatment of VZV infection to *reduce the risk of post herpetic neuralgia*
- Post exposure prophylaxis & t/t for *herpes simplex* after monkey bite

Valacyclovir, Famciclovir & Penciclovir
- T/t of initial & recurrent HSV genital infections
- Suppression of frequently recurring genital HSV infections
- Treatment of herpes zoster

Ganciclovir & Valganciclovir
- CMV retinitis in AIDS
- Suppression & prevention of CMV disease in transplant recipients

Trifluridine (topical)
- T/t of primary HSV conjunctivitis
- T/t of recurrent epithelial keratitis
- ***Acyclovir resistant mucocutaneous HSV infections in AIDS patient***Q

Foscarnet (IV)
- ***Treatment of acyclovir resistant HSV & ganciclovir resistant CMV infections***Q
- T/t of CMV retinitis in AIDS
- T/t of CMV poly radiculopathy in combination with ganciclovir

Cidofovir
- CMV retinitis in AIDS
- T/t of resistant HSV & CMV infection

DERMATOLOGY 1

DERMATOLOGY

6 SYSTEMIC DISEASES WITH PROMINENT CUTANEOUS FEATURES, PHOTOSENSITIVITY DISORDERS & CUTANEOUS DRUG ERRUPTIONS

Dermatomyositis

It is a distinctive entity identified by ***a characteristic rash accompanying, or more often preceding, muscle weakness***[Q]

Dermatological (cutaneous) manifestations

- **Heliotrope rash** is *most common* manifestation. It consists of purple-red or purple-blue discolourations of the upper eyelids; sometimes associated with ***scaling, violaceous erythema and periorbital oedema***[Q].
- **Gottron sign or papules** are **violaceous *flat topped papules (or scaly eruption) over distal interphalangeal joint*** and is ***pathognomic*** of D.M.
  [Note erythema & scaling in dorsal part of the finger can occur in SLE too; but it spares skin over interphalangeal joints.
- *Erythematous or violaceous scapy rash* can also occur on extensor surfaces of arms, legs and hands including the knees, elbows, malleoli; neck & anterior chest ('V' sign) or back and shoulders (shawl sign) and may worsen after sun-exposure. ***Erythema and scaling may be particularly prominent over elbows, knee & dorsal interphalangeal joints***[Q].
- In some patients rash is pruritic, especially on the scalp, chest and back.
- ***Periungal telangiectasia*** (dilated capillary loops at the base of finger-nails) are also characteristic; and lacy or reticular erythema may be associated with fine scaling on extensor surface of upper arms & thighs.
- The ***cuticle may be irregular (ragged cuticles), thickened and distorted and fingers may become rough & cracked, with irregular, dirty horizontal lines***[Q], resembling **mechanics hand**.
- **Poikiloderma** in areas of hypopigmentation, hyperpigmentation, mild atrophy and telangiectasia. It is rare in both SLE & scleroderma and thus serve as a clinical sign that distinguishes DM from these two diseases.

Myositis

- ***Cutaneous signs may precede or follow the development of myositis by weeks to years***[Q].
- ***At times, the muscle strength appears normal***[Q], hence the term **dermatomyositis sine myositis.** However, on muscle biopsy of such cases, significant perivascular & perimysial inflammation is seen.
- The weakness may be mild, moderate, or severe enough to lead to quadriparesis.
- **Progressive & symmetrical proximal muscle weakness** presenting as increasing difficulty with tasks requiring use of proximal muscles, such as, getting up from chair, climbing stairs, stepping on to a crub, lifting objects or combing hair
- Differences between various causes of myositis

	Dermatomyositis	Polymyositis	Inclusion body myositis
Age	Adult & childhood	> 18 years	> 50 years
Familial association	--	--	±
Fine motor movements (eg. Sewing, knitting, or writings) or Distal muscle involvement	Late	Late	Early
Facial muscle involvement	--	--	+
Falling	--	--	Common d/t early involvement of quadriceps
Course	Subacute (weeks to months)	Subacute (weeks months)	Chronic (years)

- ***Ocular muscles are spared***[Q] even in advanced untreated cases; if these muscles are' affected, the diagnosis of inflammatory myopathy should be questioned
- Sensation remains normal
- In all three forms of myopathies, pharyngeal and neck flexor muscles are often involved causing dysphagia or difficulty in holding up of the head (head drop)
- ***1/3 patients may have underlying malignancy***[Q] (eg. Ca lung, ovary or breast).

Autoantibodies in SLE, Dermatomyositis & Polymyositis

Autoantibodies in

Systemic lupus erythematosus (SLE)

Antibody	Prevalence (%)	Utility / Association
Antinuclear antibody (ANA)	98	- ***Most sensitive, best screening test***Q - Repeatedly negative test makes SLE unlikely

High disease specificity for SLE

Antibody	Prevalence (%)	Utility / Association
Anti double stranded (ds) DNA	70	- ***Most specific for SLE***Q - Correlate with *disease activity* & herald a flare of *nephritis* or *vasculitis.*
Anti - Sm	25	- ***Most specific***Q but *do not correlate* with disease activity or clinical manifestations - Most patients also have anti RNP
Anti-r-RNP (Anti ribosomal P)	20	- Correlates with depression or psychosis d/t **CNS lupus**
Anti-PCNA (proliferating cell nuclear antigen)	3	

Low disease specificity for SLE

Antibody	Prevalence (%)	Utility / Association
Anti- U1-RNP	40	Overlap (mixed) connective tissue disease (MCTD)
Anti single stranded (SS) DNA	60	Risk of SLE in patients with DLE
Anti- Ro (SS -A)	30	- Indicates risk for ***neonatal lupus with congenial heart block***Q; so should be done in women with child bearing potential & SLE - Sicca (Sjogren) syndrome, SCLE (Subacute cutaneous lupus erythematosus), ANA negative lupus - *Decreased risk for nephritis*
Anti-La (SS-B)	10	- Usually associated with anti-Ro, SCLE, Sjogren syndrome - Decreased risk for nephritis
Anti- histone	70	More common in ***drug induced lupus***Q (than SLE)
Anti- Ku	10	Overlap CTD
Anti- erythrocyte	60	Overt hemolysis
Anti-platelet	30	Thrombocytopenia
Anti neuronal (anti glutamate receptor)	60	Active CNS lupus
Anti- phospholipids (a-PL)	50	- 3 tests are available – *ELISA* for cardiolipin & B_2 glycoprotein 1 co factor (B_2G_1), and sensitive *prothrombin time by* diluted Russell venom viper test (d RVVT) - Predispose to *venous & arterial clotting, thrombocytopenia* and fetal loss (so indicated in women with child bearing potential & SLE

Idiopathic inflammatory dermatomyopathies

- **High specificity for Dermatomyositis (DM)/Polymyositis (PM)**

Autoantibody	Clinical association
Anti Jo – 1 (against *histidyl* t RNA synthetase)	*PM*Q (ASS)
- **Anti – PL- 7** (against *threonyl*- t- RNA synthetase). - **Anti PL- 12** (ag. *alanyl* –t-RNA synthetase) - **Anti – OJ** (ag. *Isoleucyl* t RNA synthetase) - **Anti- EJ** (ag. *glycyl* tRNA synthetase)	Antisynthetase syndrome (ASS)
Anti- 155 kd &/or **Se**	Classic DM
Anti- 140 kd	Amyopathic DM (?)
Anti- SRP (ag. Signal recognition particle)	Fulminant DM/PM, cardiac involvement
Anti- Mi2 (ag. helicase nuclear protein)	Shawl sign, cuticular overgrowth
Anti Fer Anti Mas Anti KJ	ag. elongation factor 1α ag small RNA ag translation factor

- **Low specificity for DM/PM**

Autoantibody	Clinical association
ANA	Clinically amyopathic DM (80%)
Anti SS DNA	*SLE*, systemic sclerosis
Anti- Ro (52 kd Ro)	Overlap with sjogren syndrome, SCLE, SLE, neonatal LE/ chronic hepatitis B
Anti- U1 RNP	Overlap with connective *tissue disease*
- **Anti PM- Scl (PM-1)** - **Anti ku** - **Anti U2 RNP**	Overlap with *scleroderma*

★ Women with child bearing potential & SLE should be screened for *aPL & anti- Ro.*

★ ANA (by immunofluorescnce), anti ds DNA, anti Sm and / or anti pL fulfills one diagnostic criteria.

Sleroderma / Systemic Sclerosis (SS)

It is a *chronic multi system* disease of *unknown etiology* that has highest case specific mortality of any of autimmune rheumatic diseases. It is characterized by *thickening of skin (Scleroderma;* distinguishing it from other connective tissue diseases), *Raynaud's phenomenon* & involvement of multiple (virtually all) internal organs, most notably *lungs, GI tract, heart & kidneys.*

Clinical features & subtypes

Feature	Limited (localized) cutaneous SS (LcSS)	Diffuse cutaneous SS (DcSS)
Raynaud's phenomenon	- Long pre-existing history precedes skin involvement - Associated with critical ischemia	Onset contemporaneous with skin involvement
Skin Sclerosis	- **Spares proximal** sites & involve fingers, forearm (distal to elbow), face - Slow progression	- **Diffuse,** also involving proximal skin i.e. upper arms, thighs, chest & abdomen (trunk) - Rapid progression
Pulmonary fibrosis	May occur Moderate	Frequent Early & severe
Pulmonary arterial hypertension	Frequent, late ,may be isolated	May occur, associated with pulmonary fibrosis
Scleroderma renal crisis	Very rare	Occurs early & more commonly (15%)
Calcinosis cutis	Frequent, prominent	May occur, mild
Others	Includes **"CREST"** (**C**alcinosis, cutis, **R**aynaud's phenomenon, **E**sophageal dysmotality, **S**clerodactyly, & **T**elangiectasia) syndrome	- Prominent inflammatory features during first 24 months - High frequency of pulmonary fibrosis, cardiac involvement & scleroderma renal crisis
Characteristic Autoanti bodies	***Anti- centromere***[Q]	- ***Anti topoisomerase (Scl-70)***[Q] - Anti – RNAP III

★ Antinuclear antibody testing shows speckled nucleolar staining with specificity for *n-RNP, fibrillarin, or PM-Scl* in overlap SS

★ Few (10%) of SS patients develop vascular, immunological & organ based fibrotic features but *lack skin sclerosis.* These are termed *systemic sclerosis sine scleroderma*

Internal organ involvement

Feature	LcSS (%)	DcSS (%)
Skin involvement	90★	100
Pulmonary fibrosis	35	65
Myopathy	11	23
Scleroderma renal crisis	2	15
Cardiac involvement	9	12
Raynaud's phenomenon	99	98
Esophageal involvement	90	80
Pulmonary artery hypertension	25	15

Autoantibodies in SS

Reactivity	Target-antigen	Frequency	Clinical association
Centro-mere	**CENP proteins**	*Lc SS*[Q] (60%) >> DcSS (2%)	Digital ischemia, limited skin sclerosis, calcinosis, severe gut disease, isolated PAH
Scl- 70	**Topoisome rase -1**	*Dc SS*[Q] (40%) >> Lc SS (15%)	Diffuse skin sclerosis, pulmonary fibrosis (ILD), cardiac involvement, scleroderma renal crisis
RNAP	**RNA polymerase III**	DcSS (25%) >> Lc SS (2%)	Diffuse skin sclerosis, hypertensive (scleroderma) renal crisis.
nRNP	U1-RNP	MCTD, 15% SS	PAH, overlap features of SLE, arthritis
	U3 – RNP (Fibrillarin)	DcSS	PAH, ILD, Scleroderma renal crisis, myositis
	PM – Scl	LcSS	Calcinosis, myositis systemic sclerosis overlap
	Th/T0	LcSS	ILD, PAH

★ Anti- fibrinolytic agents eg. D- penicillamine, relaxin, interferon γ, and anti- TGF β are of doubtful benefits.

Drug Induced Lupus (DIL)

Etiopathogenesis

- Certain drugs by **decreasing DNA methylation in Tcells** resulting in ncreased expression of genes and altered repair of DNA can induce autoimmunity and l/t DIL.
- Most common offenders include ***procanamide > hydralazine, isoniazid, chlorpromazine, carbamazapine, phenytoin and***

Clinical Presentation

- Most common serological abnormality is **positivity for antinuclear antibody (ANA) with a homologous pattern.** So almost all have ANA and most (upto 95%) have **antihistone antibodies**, but they are not specific for DIL as 50-80% of patients with idiopathic lupus erythematous have AHA and between 10-20% of ANA positive individuals develop lupus like symptoms.
- Characterized by **frequent musculoskeletal complaints (arthritis or intense arthralgia/myalgia)**, *fever, weight loss, malaise, serositis, pleura-pulmonary involvement* in more than half of patients.

*minocyclines*Q. The long list includes – **"Ma Mi/Me LiLa Is A PHD Economics In Queen's College"** i.e.

Ma Mi/Me	-	Macrodantin, Minocycline/ Methyl dopa
LiVa	-	Lithium, LaVastatin & simVastatin
Is	-	Isoniazid
A	-	Acebutalol
P	-	Procanamide, Propyl thiouracil, Propafenone, Proctolol, Phenytoin
H	-	Hydralazine, Hydrochlorthiazide, Hydantoin
D	-	D- penicillamine, Disopyramide
Economics	-	Ethosuxamide
In	-	Interferon α, Inhibitors of TNF
Queen'	-	Quinidine
S	-	Sulfasalazine
College	-	Carbamazepine, Chlorpromazine, Contraceptives

- **Renal, neurological (CNS), or vasculitic** involvement is rare. And most patients have **no cutaneous findings** of lupus **erythematosus.**

Differences from SLE (idiopathic lupus erythematosus)

- **Anti-dsDNA antibodies** (antibodies against double stranded DNA) are typically **absent** (or very rare), whereas **antisingle stranded DNA antibodies** are often **present.**
- ***Hypocomplementemia, renal, neurological & cutaneous involvement is rare***Q.
- Syndrome occurs *during therapy with certain medications,* predominantly in whites. **HLAD4** is present in 70% cases of DIL by hydralazine & micocycline.
- Clinical features & most laboratory abnormalities ***often revert towards normal when offending drug is withdrawn***Q.
- Sex ratio is nearly equal with a ***less female predilection than SLE***Q.
- Minocycline induced lupus typically occurs after 2 years of therapy and presents with a symmetrical polyarthritis, hepatitis and cutaneous findings like livedo reticularis, painful nodules on legs & non descriptional eruptions.

Difference from drug induced SCLE (subacute cutaneous lupus erythematosus)

- DI-SCLE is characterized by **widespread, non scarring papulosquamous eruption** (like psoriasis) or **annular lesions** (resembling erythema multiformae), which is often **photosensitive. Systemic involvement** (like renal, CNS, athralgia, lymphadenopathy) and fever, malaise are **absent** or mild.
- Anti-Ro (Sjogren syndrome A) antibodies are seen in many SCLE patients.
- Most common causative agents are *thiazide diuretics, calcium channel blocker, ACE inhibitors, cinarizine, and terbinafine.* Other drugs include griesofulvin, parenteral gold, piroxicam, D-penicillamine, oxprenolol, naproxen, spironolactone, sulfonyl urea, INF-β, ranitidine, carbamazapine, systemic 5FU, bupropion, acebutalol & tiotropium inhaled.

Melasma (Chloasma) or Mask of Pregnancy

- This *acquired hypermelanosis* is seen mainly on ***sun exposed skin of face in women***Q. It is more apparent following sun exposure & the affected skin is ***brown in color***Q. Melasma presents usually as ***bilateral, symmetrical & irregular shaped***Q hyper-pigmented patches affecting the ***forehead, cheeks, nose, upper lip, chin and neck***Q. The commonest type is centrofacial (65%) >> malar (on cheeks)> mandibular pattern (lower jaw). Symmetrical dark areas across the cheeks, around eyes and over forehead, give a mask like appearance.
- Many cases are attributed to ***pregnancy or combined oral contraceptive pills***Q. About 60% of pregnant women and 30% of women on OCP develop melasma. Although it may improve (fade) after delivery, it can reoccur with subsequent pregnancies. Melasma caused by OCP can still persist even after discontinuation of drug.
- The probable presumed mechanism is increased *MSH (melanocyte stimulating hormone)* & consequent stimulation of melanocyte or increase in oestrogen & progesterone. *Phenytoin or mephenytoin* may cause similar pigmentation.
- ***Chloasma is distinguishable from DLE (& SLE) by their complete absence of scaling and lack of systemic (multi-organ) involvement***Q like fever, arthritis, pleurisy, pericarditis, hepato-splenomegaly, lymphodenopathy, renal & CNS involvement.

Treatment of Chloasma

Sun protection

Sun (ultraviolet) exposure is one of the most important causative factors. So *(titanium dioxide & zinc oxide containing)* sunscreens that *block both UVA & UV-B lights* should be used.

Hypopigmenting agents

- Epidermal pigmentation is more sensitive to treatment than dermal
- **Hydroquinone** is *most effective* topical bleaching agent. It is used in **2-4%**Q concentrations (or rarely 10% in refractory cases). It also bleaches *freckles & lentigens but not café-au-lait spots or pigmented nevi.*
- **Azelaic acid** (azelex) **20%** is as effective as hydroquinone 4%. It is used to treat *acne & melasma.* It selectively affects hyperactive & abnormal melanocytes & has *minimal effects on normal pigmented skin, freckles & senile lentigens.*
- **Tretinoin (Retinin- A) 0.025 to 0.05%** concentration, enhances effectiveness of hyroquinone (by improved epidermal penetration) & azelaic acid.
- **Kligman formula** or **Triluma cream** is a combination of 4% *hydroquinone, 0.05% tretinoin and 0.01% flucinolone acetonide (steroid).*
- **Rucinol & Kojic acid**

Chemical peels

- Darker individuals are poor candidates because of high post inflammatory hyperpigmentation. It includes:
  - Trichlor acetic acid (15-30%)
  - Glycolic and (70%)
  - Alpha hydroxyl acids
- **Pulsed CO_2 laser** (first destroying the abnormal melanocytes) followed by **Q-switched alexandrite laser** selectively eliminating the dermal melanin.

Photosensitive Diseases

Photosensitivity (i.e. abnormal response to ultraviolet radiation eposure) can be divided into 6 categories

I. Acquired, Idiopathic (probably immunological photodermatosis)

- Polymorphic light eruption
- Actinic prurigo
- Hydroa vacciniforme
- Chronic actinic dermatitis
- Solar urticaria

IV. Metabolic

- ***Porphyria cutanea tarda (sporadic)*** [Q]
- ***Pellagra*** [Q]
- Kwashiorkor
- Hartnup disease
- Carcinoid syndrome

V. Neoplastic & Degenerative

- Photoaging
- Actinic keratosis
- ***Liver spots (lentigo senelis)*** [Q]
- Melanoma & nonmelanoma skin cancers

VI. Chemical & Drug photosensitivity

It may be **endogenous** (as caused by porphyrias) or **exogenous** (caused by systemic or topical chemicals). Photosensitivity induced by exogenous agents can be divided into

II. Genetic

- **DNA repair-defective disorders**
  - ***Xeroderma pigmentosa*** [Q]
  - ***Bloom syndrome*** [Q]
  - ***Cockayne syndrome*** [Q]
  - Trichothiodystrophy
  - ***Rothmund Thomson syndrome*** [Q] (probable)

Mn - **"Try Bloom & coocked O (xero) Roti"**

- **Enzymatic defect in heme synthesis** l/t elavated ***porphyrin (a known phototoxic agent)*** [Q]
  - ***Erythropoietic porphyria & protoporphyrias*** [Q]
  - Hepatoerythropoietic porphyria
  - Variegate porphyria
  - Porphyria cutnea tarda (familial)
- Others
  - Albinism
  - Kindler syndrome
  - Phenylketonuria (PKU)

III. Photoaggravated (exacerbated) dermatoses

not caused but sometimes aggravated by UV are

- Acne vulgaris (aestivale)
- ***Atopic eczema*** [Q]
- Bullous pemphigoid
- Carcinoid syndrome
- Cutaneous T cell lymphoma
- Dermatomyositis
- Disseminated superficial actinic porokeratosis
- Erythema multiformal
- Familial benign chronic pemphigus (Hailey-Hailey disease)
- Granuloma annulare
- Hartnup syndrome
- Herpes simplex
- Keratosis follicularis (Darrier's disease)
- ***Lichen planus*** [Q] (actinicus)
- ***Lupus erythematosus*** [Q] ***(Systemic i.e SLE, subacute cutaneous i.e. SCLE & discoid i.e. DLE)*** [Q]
- Lymphocytic infiltrate of Jessner
- ***Pellagra, Psoriasis, Pemphigus*** [Q]
- Pemphigus foliaceus (erythematosus)
- Pityriasis rubra pilaris
- REM (reticular erythematosus mucinosis) syndrome
- Rosacea
- Sarcoid Seborrhoeic eczema
- Smith-Lemli-Opitz syndrome
- Transient acantholytic dermatosis (Grover's disease)
- Viral infections.

Features	Phototoxicity	Photoallergy
Pathophysiology; Prevalence	**Nonimmunological** direct tissue injury; and is more common	Immune mediated **Type IV delayed hypersensitivity** response; and is much less common
Occurance after 1st exposure	Yes	No
Onset after exposure	Minutes to hours (early)	24 to 48 hours (Late)
Dose of agent needed for reaction	Large	Small
Cross-reactivity	None	Common
Diagnosis for Topical agents Systemic agents	Clinical Clinical + Phototest	Photopatch test Clinical + Phototest; possibly photopatch test
Clinical presentation	Erythema resembling exaggerated sunburn reaction that quickly desquamates or peels within several days. Edema, vesicle, bullae; burning, stinging and frequent resolution with hyperpigmentation are other features.	***Usually eczematous & pruritic rash*** [Q]**.** The clinical manifestations typically differs from those of phototoxicity in that an *intensely pruritic* eczematous dermatitis tends to predominate and evolves into lichenified, thickened, "*leathery*" changes in sun exposed areas. A small subset of patients (5-10%) may develop a persistent equisite hypersensitivity to light even when the offending drug or chemical is identified and eliminated, a condition known as persistent light reaction.
Histological features	Necrotic keratinocytes, epidermal degeneration; sparse dermal infiltrate of lymphocytes, macrophages & neutrophils	Spongiotic dermatitis, dermal lymphohistocytic infiltrate
Caustive drugs	Amiodarone, dacarbazine, fluroquinolones, 5-FU, furosemide, nalidixic acid, phenothiazines, psoralens, retinoids, sulfonamides, sulfonylureas, tetracyclines, thiazides, vinblastin	6-methyl-coumarin, aminobenzoic acid and esters, bithionol, chlorpromazine, diclofenac, fluroquinolones, halogenated salicylanilides, hypericin (st John's Wort), Musk ambrette, piroxicam, promethazine, Sulfonamides and Sulfonylureas
Type	Internal – Drugs External – Drugs, plants, food	Immediate – Solar urticavia Delayed – Drug photoallergy; Persistent light reaction /chronic actinic dermatitis

Polymorphous Light Eruption (PLE)

Clinical Presentation

- Is the 2nd most common photosensitive disorder after sunburn.
- Many affected individuals never seek medical attention because the condition is often transient, becoming manifest each spring with initial sun exposure but then subsiding spontaneously, with continuing, exposure, a phenomenon known as "**hardening**"
- Mostly present with ***often intensely pruritic erythematous papules that may coalesce into plaques in a patchy distribution on sun exposed areas of trunk & forearms***[Q].
- Morphological **skin findings remain similar for each patient with** subsequent recurrences, **significant individual variations** in skin findings are characteristic (**hence** term **polymorphous**).
- Common disorder occurring in young and middle aged persons, mostly women.
- Characterized by ***itchy papules & papulovesicles on exposed sites – particularly the forearms***. The papules are *intensely pruritic & erythematous* that may coalesce into plaques in a patchy distribution on *exposed areas of trunk ('V' area of chest), neck and forearms,* The face is usually less seriously involved.
- ***The rash develops shortly after sun exposure through out the summer & spring months; and improve in winter.*** [Q]

Diagnosis

- Diagnosis is confirmed by ***skin biopsy*** and by performing *photo-test procedures (ie photo-patch test & photo-provocation tests)* in which skin is exposed to multiple erythema doses of UV-A & UV-B. The action spectrum for PLE is usually within these portions of solar spectrum.

Prevention & Treatment

- Preventive measures include use of sunscreens & induction of hardening by cautious administration of UV-B (broad or narrow band) and/or UV-A or the use of psoralen plus UV-A (PUVA) photochemotherapy for 2-4 weeks before initial sun exposure (i.e. **prophylactic phototherapy or photo chemotherapy** at the beginning of spring may prevent occurance of PLE throughout the summer)
- Treatment of acute flare of PLE require **topical or systemic glucocorticoids**.

Lupus Erythematosus (LE)

Cutaneous manifestations of LE is usually divided into 3 main types: acute, subacute and chronic. Acute cutaneous lupus erythematosus **(ACLE)** is *almost always* a/w underlying visceral involvement (i.e. SLE). Subacute cutaneous lupus erythematosus **(SCLE)** patients meet diagnostic criteria of SLE about *50%* of the time. And chronic cutaneous lupus erythematosus **(CCLE)** also k/a discoid lupus erythematosus (**DLE**, Lupus panniculitis, chilblain lupus, & tumid lupus erythematosus) patients most often have *skin only or skin predominantly disease*. ***ACLE & SCLE are highly photosensitive & characteristically nonscarring whereas DLE causes scarring & permanent disfiguration***[Q].

ACLE

- Characterized by localized, *confluent, usually symmetrical erythema centered over malar eminences and bridging over nose* **(classic butterfly or malar rash of SLE)**. The nasolabial folds are characteristically spared, whereas forehead, chin & V area of neck can be involved.
- Erythema is often *sudden in onset* and accompanied by *edema, fine scaling and systemic involvement* (or exacerbation of systemic disease).
- While sometimes evanescent (ephemeral i.e. lasting only hours) usually last for days or few weeks. *Scarring does not occur.*
- Few patients may have generalized (widespread) morbilliform or exanthematous eruption often focused over the extensor aspects of arm & hands and characteristically sparing the knuckles (preferentially involved in dermatomyositis).

SCLE

- Initially presents as slightly scaly *erythematous macules & /or papules* that evolve into hyperkeratotic **papulo-squamous eruption** (resembling psoriasis) or **annular/polycyclic plaques** (resembling erythema multiforme).
- Lesions are characteristically *widespread, nonscarring, photo sensitive* and occur in predominantly *sun exposed areas* (i.e. back, chest, shoulders, V area of neck, extensor aspects of arm & hands; lesions are uncommon on face, flexor surface of arms & below the waist).
- Typically heal without scarring but leaving long lasting (if not permanent) vitiligo like

CCLE/DLE

- Discrete lesions are most often found on ***face, scalp & /or external ears***[Q] and on V area of neck, extensor aspect of arm, legs and trunk to lesser extent.
- It begins as *erythematous red purple macules, papules or small plaques with hyperkeratosis &* **follicular accentuation**.
- Early classical lesion typically evolve into **sharply demarcated, discoid (coin shaped) erythematosus plaques** covered by a **thick** (prominent), **adherent scale** that extend into the orifices of dilated hair follicles & occluding it (**follicular /Keratotic plugging**). When adherent scale is removed from advanced lesions, its underside shows small excrescences (horny plugs) which have occupied openings of dilated pilosebaceous canals (hair follicles). This **carpet tacking** or **tin-tack sign** is relatively specific for DLE, but can sometimes also be seen in localized pemphigus foliaceus.
- DLE lesions typically expand with erythema & hyperpigmentation at periphery sometimes with raised indurated borders. Long standing lesions develop (leave) ***hallmark central atrophy, scarring (atrophic central scarring), telangiectasia and hypopigmentation***[Q]. Characteristic peripheral hyperpigmentation is often absent in Caucasians.
- ***Irreversible, scarring alopecia***[Q] resulting from DLE differs from the reversible, non scarring alopecia of SLE.
- In face (perioral ly) DLE resolves with a striking ***acneiform (cribriform) pattern of pitted scarring***[Q]. DLE characteristically affects external ear including outer portion

Although perivascular nail fold erythema & telangiectasia can occur in ACLE, they are more common, typical & occur in more exaggerated forms in dermatomyositis.

leukoderma (grey white hypopigmentation) and telangiectasias. Pigmentary changes usually resolve completely.

of external auditory meatus. **Wide follicular pits** (sometimes with scales or blackheads) occur mainly in concha or triangular fossa of ear.

- Only 5-10% of DLE patients subsequently develop (meet the ARA criteria of) SLE. However, 25% of SLE patients develop typical discoid lesions of DLE.

ARA Diagnostic Criteria for SLE: If ≥ 4 present at any time in patient's history; the specificity is ~95% & sensitivity is ~75%

1. **Malar rash** (fixed erythema over malar eminences sparing nasolabial folds)
2. **Discoid rash** (erythematous raised patches with adherent keratotic scaling, follicular plugging and atropic scarring)
3. **Photosensitivity**
4. **Oral/Nasopharyngeal ulcerations** (usually painless)
5. **Nonerosive Arthritis** (of ≥ 2 peripheral joints with tenderness, swelling or effusion)
6. **Serositis (pleuritis or pericarditis)** documented by ECG, effusion, rub or pain.
7. **Renal disorder** (persistent proteinuria > 0.5 g/d or 3+, or cellular casts)
8. **Neurological disorder** (seizure or psychosis without other cause)
9. **Haematological disorder (hemolytic anemia with reticulocytosis or leucopenia** < 4000/μL or **lymphopenia** < 1500/μL on ≥ 2occasions or **thrombocytopenia** < 1 lack/μL in absence of offending drugs)
10. **Immunological disorders :** LE cells or **anti ds DNA antibody** or **anti Sm** antibody or **antiphospholipid antibodies** (based on a **false positive serology for syphilis** for more than **6 months** or **anticardiolipin** antibodies).
11. **Antinuclear antibody (ANA).**

Differentiating Features	ACLE	SCLE	DLE
Induration, Dermal atrophy & Folliclular plugging	-	-	+++
Pigmentary change & Hyperkeratosis	+	++	+++
Histopathology - **Thickened basement membrane & periappendageal inflammation**	-	+	+++
- Lichenoid infiltrate	+	++	+++
Lesional Lupus band	++	++	+++
Non lesional lupus band	++	++	-
ANA (antinuclear antibody & **risk for developing SLE)**	+++	++	+
Hypocomplementemia	+++	+	+
Anti-ds-DNA antibody	+++	+	-
Ro/SSA – antibody by			
ELISA	++	+++	+
Immunodiffusion	+	+++	o

Porphyria

Porphyrias – are a group of diseases that have in common inherited or acquired derangements in the synthesis of heme. Heme is an iron chelated tetrapyrrole or porphyrin, and the non metal chelated porphyrins are potent photosensitizes that absorb light intensely in both the *short (400 – 410 nm)* and the *long (580 to 650 nm)* portions of visible spectrum. Heme cannot be reutilized and must be continuously synthesized and the two body compartments with the largest capacity for its production are ***bone marrow*** and ***liver.*** The porphyrins circulate in the blood stream and diffuse into the skin, where they absorb solar energy, become photoexited, generate reactive oxygen species, and evoke cutaneous photosensitivity. This mechanism is k/a *photodynamic or oxygen dependant* and is mediated by reactive oxygen species such as singlet oxygen and superoxide anions.

Precipitated by ***drugs (eg. sulfonamide)***[Q], ethyl alcohol, estrogenic hormones, hexa chlor benzene (HCB), chlorinated phenol, iron, TCDD (2, 3, 7, 8 – Tetra chloro di benzo- p- dioxin), polychlorinated bi phenyls (PCB), herbicides (2, 4- di chloro & trichloro phenoxy acetic acid); exogenous steroids including OCP containing progestins, infection, surgery, illness & attempt to loose weight (low caloric & carbohydrate intake).

Cutaneous-Photosenstivity

- Increased **skin fragility vesicles & bullae** followed by *erosions & crusting l/t scarring*, occur predominantly in areas subjected to *repeated trauma (usually dorsa of hand)*
- Numerous small **milia** of pearly *white to yellow* colour *on fingers & hands.*
- Although skin lesions are on *light exposed area,* patients are

Erythropoietic protoporphyria (EPP)

- 2nd most common of cutaneous porphyrias (after PCT) & begins in early life. PCT is unusual before puberty & usually onset in 3rd, 4th decade.
- Characteristic **acute episode of photo sensitivity,** *including burning, stinging (smarting) & pruritis* affecting light exposed skin, esp *nose, cheeks & dorsa of hands f/b erythema, edema, urticarial* lesions & rarely purpura.
- May occur ***within minutes of sun exposure & often show seasonal variation***[Q] i.e. starting in spring,

Neuro-visceral symptoms

- Characterized by ***abdominal pain (most common ~90%), neurological & psychiatric symptoms***[Q].
- Abdominal pain is often intermittent, steady, poorly localized & spasmodic.
- *Vomiting, nausea, constipation* (ileus), decreased bowel sounds are common
- Abdominal tenderness, fever, leukocytosis are usually absent or mild because symptoms are neurological rather than inflammatory
- **Mental (psychiatric) symptoms** include

often unaware, because the acute painful burning photosensitivity so characteristic of erythropoeitic porphyrias is absent
- However, patients recognize their ***skin condition worsens in spring & summer and improve in fall & winter***[Q].
- *Mottled hyper & hypo-pigmentation* (resembling chloasma), and associated purpilish red (heliotrope) suffusion of central face involving periorbital areas (resembling plethora)
- **Non virilizing hypertrichosis** mostly pronounced on zygomatic & malar skin (monkey like face in HCB poisoning)
- *Sclerodermoid plaques*, calcification, scarring.

↓

Hepatic porphyrias a/w cutaneous photosensitivity **(PCT, VP, & HCP)**

continuing in summer & dimishing in winter.
- Lesions resolve slowly leaving *small, atrophic, waxy thickened, wrinkled skin or pitted scars*. This l/t **pathognomic' old *knuckles in a child*'** appearance and *pseudorhadages* (d/t pursing of perioral skin.)
- Severe life threating **hepatotoxicity** & *early age gall stones* occurs in small percentage of EPP. There is no *hypertrichosis, milia, sclerodermoid change, or hyperpigmentation* as in PCT, and no *erythrodontia* as in CEP. Hemolytic anemia is uncommon.

Congenital Erythropoeitic porphyria (CEP)

- *Most mutilating* cutaneous porphyria, usually develops during *first few months (infancy)* or first decade and show porphyrin deposition in bones & teeth **(erythrodontia).**
- *Skin fragility*, pink fluorescent fluid contaning *vesicle & bullae* f/b secondary infection & scarring is common. It may l/t *loss of acral tissue* (i.e. tips of ear, nose & fingers), *facial mutilation & cicatrizing alopecia.*
- Hirsutism, hyper & hypo pigmentation & eye changes may occur
- **Erythrodontia (red teeth)** of both deciduous & permanent teeth is common & virtually pathognomic.
- *Spleenomegaly , porphyrin rich cholelitheasis, fluorescent bone marrow normoblast , and fluorescent reddish pink urine* are associated features. *Hemolytic anemia* d/t short life span of RBC (36 vs 120 days) & hyperspleenism occurs.

anxiety, insomnia, depression, disorientation, ***hallucination***[Q] & paronia
- **Peripheral neuropathy** d/t *axonal degeneration* primarily affects *motor neurons of proximal muscles* (shoulder & arms) initially > focal cranial nerve > *sensory* (l/t paresthesia, pain in limb, head- neck & sensory loss) > *respiratory & bulbar paralysis* (l/t death)
- ***Seizures***[Q] can be d/t *hyponatremia* (resulting from vomiting & inappropriate fluid therapy) or neurological effect. Treatment of seizure is difficult because most anti seizure drugs can exacerbate AIP *(clonazepam may be safer than phenytoin or barbiturates)*
- **Sympathetic overactivity** may l/t tachycardia, hypertension, restlessness, tremors, excessive sweating & cardiac arrythmias causing sudden death.

|

Acute intermittent porphyria (AIP), ALAD deficiency, Heriditary coproporphyria & Varigated porphyria

Porphyrins: Clinical & Laboratory Features

Type	Enzyme		Inheri-tance	Skin Photose-nsitivity	Neuro Visceral Symptom	Urine colour	Increased precursor & /or porphyrins		
	Deficient	Activity % of normal					RBC	Urine	Stool
• **Hepatic Porphyrias**									
- 5 ALA dehydratase deficiency	ALA dehydratase	5	**AR**	-	+++		Zn-protoporphyrin	ALA, Coproporphyrin III	-
- Acute Intermittent Porphyria	HMB synthase	50	AD	-	+++	Red-purple	-	ALA, PBG, Uroporphyrin	-
- Heriditary Coproporphyria	COPRO oxidase	50	AD	+	++	N-red		ALA, PBG, Coproporphyrin III	Coproporphyrin III
- Verigate porphyria	PROTO oxidase	50	AD	++	+	N-pink-red		ALA, PBG, Coproporphysin III	Coproporphyrin III Protoporphyrin
- ***Porphyria Cutanea Tarda***[Q]	URO decorboxylase	20	AD	+++	-	Pink-red		Uroporphyrin, 7 carboxylate porphyrin	Isocoproposphyrin
• **Erythropoetic porphyrias**									
- X linked sideroblastic Anemia	ALA synthase	-	**XLR**	-	-			-	-
- Erythropoetic protoporphyria	Ferrochelatase	20-30	AD	+++	-	N	Protoporphyrin	-	Protoporphyrin
- ***Congenital Erythropoetic porphyria***[Q]	URO synthase	1-5	**AR**	+++	-	**Pink-red**	Uroporphyrin I Coproporphyrin I	Uroporphyrin I Coproporphyrin	Coproporphyrin I

Management of Porphyrias

It includes avoidance of sun light, photo protection (clothing, sunscreem etc), change of day- night rhythm, avoidance of precipitating factor and

In non acute porphyrias (PCT, EPP, CEP)

- ***Phlebotomy (venesection) is treatment of choice***Q; 400-500 ml every 2wks over 3-6 months
- **Low dose chloroquin** in patients where phlebotomy is C/I eg. presence of anemia, cardiopulmonary disorder, HIV
- **Oral beta caroteins**

★ In non acute hepato erythropoeitic porphyria, phlebotomy & low dose chloroquin (antimaliarials) are ineffective.

In acute porphyrias (AIP, VP, HCP, AADDP)

- Intensive monitoring & porphyrin measurement

Symptom	Treatment
Abdominal pain	Aspirin, Opiate- pethidine or morphine
Vomiting	Chlorpromazine, promazine, triflupromazine or promethazine
Hypertension	Propanolol
Hyponatremia	Electrolyte balance, saline infusion
Convulsions	Gabapentine
Constipation	Neostigmine

- Intravenous heme arginate or hematin and glucose

Purpura

Purpura (≥3mm) Patechial (≤ 2mm)

Occur d/t extravasation of RBC into dermis, so the lesions do not blanch with pressure

Nonpalpable

Primary cutaneous disorders (m.c)

- **Trauma**
- **Solar (actinic) purpura** (mainly on extensor forearms)
- **Steroid purpura** (secondary to potent topical steroid or endo/exogenous Cushing's syndrome)
- ***Capillaritis***Q d/t perivascular lymphocytic inflammation
  - bright red patechiae scattered in annular /coinshaped yellow brown macule
  - Found primarily on lower extremities
- **Livedoid vaculopathy**

Systemic causes

I. **Clotting disturbances**

- ***Thrombocytopenia (including ITP***Q & involve distal lower extremity)
- *Abnormal platelet function* (seen in uremia)
- *Clotting factor defect*

II. **Vascular fragility**

- ***Amyloidosis***Q
- *Ehler Danlos syndrome*
- Scurvy (flattened corckscrew hair with surrounding haemorrhage on lower extremity + gingivitis)

III. **Thrombi formation** within vessels

- **DIC**Q (triggered by viral, gram +/-, rickettsial infection, tumor & trauma)
- *Purpura fulminans* (DIC with fever & hypotension more commonly in children after varicella, scarlet fever or URTI)
- ***Monoclonal cryoglobulinemia***Q (associated with multiple myeloma, waldenstrom's macroglobulinemia, lymphocytic leukemia & lymphoma. purpura of lower extremities & haemorrhagic infarcts of finger & toes with disease exacerbation following cold exposure, increased serum viscosity.
- ***Thrombotic thrombocytopenic purpura***Q (have fever & microangiopathic hemolytic anemia)
- *Heparin induced thrombocytopenia & thrombosis*
- *Warfarin reaction / induced necrosis* (often involve areas with abundant sub cutaneous fat-breast, abdomen; buttocks, thigh, calves in females between 3- 10 days of therapy. Painful erythema becomes pruritic, then necrotic & finally adherent black eschar).

IV. **Emboli**

- *Cholesterol emboli* (usually on lower limbs of pt. with atherosclerotic vascular ds. Following anticoagulant therapy or invasive vascular procedure eg. arteriogram)
- *Fat embolism (on upper body 2-3 days after major injury*
- *Tumor or thrombus embolism* (seen in atrial myxomas & marantic endocarditis)

V. **Immune complex ds.**

- *Waldenstroms hypergammaglobulinemic purpura* (petechiae on lower extremity with exacerbations associated with prolonged standing & walking. There are circulating complexes of IgG-anti IgG molecule)
- ***Gardener –Diamond syndrome/ auto erythrocyte sensitivity***
- (Female pt. develop large ecchymoses within area of painful, warm erythema. Intradermal inj. of autologous RBC or phosphatidyl serine can recproduce lesions in some)

Palpable

I. **Vasculitis**

- ***Cutaneous small vessel (Leukcytoclastic vasculitis (LCV)***
  - etiologies include antibiotics, hepatitis C virus infection, autoimmune connective tissue disease. Lesions of LCV are circular in outline
  - ***HSP***Q (seen primarily in children & adolescents following URTI. Lesions on buttocks & lower limbs + fever, arthralgia, GI bleeding abdomen pain & nephritis)
  - ***Polyarteritis nodosa***Q (arteritis l/t irregular outline of purpura & LCV)

II. Infectious emboli (usually irregular in outline)

- ***Accute meningococcemia***Q *(primarily involve trunk, lower limbs & pressure sites and a gunmetal gray colour develops with in them + preceding URTI, fever, meningitis, DIC & deficiency of terminal components of complements)*
- ***Disseminated gonococcal infection***Q / arthritis – dermatitis syndrome (arthralgia, tenosynovitis, fever + papule, vesicopustule with central purpura or haemorrhagic necrosis found on distal extremitis)
- ***Rockey mountain spotted fever***Q *(several day h/o fever, chills, severe headache & photophobia precedes cutaneous erruption)*
- ***Ecthyma gangrenosum***Q (Pseudomonas aeruginosa is classically associated but other gram –ve rods eg. Klebsiella, E.coli. & Serratia and in immuno compromised candida & opportunistic fungi can also l/t similar lesions)

Palpable purpura

It is d/t vasculitis or vasoclusion (infective, systemic, embolic) affecting cutaneous vasculature (small & medium size):

Round /Portwine Classic palpable purpura

Lesions usually in dependent areas

Leukocytoclastic vasculitis Immune complex
- Only small vessels involved
  - Idiopathic / infection / drug-associated IgG/IgM complexes
  - ***Idiopathic IgA complexes (H-S purpura or IgA with drugs /infection)***Q
  - Subacute bacterial endocarditis (involve hands)
  - Waldenstrom hypergammaglobulinemia
  - Urticaria /Pustular vasculitis (often random localization)
- Small & medium size vessels involved
  - ***Mixed cryoglobulinemia***Q
  - ***Rheumatic vasculitis***Q (lupus erythematosus, rheumatoid arthritis, dermatomyositis)

Random lesions

Pauci-immune – Leukocyto clastic vasculitis
- ANCA (antineutrophilic cytoplasmic antibodies) associated
  - ***Wegner granulomatosis***Q
  - Microscopic polyangitis
  - Churg – Straus & (rarely)
- Others
  - Erythema elevatum diutinum (hands, feet, elbow & buttocks)
  - Sweet syndrome

Non leukocytoclastic
- Involve small vessels only
  - Erythema multiformae (acral early)
  - Pityriasis lichenoides et varioliformis acuta
  - Chronic pigmented purpura (often involve legs)
  - Waldenstrom hypergamma globulinemia
  - Urticaria lymphocytic vasculitis

Retiform purpura

- Immune complex / Pauci immune Leucocytolastic vasculitis
  - ***Henosch- Schonlein purpura (IgA vasculitis)***Q
  - ***Mixed cryoglobulinemia***Q
  - Rheumatic vasculitides
  - ***Wegner granulomatosis***Q
  - Microscopic polyangitis
  - Churg- strauss
  - Benign cutaneous ***polyarteritis nodosa***Q (ANCA –ve pauci-immune)
- Nonvasculitic
  - Livedoid vasculitis (lower legs)
  - Pernio/chill blains (finger / toes)
  - Pyoderma gangrenosum
  - Sweet syndrome

Henoch-Scholein (Anaphylactoid) Purpura Syndrome

- It is usually a *benign, self limiting and relapsing* (typically in first 3 months) *systemic vasculitis syndrome involving small vessels* (arteriole, capillary , venule) of *dermis (skin), intestine and kidney* d/t entrapment of ***IgA1 dominant immune complex***Q ***in blood vessel walls.***
- It's ***incited by upper respiratory tract infection (streptococcal or viral)***Q, drugs, food, insect bite & immunization.
- It is ***most common systemic vasculitis of children occurring predominantly in children (between 2-10 with a peak incidence at 4-7 years***Q and adolescents. However infants & adults may be involved.
- Male to female ratio of 1.5:1, peak in spring and cluster of cases d/t person to person respiratory spread is also reported. It presents with:

Skin (100%)

- ***Palpable non blanchin,g non thrombocytopenic, symmetrical purpura & splinter hemorrhage mostly on lower extremities & buttocks***Q.
- Arms, face & ears can be involved but *trunk is usually spared.*

Joint symptoms (84%)

Self limiting, non-deforming but incapacitating arthralgiaQ (>> arthritis) involves ankle, knees and dorsum of hands & feet is d/t periarticular edema.

★ In **adults,** presenting symptoms are most frequently related to skin & joints. Adults have more frequent & severe renal involvement and increased ESR; but have less frequent abdominal pain & fever.

★ Myocardial involvement in adults & scrotal swelling in children are rare presentations

GI symptoms (70% of pediatric & lesser in adults patients)

- ***Colicky abdominal pain***Q (most common)
- Nausea, vomiting, diarrhea or constipation
- ***Upper GI bleeding (epistaxis)***Q, ***& frequent passage of blood (melena) & mucous per rectim***Q.
- GI symptoms precede skin disease by upto 2 weeks and are potentially most serious & may l/t *intussuception* (usually of small bowel). Inflammation of duodenum especially 2nd part is characteristic of HSP.

Diagnosis

- Histological demonstration of ***extra (peri) vascular netrophilic infiltrates with destruction of walls of capillary & venules (leukocytoclastic vasculitis)***Q.
- **Direct immunofluorescence** shows ***IgA (mostly IgA1) and C_3 deposits about small blood vessels in skin, intestine & kidney***Q.

Renal symptoms (10-50%)

- Mostly mild glomerulonephritis (similar to IgA nephropathy) l/t *proteinuria,* & ***microscopic hematuria***Q, with RBC casts.
- It ***usually resolves spontaneously without treatment***Q.
- Rarely a progressive (necrotizing or proliferative) GN develop. The ***long term prognosis of HSP is directly dependent on the severity of renal involvment***Q.
- **Renal biopsy** provides *prognostic information;* is rarely needed for diagnosis.
- HS nephritis is m.c. form of cresentic GN.

Treatment

- **Glucocorticoid (prednisolone** 1mg /kg/ day) decrease tissue edema, arthralgia & abdominal discomfort but has ***no role in skin or renal disease***Q and in *decreasing the duration of active disease or chances of recurrence*
- Rapidly progressive GN is treated with *intensive plasma exchange* + cytotoxic drugs.

Adamantiades Behcet's disease (Behcet's Syndrome)

It is a chronic, recurrent, multi system inflammatory disorder of unknown etiology, classified as *systemic vasculitits involving all size & types of blood vessels* and characterized clinically by *recurrent oral apthous & genital ulcers, skin lesions, iridocyclitis/posterior uveltis* and arthritis, occasionally accompainied by vascular, gi, neurological or other systemic manifestation.

Clinical Features and Diagnostic Criteria

- **Recurrent oral apthous ulcer** (minor, major or hepetiform) which are usually *multiple, recurrent (at least 3 times in a year), painful, sharply marginated* with a *yellow fibrin coated base and surrounding erythema* is a defining major criteria seen in 100% cases. It usually heal *without scarring*.
- **Genital ulcers** are less recurrent and usually heal with a characteristic **scar**.
- **Skin lesions** include ***erythema nodosum like nodules***Q, superficial thrombophelebitis, pustular vasculitic lesions including pathergy lesions), sweet like lesions, pyoderma gangrenosum like lesion, palpable purpuric lesions or pseudofolliculitis acneform nodules: (both less relevant)
- **Ocular lesions: uveitis (usually posterior** or pan uveitis) also k/a **retinal vasulitis** is main ocular feature. Anterior uvetits (iridocyclitis), hypoyon etc. are other features
- Addition systemic symptoms include
- **Arthritis** i.e. nonerosive, asymmetric, sterile, migratory, seronegative - oligoarthritis
- **Epididymitis, Gastro-intestinal lesions** represented by ileocecal ulceration CNS lesions
- **Vascular lesions** include venous occulusion, thrombosis, varices, arterial occlusions and aneurysm *often being migratory and sometimes fatal*.
- **Positive pathergy test & HLA-B-51**

Pathergy Test

- It is triggering of a *significant inflammatory response by minor injury* such as venipuncture.
- It is a sufficiently specific and frequent feature of Bachet's (seen in 40% cases) which is considered diagnostic. Although it is *not pathognomic*, as it can also occur in patients with *pyoderma gangrenosum*, rheumatoid arthritis Chron's disease and genital herpes infection.
- It manifests *within 48 hours* as an hyper reactivity reaction/erythematous papule>2mm or pustule after needle prick or venipuncture or venous access.

Histopathology

- Characteristic features are *vasculitis and thrombosis.*

Treatment

- **Topical steroids** are the main stay of treatment in painful oro-genital lesions.

Kawasaki (Mucocutaneous - Lymphnode) Syndrome

It is an acute *multisystem vasculitis* of unknown etiology associated with marked activation of T cells & monocyte / macrophages.

Diagnostic Criteria

Symptom	Occurrence (%)
Fever lasting > 5 days (with spikes) plus at least 4 of the following:	100
1. *Bilateral painless bulbar non exudative conjuctival injection*Q	92
2. Oro-*pharyngeal* mucous membrane changes (≥1) - ***Cherry red (injected) or fissured lips***Q (± drying, cracking & fissuring) - Injected (red) pharynx - ***Strawberry tongue***Q (i.e. hypertrophic tongue papillae with hyperemia)	100 84 72 32
3. Extremity changes (≥1) - Erythema of palms or soles - ***Edema (non pitting) of hands or feet***Q (tenderness may limit walking & hand use) - ***Desquamation (perigenital & perineal followed by periungual, starting at the tips of finger)***Q.	 72 48 56
4. Rash – polymorphous erythematous exanthema	100
5. Acute non – suppurative cervical lymphadenopathy (≥1 node, > 1.5 cm in diameter)	72

Epidemiology

Primarily an illness of young children ranging from 7 weeks- 12 years, with ~ ***80% being younger than 5 years of age***Q. Male: female ratio is 1.5: 1.

3 - Clinical phases

1. **Acute febrile phase** *ends* with resolution of fever in *7-14 days*. It has conjunctival injection, mouth & lip changes, erythema of hand & feet, rash and cervical lymphadenopathy.
2. **Subacute phase** is from end of fever to 25 days. It has desquamation, arthralgia, arthritis & thrombocytosis
3. **Convalescent** phase from disappearance of clinical sign to normalcy of ESR (usually 6- 8 weeks after onset of illness).

Associated features / Complications

- **Cardiovascular manifestations** are ***leading cause of morbidity & mortality***Q and include myocarditis, artierial aneurysm, pericarditis, MR, AR, ventricular arrhythmias.
- ***Arthralgia & arthritis***Q
- Urethritis with sterile pyuria
- Aseptic meningitis
- Hydrops of gall bladder
- Diarrhea, vomiting or abdominal pain
- Sensorineural hearing loss
- Uveitis
- Hepatic dysfunction

Treatment

- **Treatment of choice** in KS in **first 10 days** of fever is ***intravenous gammaglobulin/ immunoglobulin (IVGG or IVIG) as a large single dose of 2gm/kg given over 10-12 hours plus high dose aspirin (80-100 mg/kg/day in four doses)***Q. It reduces risk of coronary artery disease from 20% to < <5%.
- Aspirin is reduced to antithrombotic (3-5 mg/kg/day as single dose) *in 14 days when fever* has *resolved* and can be discontinued after 6-8 weeks if Echo shows no evidence of coronary artery disease. And if abnormality is detected, low dose aspirin is *continued indefinitely*

Reactive arthritis (ReA) / Fiessenger – Leroy – Reiter syndrome

It is primarily an ***acute non- purulent, asymmetrical, additive arthritis***Q, complicating an infection elsewhere

Triggering Etiological Agents

- **Enteric infection** with *Shigella (mostly flexneri), Salmonella, Yersinia and Campylobacter* species
- **Genitourinary (Venereal) infection** (STD) with *Chlamydia trachomatis, Ureaplasma Urealyticum, & Mycoplasa genitalium*
- **HLA – B27** is positive in 50-60% of blacks & 60- 85% of whites.
- **HIV infection stage I disease** (WHO classification)
  - In blacks who are rarely HLA B27 positive, ReA is oftenly 1st manifestation of infection and often remits with disease progression.
  - In contrast, western Caucasians with HIV & spondyloarthritis are predominantly HLA B 27 positive, and arthritis flares as age advances

Etio-pathogenesis & Epidemiology

- Most of triggering organisms produce **lipopdysaccharide (LPS)** & share a capacity to attack mucosal surfaces, to invade host cells and to survive intracellularly.
- Prevalence of HLA B2 positivity is more in Shigella, Yersenia or Chlamydia infections than in Salmonella & Campylobacter infections
- ReA is most common in 18-40 years, but can occur in children (>5) & older adults.

Differences in post-enteric & post veneral ReA

- Gender ratio is *1 : 1* in ReA following enteric infection but *9 : 1 with male* predominance after venereal infections.
- Skin lesions of *keratoderma blenorrhagica* and histological evidence of *inflammation in colon & ileum* are mainly seen in venereally acquired ReA

Clinical Features

Classic History

- Careful history will elicit evidence of an ***antecedent infection of GIT or genito urinary tract, 1 to 4 weeks prior to onset of symptoms***Q
- A sizable minority may have no clinical or lab evidence of antecedent infection but may reveal
  - *A recent new sexual partner*
  - ***History of travel to endemic region***Q

Features

- **Constitutional symptoms** include fever, fatigue, malaise & weight loss
- **Musculoskeletal features**
  - ***Acute, asymmetrical, additive*** (new joints involved in 2 days-2 weeks) ***non purulent, painful, polyarthritis***Q mostly involving joints of lower extremity, esp knee *(m.c)*Q, ankle, subtalar, metatarsophalangeal & toe inter phalangeal. Wrist & fingers can also be involved
  - **Tense joint effusions** are not uncommon usually in *knee*Q.
  - **Dactylitis (sausage digit),** a diffuse swelling of a solitary finger or toe is a distinctive feature but is also seen in other *peripheral spondylo arthritis, polyarticular gout & sarcoidosis.*
  - *Enthesitis, tendinitis & fascitis* producing pain at tendoachillis, & heel (plantar fascitis).
  - Sacroilitis in 20% cases

Characteristic Triad

Mn

- **C** - ***Conjunctivitis***Q (± uveitis)
- **U** - ***Urethritis***Q (± cervicitis)
- **P** - Poly***arthritis***Q

- **Urogenital** lesions include ***urethritis***Q, prostatitis (in males) or cervicitis or salpingitis (in females.)
- **Ocular involvement** ranges from asymptomatic ***conjunctivitis***Q to blinding anterior uveitis.
- **Mucocutneous Features**
  - ***Superficial transient & often asymptomatic oral ulcers***Q (typically painful in Bechet's)
  - Characteristic skin lesion, **keratoderma blenorrhagica**, (consists of *vesicles*, that become *hyperkeratotic*, ultimately forming crust before disappearing) is ***most common on plams & soles***Q
  - **Circinate balanitis, *on glans***Q, consists of vesicles that quickly rupture to form painless superficial erosion.
  - Nail changes are common & include *onycholysis, distal yellowish discolouration & /or heaped up hyperkeratosis.*
- Rare features are cardiac conduction defects, aortic insufficiency, pleuro- pulmonary infiltrates & central or peripheral nervous system defects.

Laboratory findings & Diagnosis

- Diagnosis is clinical with no definitive test. Mild anemia, ↑ESR and C-RP (acute phase reactants), moderate leukcytosis & thrombocytopenia
- *HLA B27* association common but not absolute
- *Elevated antibodies to Yersinia, Salmonela, or Chlamydia* may be present
- PCR of 1st voided urine for chlamydial DNA is highly sensitive
- Radiological features
  - Juxtaarticular osteoporosis (early) f/b → marginal erosions & loss of joint space (late).
  - **Periostitis with reactive new bone formation** is characteristic of ReA, as it is with all spondylo arthritides
  - Spurs at insertion sites, ***asymmetrical sacroilitis and asymmetrical spondylitis with coarse & non marginal syndesmophytes***Q arising from the middle of vertebral body, a pattern rarely seen in primary ankylosing spondylitis.

Differential diagnosis

- Unlike ReA, **gonococcal arthritis** tends to involve both upper & lower extremities equally, lack back symptoms & has characteristic vesicular skin lesions. A positive gonococcal culture from skin, synovium or blood establish diagnosis of disseminated gonococcal infection but positive cultures from urethra or cervix does not exclude diagnosis of ReA. Theraputic trial of antibiotic improves gonococcal A.
- Unlike ReA, **psoriatic arthritis** is gradual in onset, primarily affects upper extremities, less commonly associated with perirthritis and usually lack mouth ulcers, urethritis or bowel symptoms.

Diagnostic criteria of **Bechet's syndrome:**

- *Recurrent oral* ulcerations *(apthous or herpetiform, atleast 3 times over 12 months period)*

+

- *Two of the following : Recurrent genital ulcerations, skin lesions, ocular lesions*

DERMATOLOGY

1

Neutrophilic & Eosinophilic Dermatomes

Neutrophilic dermatoses

Histologically, neutrophilic infiltrate appears at variable levels in epidermis, dermis & subcutaneous tissue. It encompasses 5 entitics:

1. ***Subcorneal pustular dermatosis***[Q] ***(Sneddon- Wilkinson disease)***
2. ***Acute febrile neutrophilic dermatosis***[Q] ***(Sweet's syndrome)***
3. Erythema elevatum diutinum
4. ***Pyoderma gangrenosum***[Q]
5. Neutrophilic eccrine hidradenitis

Eosinophilic Dermatoses

I. Diseases **characterized** by tissue eosinophils

- Hypereosinophilic syndromes
- Wells syndrome (eosinophilic cellulitis)
- ***Kimura disease***[Q]
- ***Granuloma faciale***[Q]
- Angiolymphoid hyperplasia with eosinophilia
- Eosinophilic pustular folliculitis (Ofuji disease)
- Eosinophilic ulcer of oral mucosa.

II. Diseases **typically associated** with tissue eosinophils

- Arthropod bites & sting
- Infestations / parasitic diseases
- Urticaria / Angioedema
- Dermatoses of pregnancy
- Bullous dermatoses eg. pemphigoid, pemphigus & incontinentia pigmenti
- Histocytic diseases eg. Langerhans cell histocytosis & juvenile xanthogranuloma
- Vasculitis eg. Churg- strauss syndrome & Eosinophilic vasculitis.
- Eosinophilic panniculitis eg. erythema nodosum etc.

Sweet Syndrome (Acute Febrile Natrophilic Dermatosis)

Sweet syndrome (Acute febrile neutrophilic dermatosis with cutaneous and systemic manifestation)

Etiology

May be idiopathic or sometimes secondary to-

- Hypersensitivity to bacterial, viral or tumor antigen
- Association with otitis media, osteomyelitis, aseptic meningitis, HIV, and infections of upper respiratory tract, urinary tract or GI system & liver
- ***Association with malignancy like myelogenous leukemia***[Q] and bowel or breast cancer.
- May be secondary to Bechet's disease, rheumatoid arthritis, inflammatory bowel disease (Crohn's & ulcerative colitis), insect bite, needle prick and pregnancy.

Clinical features

- It occurs mostly in young women & rarely in children.
- **Systemic features:** It presents with ***recurrent moderate – high fever***[Q], tiredness, headache, arthralgia, conjunctivitis & mouth ulcers
- **Cutaneous features:** Abrupt onset of raised, ***tender, edematous and erythematous plaques or nodules and targetetoid lesions with pseudovesiculation***[Q] on any area of skin.
- **Distinctive skin lesions** develop in following pattern:

  Infection (URTI/fever) → Small red bumps on back, neck, arms & face → plaques → tender & painful blister, pustules or ulcer → disappear on their own in weeks to months without medication and in days with medication.
- Anemia, leukocytosis, increased CRP & ESR.
- **Histopathology: Skin biopsy** reveals **neutrophilic perivascular infiltrates without evidence of vasculitis**[Q]. Dense diffuse neutrophilic infiltrate with **leucocytoclasis** but not vasculitis.

Diagnostic criteria

- **Major criteria** (Both are required)

1. ***Abrupt onset of painful or tender erythematous plaques or nodules occasionally with vesicles, pustules or bullae***[Q].
2. ***Histopathological evidence of a dense neutrophilic infiltrate in dermis without evidence of Leukocytoclastic vasculitis***[Q].

- **Minor criteria** (2 of 4 is required for diagnosis)

1. Preceded by a non specific upper respiratory or gastrointestinal tract infection or vaccination or associated with:
   - Pregnancy
   - ***Hemoproliferative disorders or solid visceral malignancy***[Q]
   - Inflammatory diseases such as chronic autoimmune disorders & infections.
2. Periods of ***pyrexia >38°C (100°F)***[Q] and malaise
3. Abnormal laboratory values at onset (3 of 4): ESR > 20 mm/h; positive C-reactive protein; >8000 leukocytosis; segmented nuclear neutrophils & ***> 70% neutrophils in peripheral blood***[Q]
4. ***Excellent response to treatment with systemic corticosteroid or potassium iodide***[Q].

- **Drug induced sweet's syndrome** is diagnosed by presence of both major, 2nd minor criteria and
  - Temporal relation b/w drug ingestion & clinical presentation or temporally related recurrence
  - Temporally related resolution of lesions after drug withdrawal or treatment with systemic corticosteroids.

Pyoderma Gangrenosum (PG)

Rare *chronic, recurrent, non-infectious, inflammatory, neutrophillic ulcerating skin disease* of unknown etiology characterized by neutrophilic infiltration & destruction of dermis.

Associations

- Occurs in patients with chronic underlying inflammatory or malignant disease such as ***ulcerative colitis***[Q], rheumatoid arthritis, chronic active hepatitis, Crohn's disease, IgA monoclonal gammopathy, and hematological & lymphoreticular malignancies, but in 40-50% of patients, no associated disease is found.
- *Minor cutaneous trauma (pathergy)* such as needle stick, inoculation site, insect bite precede PG in 25% cases (**pathergic phenomenon**).

Cutaneous manifestation

- Primary lesion usually single but sometimes multiple begins as tender, red macule or papule, pustule, nodule or bullae on normal appearing skin, *most commonly on leg.*
- As necrotizing inflammatory process extends peripherally, center degenerates, crusts & erodes resulting in a necrotic ulcer (i.e. ulcer with a purulent base), *alarming increase in severity of pain,* with an undermined *bluish (purple-red) edge and halo of surrounding erythema.*
- *Surrounding skin* becomes dusky red & *indurated* and develop a *zone (areola) of erythema.*

Panniculitis

It is *inflammation of subcutaneous fat (or panniculus),* may present as *subcutaneous nodules* and is frequently a sign of systemic disease. Several forms of panniculitis include *erythema nodosum, erythema induratium/nodular vasculitis, Weber Christian syndrome, lupus* profundus, lipodermatosclerosis, α_1 *anti trypsin* deficiency, factitial & fat necrosis secondary to *pancreatic disease.*

Erythema nodusum

- It is *most common type of septal panniculitis* and is considered to be a ***hypersensitivity reaction***[Q] against various etiological agents

Most common

- Group A, B hemolytic **Streptococcal infections**
- Upper respiratory tract viral infections
- ***Sarcoidosis***[Q]
- ***Inflammatory bowel disease (Crohn's & UC)***[Q]
- ***Rheumatological***[Q] & autoimmune disease including ***SLE***[Q], Reiter's Behcet's, Coeliac ds & autoimmune hepatitis
- ***Pregnancy***[Q], Malignancy, acne fulminans, hematological stem cell transplantation

Less common Associations

Infections

- ***Tuberculosis***[Q], ***Leprosy***[Q]
- Histoplasmosis, Brucellosis
- Coccidioodomycosis, Mycoplasma
- Psittaosis
- Cat scratch fever
- Yersinia gastroenteritis
- ***Salmonella gastroenteritis***[Q]
- Chlamydia trachomatis, Chalmydophilia pneumoniae, M. pneumoniae, Hepatitis B virus

Drugs

- ***Oral contraceptives***[Q]
- ***Sulfonamides***[Q]
- ***Penicillins***[Q]
- Asparmate
- Bromides
- Iodides
- Hepatitis B vaccine
- Isotretinoin,
- Imatinib mesylate

- It may occur at any age but most cases appear between 2nd & 4th decade of life with women accounting for 80% of cases

Cutaneous manifestation:

- Typical lesions consist of a ***sudden onset of bilateral symmetrical very painful/tender, erythematous, warm nodules & raised plaques usually on anterior aspect of lower extremities (typically on shins, knees & ankles)***[Q]. Less commonly other sites including face may be involved.
- The lesions are often *more easily palpated than visualized.* Nodules may coalesce to form plaques.

Erythema induratum/Nodular vasculitis

- It is *most common form of lobular panniculitis with subcutaneous (septal) vasculitis* and is considered to be a *hypersensitivity reaction* against various agents. These include bacterial (such as streptococcal, mycobacterial) infections, viral (such as hepatitis C) infections, drug (eg .propythiouracil), autoimmune colitis & colonic carcinoma.
- **Erythema induratum of Bazin** is preferred for those cases in which *etiological relationship with tuberculosis* is demonstrated and the remainder of cases are referred to as **nodular vasculitis (Whitfield erythema).**
- It manifests as ***tender, dusky erythematous often suppurative subcutaneous nodules or plaques on the posterolateral (Calf) aspect of lower legs***[Q].
- It is typically ***seen in healthy, middle aged,***

Weber Christian Syndrome/(Idiopathic) Nodular Panniculitis

Relapsing febrile non-suppurative nodular panniculitis

- *It is lobular panniculitis without vasculitis often accompanied by systemic manifestations* including fever, malaise, abdominal pain, arthritis, myalgia, weight loss) and rarely involvement of visceral fat (including heart, lungs, kidneys & liver which may l/t death)
- All ages may be affected, but it is very rare in childhood & most common in young adult females who develop crops of dull red, tender, subcutaneous nodules usually about 1-2 cm in diameter.
- Lesions are maximal on lower limbs (usually calf), although

- Initially within few days the nodules show a vivid (shiny) red or purple colour that evolves to a yellow or greenish coloration and flatten appearance (similar to an old ecchymosis or bruise), so referred to as ***erythema contusiformis.*** This transformation is characteristic of EN, making retrospective diagnosis possible.
- ***Lesions of EN never ulcerate, atrophy or scar***[Q], which is contrast to all other types of panniculitis
- Eruptions generally *last for 3-6 weeks, and recurrences are freaquent.*

Systemic manifestation:

- ***Fever, fatigue, malaise arthralgia, headache***[Q], gastrointestinal upset (abdominal pain, vomiting, diarrhoea), cough, conjunctivitis and elevated ESR/CRP, *leucocytosis* may accompany lesions.

Histology:

- **Septal panniculitis** (septal oedema with initial neutrophils/eosinophils & later histiocytes infiltration) **without vasculitis** is classical histological feature.
  Miescher's radial granuloma, which consists of small, round well defined, nodular aggregations of small, histiocytes /macrophage radially arranged around a small slit or small vessel; although is *characteristic histological marker* of *EN*, but is also seen in Sweet's syndrome, Bechet's disease, erythema induratum, & nodular lesions in systemic fibrosing dermapathy.

sometimes obese women who may have venous stasis[Q]. Patients often have thick (heavy column like) calves with erythrocyanosis, perifollicular erythema & cutis marmorata.

- Lesions may be unilateral, are often inflamed and usually adhere to skin surface, ***ulcerate and then heal slowly leaving an atrophic scar***[Q].
- Lesions mostly develop during the cold months of winter are *usually moderately tender but may be asymptomatic (indolent).*
- This course is chronic, with relapses typically occurring over several years.

trunk & face can be affected

- Many nodules eventually resolve, leaving a pigmented area or an *atrophic depression*. In few cases, there may be *ulceration/ necrosis with drainage of oily, brownish, serous fluid* eventually l/t *scarriing.*
- Term weber Christian disease should be abandoned & is best avoided.

Histological Classification of Panniculitis (P)

Septal Panniculitis	Lobular Panniculitis	Mixed septal & lobular Panniculitis	Panniculitis with Vasculitis
- Erythema nodosum - Erythema nodosum migrans (subacute nodular migratory panniculitis) - Eosinophilic panniculitis (may overlap with lobular or mixed panniculitis; show *flame figures*/fragmented eosnophilic granules; is a reactive process)	- Relapsing febrile nodular panniculitis(Weber Christian syndrome) - Idiopathic nodular panniculitis - Lipoatrophic/autoimmune/connective tissue P(Rothman Makai syndrome) - **Panniculitis a/w crystal deposition** sclerema neonatorum, ***subcutaneous fat necrosis of newborn***[Q], gout or factitial panniculitis, ***post steroidal P***[Q], calciphylaxis (inj of meperidine & pentazocine) - Enzymatic (pancreatic) panniculitis - α_1-Antitrypsin deficiency P. - Fat necrosis – cold injury (adpinecrosis frigore/Haxthausen's disease), encapsulated (nodular cystic) fat necrosis, lipomembranous (membranocystic) fat necrosis - Lymphomatous panniculitis - Cytophagic histiocytic panniculitis	- *Lupus erythematosus* (Le) profundus - *Scleroderma* (fascitis with eosinophilia) - *Connective tissue* panniculitis (overlaps with lipoatrophic P) - Subcutaneous sarcoidosis - Subcutaneous *granuloma annulare* - *Necrobiosis lipoidica* - Infective panniculitis (eg.opportunistic bacterial or fungal infections) - Physical & factitious P (eg oil granuloma/oleoma/oleogranuloma/ paraffinoma/sclerosing lipogranuloma; *idiopathic/eosinophilic sclerosing lipogranuloma*) - Sclerosing P (lipodermatosclerosis/hypodermatitis sclerodermaformis) - Fascitis-Panniculitis syndromes	- Small vessels vasculitis- leukocytoclastic vasculitis - Large vessel vasculitis- PAN, thrombophlebitis, ***nodular vasculitis (erythema induratum)***[Q] - Neutrophilic panniculitis - Oedematous scarring vasculitic panniculitis; hydroa like lymphoma

Questions

AUTOIMMUNE SYSTEMIC DISEASE

1. **Which of the following not a feature of dermatomyositis?** *(AIIMS Nov 09)*
   A. Gottren's papules ☐
   B. Periungua telangiectasia ☐
   C. Salmon rash ☐
   D. Mechanic's hand ☐
2. **True about dermatomyositis** *(PGI Nov 09)*
   A. Gottron papules ☐
   B. ANA a/w all cases ☐
   C. All cases a/w malignancy ☐
   D. Proximal muscle wasting ☐
3. **Gottron's papules or sign seen in:** *(AIIMS 93)* ☐
   A. Dermatomyositis ☐
   B. Multiple myeloma ☐
   C. Acute myeloid leukemia ☐
   D. Psoriasis ☐
4. **A 40 year old woman presented with a 8 month history of erythema and swelling of the periorbital region & papules & plaques on the dorsolateral aspect of forearms & knuckles with ragged cuticles. There was no muscle weakness. The most likely diagnosis is:**
   A. SLE *(AIIMS Nov 04, DNB 11)* ☐
   B. Dermatomyositis ☐
   C. Systemic sclerosis ☐
   D. Mixed connective tissue disorder ☐
5. **Antibody that is strongly associated with polymyositis?**
   A. Anti-jo1 *(AIIMS Nov 08)* ☐
   B. Anti-ku ☐
   C. Anti-Scl-70 ☐
   D. Anti-sm ☐
6. **Female presents with history of color change from pallor to cyanosis on exposure to cold in fingers. This condition is mostly associated with?** *(AIIMS Nov 08, DNB 05)*
   A. Scleroderma ☐
   B. Leukemia ☐
   C. Lung infections ☐
   D. Hepatosplenomegaly ☐
7. **All are manifestations of SLE except:**
   A. Lesions resemblig Chr. DLE *(PGI 98)* ☐
   B. Butterfly rash ☐
   C. Photosensitivity ☐
   D. Constitutional symptom ☐
   E. Sex ratio is nearly equal ☐
8. **True about drug induced SLE is:** *(PGI 2K, DNB 05)*
   A. CNS manifestation are common ☐
   B. Renal involvement is common ☐
   C. Antihistone antibodies are found in many ☐
   D. All with antibodies progress to lupus ☐
   E. Sex ratio is nearly equal ☐
9. **Lupus like picture is causes by all except:**
   A. Chloroquine *(AI 91, DNB 03)* ☐
   B. Procanamide ☐
   C. Hydralazine ☐
   D. Isoniazid ☐
10. **Chloroquin is indicated in treatment of**
    A. Pemphigus *(AI 92, DNB 10)* ☐
    B. Pempigoid ☐
    C. Psoriasis ☐
    D. DLE ☐
11. **All of the following drugs can lead to SLE like reaction except?** *(AIIMS May 13)*
    A. Hydralazine ☐
    B. Penicilline ☐
    C. Isoniazid ☐
    D. Sulphonamide ☐
12. **23 year old lady sony develops brown macular lesions over bridge of nose and cheek following exposure to light. The probable diagnosis is** *(AIIMS May 12, 99)*
    A. SLE ☐
    B. Acne Rosacea ☐
    C. Chloasma ☐
    D. Photodermatitis ☐
13. **A girl of 19 years with arthritis and photosensitive rash on cheeks, likely diagnosis is** *(AI 01, Bihar 03)*
    A. SLE ☐
    B. Chlosma ☐
    C. Steveris Johnson Syndrom ☐
    D. Lyme's Disease ☐
14. **The concentration of hydroqinone for treating cholasma should be-** *(AIIMS 96, DNB 98)*
    A. 1% ☐
    B. 1 to 2 % ☐
    C. 2 to 5 % ☐
    D. 10% ☐

PHOTOSENSITIVITY DISORDERS

15. **Photosensitive dermatitis is/are :** *(PGI May 2011)*
    A. Psoriasis ☐
    B. Pellagra ☐
    C. Pemphigus ☐
    D. SLE ☐
    E. Congenital erythropoietic porphyria ☐
16. **Which of the following are photosenstive diseases:**
    A. SLE *(PGI 01, DNB 99)* ☐
    B. Liver spots ☐
    C. Calcinosis cutis ☐
    D. Morphea ☐
    E. Prophyria cutanea tarda ☐
17. **Which of the following not photosensitive :** *(AI 04)*
    A. Porphyria ☐
    B. DLE ☐
    C. SLE ☐
    D. Lichen Planus ☐
18. **Exposure to sunlight can precipitate :**
    A. Chlosma *(AI, UPSC 2K, DNB 02)* ☐
    B. Discoid lupus erytyhematosus ☐
    C. Dermatitis herpatiformis ☐
    D. Lupus vulgaris ☐
19. **A 45-year-old farmer has itchy erythematous papular lesions on face, neck, 'V' area of chest, dorsum of hands and forearms for 3 years. The lesions are more severe in summers and improve by 75% in winters. The most appropriate test to diagnose the condition would be:**
    A. Skin biopsy *(AI 06)* ☐
    B. Estimation of IgE levels in blood ☐
    C. Patch test ☐
    D. Intradermal prick test ☐

PORPHYRIA

20. **Chandu 32 years male presents with abdominal pain and vomitting. He also complain of some psychiatric**

symptoms & visual hallucination. Most likely diagnosis is (AI 01, DNB 04)
A. Hypothyroidism ☐
B. Hyperthyroidism ☐
C. Hysteria ☐
D. Intermittent Porphyria ☐

21. A girl on sulphonamides developed abdominal pain and presented to emergency with seizure. What is the probable cause? (AIIMS Nov 08)
A. Acute intermittent porphyria ☐
B. Congenital erythropoietic porphyria ☐
C. Infectious mononucleosis ☐
D. Kawasaki's disease ☐

22. A 40 year old farmer with history of recurrenmt attack of porphyria complains of itching when exposed to the sun and maculopapular rashes on sun exposed area. His symptoms are exaggerated in summer. The diagnosis is :
A. Seborrheic dermatitis (AIIMS 01) ☐
B. Contact dermatitis ☐
C. Psoriasis ☐
D. Porphyrea Cutanea tarda ☐

23. Porphyrins are synthesized mainly in
A. Spleen (AIIMS 95) ☐
B. Liver and spleen ☐
C. Bonemarrow and spleen ☐
D. Liver and Bone marrow ☐

24. Porphyria cutanea tarda can be treated by: (AI 98)
A. Phlebotomy ☐
B. Heme ☐
C. Low dose chlotoquine ☐
D. Metronidazole ☐

25. Treatment of choice in the cutaneous complication of porphyria is : (Jipmer 96, PGI 01)
A. I. V dextrose ☐
B. I. V Haematin ☐
C. Beta carotene ☐
D. Calamine ☐

PURPURA

26. Non Palpable purpura is seen in A/E
A. H. S. Purpura (AIIMS 94) ☐
B. Drug induced vasculitis ☐
C. Idiopathic thrombocyto penic purpura ☐
D. Amyloid ☐

27. Palpable purpura is seen in all except:
A. Wegeners GN (PGI 99, DNB 07) ☐
B. ITP ☐
C. HSP ☐
D. Serum sickness ☐

28. Palpable pupura is seen in all conditions except
A. Cryoglobulinuria (AI 2K, DNB 06) ☐
B. H. S. Pupura ☐
C. Gaint cell arteritis ☐
D. Drug induced vasculitis ☐

29. A 42- year- old female has palpable purpura with rash over buttocks, pain in abdomen, and arthropathy diagnosis is
A. Sweet syndrome (AI 08) ☐
B. HSP ☐
C. Purpura fulminans ☐
D. Meningococcemia ☐

30. IgA deposits on skin biopsy (AIIMS May 09)
A. Henoch Schouleiln puspura ☐
B. Giant cell arteritis ☐
C. Microscopic polyangitis ☐
D. Wegener's granulomatosis ☐

31. A 5 year old child develops non blanching macules, papules and petecheal hemorrhage on lower extremities, mild abdominal pain, and skin biopsy showed IgA deposition along blood vessels and perivascular neutrophilic infiltrate. Most probably diagnosis is
A. Wegner's granulomatosis (AIIMS May 09, Nov 11) ☐
B. Poly artiritis nodosa ☐
C. Henoch Schonlein purpura ☐
D. Kawasaki disease ☐

32. Which of following is/are not the feature of Henoch-Schonlein Purpura (HSP) : (PGI Dec 08)
A. Abdominal pain ☐
B. Splinter haemorrhage ☐
C. Thrombocytopenia ☐
D. Epistaxis ☐
E. Arthritis ☐

33. All regarding HSP is true except (PGI 08)
A. Hematuria resolve without treatment ☐
B. Steroids best treat skin lesions ☐
C. Self limiting arthralgia ☐
D. Excellent prognosis ☐
E. Purpura fulminans ☐

34. 'Pinch purpura' is diagnostic of (AIIMS May 05)
A. Systemic 1° amyloidosis ☐
B. 2° systemic anyloidosis ☐
C. ITP ☐
D. Drug induced purpura ☐

35. Treatment of Kawasaki's disease? (AIIMS may 09, Nov 11)
A. IVI g ☐
B. Steroids ☐
C. Thalidomide ☐
D. Dapsone ☐

36. A 4 year old child with high fever developed toxic look, eruptions on trunk & proximal extremities, bilateral bulbar conjunctivitis without discharge and fissuring – crusting- red lips. Due to limb edema walking became difficult. She also had desquamation in perineum & finger tips with cervical adenopathy. Diagnosis is
A. PAN (UP 07, AIIMS 05) ☐
B. HSP ☐
C. Kawasaki syndrome ☐
D. Erythema infectosum ☐

37. Necrotizing lymphadenitis is seen in (AI 11)
A. Kimura's disease ☐
B. Hodgkin's disease ☐
C. Castleman's disease ☐
D. Kikuchi disease ☐

38. Which of the organisms most commonly causes reactive arthritis? (AIIMS Nov 08)
A. Ureaplasma urealyticum ☐
B. Group A beta hemolytic streptococci ☐
C. Borrelia burgdorferi ☐
D. Chlamydia ☐

39. A patient gives h/o recurrent oral ulcers. The ulcers are small with a yellow floor surrounded by an erythematous halo on lips. He also has multiple, tender nodules on shin. The probable diagnosis is
A. Pemphigus vulgaris (AIIMS Nov 11) ☐
B. Bechet's syndrome ☐
C. Herpes Labialis ☐
D. Fixed drug eruption ☐

40. A 27-year-old male had burning micturation & urethral discharge. After 4 weeks he developed joint pains involving both the knees & ankles, redness of the eyes & skin lesions. The most probable clinical diagnosis:
A. Psoriasis vulgaris (AIIMS May 05, DNB 02) ☐
B. Reiter's synd ☐
C. Bechet's synd ☐

D. Sarcoidosis ☐

41. Which of the following is not included in the triad of Reiter's syndrome : *(DNB 99, Kerala 99, CUPGEE 96)*
A. Conjunctivetis ☐
B. Urethritis ☐
C. Arthritis ☐
D. Keratoderma blenorrhagica ☐

42. A 29 years old male with a history of long leisure trip presented with right knee pain and swollen join with foreign body sensation in eye. The most probable diagnosis is
A. Sarcoidosis *(AI 2009)* ☐
B. Tuberculosis ☐
C. Reiter's disease ☐
D. Bechet's disease ☐

43. What is not seen in Reiters syndrome? *(AIIMS Nov 08)*
A. Subcutaneous nodules ☐
B. Keratoderma blennorrhagicum ☐
C. Circinate balanitis ☐
D. Oral ulcers ☐

44. True regarding reactive arthritis is all except *(PGI – 08)*
A. HLA B27 & HIV affects severity ☐
B. Dactylitis & enthesitis ☐
C. Keratoderma mostly on glans ☐
D. Asymmetrical sacroilitis ☐
E. Onycholysis & hyperkeratosis of nails ☐

45. Recurrent orogenital ulceration with arthritis is seen in
A. Bechets syndrome *(PGI 96)* ☐
B. Gonorrhoea ☐
C. Reiters syndrome ☐
D. Syphilis ☐

46. All the following are primary cutaneous diseases except:
A. Psoriasis *(AIIMS May 10, AI 09)* ☐
B. Reiter's disease ☐
C. Lichen planus ☐
D. Icthiosis/Bowen's disease ☐

NEUTROPHILIC DERMATOSES

47. All are neutrophilic dermatosis except - *(PGI June 08)*
A. Subcorneal pustular dermatosis ☐
B. Kimura disease ☐
C. Granuloma facial ☐
D. Sweet's syndrome ☐
E. Pyoderma gungrenosum ☐

48. False about sweet syndrome *(PGI Nov 09)*
A. May be a/w high fever ☐
B. Neutrophilia not present ☐
C. May be a/w hematological malignancy ☐
D. Pseudovesication ☐
E. Tender erythematous nodule / plaque. ☐

49. A child with fever had multiple skin lesions, and on microscopic examination the skin lesions are seen to have neutrophilic and histiocytic infiltration in the dermis. What is the diagnosis? *(AI 09, 11)*
A. Sweet syndrome ☐
B. Behchet's syndrome ☐
C. Pyoderma gangrenosum ☐
D. Juvenile dermatosis ☐

50. Pyoderma gangrenosum is seen in : *(TN 97)*
A. Crohns disease ☐
B. Divertuculosis ☐
C. Ulcerative colitis ☐
D. Ca. Colon ☐

CUTANEOUS DRUG ERRUPTION

51. A 27 year old sexually active male develops a vesicobullous lesion on the glans soon after taking tab paracetamol for fever. The lesion healed with hyper pigmentation. The most likely diagnosis is: *(AI 2005)*
A. Bechet's syndrome ☐
B. Herpes genitalis ☐
C. Fixed drug eruption ☐
D. Pemphigus vulgaris ☐

52. Recurrent erythematous plaques on glans penis in a 19 yrs old sexually active male which heals with residual hyperpigmentation, is suggestive of? *(AIIMS Nov 09)*
A. Apthous Balanitica ☐
B. Fixed Drug Eruption ☐
C. Herpes Gestations ☐
D. Chlamydial infective ☐

PANNICULITIS

53. Neonatal fat necrosis (subcutaneous fat necrosis of newborn) resembles: *(AIIMS May 2011)*
A. Erythema induratum ☐
B. Post-steroidal panniculitis ☐
C. Lupus panniculitis ☐
D. Lipodermatosclerosis ☐

54. Erythema nodosum is seen in all of the following excep:
A. Pregnancy *(AI 11)* ☐
B. Tuberculosis ☐
C. SLE ☐
D. Chronic pancreatitis ☐

55. Erythema nodosum is seen in all, EXCEPT: *(AIIMS 92)*
A. Rheumatoid arthritis ☐
B. Tuberculosis ☐
C. Enteric fever ☐
D. Aspirin therapy ☐

56. Erythema nodosum is seen in A/E *(AIIMS 94)*
A. Salicylate poisioning ☐
B. Typhoid ☐
C. Tuberculosis ☐
D. Leprosy ☐

57. Erythema nodosum is due to A/E: *(Jharkhand2004)*
A. Contraceptive pilles ☐
B. Barbiturates ☐
C. Penicillin ☐
D. Sulphonamides ☐

58. Erythema nodosum is not seen in:
A. Primary TB *(AIIMS 91)* ☐
B. Sulfonamides ☐
C. Giant cell arteritis ☐
D. Streptococcal Infection ☐

59. 25 yr old male having fever & malaise since 2 weeks, arthritis of ankle joint and tender erytematous nodules over the shin. Diagnosis is: *(AIIMS May 2010)*
A. Erythema nodosum ☐
B. Hansen'sdisease ☐
C. Weber- Christian disease ☐
D. Nodular Vasculitis ☐

60. Which of these statements is false for lesions of Erythema nodosum: *(MP 2004)*
A. They are considered as hypersensitivity reaction ☐
B. The skin overlying the lesions is red, smooth and shiny ☐
C. They are usually non tender ☐
D. They can be associated with tuberculosis ☐

61. A young female presents with a history of fever and nodular lesion over the shin. Histopathology reveals foamy histiocytes with neutrophilic infiltration. There is no evidence of vasculitis. Most probable diagnosis is:
A. Sweet's Syndrome *(AI 2011)* ☐
B. Erythema nodosum ☐
C. Erythema nodosum leprosum ☐
D. Behcet's syndrome ☐

Answers and Explanations:

Autoimmune Systemic Diseases

1. **C i.e. Salmon rash**
2. **A & D i.e. Gottron papules; Proximal muscle wasting**
3. **A i.e. Dermatomyositis** 4. **B i.e. Dermatomyositis**

[Ref. Harrison 17/p 2696-2703; Fitzpatrick's 7/e p-1536-1553; Roxburgh's 17/e p. 83-84, 164; Neena 3/e p. 196-95]

***Presence of characteristic periorbital erythema & edema (Helitrope rash), Gottron's papules, periungal telangiectasia, mechanics hand, shawl sign, poikiloderma (ragged cuticles) & calcinosis cutis favour the diagnosis of dermatomyositis*Q.**

5. **A. i.e. Anti Jo 1** *[Ref: Harrison's 17/e p- 2697, 2076; Fitzpatrick 7/e p. - 1528, 1539]*

Myositis specific auto antibodies include the ***antisynthetases [Jo-1, PL-7, PL-12, OJ, Mi-2, and signal recognition particle (SRP)]***Q. Whereas, *PM/Scl, Ro / SSA (Ro 52, Ro 60), and U1- RNP* represent major **myositis associated autoantibodies.**

6. **A. i.e. Scleroderma** *Ref: Harrison's 17/e p-2096-2105; Fitzpatrick 7/e p. 1553-62*

Raynaud's phenomenon (i.e. ***cold/vibration/emotional stress-exposure l/t pallor → cynosis & finally erythema***Q of digits, ear & tip of nose) is ***almost always present (along with skin sclerosis) and is often earliest feature***Q of **Systemic sclerosis (Scleroderm).** It may precede extensive skin & internal organ involvement by week-months (in diffuse SS) to years (in limited cutaneous SS).

7. **E i.e. Sex ratio is nearly equal** *[Ref: Rook's 8/e p. 51.27; Harrison 18/e 2724-31]*

- Most authors agree that *females outnumber males*Q by a **ratio of ~8:1** and 90% of SLE patients at diagnosis are **women of child bearing age (~38 years).** The condition is universal; people of all genders, ages and ethnic groups are susceptible; but SLE is **3 times more common in black people than in white.** So highest prevalence is in black women and lowest in white men.
- According to American rheumatism association diagnostic criteria of SLE, it may present with ***photosensitive, butterfly (malar) rash or discoid rash (resembling chronic DLE)*** Q and **non erosive arthritis**, oral/nasopharyngeal ulcerations, serositis, renal/neurological/hematological/ immunological disorder and ANA.
- ***Systemic constitutional symptoms like fatigue, malaise, fever, anorexia and weight loss***Q are present in 95% of patients (although these are not included in diagnostic criteria).
- ANA are positive in > 98% of patients so repeated negative tests suggests that the diagnosis is not SLE, unless other antibodies are present. **High titer Ig antibodies to Sm antigen & ds DNA are both specific for SLE** and, therefore favour the diagnosis in presence of compatible clinical symptoms . Presence of multiple autoantibodies without clinical symptoms should not be considered diagnostic for SLE, although such persons are at increased risk.
- **Nephritis** is usually the **most serious** manifestation of SLE, since nephritis & infections are the **leading causes of mortality** in 1st decade of disease. Since nephritis is mostly asymptomatic, urinalysis should be done in suspected cases. **Renal biopsy** to classify nephritis (minimal mesangial, proliferative mesangial, focal, diffuse glomerulonephritis, membranous and advanced sclerotic) is **useful in planning current and near future therapies.**

8. **C i.e. Antihistone antibodies are found** *[Ref: Rooks 8/e p. 29.21, 51.32; Harrison 18/e p. 2735; Fitzpatric 7/e p. 355-57, 361,]*

Drug induced lupus is *caused by procainamide, hydralazine, isoniazid (but not chloroquine)* Q. It is a syndrome of *positive ANA associated commonly with antihistone antibodies, fever, malaise, arthritis or intense arthralgias/myalgias, serositis, and/or rash*Q. It occurs *predominantly in whites, has less female predilection than SLE, rarely involves brain or kidneys, is rarely a/w anti ds DNA and usually resolves over several weeks after discontinuation of offending drug*Q.

9. **A i.e. Chloroquine**
10. **D i.e. DLE** *[Ref: Goodman & Gillman 12/e p. 1405]*
11. **B i.e. Penicillin (?)** *[Ref: Harrison 18/e p. 2735; Fitzpatrick 5/e p. 1919]*

***Chloroquine is used in treatment of DLE & SLE and it does not produce lupus like picture*Q.**

Chloroquine is drug of choice for malaria caused by all plasmodium ovale/malariae/knowlesi and chloroquine sensitive P. falciparum & P. vivax. Chloroqione is also useful in-

Mnemonic		Use of chloroquine
Dr	=	*DLE*
S		*SLE, Sarcoidosis*Q*, Severe polymorphous light eruption*
M		Malaria
Pandey	=	Porphyria cutanea tarda (PCT)
Has Entered	=	Hepatic (Extraintestinal) amoebiasis
In	=	Infectious mono nucleosis
Labour	=	*Lepra reaction*Q
Room	=	Rheumatoid arthritis

SLE causing Drugs

Mnemonic		
H	=	*Hydralazine*Q
I	=	*Isoniazid*Q
P	=	*Procanamide*Q, Proctolol, Penicillamine, Phenytoin
Conture	=	Carbamazapine, Contraceptive

List of **drugs inducing SLE like syndrome** (in Rook's 8/e p. 51.32) **includes hydralazine, isoniazid (isonicotinic acid hydrazide), sulfasalazine, sulphonamide, penicillamine and penicillin all**Q. Whereas, shorlists given in Fitzpatrik & Harrison does not include both sulphonamides and penicillin. I have chosen penicillin as a probable answer because **sulfonamides and sulfonylureas** (sulfanilamide; tolbutamide & chlorproparmide) are included in list of **major topical photoallergens** (Rook's 29.21)

12. C i.e. Chloasma **13. A i.e. SLE** **14. C i.e. 2-5%**

[Ref: Roxborough 18/e p. 251-52, 314; Rook's 8/e p. 51.27-51.63, 36.11, 58.25/34/35; Harrison 18/e p. 429; Neena Khanna 3/e, p-137; Thomas Habif 4/e, p-692; Fitzpatric's 7/e, p-629, 1480]

- ***Light brown butterfly rash without systemic involvement in pregnancy and on OCP***Q is seen in **chloasma.** Whereas ***erythematous (red) phostosensitive butterfly rash with multisystem (multi organ) involvement like arthritis, nephritis, Raynaud's phenomenon etc***Q is seen in SLE.
- **Hydroquinone**, the most effective topical bleaching agent is used in 2-4% *concentration* in chloasma.

Chloasma/Melasma/Mask of pregnancy	SLE
- ***Light brown macules (rash or pigmentation)***Q - ***Associated with pregnancy (most common), OCP***Q, menstrual disturbance in unmarried girls & persistent anemia - More common in **females** on bridge of nose & cheeks (malar eminence). Linear area just above eyebrows is usually involved and area between nose & upper lip and skin around eyes as a rule spared.	- ***Dusky red (erythematous) photosensitive pigmentation***Q. - Associated with ***multi-organ involvement like arthritis/arthralgia, nephritis, raynaud's phenomenon etc***Q. - More common in **females** involving bridge of nose & cheeks i.e. malar eminence (malar butterfly rash)

Photodermatitis

- In *farmers, sailors, labourer* (in professions, which keep them in sun for prolonged periods)
- ***Scally read lesions***Q in sun exposed areas

Rosacea

- Recurrent episodes of bright red erythema and hot flushes on face, mostly in females nearing their menopause, triggered by emotional tension, hot spicy food & beverages.
- Later on erythema becomes persistant and telengectasia appears on nose, cheeks and chin

Photosensitive Disorders

15. All i.e. Psoriasis, Pellagra, Pemphigus, SLE, Congenital erythropoietic porphyria
16. A i.e. SLE; B i.e. Liver spots; E i.e. Porphyria cutanea tarda
17. D i.e. Lichen Planus **18. B i.e. Discoid lupus erytyhematosus**

[Ref: Harrison 18/e p. 444-45; Rook's 8/e p. 29.9-29.22; Fitzpatrick's 7/e p. 816-34]

- **Photosensitive dermatitis (skin lesions)** are *lupus erythematosus (SLE, DLE, SCLE), porphyrias*Q (erythropoietic/hepatoerythropoietic/variegate porphyria, erythropoietic protoporphyria and *porphyria cutaneatarda*Q), *psoriasis, pellagra, pemphigus, lichen planus (actinicus), and liver spots (lentigo senelis)*Q.
- **Morphea** is localized form of scleroderma (systemic sclerosis). **Calcinosis cutis** is calcified lesions seen in scleroderma & dermatomyositis.

Photosensitivity Diseases

Genetic

- ***Porphyrias (PCT***Q – familia variegate porphyria, hepatoerythropoietic / erythro poietic / erythropoietic proto - porphyria)
- Albinism
- ***Xeroderma pigmentosa***Q
- Rothmund – Thomson syndrome, Bloom syndrome, Kindler syndrome, Cockayne's disease and phenyl ketonuria (PKU)

Metabolic

- PCT – sporadic Hartnup disease
- Kwashiorkor, pellagra and carcinoid syndrome

Photoaggravated

- *Lupus erythematosus (SLE, SCLE, DLE)*Q
- Dermatomyositis, acne vulgaris (aestivale), lichen planus actinicus, herpes simplex.

Photo allergic

- Immediate: *Solar urticaria*Q
- Delayed: Persistent light reaction / chronic actinic dermatitis, drugs.

Phototoxic

- Drugs, plants, foods

Neoplastic & Degenerative

- Melanoma & non melanoma skin cancers
- Photoaging, actinic keratosis, *lentigo senilis (liver spots)*Q

Idiopathic

- *Polymorphous light eruption*Q
- Actinic prurigo, hydroa aestivale

19. **A i.e. Skin biopsy** *[Ref: Harrison 16th/ 328 – 26]*

- Presence of ***itchy papules or papulovesicles on sun-exposed areas particularlyl of forearm with a history of seasonal variations ie more severe in summer and improved in winters***Q – for long duration suggest the diagnosis of – **Polymorphic light reaction.** Diagnosis of PLR is confirmed by ***skin biopsy and by performing photo-test procedures (i.e. photo-patch test & photo provocative tests)***Q.
- **Phototoxicity** – is a non-immunological reaction caused by photo toxic drugs – amiodarone, dacarbazine, fluroquinolones, 5-FU, furosemide, nalidixic acid, phenothiazines, psoralens, retinoids, sulfonamides, sulfonylureas, tetracyclines, thiazides, vinblastin. The usual clinical manifestations include erythema resembling a sunburn reaction that quickly desquamates, or *"peels"*, within several days. In addition, edema, vesicles and bullae may occur.
- **Photo allergy –** is immune mediated, less common reaction caused by – 6-methyl-coumarin, aminobenzoic acid and esters, bithionol, chlorpromazine, diclofenac, fluroquinolones, halogenated salicylanilides, hypericin (st John's Wort), Musk ambrette, piroxicam, promethazine, Sulfonamides and Sulfonylureas. The clinical manifestations typically differs from those of phototoxicity in that an *intensely pruritic* eczematous dermatitis tends to predominate and evolves into lichenified, thickened, *"leathery"* changes in sun exposed areas. A small subset of patients (5-10%) may develop a persistent equisite hypersensitivity to light even when the offending drug or chemical is identified and eliminated, a condition known as persistent light reaction.
- A very uncommon type of persistent photosensitivity is known as **chronic actinic dermatitis**. These patients are typically elderly men with a long history of preexisting allergic contact dermatitis or photosensitivity. They are usually exquisitely sensitive to UV-B, UV-A and visible wave lengths (ie manifest a broad spectrum of UV – hyperresponsiveness).
- *Diagnostic confirmation of phototoxicity & photoallergy* can be done by using photo test procedures. For phototoxicity & photoallergy UV-A radiation (MED = minimal erythema dose) is used. Patients with persistent light reaction characteristically show diminished threshold to erythema evoked by UV –B.
- In solar urticaria, lesions occur ***within minutes of sun exposure***, on exposed areas.

Porphyria

20. **D i.e. Intermittent porphyria** *[Ref: Kaplan Synopsis 9/e p. 275-286; CDTP p-95-113;*
21. **A. i.e. Acute intermittent porphyria** *Shorter Oxford 5/e p. 2-20; Harrison 17/e p. 2434-40]*

Acute intermittent porphyria is a ***neuro visceral syndrome*** & should be suspected whenever a patient presents with symptoms suggesting involvement of both visceral & nervous system ***precipitated by drugs eg sulfonamides etc***Q

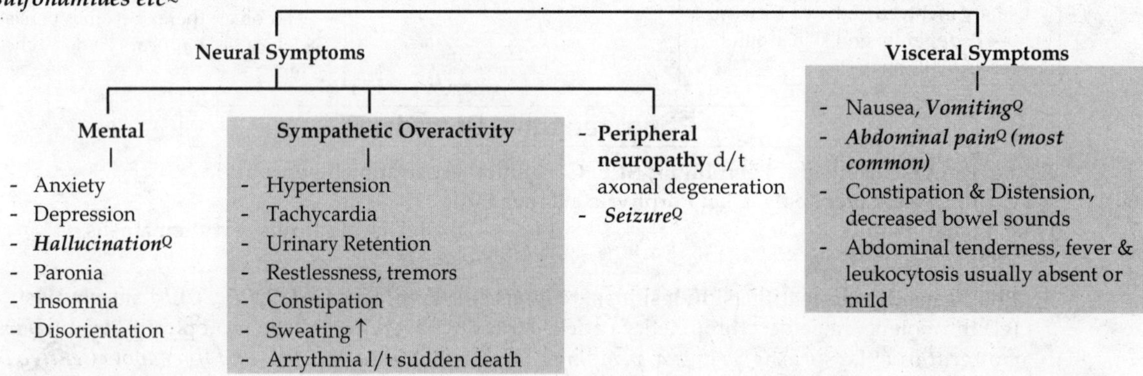

In this patient psychiatric symptoms (hallucination) & visceral symptoms (abdominal pain & vomiting) both are present leading to diagnosis of AIP.

22. **D i.e. Porphyria cutanea tarda**

Two types of porphyria are photosensitive

Porphyria cutanea tarda	Erythropoietic porphyria
- Is *most common* type of porphyria and is caused by decreased activity of enzyme *uroporphyrinogen decorboxylase.* - Two types of PCT are: (1) Sporadic or acquired type, seen in individuals ingesting ethanol or estrogens; (2) inherited type. Both forms are associated with increased hepatic iron stores. - Predominant clinical feature is a chronic photosensitivity characterized by *increased fragality of sun exposed skin, particularly areas subject to repeated trauma* such as dorsum of hands,	- Erythropoietic porphyria originate in the *bone marrow* and is d/t decrease in mitochondrial enzyme *ferrochelatase*; congenital type is d/t deficiency of *URO synthetase.* - Clinical features include an acute photosensitivity, characterized by subjective *burning and stinging of exposed* skin that often develops during or just after sun exposure. These may be skin swelling, and

forearms, face and ears. The predominant skin lesions are *vesicles and bullae,* that rupture, producing moist erosion, often with a hemorrhagic base, that heal slowly with crusting and purplish discolouration of the affected skin. *Hypertrichosis, mottled pigmentary change,* and scleroderma like induration are associated features.

- Confirmation of diagnosis is done by measurement of *urinary porphyrin excretion, plasma porphyrin assay and by assay of erythrocyte and/or hepatic uroporphyrinogen decorboxylase.*

after repeated episodes, *wax like scarring.*

- Diagnosis is confirmed by demonstration of *elevated levels of free erythrocytes protoporphyrins* Detection of *increased plasma protoporphyrin* helps to differentiate lead poisoning & iron deficiency anemia; in both of which elevated erythrocyte protoporphyrin levels occur in the absence of cutaneous photosensitivity & of elevated plasma protoporphyrin levels.

★ **Seborrhic Dermatitis:** presents with ***greasy scales & severe dandruff.*** **Cradle cap** is seborrhic dermatitis of scalp, face & groin in infant. But infant cradle cap is found in ptyriasis capititis complicated by seborrheic dermatitis.

23. **D i.e. Liver & Bone marrow**
24. **A. i.e. Phlebotomy > C. i.e. Low dose chloroquin**
25. **C. i.e. B carotene**

- **Porphyrin** are **synthesized** ***in liver and bone marrow***[Q].
- In **nonacute** porphyrias like **porphyria cutanea tarda (PCT)**, and **erythropoetic porphyrias**, treatment of choice is ***phlebotomy***[Q].
- Treatment of choice is cutaneous complication of porphyria is ***β-carotene***[Q].

Purpura

26. **A i.e. H. S. Purpura**
27. **B i.e. ITP**
28. **C i.e. Gaint cell arteritis** *[Ref: Rook's 8/e p. 49.1-49.51; 50.1-50.43; Fitzpatrick's 7/e p-1379 – 83, 1639; Harrison 18/e p. 421]*

- **Nonpalpable purpura** is seen in *clotting disturbances* like ***ITP***[Q] and platelet/ clotting factor defect; *in thrombi formation* like ***TTP,*** DIC, warfarin or heparin induced reaction; in increased *vascular fragility* like ***amyloidosis***[Q], scurvy & Ehlers-Danlos syndrome. ***Steroid purpura & capillaritis***[Q] also produce nonpalpable purpura.
- **Palpable purpura** is seen in **small vessel (or leucocytoclastic) vasculitis** like *Wegner's granulomatosis, Henoch Scholein Purpura,* Churg Strauss syndrome, microscopic polyangitis (polyarteritis), ***essential cryoglobulinaemia***[Q], cutaneous leucocytoclastic vasculitis (hypersensitivity angiitis or cutaneous necrotizing venulitis mainly affecting cutaneous post capillary venules), ***drug induced leucocytoclastic vasculitis***[Q] and ***serum sickness like reaction***[Q].

Palpable Purpura

Infectious Embolic (bacterial, fungal or parasitic)	**E**ccentric **G**eneral **M**anager **R**ocky	**E**cthyma **g**angrenosum disseminated **G**onococcal infection acute **M**eningococcemia **Rocky** mountain spotted fever
Vasculitis (leucocytoclastic **small &/or medium sized vessels)**	**W**as **P**lanning **H**is **M** **R** **C** **S**	**W**egner's granulomatosis **W**aldenstrom hypergammaglobulinemia **P**olyarteritis nodosa (**PAN**) **H**enosch **S**cholein Purpura (HSP) **M**icroscopic polyangitis **R**heumatic vasculitis **C**ryoglobulinemia (mixed) **C**hurg-**S**traus Syndrome **S**erum sickness & drug induced leucocytoclastic vasculitis

Non Palpable Purpura

Systemic

I. **Clotting disturbances** eg ITP, abnomral platelet function and clotting factor defects.
II. **Vascular fragility** eg **s**curvy, **a**myloidosis & Ehler-**D**anlos Syndrome (MN-"**SAD**")
III. **Thrombi** eg disseminated intravascular coagulation (DIC), monoclonal cryoglobulinemia, thrombotic thrombocytopenic purpura (TTP), thrombocytosis, heparin induced thrombocytopenia & thrombosis, warfarin reaction, antiphospholipid antibody syndrome, homozygous protein C & protein S deficiency
IV. Possible immune complex eg Waldenstrom hypergammaglobulinemic purpura and Gardner-Diamond syndrome (autoerythrocyte sensitivity)
V. Non infections emboli eg fat & cholesterol.

Primary Cutaneous disorders

- ***Steroid purpura***[Q]
- Solar (Senile, actinic) purpura
- Capillaritis
- Trauma
- Livedoid vasculopathy (with venous hypertension)

29. **B i.e., HSP**
30. **A.i.e. Henosch Schonlein purpura**
31. **C.i.e. Henoch Schonlein purpura**
32. **C. i.e. Thrombocytopenia**

33. B & E i.e. Steroids best treat skin lesions & Purpura fulminans
[Ref: Harrison 17/e p-2128, 335; Thomas Habif Clinical Dermatology 4/e p.645-50; Fitzpatric 7/e p. 1599-1602, 1734, 1382; Nelson 18/e p. 1043-45, 2732]

- Presence of ***palpable (non-blanching) purpura, mainly involving dependent areas such as buttocks & lower extremities in children & adolescents (<20 years)***Q along with ***arthralgia; gastrointestinal bleeding, colic abdominal pain, hematuria***Q, and histo pathological demonstration of ***extra /peri- vascular neutrophil (granulocyte) infiltrates (leukocytoclastic vasculitis)***Q with ***IgA (mostly IgA1 subtype) and C3 deposition about small blood vessels in skin, intestine and kidney***Q by immunofluorescence is diagnostic of - **Henoch – Schonlein purpura.**
- **Meningiococcemia** presents with short lived URTI, nausea, headache muscle soreness followed by → fever, obtundation, meningitis → vomiting, stupor, *hemorrhagic rash & hypotension*. Skin findings include *transient macular & papular lesions* (resembling viral exanthema) f/b *characteristic small, irregular, smudged appearance, asymmetrical petechiae* most often on extremities & trunk but can also be on head, palm, sole & mucous membrane Extensive maplike hemorrhagic lesions with central necrosis (suggilations) & bullae can develop.
- **Purpura Fulminans** is *extensive hemorrhagic* necrosis of skin d/t DIC (disseminated intravascular coagulation). It may be idiopathic (with in 10 days of *Scarlet fever or varicella*), secondary (in acute sepsis with gram +ve or –ve organism *most commonly meningococcemia*) or associated with *homozygous protein C deficiency*.

34. A i.e. Systemic primary amyloidosis *[Ref: Harrison 18/e p. 945-49]*

Pinch purpura is diagnostic of systemic primary amyloidosisQ

Skin manifestations in amyloidosis

1° Systemic amyloidosis (AA)	2° Systemic amyloidosis (AL)	Forms localized to skin
- *Pink, translucent lesion in 30% cases* - *MC in face (periorbital & perioral regions) & flexures* - *Biopsy can demonstrate amyloid deposits in dermis & blood vessel walls* - ***Petechia & parpura appear easily on minor trauma hence, PINCH PURPURA***Q	- *Rare*	- *Macular amyloidosis (upper back)* - *Lichenoid amyloidosis (usually lower extremities)* - *Nodular amyloidosis*

35. A. i.e. I.V. Immunoglobins **36. C. i.e. Kawasaki syndrome**
[Ref: Fitzpatrick 7/e p. 1626- 32; Thomas Habif Clinical Dermatology 4/e p. 474-78; Nelson 17/e p- 824, 18/e p-1041 ; Harrison's 17/e p- 2130, 2044, 1216]

Kawasaki mucocutaneous syndrome presents with ***fever (with spikes) for > 5 days, bilateral painless bulbar non discharging conjunctivitis, fissuring-crusting red lips, strawberry tongue, polymorphous erythematous eruption, desquamation-erythema & edema of extremity and acute non suppurative cervical lymphadenopathy***Q. Treatment of choice is ***intravenous gammaglobulin***Q.

37. D i.e. Kikuchi disease *[Ref: Rook's 8/e p. 33.77]*

Kikuchi – Fujmoto disease (or **Kikuchi's disease/histocytic necrotizing lymphadenitis**) presents with *painful lymphadenitis* affecting mainly cervical nodes along with fever, malaise and upper respiratory tract symptoms mostly in young women (mimicing malignant lymphoma). It may be a/w EBV (mc), parovo virus B19, HSV, HHV 6/7.

38. D i.e. Chlamydia

- **Reactive arthritis (ReA)** is most commonly triggered by ***Shigella (usually flexneri***Q > sonnei, boydii, dysenteriae) > ***Chlamydia trachomatis***Q > Salmonell, Yersinia (enterocolitica, pseudotuberculosis), Campylobacter jejuni > Clostridium difficile, Campylobacter coli, toxic E.coli > **Ureoplasma ureallyticum**, Mycoplasma genitalium > Chlamydia pneumoniae URTI
- **Most common** cause of **ReA** are ***Shigella flexneri (enteric) and Chlamydia trachomatis (genito urinary /venereal) infections***Q.

39. B i.e. Bechet's syndrome *[Ref: Fitzpatrick 7/e p. 1620-24; Rook's 8/e p. 50.56/62]*

Recurrent oral apthous ulcers (oral ulcers with yellow floor surrounded by erythematous halo) with **erythema nodosum like nodules** (multiple, tender nodules on shin) suggest the diagnois of **Behcet's syndrome.**

40. **B i.e. Reiter's syndrome** **41.** **D. i.e. Keratoderma blenorrhagica**
42. **C. i.e. Reiter's disease** **43.** **A. i.e. Subcutaneous nodules**
44. **C. Keratoderma mostly on glans** **45.** **A i.e. Becht's syndrome, C. i.e. Reiter's syndrome**
[Ref: Harrison's 17/e p- 1072, 2174, 2132, 2135, 213-14, 2153-54; Kelley's Medicine 2/e p-359; Current Rheumatology 2/e p-183; CMDT 2009 p/754-55, 758, 118; IADVL 2/e p- 1441]

- **Reiter's syndrome (reactive arthritis)** is an ***acute nonpurulent, asymmetrical, additive (poly) arthritis triggered by an infection elsewhere (like STD, enteric infection because of travel to endemic area), HIV & HLA B 27***Q. It presents with classical triad of **"CUP"** i.e. ***conjunctivitis, urethritis and polyarthritis***Q.
- ***Dactylitis (sausage digit), enthesitis, asymmetrical spondylitis & sacroilitis****, onycholysis & hyperkeratosis of nails, circinate balanitis of glans, keratoderma blenorrhagica on palms & soles and superficial asymptomatic aoral ulcers* are other features of reactive arthritis.

46. **B i.e. Reiter's disease:** *[Ref: Harrison 17th/ 2174; IADVL 2nd/1441]*

- **Reiter's disease** or **syndrome** is ***primarly a reactive polyarthritis***Q characterized by presence of non suppurative, painful, asymmetrical oligoarthritis with or without ***urethritis, ureitis, conjunctivitis, oral ulcers and secondary cutaneous involvement in form of rash***Q.
- Psoriasis, Bowen's disease (squamous cell carcinoma in situ), lichen planus and icthyosis are primary cutaneous diseases.

Neutrophilic Dermatomes

47. **B. i.e. Kimura disease C. i.e. Granuloma faciale** **48.** **B i.e. Neutrophilia not present**
49. **A i.e. Sweet syndrome** *[Ref: Thomas Habif clinical dermatology 4/e p-650-55; Fitzpatrick's 7/e p- 308; Nelson's pediatrics 17/e p- 833; Harrison 17/e p. 333]*

- ***Presence of fever and multiple tender erythematous skin lesions with neutrophilic infiltration in the dermis suggests a diagnosis of Acute Febrile Neutrophilic Dermatosis or Sweet Syndrome.***
- ***Acute febrile neutrophilic dermatoses (Sweet's syndrome), subcorneal pustular dermatoses (Sneddon-Wilkinson disease) & pyoderma gangrenosum***Q are **neutrophilic dermatoses** whereas, ***Kimura disease & granuloma fasciale***Q are **eosinophilic** dermatoses.
- **Sweet syndrome** presents with ***abrupt onset of raised, tender, edematous & erythematous plaques or nodules & targetetoid lesions occasionally with pustules, bullae or vesicles & pseudovesication, and histological evidence of dense neutrophilic infiltrate in dermis without evidence of leukocytoclastic vasculitis***Q. It may be ***associated with hematological or solid visceral malignancy and recurrent periods of moderate to high pyrexia***Q.

50. **C. i.e. Ulcerative colitis**
[Ref: Thomas Habif clinical dermatology 4/e p- 650-54; Fitzapatrick's Dermatology in general medicine 7/e p- 296-99]

Pyoderma gangrenosum occurs in both ***ulcerative colitis & Crohn's disease***Q. But ~ 50% of PG occurs in association with UC. And ~ 2% of active UC patients have PG and another 4% UC patients have erythema nodosum. *The mean duration of chronic ulcerative colitis before the appearance of erythema nodosum & PG is 5 & 10 years* respectively.

Cutaneous Drug Eruption

51. **C ie Fixed drug eruption** *[Ref: Roxburgh's 17/e p. 95; Fitzpatrick 7/e 359-60; Bahl 9/e p-270; Harrison's 17/e – p 346]*

Fixed Drug Eruption

- ***Adverse cutaneous drug reaction appearing soon after ingestion***Q (from 30 min to 8-16 hours) of offending agent in previously sensitized individuals
- Numerous drugs, including *anti-inflammatory agents (eg salicylates, NSAID's including paracetamol), phenylbutazone, phenacetin and dapsone, sulfonamides, tetracycline & mefenamic acid* may be responsible
- ***Genital & perianal skin is the most commonly involved site***Q. Nevertheless any site may be involved.
- ***Most commonly lesions are solitary***Q but they may be multiple

• Herpes genitalis

- ***Multiple, painful, bleeding non-indurated vesicles or ulcer with painful lymph-adenopathy***Q

• Pemphigus vulgaris

- ***Flaccid intraepidermal bullae***Q on upper part of body in 40 – 60 years adult with mucosal involvement.
- ***Nikolsky sign positive, row of tomb stone & accantholysis present***Q

- Lesions *evolve from macules to papules to vesicles & bullae and then erode*Q.
- Lesions *heal by residual hyper-pigmentation* Q
- *Usually asymptomatic*Q but may be pruritic, painful, or burning (when eroded)
- Lesions persist if drug is continued and resolve days to weeks after drug is discontinued
- FDE *occurs repeatedly at the same (ie fixed) site within hours, every time drug is taken and heal by residual grayish or slate colored hyperpigmentation*Q. *On rechallange, not only do the lesions recur in the same location, but also new lesions often reappears*
- Challenge or provocation/Patch test can ascertain etiology

- **Bechet's syndrome**
- Multisystemic disorder with recurrent oral & genital ulcerations with ocular involvement
- Recurrent apthous ulcerations are sine qua non for diagnosis
- Ulcers heal without leaving scars
- Genital ulcers are less common and do not involve glans and urethra

1

DERMATOLOGY

52. **B i.e. Fixed Drug Eruption** *[Ref: Fitzpatrick 7/e p.658, 1020-21, 1875-77; Rook's 8/e p. 33.14/18*

- Post inflammatory **hyperpigmentation of male genital** is caused by ***trauma, lichen planus, herpes simplex, fixed drug eruption & Bowenoid papulosis***Q. Only FDE is available in option, as herpes (pemphigoid) gestationis is not HSV infection.
- **Post inflammatory hypopigmentation** of male genital is caused by post cryo (electro/chemo) therapy, lichen planus/ sclerosis, herpes simplex, contact (condom) dermatitis, systemic sclerosis, cicatricial pemphigoid, gonococcal dermatitis, pityriasis versicolr, peyronie disease, onchocercal leopard skin, leprosy, syphilis, pseudoepitheliomatous & micaceous keratotic balanitis.
- **Bowenoid papulosis** is characterized clinically by the presence of pigmented verrucous plaques & papules primarily on genitals, & histopathologically by the presence of squamous cell carcinoma in situ changes.

Panniculitis

53. **B i.e. Post-steroidal panniculitis** *[Ref: Rook's 8/e p. 46.1/40; Andrews pediatric dermatology chap-44]*

- Histology of **poststeroid panniculitis** is very similar to that of **sub-cutaneous fat necrosis of newborn**, in that *needle shaped crystals may be found within lipocytes & histiocytes.*
- **Subcutaneous fat necrosis of newborn** occurs in infants treated acutely with high doses of systemic steroids during withdrawl. It is inflammatory process involving areas of abundant sub cutaneous fat (discrete nodules) with good prognosis. The steroid reinstituted & tapered slowly. **Scleroma neonatorum** is non inflammatory, rapidly progressive, diffuse, non tender hardening of subcutaneous tissue seen in sick infants with recurrent or persistent hypothermia. It has poor prognosis.

54. **D i.e. Chronic pancreatitis**
55. **D i.e. Aspirin therapy**
56. **A i.e. Salicylate poisioning**
57. **B i.e. Barbiturates**
58. **C i.e. Giant cell arteritis**
59. **A i.e. Erythema nodosum**
60. **C i.e. They are usually tender** *[Ref: Rooks 8/e p. 50.82-86, 46.13/15/24, 31.10/24, 50.31; Harrison 17/e p. 332-33; Robbins 7/e p-1265; Neena 3/e p-160-62; Fitzpatrick 7/e p. 572-74, 584-85, 1791]*

Erythema nodosum is seen in **"SIT Replay"**

S	*Sarcoidosis*Q, *Streptococci group A β hemolytic*Q, *Salmonella gastroenteritis (enteric fever/ typhoid)*, *Sulfonamides*Q, *Syphilis*, *SLE*Q
I	*Inflammatory bowel disease i.e. ulcerative colitis & Chron's disease*Q
T	*Tuberculosis*Q, *Typhoid*Q
Re	*Rheumatological & autoimmune diseases*Q as SLE etc
Pe	*Penicillin*Q, *Pregnancy*Q
Le	*Leprosy*Q

- **Erythema nodosum** is a symptom complex characterized by ***tender, erythematous non ulcerating nodules that appear most commonly on the extensor surface (shin) of the lower legs***Q with systemic symptoms (fever, malaise etc).
- **Erythema induratum (nodular vasculitis)** presents with ***asymptomatic/moderately tender erythematous suppurative nodule/ plaque on postero lateral aspect (or calf) of lower leg in healthy middle aged obese women having thick (heavy column like) calves***Q. Lesions ulcerate & heal with atrophic scar.
- **Nodular panniculitis** presents with ***systemic manifestation***Q with crops of dull red, tender ***nodules maximal on lower limbs (usually calf) which may ulcerate with drainage of oily brownish serous fluid eventually l/t atrophic scarring***Q.

★ **Erythema nodosum leprosum** is a/w treatment in lepromatous leprosy (Hensen's disease). ***Involvement of both upper & lower extremities is the rule***Q & facial lesions occur in half of the patients.

★ **Urticarial vasculitis** eruptions are *generalized wheals or erythematous plaques with central clearing* & often accompanied by *painful or burning sensation. Lesions last for 24 hours* unlike usual urticarial lesions which clear quickly. Malaise, fever, arthragia, nephritis occur frequently.

61. **B i.e. Erythema nodosum** *[Ref: Fitzpatrick's 7/e p. 573; Springer InflamatoryDematoputhology: 2010/125]*

History of fever and nodular lesions with neutrophillic infiltration and absence of vasculitis may be seen in Sweet's syndrome and Erythema nodosum. Presence of histiocytic infiltration however is rare/uncommon in Sweets syndrome and more typical of Erythema nodosum. ***Erthema nodosum is therefore the single best answer amongst the options provided.***

Feature	Erythema Nodosum	Erythema nodosum leprosum	Sweet Syndrome
Neurtrophilic Infiltration	*Present*	*Present*	*Present*
Histiocytic infiltration	*Present*	*Present*	*Rare*
Vasculitis	*Absent*	*Present*	*Absent*

Histopathology of Erythema Nodosum (EN)

- EN is a stereotypical example of a ***mostly septal panniculitis with no vasculitis***Q (classical feature). Early lesions show *septal edema (thickening) with inflammatory cells (lymphohistocytic infiltrate* with an admixture of *neutrophil and eosinophil*). As in other panniculitis, the composition of inflammatory infiltrate in the septa varies with age of EN lesion, with neutrophils being predominant cells in early lesions, whereas histiocytes and small granulomas are seen in late stage lesions.
- Inflammation is typically concentrated at *periphery of septae* and extends (spreads) to periseptal areas into surrounding fat lobules between adipocytes. In late stage, older lesions demonstrate *markedly widened septae* with granulation tissue at the interface b/w seta and fat lobule, peripheral fibrosis, inflammation extending into peripheral regions of fat lobules and predominantly lymphohistocytic lobuler infiltrate (i.e. **lipidrich macrophages with a foam cell appearance**). Macrophage without phagocytosed lipid surround multinucleated giant cells, forming granulomas. With time the lesions resolve *without atrophy or scarring of involved septae.*
- **Miescher radial granuloma**, which consists of a small, round, well defined nodular aggregation of small histiocytes (i.e cluster of macrophages) radially arranged around a minute central slit; is although characteristic of EN, they are also seen in *erythema induratum, nodular lesions in systemic fibrosing dermopathy, Sweet's syndrome, and Bechet's disease.*
- In older lesions of EN, histiocytes, coalesce to form *multinucleated giant cells,* many of which still keep in their cytoplasm a **stellate central cleft** reminiscent of those centers of Miescher radial granuloma.

Erythema Nodosum Leprosum (ENL)

- **Erythema nodosum leprosum (ENL)** is not EN occurring in leprosy; infact it is leprosy specific response which has some features in common with EN. It occurs in patients with *multibacillary (LL and BL) disease, before, during or after chemotherapy*. Attacks are *acute* initially but may be prolonged, recurrent or quiet and insidious eventually. It most commonly manifest as ***crops of painful and tender, bright pink-red; dermal and subcutaneous-nodules arising in clinically normal skin usually on face and extensor surfaces of limbs***Q. Involvement of both upper and lower extremities is the rule and face is involved in 50% patients. Lesions may be targetoid, vesicular, pustular, ulcerative or necrotic and associated with *fever, anorexia, and malaise.* Arthralgias and arthritis are more common. Neuritis, lymph adenitis, ochitis/epididymitis, uveitis/iritis, and myositis, neutrophilic leucocytosis, abrupt fall in haematocrit and *diagnostic dramatic response to thalidomide* is seen.
- The signature cell of ENL is neutrophil which may be abundant, scant or absent in old lesions. In type 2 reactions, *foamy macrophage and polymorphs (neutrophil) infiltrate the granuloma* and there is **vaculitis and macrophage degeneration** together with **breakdown of foam cells**. Other features include increase in lymphocytes, a thickened epidermis, a lobular panniculitis, and vasculitis (un common). The usual histological pattern is *"bottom heavy infiltrate"* Preferring the deep dermis and sucutis.

7 LEPROSY (HENSEN'S DISEASE)

Etiology & Microbiology

- **Mycobacterium (M) leprae** is an *obligate intracellular, gram positive, acid fast, non-cultivable, non toxic bacillus* that is confined to *humans, armadillos and sphagnum moss.*
- Genome of M. leprae is *shorter* (3.27 mega bases) than M. tuberculosis (4.41 Mb) and lesser (only 1605) genes encode for protein (whereas M.tuberculosis uses 91% of its genome to encode 4000 proteins). Both share 1439 genes. Because of **reductive evolution (gene deletion and decay)**, M. leprae lost genes for catabolic and respiratory pathways; transport systems; purine, methionine, and glutamine synthesis; and nitrogen regulation, which explains the *failure to cultivate the organism and its obligatory intracellular environment.*
- M. leprae is nontoxic (i.e. produces no known toxins), like Treponema palladium and the clinical manifestations of leprosy being produced by host's response to bacteria or by accumulation of enormous numbers of bacteria. It grows at 30-33°C with a doubling time fo 12 days (~2 weeks) and remaining viable in environments for upto 10 days.
- M. leprae grows best in ***cooler tissues like skin, peripheral nerves, anterior chamber of eye, upper respiratory tract an testis***Q, sparing warmer areas of skin (like axilla, scalp, groin and midline of back).
- **Phenolic glycolipid (PGL) I** is a major species specific and immunogenic constituent of highly nonpolar outer layer of bacillus complex cell wall, which is detected in serological tests. Entery into nerves is mediated by the binding of species specific unique *trisaccharide in PGL I to laminin 2 in basal lamina of schwann cell axoans*, providing a rationale to the fact that M. leprae is the ***only bacterium to invade peripheral nerves***Q.
- **Morphological index (MI)**, is a measure of number of acid fast bacilli (AFB) in skin scarpings that stain uniformly bright and it correlates with viability. In untreated patients only 1% of M. leprae are viable.
- **Bacteriological index (BI)**, or biopsy index quanitifies M. leprae in tissue or smears. Bacteriological index (BI), a *logarithm measure of density of M. leprae in dermis*, may be as high as 4 to 6+ in untreated patients and fall by 1 unit per year during effective antimicrobial therapy; the rate of decrease is independent of relative potency of therapy. BI of 6 is ≥1000 bacilli/oil immersion field; BI of 5 is 100 – 1000/OIF; BI of 4 is 10-100/OIF; BI of 3 is 1-10/OIF; BI of 2 is 1 bacillus/ 1 to 10 OIF; BI of 1 is 1 bacillus/10 to 100 OIF; and BI of O is no bacilli in 100 OIFs.
- BI of 6 indicates 10^9 bacilli per gram of granuloma tissue whereas a BI of O, may have 10^3 bacilli per gram.
- A patient is **paucibacillary** if no AFB are found in tissue or smear, and to be **multibacillary** if one or

Ridley's Granulomatous Spectrum

Ranging from high to low resistance as being mediated by a **type IV** immunological reaction, **cell mediated immunity (CMI)** or **delayed type hypersensitivity (DTH)**.

- High Type IV CMI, DTH & resistance	**TT ← BT ↔ BB ↔ BL ↔ LLs LLp**	**- Low Type IV CMI, DTH & resistance**
- Lepromin test positive	**← Gradual increase of CMI,-DTH, - Resistance & lepromin test positivity**	**- Lepromin test negative**

Clinical-Bacteriological-Patho-Immunological Spectrum of Leprosy

Ridley-Jopling Classification of leprosy is based on **clinical** (skin & nerve involvement), **bacteriolocgical** (bacteriological index, morphological index), **pathological** and **immunological (**lepromin test) criteria. It divides leprosy in TT (tuber culoid), BT (Borderline tuberculoid), BB (mid border line), BL (borderline leprotous) and LL (lepromatous leprosy).

Feature	Tuberculoid (TT,BT) Leprosy	Borderline (BB,BL) Leprosy	Lepromatous (LL) Leprosy
Skin lesions **Number**	1-10 (few)	Intermediate between BT and LL	Hundreds, confluent **(multiple)**
Distribution	Asymmetrical, anywhere		**Symmetrical**, avoiding spared areas
Edge and clarity	**Defined edge** (elevated borders), markedly hypopigmented		Vague edge (**poorly marginated**). Slight hypopigmentation
Description of skin lesion	One or few (≤10) sharply defined, asymmetric, annular macules or plaques with a tedndency to ward central clearing, elevated boders	Ill defined plaques with an occasional sharp margin, few or many in numbers	Symmetrical, ill defined (poorly marginated) multiple infiltrated nodules and plaques or diffuse infiltration; X-anthoma like or dermatofibroma papules; ***leonine facies***Q and eyebrow alopecia
Nerve lesions **Anesthesia**	**Early, marked, defined**, localized to skin lesions or major peripheral nerve	Anesthetic or hypesthetic skin lesions; nerve trunk palsies, at times symmetrical	Hypesthsia is a **late** sign, initially **slight, ill defined**, but extensive over cool areas of body (acral, distal, symmetric anaesthesia common)
Atutonomic loss	**Early** in skin and nerve lesions		**Late**, extensive (as for anesthesia)

more AFB are found.

- A person having **1-5 skin lesions &/or only one nerve involvement** is a case of **paucibacillary leprosy**; whereas **6 or more skin lesions and/or more than one nerve involvement** is a case of ***multibacillary leprosy***[Q].
- Rising MI or BI suggest *relapse or perhaps drug resistance* (if patient is being treated).Drug resistance can be confirmed or excluded in mouse model of leprosy by *recognition of mutant gene*.

Transmission

- Multiple, uncertain routes like *nasal droplet injection* (>10^{10} AFB in sneeze of untreated lepromatous patient), *contact with infected soil*, and even insect vectors (bedbugs and mosquitoes), and direct *dermal inoculation* (tattooing) have been considered the prime candidates.
- ***Skin to skin contact is generally not considered an important route of transmission***[Q].
- In endemic countries (like India) 50% of leprosy patients have a history of intimate contact with an infected person (often a household member) while in non endemic countries it is only 10%
- A household (intimate) contact carries an eventual risk of disease acquisition of 10% in endemic as opposed to only 1% in non-endemic areas.

H/O intimate (household infected contact)	Endemic area	50%
	Non endemic	10%
Risk of disease aquisition in intimate contact	Endemic	10%
	Non-endemic	1%

- **Incubation period** is generally 5-7 years (but may be 2 to 40 years) b/o long doubling time.

Nerve enlargement	**Marked**, in a **few** nerves near lesions; **nerve abscesses** most common in BT		Slight but late widespread
Mucosal and systemic involvement	Absent	-	Common, severe during type 2 lepra reactions
M. leprae (number)	Not detectable		Numerous in all affected tissues
Acid fast bacilli (BI)	0-1+	3-5+	4-6+
Langerhans giant cells	1-3+	-	-
Leporomin skin test	+++ (3+)	-	-
Lymphocytes	2+	1+	0-1+
Macrophage differentiation	**Eithelioid**	Epithelioid in BB; usually differentiated, but may have foamy changes in BL	**Foamy** change is a rule; but may be undifferentiated in early lesions
Lymphocyte transformation test	Generally positive	1-10%	1-2%
M.leprae PGL-1 antibodies	60%	85%	95%
CD4+/CD8+ T-cell ratio in lesions	1.2	BB (not tested); BL (0.48)	0.50

Diagnosis of Leprosy

1. **Clinical examination**
   - *Sensory testing*[Q]
   - Peripheral nerve examination
2. Demonstration of acid fast bacilli
   - In skin smear prepared by ***slit & scrape method***[Q]
   - Nasal swabs by modified ***ziehl – nelson method***[Q]
3. **Nerve biopsy**
4. Foot pad culture (in mouse)
5. *IgM antibodies to PGL – 1* support diagnosis only in lepromatous patients not in tuberculoid leprosy.
6. *Skin biopsy*[Q]*/ FNAC*[Q]: In **tuberculoid** leprosy, *lesional area*, preferably the *advancing edge* must be biopsied, because normal appearing skin does not have pathological features. In **lepromatous** leprosy *nodules, plaques and indurated* areas are optimal biopsy sites, but biopsies of normal appearing skin are also generally diagnostic.
   - ***Periappendigial lymphocytosis***[Q] **&**
   - ***Virchow (lepra / foam) cells***[Q] are diagnostic
   - Useful in ***indeterminate leprosy*** & differentiating it from other granulomatous lesion.

Lepromin Test

- Lepromin is a crude, semi-standardized preparation of *heat killed M. leprae bacilli* from a lepromatous nodule or infected armadillo liver. Lepromin, 0.1 ml is injected intradermally & reaction is read at *48h* **(Fernandez reaction)** or *3-4 weeks* (**Mitsuda reaction**). The Fernandez response indicates *delayed hypersensitivity* to the *soluble components* of lepromin whereas, Mitsuda reaction is a *granulomatous response* to particulate antigenic material. ***Neither reaction of lepromin test is diagnostic***[Q]. Two draw backs that stand in the way of lepromin test being used for diagnosis are:
  - Positive lepromin test (both reactions) in people with no evidence of leprosy
  - Negative results in lepromatous (LL) and near lepromatous (BL, BB) cases.
- It is ***strongly positive in patient with good CMI i.e. tuberculoid type***[Q] and gets weaker as one passes through the spectrum of the lepromatous end, the typical lepromatous case is lepromin negative indicating a failure of CMI. ***All TT are strongly and most (85%) BT are weakly positive***[Q] (≥3 mm induration at 21 days), and ***BB, BL and LL are negative (<3mm)***[Q]. The response is unpredictable in indeterminate leprosy.
- It is useful in evaluating-
  1. ***Cell mediated immunity status***[Q] of patient
  2. ***Prognosis***[Q]
  3. ***Classification of leprosy***[Q]

Clinical and Histological presentation of Leprosy

Tuberculoid Leprosy (TT & BT)

- One or few, well demarcated, ***asymmetrical, hypersthetic, nonpruritic, hypopigmented macule***[Q] ***or plaques*** with spreading erythematous; copper colored or purple and raised, clear cut edges sloping towards a flattened & hypopigmented centre; the central area atrophic & depressed. Fully developed lesions are anesthetic & devoid of normal skin organs (sweat glands & hair

Lepromatous Leprosy (LL & BL)

- Numerous, ***wide spread, B/L symmetrical skin coloured or slightly erythematous papule, nodule, raised plaques***[Q] or diffuse dermal infiltration.
- *Nerve involvement* (enlargement & damage) tends to be *symmetrical* and are *more* insidious but ultimately *more extensive*
- *In **untreated LL** patients , lymphocytes fail to recognize either M. laprae or*

follicles), dry, scaly & anhidrotic
- ***Asymmetrical enlargement of one or few peripheral nerves***Q (mostly ulnar, posterior auricular, posterior tibial, peroneal) with *hyperesthesia & myopathy*
- *T- cells breech perineurium, and destruction of schwann cells and axons may be evident, resulting in fibrosis of the epineurium,* ***replacement of endoneurium with epithilial granulomas***Q*, & occasionaly caseous necrosis. Such invasion & destruction of nerves in dermis by T – cells are pathognomic for leprosy.*
- Circulating lymphocytes *from patients with tuberculoid leprosy, readily* recognize M. leprae & its constituent proteins, *and patients have* **positive lepromin skin tests**Q.
- *There is a* 2 : 1 **predominnce of helper CD4 + over CD8 + T- lymphocytes**Q
- *Tuberculoid tissues are rich in m-RNAs of proinflammatory TH1 Family of cytokines :* ***interleukin (IL) – 2 interferon γ (IFN - γ)***, *and* **TL – 12**Q*; in contrast IL – 4 , IL – 5 , and IL – 10 mRNAs are scarce.*

its protein constituents , and **lepromin tests are negative**Q. *This loss of protective cellular immunity appears to be antigen specific as patients are* not unusually susceptible to opportunistic infections, *cancer or AIDS & maintain delayed type hypersensitivity against candida, trichophyton, mumps, tetanus toxoid & even purified derivative of tuberculin. At times M-laprae specific anergy is reversible with effective chemotherapy.*
- *In LL tissue, there is* ***2 : 1 ratio of CD 8+ to CD4 + T- lymphocytes***Q.
- *LL tissue demonstrate a* TH2 cytokine profile, *being* **rich in mRNAs for IL4, IL-5 and IL-10**Q *and poor in those for IL2, IL-12 & IFN - γ*
- *Cytokines mediate a protective tissue response in leprosy, as infection of IFN γ or IL-2 into lepromatous lesions causes a loss of AFB & histological conversion toward a tuberculoid pattern.*
- *In LL, bacilli are numerous in skin (form globi) and peripheral nerves where they intially invade Schwann cells, resulting in foamy degenerative myelination & axonal degeneration and later in Wallerian degeneration. Bacilli are plentiful in circulating blood & in all organ systems* **except central nervous system, ovaries and lungs**Q
- *In Caribbean & mexico LL without visible skin lesion but with diffuse dermal infiltration and thickned dermis is termed* ***diffuse lepromatosis.***

Polar Tuberculoid (TT)	Borderline Tuberculoid (BT)	Borderline Leprosy (BB)	Borderline Lepromatous (BL)	Lepromatous Leprosy (LL)
- **Strong immunity** is manifested by *spontaneous cure and absence of downgrading;* but antibiotic therapy is recommended. - Skin lesions are often **solitary,** non-infectious with an upper limit of **10cm** diameter (in TT denovo) but may be *multiple (usually <3)* in those who upgrade to TT from BT. - Typical lesion is *firmly indurated, elevated, erythematous, scaly, dry, hairless, hypopigmented, characteristically hypesthetic and anhidrotic plaque,* often assuming an *annular* configuration secondary to *peripheral propagation and central clearing.* The border of plaque or both borders of annulus are sharply marginated. - **Histology**: *Small tubercles (i.e. tuberculoid*	- Immunological resistance is strong enough to restrain the infection (i.e. the disease is limited and bacillary growth retarded), but the host response is insufficient to self cure (i.e. the **disease does not heal spontaneously**). - It is some what unstable i.e. resistance may increase upgrading to TT, or decrease, downgrading to BL. - Primary skin lesions are plaques and papules or annular lesions (which may be incomplete) with ***sharply marginated satellite papules***Q. In contrast to TT, typically there is **little or no scaling, less erythema, less induration and less elevation, but lesons may become much larger (> 10cm),** a single lesions sometimes involving an entire extremity. **Multiple,**	- It is immunological mid point (zone), being most unstable area, with patients quickly up or down grading. - Characteristic skin lesions are 1. Classical **annular lesions** with sharply marginated interior and exterior margins, **well defined centres** contrasting with spreading erythematous infilteration. **2. Plaques with punched out appearance** 3. Large plaques with islands of clinically normal skin within the plaque, giving a **swiss cheese appearance** or **classic dimorphic lesion.** - Skin lesions are intermediate in number between those of two polar types. Because of instability, it is the rarest type. - **Histology:** Diffuse epitheliod cell granuloma with very scanty lymphocytes and no giant cells; the papillary zone is clear, nerves are slightly swollen by	- Resistance is too low to significantly restrain bacillary proliferation but still sufficient to induce tissue destructive inflammation, especially in nerves. Thus BL patients have worst of both worlds. - Classic **borderline** or **dimorphic lesion** (one having both morphologies) is most characteristic which is an indurated and elevated annular plaque that has a well defined tuberculoid interior margin but a poorly defined lepromatous exterior margin. - Poorly or sharply marinated plaques with **punched out or swiss cheese** sharply maginated areas of normal skin in the interior of plaque are also characteristic. - Annular and	- ***Lack of cell mediated immunity***Q against M. leprae permits unrestricted bacillary replication and **widely disseminated multiorgan disease**. In addition bacilli are plentiful in circulating blood and in all organ systems ***except the lungs and central nervous system***Q (Harrison). However, patients are afebrile and there is *no evidence of major organ system dysfunction.* - **Diffuse dermal infiltration** is always present (usually) subclinically but may go unnoticed by patient who after complains of other early symptoms like *nasal stuffiness, discharge and epistaxis and edema of legs and ankles* d/t increased capillary stasis and permeability. - Dermal sign sinclude macules, papules, nodules, raised plaques or diffuse dermal infiltration. **Symmetrically distributed,** poorly defined nodules (up to 2cm) are the most common lesions. Lesions may be anywhere apart form hiary **scalp, axillae, groins and perineum** (regions of skin with the highest temperature). Diffuse dermal infiltration (non-nodular LL) is always present subclinically and is manifested *by enlargement of (pendulous) ear lobes, widening of nasal root, and fusiform selling of fingers.* - Late manifestations include **leonine facies** (lines of forehead become deeper as the skin thicknes), **Madarosis** (eyebrows and eye-lashes become thinned or lost initially the lateral margins only progressing to medially), **saddle nose** (nose misshapen and may collapse d/t septal perforation and loss of anterior nasal spine), *hoarse voice,* the *upper incisor* teeth loosen or fall out, *pendulous earlobes* and dry scaling (icthyotic) skin particularly on feet. - In mexico, 90% cases are lepromatosis. **Diffuse lepromatosis** with *diffuse thickened dermal infiltration but without visible skin lesions* is found almost exclusively in western Mexico and Caribbean.

granuloma surrounding neurovascular elements) with large lymphocytic mantles (in denovo lesions); along with *abundant Langhans giant cells and exocytosis into epidermis* (in upgrading lesions). Only type in which granuloma invades papillary zone and may even erode epidermis but acid fast bacilli (AFB) are not seen.
- Not infections and not a/w lepara reactions.
- **Most common type in India**Q and Africa but (virtually absent in south east Asia.

asymmetric lesions are the rule, but solitary lesions are not rare.
- **Impaired sensation** in skin lesions is the rule. Nerve trunk enlargement or palsies, usually asymmetrical and affecting no more than 2 nerves are common. Nerve abscesses are more common in males.
- Most common type in sough east Asia. **Associated with type I (but not type II) lepra reaction.**
- **Histology**: Epitheloid cell granuloma is more diffuse (lymphocyte mantles are loss well developed) than in TT with a free but narrow papillary zone. Giant cells tend to be foreign body rather than Langhans cells (which are less common or absent). Any exocytosis is focal and dermal nerves are moderately swollen by cellular infiltrate or only show schwann cell proliferation. **AFB** and plasma cells are absent or scanty; if present delayed **type hypersensitivity jopling's type I reactions;** Upgrading, Reversal or Downgrading reactions should be suspected.

cellular infiltrate, and AFB are present in moderate numbers.

Indeterminate Leprosy

- Early and transitory stage (lesion) of leprosy, appearing before the host makes a definitive immunological commitment to curve or to an overt granulomatous response, and histologically there is a scattered nonspecific histiocytic and lymphocytic infiltration with some concentration around skin appendages.
- ***Clinically present as hypopigmented macule or patch with or without sensory defecit and AFB***Q, if found, are present in **very small numbers (may be single within dermal nerve but never rich).**
- May last for months or years before giving way to one of determinate type.

Pure neuritic Leprosy

- Presents with asymmetrical involvement of peripheral nerve trunks and no visible skin lesions.
- It is non-infectious, slit smear negative, seen most frequently, but not exclusively, in India and Nepal where it accounts for 5-10% of patients.

plaque lesions are a symmetric abut poorly defined lepromatous like papules and nodules are roughly symmetric. Lesions in BL are usually multiple (numerous) and widespread.
- **Nerve trunk palsies** have their **highest** prevalence in BL disease, ranging from no involvement to sensory-motor deficits in all four extremities. ***Symmetrical involvement of bilateral ulnar and median nerve is characteristic***Q.
- **Histology**: Classic response is *dense lymphocytic infiltrate* confined to the space occupied by macrophages, *lamination of perineurium with a lymphocytic infiltrate* (pattern of chronic iflammation), foamy or undifferentiated macrophages. AFB are easily found. The formation of *small granulomas* is characteristic which may **abut** stands of normal looking but heavily bacillated Schwann cells.

- **Histoid lesions** are distinctive round, regular, cutaneous nodules that stand out on normal skin and are ***characteristic of relapse after treatment***Q.
- Nerve enlargement and damage tend to be *symmetric, more insidious but ultimately more extensive* than in tuberculoid leprosy (and result from actual bacillary invasion). LL patients have acral, distal, symmetric peripheral neuropathy and nerve trunk enlargement.
- **Ocular (anterior chamber) involvement** cause keratitis, iridocyclitis and iris atrophy. **Testicular involvement** mainifested as ***elevated FSH and LH levels, impotence, infertitity (sterility) loss of libido and testicular sensation, atrophy and gynaecomastia***Q. **Upper respiratory tract** involvement form tip of nose to vocal cord present as rhinitis, septal perforation, nasal collapse, and hoarseness from vocal cord nodules. **Liver, spleen, lymph nodes and bone marrow** involvement is common but clinically evident injury is rare
- When borderline leprosy downgrades to subpolar (LLs) it can be differentiated form polar lepromatous (LLp) because, in addition to typical lepromatous skin lesions there are several asymmetrical thickened nerves and ≥1 typical bordline skin lesions. Damage to structures other than skin and nerves will not be manifest clinically in borderline leprosy.
- **Histology:** Thinning of epidermis, and flattening of rate ridges above a ***clear (free) subepidermal grenz zone***Q. *The papillary layer* of dermis appears as *clear band* whilst *deeper* in dermis lies *diffuse leproma* consisting of dense, uniform, *foamy macrophage infiltrate*, with a addition of few pseudo follicular aggregates of lymphocytes, plasma cells and mast cells. ***The dermis contains enormous number of AFB, singly or in clumps (globi)***Q. There is ***asymptomatic bacillation of Schwann cells l/t foamy degeneration***Q. Demyelinaton, damage and destruction of axis cylinder are prominent features l/t Wallerian degeneration. ***Despite large numbers of bacilli in nerve there is only a small inflammatory response***Q; ultimately the nerve fibroses and hyalinized. In LLs there is an ***onion skin perineurial lamination* but not infiltration.** In LLp perineurium is undisturbed.
- *Diffuse erythema* becoming worse on exposure to sun; Mucous membrane involvement & ulceration; Regurgitation due to perforation of palate.

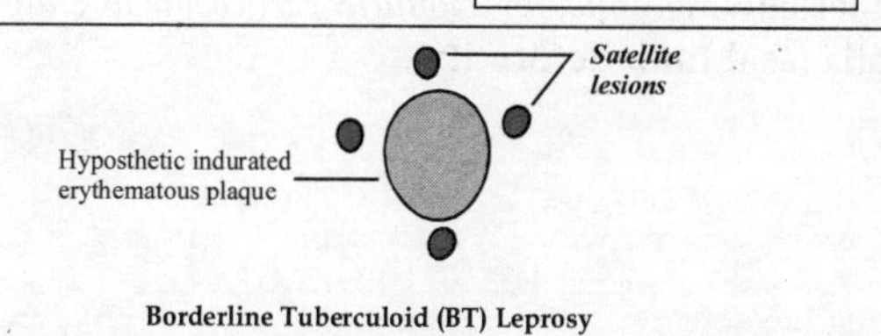

Borderline Tuberculoid (BT) Leprosy

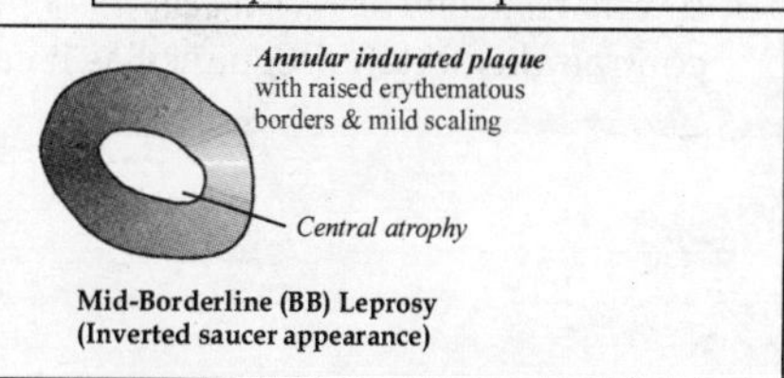

Mid-Borderline (BB) Leprosy (Inverted saucer appearance)

DERMATOLOGY 1

Reactional States

Jopling's Type I Lepra Reactions (Down grading & Reversal Reactions)

- Occur in almost 50% patients with ***borderline forms of leprosy***Q but not in polar disease
- Reversal reactions often occur in first month or year after initiation of therapy, but may develop several years there after.
- Clinical presentation is:
  - ***Signs of inflammation in previous lesions***Q (macules, papules & plaques)
  - Appearance of new skin lesions
  - ***Neuritis***Q
  - Fever – generally low grade
- The most commonly involved nerve trunk is ***ulnar nerve at elbow***Q f/b *posterior tibial / peroneal & posterior auricular nerves.*
- If patient with affected nerves is not treated *promptly with glucocorticoids*, irreversible nerve damage may result in as little as 24 hours.
- It is ***type IV delayed hypersensitivity reaction***Q.
- Edema is most characteristic microscopic feature, whose diagnosis is primarily clinical.
- Reversal reactions are typified by *TH1 cytokine profile*, with an ***influx of CD4+ helper cell, and increased level of IFN -γ & IL -2***Q. and large number of T- cells bearing γ/δ receptors – a unique feature of leprosy
- **Treatment**
  - ***Continuation of antileprotic drug*** Q
  - ***Analgesics (NSAIDs)***Q
  - ***Drug of choice is corticosteroid***Q (indicated in lesions at *cosmetically important site as face*, lesions with intense inflammation that pose a threat of ulceration, and cases in which neuritis is present)
  - ***Thalidomide is ineffective and has no role***Q; *Clofazimine* (200 – 300 mg/ d) is of questionable benefit
  - Rest & splintage of affected limb.

Jopling's Type II Lepra Reactions (Erythema Nodosum Leprosum, ENL)

- Occurs exclusively in patients near the ***Lepramatous end of the leprosy spectrum (BL & LL)***Q, affecting ~ 50% of this group.
- In 90% of cases, it *follows the institution of chemotherapy*, generally within 2 years. (i.e. in only 10% it occurs before diagnosis & start of treatment)
- Clinical features are:
  Involvement of both upper & lower extremities is the rule & facial lesion occur in half of the patientsQ. Of the other organs involved, *arthralgias & arthritis are more common.*
  - *Crops of painful erythematous papules*, that resolve spontaneously in a few days to a week but may recur, (m.c.)
  - ***Malaise & fever***Q that can be *profound*
  - **Neuritis, lymphadenitis, uveitis, iritis orchitis/epididymitis & glomerulonephritis,** anemia, leukocytosis & abnormal LFT (particularly ↑ amino transferase levels)
  - May have single bout of ENL or chronic recurrent mainfestations ENL may result in *death* (rarely)
- Skin biopsy of ENL papule reveals *vasculitis* or *panniculitis*, (sometimes with many lymphocytes but characteristically with polymorpho-nuclear leukocytes as well.)
- ***TNF seems to play central role in ENL***Q and its levels are increased.
- It is thought to be ***type III hypersensitivity jerish – herxheimer arthus type***Q reaction d/t immune complex deposition, given its T_{H2} *cytokinin* profile and *high levels of IL –6 & IL – 8*
- However, in ENL tissue, the presence of *HLA – Dr* framework of epidermal cells – considerd a marker for delayed type hypersensitivity response – and evidence for *higher levels of IL-2 & IF-γ* than are seen in polar lepromatous disease suggest an alternative mechanism.

Stage	Treatment
Mild (i.e. without fever or other organ involvement, with occasional crops of only a few skin papules)	- Antipyeritc / NSAIDs alone
Moderate – Severe (many skin lesions, fever, malaise and other tissue involvement)	- *Glucocorticoids*Q (brief 1-2 wk course) - *Clofazimine*Q (causes dose reduction of steroid)
If despite two courses of glucocorticoid therapy ENL appears to be **recurring & persisting**	- ***Thalidomide***Q ***(100 – 300 mg nightly)*** - ***S/E is phocomelia***Q So C/I in pregnancy

Thalidomide 100-300 mg is most efficicacious (gold standard drug for ENL) and has dramatic action probably d/t its *reduction of TNF levels, and IgM synthesis* and its slowing of *polymorhonuclear leucocyte migration.* But it is contraindicated in pregnancy as it causes **phocomalia (seal limb deformity).**

Lucio's Phenomenon

- Seen exclusively in patients from Caribbean & Mexico who have the diffuse lepromatous form of leprosy (mainly in untreated) – **Latapi lepromatosis (Lucio leprosy)**
- Patients develop recurrent crops of large sharply marginated, ulcerative lesions – esp. on lower extremity that may be generalized, and when so are frequently fatal as result of 2° infection & septic bacteremia.
- Histology shows ischemic necrosis of epidermis & superficial dermis, heavy parasitism of endothelial cells with AFB, and endothelial proliferation and thrombus formation in larger vessels of deeper dermis.
- Like ENL, it is mediated by immune complex
- Treatment
  - ***Neither steroids nor thalidomide is effective***Q
  - Optimal wound care & therapy for bacterimia are indicated
  - In severe cases, ***exchange transfusion (plasmapheresis) is useful.***

Antimicrobial Regimens for Treatment of Leprosy

Leprosy form	More Intensive Regimen	WHO Regimen (1982)		Duration of Treatment	Follow-up
		Monthly supervised	Daily self administered		
Multibacillary (lepromatous) - Patients with demonstrable **AFB in dermis** in skin smear (old definition) - **≥ 6 skin lesion** (new)	- **Rifampicin (600mg/day)** for **3 years** plus **dapsone (100mg/d)** indefinitely throughout life	- **Rifampicin (600mg)** plus - **Clofazimine (300mg)**	- **Dapsone (100mg) Plus** - **Clofazimine (50mg)**	Initally recommended **2years** of until smears become **negative (~5 years)** but now course is reduced to **1 year**	**5 Year**
Paucibacillary (Tuberculoid) - Patients without demonstrable AFB in dermis (old) - < 6 skin lesion	- **Dapsone (100mg/d)** for 5years	**Rifampicin (600 mg)**	**Dapsone (100mg)**	6 months	**2 years**
Single lesion Paucibacillary		- **Single dose of ROM** i.e. **rifampiocin (600 mg), ofloxacin (400mg)** and **minocycline (100 mg)**			

Questions

1. **Normal commensal of skin are** *(PGI June 09)*
   A. Staphylococcus aureus ☐
   B. Candida ☐
   C. Propioni bacterium acnes ☐
   D. Diptheria ☐
   E. Streptopyogenes ☐

Clinical Presentation and Types

2. **The Redley-Joplilng classification for leprosy is based on which of the following parameter?** *(AIIMS May 13)*
   A. Clinical, bacteriological, immunological ☐
   B. Histopathological, clinical, therapeutic ☐
   C. Histopathological, epidemiologica, therapeutics ☐
   D. Histopathological, clinical, epidermiological ☐
3. **Most common type of leprosy in India:** *(PGI 97)*
   A. BT ☐
   B. TT ☐
   C. LL ☐
   D. BL ☐
4. **Skin (cutaneous) smear is negative in which leprosy**
   A. Indeterminate *(PGI May 12, 04) (AI 97)* ☐
   B. Neuritic ☐
   C. Lepromatous ☐
   D. Borderline ☐
   E. Lupus erythematosus, Lichen planus ☐
5. **Single lesion in skin is seen in which type of leprosy:**
   A. TT *(AI 93)* ☐
   B. BT ☐
   C. BL ☐
   D. LL ☐
6. **A single hypopigmented anesthetic patch with satellite lesion on forearm, likely diagnosis is :** *(AIIMS 94)*
   A. Inderterminate leprosy ☐
   B. Tuberculoid leprosy ☐
   C. Neuritic leprosy ☐
   D. Lupus Vulgaris ☐
7. **Satellite Lesion are seen in:** *(AI & AIIMS 99)*
   A. Tuberculoid Leprosy ☐
   B. Lepromatous Leprosy ☐
   C. Borderline Tuberculoid Leprosy ☐
   D. Histoid Leprosy ☐
8. **Inverted saucer shaped lesion is found in** *(AIIMS 95)*
   A. Lepromatous leprosy ☐
   B. Tuberculoid leprosy ☐
   C. Borderline leprosy ☐
   D. Indeterminate leprosy ☐
9. **Characteristic feature of borderline leprosy**
   A. Inverted saucer lesion *(AIIMS May 12)* ☐
   B. ENL ☐
   C. Hypopigmented macule & plaques all over body ☐
   D. Glove & stocking anesthesia ☐
10. **A 45 year old male had multiple hypoaesthetic mildly erythematous large plaques with elevated margins on trunk and extremities. His ulnar and lateral popliteal nerves on both sides were enlarged. The most probable diagnosis is:** *(AIIMS Nov 03)*
    A. Lepromatous leprosy ☐
    B. Borderline leprosy ☐
    C. Borderline tuberculoid leprosy ☐
    D. Borderline lepromatous leprosy ☐
11. **A patient with multiple hypopigmented & hypesthetic patches on lateral aspect of forearm with abundance of AFB and granulomatous inflammation on histology. The diagnosis is** *(AIIMS May 12)*
    A. Tuberculoid leprosy ☐
    B. Indetermediate leprosy ☐
    C. Borderline leprosy ☐
    D. Lepromatous leprosy ☐
12. **An 8-year old boy from Bihar presents with a 6 month h/o an ill defined hypopigmented slightly atrophic macule on the face. The most likely diagnosis is:**
    A. Ptyriasis alba *(AI 05, DNB 01)* ☐
    B. Indeterminate leprosy ☐

C. Morphacea
D. Calcium deficiency

13. 8 year old boy from Tamil Nadu presents with a white, non anaesthetic, non scaly hypopigmented macule on his face, likely diagnosis is : *(AI 01, AIIMS 98)*
A. Pityriasis alba
B. Pityriasis versicolour
C. Indeterminate leprosy
D. Neuritic leprosy

14. All lesions are seen in leprosy except *(AI 97)*
A. Erythematous Macule
B. Hypopigmented patch
C. Vesicles
D. Flat & raised patches

15. All are features of lepromatous leprosy except: *(TN 96, AIIMS 94)*
A. Gynaecomastia
B. Madarosis
C. Saddle nose
D. Perforating Ulcer

16. Commonest nerve involved in leprosy is: *(AIIMS 94)*
A. Ulnar
B. Median
C. Radial
D. Sciatic

17. In leprosy nerves commonly involved are: *(PGI 97)*
A. High ulnar, low median
B. High median, low ulnar
C. Triple nerve palsy
D. High radial, low median

18. Earliest sensation to be lost in Hansens disease is: *(UP 98, DNB 96)*
A. Pain
B. Touch
C. Vibration
D. Temperature

19. In Leprosy which of the following is not seen: *(PGI 2K, DNB 03)*
A. Abnormal EMG
B. Voluntary muscle wasting
C. Decreased Proprioception
D. Decreased response to tactile sensation
E. Increased response to tactile sensation

20. Leprosy do not involve: *(PGI 98)*
A. CNS
B. Testis
C. Skin
D. Cornea

21. Leprosy affects all organs except *(AIIMS May 10)*
A. Eyes
B. Nerves
C. Uterus
D. Ovary

22. Tuberculoid leprosy is characterised by- *(Jipmer 92) (DNB 99, CMC 98)*
A. Non caseating granuloma in nerve
B. Sub epidermall free zone
C. Bacilli in skin
D. Skin caseation

23. All are true lepromatous leprosy except- *(TN 96, CMC 02)*
A. Presence of globi
B. Subepidermal free zone
C. Decreased cell mediated immunity
D. Presence of granulomas subdermally

24. Skin biopsy in leprosy is characterizedby: *(AI 97)*
A. Pariappendegial bacilli
B. Pariappendegeal lymphocytosis
C. Perivascular lymphocytosis
D. All of above

25. Cellmediated immunity is maximum suppressed in *(AIIMS 93)*
A. BT
B. LL
C. TT
D. Indeterminate

26. Virchow's cells are seen in: *(DNB 97, UP 95)*
A. Henoch scholein purpura
B. Toxic Epidermal necrolysis
C. Congenital Syphilis
D. Leprosy

27. Lepromin test is used for: *(AIIMS Nov 08)*
A. Diagnosis
B. Treatment
C. Prognosis
D. Epidemiological investigation

28. The following test is not used for diagnosis of leprosy : *(AIIMS May 06, CMC 09)*
A. Lepramin test
B. Slit skin smear
C. Fine needle aspiration cytology
D. Skin biopsy

29. Not true about lepromin test is *(AIIMS May 10)*
A. It is diagnostic
B. Negative in infants < 6 months
C. Used to classify
D. BCG vaccination may convert negative to positive

30. Lepromin test is positive in which leprosy *(AIIMS 2K, DNB 03)*
A. Lepromatous
B. Indeterminate
C. Histoid
D. Tuberculoid

31. A 16 year old student reported for the evaluation of multiple hypopigmented macules on the trunk and limbs. All of the following tests are useful in making a diagnosis of leprosy, except: *(AIIMS Nov 03)*
A. Sensation testing
B. Lepromin test
C. Slit smears
D. Skin biopsy

Reactional States

32. A 27-year-old patient was diagnosed to have borderline leprosy and started on multibacillary multi-drug therapy. Six weeks later, he developed pain in the nerves and redness and swelling of the skin lesions. The management of his illness should include all of the following, except: *(AIIMS 04)*
A. Stop anti-leprosy drugs
B. Systemic corticosteroids
C. Rest to the limbs affected
D. Analgesics

33. Reversal lepra reaction shown no response to : *(Jipmer 95, DNB 92)*
A. Cloafazimine
B. Chloroquine
C. Glucocorticoids
D. Thalidomide

34. DOC in type I lepra reaction with severe neuritis *(AI 95)*
A. Thalidomide
B. Clafazamine
C. Dapsone
D. Systemic Corticosteroid

35. Treatment of Acute neuritis in Lepra I reaction is A/E: *(AI 94)*
A. Dapsone
B. Steroid
C. Thalidomide

D. Incision and Drainage ☐

36. **Best meathod of treatment of ulner never abscess in case of leprosy is:** *(AIIMS 96)*
A. High does of steroid ☐
B. Incision and drainage ☐
C. Thalidomide ☐
D. High does of clofazamine ☐

37. **The main cytokine, involved in erythema nodusum leprosum (ENL) reaction is:**
A. Interleukin – 2 *(AIIMS May 2006)* ☐
B. Interferon – gamma ☐
C. Tumor necrosis factor- alpha ☐
D. Macrophage colony stimulating factor ☐

38. **ENL is seen in which form of leprosy:**
A. Indeterminate *(PGI 05, 04, May 11, AIIMS 92)* ☐
B. BT ☐
C. LL (lepromatous leprosy) ☐
D. BL ☐
E. TT ☐

39. **Manifestation of ENL includes all of the following except:** *(PGI Dec 05, DNB 08)*
A. Pancreatistis ☐
B. Fever ☐
C. Hepatitis ☐
D. Arthritis ☐
E. Cutaneous nodules ☐

40. **Drug of choice in Erythema Nodosum Leprosum (type II lepra reaction):**
A. Steroid *(AI 08, AIIMS 92)* ☐
B. Thalidomide ☐
C. Clofazimine ☐
D. Aspirin ☐

41. **Thalidomide is drug of choice for:** *(AI 99)*
E. Lepra I reaction ☐
A. Lepra II reaction ☐
B. Both ☐
C. Nerve Abscess ☐

42. **The daily dose of thalidomide for controlling E.N.L. is :**
A. 100 mg *(PGI 98, DNB 91)* ☐
B. 200 – 300 mg ☐
C. 500 mg ☐
D. 1000 mg only ☐

43. **The following drug is not used for the treatment of type II lepra reaction** *(AIIMS May 06, CMC 08)*
A. Chloroquin ☐
B. Thalidomide ☐
C. Cyclosporine ☐
D. Corticosteroids ☐

Drugs and Management of Leprosy

44. **The most effective drug against M. leprae is:** *(AI 03)*
A. Dapsone ☐
B. Rifampicin ☐
C. Clofazamine ☐
D. Prothionamide ☐

45. **Most potent anti-leprotic drug is:** *(AIIMS 97)*
A. Rifampcin ☐
B. Dapsone ☐
C. Clofazimine ☐
D. Norflox ☐

46. **The first line antileprosy drugs include all except-**
A. Dapsone *(PGI 97, Delhi 03)* ☐
B. Thiacetazone ☐
C. Clofazimine ☐
D. Rifampicin ☐

47. **Antileprotic drug also used in lepra reaction is:**
A. Rifampcin *(AIIMS 97)* ☐
B. Dapsone ☐
C. Ciprofloxacin ☐
D. Clofazimine ☐

48. **Dose of Dapsone is -** *(AI 88, DNB 98)*
A. 1-2 mg/kg ☐
B. 5 mg/kg ☐
C. 10 mg/kg ☐
D. 20 mg/kg ☐

49. **One of the following is a side effect of clofazimine used in leprosy therapy-**
A. Hyperpigmentation *(AI 96, DNB 97)* ☐
B. Erythema ☐
C. Discoloration of body secretions ☐
D. Macular rash ☐

50. **Skin pigmentation & icthyosis like side effects are seen in:** *(AI 96)*
A. Rifampcin ☐
B. Clofazimine ☐
C. Dapsone ☐
D. Steroid ☐

51. **Control of TB and leprosy is by:** *(Kerala 94)*
A. Isolation of cases ☐
B. Specific protection ☐
C. Early diagnosis and treatment ☐
D. Elimination of reservoirs ☐

52. **Multidrug therapy is given for** *(AI 94)*
A. Syphilis ☐
B. Leprosy ☐
C. Herpetiformis ☐
D. Icthyosis Vulgaris ☐

53. **WHO regime for paucibacillary leprosy:** *(AI 96)*
A. 100 mg Dapsone daily + Rifampcin monthly (600 mg) ☐
B. Dapsone daily + Rifampcin daily ☐
C. Dapsone + Rifampcin + Clofazemine daily ☐
D. Rifampcin + Clofazamine daily ☐

54. **Duration of treatment in pauci bacillary leprosy is**
A. 6 months *(Jipmer 93)* ☐
B. 9 months ☐
C. 2 years ☐
D. Till sumptoms subside ☐

55. **Average duration of treatment in multibacillary leprosy is** *(AIIMS 93)*
A. 1 year ☐
B. 2 year ☐
C. 3 year ☐
D. Life long ☐

56. **Thalidomide is not used in** *(AIIMS May & Nov. 08)*
A. ENL ☐
B. Bechet's syndrome ☐
C. HIV associated Oral ulcers ☐
D. HIV associated neuropathy ☐

57. **All are true statement regarding leprosy except:**
A. Paucibacillary leprosy means person having 1-5 skin lesions &/or only one nerve involvement ☐
B. Regular MDT means patient received 2/3rd of month of treatment schedule *(PGI May 12)* ☐
C. Lepra reaction if not treated can lead to permanent deformities ☐
D. Immunoprophylaxis have no role in leprosy ☐

Answers and Explanations:

1. **B, C i.e. Candida; Propioni bacterium acnes** *[Ref: Jawetz Microbiology 13/e p-260; Neena Khanna 4/e p-241]*

Resident flora (normal commensal) of skin consists of permanently present mixture of several non pathogenic microorganisms. It includes :

- Coagulase negative ***Staphylococcus epidermidis (not coagulase positive staphylococcus aureus)***[Q] and peptococcus.
- Diptheroid bacilli which may be aerobic (eg **Corynebacterium minutissimum**) or anerobic (eg ***propionibacterium acnes)***[Q].
- Brevibacterium, α hemolytic streptococcus (S.viridians), enterococci (S. fecalis), gram –ve Coliform bacilli & acine tobacter' (Harellea) and acid fast non pathogenic mycobacterium (in areas rich in sebaceous secretion eg external ear & genitalia).
- Fungus such as **candida** and yeast eg **Malassezia.**

Clinical Presentation and Types

2. **A i.e. Clinical, bacteriological, immunological** *[Ref: Fitzputrick's 8/e p. 2253-61; Neena Khanna 4/e p 257]*

Ridley-Jopling classification of leprosy is based on **clinical** (skin & nerve involvement), **bacteriolocgical** (bacteriological index, morphological index), **pathological** and **immunological (l**epromin test) criteria. It divides leprosy in TT (tuber culoid), BT (Borderline tuberculoid), BB (mid border line), BL (borderline leprotous) and LL (lepromatous leprosy).

3. **B i.e. TT**
4. **B i.e. Neuritic** *[Ref:Harrison 18/e/ 1359-65;Rooks 8/e p 32.1-32.20;Fitzpatrick's 7/e p.1786-96; Roxburgh's 18/e p 49-50;]*

Leprosy Type	Slit Smear & Infectivity
Neuritic	*Negative*[Q]
Tuberculoid	- AFB may be found from margin - Not infective usually
Borderline	- AFB may be found - Infective
Lepromatous	- Teeming with AFB - Infective
Indeterminate	- Slit smear & lepromin test is ±

Country	Most common type of leprosy
India, Africa	**TT (Polar tuberculoid)**[Q]
Southeast Asia	BT (Borderline tuber culoid)
Mexico, Caribbea	Lepromatous (LL>BL)

5. **A i.e. TT**
6. **B i.e. Tuberculoid Leprosy (Nearest answer)**
7. **C i.e. Borderline tuberculoid leprosy**
8. **C i.e. Border line leprosy**
9. **A i.e. Inverted saucer lesion**
10. **D i.e. Border line lepromatous leprosy**
11. **C i.e. Border line leprosy**

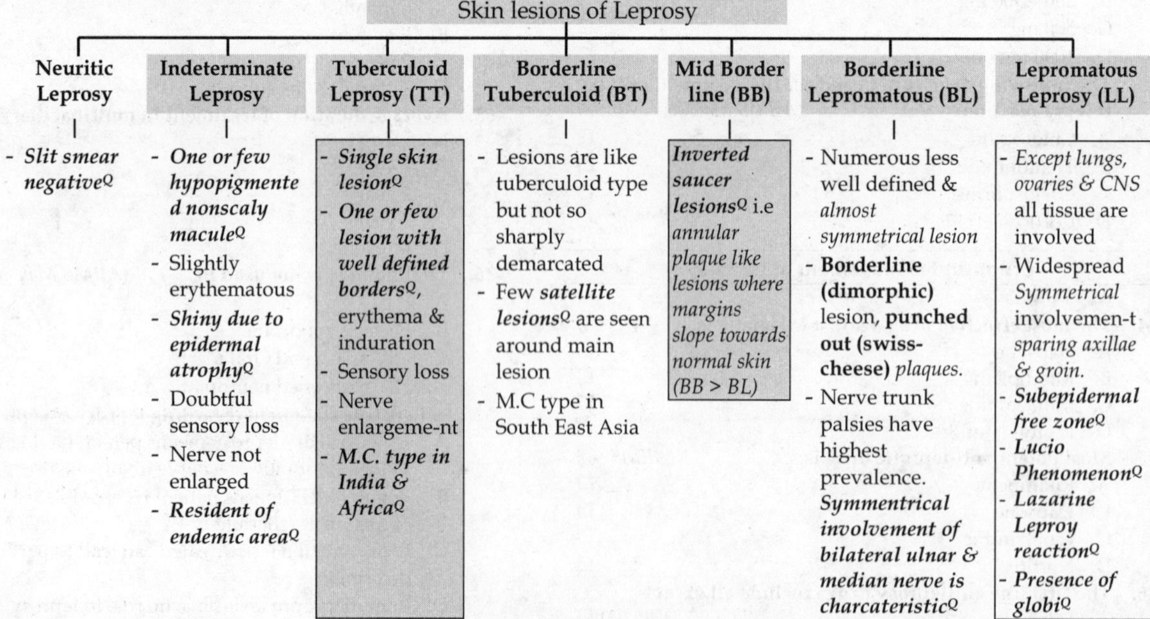

Skin lesions of Leprosy
Neuritic Leprosy
- Slit smear negative[Q]
Indeterminate Leprosy
- One or few hypopigmented nonscaly macule[Q]
- Slightly erythematous
- Shiny due to epidermal atrophy[Q]
- Doubtful sensory loss
- Nerve not enlarged
- Resident of endemic area[Q]
Tuberculoid Leprosy (TT)
- Single skin lesion[Q]
- One or few lesion with well defined borders[Q], erythema & induration
- Sensory loss
- Nerve enlargement
- M.C. type in India & Africa[Q]
Borderline Tuberculoid (BT)
- Lesions are like tuberculoid type but not so sharply demarcated
- Few satellite lesions[Q] are seen around main lesion
- M.C type in South East Asia
Mid Border line (BB)
Inverted saucer lesions[Q] i.e annular plaque like lesions where margins slope towards normal skin (BB > BL)
Borderline Lepromatous (BL)
- Numerous less well defined & almost symmetrical lesion
- Borderline (dimorphic) lesion, punched out (swiss-cheese) plaques.
- Nerve trunk palsies have highest prevalence. Symmentrical involvement of bilateral ulnar & median nerve is charcateristic[Q]
Lepromatous Leprosy (LL)
- Except lungs, ovaries & CNS all tissue are involved
- Widespread Symmetrical involvemen-t sparing axillae & groin.
- Subepidermal free zone[Q]
- Lucio Phenomenon[Q]
- Lazarine Leproy reaction[Q]
- Presence of globi[Q]

12. **B i.e. Indeterminate leprosy** **13.** **C i.e. Indeterminate leprosy**

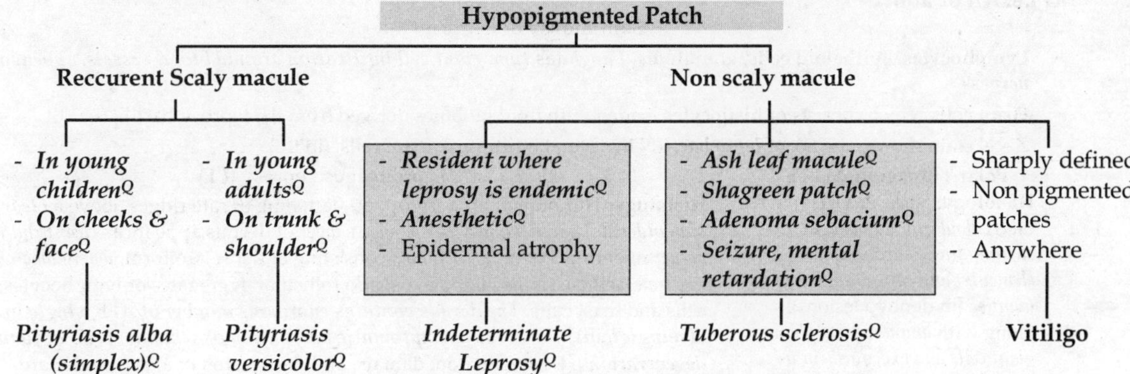

14. **C i.e. Vesicles** **15.** **None > D i.e. Perforating Ulcer**

- **Leprosy and acquired syphilis** are ***not vesico-bullous disorders***Q (i.e. there is no vesicle and bullae formation, which can be seen in **congenital syphilis**).
- **Neuropathic / Trophic /Perforating / Plantar – ulcer** is a frequent **complication (not clinical feature) of lepromatous leprosy**Q *because sensory impaiment appears before motor weakness and patient continues to miisuse his feet and hands.*

16. **A i.e. Ulnar nerve** **17.** **A i.e. High ulnar & low median**
18. **D. i.e. Temerature** **19.** **C i.e. Decreased proprioception**

[Ref: Harrison's 18/e p. 1383; Fitzpatrick's 7/e p-1788; Rooks 8/e p.32.13]

- Nerves commonly involved in leprosy are:
  1. ***Posterior tibial (most common)***Q.
  2. ***Ulnar (2nd most common, most commonly l/t abscess)***Q
  3. Peroneal/lateral popliteal
  4. Median & Facial
  5. Posterior auricular
  6. Supra orbital, supraclavicular, digital
- ***Posterior tibial is the most frequently affected nerve f/b ulnar***Q, median, lateral popliteal and facial. ***Ulnar & median nerve lesions are usually low***Q, causing small muscles but not deep flexor weakness, & anesthesia of two halves of hand (Rook – 32.13)
- The most commonly affected nerve trunk is ***ulnar nerve at elbow***Q. Insensitivity affects fine touch, pain and heat receptors ***but generally spares position & vibrating appreciation***Q *(Harrison 1383)*
- Generation time of lepra bacilli is **12 – 13 days.** Maximum no. of bacilli is shed in **nasal secretions.** *Virchow cells* are diagnostic. **Lepra cells (Foam cells)** are large *undifferentiated histiocytes*Q. Ist involved is **Schwann cell.** Ist sensation lost is **temperature** & pain.
- ***Propioception is carried by Goll & Burdech tract (posterior column) which is not involved in leprosy***Q. ***Temperature & pain***Q lost earlier than touch & pressure. Leprosy mainly affects *peripheral nerves, eventually l/t muscle wasting.* ***Myopathy, muscle wasting may l/t abnormal EMG***Q.

20. **A i.e. CNS** *[Ref: Rooks 8/e p. 32.12-13; Fitzpatrick 7/e p. 1790; Harrison 18/e p. 1362;*
21. **C i.e. Uterus** *Blastein pathology of female genital tract 5/e p-681]*

- In lepromatous leprosy (LL) bacilli are plentiful in circulating blood and widely disseminated ***in all organ systems except the lungs and central nervous system***Q *(Harrison 18/1362)*
- **Leprosy** affects ***nerves (posterior tibial > ulnar), eyes***Q (lagopthalmos, corneal insensitivity, ulcer, uveitis, iritis, blindness), ***testis***Q (↑FSH/LH, decreased testosterone, aspermia/hypospermia, impotence & infertility),larynx (hoarseness d/t vocal nodule), nose (rhinitis, septal perforation, nasal collapse), kidney, liver, spleen, peripheral lymph nodes, bone marrow, bone (osteoporosis, cyst, fracture) and nails.
- Skin lesions may be anywhere apart from *hairy scalp, axillae, groins and perineum* (regions of skin with highest temperature)- *Rook's 8/e p. 32.10*
- Female genital tract is rarely involved in leprosy. But when involved ***ovary is the commonest site to be involved***Q causing ↑FSH/LH/prolactin and infertility due to ovarian failure.
- Pregnancy precipitates leprosy b/o altered immunity. When *pregnant*, LL and BL patients are predisposed to develop *ENL d/t reduced immunity*, but *post-partum* they are predisposed to develop *DTH reaction (Jopling's type I reaction;* upgrading, reversal or downgrading) d/t restored immunity.
- Untreated lactating BL and LL mothers have *viable bacilli in their milk*, but no risk has been identified in infants ingesting such bacilli. Dapsone in mother's mother's milk may produce hemolysis in the baby (Fitzpatric-1790).

22. **A. i.e. Non caseating granuloma in nerve** 23. **D. i.e. Presence of granulomas subdermally**
24. **D i.e. All of above**

Skin Biopsy of Leprosy

- **Lymphocytes, epitheloid cells, granuloma,** ***Langhans type giant cell infiltration around blood vessels, appendages & nerves***Q
- **Foam cells** which consists of **histiocytes** loaded with lipid globules derived from the leprosy bacilli; (in LL)
- Z – N stain show large no. of ***lepra bacilli***Q in dermal infiltrate & foam cells. (in LL)

Polar Tuberculoid (TT)	Lepromatous Leprosy (LL)
- **Histology**: *Small tubercles (i.e. tuberculoid granuloma surrounding neurovascular elements) with large lymphocytic mantles* (in denovo lesions); along with *abundant Langhans giant cells and exocytosis into epidermis* (in upgrading lesions). Only type in which granuloma invades papillary zone and may even erode epidermis but acid fast bacilli. AFB are not seen.	- **Histology:** Thinning of epidermis, and flattening of rate ridges above a ***clear (free) subepidermal grenz zone***Q. *The papillary layer* of dermis appears as *clear band* whilst *deeper* in dermis lies *diffuse leproma* consisting of dense, uniform, *foamy macrophage infiltrate*, with a addition of few pseudo follicular aggregates of lymphocytes, plasma cells and mast cells. ***The dermis contains enormous number of AFB, singly or in clumps (globi)*** Q. There is ***asymptomatic bacillation of schwann cells l/t foamy degeneration***Q. Demyelinaton, damage and destruction of axis cylinder are prominent features l/t Wallerian degeneration. ***Despite large numbers of bacilli in nerve there is only a small inflammatory response***Q; ultimately the nerve fibroses and hyalinized. In LLs there is an ***onion skin perineurial lamination*** but not infiltration. In LLp perineurium is undisturbed. - *Diffuse erythema* becoming worse on exposure to sun; Mucous membrane involvement & ulceration; Regurgitation due to perforation of palate.

Immunity and Tests

25. **B i.e. LL**

- Least CMI/Host Resistance (CMI max suppressed)
- Lepromin Test most negative

→ LL

BL

BT

Gradual increase of CMI & Lepromin positivity

- Lepromin test most positive
- CMI maximum (least suppressed)

→ TT

From tuberculiod type (TT) to lepromatous leprosy (LL), there is ***gradual decrease in cell mediated immunity (CMI) and lepromin test positivity***Q (i.e. it becomes negative).

26. **D. i.e. Leprosy** 27. **C. i.e. Prognosis**
28. **A i.e. Lepromin test** 29. **A i.e. It is diagnostic**
30. **D i.e. Tuberculoid** 31. **B i.e. Lepromin test**

Lepromin test has no diagnostic value; it has only prognostic significanceQ as it tells about *cell mediated immunity & classify the type of disease.* ***Lepromin test is most positive in TT because cell mediated immunity is least suppressed***Q

Reactional States

32. **A i.e. Stop Anti leprosy drugs** 33. **D. i.e. Thalidomide**

- Appearance of new skin lesions or signs of inflammation (e.g. redness and swelling etc.) in prevous lesions, neuritis (e.g. nerve pain) and low grade fever in borderline forms of leprosy suggest the diagnosis of Jopling's type I (delayed type IV hype/sensitivity) reaction. If type I lepra reaction *preceeds the initiation of* appropiate antimicrobial *therapy* it is k/a **down grading reaction** & the case becomes histologically more lepromatous. When it occurs *after initiation of therapy,* it is termed as **reversal reaction** & the case becomes more tuberculoid.
- This is presentation of lepra reaction (type I – reversal) & in any case of lepra reaction antileprotic drug is not stopped.
- **Thalidomide** is ***ineffective and has no role in type I lepra (downgrading and reversal) reactions***Q.

34. **D i.e. Systemic corticosteroid** 35. **D i.e. Incision & drainage; C i.e. Thalidomide**
36. **B i.e. Incision & Drainage**

Condition	Treatment of choice	Accessory treatment
Neuritis in leprosy	*Corticosteroid*Q	Antileprotic drugs (ALD)
Nerve abscess in leprosy	***Incision & drainage***Q	***f/b ALD & steroid***
Type I Lepra reaction Type II lepra reaction	***Corticosteroid***Q ***Corticosteroid***Q	
Recurring & persistent Type II lepra reaction	***Thalidomide***Q	

- *Incision and Drainage of abscess* followed by *anti leprotic treatment* and *glucocorticoids* is done for nerve abscess in leprosy.
- Controversial question. In type I lepra reaction, thaladomide has no role but incision & drainage is done in nerve abscess not in acute neuritis.

37. C i.e. Tumor necrosis factor
38. C, D i.e. LL, BL
39. A, D i.e. Pancreatitis, Arthritis
40. A i.e. Steroid
41. B i.e. Lepra II reaction
42. B. i.e. 200 – 300 mg
43. C i.e. Cyclosporin

- ***Elevated levels of circulating tumor necrosis factor (TNF) have been demonstrated in ENL; thus TNF may play a central role in the pathobiology of this syndrome***Q.
- Erythema nodosum leparosum (ENL, Jopling's type II reaction), is a ***type III hypersensitivity that occurs exclusively in BL, LL which usually follows therapy***Q but may precede therapy. Clinical features include Painful erythematous papules (MC), Fever, malaise, Neuritis, Lymphadenitis, Uveitis, Orchitis, Glomerulonephritis, Anemia, Leukocytosis, and Abnormal liver function test (increased aminotransferase).

	Lepra Reactions		
	Jopling's Type I- downgrading and upgrading (reversal)	**Jopling's Type II Erythema nedosum lepresum (ENL)**	**Lucio Phenomenon**
Hypersensitivity Type	**Type IV** (i.e. DTH)	**Type II** (i.e. Jarisch-Herxheimer)	**Type III**
Found in	- Almost 50% of patients with ***borderline forms of leprosy***Q but not in patients with pure lepromatous disease (Harrison) - Most common in **BL** but not rare in LLs, BB or BT patients (Fitzpatric) - Occur in borderline disease (Rooks)	Exclusively near ***lepromatous end of leprosy spectrum (LL>BL)***Q in patients with multibacillary disease spontaneously (roseolar leprosy) or whilst on treatment.	**Diffuse lepromatosis** form of lepromatous leprosy (LL) in Caribbean and Mexico region (**Latapi lepromatosis**)
Thalidomide (100.300mg nightly)	*No role*Q (Ineffective)	***Most effective and gold standard***Q; used in recurring and persisting cases (when 2 courses of **steroid fail**)	Neither steroid nor thalidomide is effective (no role)
Drug of Choice	*Corticosteroid*Q	Corticosteroid	Exchange transfusion

Treatment of Reactions

- ***It is important not to stop anti – leprosy drugs in patients who develop lepra reactions***Q.
- Managment plan according to severity

	Type I Lepra reaction	Type II Lepra reaction (ENL)
Mild	- NSAIDs	- NSAIDs
Moderate	- NSAIDs - ***Oral corticosteroids***Q	- NSAIDs - ***Thalidomide***Q - ***Chloroquin***Q - ***Clofazimine***Q
Severe	- NSAIDs - Oral corticosterioids	- Thalidomide - ***Corticosteroids***Q (For impending nerve damage, orchitis, necrotic ENL) - ***Parenteral antimany***Q

✶ **Thalidomide** is now approved by FDA for treatment of ENL. This drug is *sedating* and extremely ***teratogenic***Q, and ***should never be taken by anyone who is or may become pregnant***Q. Physicians wishing to prescribe thalidomide must register with the *System for Thalidomide Education and Prescription Safety (S.T.E.P.S).* at 1 – 888 – 423- 5436 *(Celgene corporation)*; the sole *exceptions* to this registration requirement are *physician at Hansen's disease clinics* that are receiving medication support from the national Hansen's disease program.

Drugs and Management of Leprosy

44. B ie Rifampcin
45. A i.e. Rifampcin
46. B. i.e. Thiacetazone
47. D i.e. Clofazamine
48. A. i.e. 1-2 mg/kg
49. A i.e. Hyperpigmentation C i.e. Discolouration of body secretions
50. B i.e. Clofazimine *[Ref: Goodmen and Gilman's 12/e p – 1563-64, 1560, 1567; Fitzpatric 7/e p. 2154-57]*

- **Rifampin (rifampcin)** is the ***most bactericidal (leprocidal)***Q drug in current regimens. Because of high kill rates and massive release of bacterial antigens, rifampin is *not given during a reversal reaction or in erythema nodosum leprosum.*
- **Dapsone** and **clofazimine** are ***only bacteriostatic (leparostatic)***Q. These along with rifampicin are first line antileprotic drugs.
- **Clofazimine** is a fat soluble riminophenazien ***dye with leprostatic and anti-inflammatory properties***Q. Its anti-inflammatory effects are ***used in treatment of reversal reactions and ENL***Q. Side effects include GI problems (abdominal pain, diarrhoea, nausea and vomiting; crystal deposits in intestinal mucosa, liver, spleen and abdominal lymph nodes), ***reddish brown discoloration of body secretions, eye, exposed skin and hair and dryness and itching of skin (icthyosis)***Q.
- **Dapsone (DDS, 4'-diamino-diphenylsulfone)**, a structural analog of PABA, is a *competitive inhibitor of dihydropteroate synthase* (fo/p1/p2) I folate pathway, which is a reason of its broadspectrum activity with *antibacterial, anti-protozoal, and antifungal effects.* It has anti-inflammatory and free radicle scavenger action, it inhbits neutrophil myeloperoxidase and lysosomal enzyme activity, respiratory burst and neutrophil migration.

Dapsone

Dose and side Effects

- Dose is ***1-2mg/kg***Q and half life is **>*24 hours***Q. Clinical response is seen at doses ranging from 25-200mg/day (but rarely requiring 300mg/d.) Doses of **≤ 100mg** in healthy persons and **≤ 50mg** in healthy individuals with a G6PD deficiency do not cause hemolysis. Sulfones tend to be retained in *skin, muscle and especially in lever and kidney* for upto *3 weeks*. Intestinal reabsorption of sulfones excreted in bile contributes to long term retention in blood stream.
- G6PD protects RBCs against oxidative stress. Dapsone an oxidant ***causes severe hemolysis (l/t haemolytic anemia most common side effect)***Q in patients with G6PD deficiency. Hemolysis and methemaglobinemia develops in almost every individual treated with 200-300mg of dapsone per day.
- **Methemoglobinemia**Q also is common and may be severe in NADH-dependent methemoglobin reductase deficiency.
- Idiosyncratic or allergic like **distal peripheral neuropathy (almost always motor** occasionally with a sensory component); which is reversible with dose decrease or discontinuation. **Sulfone syndrome** (Mono nucleosis like hypersensitivity) usually develops between 2 and 7 weeks after starting drug and inevitably includes the **triad of fever, rash (exfoliative or SJ like) and hepatitis.** Agranulocytosis, leukopenia severe hypoalbuminea are other S/Es.

Theraputic uses

- **Infections**: DDS is effective against **M.leprae**, MAC, M.kanssii bacteria; **plasmodium falciparum and toxoplasma gondii** parasites; and **pneumocystic** jiroveci fungus and so is used in
  - *Leprosy*Q
  - *Malaria*Q (combined with chlor proguani)
  - *Actinomycosis*Q, rhinosporidosis, P. jiroveci infection and prophylaxis, and P. Carinii pheneumonia prophyloxis in sulfa allergic immuno compromised patients, and for T. gondii prophylaxis.
- Non-infections diseases with consistent response to dapsone include
  - *Dermatitis herpetiformis (drug of choice)*Q
  - Erythema elevatum diutinum, linear immunoglobuline A dermatosis/chronic bullous dermatosis of childhood and bullous eruption fo SLE.
- Other non-infectious conditions in which DDS has found sporadic (less rapid, regular or predictable) success have a unifying feature of having **granulocytes (neutrophils or eosinophils)** as the predominant infiltrating cell. Examples are:
  - **Collagen vascular disease** e.g. RA, rheumatoid papules, relapsing plychondritis, subacute cutaneous lupus erythematosus, chronic cutaneous lupus, lupus profundus; various vasculitides including cutaneous PAN, HS purpura, chronic leukocytoclastic vasculitis without internal organ involvement and Bechet syndrome.
  - **Autoimmune diseases** e.g. steroid resistant or dependent ITP, bullous pemphigoid, cicatricial (mucous membrane) pemphigoid, particularly in early inflammatory phase of ocular disease, sobcorneal pustular dermatoses, pemphigus vulgaris/foliaceaous and urticarial vasculitis.
  - Inflammatory conditons like acne vulgaris and acne conglobate (but is not recommended).

51. **C. i.e. Early diagnosis & treatment**
52. **B i.e. Leprosy**
53. **A i.e. 100 mg Dapsone daily + Rifampcin 600 mg monthly**
54. **A. i.e. 6 months**
55. **A i.e. 1 year**

- **Control of leprosy and tuber culosis (TB)** is done by ***early diagnosis and treatment with multidrug therapy***Q
- **WHO regimen for paucibacillary** leprosy is ***dapsone 100mg daily unsupervised + rifampicin 600mg monthly supervised for total duration of 6 months***Q and followup upto 2year.
- WHO regimen for *multibucillary leprosy is dapsone (100mg) and clofazimien (50mg) daily self-administered + rifapian (600mg) and clofazimine (300mg) monthly supervised for 1 year* duration (new recommendation) and follwoup upto 5years.

56. **D i.e. HIV associated neuropathy** *[Ref: Harrison 17/e p-2132, 2148, 671, 675, 705, 1037, 2659; Fitzpatrick's 7/e p. 2234; Goodman & Gillman 12/e p. 1741-42]*

Peripheral neuropathy is a dose limiting toxicity of thalidomide & not a therapeutic indicationQ. It causes painful sensory ganglionopathy & axonal neuropathy.

Indications of Thalidomide

- ***Erythema nodosum leprosum (ENL)***Q: Only FDA approved use for treatment of **cutaneous manifestations of moderate to severe ENL** and for maintenance therapy for prevention and suppression of cutaneous manifestations of ENL recurrence.
- ***Severe, recurrent apthous stomatitis***Q, especially in AIDS patients is common off label use.
- ***Behects syndrome***Q
- Chronic graft versus host disease.

★ HIV associated colitis and wasting, multiple myeloma, myelodysplasia, chronic idiopathic myelofibrosis, glucocorticosteroid refractory fistulosis-Chron's disease, sarcoidosis, prurigo, stomatitis are other rare uses.

57. **D i.e. Immunoprophylaxis has no role in leprosy**
[Ref: Park 21/e p. 290-99; Harrison 18/e p. 1366; Fitzpatrick's 8/e p. 2253-62]

- A person having **1-5 skin lesions &/or only one nerve involvement** is a case of **paucibacillary leprosy;** whereas **6 or more skin lesions and/or more than one nerve involvement** is a case of ***multibacillary leprosy***Q.
- **Because of peripheral nerve trunk involvement,** if lepra reactions are not treated promptly & adequately, such reactions ***can result in permanent deformities***Q.
- **Regular multi drug treatment** means ***patient has received MDT for atleast 2/3rd of the months in treatment schedule***Q. Eg 12 month regular treatment implies that patient had at least 8 full months of combined therapy during 12 months period.
- **Immunoprophylaxis i.e. vaccination at birth with BCG** either alone or in combination of with other vaccines (from killed M. Leprae or atypical mycobacterium) has protective efficacy from 30-80%. High BCG vaccination coverage remains an important contribution in reducing the disease burden of leprosy. The addition of heat killed M. leprae to BCG does not increase vaccine efficacy.

8 SKIN TUBERCULOSIS & OTHER BACTERIAL INFECTIONS

Classification of Cutaneous Tuberculosis

	Host Immune status	Clinical Disease	Comment
Exogenous infection	**Naïve**	**Primary Inoculation TB (Tuberous chancre, tuberculous primary complex)**	TB chancre & affected regional lymph nodes constitute primary skin complex
	Immune[Q]	**Tuberculosis verrucosa cutis (Warty TB)** = 2nd m.c.in tropics	Pauci bacillary disorder caused by ***exogenous re-infection (inoculation) in previously sensitized individual with high immunity***[Q].
Endogenous spread	**High**	**Lupus vulgaris**	*Extremely chronic, progressive* form, developing in individuals with moderate immunity & high degree of tuberculin sensitivity.
		Scrofuloderma (TB colliquativa cutis) = most common in tropics	Subcutaneous TB l/t *cold abscess formation* & secondary breakdown of overlying skin. It ***represents contiguous involvement of skin overlying another site of infection (eg. TB lymphadenitis, TB of bones & joints, or tuberculous epididymitis)***[Q].
	Low	- **Acute miliary TB** (TB cutis miliaris disseminate) - **Metastatic tuberculous abscess** (TB Gumma) - **Orificial TB** (TB ulcerosa cutis et mucosae)*	★ TB of orificial mucous membranes caused by auto-inoculation of mycobacterium from far advanced progressive TB of internal organs (eg. pulmonary, intestinal or rarely genitourinary TB)
TB d/t Bacilli Calmette-Guerin (BCG)	Naïve	- Normal primary complex like reaction - Perforating regional adenitis - Post vaccination lupus vulgaris	
Tuberculids True	Not clear	- ***Lichen scrofulosorum***[Q] - ***Papulonecrotic tuberculid***[Q]	Mycobacterium tuberculosis / bovis play a *significant role*
Facultative		- Nodular –vasculitis (Erythema induratum of Bazin - Erythema nodosum	Mycobacterium tuberculosis/bovis may be one of several pathogenic factors.

Lupus Vulgaris

- **Lupus vulgaris** is a *postprimary, paucibacillary, extremely chronic, progressive form of cutaneous tuberculosis* occurring in individuals with *moderate immunity* and *high* degree of *tuberculin sensitivity*. It is caused by hematogenous, lymphatic or contiguous spread from elsewhere in body.
- **Lupus vulgaris** initial lesion is *small, reddish brown flat plaque (macule or papule) of soft or friable, almost gelatinous consistency*. Slow evolution of lesion, long duration course (over 1 to 3 decades) and ***diagnostic apple jelly nodules revealed by diascopy are highly characteristic***[Q].
- Progression is characterized by *elevation*, infiltration and a *deeper brownish color and formation of plaque*. The lesion grows by slow peripheral extension to become ***gyrate or discoid in shape with areas of atrophy***[Q]. Involution in one area with expansion in another often result in a gyrate outline border and give LV lesion a characteristic appearance – ***central atrophy and serpiginous edge***[Q]. **Atrophic scarring** with or without prior **ulceration**, is characteristic, as is recurrence within a scar. Fibrosis may be pronounced and mutilating.
- There is usually a **single lesion**, except in disseminated forms (particularly after measles- k/a **lupus postexan thematicus**).
- In Europe 80-90% lesions are on **head and neck**, particularly around nose>check, earlobes or scalp; rarely on arms and legs and uncommonly on trunk. In **India and developing countries** lesions are ***often on lower limbs, buttocks and trunk***[Q].

Tuberculosis verrucosa cutis / Warty Tuberculosis

Definition and Pathogenesis

- It is an *indolent, warty, plaque like paucibacillary* form of cutaneous TB caused by *exogenous re-infection (inoculation)* in previously sensitized individuals with *high immunity.*
- Lesions arise in three ways-1) accidental inoculation in professionals like physicians, pathologist, postmortem attendents handling infectious material (thus k/a anatomist's or prosector's warts, verruca necrogenica); 2) ***inoculation at sites of minor wounds, from sputum by sitting on ground or walking barefoot in children & farmers***[Q]; 3) or rarely from patients own sputum (autoinoculation).

Histopathology

- Striking **pseudo epitheliomatous hyperplasia** with marked hyperkeratosis, a dense inflammatory infiltrate, and *abscess in superficial dermis* or within the pseudoepitheliomatous rete pegs.

Clinical Features

- Lesions usually occur on areas exposed to trauma and to infected material i.e. hands in western countries & professionals and **lower extremities (knees, ankle and buttock)** ***in Asia, children & Farmers***[Q]
- Lesion starts as a *small, asymptomatic, indurated, warty papule* or papulopustule with a slight inflammatory *purple areola (halo).* Slow growth and irregular peripheral expansion lead to the development of **hyperkeratotic verrucous plaque** with a **serpiginous outline** with finger like projections. The color is purple, red or brown. The **central** may involute, leaving **white atrophic scar.** Exudative fissures chischarging pus extend into underlying brownish red to purplish infiltrated base.
- Lesion usually is ***solitary***[Q], but very rarely multiple lesions with sporotrichoid spread may be seen. Regional lymph nodes are rarely affected.

Tuberculides

Definition	Classification	
- In contrast to true tuberculosis, tuberculids are explained as a ***hypersensitivity reaction to Mycobacterium tuberculosis or its products in a patient with significant immunity***[Q].	**True Tuberculides** (M.tuber culosis / bovis appear to play a significant role)	• Micropapular – **Lichen** ***scrofulosorum***[Q] • Papular – *Papulonecrotic tuber culide* • Nodular – *Erythema induratum of Bazin / Nodular tuberculide*
- The main features are *a positive tuberculin test*, evidence of *manifest or past tuberculosis* and a *positive response to antituberculous therapy* - There is virtually always *absence of bacilli in skin biopsy* specimens & culture, although PCR has detected mycobacterial DNA in some forms - Several conditions once thought to represent tuberculides are now classified as variants of rosacea.	**Facultative Tuberculides** (M. tuberculosis / bovis may be one of the several etiopathogenic factors	• ***Erythema nodosum***[Q] • Erythema induratum (Nodular Vasculitis)
	Nontuberculides (formerly designated tuberculides; there is no relationship to tuber- culosis)	• Lichenoid tuberculid • Rosacea like tuberculid • Lupus miliaris disseminatus faciei

Pyodermas

Pyodermas are ***cutaneous bacterial infections***[Q] (of skin) and are mostly caused by *S. aureus or group A streptococcus.* **Primary pyodermas** occur without any predisposing cause (i.e. are idiopathic) in normal skin. Whereas **secondary pyodermas** occur in conditions predisposing bacterial colonization like atopic dermatitis, ectoparasite / fungal infections, miliaria (causing breech in skin continuity), diabetes mellitus (IDDM), dialysis (hemo or peritoneal), IV drug use, liver dysfunction, HIV, prolonged steroid use, cancer, hypothyroid, hypoadrenocorticism (decreasing immunity). It can be classified into

Non follicular

I. Digital infections

- Staphylococcal **paronychia** (proximal nail fold)
- Stap. **whitlow (Felon)** of bulbous distal end of finger
- Blistering distal dactylitis (staph)

II. Intertriginous infection

- Intertrigo, vulvovaginitis & perianal cellulites (by group A streptococci)
- Perianal dermatitis (by staph)

III. Skin infections

Localized

- Superficial
  - ***Impetigo***

Spreading or Invasive

- **Superficial- Erysipelas** is superficial cutaneous

Follicular

Pyoderma that begins within the hair follicle; caused mostly by Staph. aureus

I. Folliculitis

1. **Superficial folliculitis (follicular or Bockhart impetigo)**, blepharitis
   - Periporitis staphylogens is secondary infection of miliaria of neonates by S. aureus.
   - Non-infectious, inflammatory, follicular disorders viz. pseudofolliculitis barbae, folliculitis keloidalis (or acne keloidalis nuchae), perifolliculitis captis, irritant folliculitis must be differentiated.
2. **Deep folliculitis** like ***sycosis barbae and lupoid sycosis***[Q] (deep, chronic, circinate form of sycosis barbae) are a/w perifollicular inflammation.

1

DERMATOLOGY

*contagiosa*Q
- **Bullous impetigo**Q (pemphigus neonatorum or Ritter disease)

• Deep
- *Ecthyma*Q
- Botryomycosis

cellulitis with marked dermal lymphatic vessel involvement l/t erythema & peau d orange appearance. It is mostly caused by group A β hemolytic streptococci (GAS) rarely by S. aureus.

• **Deep-Cellulitis** Extends deeper into dermis & subcutaneous tissue; caused mostly by S.aureus & GAS

II. Perifollicular Abscess

1. **Furuncles (Boil)** is deep seated inflammatory nodule arising around hair follicle, from a preceding superficial folliculitis & evolving into an abscess

2. **Carbuncle** is more extensive deeper, larger serious, painful lesion develop when multiple closely set furuncle coalesce and suppurate. patient appear quite ill with fever & malaise.

1

DERMATOLOGY

Questions

Skin Tuberculosis

1. **Tuberculosis verrucosa cutis is a form of:**
   A. Tuberculid *(DNB 07, SGPGI 05)* ☐
   B. Primary tuberculosis ☐
   C. Postprimary tuberculosis with good resistance ☐
   D. Post primary tuberculosis with poor resistance ☐
2. **Most common type of cutaneous T.B. is:** *(PGI Dec 06)*
   A. Lupus vulgaris ☐
   B. Scrofuloderma ☐
   C. T.B. verruca cutis ☐
   D. Erythema induratum ☐
3. **Skin (cutaneous) manifestations of T.B.** *(PGI May 12, 04)*
   A. Lupus vulgaris ☐
   B. Lupus pernio ☐
   C. Scrofuloderma ☐
   D. Butcher warts ☐
   E. Lupus erythematosus, Lichen planus ☐
4. **Tuberculosis of skin is called as** *(AIIMS 98, SGPGI 04)*
   A. Lupus Vulgaris ☐
   B. Lupus Pernio ☐
   C. Lupus profundus ☐
   D. Scrofuloderma ☐
5. **True about lupus vulgaris-** *(PGI Dec 04)*
   A. Apple jelly nodule at root of nose ☐
   B. TB of skin & mucosa ☐
   C. Also knownas scrofuloderma ☐
   D. ATT is helpful ☐
6. **A 12 year old boy had a gradually progressive plaque on a buttock for the last 3 years. The plaque was 15 cm in diameter, annular in shape, with crusting and induration at the periphery and scarring at the center. The most likely diagnosis.**
   A. Tinea corporis *(AIIMS Nov 03)* ☐
   B. Granuloma annulare ☐
   C. Lupus vulgaris ☐
   D. Borderline leprosy ☐
7. **An 8 year old boy present with well defined annular lesion over the buttock with central scarring that is gradually progressive over the last 8 months. The diagnosis is:**
   A. Annular psoriasis *(AIIMS 01)* ☐
   B. Lupus Vulgaris ☐
   C. Tinea Corporis ☐
   D. Chronic granulomatous disease ☐
8. **A young boy presented with a lesion over his right buttock which had peripheral scaling and central clearing with scarring. The investigation of choice would be:**
   A. Tzank smear *(AIIMS 01)* ☐
   B. KOH preparation ☐
   C. Biopsy ☐
   D. Sabourad's agar ☐
9. **Apple-jelly nodules is/are seen in:** *(PGI Nov 2010)*
   A. Lupus vulgaris ☐
   B. DLE ☐
   C. Lichen planus ☐
   D. Psoriasis ☐
10. **20 year old male from Jaipur with erythermatous lesion on cheek with central crusting likely diagnosis is:** *(AI 01)*
    A. SLE ☐
    B. Lupus Vulgaris ☐
    C. Chillblain ☐
    D. Cutaneous Leishmaniasis ☐
11. **A farmer has a single warty lesion on leg. Which of the following could be most likely lesion:** *(AIIMS Nov 2010)*
    A. Verruca vulgaris ☐
    B. Tuberculosis verrucosa cutis ☐
    C. Mycetoma ☐
    D. Lichen planus hypertrophicus ☐
12. **Cutaneous (skin) Tuberculosis secondary to underlying tissue eg lymph node is called as***(AI 99, AIIMS 98, PGI 04)*
    A. Lupus Vulgaris *(DNB 01)* ☐
    B. Scrofuloderma ☐
    C. Spina Ventosa ☐
    D. Tuberculous Verrucosa Cutis ☐
13. **Tuberculides are seen in** *(AIIMS May 07)*
    A. Lupus vulgaris ☐
    B. Scrofuloderma ☐
    C. Lichen scrofulososum ☐
    D. Erythema nodosum ☐
14. **Which of the following is /are tuberculides**
    A. Lichen scrofulosorum *(PGI June 07, 2K, DNB 03)* ☐
    B. Lichen nichidus *(AIIMS Nov 06)* ☐
    C. Lichen aureus ☐
    D. Erythema nodosum. ☐

15. Involvement of sweat gland, dermal appendages, and hair follicles with epitheloid granuloma are typical features of which of the following? *(AI 09, DNB 11)*
A. Lichen Scrofulosum ☐
B. Miliary TB ☐
C. Papulonecrotic type ☐
D. Lupus vulgaris ☐

16. Mycobacterium causeing skin ulcer: *(PGI 02)*
A. M.smegmatis ☐
B. M.scrofulaceum ☐
C. M.ulcerans ☐
D. M.fortuitum ☐
E. M.marinum ☐

17. Skin hazards of swimming are : *(PGI 01)*
A. Verrucae ☐
B. Pyoderma gangrenosum ☐
C. M. marinum infection ☐
D. M.ulcerans infection ☐

18. Epitheliod granuloma is characterstic of *(AIIMS 94)*
A. Sarcoidosis ☐
B. Eosinohilia ☐
C. T.B. ☐
D. Mycosis Fungoides ☐

Other Bacterial Infections

19. Staphylococcal infection causes all disease execept:
A. Impetigo *(AI 97)* ☐
B. Erysipelas ☐
C. Ecthyma ☐
D. Scaldy Skin Syndrome ☐

20. Toxic shock syndrome is caused by *(AI 93)*
A. Staphylococcal infection ☐
B. Streptococcus ☐
C. Pseudomonas ☐
D. E. Coli ☐

21. False statement about impetigo *(PGI 01)*
A. Mostly caused by staphylococcus or streptococcus or both ☐
B. It predisposes to glomerulonephritis ☐
C. Produces scar on healing ☐
D. Erythromycin is drug of choice ☐
E. It is infectious lesion ☐

22. Commonest skin infection in children is - *(AI 89)*
A. Scabies ☐
B. Impetigo contagiosa ☐
C. Molluscum contagiosa ☐
D. Warts ☐

23. Impetigo contageosa most commonly due to :
A. Group B Streptococcous *(JHARKHAND – 2004)* ☐
B. Staphylococcus ☐
C. Moniliasis ☐
D. Streptococcus Viridans ☐

24. 'Honey colored' crusts are characteristic of :
A. Nummular eczema *(Jipmer 79, PGI 81)* ☐
B. Impetigo ☐
C. Herpes zoster ☐
D. Cutaneous diptheria ☐

25. True about Impetigo is: *(PGI June 08)*
A. Contagious ☐
B. Bacterial infection ☐
C. Non contagious ☐
D. Honey coloured cast ☐
E. Viral infection ☐

26. Erysipeloid is transmitted by : *(PGI 99)*
A. Droplet ☐
B. Feco-oral ☐
C. Mosquito bite ☐
D. Contact with animal ☐

27. Staphylococcus causes A/E:: *(PGI 99)*
A. Scarlet fever ☐
B. TSS ☐
C. Carbuncle ☐
D. Sycosis barbae ☐

28. Desquamation of skin occurs in *(PGI Nov 11)*
A. Erythema infectiosum ☐
B. Kawasaki disease ☐
C. Scarlet fever ☐
D. Toxic shock syndrome ☐
E. Infectious mononucleosis ☐

29. Which of these statements is false for Erytherma marginatum : *(MP 04, DNB 06)*
A. Lesions are serpiginous ☐
B. Characteristically it is an evanescent ☐
C. Rash worsens on application of heart ☐
D. Rash is itchy ☐

30. After 3 days of fever patient developed maculo erythematous rash lasting for 48 hrs diagnosis is: *(AI 02)*
A. Fifth disease ☐
B. Rubella ☐
C. Measles ☐
D. Roseola infantum ☐

31. Primary pyodermas are: *(PGI May 2011)*
A. Impetigo contagiosa ☐
B. Ecthyma ☐
C. Furncle ☐
D. Pyoderma gangrenosa ☐
E. Impetigo herpetiformes ☐

32. Which of the following are bacterial infection of skin-
A. Pyoderma gangrenosum *(PGI June 05, DNB 04)* ☐
B. Piedra ☐
C. Impetigo contagiosa ☐
D. Impetigo herpetiformis ☐
E. Ecthyma ☐

Answers and Explanations:

Skin Tuberculosis

1. **C i.e. Postprimary tuberculosis with good resistance:** *Ref: Fitzpatrick's 7/p 1768-74*

***Tuberculosis verrucosa cutis is postprimary tuberculosis with good resistane*Q.**

2. **A i.e. Lupus vulgaris**
3. **A & C i.e. (Lupus vulgaris) & (Scrofuloderma)**

- *Butcher's wart is caused by HPV-2 & HPV – 7*Q
- Different types of skin tuberculosis are: ***Lupus vulgaris*Q (Apple-jelly nodules** are seen), lupus miliaris disseminata faciei, ***lichen scrofulosorum*Q, *scrofuloderma*Q** (skin T.B. secondary to underlying structure), tuberculosis verrucosa cutis, tuberculosis cutis orificalis (T.B. of orifices as oral, anal, urogenital), papulo necrotic tuberculids, ***erythema nodosum*Q**, erythema induratum, acne agmination, rosea like lesion.

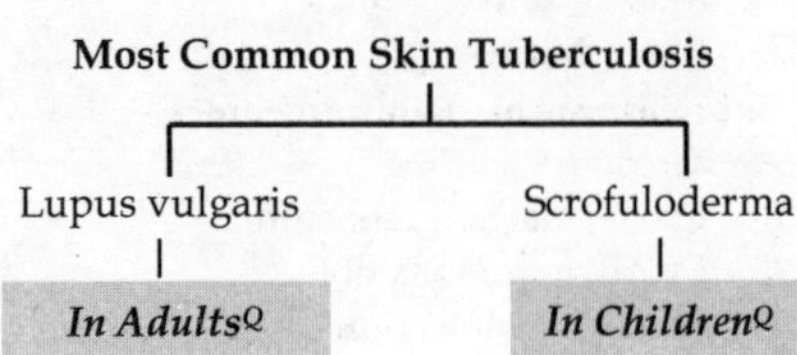

4. **A i.e. Lupus vulgaris** *[Ref: Rook's 8/e p. 31.16-20; Fitzpatrick's 7/e p-1769-72; Roxburgh 18/e p.47-49]*
5. **A i.e. Apple jelly nodule at root of nose; B i.e. TB of skin and mucosa; D i.e. ATT is helpful**
6. **C i.e. Lupus vulgaris** 7. **B i.e. Lupus vulgaris** 8. **C i.e. Biopsy**

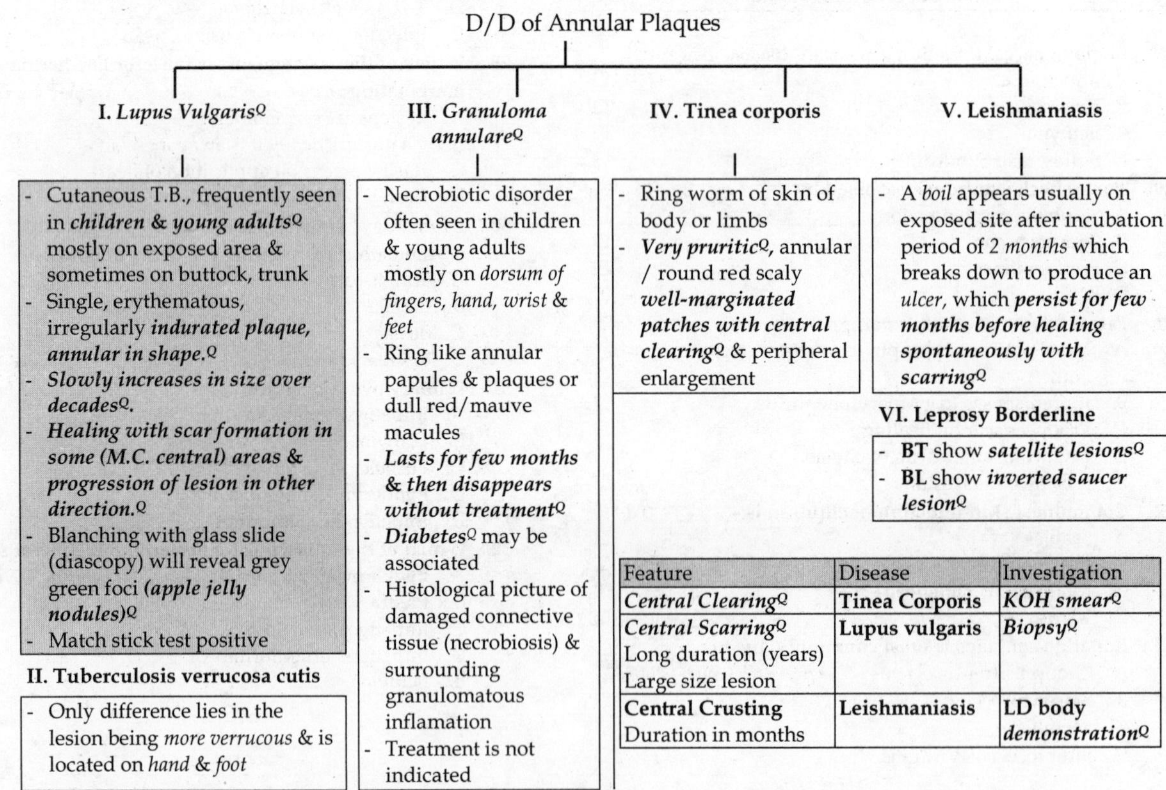

Feature	Disease	Investigation
*Central Clearing*Q	**Tinea Corporis**	*KOH smear*Q
*Central Scarring*Q Long duration (years) Large size lesion	**Lupus vulgaris**	*Biopsy*Q
Central Crusting Duration in months	**Leishmaniasis**	**LD body *demonstration*Q**

- ATT is helpful in both lupus vulgaris and scrofuloderma.
- In annular psoriasis -lesion contain loosely adeherant silvery scales and there is no scarring. For Tinea corporis -8 months time duration is very long and itching is very important complaint which is not mentioned.

9. **A i.e. Lupus vulgaris** *[Ref: Rook's 8/e p. 31.7; Fitzpatrick's 7/e p. 30, 39, 1486-87, 1771, 2004]*

- **Apple jelly sign** is production of yellowish hue from pressure with a glass slide **(diascopy)** on a ***granulomatous inflammatory lesions like tuberculosis (lupus-vulgaris), sarcoidosis, leishmaniasis*Q.**

- Most common cutaneous presentation of sarcoid is 2 to 5 mm papule often have a translucent **red-brown or yellow brown color (like apple jelly)** that is accentuated with diascopy (which also appreciates the nodular quality of underlying granuloma). The ***apple jelly appearance and nodules are specific but not pathognomic for sarcoidosis***[Q], as other granulomatous skin conditions such as ***lupus vulgaris***[Q] may exhibit similar diascopic properties.
- Erythematous, scaly papules, ofter with **apple jelly appearance** at the borders of a completely or partially healed lesion are characteristic of **leishmania recidiva cutis/leishmania residivans** (a rare form of chronic cutaneous leishmaniasis caused mostly by L.tropica in old world and rarely L.braziliensis in new world). Reactivation of dormant infection (after upto 15 years) accounts for most of cases, but reinfection with different stain may occur. It may also complicate vaccination with a live strain of leishmania.

10. **D i.e. Cutaneous Leishmaniasis**

Cutaneous Leishmaniasis	Chillblains	Lupus Vulgaris	SLE
- Found in North Africa, South America, ***North West Rajasthan***[Q] - After incubation pd. of 2 months, a boil appears on exposed site (***Baghdad Boil***[Q]); which breaks down to produce ulcer (***oriental sore***[Q]), which heals spontaneously in few months - Characterstic lesion has ***central depression, crusting & surrounded by raised indurated border***[Q]	- Occur in *damp cold* - Mostly affects ***finger & toes***[Q] - Dusky red or mauve swelling may be *painful & itchy*	- Slowly progressive *single, erythematous irregularly indurated plaque* which may ulcerate in some areas - *Healing with scar formation in some areas & progression in other areas* - ***Slowly increases in size over one, two or three decades***[Q]	- More common in ***females***[Q] - M.C. involve area exposed to sunlight i.e. *involvement of bridge of nose & cheecks* is ***a characteristic feature***[Q] - ***Associated with involvement of other organ system***[Q]

11. **B i.e. Tuberculosis verrucosa cutis** *[Ref: Novak 253-56; Rook's 8/e p. 31.12-31.13, 33.43, 41.10, 41.7; Neena Khanna 4/e p. 269, 253-56; Fitzpatrick 7/e p. 247, 1914]*

- **Tuberculosis verrucosa cutis** usually presents as **single**, indolent verrucous (warty) papule/nodule with a serpiginous edge, indurated base, erythematous areola, central scarring and serous /pus discharging clefts and fissure ***on trauma prone sites leg and hands***[Q].
- Whereas, *lichen planus hypertrophicus* lesions are ***multiple, bilaterally sympetrical and itchy***[Q] mostly on shins and ankle. **Verruca vulgaris (common warts)** are usualy asymptomatic multiple warty lesions on back of hand & fingers. **Mycetoma** is characterized by ***multiple draining sinuses***[Q].

12. **B i.e. Scrofuloderma**

Skin T. B.

- **Scrofuloderma**: Skin TB ***secondary to underlying lymph node joint, bone, etc.***[Q]
- **Lupus Vulgaris**: Skin TB with ***no underlying active focus***[Q]
- **T.Verrucosa Cutis**: TB Bacilli is *accidently inoculated* into integument, seen in TB patient, pathologist, veterinary surgeons. No underlying focus (like lupus but more verrucous)
- **Tuberculosis cutis orificalis**: This type involves mucosa & skin. ex - Oral mucosa in Pulmonary T.B.
  - Anal region in Gastrointestinal TB
  - Urogenital Mucosa in Renal TB

13. **C i.e., Lichen scrofulosorum** *[Ref: Rook's 7/e p. 28.11, 28.20; Fitzpatrick's 7/e p-1769-74, 272]*
14. **A i.e., Lichen scrofulosorum > D i.e., Erythema nodosum**
15. **A i.e. Lichen scrofulosorum**

- **Tuberculids** is *hypersensitivity reaction to mycobacterium tuberculosis,* where the evidence of etiology is not definite but show tubercular granuloma on histology & a positive response to antitubercular treatment.
- ***Lichen scrofulosorum & papulonecrotic tuberculide*** *are two definite (true) tuberculides*[Q].
- **Papulonecrotic** variety is most common and clinically present with *chronic, recurrent, symmetrical, necrotizing eruption of papules* arising in crops and primarily involving arms & legs. A hallmark is that lesion heals with *varioliform scarring.*
- **Lichen scrofulosorum** is an uncommon asymptomatic lichenoid eruption of minute (0.5-3mm) papules occurring in children and adolescents with strongly positive tuberculin reaction. ***It mainly involves perifolicular distribution on abdomen, chest, back & proximal limbs***[Q]. A **hallmark** is that ***superficial epitheloid dermal granulomas surround hair follicles and sweat ducts and may occupy several dermal papillae***[Q].

16. C i.e. M. ulcerans; E i.e. M. marinum

Skin Ulcer producing Mycobacterium

Species	Lesion
M. ulcerans	***Buruli Ulcer***Q
M. marinum	***Swimming pool granuloma***Q, which breaks down to indolent ulcer
M. tuberculosis	***Lupus vulgaris***Q Scrofuloderma etc.

✶ M. scrofulaceum l/t cervical adenitis in children.

17. A i.e. Verrucae; C i.e. M. marinum infection

Skin hazards of swimming

Causative agent	Disease
Mycobacterium marinumQ	**Swimming pool granuloma**
Schistosoma mansoniQ ***S. japonicum***Q	**Swimmer's itch**
AdenovirusQ Planter warts	**Swimming pool conjunctivitis** **Verrucae** (rare)

✶ **Pyoderma gangrenosum** is a rare serious *ulcerative disorder* of skin d/t serious underlying systemic disorders as *ulcerative colitis, crohn's ds. rheumatoid arthritis or myeloma.* Skin ulcers are – blue – mauve, *dinner plate* shaped *with undermined margins.*

18. A i.e. Sarcoidosis

Lupus pernio and epitheliod granulomaQ are charecteristic of **Sarcoid**

Other Bacterial Infections

19. B i.e. Erysipelas

20. A i.e. Staphylococcal infection

[Ref: Fitzpatrick's Dermatology in General Medicine 6/e p-1876-88; Rooks Textbook of Dermatology 7/e p.27.8-40]

- **Staphylococcal infections**

  1. ***Toxic shock syndrome***Q (in IUCD users)
  2. ***Scalded skin syndrome***Q
  3. Food poisioning (symptoms b/w **2-6 *hours***Q of ingestion)
  4. Bullous impetigo
  5. Nonstreptococcal scarlentiform eruption (staphylococcal scarlet fever)
  6. ***Sycosis barbae & nuchae***Q

- **Nonbullous impetigo & Cellulitis** are more commonly caused by **β-Hemolytic streptococci**Q.

21. C i.e. Produce scar on healing; D i.e. Erythromycin is drug of choice

22. B i.e. Impetigo contagiosa

23. B i.e. Staphylococcus

24. B i.e. Impetigo

25. A. i.e. Contageous, B. i.e. Bacterial infection, D. i.e. Honey coloured crust

[Ref: Davidson 19/e P-23, 24; Fitzpatrick's 7/e p-1695-99; Harrison 17th/317, 877; Neena Khanna 3/e p. 209-10; Rooks 8/e p.30.14-30.16]

Impetigo (Pyoderma)

- It is a **contiguous, superficial pyogenic** infection of skin. Pyodermas are infections in **epidermis, just below the stratum corneum or in hiar follicles.** Two main clinical forms are
  1. **Bullous impetigo** accepted as staphylococcal disease (by S. aureus) mostly.
  2. **Nonbulous impetigo (or impetigo contagiosa or Tilbury Fox)** may be cause by **Staphylococcus aureus** (most common); by group **A-β haemolytic streptococci** (mainly in developing nations) or by both.
- Pre school and young school age ***children are most commoly affected***Q. Although over-crowding (living in barracks), poor hygiene and existing skin disease especially scabies, predispose to infection. ***It most commonly affects children and is most common bacterial infection of children***Q. It occurs in all age including adults and neonates (called **pemphigus neonatorum**). It spread by close cantact (contageous).
- In nonbulous impetigo, the initial lesion is a very thin walled *vesicle on an erythematous base* which ruptures so rapidly that its seldom seen. The exuding serum dries to form ***yellowish brown (golden or honey coloured) crusts***Q, which are usually thicker and dirtier in strptococal form. Gradual, irregular, peripheral extension occurs without central healing. Multiple lesions may coalesce, crusts eventually dry and separate to leave erythema, which fades **without scarring**. Lesions are usually ***not painful, heals without scarring***Q, no fever and patient is not ill. Characteristic feature is ***honey clored crust and neutrophils beneath stratum***Q corneum.
- Face (esp around nose and mouth) and limbs are most commonly affected but scalp (in tinea capitis) and other body parts (in atopic dermatitis and scabies) are involved also. Lesions cure spontaneously in 2-3 weeks.
- In **Bullous impetigo**, the bullae are less rapidly ruptured, are much larger (1-2cm) and persist for 2-3 days. After rupture thin, flat brownish crusts are formed. *Central healing and peripheral extension* may give rise to circinate lesions.
- **Streptococal impetigo** may l/t ***post streptococcal acute glomerulonephritis (AGN)***Q, Scarlet fever, urticaria and erythema multiforme complications. ***Rheumatic fever is not a complication of streptococcal impetigo***Q.
- Treatment include ***oral dicloxacillin or cephalexin***Q and ***topical mupirocin or sodium fusidate***Q.

26. D i.e. Contact with animals *[Ref: Behl 6/e P-161; Fitzpatrick's 6/e p-1876-88; Rooks 7/e p.27.8-40]*

- **Erysipeloid** is caused by *Erysipelothrix rhusiopathiae & Bacillus erisepeletus,* is most often associated with **fish & swine** & causes cellulitis primarily in fishmongers & bone renderers.
- It is ***transmitted by contact with animals***Q.

27. A i.e. Scarlet fever

- ***Scarlet fever and erysipelas are streptococcal infections (not caused by staphylococcus)*Q.**
- **Scarlet fever** is caused by ***Group A streptococcus*Q**
- **Erysipelas** is acute inflamation of lymphatics of skin caused by ***β Hemolytic - streptococci*Q**
  - There is sudden onset of well marginated painful & swollen erythematous area usually on the ***face or lower limb.*Q** There may be haemorrhage & blisters.
  - Milian's ear sign is positive.
- **Ecthyma**
  - Varient of impetigo with punched out lesions generally on lower extremity.
- **Scalded Skin Syndrome**
  - Caused by **Exfoliative Toxin (ET) or Exfoliatin**Q elaborated by ***Staphylococcus.*Q**
  - Severe form of SSS is known as:
    Ritter's disease in ***new born*Q**
    Toxic Epidermal Necrolysis (TEN) in ***older*Q** individuals
- **Carbuncles & Furuncle (Boils)**
  - ***Staphylococcus aureus infection of hair follicle*Q**
- **Sycosis barbae & Sycosis nuchae**
  - Deep **Staphylococcus aureus** infection of hair follicles.
  - Asymptomatic or Painful & tender erythematous papules & pustules situated around coarse terminal hairs in **beard (S. barbae) & back of neck (S. nuchae).**

28. B i.e. Kawasaki disease; C i.e. Scarlet fever; D i.e. Toxic shock syndrome
[Ref: Harrison 18/e p. 150-56; Fitzpatrick 7/e p. 31]

Desquamation (scaling) is skin peeling or shedding of outermost *layer of stratum corneum (normal turnover time is 27 dyas). Scarlet fever, staphylococcal scalded skin syndrome, SJS, TEN, toxic shock syndrome, exfoliative erythroderma, Kawasaki disease and DHS/DRESS*Q lead to **confluent desquamative erythemas.**

Diseases associated with Fever and Rash

Centrally distributed maculopapular eruptions

- Acute meningococcemia, primary HIV infection
- **Drug induced hypersensitivity syndrome (DIHS)/ drug reaction with eosinophila and systemic symptoms (DRESS)**
- **1st disease /Rubeola/Measels** (by *paramyxovirus*Q; cause ***Koplik's spot*Q)**
- **3rd disease/Rubella/German measles** (by Toga virus; l/t **Forschheimer spots)**
- **5th disease/Erythema infectiosum** (by human parvovirus B19; l/t ***slapped cheeks appearance and gloves and socks syndrome*Q**)
- **6th disease/Roseola/Exanthem subitum** (by huma herpes virus 6)
- Infectious mononucleosis (by Epstein barr virus)
- Drug induced and viral (Echo and coxsackieviruses) exanthemas
- Epidemic typhus/Brill-Zinsser disease (by Rickettsia prowazeki)
- Endemic (Murine) typus (by R. Typhi)
- Rickettsial spotted fevers (by R. conori, Boutonneuse fever = R. australis = North Queensland tick typhus, R. Sibirica = Siberian tick typhus)
- Human monocytotropic ehrlichiosis (by Ehrlichia chaffeensis)
- Leptospirosis (by leptospira interrogans)
- ***Lyme disease (Borrelia burgdoferi*Q**; l/t erythema migrans and multiple secondary erythema migrans)
- Southern tick associated rash illness/**STARI**, Master's disease (by Borrelia lonestari; l/t smaller erythema migrans)
- **Typhoid fever** (by salmonella typhi; l/t ***rose spots*Q** on trunk)
- Relapsing fever (Borrelia); Rat bite fecer/Sodoku (by spirillum minus)
- Dengue fever (by Dengue-flaviviruses)
- ***Rheumatic fever/Erythema marginatum (Group A streptococcus)*Q**

Peripheral Erruptions

- Chronic meningococcemia, disseminated gonococcal infections, human parvo virus B-19 infection
- Secondary syphilis (T.pallidium), Bacterial endocarditis (strepto/staphylococcal etc).
- ***Rocky mountain spotted fever (Rickettsia ricketsii)*Q**, Chikungunya fever (chikungunya virus),***Hand-foot-and mouth disease (Coxsackievirus A16)*Q**
- Rat bite fever/Haverhill fever (streptobacillus moniliformis)
- Erythema multiforme (infection, drug etc.)

Confluent DesquamativeErthemas

- ***2nd disease/Scarlet fever*Q** (by group A streptococcus pyrogenic exotoxins A,B,C)
- ***Toxic shock syndrome*Q** (by GAS pyrogenic exotoxin A/B or M; S.aureus toxic shock syndrome toxin 1, enterotoxin B or C)
- **Staphylococcal scalded skin syndrome** (S. aureus phage group II)
- Exfoliative erythroderma syndrome (underlying psoriasis, eczema, drug eruption, mycosis fungoides)
- DIHS/DRESS (aromatic anticonvulsants, minocycline, sulfonamides)
- **Stevens-Johnson syndrome (SJS), toxic epidermal necrolysis =TEN** (drugs e.g. allopurinol, anticonvulsant, antibiotics etc. in 80% cases; infection)
- ***Kawasaki disease*Q** (idiopathic)

Vesicobullous/Pustular Erruptions

- SSSS, TEN, DIHS/DRESS, Handfoot mouth Syndrome
- **Varicella/chicken pox** (by varicella zoster virus; dewdrops on rose petal appearance)
- Hot tub folliculitis or hot foot syndrome (Pseudomonas aeruginosa)
- **Variola/small pox** (by variola major vivus)
- Primary HSV infection; disseminated herpes virus infection (VZV or HSV);

- SLE, Still's disease (both autoimmune)
- African trypanosomiasis (Trypanosoma brucei rhodesiense/gambiense)
- Arcanobacteria pharyngitis (Corynebacterium/arcanobacterium-hemolyticum)
- Rickettsial pox (R. akari); Ecthyma gangrenosum (P.aeruginosa, other gram-ve rods, fungi)
- Acute generalized eruptive pustulosis (drugs, viral); disseminated vibrio vulnificus infection

29. **D i.e. Rash is itchy**

These rashes in Erytherma marginatum are transient, migrating from place to place, non-pruritic, not indurated and blanch on pressure. Q

Erythema Marginatum

- It is one of the *major criteria for diagnosis of rheumatic fever*
- Extermely rare in Indians
- It is an ***evanescent macualar eruption with rounded or serpiginous borders.*** Q
- These are ***erythematous pink rashes with a clear center and round or serpiginous margin.*** Q
- Not raised above the skin.
- They are ***brought on by application of heat*** Q.
- *Most commonly seen on the trunk and proximal parts of extremities, but never on face.*

30. **D i.e. Roseola infantum** *[Ref: Harrison's 14/e P-1159; 15/e P-96]*

	Roseola infantum / Exanthema subetum / Sixth disease	Erythema Infectiosum (Fifth disease)	Rubella / Third disease	Rubeola / First disease (Measles)
Eto	**HHV – 6**	**Human parvo virus B-19**	**Toga virus**	Paramyxovirus
C/F	• Affects < 3 yrs old child - **Maculopapular lesions sparing face** - **Resolve with in 2 days (48 hrs)**	- Involves mostly 3-12 years age group - Bright **red slapped cheek appearance** f/b diffuse lacy reticular rash that waxes and wanes over 3 weeks.	- **Forchheimers spots** - Spreads from hair line down-ward & cleaning as it spreads	- Koplik's spots - Discrete lesions that become confluent as rash spreads from hair line downwards sparing palms and sole, lasts >=3 days

31. **A i.e. Impetigo contagiosa; B i.e. Ecthyma; C i.e. Furncle** *[Ref: Fitzpatrick's 7/e p. 1694-1709, 706, 296-302, 959; Rook's 8/e p. 5.7, 2.13, 43.13, 50.64; Neena Khanna 4/e p. 244]*

- **Pyoderma gangrenosum** (PG) is non infectious neutrophilic dermatosis commonly associated with underlying systemic disese like UC; Chrons etc. **Pyostomatitis vegetans**, malignant pyoderma, superficial vegetative granulomatous pyoderma, ulcerative/pustular/bullous erruptions of UC are variants of PG.
- **Pyoderma faciale** also k/a **rosacea fulminans** or **rosacea conglobata** occurs mainly in adult women (in 20s) and is characterized by sudden, severe eruption of confluent papules, nodules, pustules, cystic swellings which may be interconnected by draining sinuses usually confined to face, involving checks, chin, nose & forehead within a background of diffuse facial erythema. Comedones are usually absent or inconspicuous, as are other features of acne vulgaris or rosacea (& yet unclear whether this is a variant of these or a seperate entity). Some cases may develop during pregnnacy or medication (interferon α-2B & ribavirin therapy for hepatitis C)
- **Impetigo herpetiformis** is ***variant of pustular psoriasis*** Q attributed to hormonal alterations ***during pregnancy (generally during 3rd trimester)*** Q. Absence of positive family history, abrupt resolution of symptoms at delivery and a tendency to only recur during subsequent pregnancies distinguish this from generalized pustular psoriasis.
- ***Impetigo contagiosa*** Q, bullous impetigo, ***ecthyma*** Q, botryomycosis, superficial folliculitis (follicular or Bockhart impetigo), ***folliculitis (sycosis barbae)*** Q, ***furncle (boil)*** Q, carbuncle, blistering distal dactylitis and paronychia are **superficial primary pyodermas** caused by staph.aureus. Whereas, impetigo, ecthyma, blistering distal dactylitis (in nonintertriginous skin) and **intertrigo**, vulvovaginitis & perianal cellulitis (in inter triginous skin) are superficial primary **pyodermas** caused by group A streptococci. ***Pyoderma gangrenosum, pyoderma faciale & impetigo herpetiformis are not pyodermas*** Q.
- **Trichomycosis axillaris & pubis** is a bacterial (aerobic corynebacterium) not fungal infection of hair shaft. **Erythrasma** is superficial bacterial infection of skin caused by ***corynebacterium minutissimum*** Q.

32. **C i.e. Imetigo contagiosa; E i.e. Ecthyma**

- **Piedra** is a fungal infection of hair. **Pyoderma gangrenosum** is a rare, serious ulcerative disorder that is often d/t serious underlying systemic disease eg *ulcerative colitis, chron's disease, rheumatoid arthritis or myeloma* etc.
- Impetigo herpetiformis is the synonym of generalized pustular psoriasis of pregnancy.

9 FUNGAL INFECTIONS

Fungal Infections of Skin

Superficial	Deep
- Pityriasis - ***Tinea (corporis, cruris, pedis, capitis, unguum)*** [Q] - Candidiasis	- Histoplasmosis - Cryptococcosis - Coccidiomycosis - ***Sporotrichosis*** [Q] - Blastomycosis - ***Madura Foot*** [Q] - Actinomycosis

Stains used to identify Fungi

Periodic Acid Schiff (PAS)
- *Stains fungal tissue Red*
- *Stains both living and dead fungi*

Methenamine Silver Stain (Grocott's and Gomori's stain)
- *Stains fungal tissue Black*
- *Stains only living fungi*

Special stains	Tissue constituent (used to identify)	Appearance
Periodic acid-Schiff (PAS)	***Glycogen (diastase sensitive)*** ***Fungal wall (Neutral Polysaccharides)***	***Magenta red*** ***Red***
Grocott's	***Fungus wall (neutral mucopolysaccharide)***	***Black***
Gomori's (Methanamine Silver)	***Bacteria*** ***Gram +ve*** ***Gram –ve***	 ***Blue violet*** ***Red/ Pink***
Alizarin Red	***Clacium salts***	***Red***
Von Kossa	***Calcium salts***	***Brown/Black***
Masson's trichome	***Collagen*** ***Muscle + fibrin***	***Green*** ***Red***
Van Gieson	*Collagen* *Muscle, nerve*	*Red* *Yellow*
Congo red	*Amyloid*	*Red with green birefringence*
Acid orcein-Giemsa	*Elastic fibre* *Collagen* *Melanin* *Haemosiderin* *Amyloid* *Mast cell granules*	*Dark brown* *Pink* *Black* *Green/Yellow* *Light blue* *Purple*
Aldehyde fuschin	*Elastic fibre*	*Purple*
Gomori's Trichome	*Reticulum*	*Black*
Alcian blue (pH 4.5, 0.5)	*Acid Mucopolysaccharides*	*Blue*
Toludine blue	*Acid Mucopolysaccharides*	*Metachromatic purple including mast cells*
Perl's Prussian blue	*Iron (haemosiderin)*	*Blue*
Masson's Fontana	*Melanin*	*Black*
Ziehl-Nelson/Wade-Fite	*Acid-fast bacilli*	*Red*

Dermatophytosis or Ring Worm (Tinea) Infection

Dermatophytes include a group of fungi (*ring worm*) that under most conditions have the ability to ***infect & survive only on dead keratin; that is the superficial topmost layer of skin (stratum corneum or keratin layer), hair and nails*** [Q]. They *cannot survive on mucosal surfaces* (eg mouth or vagina) where the keratin layer does not form. Deep invasion and multisystem dissemination is very rarely seen in immunocompromized hosts. The ring worm fungi belongs to 3 genera:

Trichophyton	Microsporum	Epidermophyton
- Infects skin, hair & nail. - Several infecting species include **Trichophyton rubrum/ mentangrophyte /violaceum /verrucosum / & schoenleini**	- ***Infects skin and hair but does not involve nails*** [Q] - *Several infecting species include Microsporum audounii, M. gypseum* (most virulent geophilic i.e. earth loving = originating in soil, l/t occasional epidemic spread), and *M. cains* (zoophilic = found on animals)	- ***Infect skin & nails but does not involve hair*** [Q] - Only infecting species is *Epidermophyton floccosum.*

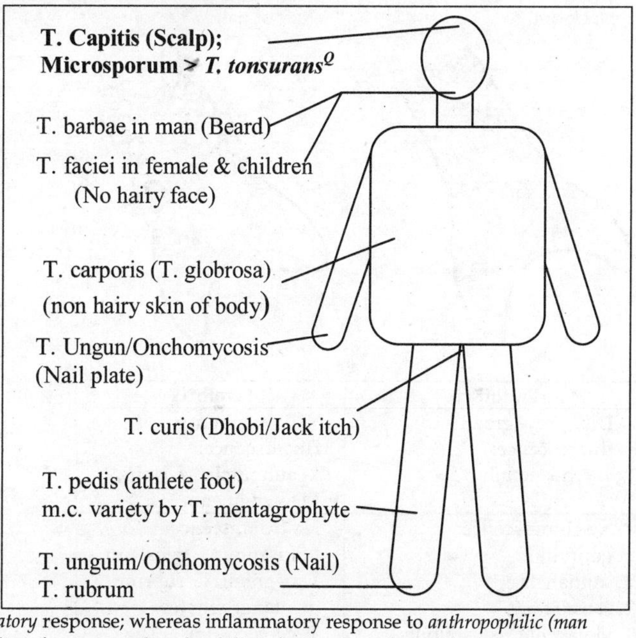

T. Capitis (Scalp); Microsporum > *T. tonsurans* [Q]

T. barbae in man (Beard)

T. faciei in female & children (No hairy face)

T. carporis (T. globrosa) (non hairy skin of body)

T. Ungun/Onchomycosis (Nail plate)

T. curis (Dhobi/Jack itch)

T. pedis (athlete foot) m.c. variety by T. mentagrophyte

T. unguim/Onchomycosis (Nail) T. rubrum

★ In general, *geophilic* & *zoophilic* dermatophytes elisit a brisk *inflammatory* response; whereas inflammatory response to *anthropophilic (man loving)* fungi is usually mild. But unlike sporadic geophilic & zophilic infections, anthrophophilic infections are *often epidemic* in nature.

★ **Microsporidium* is a *spore forming protozoa.*

Tinea Capitis

It is dermatophytosis of *scalp and associated hair*

Epidemiology

- ***Most commonly found in pre-pubertal children between 3 and 14 years of age***Q.
- May be caused by any pathogenic dermatophyte from ***genera Trichophyton and Microsporum excepting T. concentricum***Q. It is ***not caused by dermatophyte of genera epidermophyton.***Q
- ***Most common cause worldwide is M. canis, whereas in US, T. tonsurans (large spored endothrix) is most prevalent***Q f/b M. canis (small spored endothrix). (Fitzpatric- 1811) .
- ***M. canis is most common cause of Tenia capitis***Q (Roaburg); T. tonsurans is mot common cause of T. capitis in US since 1950's (Habif) .
- Even after sheding, hairs may harbor infectious organism for > *1 year.*

Pathogenesis

Hair involvement may be of:

Endothrix pattern	Ectohrix pattern
- Fungus *grows completely within the hair shaft,* replacing the intrapilary keratin, ***leaving the cortex (cuticle surface) intact***Q. The hyphae within the hair are converted to arthrocoinidia (spores). - As a result, hair is very fragile and breaks at the surface of scalp, where the support from follicular wall is lost, leaving behind a tiny black dot.	- Infection establish in perifollicular stratum corneum, spreading around & into the hair shaft of mid to late anagen hairs before descending into follicle to penetrate the cortex of hair - Cortex (cuticle surface) is breached and arthospores (& hyphae) are located both on inner side & outer shaft of hair.

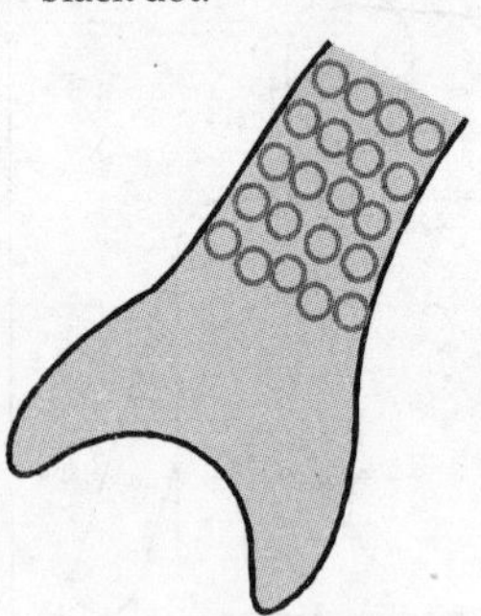

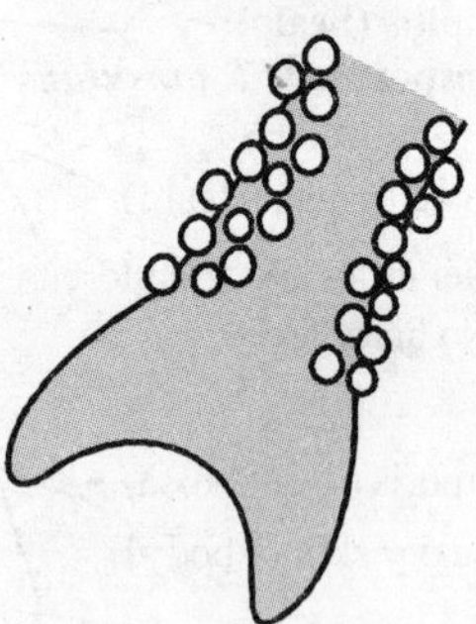

Endothrix	Ectothrix
- **Dull grey- green fluorescence:** T. schoenleinii	- **Yellow-green fluorescence:** M.audouinii, ***M. canis,***Q M.ferrugineum
- **No fluorescence**: T. gourvillii, T. soudanense, ***T. tonsurans***Q, T. violaceum, T. yaoundei	- **No fluorescence:** M.fulvum, M. gypseum, T.megninii, T: rubrum, T. mentangrophytes, T. verrucosum

- Alopecia areata and Tinea captis (mostly) leads to non-cicatric alopecia which can be differentiated by-

Clinical patterns

1. Non-inflammatory Human or Epidemic (seborrheic /scaly) type

- Most common & most difficult to diagnose because it resembles dandruff (or seborrhea) d/t *prominent scaling.*
- Most commonly caused by anthropophillic ectothrix eg. *M. audouinii or M. canis* f/b M. ferrugineum & T. tonsurans.
- Hairs turn *gray & lusterless* secondary to sheath of anthroconidia & ***breaks of just above the level of scalp l/t large, well defined, round, hyperkeratotic , scaly plaque of alopecia (gray patch type) usually on occiput***Q giving the appearance of **mowed wheat field**
- Inflammation is minimal. Often there is adenopathy & no hair loss.
- Culture is often necessary because only 30% have positive KOH examination

2. Inflammatory (Kerion) type

- It is hypersensitivity reaction to infection usually seen with zoophilic or geophilic *M. cannis & M. gypseum* > M. audouinii, M. nanum, T. mentagrophytes, T. schoenleinii, T. tonsurans, T. verrucosum
- Ranges from pustular folliculitis to **kerion**, which is ***boggy inflammatory tender mass studded with broken hairs, follicular orifice oozing with pus & easily pluckable hair***Q.
- ***Pruritis, pain, fever, occipital & posterior cervical lymphadenopathy & scarring alopecia may occur***Q.

3. Black dot

- Caused by anthropophillic endothrix ***T. tonsurans & T. violaceum***Q
- It is *least inflammatory* form resembling scaly variety but with less scaling, itching ; & *hair are broken at or below that scalp* surface resulting in <2 mm long stump and l/t **black dot appearance**.

4. Favus or Tinea favosa

- T. schoenleinii is the most common cause of human favus f/b T. violaceum, and M. gypseum.
- It is a chronic infection of scalp, glabrous skin, & /or nails characterized by **thick yellow honey comb crust (Scutula)** within the hair follicles which l/t scarring alopecia.

Investigation

- Diagnosis is made by first examining scale & hair on **microscope slide in potassium hydroxide (KOH) wet mount**. It is the ***single most important test for diagnosis***Q.
  Although it does not tell about species & susceptibility.
- **Culture** is *usually not necessary* to know the species because the same agent is active against all of them. Culture medium used are *DTM (dermatophyte test medium), sabouraud's dextrose agar* & mycosel agar. DTM is less accurate in species identification b/o presence of dye. Sabouraud's agar, which does not contain antibiotics, allows growth of most fungi. This makes it useful for nail infections because detection of non-dermatophytes is desirable in nail infection. **Mycosel aged** is modified subouraud's that contain cycloheximide & chloramphenicol to prevent growth of bacteria & saprophytic fungi; the dextrose content is lowered & pH raised to allow for better growth of dermatophytes *making it best for evaluation of hair tenia* because only dermatophytes cause hair tenia. Culture results become positive in 1-2 weeks.
- **Wood's lamp examination** (>365 nm) produce *blue-green (yellow-green)* fluorescence with *M. cannis, M. audouinni & M. ferrugineum;* and *dull (pale) grey-green fluorescence* with *T. schoenleinii.*

Tinea Captis	Alopecia aerata
- More common in *children*Q - *Itching & scales present*Q - Exclamation mark (!) not formed but stumps of broken hair are numerous.	- In *Adults*Q - *Absent*Q - Stumps are exclamation mark shaped (!) but scanty.

Treatment

- **Oral Griesofulvin** (20-25 mg/kg/day) is *drug of choice*Q. Other systemic options are fluconazole, itraconazole & terbinafine.
- Topical ketoconazole, povidone iodine, Zn pyrithione & selenium sulfide are only adjuvant treatment.

Onychomysis & Tinea Unguium

- **Onychomycosis** (most prevalent nail disease) is any infection of nail caused by dermatophyte or non dermatophyte fungi or yeast. However, **Tinea unguium** refers strictly to ***dermatophyte infection of nail plate***Q.
- Dermatophytes cause the great majority of onychomycosis. Tinea unguium is caused predominantly by ***T. rubrum (most common, 70%)***Q, *T. mentagrophytes (20%), T. tonsurans & E. floccosum.*

Treatment

Depends on severity, causative agent & matrix involvement

Without nail matrix involvement

Topical treatment alone can be sufficient

- **Ciclopirox** applied daily for 48 weeks is effective against Tinea unguium, candida, & some molds. It avoids risk of drug interaction, an important consideration for chronic therapy in older population.
- **Amorolfine** is effective against dermatophytes, yeasts & moulds when applied once weekly.

With nail matrix involvement

Oral antifungals may be used for *refractory, severe, or non- dermatophytic onychomycosis*, or when shorter treatment regimen, or higher chances for clearance or cure is desired.

- **Terbinafine** is the ***most effective oral t/t***Q for fungally infected toe nails available today. It is effective against dermatophytes, Aspergillus, Scopulariopsis (± candida) when given 250 mg daily for 6 weeks (in finger nails) or 12 weeks (toe nails).
- **Itraconazole** is fungistatic against dermatophytes, non dermatophytes & yeasts at 400 mg daily for 1 week/month pulse dose or 200 mg daily continuous dose for 2 months (finger nails) or 3 months (toenails) .
- **Fluconazole** is fungistatic against dermatophytes, some non dermatophytes & candida at 150-300mg once /week for 3 - 12 months
- **Griesofulvin** is ***no longer considered standard treatment***Q for onychomycosis & T. unguium because of its adverse effects, drug interactions, prolonged t/t course & low cure rates.

Tinea Pedis & Tinea Manus

It is *most common type of dermatophytosis* caused predominantly by ***T.rubrum (most common), T. mentagrophytes & E. flocossum***Q. Tinea pedis is infection of feet whereas Tinea manus affects hands (palmar & inter- digital areas). It presents in 4 forms:

Chronic intertriginous (inter digital) type (Athelete's Foot)

Most common type, begins as erosion, scaling & erythema of web space particularly b/w lateral 3 toes ***(most commonly between 4th & 5th toe)***Q. Warm moist environment (in shoes) l/t ***maceration, soggy-hyperhidrosis & itching (pruritis)***Q.

Chronic hyperkeratotic : Moccasin type

- Mostly caused by *T. rubrum* and usually involve ***two feet and one hand or two hands and one feet (syndromes)***
- Entire sole & palm is covered with a fine, silvery white scale. The skin is pink, tender & pruritic.

Vesicobullous type / **Acute ulcerative type**

- Vesico-bullous type is caused by *T. mentagrophyte.* Coinfection with gram-ve l/t purulent ulceration.
- A second wave of itchy sterile vesicles follow shortly in same areas or distant sites d/t allergic response to fungus & is k/a **dermatophytid** or **id reaction.**
- Cellulitis, lymphangitis, lymphadenopathy & fever are usually
- Rarely reported in children (mostly d/t *T. rubrum*)

Tinea Cruris/ Jack itch / Dhobi Itch

- It is *2nd most common* dermatophytosis world wide *involving groin, pubic, perineal – perianal skin and genitalia.* It is ***3 times more common in males than in females, and adults are affected more commonly***Q than children.
- ***Most tenia cruris is caused by Trichophyton rubrum***Q (in India & world wide) and *epiderophyton floccosum* (most often responsible for epidemics) > T. mentagrophytes & T. verrucosum. Warm, moist environment is predisposing factor.
- Lesions are ***mostly unilateral***Q *& begins in crural fold. A half moon shaped plaque* forms as a ***well defined scaling***Q, & sometimes a vesicular border advances out of crural fold onto the thigh. The skin within the border turns red-brown, is less scaly & may develop red papules. ***Involvement of scrotum & genitalia is unusual***Q – unlike **Candida**; which is ***more extensive, often bilateral, involve scrotum and show typical fringe of scale at border and satellite pustules.***Q
- E. floceosum infection is most often limited & show *central clearing*Q. In contrast, T. rubrum infections are often coalescent with extension to pubic, perineal, buttock & lower abdominal areas.

Tinea Corporis (Glabrosa) or Circinata

Tinea Corporis (Glabrosa or Circinata)

- It is dermatophytoses of glabrous (hairless) skin except the palms, soles & groin. It invoves face (excluding beard in men), trunk & limb and hence called Tinea corporis (ringworm of body).
- Most commonly caused by ***Trichophyton rubrum***Q, T. mentagrophyte, M. canis, & T. tonsurans. T. rubrum & T. verrucosum l/t additional follicular involvement. **Tinea imbricata** is caused by T. concentricum. **Tinea corporis gladiatorum** (in wrestlers d/t minor trauma, skin to skin contant) is caused by T. tonsurans.
- **Classical presentation** is *itchy* ***annular or serpiginous lesion with a well defined, irregular, erythematous and vesicular border with scale across the entire border***Q. Raised border advances centrifugally in all directions. The ***central of lesion may exhibit clearing***Q and become brown or hypopigmented and less scaly as the active border progresses outward.
- Tinea imbricata shows wide spread, multiple concentric, polycyclic scaly lesions with minimal inflammation & no (to little) vesiculation. Whereas concentric vesicular ring suggests. **Tinea incognito** caused by T. rubrum. **Majocchi granuloma** is caused by T. rubrum in women who shave their legs. It occurs when fungal hyphae invade hair & hair follicles and appear as folliculocentric papules.
- It is differentiated from pityriasis rosea by the fact that scaly ring of pityriasis rosea does not reach the edge of red border (as it does in tinea), rapid onset and localization to trunk (in p. rosea).

Type	Affected body part	Causative agent
Tinea corporis (glabrosa)	Skin of ***body or limbs***Q (usually non hairy)	***Trichophyton rubrum***Q
Tinea cruris (Dobhi/Jack itch)	***Groin***Q, perineum, thighs, scrotum (least & late involvement)	***Trichophyton rubrum (most common cause in India)***Q, Epidermophyton floccosum (most common cause in Western countries)
Tinea capitis	***Scalp***Q	***Microsporium canis***Q (m.c.) T. schoenleini T. tonsurans
Tinea pedis (Athelete foot)	***Feet***Q, m.c. 4th web space	T. rubrum ***T. mentagrophytes***Q E. floccosum
Tinea manuum	***Palms***Q	T. rubrum
Tinea unguium / Onchomycosis	***Nail plates***Q> ***nail bed***Q	T. rubrum T. mentagrophyte E. floccosum

Dermatophytosis (Tinea) Treatment

- Noninflammatory lesions of trunk, groin, hand, feet and sole → **Topical** Clotrimazole, Mi/keto /E.conazole Naftifine, Terbinafine, ***Ciclopirox oleamine***Q
- Hyperkeratotic lesion of palm → **Whit field's Ointment** initially to thin the keratin f/b topical Antifungals
- • Moderately severe ring worm • **Scalp, Beard, Nail bed involvement** → **Systemic therapy** Itraconazole, Terbinafine, Griseofulvin

Drug of choice in Dermatophytosis

- Ordinary ring worm of hairy skin → Local – ***Imidazole containing cream***Q (as Miconazole, Econazole, clotrimazole etc)
- - ***Tinea ungum***Q - T. capitis - Multiple area involvement - Failed topical t/t → ***Griseofulvin***Q

Griseofulvin

- **Griseofulvin** causes *abnormal metaphyseal configuration,* unlike typical **mitotic inhibitors (colchicines & vinca alkaloids),** it does not cause metaphase arrest.
- It is active against most dermatophytes including Trichophyton, Microsporum, Epidermophyton, but ***not against Candida, fungus causing deep mycosis & pityriasis versicolor***Q.
- It is ***ineffective topically***Q can be used systemically only

Infected part	Duration of t/t
Skin	3 weeks
Palm & soles	4-6 weeks
Finger nails	***4-6 months***Q
Toe	8-12 months

Candidiasis (Moniliasis)

It is infection caused by yeast like fungus – Candida albicans (m.c.) or other members of genus candida. It only ***infects the outer layers of epithelium of mucous membrane and skin (stratum corneum) usually***Q. Internal systemic infections are rare.

Predisposing factors

- *Pregnancy, diabetes*Q
- Oral contraceptives, antibiotic therapy
- Skin maceration, topical steroid therapy
- Immunodeficiency d/t AIDS, cushing's syndrome etc.

Primary lesion

- Is a *pustule*Q, the content of which disset horizontally under the stratum corneum & peel it away resulting in *red, denuded, glistening surface, with a long cigarette paper like scaling advancing border.*
- Infected mucous membranes accumulate scales & inflammatory cells & produce ***characteristic white or yellow-white curdy material***Q.
- Pustules form but become macerated under apposing skin & develop into red papule or moist glistening plaque with a ocean wave shaped fringe of macerated moist scale at border.
- Pinpoint ***satellite vesico-pustules outside the advancing border is important diagnostic feature***Q

Type	Lesion involve
Intertrigo	*Body folds of obese* where skin touches skin (intertriginous area) eg. under pendulous breast, & abdominal folds, in axilla & groin.
Diaper- rash	*Under wet diaper in infants,* a pseudo intertriginous area is created
Perleche	*Angular cheilitis & stomatitis*
Thrush	***Usually buccal, creamy curd like pseudomembranous***Q
Candida miliaria	*Back in bed ridden patients*
Erosio interdigitalis blastomycetica	Interdigital candidal or polymicrobial infection l/t ***thickness, erosion & discolouration***Q
Balanoposthitis vulvo-vaginitis	

A white patch on tongue may also be seen in Lichen planus, however, Lichen Planus lesions are not creamy/curd like and are typically described as having a 'Lace Like' pattern.

Feature	Candidiasis (Thrush)	Lichen Planus
Appearance	- White curd like (creamy) discrete or confluent patches (pseudomembrane) - Can be scrapped revealing a red raw mucosal surface	- White sharply defined lace like striae or patches often interspersed with papules. - Cannot be easily separated.
Other features	- Associated glossitis	- Associated typical skin lesions (Wickham's striae)
Diagnosis	- KOH smears for yeasts	- Biopsy
Treatment	- Antifungals (eg Fluconazole)	- Local steroids

Treatment

- ***Amphotericin B (drug of choice)***Q & **Caspofungin** are used for treating disseminated candidiasis.
- ***Griseofulvin & terbinafine are not effective***Q
- **Oral preparations** include fluconazole, itra conazole & ketoconazole. **Fluconazole** is preferred ***first line drug for candida vaginitis and for prophylaxis & t/t of localized & systemic candida albicans infection***Q.
- **Topical agents** are safe in pregnancy and include: clotrimazole, nystatin, miconazole, butoconazole, teraconazole, tioconazole; and gentian violet & boric acid.

Actinomycosis

Induration, ***sinus formation***Q **&** ***relapse***Q are *clinical hallmark of actinomycosis*

- *Actinomyces isreli* is causative agent.
- ***Oral-cervico-facial type***Q is most common variety.
- ***Lower jaw***Q is most common site to be involved.
- ***Induration, sinus formation & relapse***Q are clinical hallmark of actinomycosis.
- Drug of choice is ***Penicillin-G***Q

Antifungal Drugs

Antibiotics
- Polyenes:
  1. *Amphotericin B,*
  2. *Nystatin*
  3. *Natamycin*
  4. *Hamycin*
- Hetrocyclic benzofurans;
  - Greisofulvin

Antimetabolite
- 5- Flucytosine (5 FC)

Allglamienes
- Naftifine
- Terbinafine
- Benzyamines
- Butenafine

Azoles
- **Imidazole:**
  - Clotrimazole
  - Econazole
  - Ketoconazole
  - Miconazole
  - Oxconazole
  - Sertaconazole
  - Sulconazole
- Triazole
  - Fluconazole
  - Itraconazole
  - Voriconazole

Other
- Tolnaftate
- ***Ciclopirox olamine***Q
- ***Undecylenic acid***Q
- Benzoic acid
- Butenafine
- Quiniodochlor
- Potassium iodide
- Sodium thiosulfate

Ultra Violet Waves & Wood's Lamp

There are 3 segments of UVR

UV-C /short wave UV-radiation
- 250-280 nm
- **Filtered by ozone layer** & would only become biologically important if the ozone layer becomes seriously depleted
- Circulating lymphocytes are most sensitive to UV-C

UV-B / medium wave UV-radiation
- **280-320 nm**
- ***Mainly responsible for sunburn, suntan, skin cancers***Q (mainly 290 nm)
- **Medically most important UV Rays**

UV-A /long wave UV-radiation
- **320-400 nm**
- ***Wood's lamp***Q produce long wave UVR (360 nm)
- **Used in photo-chemotherapy (PUVA)**Q

Disease	Colour
*Tinea capitis*Q	*Light/yellow-green*Q
Tinea/*Pityriasis versicolor*Q	Apple-green / golden-yellow
Pseudomonas infection	Greenish white / pale blue
Psoriasis	Pale blue
Tuberous sclerosis	Blue white (Ash leaf spots)
Vitiligo	Total white
*Erythrasma*Q *(corynebacterium minutissimum)*	*Coral red/pink*Q
*Porphyria cutanea tarda*Q	*Red/Pink urine*Q

★ Wood's lamp filter is made up of ***NiO_2 & Si***Q. On wood's lamp examination:

DERMATOLOGY 1

1

DERMATOLOGY

Questions

1. **Which of the following are fungal infection of skin-** *(PGI June 05)*
   A. Sporotrichosis
   B. Molluscum contagiousm
   C. Madura foot
   D. Tinea
2. **Which of the following stains is used to study fungal morphology in tissue sections** *(AI 10)*
   A. PAS
   B. Von- kossa
   C. Alizarin Red
   D. Masson's Trichrome

Dermatophytosis

3. **Dermatophytes** are: *(PGI 06, 03)*
   A. Sporothrix
   B. Tinea versicularis
   C. Microsporidium
   D. Trichophyton rubrum
   E. All of the above
4. **Dermatophytes infection to:** *(Bihar 06, DNB 09)*
   A. Superficial
   B. Subdermal
   C. Subfascial
   D. Muscular
5. **Ring worm fungi live in** *(AIIMS 1992, UP 97)*
   A. Stratum Corneum
   B. Dermis
   C. Prickle Cell layer
   D. Basal Cell layer
6. **Which does not cause Tinea Capitis**
   A. Epidermophyton *(AIIMS 1994, 92, 97)*
   B. Microsporum
   C. Trichophyton Rubrum
   D. Trichophyton Violaceum/Schoenleinii
7. **Most common organisim causing T. capitis is**
   A. Trichophyton tonsurans *(AI 01, DNB 03)*
   B. Microsporum
   C. Epidermophyton
   D. Candida albicans
8. **Black dot ring worm is caused by-** *(PGI 99, AIIMS 95)*
   A. Microsporon
   B. Trichophyton
   C. Epidermophyton
   D. Candida
9. **Karion is seen in** *(AIIMS 1998)*
   A. Candida infection
   B. Trichomoniasis
   C. Pityriasis
   D. Dermatophystosis
10. **An 8 yr old boy presents with boggy swelling and easily pluckable hair, Diagnosis is** *(AIIMS 1998)*
    A. Tinea capitis
    B. Alopecia areata
    C. Tuberculorid leprosy
    D. Pityriasis alba
11. **A 8 year old child has localized non cicatrial alopecia over scalp with itching and scales. The diagnosis is :**
    A. Tinea Barbae *(AIIMS 1993)*
    B. Alopecia areata
    C. Tinea Capitis
    D. Lichen planus
12. **A 10-yr-old boy presented with painful boggy swelling of scalp, multiple sinuses with purulent discharge, easily pluckable hair, and lymph nodes enlarged in occipital region. Which one of the following would be most help ful for diagnostic evaluation?** *(AIIMS May 13, 09, AI 01)*
    A. Biopsy and Giemsa staining
    B. Bacterial culture
    C. KOH mount
    D. Patch test, Gram staining & Tzank smear
13. **An eleven year old boy is having tinea capitis on his scalp. The most appropriate line of treatment is:** *(AI 2003)*
    A. Oral griseofulvin therapy
    B. Topical griseofulvin therapy
    C. Shaving of the scalp
    D. Selenium sulphide shampoo
14. **Tinea ungum effects** *(AI 1995)*
    A. Nail fold
    B. Nail plate
    C. Joints
    D. Inter digital space
15. **Treatment of tinea unguium-** *(PGI June 05)*
    A. Fluticasone
    B. Itraconazole
    C. Oleamine oil
    D. Turbinafin
    E. Neomycin
16. **Ciclipirox Oleamine is used in :** *(AP 96, DNB 98)*
    A. Dermatophytosis
    B. Acne
    C. Psoriasis
    D. Lichen Planus
17. **DOC for Tenia Ungum** *(AI 93, UP 05, DNB 02)*
    A. Ampthotericin B
    B. Miconazole
    C. Gresiofulvin
    D. Nystatin
18. **Grisefulvin given for the treatment of fungal infection in the fingure nail dermatophytosis for how much duration**
    A. 4 weeks *(AI 02, CMC 05)*
    B. 6 weeks
    C. 2 months
    D. 3 months
19. **Not used topically** *(AI 95)*
    A. Nystatin
    B. Ketoconazole
    C. Griseofulvin
    D. Micronazole
20. **Grisofulvin is used in all except** *(AIIMS 90)*
    A. Tinea Capitis
    B. Tinea Versicolor & Candida
    C. Tinea Corporis
    D. Tinea Ungium
21. **Regarding Athelete's foot which us correct:**
    A. 4th tow web is commonly involved
    B. Severe itching *(PGI 96, Kerala 97)*
    C. Caused by trichophyton mentagrophyte
    D. Hyperhydrosis is present
    E. All of the above
22. **Dhobi's itch is:** *(Jipmer 92, DNB 94)*
    A. Tinea corfioris
    B. Tinea cruris
    C. Tinea barbae
    D. Tinea capitis

23. **Most common age group to suffer from T. Cruris**
A. Infant *(AIIMS 91)* □
B. Male child □
C. Adult male □
D. Adult female □

24. **A 22 years old male patient presents with a complaints of severe itching and white scaly lesions in the groin for past month. Which of the following is most likely to be the causative agent** *(AIIMS Nov 03, Jipmer 05)*
A. *Trichophyton rubrum* □
B. *Candida albicans* □
C. *Candida glabrata* □
D. *Malassezia furfur* □

25. **A 36 years old factory worker developed itchy annular scaly plaques in both groins. Application of a carticosteroid ointment led to temporary relief but the plaques continued to extend at the periphery. The most likely diagnosis is:** *(AI 05, CMC 07)*
A. Erythema annulare centrifugam □
B. Granuloma annulare □
C. Annular lichen planus □
D. Tenia cruris □

26. **Tinea incognito is seen with:** *(PGI 99, Calcutta 02)*
A. Steroid treatment □
B. 1% BHi3 □
C. 5% permethrin □
D. Antibiotics □

27. **A 30 yr old female presents with history of itching under right breast. On examination annular ring lesion was present under the breast. The diagnosis is:** *(AIIMS May 02)*
A. Trichophyton rubrum □
B. Candida albicans □
C. Epidermophyton □
D. Microsporum □

28. **The test likely to help in diagnosis of a patient who presents with an itchy annular plaque on the face is:**
A. Gram's stain *(AI 2003)* □
B. Potassium hydroxide mount □
C. Tissue smear □
D. Wood's lamp examination □

29. **Which of the following drugs is not antifungal?** *(AI 08)*
A. Capofungin □
B. Undecylenic acid □
C. Ciclopirox □
D. Clofazimine □

30. **An otherwise healthy male presents with a creamy curd like white patch on the tongue. The probable diagnosis is**
A. Candidiasis *(AI 2010)* □
B. Histoplasmosis □
C. Lichen Planus □
D. Aspergillosis □

31. **Commonest fungal infection of the female genitalia in diabetes is:** *(Karnataka 98, DNB 2K)*
A. Cryptococcal □
B. Madura mycosis □
C. Candidial □
D. Aspergellosis □

32. **A washerman presents with thickness erosion & discolouration of web spaces of toes diagnosis is:**
A. Psoriasis □
B. Tinea Unguum □
C. Both □
D. Candidiasis □

33. **Drug of choice in systemic candidiasis is:** *(Jipmer 93)*
A. Amphotericin □
B. Griseofulvin □
C. Nystatin □
D. Ketoconazole □

34. **About dermatophytes all are true execpt**
A. Candida albicans usually cause systemic infection □
B. Dermatophytes involve superficial layers of skin □
C. Microsporum doesn't involve nail *(AIIMS 1993)* □
D. Epidermophyte doesn't involve hair □

35. **Discharging sinus is seen in** *(AI 96)*
A. Syphillis □
B. Herpes □
C. Actinomycosis □
D. Molluscum Contagiosum □

36. **Linear lesion is seen in:** *(PGI 97)*
A. Sporotrichosis □
B. Lichen planus □
C. Psoriasis □
D. Pemphigus □

37. **Wavelength of light produced by wood's Lamp is -**
A. 320nm *(PGI 99, AIIMS 01)* □
B. 360 nm □
C. 400 nm □
D. 480 nm □
E. 760-800 nm □

38. **The range of light which causes maximum skin damage is-** *(JIPMER 98, AIIMS 99)*
A. 360-400 nm □
B. 290-360 nm □
C. 240-290 nm □
D. 760-800 nm □

39. **Medically most important form of UV radiation is -** *(AI 99)*
A. UV-A □
B. UV-B □
C. UV-C □
D. None of the above □

40. **The wood's lamp filter is made of -** *(AIIMS 99, PGI 2K)*
A. Tin and chromium oxied □
B. Nickel oxide and silica □
C. Copper oxide and Barium oxide □
D. Zinc oxide □

41. **A pinkish red Flurorescence of urine with wood's Lamp is seen in** *(JIPMER 99,PGI 2K)*
A. Lead poisoning □
B. Porphyria cutanea tarda □
C. Erythromelagia □
D. Acrocyanosis □

42. **Coral red-fluorescence wood's Lamp seen in-**
A. Porphyria cutanea tarda *(PGI 98, AIIMS 2K)* □
B. Erythrasma □
C. Livedo-reticulris □
D. Hypomelanosis □

43. **Wood's lamp light is used in the diagnosis of :**
A. Tinea capitis *(AIIMS May 02)* □
B. Candida albicans □
C. Histoplasma □
D. Cryptococcos □

44. **Uses of woods light includes :** *(AI 99)*
A. Urine examination in porphyria □
B. Examination of hair in T. capitis □
C. Selerema □
D. All □

45. **Woods lamp examination is used in diagnosis of:**
A. Erythrasma *(PGI May 12)* □
B. Lichen planus □
C. Psoriasis □
D. P. versicolor □
E. T. capitis □

Answers and Explanations:

1. **A i.e Sporotrichosis; C i.e. Madura foot; D i.e. Tinea** *[Ref: Roxburg 17th/37]*

***Tinea, Madura foot & sporotrichosis are fungal infections of skin but molluscum contagiosum is a pox viral skin infection*Q.**

2. **A i.e PAS** *[Ref: Ananthnarayanan 8th/601; Rook's 8th/10.8; Fundamentals of Pathology of Skin 3rd/ 8,9,10,11]*

The periodic Acid Schiff (PAS) stain is a valuable method for the demonstration of fungal elements in tissues. *Von Kossa stain and Alizarin Red are used to identify calcium, while Masson's Trichrome is used to identify collagen, muscle and fibrin.*

Dermatophytosis

3. **D i.e. Trichophytorubrum C i.e. Microsporum**
4. **A. i.e. Superficial** *Ref: Fitzpatrick's 7/e p-1807-19; Thomas Habif 4/e p-409-15; PN Behi 10/e p-164-66,171,176*
5. **A i.e. Stratum corneum**

- **Dermatophytosis** is caused by ***trichophyton, epidermophyton & microsporum*Q**; and it infects ***superficial topmost layer of skin (stratum corneum or keratin layer), hair and nails*Q**.
- **Cutaneous mycosis (Tenia or Ring worm or Dermatophytosis)** ***infect stratum corneum, hair & nails*Q** and do not penetrate living tissues.

6. **A i.e. Epidermophyton** 7. **B i.e. Microsporum** 8. **B. i.e. Trichophyton**
9. **D i.e. Dermatophytosis** 10. **A i.e. Tinea capitis** 11. **C i.e. Tinea Captis**
12. **C i.e. KOH mount** 13. **A i.e. Oral griseofulvin**

Ref: Fitzpatrick's 7/e p- 1811-14; Thomas Habif 4/e p- 427-33; Jawetz 22/e p- 528; Greenwood's microbiology 16/e p-574; Roxburgh's 17/e p-41; Neena Khanna 3rd/e p-243-50; Harrison's 17/e p-318]

- **Tenia capitis** is ***most commonly caused by Microsporum canis*Q > *Trichophyton tonsurans*;** and ***never caused by Epidermophyton*Q** as it does not involve hair. It presents with ***localized non-cicatrial (mostly) alopecia, itching, scaling with or without boggy swelling of scalp & easily pluckable hair*Q**. Tenia capitis is diagnosed by ***potassium hydroxide (KOH) wet mounts of hair & scale*Q *and treated by griseofulvin*Q**.
- **Griseofulvin is used systemically only** for dermatophytosis, **it is ineffective topically.** *It is the drug of choice for treatment of tinea requiring systemic therapy.* ***Griseofulvin has no role in treatment of Tinea versicolar & candida.*Q**

14. **B i.e. Nail plate** 15. **B i.e. Itraconazole; D i.e. Turbinafin**
16. **A i.e. Dermatophytosis** 17. **C i.e. Griseofulvin**
18. **D i.e. 3 months** *[Ref: Roxburg 17th/42, 43; Fitzpatrick's 7/e p- 1817-20; Thomas Habif clinical dermatology 4/e p- 413-16; Pasricha 4/e p-118*

Tinea unguium is ***dermatophyte infection of nail plate*Q**. It is treated by ***topical ciclopiro oleamine & amorolfine*Q** (in cases without nail matrix involvement) and/or ***oral terbinafine, itraconazole, fluconazole and griseofulvin*Q** (in cases with nail matrix involvement).

19. **C i.e. Griseofulvin** 20. **B i.e. Tinea versicolor & candida**

Griseofulvin is ***ineffective topically and used systemically only for dermatophytosis*Q**. It is used for **4-6 *months*Q** in tinea ungum (finger nail) infection. It is ***not active against candida, fungus causing deep mycosis and pityriasis versicolor*Q**.

Condition	DOC
Systemic Fungal infection	*Amphotericin B*Q
All Dermatophytes (All Tinea except Tinea Versicolour)	*Griesofulvin*Q

21. **E i.e. All of the above** *Ref: Fitzpatrick's 7th/e p- 1815-16; Thomas Habif 4th/e p- 425,413-15*

Athelete's foot (tinea pedis) most commonly affects ***4th toe web*Q**. It is caused by ***T. rubrum (mc)/ mentagrophytes & E.flocossum*Q** and presents with ***hyperhidrosis & severe itching*Q**.

22. **B. i.e. Tinea cruris** 23. **C i.e. Adult male** 24. **A i.e. Trichophyton rubrum**

[Ref: Fitzpatrick's 7/e p 1815; Thomas Habif 4/e p. 417; Roxburgh's 17/e 37-40, 116; Pasricha 4/e 114, 115-124]

Tinea cruris (dhobi itch) most commonly affects ***adult males***Q.

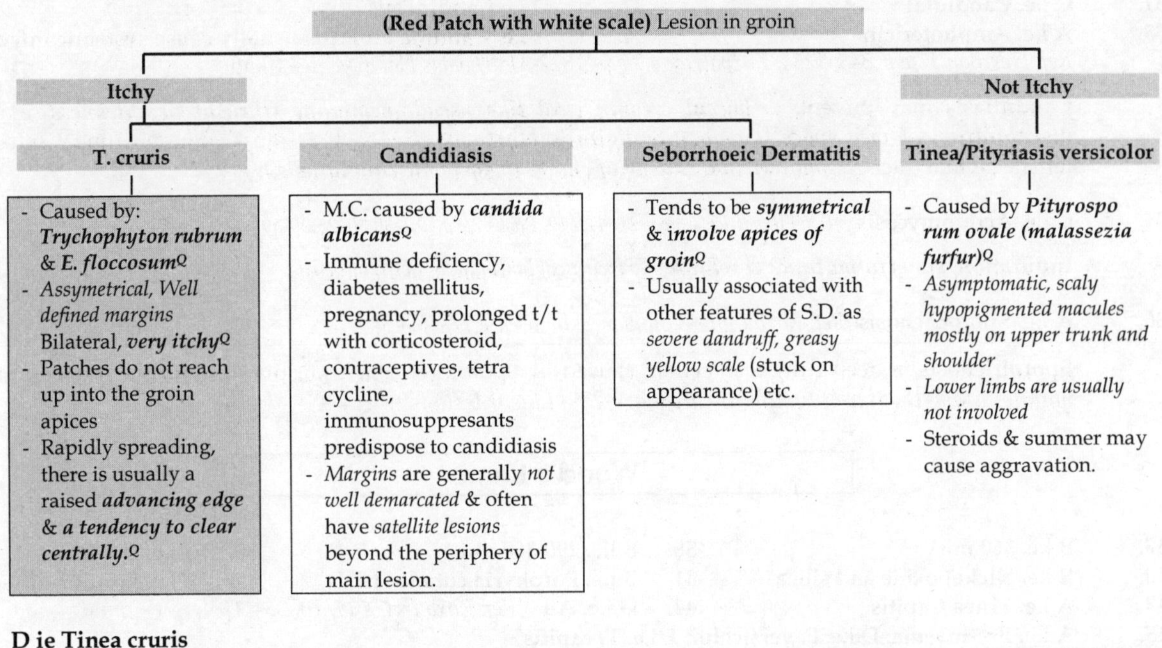

(Red Patch with white scale) Lesion in groin
Itchy
Not Itchy
T. cruris
Candidiasis
Seborrhoeic Dermatitis
Tinea/Pityriasis versicolor
- Caused by: Trychophyton rubrum & E. floccosumQ
- Assymetrical, Well defined margins Bilateral, very itchyQ
- Patches do not reach up into the groin apices
- Rapidly spreading, there is usually a raised advancing edge & a tendency to clear centrally.Q
- M.C. caused by candida albicansQ
- Immune deficiency, diabetes mellitus, pregnancy, prolonged t/t with corticosteroid, contraceptives, tetra cycline, immunosuppresants predispose to candidiasis
- Margins are generally not well demarcated & often have satellite lesions beyond the periphery of main lesion.
- Tends to be symmetrical & involve apices of groinQ
- Usually associated with other features of S.D. as severe dandruff, greasy yellow scale (stuck on appearance) etc.
- Caused by Pityrospo rum ovale (malassezia furfur)Q
- Asymptomatic, scaly hypopigmented macules mostly on upper trunk and shoulder
- Lower limbs are usually not involved
- Steroids & summer may cause aggravation.

25. **D ie Tinea cruris**

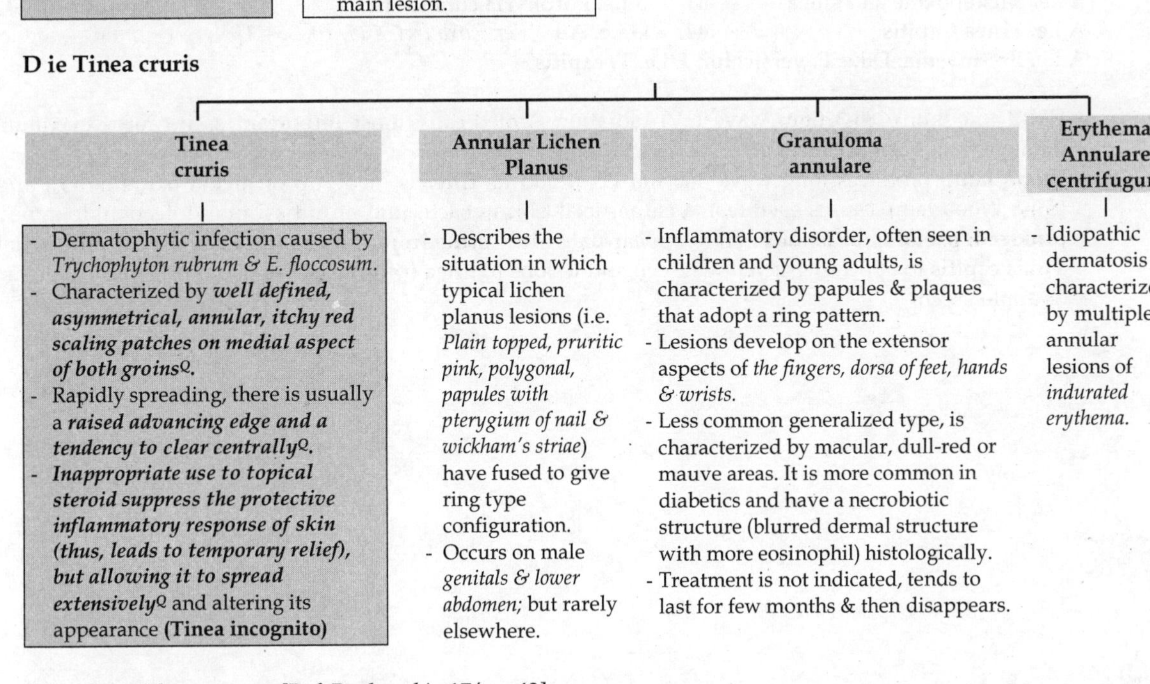

Tinea cruris
Annular Lichen Planus
Granuloma annulare
Erythema Annulare centrifugum
- Dermatophytic infection caused by Trychophyton rubrum & E. floccosum.
- Characterized by well defined, asymmetrical, annular, itchy red scaling patches on medial aspect of both groinsQ.
- Rapidly spreading, there is usually a raised advancing edge and a tendency to clear centrallyQ.
- Inappropriate use to topical steroid suppress the protective inflammatory response of skin (thus, leads to temporary relief), but allowing it to spread extensivelyQ and altering its appearance (Tinea incognito)
- Describes the situation in which typical lichen planus lesions (i.e. Plain topped, pruritic pink, polygonal, papules with pterygium of nail & wickham's striae) have fused to give ring type configuration.
- Occurs on male genitals & lower abdomen; but rarely elsewhere.
- Inflammatory disorder, often seen in children and young adults, is characterized by papules & plaques that adopt a ring pattern.
- Lesions develop on the extensor aspects of the fingers, dorsa of feet, hands & wrists.
- Less common generalized type, is characterized by macular, dull-red or mauve areas. It is more common in diabetics and have a necrobiotic structure (blurred dermal structure with more eosinophil) histologically.
- Treatment is not indicated, tends to last for few months & then disappears.
- Idiopathic dermatosis characterized by multiple annular lesions of indurated erythema.

26. **A i.e. Steroid treatment** *[Ref: Roxburgh's 17/e p. 42]*

Tinea incognito is extensive ring worm infection with atypical appearance due to ***inappropriate use of steroids.***Q

27. **A i.e. Trichophyton rubrum** 28. **B i.e. KOH mount**

Ref: Thomas Habif 4/e p-420-22; Fitzpatrick's 7/e p-1814; Roxburgh's 17/e P- 39-43; Pasricha 4/e p-114

Trichophyton rubrum is most common cause of ***tinea corporis (body), t. cruris, t. pedis, t. manuum & t.unguium***Q. Diagnosis is made by **KOH wet mount.**

29. **D i.e., Clofazimine**

Capsofungin, an echinocandin, is a *cell wall* antagonist that *blocks glucan synthetase.* It's an *intravenous drug* used in treatment of *aspergillosis or candidosis (resistant species).*

Ciclopirox and **undecylenic acid** are antifungal but clofazimine is not.

30. **A i.e. Candidiasis**
31. **C i.e. Candidial**
32. **D i.e Candidiasis**
33. **A i.e. Amphotericin**
34. **A i.e. Candida albicans usually cause systemic infection**

Ref: Harriion 17/e p. 345, 1254; Fitzpatrick's 7/e p- 1822-31; Thomas Habif 4/e p- 440-50

Candidiasis may present as ***buccal creamy curd like pseudomembrane (thrush) or thickness, erosion & discoloration of web space (erosio interdigitalis blastomycetica)***Q. It is most common fungal infection of female genital tract. ***Amphotericin B is drug of choice in systemic candidiasis***Q.

35. **C i.e. Actinomycosis** *[Ref: Fitzpatrick's 6/e p-2164-2212; Rooks 7/e p.30.1-30.30, 25.20-39]*

Induration, ***sinus formation***Q **&** ***relapse***Q *are clinical hallmark of actinomycosis*

36. **A i.e. Sporotrichosis** *[Ref: Roxburgh's-Common Skin disease 17/e p. 43]*

Sporotrichosis, a deep fungal infection, caused by sporothrix schenckii, may produce a ***series of inflamed nodules along the line of lymphatic drainage.***Q (ie ***Linear lesions***Q)

Wood's Lamp

37. **B i.e. 360 nm**
38. **B i.e. 290-360 nm**
39. **B i.e. UV-B**
40. **B i.e. Nickel oxide and silica**
41. **B i.e. Porphyria cutanea tarda**
42. **B i.e. Erythrasma**
43. **A i.e. Tinea Capitis**
44. **D i.e. All** *[Ref: Roxburgh's 17/e p. 38-41]*
45. **A i.e. Erythrasma; D i.e. P. versicolor; E i.e. T. capitis**

- **UV-B** (medium/**280-320nm** wave UV) radiation is **medically most important** as it causes **maximum skin damage (tan, burn & cancers).**
- **Wood lamp** produces **long wave 360 nm UVR** and its **filter** is made up of **nickel oxide (NiO_2) and silica (Si)**Q. Wood lamp causes **erythrasma** (superficial **Corynebacterium minutissimum** infection) to appear **coral pink-red; pseudomonas** infection to appear **pale blue; urine in porphyria (PCT)** to appear **pink-red; hair in Tinea capitis** to appear light yellow green and lesions in **tinea (pityriasis) versicolor** to appear golden yellow or apple green.

10 SCABIES

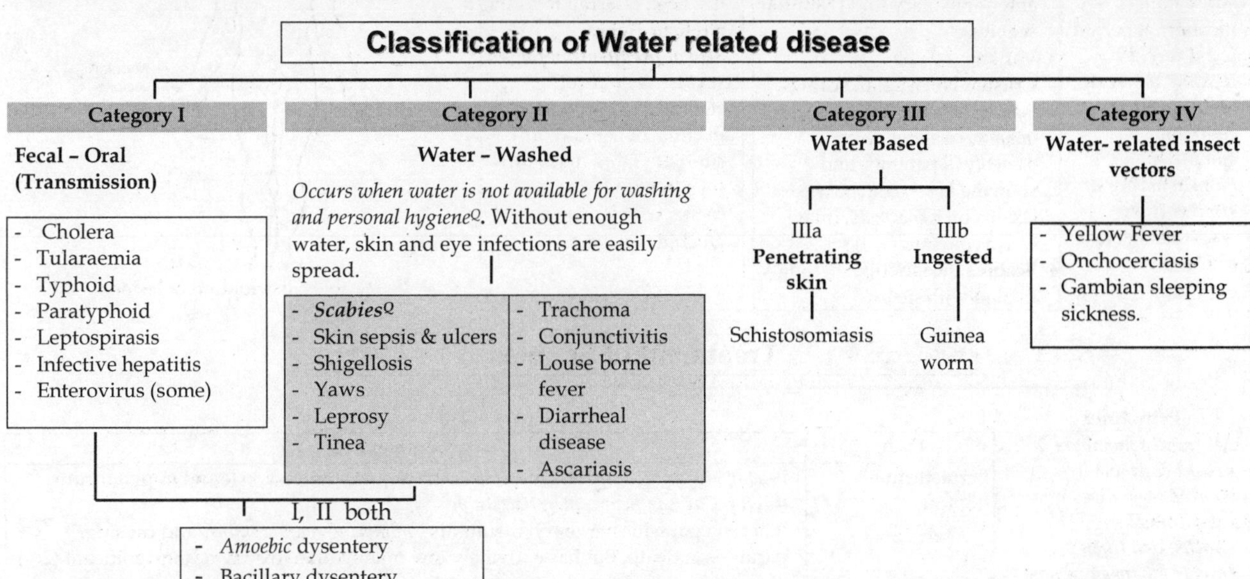

Also know:

Biological (Water borne disease)
1. Due to infective agent a. Viral-hepatitis: Polio, Rota virus b. Bacteria: Cholera, Typhoid, E.coli diarrhoea c. Protozoa: Amoebiasis, Giardiasis d. Helminth-Round/Thread worm hydatid ds. e. Leptospiral well's disease 2. Due to Aquatic Host a. Snail: Schistomiasis b. Cyclops c. Guinea worm d. Fishtape worm

Chemical
Due to pollutants

* **Other Water Related disease**
  I. d/t disease carrying insects breeding in or near water.
  II. Dental health d/t fluorides
  III. Cynosis in infant (Methaemoglobinemia) d/t high nitrate content in water.
* **Water based diseases** are *Electrolyte imbalances*.

Scabies

Epidemiology

- Infestation caused by ***Acarus / Sarcoptes scabie***Q
- Usually a disease of children, with no gender predilection, & mainly involving lower socio economic strata living in poor hygiene & crowding.
- Transmitted by *close physical contact* from

Morphology of lesions & variants

- Primary lesions are of three types:
  - **Burrow** : is the ***serpentine (S-shaped) path traversed by parasite in stratum corneum***Q. ***It is pathognomic lesion***Q
  - **Papules** & papulo – vesicles: are d/t hypersensitivity to the mite
  - Fine pin head size follicular papules.
- Secondary lesions
  - **Pustules** d/t 2° infection is one of commonest form of presentation
  - **Eczematized exudative**

Site of predilection

- ***In adults web of fingers***Q, flexure aspect of wrist, ulnar aspect of forearm, anterior axillary fold, umbilicus, periumbilical fold, ***genitals***Q *(penis & scrotum in males, nipple & areola in females)*, upper thigh, lower part of buttocks
- Back is rarely affected
- ***Scalp, face, palms & soles are characteristically spared in adults***Q.
- In **infants**, ***scalp, face, palms and soles are***

Treatment

Drug of choice	***Permethrin***Q (1st) ***BHC***Q (2nd)
Oral drug (only)	***Ivermectin***Q
Other drugs	***Benzyl benzate***Q 25% ***Crotamiton***Q 10% Malathion Monosulfiram
In 2° infection	IV antibiotics

- Scabicides should be applied to the whole body (below jaw line in adults) ***to all members of family whether symptomatic or not***Q
- Itching may last for several days & does not require retreatment with scabicide. Antihistamines are usually adequate
- *Ordinary laundering of cloths & bed linen.* Mites

human to human or from pets to human. Thus there are often *several cases in same house hold*Q - *Incubation period is 2-4 weeks*Q - *Itching' worse at night, is most common symptom*Q - *Family hstory of similar itchy eruptions in close contact*Q	**crusted lesions**, in *infants & children* are predominant lesions - **Nodular lesions** are seen on *scrotum*Q (m.c.), groin, and anterior axillary fold (**Nodular scabies**) • Variants / Type - **Crusted Norwegian scabies**, is *most severe*Q form seen in *immuno compromised or mentally ill* patients, and showing *hyperkeratotic crusted* lesions on *whole body*. (may cause epidemic) - **Scabies incognetio** is wrongly treated with *steroids*.	*typically involved*Q. - An anatomical circle, encompassing the axial, elbow flexures, wrists, hands, and genital region has been referred to as the **circle of Hebra.** - *Site of predilection for scabies is circle of Hebra*Q. Scabies & scabies in circle of hebra (both) simulate sabra dermatitis seen in prickly pears (eg. cactus with spines & glochids) pickers.

any way die in unworn clothes in ~ 7 days.

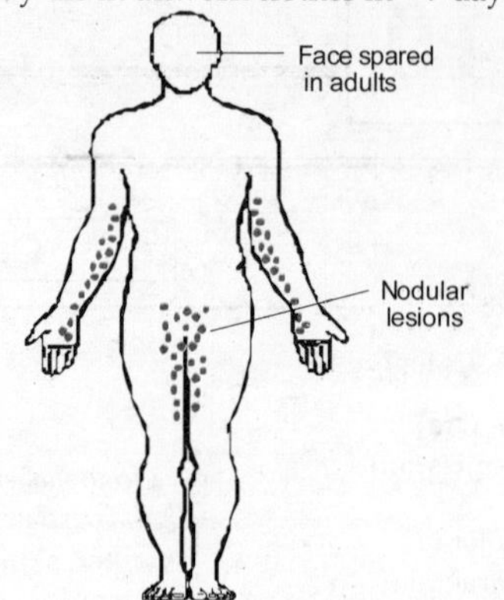

Scabies distribution of lesions

Treatment of Scabies

Principles

- *All family members & sexual contacts are treated regardless of symptoms*Q.
- *Cloths, bed linen & towels etc. used in past 5 days, should be washed & dried in hot cycle or be dry cleaned*Q
- Because the mite can live upto *3 days off skin*, carpets & upholstery should be vaccumed.
- *Pets do not need to be treated*Q because they do not harbor the human mite.
- **In adults,** topical scabicides should be applied to the entire skin surface, *excepting the face & scalp*, with special attention to intertrigenous areas, genitals, periungal regions & behind the ears.
- In **children** & those with **crusted scabies,** the *face & scalp should* also be treated.
- Patient must be informed that even after adequate scabicidal therapy, the *rash and pruritis may persist for upto 4 weeks*, otherwise they may think t/t was unsuccessful & inappropriately overuse medication.

Drugs used

Drug	Comment
Permethrin 5% (topical)	- Is *synthetic* pyrethroid modeled after the natural insecticide found in pyrethrum flower, *Chrysanthemum cinerariaefolium* - It acts on parasitic nerve cell membrane, *inhibiting sodium influx*, and causing paralysis & death. But has extremely low mammalian toxicity d/t insignificant (2%) absorption. - ***Drug of choice for treatment of scabies in children & adults of all age***Q. - It is contraindicated in infants < 2 months of age (d/t lack of safety data) and is *category B drug* (i.e. used with caution) *in pregnant & breast feeding women.* - Itching & stinging is major S/E and is also useful in pediculosis capitis /pubis, mite infestation including cheyletiella & as insect repellant.
γ- Benzene -hexa chloride/ Gammexene (Hexachlorocyclohexane or Lindane) 1% topical	- It is a cholinesterase inhibitor chlorinated hydrocarbon pesticide with CNS stimulant effect producing seizure & death in scabies & lice mite. - High (10%) absorption from intact skin, accumulation in fat & binding to brin tissue causes ***CNS toxicity, muscle spasm, seizure, & aplastic anemia l/t USFDA recommendation that BHC only be used as second line agent***Q. - It should be **avoided (C/I)** ***in children < 3 years, pregnant (category C) or breast feeding women***Q, patients with *seizure disorder* or over- broken *(acutely inflamed or raw)* skin, patients with *HIV or acquired immunodeficiency* syndrome, children weighing *< 50 kg or premature, emasciated or mal nourished children.*
Crotamiton (Crotonyl – N-ethyl-O- toludine) 10% topical	- *Antipruritic* quatities, but is *less effective* - Used for scabies (not lice). It is approved for infants & children but is pregnancy category C.
Precipitated sulfur (5-10% topical)	- ***Safe in children < 2months and during pregnancy***Q. But messy to apply, has unpleasant odour, and causes dryness.
Benzyl benzoate 10% topical	Not used in USA
Ivermetin 200μg/kg oral	- It is an antiparasitic agent used for *treatment and prevention of onchocerciasis (river blindness) & other filarial diseases.* - It is the ***only drug effective orally in scabies & lice (pediculosis)***Q. - Single oral dose can be repeated in 10-14 days, is highly effective particularly in crusted or resistant cases (when combined with topical agent). - It *inhibits glutamated (GABA) gated - chloride ion channels* found in peripheral nervous system (PNS) of invertebrates l/t increased permeability of cell membrane to Cl^- ion with hyperpolarization of nerve & /or muscle cells resulting in paralysis & death of parasite. In mammals these receptors are confined to CNS and normally the drug does not cross blood brain barrier. - Therefore, drug should not be used in conditions where BBB may be disrupted eg. *children < 5 years age or weighing <15 kg, or during pregnancy or lactation* - Discovered in ferments of soil actinomycete streptomyces avermitilis, structurally similar to macrolidic antibiotics but with no antibacterial activity.

★ **Systemic antibiotics** are used for ***secondary infections***Q. *Topical steroid, antihistamines* and if necessary *systemic steroids (short course)* are prescribed for **pruritis**. Systemic steroids are also useful in severe eczamatization (i.e. exudation & crusting).

Questions

1. **Scabies, an infection of the skin caused by Sarcoptes scabiet, is an example of:**
   A. Water borne disease *(AIIMS Nov 02)* ☐
   B. Water washed disease ☐
   C. Water based disease ☐
   D. Water related disease ☐

2. **Incubation period of scabies is:** *(Calcutta 2K, DNB 04)*
   A. 7 days ☐
   B. 2 weeks ☐
   C. 4 weeks ☐
   D. 2-3 days ☐

3. **Characteristic lesion of scabies is-** *(Kerala 87, Bihar 03)*
   A. Burrow *(UPSC 04)* ☐
   B. Fissure ☐
   C. Vesicle ☐
   D. Papule ☐

4. **The burrows in scabies is in the** *(KA 98, Kerala 90)*
   A. Straum germination ☐
   B. Straum corneum ☐
   C. Malphigian layer ☐
   D. Dermis ☐

5. **Most severe form of scabies-**
   A. Norwegian scabies *(AP 98, UPSC 96, DNB 01)* ☐
   B. Neular sabies ☐
   C. Animal scabies ☐
   D. Genital ☐
   E. Generalised scabies ☐

6. **Nodular scabies is found in** *(AIIMS 97)*
   A. Web space of finger ☐
   B. Axilla ☐
   C. Abdomen ☐
   D. Scrotum ☐

7. **Circle of hebra is associated with:** *(PGI June 08)*
   A. Syphilis ☐
   B. Scabies ☐
   C. Leprosy ☐
   D. Lichen planus ☐

8. **Scabies in children differs from that in adults in that it affects** *(Jipmer 2K, DNB 09)*
   A. Webspace ☐
   B. Face ☐
   C. Genitalia ☐
   D. Axilla ☐

9. **Adult scabies is characterized by-**
   A. Involve palm & soles *(PGI Dec 04)* ☐
   B. Involve face ☐
   C. Involve anterior abdomen ☐
   D. Involve web space ☐
   E. Involve genitalia ☐

10. **A 9 month old child has multiple itchy papulovesicular lesions on face, trunk, palm & sole. Similar lesions are also seen in the younger brother. Which of the following is most possible diagnosis?**
    A. Papular urticaria *(AIIMS Nov 02, 95, 96)* ☐
    B. Scabies ☐
    C. Atopic dermatitis ☐
    D. Allergic contact dermatitis ☐

11. **An infant presented with itchy eczematous crusted lesions with exudation on palm, sole, glans penis and face. All are true except:** *(PGI 02)*
    A. Family should be examined ☐
    B. Only patient needs drug treatment ☐
    C. All clothing & linen should be discarded or burnt ☐
    D. Distribution of lesion help in diagnosis making. ☐
    E. Drug should be applied to affected areas for whole day ☐

12. **An infant presenting with itchy lesions over groin and prepuce all is indicated except** *(AI 01)*
    A. Bathe & apply scabicidal solution ☐
    B. Treatment of all family members ☐
    C. Dispose all clothes by burning ☐
    D. IV antibiotics ☐

13. **An 8-month old child presented with itchy, exudative lesions on the face, palms and soles. The siblings also have similar complaints. The treatment of choice is such a patient is:** *(AI 03)*
    A. Systemic ampicillin ☐
    B. Topical betamethasone ☐
    C. Systemic prednisolone ☐
    D. Topical permethrin ☐

14. **The drug used for scabies is/are** *(AI 88)*
    A. Sulphur ointment ☐
    B. Benzyle benzoate ☐
    C. Gamma benzene hexachloride ☐
    D. Crotamiton ☐
    E. All of the above ☐

15. **Ivermectin in indicated in the treatment of :**
    A. Syphilis *(AIIMS May 2006)* ☐
    B. Scabies ☐
    C. Tuberculosis ☐
    D. Dermatophytosis ☐

16. **Permethrin is used in treatment of** *(AI 99)*
    A. Scabies ☐
    B. Leprosy ☐
    C. Body Louse ☐
    D. Leishmaniaris ☐

17. **Drugs/treatment used in scabies are all except**
    A. Crotamiton *(PGI May 12, 11)* ☐
    B. Permethrin ☐
    C. Lindane, Benzyl benzoate ☐
    D. Gammexene (BHC); Washing of clothes ☐
    E. Tacrolimus ☐

18. **A 6 month old infant presented with multiple erythematous papules & exudative lesions on the face, scalp, trunk and few vesicles on palms and soles for 2 weeks. His mother has H/o itchy lesions. The most likely diag is:**
    A. Scabies *(AIIMS May 12, May 05, AI 06)* ☐
    B. Infantile exzema (atopic dermatitis) ☐
    C. Infantile seborrheic dermatitis ☐
    D. Impetigo contagiosa ☐
    E. Seborrheic dermatitis ☐

Answers and Explanations:

1. **D i.e. Water related disease** *[Ref. Park 17/e p. 494; Fitzpatrick's 6/e p-2283-85]*

   Scabies is **water washed (category II) water related disease.**

2. **C. i.e. 4 weeks** 3. **A i.e. Burrow** 4. **B. i.e. Stratum corneum**
5. **A i.e. Norwegion scabies** 6. **D i.e. Scrotum** 7. **B. i.e. Scabies**
8. **B. i.e. Face** 9. **A i.e. Involve palm & soles; D i.e. Involve web space; E i.e. Involve genitalia**
10. **B i.e. Scabies** 11. **A i.e. Family should be examined; C i.e. All clothing & linen should be discarded or burnt; E i.e. Drug should be applied to affected areas for whole day**
12. **D i.e. IV antibiotics** 13. **D i.e. Topical permethrin**
14. **E. i.e. All** 15. **B i.e. Scabies** 16. **A i.e. Scabies**
17. **E i.e. Tacrolimus** *[Ref: Neena Khanna 3/e p. 294-97; Pasricha 3/e p. 70; Behl 10/e p. 178-81; Fitzpatrick's 7/e p-2133-2063, 2029-32; Thomas Habif Dermatology 4/e p. 497-505]*

Scabies

Causative agent	*Sarcoptes scabie*[Q]
Most common complaint	Itching (Family history is found i.e. other family members are usually involved)
Lesion	Papule / Vesicle / Burrow
Pathognomic lesion	S shaped *burrow in stratum corneum*[Q]
Most common Involved site	- **Inter digital space**[Q] - ***Anterior wrist***[Q] - Ulnar border of hand
In Infants (& elderly) also involves	- ***Scalp, Face, Neck***[Q] - ***Palms & Soles***[Q] - ***Penis involvement*** - ***Eczematization***
Nodular scabies involve	*Scrotum*[Q]
Norwegian/ Crusted Scabies	- ***Most severe form***[Q] - Found in old, malnourished, immuno suppressed patients - Involve whole body
Scabies Incognetio	- Is wrongly treated with Steroids
Drugs ***All family members & contacts treated and clothings/linen washed***[Q]	- *Permethrin*[Q] is drug of choice in children (except < 2 months), adults and used with caution in pregnancy & breast feeding women. - 1% *gammexene or lindane*[Q] (2nd choice) - Crotamiton - Precipitated sulfur (safe in < 2 months children & during pregnancy) - Benzyl benzoate - ***Ivermectin***[Q]

★ **Tacrolimus** (a calcineurin inhibitor & immunomodulator) is used in vitiligo, atopic dermatitis and rosacea (but not scabies)

D/D of Itchy Papulo-vesicular lesions

Scabies	Infantile /Atopic eczema
Close contacts have typical lesions of scabies[Q]	***H/O Asthma + family members give h/o atopy***[Q]
Papulovesiculations on palms & soles in infants[Q]	***Palms & soles spared***[Q] though may show hyperlinearity
- Mostly involve ***palms, inter digital area of fingers***[Q], flexural creases & over the elbows etc. - ***Head & neck are involved in infants only***[Q]	Mostly involve ***face***[Q], ***popliteal fossae, antecubital fossae, wrist***[Q] ***i.e. face & flexures***[Q] of infant to young adult
Intense itching with minor physical signs	Itching made worse by ***sundry (in rainy seasons)***[Q], changes in temperature etc
Burrows & demonstration of female scabies mite are pathognomic[Q].	- ***Excoriation, Lichenification, Hyperlinear palms, Denny morgan folds***[Q], ***white dermatographism***[Q] are seen - Associated with other allergic disorders like ***urticaria***[Q]; asthma, rhinitis, hay fever, alopecia & ***susceptibility to skin infection***[Q],

18. **A ie Scabies**

- The diagnosis is scabies, which is characterized by **severe itching** and diffusely scattered papular and papulo-vesicular lesions which may appear on all parts of body except the face. It is common to find **other individuals especially children** staying in same house also **showing similar features.**
- **In infants, eczematization is very common** and it leads to **exudation and crusting** especially on the wrist and ankle. Secondary infection leads to **pustule, crust fever and lymphadenopathy.**
- Involvement of palm & soles, duration of < 6 weeks (2 weeks) and presence of same lesions in mother, favour the diagnosis of scabies.

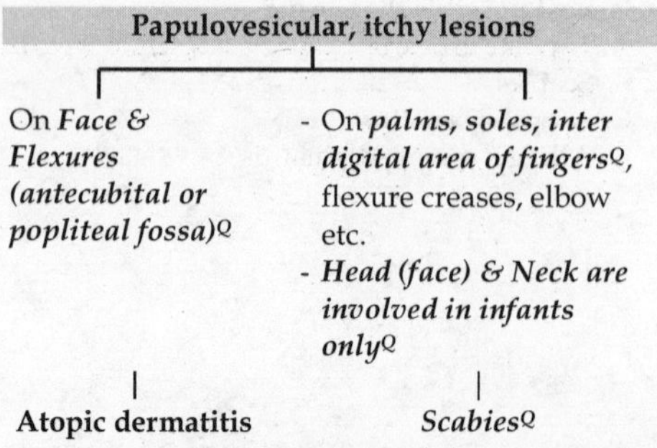

Scabies

- *Intense itching* even in presence of minor physical signs
- The physical sign are essentially those of eczema & effects of scratching.
- *Vesicles* are seen but *excoriations* and prurigo-like *papules* are more common.
- *Pathognomic lesion is burrow or run* (in stratum corneum); which is a tiny, raised, linear or serpiginous white mark.
- The best sites to find burrows are *palms & interdigital areas of fingers, flexural creases* and over the elbows.
- Other common sites of involvement are – anterior axillary fold, buttock fold, areola of breast, lower abdomen, *genitalia,* knees, ankle and *soles.*
- ***Head and neck is involved in infants only.***
- ***Same type of lesion may also present in family members.***
- ***Positive family or social history with itching contacts***

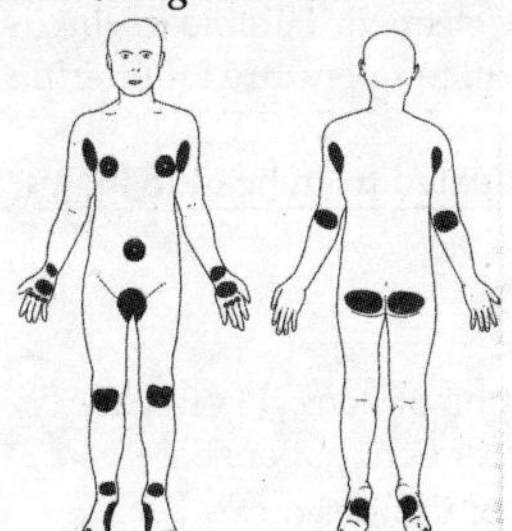

- Finding of mite or egg by pin or by examining skin scrapings or a skin surface biopsy taken with cynoacrylate glue, confirms diagnosis.

Atopic Dermatitis/Infantile Eczema

- ***Extremely itchy***[Q]***, erythematous papular or papulo-vesicular lesions mostly on face and flexures (popliteal fossa, antecubital fossae & wrist)*** of infant, children, adolescent & young adult
- Itching made worse by ***change in temperature, sundry (rainy season)*** etc.
- Perpetual rubbing & scratiching I/t *excoriation, lichenification,* hyperlinear palms & ***Denny morgan fold*** (crease lines just below eyes) .
- ***Personal or family h/o of atopy (eg asthama, hay fever, rhinitis, urticaria***[Q]) present
- ***Clinical course lasting longer than 6 weeks***[Q]
- Course marked by exacerbation & remission
- May be associated with alopecia areate & ***susceptibility to skin infection***

Seborrheic Dermatitis

- ***Infantile S.D. may be evident within first few weeks of life (usually < 3 months)***[Q]. It involves scalp (*cradle cap*), face or groin.
- It is rarely seen in children beyond infancy but becomes evident again during adult life.
- Lesions are characterized by *greasy scales* overlying erythematous patches or plaques
- Reddened itchy patches may become either scaly or crusted & exudative.
- The most common location is *scalp* where it may be recognized as severe *dandruff.*
- Other sites are eyebrows, eyelids, glabella, and nasolabial folds.
- Scaling of external auditory canal is common & mistaken as fungal infection. Retroauricular areas often become macerated & tender.
- May be associated with Parkinson's disease, cerbro-vascular accident & HIV infection.
- Rarely groin, axilla central chest, sub mammary folds & gluteal cleft may also be involved.

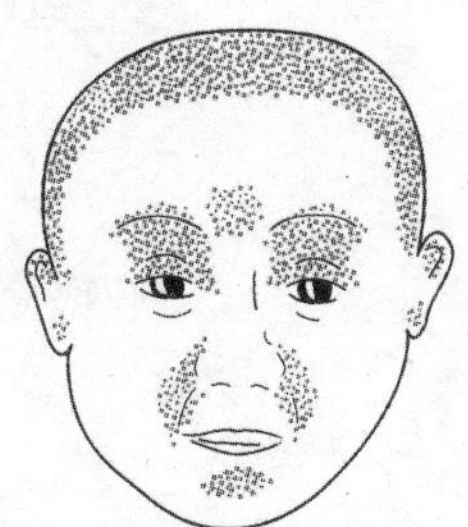

Frequently affected sites in seborrhoeic dermatitis

Impetigo contagiosa

- Contagious superficial skin infection caused by staph. aureus (mostly)
- *Red, sore* areas, which may blister, appear on exposed skin
- *Yellowish gold curst* surmounts the lesion
- It is mostly a disorder of *prepubertal children*
- May be associated with *glomerulo-nephritis,*

11 PEDICULOSIS (Louse)

Types of Pediculosis

- **Pediculosis Capitis (Head Louse)**
  Involves scalp
- **Pediculosis (Phthiriasis) Pubis/ or Pubic / Crab Lice**
  *Is a STD*Q
- **Pediculosis Corporis (Clothing/Body Lice)**
  - Causes *vagabond disease*Q
  - Lice does not resides on skin rather it resides on under clothing, except when feeding
  - **It is the clothing, not the patient, which requires treatment**. The most important treatment of body lice is disinfection of all clothing and bedding. However the patient should also be treated from head to toe with a topical insecticide or oral ivermectin.

Treatment

Head Lice (P. Capitis)	Topical (Shampoo or lotion) of - **Permethrin 1%-5% or malathion** 0.5% overnight application are **drug of choice** but not approved for children < 6yrs - **Carbaryl** 0/5% (Carcinogen) - **Lindane** 1% topically for 4 minutes (USFDA black box warning) - **Ivermectin** of 10 minutes - Phenothrin 10%, **DDT, BHC 1%** (Gamma benzene hexachloride or gamexine effective against nits, larvae & adults), **benzyl benzoate** (effective against larvae & adults) - **Oral Ivermectin** 200 mg/kg on day 1,8 and 15 is more effective than topical malathion, has very good efficacy on adult lice, not ovicidal; **not recommended for pregnant females and children < 15 kg** ★ Both malathion & ivermectin are prescriptional products only
Crab (Pubic) lice	- Same treatment as of head lice - All sexual contacts should be treated
Body (Clothing) Lice	- ***Destruction &/or disinfestations of all clothes & beddings of the infected individual, family members, & close contacts*Q are necessary** - Beds & clothings should be burned or sprayed with lice sprays, or fumigated, machine washed in hot water & dried on high heat or dry cleaned. Tumble drying is most effective means although high temperature laundering & dry cleaning are also effective. - Patient should be treated from head to toe by above drugs

Questions

1. **Vagabond's disease is** *(Calcutta 2K, DNB 01)*
   A. Pediculosis corposis ☐
   B. Scabies ☐
   C. Eczema ☐
   D. Ringworm ☐
2. **TOC for pediculosis corporis is** *(AIIMS 98)*
   A. 3 application of BHC ☐
   B. 4 application of BHC ☐
   C. Disinfection of all clothes and beddings ☐
   D. DDT application ☐
3. **TOC in pediaculosis corporis is** *(AIIMS 93)*
   A. 3 applications of Gama Benzene Hexa Chloride ☐
   B. One application of Benzyl Benzoate ☐
   C. 4 application of Benzyl Benzoate ☐
   D. Disinfection of Clothes only ☐
4. **Drug used for pediculosis is/are:** *(PGI May 13)*
   A. Malathion ☐
   B. Permethrin ☐
   C. Ivermectin ☐
   D. Diethylcarbazine ☐
   E. Nitrate ☐

Answers and Explanations:

1. **A. i.e. Pediculosis corporis**
2. **C i.e. Disinfection of all clothes & beddings**
3. **A i.e. 3 applications of Gama Benzene Hexa Chloride**
4. **A, B, C i.e. Malathion, Permethrin, Ivermectin**

[Ref: Harrison 18th/3578; Rook's 8/p. 38.15/20; Fitzpatrick's 8/e p. 2573-78; Pasricha 4/e p. 140; Roxburgh's 17/e p. 63; Neena 4/e p. 339]

- In P. corporis, louse usually resides in clothes so for diagnosis lice should be sought in the clothes especially under the seams of under clothes. ***Treatment is directed mainly towards disinfection of all clothes and bedding.***Q *Local calamine or corticosteroid application with oral antihistaminic gives symptomatic relief.*
- ***Treatment of T carporis is disinfection of all clothes + local application of pediculocide drug (not only disinfection of clothes).*** Q
- **Drugs used for pediculosis** are pyrethrins, synthetic pyrethroids (**permethrin** & phenothrin); **malathion,** carbaryl, lindane, DDT, BHC, Benzyl benzoate and **ivermectin** (all topical except ivermectin which is both topical and oral).

12 VENEREAL (SEXUALLY TRANSMITTED) DISEASE

Warts

Clinical lesion	Human Papilloma Virus (HPV) type
Deep plantar/palmar (myrmecia) wart/V. plantaris	**1** (m.c), 2, 4, 60 (l/t plantar epidermoid cyst)
Mosaic wart	2
Common wart (of hands & fingers) / **Verruca vulgaris** (most common type)	**2** (m.c), 4 > 27, 29
Plane wart (Verruca plana)	3, 10 > 28, , 41*, 49 (flat wart in EV)
Epidermodysplasia verruciformis (EV)	5*, 8*, > 9, 12, 14*, 15, 17, 19, 20*-25, 36-38, 47, 50, 51
Laryngeal papilloma	***6, 11***Q, 30 (Laryngeal carcinoma)
Ano-genital wart (condyloma accuminata)/ Veneral wart	- ***6, 11***Q (low onchogenic), 30, 42, 43 - 16, 18, 31, 33, 35, 39, 40, 45, 51-60 are high onchogenic potential & may l/t cervical / penile / vulval - intraepithelial neoplasia (CIN, PIN, VIN)
Butcher's wart	7Q

*Risk of squamous cell carcinoma

***Buschke – Lowenstein tumor** in HPV 54 l/t massive warts

Histopathology

- ***Acanthotic & hyperkeratotic epidermis*** *with papillomatosis and parakeratosis.* In flat warts acanthosis & hyperkeratosis is less and papillomatosis & parakeratosis is absent
- **Koilocytotic cells or Koilocytes** are large keratinocytes with an eccentric, pyknotic nucleus surrounded by ***a perinuclear halo.*** *Koilocytes are characteristic of HPV papillomas & there presence in papanicolau (Pap) smear represent hallmark of HPV infection*Q.
- Epidermal thickening with particular increase in granular cell layer, which shows a characteristic ***basophilic stippled appearance***Q. Anogenital warts may lack granular layer.
- The granular & upper spinous cell layers contain cells with **perinuclear**

Treatment

Topical agents for chemical cautery

- ***Salicytic acid*** **(12- 26%) &** ***lactic acid*** **(4-20%): t/t of 1st choice for common & plantar warts but not suitable for anogenital & facial skin.** Efficacious in *young children* who do not tolerate other modalities.
- *Caustics trichloracetic acid , mono chloracetic acid, $AgNO_3$*
- *Glutaraldehyde* (10%): brown discoloura-tion & skin hardening limits acceptability on hands, but is useful on feet
- *Retinoic acid*: to treat plane warts in children
- *Formalin* : for plantar warts
- *Cantharidin* : extract from green blister beetle
- ***Podophyllin (15%), podophyllotoxin (0.5%) are used in t/t of anogenital warts***Q, as they are more effective on mucosal than keratinized surfaces. It is anti mitotic, disrupting the formation of spindle on which chromosomes align at mitosis. It should *not be used on exceptionally large or bleeding area,* where it can l/t intrauterine death, vomitting, diarrhoea, liver / renal damage, peripheral neuropathy, bone marrow suppression, coma, death d/t systemic absorption. *Oral ingestion* has similar effects. It is ***contraindicated in pregnancy***Q
- **5-flurouracil (5-FU) :** to treat *genitals & cutaneous* warts with occlusion in t/t of plantar wants. S/ ε are onycholysis, hyperpigmentation, erythema & erosion.
- *Cidofovir* (*S* / ε pain & ulceration)

Oral Retinoids

Etretinate is useful in extensive & hyperkeratotic warts in immuno compromised patients eg sarcoidosis & CLL.

Intralesional injection

- *Bleomycin* (*S* / ε is extensive tissue necrosis, C/I in pregnancy)
- 5-FU (new)
- Candidal extracts, cidofovir
- Recombinant human interferon (*IFN*) in refractory genital warts

Photodynamic therapy

- Systemic / topical *aminolaevulinic acid* to treat common wart & laryngeal papillomatosis.

Immunotherapy

- **Contact sensitization:** *Induction of allergic contact dermatitis with* dinitrochloro benzene (mutagenic) ropenone (DPC) & squaric acid dibutylester *against wart*
- **Cimetidine** causes resolution of cutneous (plane & common) warts, particularly in *children following failed contact sensitization.*
- **Interferon** may reduce warts in laryngeal papillomatosis & EV, which recur when therapy is stopped.
- **Topical immunomodulation:** *Imiquimod (5%)*Q is used for *resistant cases* or **patients with extensive lesions**. This has to be used with care as it also induces an inflammatory response in patients who have back ground dermatitis. It should not be used in patients who have benign **vulval, aphthous ulcer**.

  *Imiquiod & low dose retinoids may reduce development of cutaneous malignancies in renal transplant recipients.

  ***Topical immunomodulation by imiquimod* (5%), *a potent stimulator of proinflammatory cytokines release* which acts by activation of Toll like receptors 7 & 8, is *approved for treatment of genital warts*Q.**

Antiviral therapy

- Cidofovir: topical & intralesional injection is extremely effective in plantar, anogenital & laryngeal warts. Grade III CIN / VIN/PIN also respond.

Surgical method (successful where lesions are few or filliform)

- Curettage & cautery / electrocoagulation / diathermy
- **Cryotherapy with liquid nitrogen** (or carbon dioxide snow): In **pregnancy,** ***only cryotherapy or destructive techniques with cautery or hyfrecation can be used safely***Q
- Laser (CO_2) / hyfrecation/ topical trichloro acetic
- Infrared coagulatory
- Local head by Nd: VAG laser
- Radiotherapy

Psychological methods

- Hypnosis

vacuolization in plane warts and show a characteristic *basket weake like hyper keratosis with many large clear cells in EV.*
- Thick bands of elongated *rette ridges extend extensively into the highly vascular dermis.*

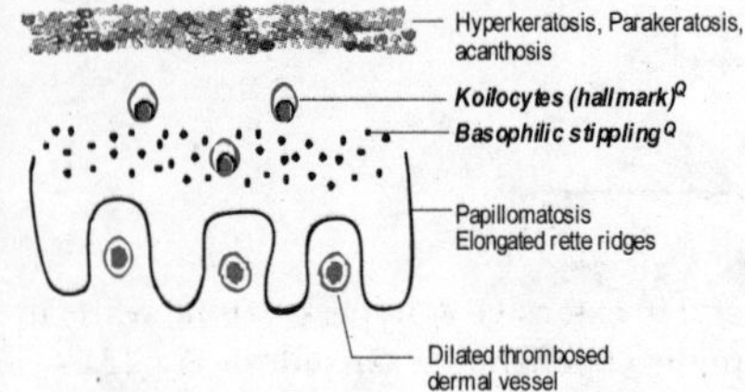

Prevention of HPV

- No approach prevents transmission of nongenital warts. However a prophylactic HPV vaccine *prevents genital HPV infection.* The non infectious vaccine is based on observation that L_1 protein when expressed in cells, self assemble to form *virus like particles (VLPs)* that morphologically resemble capsids.
- *Intramuscular* L_1 VLP vaccine induces > *99% seroconversion*, confer close to 100% protection in women against the development of lesions attributable to genital HPV types in vaccine, and induces serum neutralization antibody titers that are ≥40 times than those that develop after natural infection.
- Despite its high level of efficacy in preventing HPV infection its has no therapeutic activity. Its protection is largely type specific which means that most infections caused by HPV types other than those in HPV vaccine will not be prevented.
- However, HPV-6 and – 11 cause ~ 90% of genital warts, whereas HPV-16 and – 18 cause about 70% of cervical cancer. Thus the
  - **Quadrivalent vaccine** (for **HPV-6,-11, 16, and 18**) approved by USFDA in 2006 for girls & women ages 9 to 26 years, has the potential to drastically reduce the incidence of genital warts & to protect against majority of HPV infections that l/t cervical cancer.
  - **Bivalent vaccine** (against **HPV-16 and 18**) is also being developed commercially, primarily as a *vaccine to prevent cervical cancer.*

Podophyllin resin & Podophyllotoxin

- **Podophyllin** is a crude resin ***derived from either American mandrake (may apple), Pedophyllum peltatum or Indian podophyllum, P. emodi plants***Q. Podophyllin is produced as *10-40% ethanolic or benzoin* crude extract. *Composition is not standardized* and contain a mixture of *podophyllotoxin, α & β peltatin*, des oxypodophyllotoxin, dehydropodophyllotoxin etc. Its *most potent active ingredient- podophyllotoxin*, rapidly crystallizes out, l/t a short shelf life.
- **Podophyllotoxin (podofilox)** is *purified active extract of podophyllum* resin with *antineoplastic & antiviral activity.* Both podophyllin & podophyllotoxin bind *tubulin* (a microtubule protein of mitotic spindle) & epidermal *mitosis is inhbited in metaphase.* Both are used in treatment of ***ano-genital warts***Q, but are ineffective for common warts & plantar warts.
- *Patient administered podophyllotoxin* is more effective, less toxic, require less dose & is less costly as compared to *physician applied podophyllum*, although ***relapse rates are high with both treatments***Q. Thus multiple cycles of treatment are often necessary.
- After excessive podophyllin t/t of large anogenital wart, subdermal injection or accidental ingestion, systemic toxicities including *CNS & respiratory depression* develop. *Local side effects* such as erythema, erosions, tenderness & rarely scarring and depigmentation develop with both. Depending on ***individual variations***Q of local response, podophyllin may remain on wart for 8- 12 hours on subraquent applications, if there was no or little inflammation after 1st treatment.
- ***Because of teratogenic (mutagenic) potential, both podophyllin & podophyllotoxin are contraindicated in pregnancy***Q.

Lymphogranuloma Venereum / LGV

Etiology

- **Lymphogranuloma venerum (LGV)** is an invasive systemic STD that is caused by ***Chlamydia trachomatis serovars*** L_1, L_2 ***and*** L_3Q, which, unlike the oculogenital D-K strains that cause mucosal disease, invade and damage lymphatics.

Clinical Presentation

- LGV occurs in 3 stages. LGV begins (primary stage) as a **small painless papule** that tends to form **transient herpetiform ulcer** at the site of inoculation, often escaping attention. ***This asymptomatic ulcer is most often unnoticed, heals rapidly and usually leaves no scar***Q.
- The **secondary stage** that occurs 2-6 weeks after exposure and classically described as **inguinal syndrome** is the most common

Investigation & Diagnosis

- **Diagnostic method of choice** is **nucleic acid amplification test (NAATs)**. Sample of choice is *cervical swab* (in symptomatic women undergoing pelvic examination), *self collected vaginal swab* (in screening of asymptomatic women), and *urine* (in out reach screening and in males). Because NAATs measures nucleic acids instead of live organisms, it may continue to yield a positive result until as long as 3 weeks after therapy, when viable organism have actually been eradicated. So it should not be used as test of cure until after 3 weeks. Diagnosis can be confirmed by *real time PCR assays for LGV specific DNA.*
- Serological test of choice is microimmunofluorescence (MIF) antibody testing to L-serovar. MIF titre > 1: 128 is strongly

presenting picture in heterosexuals. It is characterized by painful inguinal lymphadenitis and associated constitutional symptoms.

- The lymphadenopathy is **tender, initially unilateral & discrete** but progressive periadenitis results in ***a matted mass of fluctuant & suppurative nodes (bubos) with fistulae formation***Q. The overlying skin becomes fixed, inflamed, & thin with multiple draining fistulas. Palpable enlargement of ipsilateral femoral (iliac) and inguinal lymph nodes separated by inguinal ligament produces ***sign of the groove***Q – although it is not specific. In homosexual men the secondary stage presents as **anorectal syndrome**.
- **Tertiary stage** occurs many years after initial stage and manifestations result from *fibrosis and lymphatic obstruction* and include ***elephantiasis of external genitalia***Q, ***esthiomine***Q (rectal & vaginal strictures), rectovaginal & urethral fistulae scarring etc.

suggestive of LGV but serological testing lack sensitivity in early infections. Complement fixation (CF) tests (> 1: 64) support diagnosis but lack sensitivity & specificity and now are rarely employed. **Frei-intradermal hypersensitivity test** is now only of historical interest.

Treatment

- A course of **tetracycline / doxycycline**Q **/ minocycline / erythromycin / fluoroquinolone** (for 7 days – Harrison / 21 days - Rooks) or single dose of ***azithromycin***Q can be used for uncomplicated chlamydial infections. Although not approved by FDA, all except fluoroquinolone appear to be safe in pregnancy. However, **amoxicillin** can also be given to pregnant women. Treatment of sex partner is recommended.

Donovanosis (Granuloma Venereum/ Ingunale)

Etiology

- **Donovanosis** is a chronic, progressive, STD of low infectivity, caused by gram negative ***Klebsiella granulomatis comb nov (calymmatobacterium or donovania granulomatis)***Q.

Clinical Picture

- Initial lesion is a papule or subcutaneous nodule that ulcerates. The typical lesions which may be multiple are ***large beefy red, nontender granulomatous ulcer that bleeds readily when touched***Q and gradually extend. However 1) hypertrophic (verrucous) ulcer with a raised irregular edge; 2) a necrotic, offensive smelling ulcer causing tissue destruction, and 3) sclerotic or cicatrical lesion with fibrous & scar tissue also occur. *Genitals* are most commonly (90%) affected; the most common sites are *coronal sulcus or inner penile prepuce, frenum & glans* in men and *labia minora & fourchette in women.*
- ***Lymphadenopathy is unusual but subcutaneous extension of granulomas may mimic enlarged inguinal lymphnodes (pseudo bubos)***Q. Complications include **pseudo-elephantiasis** (resulting from persistent granulomas, which may constrict lymphatics by genital scarring), *neoplastic changes* and stenosis of urethra, vagina and anus.

Investigation & Diagnosis

- Diagnosis is made by **microscopic identification of Donovan bodies** in smear, which can be seen in large, mononuclear (Pund) cells as gram negative intracytoplasmic cysts filled with deeply stained bodies showing **bipolar staining (safety pin appearance).** These cysts rupture & release infective organism.
- A **PCR analysis with a calorimetric detection** system can now be used in routine diagnosis.

Treatment

- **Azithromycin** is ***drug of choice***Q. Erythromycin, ***doxy/tetracycline***Q, cotrimoxazole, ciprofloxacin/norfloxacin, ceftriaxone and ***aminoglycosides (eg gentamycin)***Q are also effective.

Differences

LGV	Donovanosis
Matted, fluctuant, suppurative **lymphnodes** with fistula (discharging sinus), **Bubos, Elephantiasis** of genitalia, **Esthiomine** (rectal & vaginal strictures) and **Groove sign**	No lymphnadenopathy, **pseudo-bubo; pseudo-elephantiasis** of genitalia

Chancroid (Soft chancre, Ulcus molle, Ducrey's Disease)

Etiology

- Soft chancre is caused by ***Haemophilus ducreyi***Q, a gram negative, facultative anaerobic coccobacillus that require hemin (X) factor for growth. However, r – RNA analysis suggest that it is more closely linked to the *Actinobacillus cluster of Pasteurellaceae.*

Clinical Presentation

- Initial lesion – a ***soft papule with surrounding erythema (& without prodromal symptoms) appears after a short incubation period of 3 to 7 days, rarely more than 10 days***Q. In 2-3 days the papule evolve into **micropustules (but not vesicles)** resembling folliculitis, which spontaneously ruptures and forms a **sharply circumscribed, generally non-indurated ulcer**. The lesions are **usually multiple**, upto 1 cm in diameter, have ***ragged & undermined edges***Q, and have a purulent base

Investigation & Diagnosis

- Diagnosis: **Direct examination of clinical material by Gram or Giemsa stain** shows characteristic (but not pathognomic) ***shoal/school of fish or rail road track appearance***Q. But this has low sensitivity & specificity.
- Primary tool for accurate diagnosis of chancroid currently relies on **culture of H.ducreyi from** the lesion.
- However recently developed **multiplex PCR assay for simultaneous amplification of DNA**

1

DERMATOLOGY

covered by necrotic yellow-gray exudates and granulation tissue that *bleeds easily on manipulation*Q. In contrast to those of syphilis, chancroid ulcers are ***usually painful, tender and not indurated (i.e. soft)***Q. Little or no inflammation of surrounding skin is evident. Most lesions are found on prepuce, frenulum or glans (in males) and vulva esp on fourchette, labia minora & vestibule (in females).

- **Painful, tender, enlarged inguinal lymphadenitis (bubo)** occurs in half of patients within 2 weks of primary lesion. Mostly it is *unilateral, with typical erythema of overlying skin,* and may frequently become **suppurating bubo or fluctuant inguinal abscess** which may rupture spontaneously.

targets from H.ducreyi, Treponema pallidum & herpes simplex type 1 and 2 has a resolved sensitivity & specificity for H. ducreyi of 98.4% and 99.6%. When commercially available, it will be a useful diagnostic tool to identify the etiology of genital ulcers.

Treatment

- **Azithromycin** (single oral dose) or **ciftriaxone** (single IM dose) or **ciprofloxacin** (oral 3 days) or **erythromycin** (oral 7 days).

Diseases, Causative Organism and Treatment

Disease	Causative Organism
Donovanosis / Granuloma inguinale (venerum)	*Calymmatobacter (donovanian) granulomatis*Q
L.G.V. / L.G.I.	*Chlamydia trachomatis*Q-L_1, L_2 **(m.c.)**, L_3
Chancroid	**Haemophyllus ducrey**Q (m.c.) **Herpes hominis virus**Q B. melangiogenicus, Staph., Strepto corynebacterium & N. gonorrhea
Condylomata acuminate (Genital warts)	*Human papilloma virus*Q (HPV) type 6, 11, 16, 18
Chancre (Syphilis)	*Treponema pallidium*Q
Endemic (Non veneral) Syphilis	
Yaws	**T. pertenue**Q
Pinta	**T. caratenum**Q
Gonorrhea	*Nisseria gonorrhea*Q
Erysipelas	*β Hemolytic streptococcus*Q
Impetigo Contagiosa	*Staphylococcus aureus*Q f/b *β Hemolytic Group-A-Streptococcus*Q
Scarlet fever	*Group A – streptococci*Q

STD	Drug of Ist choice
Gonorrhoea - *Non penicillinase producing* - *Penicillinase producing*	- Amoxy/Ampicillin, *Procaine penicillin G*Q. (old) - *Ceftriaxone*Q, *cefixime* (new)
Syphilis - Early (Primary, Secondary & latent) & Late - Neurosyphilis	- *Benzathine Penicillin G*Q / Procaine Pen. G - Aqueous Pen. G / Aqueous Pen. G procaine
LGV (Chlamydia trachomatis)	- *Doxycycline*Q - *Azithromycin*Q
Donovanosis / Granuloma inguinale (Calymm. granulomatis)	- *Azithromycin*Q *(1st)* - *Doxy / Tetra-cycline*Q
Chancroid (H. ducreyi)	- *Ceftriaxone*Q - *Azithro / Erythromycin*Q - *Cotrimoxazole*Q
Herpes	- *Acyclovir*Q
Trichomonas vaginalis	- *Metronidazole*Q */ Tinidazole* - Treat male partner also if recurrent

Syphilis

Natural Course of syphilis

Early Syphilis

- Infection is less than *2 years* (24 months) old
- Lesions are *teeming with T. pallidium*
- Patient remains *highly infectious*.
- ***Relapse usually occurs in early syphilis***Q, particularly in irregulary or inadequately treated case. The relapse may take any of the following form.

1. Serological relapse : VDRL test becomes positive in higher titers than before.
2. Mucocutaneous relapse: ***Reccurence of the chancre in its original place (chancre redux)***Q, or recurrence of mucocutaneous lesion, both showing treponema pallidium in the serum.
3. Osseous – relapse : occurence of osteitis & periosteitis.
4. Neuro – relapse : in form of asymptomatic neuro – syphilis.

Clinical presentation

Congenital Syphilis

- **Early Congenital Syphilis**
  - *Snuffles (Rhinitis)*Q is earliest feature
  - ***Lesions are vesico-bullous***Q
  - On mucosa, *snail track ulcers*
- **Late Congenital Syphilis**
  - ***Hutchinson triad***Q ***i.e. interstial keratitis (IK) + 8th nerve deafness + Hutchinson's teeth***Q

Acquired Syphilis

- **Primary Syphilis**
  - ***Painless, Indurated, nonbleeding, usually* single punched out ulcer (hard chancre)**Q
  - Painless, rubbery shotty lymphadenopathy
- **Secondary Syphilis**
  - Protean manifestation include **mucocutaneous lesions and generalized nontender**, painless, discrete, mobile, rubbery **lymphadenopathy.**
  - Skin rash is the commonest feature and consists of *macular (roseolar) syphilide, papular* (basic lesion of 2° syphilis), *papulosquamous* and occasionally *pustular syphilides;* and often ≥1 form is present simultaneously. Initial lesions are

5. Ocular – relapse : occuring as iritis, iridocyclitis or neuro – retinitis
6. Visceral relapse as hepatitis.
7. An apparently healthy mother with negative serology giving birth to a syphilitic chid; or infection in the sex parther, without any clinical or serological relapse in the patient.

Late Syphilis

- Infection is more than 24 months old
- T. pallidium are sparse
- Lesions are not infectious.

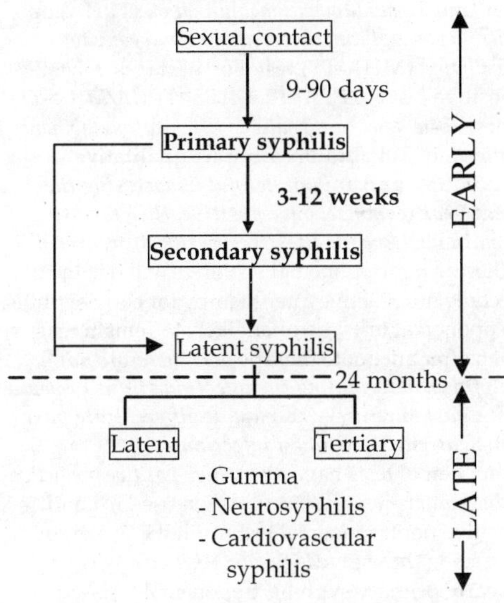

Latent Syphilis

- It is described as the ***asymptomatic stage***Q of syphilis in a patient with a definite history, revealing the contraction of the disease, but exhibiting only a ***reactive serology. (serologically positive)***Q.
- It occurs between secondary & tertiary stage of syphilis.
- It can be subdivided in to 2 stages:

1. **Early latent (relapsing) syphilis**: Occuring during first 2 years & 25% of patients developing *chancre redux*.
2. **Late latent (non relapsing) syphilis**: Occuring after 2 years & showing no relapse.

- It may either progress and develop signs & symptoms of late tertiary syphilis (in 1/3rd cases), or persist as latent syphilis or have a spontaneous cure.

Treatment

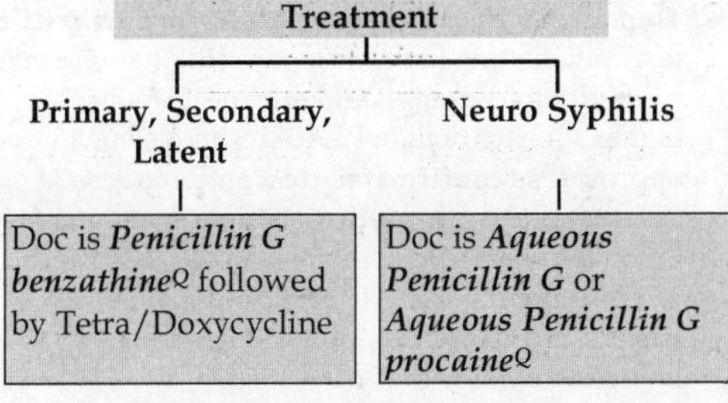

(pegged central upper incisors)

- **Hutchinson's teeth** (i.e. **upper central incisor** are **conical, peg or barrel shaped**, with a degree of **notching at the free margin**; they may be well *separated* and *coverage or diverge* described as **screwdriver teeth**) are d/t defective development of permanent teeth buds and often a/w abnormalities of upper jaw.
- **Mulberry (usually first) molar** has a flat occlusive surface with only poorly enameled rudiments of usual caps.
- Borad based, **saddle backed nose, dish face.**
- ***Sabre tibia***Q
- Bull dog's jaw (protusion of jaw)
- ***Rhagades***Q (linear fissure at corner of mouth, nares, perianal ores)
- ***Frontal bossing of parrot***Q (parrot's node on skull), **pepper & salt fundus** d/t scarred choroiditis & optic atrophy.
- **Higaumenakis sign** (periostitis l/t U/L enlargement of sternal end of clavicle)

asymptomatic, nonitchy, subtle (i.e. patient unaware of it), **symmetrical, pale coppery red or pink, discrete macules** distributed on trunk and proximal extremities; these macules progress to firm, round/oval, **shiny papules** that are ***distributed widely and that frequently involves the palm and soles***Q. It progresses to papuloquamous syphilide that quickly ***(easily) shed thin layer of scale***Q. Rarely depigmented spots on hyperpigmented background on back or sides of neck (i.e. **leukoderma syphiliticum** or **necklace of Venus**) or severe necrotic lesions (**lues maligna**, mostly in HIV), or papules forming a line along the hair margin (**corona veneris**), or a large central papule surrounded by small satellite pupules (**corymbose syphilides**) or tender **fissured-split papules** on angle of mouth and free margin of prepace may be seen.

- **Papules** enlarge to produce **broad, moist, gray-white** or pink, **hypertrophied** coalesced, higly infectious lesions k/a ***condylomata lata in warm moist, intertriginous areas (commonly perianal area, vulva and scrotum)***Q.
- Painless, superficial, **sivery-gray mucosal erosions (mucosal patches)** surrounded by a red periphery and involving ***oral and genital mucosa*** may occur. ***Moth eaten alopecia***Q may occur.
- Constitutional symptoms accompanying or preceding include sore throat, fever, weight loss, malaise, anorexia, headache, meningismus. Less common complications include hepatitis, nephropathy, gastrointestinal involvement (hypertrophic gastritis, patchy proctitis or rectosigmoid mass), arthritis, periostitis, optic neuritis; irits/uveitis, nephrotic syndrome and proteinuria.

- ***B/L symmetrical asymptomatic***Q localized or diffuse ***mucocutaneous lesion***Q *(macule,* papule, papulosquamous & rarely pustule)
- ***Rashes are coppery red, symmetrically distributed and do not itch***Q.
- Non tender generalized lymphadenopathy
- Highly infectious ***condylomata lata***Q, in warm moist interiginous body areas.
- *Moth eaten alopecia*
- Arthritis, Proteinuria

- **Tertiary Syphilis**

- ***Gumma***Q
- Neurosyphilis/Tabes dorsalis
- Ostitis, periostitis
- Aortitis, aortic insufficiency, coronary stenosis.

★ Gumma is a well defined, punched out ulcer with wash leather slough.

DERMATOLOGY

1

Laboratory Diagnosis and Evaluation

Demonstraton of organism (for research purpose mostly)

- T. pallidum spirochete cannot be cultured and **dark field microscopy** (silver stains such as warthin-starry), **direct immuno fluorescence antibody staining of T. pallidium (DFA-TP test)** and treponemal immobilization test **(TPI)** have been used to identify spirochete in sample.
- More sensitive new tests are **PCR** and **RNA amplification** (more sensitive than PCR) and positive results are indicative of living organism.

Serological Tests

Are of 2 types; both types reactive in persons with *any treponemal infection, including yaws, pinta and endemic syphilis.* No test can differentiate one treponematosis from another.

Non-treponemal (reaginic) tests

- 4 tests are available that use venereal disease research laboratory (**VDRL**) **antigen (a cardiolipin-lacithin-cholesterole antigen complex)** and include **VDRL test**, unheated serum regain **(USR) test**, rapid plasma reagin **(RPR) test** and toluidine red unheated serum test **(TRUST)**. Out of these VDRL and RPR tests are most widely used.
- These **quantitative** non-treponemal **antibody tests measure IgG and IgM** directed against VDRL antigen complex and are ***useful in assessing response to treatment***Q.
- RPR and VDRL are ***recommended for screening***Q *or for quantitation of serum antibody*. The ***titer reflects disease activity***Q, being nonreactive initially (1-4 weeks), rising during the evolution of early syphilis and after exceeding 1:32 in secondary syphilis (highest titers). After therapy for early syphilis, a **persistent fall by 4 folds** or 2 dilutions or more (e.g: a decline from 1:32 to 1:8) is considered an **adequate response** to treatment. Patients with HIV or **h/o prior syphilis** are less likely to become nonreactive to VDRL/RPR test.
- VDRL titers do not correspond directly to RPR titres; so sequential quantative testing (as for response to treatment) must always use a single test.
- Few (1%) patients with high titers show **prozone phenomenon** – i.e. undiluted serum gives nonreactive (negative) or weakly reactive results (b/o antibody exess and/or blockinig antibodies), whereas test is reactive with diluted serum.

RPR test

*Test of choice for rapid serological diagnosis in a clinical setting*Q (easy, automated and uses unheated serum). Also useful in *determining which patient will benefit from CSF examination.*

VDRL test

Standard test for examining CSF; CSF-VDRL test is *highly specific* and when reactive is considered **diagnostic of neurosyphilis**; however, it is *insensitive* and may be nonreactive even in cases of symptomatic neurosyphilis. It's sensitivity is highest in meningovascular syphilis and paresis. A *non reactive FTA-ABS test on CSF is used to rule out asymptomatic neurosyphilis* and *measuring CXCL-13* in CSF distinguish between nerurosyphilis and HIV related CSF abnormalities.

3 Must remember Clinical uses of Serological test

- Screeing or diagnosis = **RPR or VDRL**
- Quantitative measurement of antibody to assess clinical syphilis activity or to monitor response to therapy = **RPR or VDRL**
- Confirmation of syphilis in a patient with a reactive RPR or VDRL test = **FTA - ABS, TPPA, EIA**

Evaluation for Neurosyphilis

- CNS involvement is detected by *CSF pleocytosis* (>5WBC/μL in non HIV and >20 WBC/μL in HIV patients), *increased CSF protein concentration* (>45 mg/dl)- both nonspecific, and highly specific *CSF VDRL test.*
- **Reactive CSF VDRL is diagnostic of neurosyphilis**; however, it is insensitive and may be nonreactive even in symptomatic neurosyphilis CSF-FTA-ABS is more often reactive in all sage but reactivity may be d/t passive transfer of serum antibody into CSF. However, a **non reactive CSF-FTA-ABS test is used to rule out neurosyphilis**; and measuring CXCL-13 in CSF can distinguish b/w neurosyphilis and HIV related CSF abnormality.

Treponemal (Specific) tests

- It *include the T.pallidum particle agglutination* **(TPPA)**, *fluorescent treponemal antibody absorption* **(FTA-ABS) test** and *T.pallidum haemagglutination* **(TPHA)** or *micro-haemagglutination assay for atnitbodies to T.pallidum* **(MHA-TP) test.** For all stages, most sensitive test is ***TPPA>FTA-ABS>TPHA/MHA-TP***Q.
- These tests *detect antibodies to native or recombinant antigens* of T. Pallidum. They are **qualitative** procedures and are ***not helpful in assessing the treatment response; once positive, they tend to remain positive for life, irrespective of treatment***Q.
- Whereas nontreponemal test titers will decline or become nonreactive after therapy for early syphilis, treaponemal tests are often likely to remain reactive even after adequate therapy and ***therefore not helpful in determining the infection status of person with past syphilis***Q ***(i.e. cannot differentiate past from current T.pallidum infection)***Q.
- Treponemal tests have a *very high positive predictive value for diagnosis of syphilis,* when used to confirm positive nontreponemal test result. However, in screening these give *high false positive results.*
- In early primary syphilis, treponemal tests are slightly more sensitive (85-90%) then non-treponemal tests (80%); however, both may be non reactive. So in primary syphilis *sensitivity is increased either by FTA-ABS or simply repetition of VDRL test* after 1-2 weeeks if initial VDRL is negative.
- VDRL & RPR titers and sensitivity may decline in untreated persons with *late latent or late syphilis,* but treponemal test remain sensitive in these stages. ***So negative TPPA or FTA ABS excludes diagnosis of present and past syphilis***Q except in very early stage (or ? neurosyphilis).
- **Sensitivity** of serological test in untreated syphilis

Test	Primary	Secondary	Latent	Tertiary
VDRL	74 (74-87)	100	95 (88-100)	71 (37-94)
FTA-ABS	84 (70-100)	100	100	96
MHA-TP	76 (69-90)	100	100	94

- Treponemal **immuno chromatographic strip (ICS)** test and enzyme immune assays **(EIA)** are based on reactivity to recombinant antigens. EIAs has a higher specificity than FTA-ABS and is now approved as **confirmatory test** and b/o ease of automation is now used as a **single screening test** (as an alternative to combined VDRL/RPR and TPHA screen). However to differentiate b/w current and treated syphilis or false reactivity following algorithm is used.

- Indication of **CSF examination** in adults is indicated.

All patients	Additional indication in HIV
Signs and symptoms of **CNS involvement** (e.g: meningitis, cranial nerve dysfunction, altered mental status, hearing loss, ataxia, loss of vibration sense), **ophthalmic** disease (e.g. uveitis, iritis, pupillary abnormalities) or **suspected treatment failure** or **RPR or VDRL titer ≥ 1:32** (11 and 6 folds higher in HIV and non HIV persons respectively).	**CD 4+** T cell count **<350/μL** or all HIV cases (some experts).

- ***Activity of (asymptomatic or symptomatic) neurosyphilis correlates best***[Q] with CSF pleocytosis, which provides the ***most sensitive index of response to treatment***[Q].

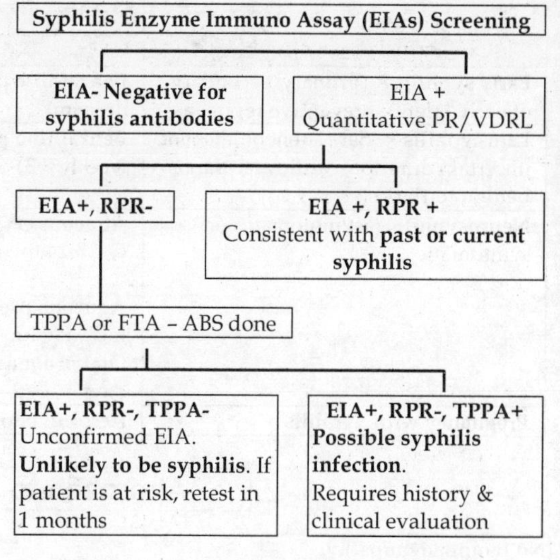
Syphilis Enzyme Immuno Assay (EIAs) Screening
EIA- Negative for syphilis antibodies
EIA + Quantitative PR/VDRL
EIA+, RPR-
EIA +, RPR + Consistent with past or current syphilis
TPPA or FTA – ABS done
EIA+, RPR-, TPPA- Unconfirmed EIA. Unlikely to be syphilis. If patient is at risk, retest in 1 months
EIA+, RPR-, TPPA+ Possible syphilis infection. Requires history & clinical evaluation

Evaluation of Congenital Syphilis

Both infected and non-infected newborns of mothers with *reactive serological tests* may themselves have reactive tests b/o transplacental transfer of IgG antibody. *Neonatal IgM antibody detection* is useful (but not available) test. So if

Asymptomatic infants born to women treated adequately with **pencillin during 1st or 2nd trimester.**

Monthly quantitative non treponemal tests to monitor for adequate reduction in antibody titers. **Rising or persistent** titers indicate infection and require treatment.

- Treatment status of seropositive mother is unkown;
- Mother has received inadequate or nonpenicillin therapy or has **received penicillin in 3rd** trimester or
- Infant may be difficult to follow

Infant should be treated at birth

★ In **secondary syphilis,** all tests are ***100% sensitive***[Q] but most commonly used test is VDRL. **Earliest** test to become positive is ***FTA-ABS***[Q]. Most **specific** test is **TPI > FTA-ABS.**

Test	Type
VDRL	***Slide flocculation Test***[Q]
Khan Test	***Tube Flocculation Test***[Q]
Waserman Reaction	***Complement fixation Test***[Q]

Treatment of Syphilis

- **Parenteral Penicillin G** is the ***drug of choice for all stages of syphilis***[Q]; however, the preparation, dosage and duration of treatment depends on stage and manifestation of disease. *Penicillin is the most effective treponemicide,* inexpensive, easy to administer and has few side effects. T. pallidum is killed by *very low concentration of penicillin G (> 0.03 U/mL for at least 10 days),* although a *long period of exposure* is required b/o the unusually slow rate of multiplication of organism. There is ***no evidence of penicillin resistance in T.pallidum***[Q]. Parenteral (injectable) penicillin is preferred to oral preparations b/o patient compliance and gi absorption uncertainty.
- A single intramuscular **(im) dose 24 lacks U (2.4MU) of benzathine penicillin G** (BPG) maintains effective serum levels for about 2 weeks and is *recommended 1st line therapy for most cases.* In comparision a single im dose of **6 lack U – aqueous procaine penicillin G** (APPG) maintains an effective serum concentrations for at least 24 hours.
- **Preventive regimen and early syphilis (primary, secondary or early latent)** require BPG single dose (Harrison)/ BPG on day 1 and 8 or APPG daily ×10. Whereas, **late syphilis (late latent** or latent of uncertaion duration, **cardiovascular syphilis** or **benign tertiary)** require BPG weekly for 3 weeks (on day 1, 8 and 15) i.e total dose of 7.2 million units (Harrison) or APPG daily × 17 *(Rooks).*
- The penetration of APPG **into CSF- (and aqueous humor)** is poor, that of erythromycin is poorer and that of BPG is poorest. So **benzathine penicillin G** (even in doses of upto 7.2 million units), does not produce detectable concentrations in CSF and ***should not be used for treatment of neurosyphilis***[Q], as asymptomatic cases may relapse into symptomatic neurosyphillis following treatment. For **neurosyphilis**, administration of **intravenous (IV) aqueous crystalline penicillin G (aqueous crystalline benzyl penicillin G) or im aqueous procaine penicillin G plus oral probenecid** for 10-14 days is recommended
- ***Penicillin is the only recommended agent for treatment of syphilis in pregnancy***[Q]. If the patient has a documented penicillin allergy, ***desensitization and penicillin therapy should be given***[Q].
- **For congenital syphilis,** iv aqueous crystalline penicillin G (ACBPG or benzyl penicillin sodium) or im aqueous procaine penicillin G are recommended.
- **Other effective antibiotics in syphilis are tetracyclines and cephalosporin; septinomycin and aminoglycosides (only in very large doses).**But the **sulfonamides and quinolones are inactive.**

Syphilis stage (CSF normal or not examined)★	Treatment of choice	
	No penicillin allergy	Confirmed penicillin allergy
Early syphilis★ (primary, secondary of early latent); preventive regimens	**Benzathine penicillin G** (2.4 mU single dose im)	Tetracycline (500mg PO quid) or doxycyline (100 mg PO bid) for 2 weeks.
Late syphilis★ (late latent or latent of uncertain duration, **cardiovascular** or **benign tertiary**)	**Benzathine penicillin G** (2.4mU im weekly × 3)	**Non HIV** patient: Above regimen for 4 weeks **HIV** patient: **Desensitization** and treatment with penicillin
Neurosyphilis (asymptomatic or symtomatic)	**Aqueous crystalline (benzyl)penicillin** G (18-24 mU/day IV for 10-14 days) Or **Aqueous procaine penicillin G** (2.4 mU/day im) plus **Oral probenecid** (500mg qid) for 10-14 days	Dsensitization and treatment with penicillin
Pregnancy with Syphilis	According to stage	Desensitization and treatment with penicillin.

Approach to a case of STD (Genital Ulcer)

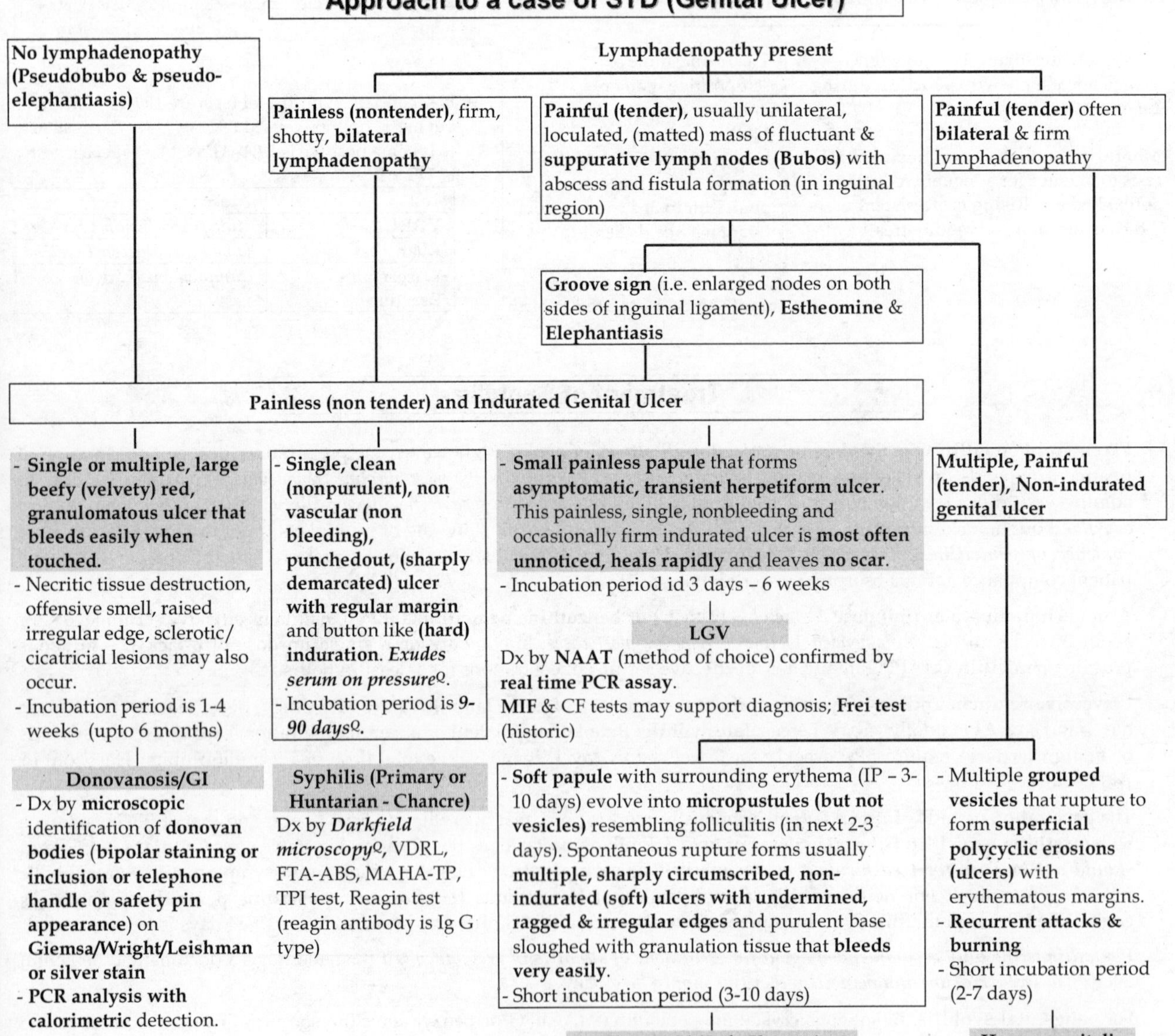

No lymphadenopathy (Pseudobubo & pseudo-elephantiasis)
Lymphadenopathy present
Painless (nontender), firm, shotty, **bilateral lymphadenopathy**
Painful (tender), usually unilateral, loculated, (matted) mass of fluctuant & **suppurative lymph nodes (Bubos)** with abscess and fistula formation (in inguinal region)
Painful (tender) often **bilateral** & firm lymphadenopathy
Groove sign (i.e. enlarged nodes on both sides of inguinal ligament), **Estheomine** & **Elephantiasis**
Painless (non tender) and Indurated Genital Ulcer
- **Single or multiple, large beefy (velvety) red, granulomatous ulcer that bleeds easily when touched.**
- Necritic tissue destruction, offensive smell, raised irregular edge, sclerotic/ cicatricial lesions may also occur.
- Incubation period is 1-4 weeks (upto 6 months)
Donovanosis/GI
- Dx by **microscopic** identification of **donovan bodies (bipolar staining or inclusion or telephone handle or safety pin appearance)** on **Giemsa/Wright/Leishman or silver stain**
- **PCR analysis with calorimetric** detection.
- **Single, clean (nonpurulent), non vascular (non bleeding), punchedout, (sharply demarcated) ulcer with regular margin** and button like **(hard) induration.** ***Exudes serum on pressure***[Q].
- Incubation period is ***9-90 days***[Q].
Syphilis (Primary or Huntarian - Chancre)
Dx by ***Darkfield microscopy***[Q], VDRL, FTA-ABS, MAHA-TP, TPI test, Reagin test (reagin antibody is Ig G type)
- **Small painless papule** that forms **asymptomatic, transient herpetiform ulcer.** This painless, single, nonbleeding and occasionally firm indurated ulcer is **most often unnoticed, heals rapidly** and leaves **no scar.**
- Incubation period id 3 days – 6 weeks
LGV
Dx by **NAAT** (method of choice) confirmed by **real time PCR assay.**
MIF & CF tests may support diagnosis; **Frei test** (historic)
Multiple, Painful (tender), Non-indurated genital ulcer
- **Soft papule** with surrounding erythema (IP – 3-10 days) evolve into **micropustules (but not vesicles)** resembling folliculitis (in next 2-3 days). Spontaneous rupture forms usually **multiple, sharply circumscribed, non-indurated (soft) ulcers with undermined, ragged & irregular edges** and purulent base sloughed with granulation tissue that **bleeds very easily.**
- Short incubation period (3-10 days)
Chancroid (Soft Chancre)
Dx by **shoal or school of fish/ rail road track appearance** on gram/ giemsa staining and microscopic examination (only suggestive); **culture** of H. ducreyi (primary tool); or Multiplex PCR assay.
- Multiple **grouped vesicles** that rupture to form **superficial polycyclic erosions (ulcers)** with erythematous margins.
- **Recurrent attacks & burning**
- Short incubation period (2-7 days)
Herpes genitalis

Questions

Warts

1. **Verrucosa Vulgaris is caused by :**
   A. HPV (Bihar 04, DNB 05) ☐
   B. EBV ☐
   C. CMV ☐
   D. HIV ☐
2. **Genital Warts (condyloma accuminata) are most commonly caused by which of the following serotypes of HPV?**
   A. HPV 6 *(AIIMS May 08, 04, 03)* ☐
   B. HPV 16 ☐
   C. HPV 18 ☐
   D. HPV33 ☐
3. **Myrmecia warts are-** *(Jipmer 98, DNB 97)*
   A. Planer wart ☐
   B. Plantar wart ☐
   C. Verrucous wart ☐
   D. Palmer wart ☐
4. **All are true regarding viral warts except**
   A. Basophilic stippling *(PGI 97)* ☐
   B. Koilocytes are characteristic ☐
   C. Spontaneous regression common in children ☐
   D. Perinucear vacuolization. ☐
   E. Verruca vulgaris is associated with HPV7 ☐
5. **Immunomodulator used in treatment of genital warts is**
   A. ATRA *(AI 08)* ☐
   B. Podophyllin ☐
   C. Imiquimod ☐
   D. Prednisolone ☐
6. **Podophylline is used in treatment of**
   A. Plantar warts *(AIIMS 92, 94, 02, 04)* ☐
   B. Palmar warts ☐
   C. Comdylomata accuminata (Genital wart) ☐
   D. Condylomata lata ☐
7. **Regarding podophyllin resin which of following statement is true:** *(PGI Dec 08)*
   A. Dervied from plant source ☐
   B. Safe in pregnancy ☐
   C. Teratogenic ☐
   D. High recurrence rate of wart after podophyllin resin treatment ☐
   E. Individual variation in response rate ☐
8. **Treatment of choice for genital warts in pregnancy?**
   A. Salicylic Acid with Lactic Acid Solution ☐
   B. Podopylin *(AIIMS Nov 09)* ☐
   C. Imiqimod ☐
   D. Cryotherapy ☐
9. **HPV vaccine is:** *(AIIMS Nov 09)*
   A. Monovalent ☐
   B. Bivalent ☐
   C. Quadrivalent ☐
   D. Bivalent and quadrivalent ☐

Gonorrhea

10. **Gonococcus is -** *(DNB 99, PGI 96, Kerala 98)*
    A. Extracellular gram positive ☐
    B. Intracytoplasmic gram postive ☐
    C. Intracytoplasmic gram negative ☐
    D. Intra nuclear gram positive ☐
11. **The commonest venereal disease in India is-**
    A. Gonorrhoea *(DNB 97, AIIMS 98, TN 99)* ☐
    B. Syphilis ☐
    C. Chancroid ☐
    D. LGV ☐
12. **The main feature of gonorrhoea is-** *(Karnat 98, DNB 01)*
    A. Purulent discharge per urethra ☐
    B. Inguinal adenitis ☐
    C. Ulcer over glans penis ☐
    D. Rashes ☐
13. **Gonococcus resistant structure is** *(AI 98, 96)*
    A. Urethra ☐
    B. Testis ☐
    C. Fallopian Tube ☐
    D. Ampulla of cervix ☐
14. **M.C. cause of Nongonococcal Urethritis**
    A. Chlamydia *(AIIMS 92)* ☐
    B. Mycoplasma ☐
    C. Trichomonas ☐
    D. Gram negative rod ☐
15. **The syndromic management of urethral discharge includes treatment of:** *(AI 03)*
    A. Neisseria gonorrhoeae and herpes genitalis ☐
    B. Chlamydia trachomatis and herpes ganitalis ☐
    C. Neisseria gonorrhoeae and Chlamydia trachomatis ☐
    D. Syphilis and chancroid ☐
16. **TOC for penicillin resistant gonorrhoea** *(AIIMS 98)*
    B. Ciprofloxacin ☐
    C. Ceftriaxone ☐
    D. Streptomycine ☐
    E. Erythromycin ☐

Lymphogranuloma Venereum

17. **LGV is caused by** *(AIIMS 99, PGI 98, Kerala 99, Bihar 05)*
    A. Chalamydia trachomatis *(DNB 06)* ☐
    B. Haemophylus ducrei ☐
    C. HTLV type II ☐
    D. Donovanosis granulomatis ☐
18. **Genital ulcer is seen in A/E:** *(AIIMS 97, PGI 97)*
    A. Granuloma inguinale ☐
    B. Syphillis ☐
    C. LGV ☐
    D. Donovanosis ☐
19. **Bubos with multiple sinuses discharging into inguinal lymph nodes are seen in:**
    A. Chancroid *(AI 94)* ☐
    B. Granuloma Inguinale ☐
    C. LGV ☐
    D. Syphilis ☐
20. **Sign of Groove is found in -** *(AI 98)*
    A. Chancroid ☐
    B. Granuloma inguinale ☐
    C. LGV ☐
    D. Syphilis ☐
21. **Genital elephantiasis is caused by:** *(AI 02)*
    A. Donovanosis ☐
    B. Congenital syphilis ☐
    C. Herpes genaitalis ☐
    D. Lymphogranuloma venerum ☐
22. **Esthiomine is seen in-** *(AP 98, DNB 99)*
    A. Chancroid ☐
    B. Syphilis ☐
    C. LGV ☐
    D. Gonorrhoea ☐
23. **Frie test is done in** *(AI 96)*
    A. Donovanosis ☐
    B. LGV ☐
    C. Syphillis ☐
    D. Leprosy ☐

24. DOC for LGV *(AIIMS 93, Karnataka 94)*
A. Doxycycline ☐
B. Ampicillin ☐
C Erythromycin ☐
D. Ceftriaxone ☐

Donovanosis

25. Donovanosis/granuloma venerum is caused by *(AI 97, 06)*
A. Calymatobacter granulomatis ☐
B. T. pertenue ☐
C. Chlamydia Trachomatis ☐
D. H. ducreyi ☐

26. Pseudo Bubo is seen in *(AIIMS 95, AI 96)*
A. Chancroid ☐
B. LGV ☐
C. Donovanois ☐
D. Syphillis ☐

27. Lymphadenopathy is seen is A/E *(AI 95)*
A. Syphlis 1st Stage ☐
B. Donovanosis ☐
C. LGV ☐
D. Chancroid ☐

28. A 30 year old male patient has a large, spreading and exuberant ulcer with bright red granulation tissue over the glands penis. There was no lymphadenopathy. The most likely causative organism is; *(AIIMS Nov 03)*
A. Treponema pallidum ☐
B. Herpes simplex virus type 1 ☐
C. Herpes simplex virus type 2 ☐
D. Calymmatobacterium granulomatis ☐

29. Safety pin appearance is shown by- *(AI 89)*
A. Hemophilus ducreyi ☐
B. Chalmydia ☐
C. Donovani granulomatis ☐
D. Mycoplosma ☐

30. Treatment of granuloma inguinale is- *(AI 97, 93)*
A. Tetracycline ☐
B. Sulphanomide ☐
C. Streptomycin ☐
D. Pencillin ☐

31. Drug of choice for Granuloma venereum-
A. Sulphomamides *(DNB 99, AP 95, UPSC 98)* ☐
B. Streptomycin ☐
C. Pencillin ☐
D. Erthromycin ☐
E. Gentamycin ☐

32. Streptomycin is useful in treatment of
A. Granuloma venerum *(AIIMS 90)* ☐
B. LGV ☐
C. Syphillis ☐
D. Chancroid ☐

Chancroid

33. Chanroid is caused by- *(AI 95, UP 96)*
A. Hemophilus ducrey's ☐
B. Hemojphilus vaginalis ☐
C. Trachoma virus ☐
D. Treponima pallidum ☐

34. Chancroid may be caused by: *(AI 99)*
A. T. pallidium ☐
B. G. donovani ☐
C. Chlamydia Trachomatis ☐
D. Herpes Hominis Virus ☐

35. Reliable test for chancroid detection- *(AP 98, AI 98)*
A. Skin test *(DNB 02)* ☐
B. Biopsy ☐
C. Grams stained smear ☐
D. Clinical examination ☐

36. School of fish appearance is shown by: *(AI 98)*
A. Hemophilus ducreyi ☐
B. Gonococcus ☐
C. Chlamydia ☐
D. Donovania granulomatis ☐

37. DOC in chancroid is *(AIIMS 98, AP 98, UP 99)*
A. Tetracycline ☐
B. Doxycycline ☐
C. Erythromycin ☐
D. Streptomycin ☐

38. 20 year old male lalu develops multiple tender bleeding, nonindurated ulcer over prepuce and glans which are painful along with suppurative lymphadenopathy, 5 days after having sexual interc-ourse with a sex worker, most probable disease is
A. LGV *(AIIMS 96, 93, 94)* ☐
B. Herpes genitials ☐
C. Molluscum Contagiousm ☐
D. Chancroid ☐
E. Donovanosis ☐

39. Multiple necrotic ulcers in prepuce of penis with tender, suppurative inguinal nodes is caused by- *(AIIMS 94)*
A. Chalmydia ☐
B. Hemophilus ducreyi ☐
C. Herpes simplex ☐
D. Syphilis ☐

40. A man having multiple, painful, indurated, undermined, sloughed edged glans which occurred 5 days after exposures; most likely diagnosis is
A. Chancroid *(AI 08)* ☐
B. Primary chancre ☐
C. Herpes genitalis ☐
D. LGV ☐

41. Painful lymphadenopathy is seen in:*(PGI 02)*
A. Donovanosis ☐
B. Syphilis ☐
C. Chancroid ☐
D. Herpes simplex ☐
E. Gonorrheea ☐

42. A 30 year old male presented with ulcerative lesion on glans penis. Wright- Giemsa stain showed 1-2 rounded structure in macrophage vacuoles. What is the etiology
A. Chlamydia trachomatis *(AIIMS May 10)* ☐
B. N. gonorrhoea ☐
C. H. ducreyi ☐
D. Calymatobacterium granulomatis ☐

43. 19 years male develops painless penile ulcers 9 days after sexual intercourse with a professional sex worker likely diagnosis is:
A. Chancroid *(AI 01)* ☐
B. Herpes ☐
C Chancre ☐
D. Traumatic ulcer ☐

44. A 23-year-old male had unprotected sexual intercourse with a commercial sex worker. Two weeks later, he developed a painless, indurated ulcer on the glans which exuded clear serum on pressure. Inguinal lymph nodes in both groins were enlarged and not tender. The most appropriate diagnostic test is: *(AIIMS 04)*
A. Gram's stain of ulcer discharge ☐
B. Darkfield microscopy of ulcer discharge ☐
C. Giemsa stain of lymph node aspirate ☐
D. ELISA for HIV infection ☐

45. A 24 year old male presents to a STD clinic with a single painless ulcer on external genitalia. The choice of laboratory test to look for the etiological agent would be:
A. Scrappings from ulcer for culture on chocolate agar with antibiotic supplement. *(AIIMS May 03)* ☐

B. Serology for detection of specific IgM antibodies. ☐
C. Scrappings from ulcer for dark field microscopy. ☐
D. Scrappings from ulcer for tissue culture ☐

46. Painful genital ulcer is/are seen in: *(PGI May 12)*
A. Chancroid ☐
B. Lymphogranuloma venereum ☐
C. Primary syphilis ☐
D. Herpes ☐
E. Granuloma inguinale ☐

Syphilis

47. 'Chancre redux' is a clinical feature of:
A. Early relapsing syphilis ☐
B. Late syphilis *(AIIMS May 06)* ☐
C. Chancroid ☐
D. Recurrent herpes simplex infection ☐

48. Primary bullous lesions is seen in which type of syphilis
A. Primary *(AI 94)* ☐
B. Secondary ☐
C. Tertiary ☐
D. Congential ☐

49. Characteristic feature of early congenital syphilis is:
A. Microcephaly *(PGI 99)* ☐
B. Saddle nose ☐
C. Interstitial keratitis with saber skin ☐
D. Vesicular rash with bulla over palms and soles ☐

50. Hutchison's syphilitic traid includes all except *(AI 98)*
A. Associated with congenital syphilis ☐
B. Notched incissor teeth ☐
C. Nerve deafness ☐
D. Interstitial Keratitis ☐
E. Associated with CVS anomalies ☐

51. Sabre Tibia *(AI 93)*
A. Scury ☐
B. Rickets ☐
C. Leprosy ☐
D. Syphilis ☐

52. A boy with multiple bullous lesions over trunk and periostitis on x-rays. What should be the next investigation *(DNB 10, AIIMS Nov 11)*
A. VDRL of mother & child ☐
B. PCR for maternal TB ☐
C. HBsAg screening ☐
D. ELISA of mother and Child ☐

53. A 40 year old female presented with numerous, nonitchy, erythematous scaly papules (lesions) on trunk, with few oral white mucosal plaques. She also had erosive lesions in perianal area. The probable diagnosis is *(AI-12)*
A. Psoriasis ☐
B. Secondary syphilis ☐
C. Lichen planus ☐
D. Disseminated candidiasis ☐

54. In secondary syphilis all are seen except: *(PGI 98)*
A. Condyloma lata ☐
B. Interstitial keratitis ☐
C. Arthritis ☐
D. Proteinuria ☐

55. Early eruption of secondary syphilis are all except-*(AI 98)*
A. Intensely pruritic ☐
B. Papular / maculo papular eruption ☐
C. Symmeterical ☐
D. Plemorphic ☐

56. Not true of secondary syphilis *(AIIMS 96, 97, 98, AI 91)*
A. May be asymptomatic ☐
B. Usually involve palms & soles ☐
C. Lymphadenopathy ☐
D. Vesicular Bullous lesions ☐

57. Condylomata latae are seen in *(AIIMS 98, AIIMS 99)*
A. Congential syphilis ☐
B. Primary syphilis ☐
C. Secondary syphilis ☐
D. Tertiary syphilis ☐

58. In secondary syphilis, true about rash is *(PGI 98)*
A. Pruritic ☐
B. Vesicular ☐
C. Asymptomatic ☐
D. Tender ☐

59. Secondary syphilis manifested by *(PGI 03)*
A. Painless lymphadenopathy ☐
B. Pruritic rash ☐
C. Mucosal erosion ☐
D. Asymptomatic rash ☐
E. Mostly asymptomatic ☐

60. A 23-yeard-old college student has asympt-omatic and hyperpigmented macules on both palms for three weeks. The most appropriate diagnostic test is: *(AIIMS 04)*
A. Veneral Diseases research Laboratory (VDRL) test. ☐
B. Skin biopsy ☐
C. Serum cortisol levels ☐
D. Assay for arsenic in skin, hair & nails ☐

61. Treponema pallidum isolation from CSF is maximum in which stage of syphilis? *(AIIMS May 09)*
A. Primary syphilis ☐
B. Secondary syphilis ☐
C. Tertiary syphilis ☐
D. Tabes dorsalis ☐

62. True about syphilis is A/E: *(AI 98)*
A. VDRL is sensitive but not specific ☐
B. Infection leads to life long immunity ☐
C. IgM & IgA ☐
D. T. pallidium when inoculated in rabbit produce progressive disease. ☐

63. A patient has syphilis since 2 year. CSF examination was done & treatment started. Which of the following test is most useful in monitoring treatment *(AIIMS Nov 09)*
A. TPI ☐
B. VDRL ☐
C. FTA ☐
D. Dark ground microscopy ☐

64. Most specific test for syphilis *(AIIMS May 10)*
A. VDRL ☐
B. RPR ☐
C. FTA-Abs ☐
D. Kahn's test ☐

65. Test not used for diagnosis of syphilis
A. VDRL *(AI 93)* ☐
B. TPI ☐
C. Reagin Test ☐
D. Frei Test ☐

66. DOC in primary syphilis is *(AI 92)*
A. Corticosteroid ☐
B. Oral Penicilline ☐
C. Benzathine Penicilline ☐
D. Crystalline Penicilline ☐

67. A young man presents with asymptomatic macules and erythematous painless lesion over glans with generalized lymphadenopahty. Treatment of choice in this condition: *(AIIMS Nov 12)*
A. Ceftriaxone ☐
B. Benzathine penicillin ☐
C. Acyclovir ☐
D. Fluconazole ☐

68. Jarisch Herxheimer reaction is commonly seen in:
A. Early syphilis *(DNB 03, SGPGI 05, PGI 98)* ☐
B. Late congenital syphilis ☐

C. Latent syphilis ☐
D. Syphilis of cardiovascular system ☐

69. **Not transmitted sexually** *(AI 92)*
A. Syphilis ☐
B. T. pertenue ☐
C. Candida ☐
D. Gonorrhoea ☐

70. **Incorrect Statement is** *(AI 92)*
A. VDRL titre decreases with treatment ☐
B. VDRL becomes positiv after 21 days of infection ☐
C. FTA-ABS is earliest & most sensitive test ☐
D. Yaws & Pinta can be differentiated by serological tests ☐

71. **A young man presents to the emergency department with a maculopapular rash 2 weeks after healing of a painless genital ulcer. The most likely etiological agent is** *(AI 11)*
A. Treponemapallidum ☐
B. Treponemapertunae ☐
C. Chalmydia Trachomatis ☐
D. Calymatobacter granulomatis ☐

72. **Drug of choice for syphilis in a pregnant women** *(AI-12)*
A. Azithromycin ☐
B. Penicillin ☐
C. Tetracycline ☐
D. Ceftriaxone ☐

73. **All is true about syphilis except** *(DNB 11, PGI May 12)*
A. Seropositive infant not treated at birth if mother received penicillin in 3rd trimester ☐
B. For neurosyphilis FTA-ABS is sensitive; VDRL diagnostic but CSF pleocylosis is best treatment response guide. ☐
C. HIV patients are less likely to become VDRL nonreactive after treatment ☐
D. EIA+, RPR+, indicate past or current infection ☐
E. Sulfonamides and quinolones are 2nd line drugs ☐

Other

74. **Treatment of both partners is recomended in A/E :**
A. Candida infection *(PGI 99)* ☐
B. Gardenella ☐
C. Herpes ☐
D. Trichomonas vaginalis ☐

75. **Recurrent balanoposthitis seen in :** *(PGI 02)*
A. DM ☐
B. Herpes simplex ☐
C. Smoking ☐
D. Alcohol ☐
E. Bad hygiene ☐

76. **Genital ulcer is/are caused by:** *(PGI Nov 2009)*
A. Human papilloma virus ☐
B. Herpes simplex virus ☐
C. HIV ☐
D. Treponema pallidum ☐
E. Lymphogranuloma venereum ☐

77. **Syndromic Management of genital ulcer syndrome in India includes** *(AIIMS Nov 11)*
A. Chancroid and Primary chancre ☐
B. Chancroid and herpes simplex ☐
C. Chancroid, Primary Chancre and herpes simplex ☐
D. Herpes simplex and primary chancre ☐

Answers and Explanations:

Warts

1. **A i.e. HPV**
2. **A i.e. HPV – 6**
3. **B i.e. Plantar wart**
4. **E i.e., Veruca vulgaris is associated with HPV7**
5. **C i.e. Imiquimod**
6. **C i.e. Condylomata accuminata**
7. **A. i.e. Derived from plant source C. i.e. Teratogenic D. i.e. High recurrence rate of wart after podophyllin resin treatment E. Individual variation in treatment**
8. **D i.e. Cryotherapy**
9. **D i.e. Bivalent and quadrivalent**

[Ref: Harrison 17th p. 319, 1117; Thomas Habif 4/e p. 340; Katzung 8/e P-1059; CMDT 2009 P-128; Roxburgh's 17/e 55; Fitzpatrick's 7/e p-1914-22; Rooks 7/e p. 25.35-25.49, 30.1-30.30, 25.20-39; Neena Khanna 2/e p. 228-31]

- **Warts** are most common virus induced tumors, caused by ***human papilloma virus (HPV)***Q. It shows **Koebner's phenomenon.**
- **Verruca vulgaris** (the most common variety of wart which involves hands & fingers) is caused by **HPV 2 (mc)**, 4> 27, 29; **Myrmecia warts (or deep plantar warts / verruca plantaris)** is caused by **HPV 1**; and **ano-genital (veneral) wart** or **condyloma accuminata** is caused by ***HPV 6, 11***Q (in 90% cases).
- Acanthotic & hyperkeratotic epidermis with large keratinocytes (i.e. **koiliocytes** with pyknotic, eccentric nucleus & **perinuclear halo**), **basophilic stippling** and **perinuclear vacuolization** are seen in histopathology of warts.
- ***Immunomodulator (topical imiquimod 5%), podophyllin (15%), podophyllotoxin (0.5%) and trichloroacetic acid***Q are used only in **veneral (genita) warts or condyloma accuminata.** Podophyllin resin is derived from plant source and because of teratogenic potential, both podophyllin & podophyllotoxin are contraindicated in pregnancy. Podophyllins are more affective on mucosal than keratinized surface, has individual variation in response and high recurrence.
- In **pregnancy**, ***only cryotherapy or destructive techniques with cautery or hyfrecation can be used safely for warts***Q.

Treatment of Wart

1. **Cryotherapy with liq.** N_2 (most useful & convenient method) or solid CO_2
2. Intracutaneous injection of cytotoxics as Bleomycin & recombinant interferon
3. Curettage & Cautery

Chemical Cautery

1. ***20% Podophyllin or glutaraldehyde***Q **(drug of choice)**
2. Salicylic Acid (10-20%)
3. Lactic Acid (5-40%)
4. ***Imiquimod***
5. ***Tricholoroacetic acid***Q (drug of choice in women & esp ***pregnancy***Q as podophyllin is C/I in pregnancy)

- **Human papilloma virus vaccine** is a ***quadrivalent***Q version of vaccine composed of L_1 *protein VLPs (virus like particles) from HPV-6,- 11,- 16 and - 18.* Its **bivalent** form is against HPV -16 & -18.

Type of Wart	T/t / Drug of choice
Condylomata accuminata (Veneral wart)	***Podophyllin***Q
Veneral wart in pregnancy	***Cryotherapy***Q ***(TOC)*** ***Trichloroacetic acid***Q (1st) ***Imiquimod***Q (2nd)
Massive wart (Buschke Loweinstein Syndrome)	***Cryo surgery***Q

1

Gonorrhea

10. **C i.e. Intracytoplasmic gram negative**
11. **A i.e. Gonorrhoea**
12. **A i.e. Purulent discharge per urethra**
13. **B i.e. Testis**
14. **A i.e. Chlamydia**
15. **C i.e. Neisseria gonorrhoeae and Chlamydia Trachomatis**
16. **B i.e. Ceftriaxone**

[Ref: Harrison 18/e p. 1220-27, 1423; Rooks 8/e p. 31.24-34.38; Fitzpatrick 7/e p. 2212]

- **Neisseria gonorrhea** is a ***gram negative, aerobic, non-motile, non-sporeforming, diplo/mono-cocci***Q, exclusively a human pathogen that principally infects host columnar epithelium. It is *oxidase positive* like other Neisseria species, from which it is distinguished by their ability to grow on selective media & to *utilize glucose but not maltose, sucrose or lactose.*
- ***Gonorrhoea is, the second most common (after Chlamydia trachomatis which is the most common) genital / sexually transmitted infection in US, UK and other developed countries***Q (Harrison 1442; Rook's 34.24). The incidence of ***gonorrhea is higher in developing countries***Q than industrialized nations predominantly affecting young, nonwhite, unmarried, less educated urban population. (Harrison 1220)
- ***Chlamydia trachomatis is the most common cause of non gonococcal urethritis (NGU) and postgonococcal urethritis (PGU)***Q. PGU refers to NGU developing in men 2-3 weeks after treatment of gonococcal urethritis with single doses of agents such as penicillin or cephalosporins which lack activity against Chlamydia. In US ***most of acute urethritis cases are NGU and C. trachomatis is implicated in most (30-50%) of these cases***Q. The other causes of NGU are *Ureaplasma urealyticum, Mycoplasma genitalium, Trichomonas vaginalis and herpes simplex virus (HSV).*
- Gonorrhoea is a STD which commonly manifests as ***cervicitis (primary site of infection in females), urethritis (most common/primary site of infection in males presenting as rapid onset severe burning dysuria with profuse purulent discharge)***Q, proctitis & conjunctivitis. If untreated it can l/t local complications such as endometritis, ***salpingitis, tuboovarian abscess***Q, bartholinitis, peritonitis and perihepatitis (Fitz-Hugh Curtis Syndrome) in females; peri urethritis and ***epididymitis***Q in male patients and ophthalmia neonatorum in new borns. Disseminated gonococcemia is uncommon & l/t skin lesions, tenosynovitis, arthritis and in rare cases endocarditis & meningitis.

Feature	Gonococcus	Syphilis
Infect / Involve	***Epididymis***Q	***Testis***Q
Resistant structure (not involve)	***Testis***Q	***Epididymis***Q
Infection spread through	Urethrae (i.e. Epididymis is involved & testis is spared)	Blood (i.e. testis is involved & epididymis is spared)

- ***Because of ascending spread of infection testis is spared or (uncommonly) last to be involved***Q only after urethritis, prostatitis, epididymitis in gonorrhea.
- Single dose regimens of 3rd ***generation cephalosporins ceftriaxone (IM) and cefixime (oral) are the mainstays of therapy***Q for uncomplicated gonococcal infection of urethra, cervix, rectum, or pharynx. **Septinomycin** is an alternative (2nd) regimen for uncomplicated gonococcal infections in *penicillin allergic patients.* All 3 drugs are suitable for pregnant & breast feeding women.
- The new management for complaints of urethral discharge involves a ***combined modality of treatment for N. gonorrhea and C. trachomatis***Q as most cases are d/t coinfection with both pathogens and incorporate an agent eg. **azithromycin or doxycycline** that is effective agenist chlamydial infection. Pregnant women who should not take doxycycline, should receive concurrent treatment with a **macrolide** antibiotic for possible chlamydial infection.

Diagnosis	1st line treatment of choice	Alternative regimens
Uncomplicated gonococcal infection of cervix, urethra, pharynx or rectum	***Single dose ceftriaxone (IM) or cefixime (oral)***Q + Single dose **azithromycin** or **doxycycline** (oral) for Chlamydia if not ruled out	Single dose IM ceftizoxime or cefotaxime or septinomycin or cefotetan or cefoxitin + single dose oral probenecid (with last 2 drugs)

Lymphogranuloma Venereum

17. **A i.e. Chlamydia trachomatis**
18. **C i.e. LGV**
19. **C i.e. LGV**
20. **C i.e. LGV**
21. **D i.e. Lymphogranuloma venerum**
22. **C i.e. LGV**
23. **B i.e. LGV**
24. **A i.e. Doxycycline**

[Ref: Harrison 18/e p. 1425-28; Rooks 8/e p.34.32-34.33]

Donovanosis (Granuloma venerum / ingunale)

25. **A i.e. Calymatobacter granulomatis**
26. **C i.e. Donovanosis**
27. **B i.e. Donovanosis**
28. **D i.e. Calymmatobacterium granulomatis**
29. **C i.e. Donovani granulomatis**
30. **A i.e. Tetracycline**
31. **D i.e. Erythromycin**
32. **A i.e. Granuloma venerum**

[Ref: Harrison 18/e p. 1320-21; Rooks 34.30-34.40]

Common Features of different STDs

Gonorrhoea

- Caused by *Nisseria gonorrhea, an* ***intracytoplasmic gram negative bacteria***Q
- It means *flow of seeds*
- ***Most common veneral disease in India***Q
- Most common feature is purulent discharge per urethra
- ***Testis is spared and epidydimis is involved***Q
- DOC is ***procaine penicillin***Q (old), ***ceftriaxone/cefixime***Q + azithromycin / doxycycline (new)

Lymphogranuloma venereum (LGV)

- A = ***Asymptomatic or no genital ulcer***Q. Painless non bleeding ulcer (if present) with Painful matted lymph node.
- B = ***Bubo***Q formed (matted lymphnodes)
- C = ***Chlamydia trachomatis***Q type L-I, II, III is causative agent
- D = DOC is ***Doxycycline***Q / tetra or mino-cycline/erythromycin > azithromycin
- E = ***Esthiomine***Q (Vaginal & Rectal Stricture and elephantiasis of vulva) seen.
- F = Fistulas, ***Frei's Test***Q done for diagnosis (not used now) is intradermal test to demonstrate hypersensitivity to *chlamydia, the causative agent of LGV.*
- G = ***Groove sign***Q (enlarged lymph nodes on both sides of inguinal ligament) present.

Donovanosis/ Granuloma venereum (inguinale)

- Caused by ***calimotobacter (donovania) granulomatis***Q (Klebsiella granulomatis), a gram –ve organism
- C/P is ***Painless bleeding ulcer*** with ***Pseudo Bubo.***Q
- Best diagnosed by ***Microscopy***Q by demonstrating -
  1. ***Donovan bodies***Q
  2. ***Safety pin appearance***Q (bipolar staining)
- ***Treatment of choice is azithromycin***Q > erythromycin (both used in pregnancy also), ***doxy/tetra cycline***Q, cotrimoxazole > aminoglycoside.

Chancroid

- **Chancroid** is caused by ***Haemophyllus ducrey (most common), Hereps Hominis virus etc***Q.
- It presents with multiple ***painful, bleeding, nonindurated (soft) ulcer and fluctulant suppurative painful lymphadenopathy***Q.
- Diagnosed by ***Gram staining***Q
  1. *Gram-ve cocco-baccili* (H. ducreyi)
  2. ***Rail road (Shoal or School of fish) appearance***Q
- **Drug of choice** is single dose **azithromycin/ ceftriaxone/ ciprofloxacin** or erythromycin for 7 days.

Chancroid (Soft chancre, Ulcus molle, Ducrey's Disease)

33. **A i.e. Hemophilus ducreyi**
34. **D i.e. Herpes virus - hominis**
35. **C i.e. Grams stained smear**
36. **A i.e. Hemophilus ducreyi**
37. **C i.e. Erythromycin** *[Ref: Harrison 18/e p. 1230-31, 1107-9; Rooks 8/e p. 34.34-34.35; Fitzpatrick 7/e p. 1983-86]*

Distinguishing Features of Genital Ulcers

Features	Syphilis (1°chancre)	Chancroid (soft chancre)	Lymphogranuloma Venereum	Donovanosis Granuloma venerum/inguinale)	Herpes genitalis
Causative agent	*Treponema pallidium*[Q]	*Haemophilus ducreyi*[Q]	*Chlamydia trachomatis*[Q] (L_1,L_2,L_3)	*Calymmatobacterium granulomatis*[Q]	*Herpes simplex virus type II*[Q] (rarely type I)
Incubation period	***9 – 90 days***[Q]	1 – 7 days rarely > 10 days	3 days – 6 weeks	1-4 weeks (upto 6 months)	2-7 days
No. of attacks	Only one (1)	1 or 2	Only one (1)	Only one (1)	**Reccurent**
No. of lesions	Usually 1	Usually ***multiple***[Q] may coalesce	Usually 1	Variable	***Multiple***[Q], may coalesce
Early 1° lesion Diameter Depth Edges	Papule 5-15 mm Superficial or deep Sharply demarcated, elevated, round or oval	Pustule Variable **Excavated** **Undermined, ragged, *sloughed***[Q] ***irregular***	Papule, pustule 2-10 mm Superficial or deep Elevated, round or oval	Papule Variable **Elevated** ***Elevated, irregular*** **serpiginous**	***Vesicle***[Q] 1-2 mm Superficial **Erythematous**
Base	***Smooth, non-purulent, non-vascular***[Q] (relatively)	***Purulent, bleeds easily***	Variable, nonvascular	***Red & velvety (beefy red), bleeds easily with exuberant granulation tissue***[Q]	Serous, erythematous, nonvascular.
Induration	***Firm***[Q]	***Soft***[Q] (mostly)	Occasionly firm	***Firm***	None
Pain	***Uncommon***[Q]	***Usually very tender***	Variable	**Uncommon**	Frequenctly ***tender***[Q]
Lymphadenopathy	***Firm, non tender, shotty, bilateral***[Q]	***Tender, may suppurate, loculated, usually unilateral (Bubo)***	Tender, may suppurate, loculated, usually unilateral (Bubo)	**No *lymphadenopathy pseudobuboes***[Q] ***(subcutaneous nodules in inguinal region, may ulcerate)***	Firm, tender, often *bilateral*
Diagnosis	- ***Dark field microscopy***[Q] - Serologicaltests	- Clinical *features* - Gram staining (gram –ve cocco-baccili with rail road appearance)	- Demonstration of LGV as elementary & inclusion bodies - ***Frie's test***[Q] - Hyper gamma-globulinemia - Complement fixation +ve	- On tissue *smear & histopathological microscopy using* ***Giemsa, Wrights or Silver stain or Leishman Stain*** 1. Gram negative C. granulomatis may be seen within characteristic large mono nuclear cell as **Donovan bodies** 2. ***Donovan bodies are seen in vacuolated cytoplasm of large mono nuclear cells as bipolar inclusions***[Q] **(safety pin or telephone handle appearance)** measuring 1 to 2 μm x 0.5 to 0.7 μm.	- Multinucleated giant cell on Tzank smear - Culture is confirmatory
Drug	- *Benzathine/procaine* penicillin in all except neurosyphilis & congenital syphilis in which *crystalline penicillin (aqueous benzyl penicillin)* is used - In penicillin sensitive patient, Tetracycline or erythromycin is used	- *Azithro/ erythromycin* - Ciftriaxone - Ciprofloxacin	- ***Doxy / tetra cycline***[Q] - Erythromycin	**Doxycycline**[Q]/ ***tetracycline*** Azithromycin / erythromycin (in pregnancy)	***Acyclovir***[Q]

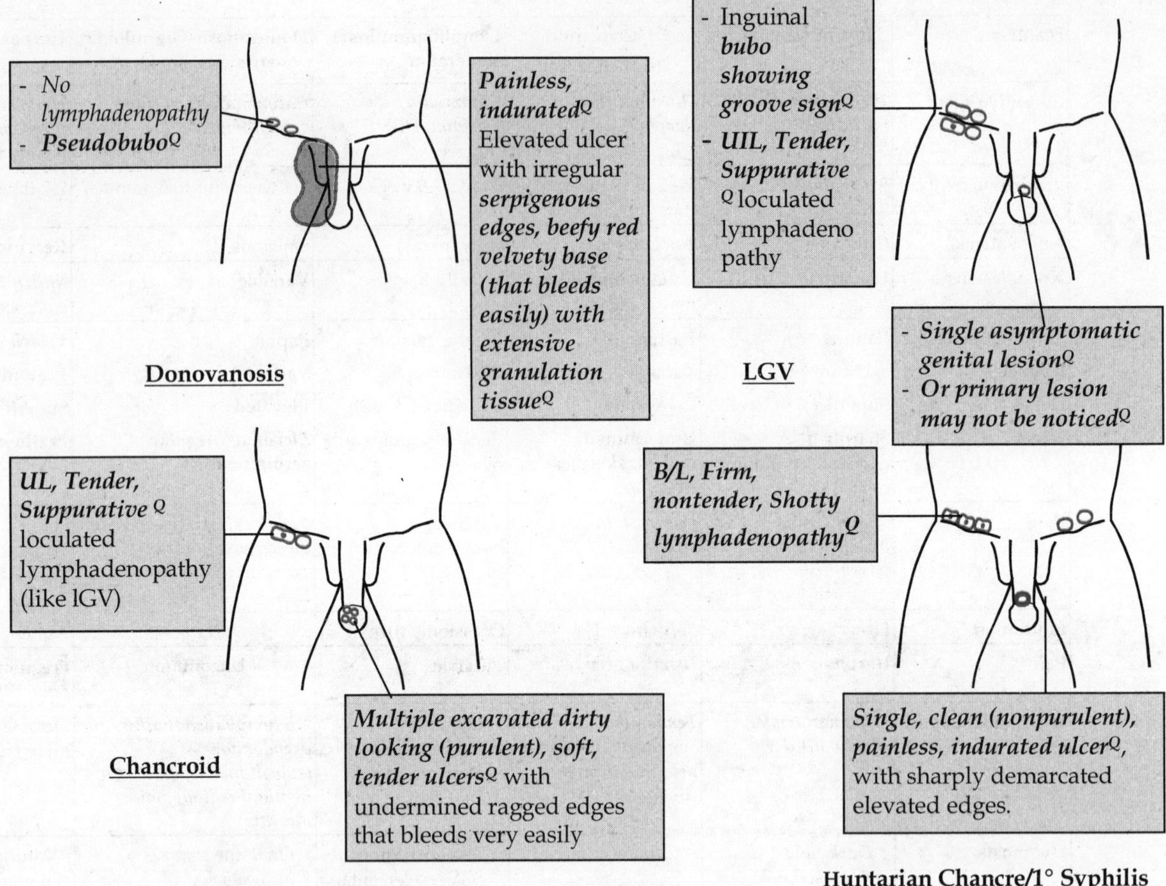

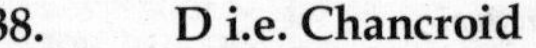

38. **D i.e. Chancroid**
39. **B i.e. Hemophillus**
40. **A i.e. Chancroid**
41. **C i.e. Chancroid; D i.e. Herpes Simplex**
42. **D i.e. Calymatobacterium granulomatis**
43. **C i.e. Chancre**
44. **B i.e. Dark field microscopy of ulcer discharge**

Approach to a case of STD on basis of lymphadenopathy

*No Lymphadenopathy*Q */Pseudo Bubo*Q

*Donovanosis*Q*/Granuloma inguinale*

- Caused by *calymmatobacterium granulomatis*Q
- ***Bleeding (red granulation tissue), painless, indurated ulcer***Q mostly involving genitalia (90%), inguinal (10%) & anal (5%) region
- ***Pseudobubo***Q is seen
- *Genital swelling* especially of labia ***(pseudoelephantiasis)***Q is seen
- Best diagnosed by ***microscopy***Q by demonstrating ***Donovan bodies***Q or ***Safety pin appearance***Q within large mononuclear cells in smear or biopsy sample.
- Doc is ***Doxy/tetracycline***Q
- In **pregnancy** doc is ***azithromycin /erythromycin***Q

Lymphadenopathy present

Painless Lymphadenopathy

*Syphilis*Q

- ***Painless, indurated, non-bleeding***Q, usually *single* punched out ulcer **(hard chancre)**
- Lymph nodes are rubbery and painless
- Caused by ***Treponema palladium***Q
- Diagnosed by ***Dark field microscopy***Q, ***FTA-ABS (most sensitive test***Q, ***earliest test to become positive***Q***) VDRL or RPR titer***Q ***(determine response to treatment as they become negative), TPI (most specific test***Q***)***, MAHATP (TPH; 2nd most sensitive test)
- ***Penicillin G***Q is drug of choice for all stages of syphilis

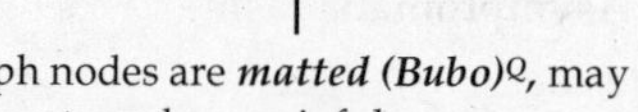

LGV[Q]

- Lymph nodes are ***matted (Bubo)***[Q], may suppurate and are painful
- ***Asymptomatic, single, painless*** (mostly) & ***non-bleeding macule/ulcer***[Q]
- Caused by ***Chlamydia trochomatic*** – L_1, L_2, *(M.C.)*, L_3[Q] strains
- Dx by direct microscopic examination of giemsa stained cell scrapings for inclusion/elementary bodies culture of organism, detection of chlamydial antigen by ELISA, detection of antibody in Serum.
- **Esthiomine** (vaginal & rectal strictures and **elephantiasis** of vulva), **Frei's test** and **groove sign** is seen)
- Drug of choice is ***doxy/tetra-cycline***[Q]

Chancroid[Q]

- Lymph node are fluctuant & spontaneously rupture & suppurate
- ***Ulcers develop within 7 days, are multiple painful, non indurated and bleeding***[Q] **(soft chancre)**
- Caused by ***Haemophilus. ducreyi***[Q]
- Dx by G***ram staining***[Q] (gram negative coccobacilli, ***school of fish***[Q] and ***rail road appearance***[Q]) & *culture of organism*
- Doc is ceftriaxone, Azithro/Erythromycin, ciprofloxacin

Herpes[Q]

- Ulcers are multiple, painful, non indurated & bleeding
- Characteristic multiple vesicular lesions make diagnosis easy
- Dx made by culture or demonstration of HSV antigen
- ***Acyclovir***[Q] is drug of choice

45. C i.e. Scrappings from ulcer for dark field microscopy

So if we concentrate on Painless ulcer

1. Painless (bleeding) ulcer without lymphadenopathy = ***Donovanosis***[Q]
2. Painless (non bleeding) ulcer with Painless lymphadenopathy = ***Syphilis***[Q]
3. Painless (non bleeding) ulcer with Painful (suppurative) lymphadenopathy = **LGV**[Q]

So this might be a case of syphilis (more common diagnosis) or donovanosis; & so the answer is darkfield microscopy.

46. A i.e. Chancroid; D i.e. Herpes

Genital ulcers are painful & *chancroid (soft chancre) and herpes genitalis*[Q]; whereas **painless** in **LGV, donovanosis (GI) and syphilis (primary or Huntarian chancre).**

Syphilis

47. A i.e. Early relapsing syphilis
48. D i.e. Congenital Syphilis
49. D i.e. Vesicular rash with bulla over palms & soles
50. E i.e. Associated with CVS anomalies
51. D i.e. Syphilis *[Ref: Behl & Aggarwal 10/e P – 236, 231; Fitzpatrick's 6/e p-2164-2212; Rooks 8/e p.34.1-34.20]*

- **Recurrence of the chancre in its original place due to relapse (not re-infection) in early syphilis**[Q] is called **chancre redux.**
- **Vesico – Bullous lesion** are charcterstically seen in early ***congenital syphilis***[Q] & not found in other stages of syphilis.

Lesions	Found in
Bulla & Vesicles	***Congenital syphilis***[Q]
Condylomata latae	***Secondary syphilis***[Q]
Condyloma – accuminata	**Genital/Veneral warts**[Q]

- ***Interstitial keratitis, along with 8th nerve deafness & hutchinson's teeth (pegged central upper incisors)***[Q] – form **Hutchinson's triad**; which is seen in **late congential syphilis.** *Sabre tibia*[Q], saddle nose, mulberry molars, bull dog jaws, frontal bossing of parrot and rhagades are other features of late congenital syphilis.

52. A i.e. VDRL of mother & child

Vescobullous lesion with periostitis[Q] indicate **congenital syphilis;** so **VDRL** shoud be done.

53. B i.e. Secondary syphilis *[Ref: Harrison 18/e p. 1392]*

Secondary syphilis presents with ***generalized, symmetrical, nonitchy, coppery red maculoppular lesions (± scales) on trunk, extremities and even palm and soles***[Q]***. Oral and genital superficial mucosal erosion (patches) are painless silver-gray***[Q] surrounded by red periphery. And warm, moist, intertriginous areas (such as perianal area, vulva and scrotum) show large, ***hypertrophic, coalesced gray-white, highly infections papules (Condylomata lata)***[Q].

54. **B i.e. Interstitial Keratitis** 55. **A i.e. Intensly pruritic**
56. **D i.e. Vesicular lesions** 57. **C i.e. Secondary Syphilis**
58. **C i.e. Asymptomatic**
59. **A i.e. Painless lymphadenopathy; C i.e. Mucosal erosion; D i.e. Asymptomatic rash**

Secondary Syphilis

Hallmark lesion	Other findings	Not found
- *Asymptomatic*[Q] - *B/L Symmetrical*[Q] *pleomorphic*[Q] - *Maculo-papular rash on palms & soles*[Q] - Nontender lymphadenopathy	- *Condylomata lata*[Q] - Moth eaten alopecia - Arthritis - Proteinurea	- *Vesico-bullous lesion*[Q] - *Intense pruritis*[Q] - *Interstitial keratitis*[Q]

60. **A i.e. Veneral Disease Laboratory (VDRL) Test**

- Estimation of cortisol levels are not indicated as only skin lesions without other symptoms is disfavouring adrenal pathology. Assay of arsenic is not required as arsenic poisoining will always present with systemic symptoms. Skin biopsy is not indicated as only presentation is hyperpigmented macules.
- So the answer is straight forward – As secondary syphilis usually presents with B/L symmetrical asymptomatic macules & the investigation required is VDRL.

61. **B. i.e. Secondary syphilis > A** *[Ref: Harrison's 17/e p- 1040-41; Fitzpatrick 7/e p. 1968-74]*

Treponema palladium has been recovered from CSF during primary & secondary syphilis in 30% of cases[Q].

62. **B/C. i.e. Infection leads to life long immunity; IgM & IgA**
63. **B i.e. VDRL** 64. **C i.e. FTA-Abs** 65. **D i.e. Frie – test**

- Most specific test is *TPI > FTA –ABS*[Q]
- Non treponemal test becomes non reactive after t/t; the **Treponemal test** often *remain reactive* **& therefore *not helpful in determining the infection status of person with past syphilis*** [Q]**. Response to treatment in early syphilis** is seen by ***sequential VDRL or RPR titer***[Q] as they become negative after treatment. **CSF-VDRL** is **highly specific but insensitive test**; may be nonreactive in symptomatic progressive neuro syphilis. It's sensitivity is highest in *meningovascular syphilis & paresis*.

Investigation & Laboratory Diagnosis of Syphilis

- ***Dark field microscopic examination***[Q] of exudates is sufficient for making diagnosis if it demonstrates organism.
- Direct fluorescent antibody T. pallidium *(DFA-TP) Test*[Q]
- Teponemal Immobilization Test *(TPI)*[Q]

★ Also remember:

- In **primary syphilis, sensitivity** is increased either by **FTA-ABS test** or simply **repetition of VDRL after 1-2** weeks if initial VDRL is negative.
- In **early primary syphilis,** the detection of antibody can be maximized either by **FTA-ABS test** or simply by **repetition of VDRL after 1-2 weeks** if the initial VDRL is negative.
- Non treponemal test becomes non reactive after t/t; the **Treponemal test** often *remain reactive* & **therefore *not helpful in determining the infection status of person with past syphilis.***[Q]
- In **secondary syphilis,** all tests are ***100% sensitive***[Q] but most commonly used test is VDRL
- In all stage most sensitive test is *FTA-ABS > MHA-TP*[Q]. In **primary & tertiary** syphilis sensitivity order of test is **FTA-ABS > MAHA-TP (TPH) > VDRL**
- **Earliest** test to become positive is *FTA-ABS*[Q]
- **Response to treatment in early syphilis** is seen by ***sequential VDRL or RPR titer***[Q] as they become negative after treatment.

- **Serological tests –** these are of two types & both type of tests are ***reactive/(positive) for any treponemal infection***[Q] ***including yaws, pinta & endemic syphilis***[Q]

Non Treponemal test	Treponemal test
- **Sensitive** & used for screening. **RPR & VDRL** are equally ***sensitive for initial screening***[Q] - Titer reflects activity of disease. **Fall** of 2 dilution (4 folds) ***following treatment is evidence of adequate response to t/t.***[Q] - Measures *IgG & IgM*[Q] directed against cardiolipin – lecithin – cholesterol – antigen complex - ***With treatment, titerfalls***[Q] which is evidence of adequate response to treatment - ***Reactive in any treponemal infection including Yaws, Pinta***[Q]	- **More secific tests** used for confirmation of reactive non treponemal test - **Non treponemal test become *non reactive (negative) after treatment***[Q], the **treponemal tests** often remain ***reactive after therapy & therefore not helpful in determining the infection status of person with past syphilis.***[Q] *FTA-ABS*[Q] · *MHA-TP*[Q] · *TPHA* (MHA-TP) Now replaced by ***serodia-TPPA test***[Q], which is more sensitive in primary syphilis

- Most **specific** test is **TPI > FTA-ABS**
- Negative TPH excludes diagnosis of present & past syphilis except in very early stage & neurosyphilis.
- **Nonreactive (-ve) CSF-FTA test** is used to ***rule out neurosyphilis***[Q]
- VDRL test becomes positive after 3-5 weeks of infection and 7-10 days of chancre.
- **CSF-VDRL** is **highly specific but insensitive test**; may be nonreactive in symptomatic progressive neuro syphilis. It's sensitivity is highest in *meningovascular syphilis & paresis.*

Test	Type
VDRL	***Slide flocculation Test***[Q]
Khan Test	***Tube Flocculation Test***[Q]
Waserman Reaction	***Complement fixation Test***[Q]

& endemic syphilis.

- ***VDRL titer do no correspond directly to RPR***[Q], so sequential quantative testing (for response of t/t) must employ single test.

VDRL[Q] — ***Standard test with CSF***[Q]

Rapid Plasma Reagin (RPR) Test[Q] — ***Test of choice for rapid-serological diagnosis in clinical setting or office***[Q]

Sensitivity of Serological tests in untreated syphilis

Test	Primary	Secondary	Latent	Tertiary
VDRL	74 (74-87)	100	95 (88-100)	71 (37-94)
FTA-ABS	84 (70-100)	100	100	96
MHA-TP	76 (69-90)	100	100	94

66. **C i.e. Benzathine penicillin**

67. **B i.e. Benzathine penicillin** *[Ref: Fitzpatrick's 8/ep 2473-90; Rooks 5/e p. 34.1-34.37]*

Presence of **asymptomatic macules** (non itchy, symmetrical, coppery red, round/oval roseolar rash of no substance k/a macular syphili) with **generalized lymphadenopathy** (painless, rubbery, discrete, mobile lymph nodes occurs in 50% cases of secondary syphilis) after a **painless erythematous, clean, hard and button like ulceration with sharply demarcated, regular, raised and indurated borders over glans (Hunterian chancre or ulcus durum or hard ulcer of primary syphilis)** in young adult indicates diagnosis of **secondary syphilis. CDC-Recommended treatment (drug of choice) for primary, secondary and early latent syphilis (in both HIV infected & uninfected patients) is parenteral (intramuscular) Benzathine penicillin G, 2.4 million units** in a single dose. Pregnant women who are enicillin allergic must be desensitized to and treated with penicillin which is the only drug known to cross placenta & treat infection in fetus.

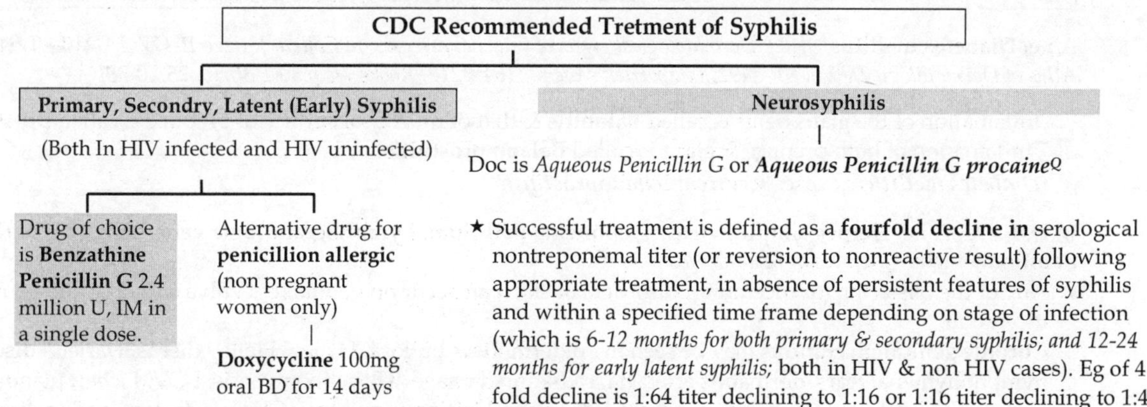
CDC Recommended Tretment of Syphilis
Primary, Secondry, Latent (Early) Syphilis
(Both In HIV infected and HIV uninfected)
Drug of choice is Benzathine Penicillin G 2.4 million U, IM in a single dose.
Alternative drug for penicillion allergic (non pregnant women only)
Doxycycline 100mg oral BD for 14 days
Neurosyphilis
Doc is Aqueous Penicillin G or Aqueous Penicillin G procaineQ
★ Successful treatment is defined as a fourfold decline in serological nontreponemal titer (or reversion to nonreactive result) following appropriate treatment, in absence of persistent features of syphilis and within a specified time frame depending on stage of infection (which is 6-12 months for both primary & secondary syphilis; and 12-24 months for early latent syphilis; both in HIV & non HIV cases). Eg of 4 fold decline is 1:64 titer declining to 1:16 or 1:16 titer declining to 1:4 or lower.

68. **A i.e. Early syphilis**

Jarisch – Herxheimer – Reaction, consisting of fever & constitutional symptoms may ***follow the treatment of syphilis***[Q] most commonly in secondary syphilis > primary syphilis > Early latent syphilis.

69. **B i.e. T. pertenue** *[Ref: Fitzpatrick's 6/e p-2164-2212; Rooks Textbook of Dermatology 7/e p.30.1-30.30, 25.20-39]*

Yaws (T. pertenue) & Pinta (T.caronetum) are ***non veneral (not transmitted sexually)***[Q]***. These can't be differentiated from Syphilis by Serological tests***[Q].

70. **D i.e. Yaws & Pinta can be differentiated by serological tests**

- **Yaws & Pinta cannot be differentiated serologically.**
- With T/t **VDRL or RPR titer decrease** so they are **used to see the response of trearment.**

- VDRL becomes positive after **3 - 5 weeks of infection**
  7 - 10 days of chancre
- **FTA-ABS** is **earliest** to become positive and **most sensitive** test
- **TPI > FTA - ABS** is **most specific test.**

71. A i.e. Treponema pallidum

Development of **nonpruritic maculopapular rash (secondary syphilis) two weeks after** heeling of **painless genital ulcer (primary syphilis) suggest Treponema pallidum** as an etiological aget.

Primary Syphilis		Secondary Syphilis
Painless, indurated, nonbleeding, usually single punched out **genital ulcer (hard chancre)** with painless, ruberry, shotty lymphadenopathy.	After **few weeks to few months;** dissemination of T. pallidum → producers systemic symptoms	- **Mucocutaneous maculo-papular rash** (B/L symmetrical but never vesicular) - Condylomata lata, moth eaten alopecia

72. B i.e. Penicillin *[Ref: Rook's 8/e p. 34.22/23; Harrison 18/e p. 1386-87]*

Penicillin is the only recommended agent for treatment of syphilis in pregnancy[Q]. If the patient has a documented penicillin allergy, *desensitization and penicillin therapy* should be given.

73. A i.e. Seropositive infant not treated at birth if mother received penicillin in 3rd trimester; E i.e. Sulfonamides and auinolones are 2nd line drugs

Others

74. C i.e. Herpes > A i.e. Candida infection *[Ref: Fitzpatrick's 6/e p-2164-2212; Rooks 7/e p.30.1-30.30, 25.20-39]*

STD	Required **T/t of Sexual partner**
Herpes	- **None** ie Avoid sex & use condomes
Candida	- **None; ie only topical t/t if** Candidal dermatitis of penis is detected
Bacterial Vaginosis (ex. gardnerella)	- T/t given only when STD present - T/t of parterner does not prevent recurrance of ds.
Trichomonas vaginalis	- Sexual partner *is always treated*[Q] as it reduces risk of recurrance reservoir.

75. A i.e. Diabetes mellitus *[Ref: Dermatological signs of internal diseases by Collen, Jorizzo P-177; IADVL- Textbook & Atlas of Dermatology 2/e Vol I P-1492; Fitzpatrick's 6/e p-2164-2212; Rooks 7/e p.30.1-30.30, 25.20-39]*

- Inflamation of the glans penis is called **Balanitis** & that of mucousal surface of prepuce is called **prosthitis.** Inflamation of both prepuce & glans is called **Balano prosthitis**.
- ***Diabetes mellitus***[Q] causes ***recurrent balanoprosthitis***[Q]

76. B, D, E > C, A i.e. Herpes simplex virus, Treponema pallidum, Lymphogranuloma venereum > HIV, Human papilloma virus *[Ref: Nena Khanna 3/ed p-280]*

- Any of the blistering (or ulcerating) disorders of skin can occur on genital (eg. vulva & vaina) and cause ulceration.
  Chronic genital ulcerations may be seen in epidermolysis bullosa, Hailey- Hailey diseas, Darier's disease, nymphohymenal tears, dermatitis artefacta, radiation damage, TB, actinomycosis, LGV, Lichen planus, LS, lupus erythematosus, pyoderma gangrenosum, hidradenitis suppurativa, Crohn's disease, and malignancy (squamous, basal cell, melanoma & Langerhans cell histocytosis)
- Common causes of genital ulcers ***include syphilis (T. palladium), LGV***[Q], chanchoid, donovanosis & ***herpes genitalis (HSV-II)***[Q]. But HIV and HPV may also l/t genital ulcers.

77. C i.e. Chancroid, Primary Chancre and herpes simplex *[Ref: Neena Khanna 4/e p. 322, 300]*

STDs presenting with ***genital ulcers include herpes genitalis (by HSV typeII), primary syphilis (primary chncre), chancroid and donovanosis***[Q]. And syndromic management of genital ulcers include if **vesicle or multiple painful ulcers.**

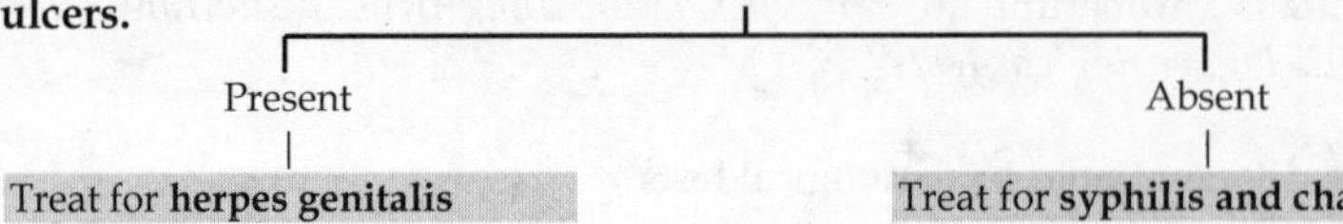

13 GENODERMATOSES & DEFICIENCY DISEASES

Xeroderma Pigmentosa

- It is an ***autosomal recessive genodermatoses with cellular hypersensitivity to ultraviolet radiation***Q & certain chemical agents including drugs (psoralens, chlorpromazine), carcinogens (benzo [α] pyrene derivatives found in cigarette smoke) and cancer chemotherapeutic agents (cisplatin, carmustine)
- UV rays & chemicals damage DNA d/t production of covalent linkage between adjacent pyrimidines. Normally damaged DNA is repaired by ***nucleotide excision & repair (NER) pathway but in XP, NER is defective***Q. So clinical presentation includes:

Skin involvement

- ***Photosensitivity is hallmark***Q of the disease, causing *acute sunburn* reaction on minimal UV exposure and numerous *freckle-like hyperpigmented* macules – predominantly on sun exposed areas in children
- **Dry** parchment like **pigmented skin**, hence the name XP.
- > 1000 fold ***increased risk of cutaneous basal cell carcinoma, squamous cell carcinoma or melanoma***Q in <20 years of age.
- 10-20 fold increase in internal neoplasms eg. brain, spinal cord, lung, testis, leukemia etc.
- ***Premature death***Q.

Ocular involvement

- Lid develop hyperpigmentation , loss of lashes, skin atrophy, ectropion, & cancers
- *Conjuctival infection* l/t photophobia
- Keratitis l/t corneal opacification & vascularization.

Neurological involvement

- Mild eg. hyporeflexia or severe eg. mental retardation, sensorineural deafness, spasticity & seizures.
- **Dc Sanctis – Cacchione syndrome** is most severe form with skin & ocular involvement plus microcephalus, mental retardation, low IQ, hypo or a-reflexia, choreoathetosis, ataxia, spasticity, Achilles tendon shortening & eventually l/t quadriparesis, dwarfism & immature sexual development.

Incontinentia Pigmenti / Bloch-Sulzberger Syndrome

- It is ***X- linked dominant***Q disorder d/t *mutation of NEMO* [nuclear factor kB (NF-kB) essential modulator] gene in chromosome Xq28. NF-kB protects against tumor necrosis factor induced apoptosis.
- ***Primarily females are affected***Q as it is believed to be embryonically lethal in majority of males.
- Typical cutaneous **linear lesions along lines of Blaschko,** follow 4 stages, which may sometimes overlap

	1 Vesicular stage	2 Verrucous stage	3 Hyper pigmented stage	4. Hypopigmented (atrophic) Stage
Timming	Lesions *present at birth or shortly* there after in first few (usually 2) *weeks* and resolve within several months.	Lesion develop *between 2-8 weeks* & resolve over weeks to months.	Lesions develop *within first few months* of life & resolve slowly by *adolescence*	Usually develop during adolescence and persist into adulthood. But rarely may start in infancy
Prevalance	90-95% of patients	70-80%	90-98%	30-75%
Lesion	Lesion consists of **linear streaks & plaques of erythematous (red) vesicles & papules on an erythematous base.** Predominantly on extremities but may also occur on trunk or on head & neck	*Thickened, warty appearing linear & whorled plaques on an erythematous base* *Usually on extremities & trunk* but may also be on head & neck	***Brown or slate grey hyperpigmentation appears in linear streaks, whorls, flecks & reticulated patches***Q. ***Hyperpigmentation usually involve & is most pronounced on trunk***Q, but may also involve the extremeties, skin folds or head & neck. *Axilla & groin* are invariably affected. The sites of involvement are *not necessarily those of preceding* vesicular & warty lesions. Pigmentation persists throughout childhood, begin to fade by early adolescence and often disappear by age 16.	***Anhidrotic, hairless, atrophic, hypopigmented linear patches or streaks***Q develop as a late manifestation. Usually seen on ***the calves of lower extremities***Q
Histology	Epidermal edema & eosinophil filled intradermal vesicles Blood eosinophilia as high as 65%	Epidermal hyperplasia hyperkeratosis & papillomatosis	1. *Vacuolization & degeneration* in epidermal *basal cell layer* 2. Extensive deposits of *melanin in basal cell layer & dermis* 3. Melanin laden macrophage	1. Thinner epidermis 2. Decreased or absent skin appendages in dermis (l/t hypopigmentation) 3. Normal or rarely decreased number of melanocytes.
Pathophysiology	Number of NEMO deficient cells decreases d/t apoptosis (and normal cells increase). Hence the *vesicular & inflammatory stage* ends.	*Hyper proliferation* is d/t proliferation of normal NEMO keratinocytes l/t dry *hyperkeratotic verrucous plaques.*	*Incontinence of melanin* pigment from epidermis into dermis l/t *hyperpigmentation,*	Hypopigmentation is d/t *dermal scarring*

★ May be associated with ocular, dental (delayed & abnormal), skeletal and CNS (microcephaly, mental retardation, seizures) anomalies.

- **Incontinenta pigmenti** *primarily involving skin*Q with neurological, *ophthalmic and dental manifestations in few (not all) cases*Q. Manifestations include-

Skin (Cutaneous)

- Four stages of linear vesicular, verrucous, hyperpigmented and hypopigmented-atrophic lesions along Blaschko lines, in **30-95% cases**
- Abnormal dermatoglyphic patterns
- Hair changes include *scarring alopecia* (in 30-40%), sparse hair in early childhood, & lusterless, wiry and coarse hair later, or rarely hypoplasia or absence of eyebrows & eyelashes.
- Nail changes occur in **7-40%** cases and include *nail dystrophy* (which ranges from mild pitting & ridging of nail plate to hyperkeratosis and onycholysis) and *can improve* with age.
- Usually involve multiple finger nails, more than toe nails.
- Subungal & periungal keratotic tumors with pain, bony deformity & lytic lesions involving underlying phalanges may be seen in older children & adults.

Extracutaneous Features

Dental (80-90%)

- Seen in **80%** patients and involve both deciduous & permanent teeth.
- Delayed dentition, partial adontia, & conical or pegged teeth are most common findings
- Anomalies are *permanent* and thus serve as useful diagnostic aid in older patient.
- Delayed eruption of teeth
- Hypo (micro) dontia
- Partial adontia
- Cone- or peg-shaped teeth
- Absence of teeth in apparently unaffected first degree relatives
- Micro/pro-gnathhia

Bone (30-40%)

- Skull and palatal defects
- Hemiverterbra, spina bifida, scoliosis
- Syndactyly, acheiria (congenital absence of hands)
- Extra ribs

Hematological

- Blood eosinophilia (in acute skin inflammatory stage)
- Neutrophil and lymphocyte dysfunction

Neurological/ CNS (30-40%)

- Seen in **30%** patients & often manifest within neonatal period.
- *Seizure* is the most common manifestation.
- Other features d/t microvascular vaso oclusive ischemia include developmental delay, mental retardation, ataxia, spastic paralysis, microcephaly, cerebral atrophy, porencephaly, hypoplasia of corpus callosum and periventricular cerebral edema.
- Mirocephaly, mental retardation,
- Motor delay, spastic paralysis, seizures, ataxia
- Hydrocephaly, hyperactivity, encephalopathy.

Immunological, Hair, Nails

- Altered Immunological reactivity
- Scarring alopecia
- Onychodystrophy (nail dysplasia), subungal keratotic tumor.

Ophthalmological/ Ocular (20-35%)

- *Seen in 20-35% of patients and involvement is commonly asymmetrical*Q.
- Become evident within first few weeks to months of life.
- ***Retinal vaso occlusive ischemia is primary mechanism***Q l/t retinal detachment, proliferative retinopathy, fibrovascular retrolental membranes, foveal hypoplasia, vitreous hemorrhages and atrophy of ciliary body.
- Non retinal manifestations include strabismus, optic nerve atrophy, conjuctival pigmentation, micropthalmia, keratitis, cataract, iris hypoplasia, nystagmus & uveitis
- Permanent blindness develop in 70%.
- Asymmetrical retina pigmentary changes with **mottled diffuse hypopigmentation** and abnormal peripheral retina vessels with areas of non perfusion (i.e **avascularity of peripheral retina) are pathognomic.**
- Retinal detachment, proliferative retinopathy, fibrovascular retinal membrane
- Micropthalmos, optic atrophy, cataracts, retrolental mass (Pseudoglioma or retinoblastoma with intraocular calcification), leukocoria, band keratopathy, blindness.
- Strabismus, congenital glaucoma, blue sclera.

Neurofibromatoses (NF)

It is **phakomatoses** (neuro ectodermatoses or neurocutaneous disorder) involving skin & nervous system. It is of several types.

NF type 1 (Von Reckling hausen disease)

- ***Autosomal dominant***Q disorder d/t mutation of tumor suppressor NF-1 gene on long arm of *chromosome 17*; that encodes ***neurofibromin protein***, which modulates signal transduction through RAS- GTP ase pathway. Neurofibromin is a *negative regulator of RAS* and is found in *neurons, oligodendrocytes & non- myelinating Schwann cells.*
- **Diagnostic criteria**: ≥ 2 of 7
  1. **Six or more (≥6) cafe – au- lait macules > 5 mm** in greatest diameter in *prepubertal* and **> 15 mm** in *post pubertal* individuals.
  2. **Two or more (≥2) neurofibromas** of any type or one or more (≥1) **plexiform neurofibroma**
  3. ***Freckling in axillae or inguinal area***Q
  4. Optic glioma

NF type 2

- ***Autosomal dominant***Q disorder d/t mutation of tumor suppressor NF_2 *gene* on *chromosome 22q*, which encodes membrane related protein **merlin (schwannomin or neurofibromin-2)**.
- It is characterized by ***bilateral vestibular schwannomas***Q, other Schwannomas (dorsal root of spinal cord, peripheral & cranial nerves), meningiomas (intracranial, intraspinal & optic nerve sheath), **ependymomas & gliomas** of CNS, and ***juvenile posterior sub capsular cataract***Q
- Retinal hamartomas, epiretinal, membranes & optic nerve sheath meningioma are other ophthalmic

5. Two or more (≥2) ***iris –lisch nodules***Q
6. A distinctive osseous lesion such as
   - Sphenoid wing dysplasia or
   - Congenital bowing or
   - Thinning of long bone cortex (with or without pseudoarthrosis)
7. First degree relative (parent, sibling or offspring) with NF-1 by above criteria.

- Complications include: ***Scoliosis***Q, *localized bony overgrowth, vasculopathy* affecting any artery (causing renal artery stenosis & hypertension, cerebral infarct, bleeding aneurysms & intermittent claudication), *intelligence & learning disabilities* (eg. visual – perceptual defecits & verbal disabilities, ADH, low IQ – 5-10 points) and ***unidentified brigh objects (UBO)*** or **Foci of abnormal signal intensity (FASI)** in internal capsule, basal ganglia, cortex, cerebellar hemisphere, optic tract & brain stem an T-2 weighted images of MRI (d/t myelin vacuolization & ↑ water content; present in children but disappear with age).
- Cancers eg. pheochromocytoma, rhabdomyosarcoma, somatostatinomas of duodenum & ampulla of vater & GI stromal tumors etc. are increased.

findings

- *Children* are more apt to present with a *non- 8th nerve tumor* such as optic nerve sheath meningiomas.
- Less common but more morbid (than N-F1) presenting with hearing loss, tinnitus, loss of balance, paralysis, café-au-lait (<6 usually), and cutaneous Schwannoma & neurofibromas.
- **Diagnostic criteria: If any one is present**
  1. ***Bilateral vestibular schwannomas***Q
  2. *1st degree relative with NF2 and unilateral vestibular schwannoma* or *any 2* or following; *meningioma, glioma, neurofibroma, Schwannoma or posterior subcapsular lenticular opacities* (cataract)
  3. Unilateral vestibular schwannoma & any 2 of following : meningioma, glioma, neurofibroma, schwannoma or posterior subcapsular lenticular opacities (cataract)
  4. Multiple (≥2) meningiomas & unilateral vestibular schwannoma and any 2 of following: Schwannoma, glioma, neurofibroma, cataract.

CALM / Café' au lait Macules

- It is localized hyperpigmentation due to local increase in pigment production.
- It is *most commonly seen in – neurofibromatosis and Mc Cune – Albright syndrome;* but can also be associated with pulmonary stenosis (Watson syndrome), tuberous sclerosis, **LEOPARD [L**entigines; **E**CG abnormalities – primary conduction defects; **O**cular hypertelorism; **P**ulmonary stenosis and subaortic valvular stenosis; **A**bnormal genitalia – (cryptorchidism, hypospadias); **R**etardation of growth; and **D**eafness (sensoirineural)**]** syndrome (in leopard syndrome hundreds of lentigines develop during childhood and are scattered over the entire surface of body) and MEN (multiple endocrinal neoplasia).
- CALM are flat, uniformly light brown in colour, and can vary in size form 0.5 to 12 cm. 80% of patients with **type I NF** will have *six or more CALM measuring ≥ 1.5 cm in diameter.* In comparison with NF, that CALM in patients with Mc Cune Albright syndrome [Polyostotic fibrous dysplasia, with precocious puberty in females] are usually larger, more irregular in outline, and tend to respect midline.
- **Neurofibromatosis type I (Von Reclinghausen's disease)** is characterized by ***cutaneous neurofibromas, pigmented lesions of skin called café au lait spots, frecking in non exposed areas such as axilla, hamartomas of the iris termed Lisch nodules and pseudoarthrosis of tibia.*** Neurofibromas are benign peripheral nerve tumors composed of proliferating Schwann cells and fibroblasts. Neurofibromas are clinically seen as soft papules or nodules that exhibit the "button hole" sign, that is, they invaginate into the skin with pressure in a manner similar to hernia. Neurofibromas are asymptomatic, unless they grow in an enclosed space.

Tuberous Sclerosis / Bourneville's Disease

- It is ***autosomal dominant***Q disorder occurring with equal frequency in different sexes, races & ethnicities. **Sporadic disease** (d/t new mutation) occurs in 2/3 and hereditary transmission in 1/3 cases.
- It presents with classical **Vogt's triad** of ***epilepsy, mental retardation and adenoma sebaceum (angiofibroma)***Q. Hence the disease is also k/a acronym **Epiloia** (i.e. **Epi** = Epilepsy, **loi** = low intelligence, **a** = adenoma sebaceum)
- Clinical features include :

Cutaneous lesions

Adenoma sebacium (Angiofibroma of face)

- Is *most common manifestation* (~ 90%)
- Reddish brown (pink- yellow) *smooth dome shaped papules* with fine *telangiectasia* located symmetrically on *nasolabial folds, cheeks, chin (central face)* and occasionally on forehead, scalp & ear.
- Location & colour suggest origin from sebaceous glands but these actually are benign hamartomas of fibrous & vascular tissue (angiofibroma)

Oral lesions

- **Multiple dental enamel pitting** in upto 100% patients
- Oral fibromas

Neurological lesions

- Cerebral lesions include ***subependymal nodules, subendymal giant cell astrocytoma and cortical tubers***Q ***(which may calcify)***
- Manifest as ***seizures (infantile spasm), mental retardation***Q, hydrocephalus, behaviour disorders & ***delayed milestones***Q.

- Rare at birth, may appear by ages 2 – 5 and proliferate in puberty.

Hypomelanotic macules (Ash leaf, Stippled or Confetti shaped spots)

- *Appear at birth or shortly there* after to be observed in ~ 90% of children making it ***most useful in early diagnosis***[Q]
- Can be located anywhere but tend to occur **on *trunk & buttocks.*** When located on scalp, cause *poliosis*.
- Are often ***off white and biopsy shows melanocytes***[Q] differentiating it from completely depigmented vitiligo.
- Confetti shaped skin lesion occurs on legs below knees or on forearms and consists of multiple hypopigmented macules (2- 3 mm diameter).

Shagreen patch

- Firm or rubbery *irregular plaque of 1-10 cm* with a colour of surrounding skin, pink or yellow brown
- Surface may appear *bumpy with coalescing papules & nodules* (leathery cobble stoned) or may have **orange peel appearance**.
- Most commonly found *on **lower back & buttocks (lumbo-sacral region)***[Q] or less commonly on thighs.

Ungual fibromas or **Koenen's tumor**

- More common on toes than on fingers
- Arise from under the proximal nail fold (**periungal fibroma**) and under nail plate (subungal fibromas)

Fibrous facial plaque

- It is irregular connective tissue nevus of normal skin, red or hyperpigmented colour.

Other skin lesions

- **Molluscum fibrosum pendulum** (skin tags or multiple fibroepithelial polyps),
- ***Café – au- lait macules (<6)***[Q], appendageal tumors (trichoepitheliomas, syringocyst adenomas), lipomas, fibromyolipomas & neurofibromas.

★ **Iris nodule** is ***a feature of neurofibromatosis not tuberous sclerosis***[Q]

Benign neoplasms

- ***Cardiac rhabdomyoma***[Q] causing Wolff- Parkinson-White syndrome
- ***Angiomyolipoma of kidney***[Q], liver, pancreas etc.
- **Lymphangio leiomyomatosis** (LAM), multi focal micronodular pneumocyte hyperplasia & clear cell tumor of lung
- ***Retinal astrocytic hamartomas***[Q] & opaque multinodular mulberry lesions
- Rectal polyp
- Astrocytoma & ependymoma
- **Hamartomas** of skin, brain, kidney, heart, retina etc.

Cystic lesions

- ***Multiple renal cyst***[Q]
- Bone cyst

Mnemonic = "**MASK**"

M
- Multiple renal cyst
- Multiple dental enamel pitting
- Molluscum fibrosum pendulum (Multiple fibroepithelial polyps)
- Mental retardation

A
- Ash leaf hypomelanotic macules
- Adenoma sebaceum (Angiofibroma of face)
- Angiolipoma & Astrocytoma

S
- Shagreen patch
- Subependymal nodule, & giant cell astrocytoma

K
- Koenen's ungula fibromas

Causes of Icthyosis

Metabolic disorders

Lipid metabolism

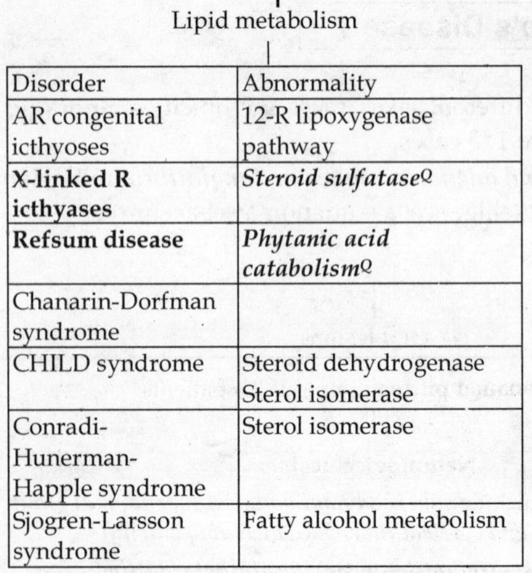

Disorder	Abnormality
AR congenital icthyoses	12-R lipoxygenase pathway
X-linked R icthyases	***Steroid sulfatase***[Q]
Refsum disease	***Phytanic acid catabolism***[Q]
Chanarin-Dorfman syndrome	
CHILD syndrome	Steroid dehydrogenase Sterol isomerase
Conradi-Hunerman-Happle syndrome	Sterol isomerase
Sjogren-Larsson syndrome	Fatty alcohol metabolism

- **Ca^{++}- dependent ATPase** abnormality
  - Darier disease
  - ***Hailey –Haiely disease (Benign familial chronic pemphigus)***[Q]
- **Transcription defect**
  - Trichothiodystrophy
- **Gap junction protein: Connexin (intercellular communication) defect**
  - Erythrokeratodermia variabitis
  - KID (keratitis, icthyosis, deafness) syndrome
  - Vohwinkel syndrome
  - PPK with deafness
- **Protein metabolism defect**
  - Netherton syndrome (protease inhibitor)
  - Papillon Lefevre syndrome (protease defect)

Acquired

- Leprosy
- Clofazimine
- ***Hypothyroidism***[Q]
- Nutritional deficiencies
- Sarcoidosis
- ***Lymphoma***[Q]
- ***AIDS***[Q]

Feature	Ichthyosis vulgaris	Icthyosis nigra	Lamellar icthyosis	Nonbullous icthyosiform erythroderma
Inheritance	***Autosomal dominant***Q i.e. an affected parent	***X linked recessive i.e. only males are affected***Q	***Autosomal recessive***Q i.e. parents are unaffected in most & consanguinity (familial marriage) is present.	
Gender	Both sexes	*Males*Q (mostly)	Both sexes	Both sexes
Onset	In 1st *few years*	At birth	At birth	At birth
Course	May improve at adolescence	Persists throughout life	Persists life long	Persists life long
Character of scales	Small & branny	***Large, adherent & brown to black***Q (hence **icthyosis nigra**)	Presence of **collodion membrane** at birth which is shed over a period of weeks Large brown adherent thick pasted (plate like) scales Erythema is minimal or absent, but when present *usually on face*	**Presence** of **collodion membrane** at birth which is shed over a period of weeks Small branny scales *Marked generalized erythema*
Site of predilection	- Mainly extensors - ***Flexures spared***Q	*Generalized* *Flexures encroached*Q	**Generalized** Flexures encroached & show continuous linear rippling	**Generalized**
Associated with	Hyperlinear palms & soles Keatosis pilaris Atopic diathesis	***Cryptorchidism***Q Corneal opacity (comma shaped)	Palmoplantar keratoderma (PPKD) is frequent Heat intolerance Ectropion, eclabium & crumpled ears	PPKD **less** frequent Heat intolerance
Defect	FLG gene Absence of filaggrin	STS gene ***Steroid sulfetase defeciency***Q l/t accumulation of cholesterol sulfate	Abnormal genes encoding for *transglutaminase 1, SNARE, icthyin, arachidonate lipoxygenase 3 & arachidonate 12 lipoxygenase R pathways* etc.	
Histopathology	Hyperkeratosis with ***reduced or absent granular layer***Q	Hyperkeratosis ***with hypergranulosis***Q	Hyperkeratosis, *acanthosis*, may show- parakeratosis	

Palmoplantar – Keratodermas (PPKs)

PPKs are a heterogenous group of disorders characterized by ***abnormal thickening of plans and soles***Q. It may be 1) **diffuse** (involving whole of plam or sole); 2) **focal** (in which large, compact keratin masses develop at sites of recurrent firiction); 3) **punctuate** (tiny rain drop keratos in creases or whole surface develop); 4) **transgradient** (extends beyond pp skin to pressure points on fingers, kuckeles or else where); 5) **complex** (a/w lesions of nonvolar skin, hair, nails, teeth and/or sweet glands including ectodermal dysplasias); and 6) **syndromic** (a/w abnormalities of other organs viz deafness, cardiomyophathy and cancer). PPKs may be.

Congenital

- Diffuse epidermolytic (Vorner's)/or nonepidermolytic (Thost-Unna) PPK
- Transgredient Keratodermas
  - Loricrin K (Camisa's/Varient Vohwinkel's syndrome/mutilating keratoderma with icthyosis)
  - Greither's syndrome, Sybert's K
  - Huriez syndrome (K with scleroatrophy)
  - Mal de meleda (KPP transgrediens/acroerythrokeratoderma)
  - Olmsted's syndrome (congenital PP and perioral severe cicatrizing K)
- Focal Keratodermas (Wachter's K/PPK varians)
- Pachyonychia congenital (Jackson-Lawler/Jadassohn-Lewandowsky syndrome)

Acquired

- Keratodermas caused by other dermatosis
  - ***Psoriasis***Q (scalloped margins = Festonne, Caro-Senear lesions = depressed plaques on sides of fingers and involvement of kunckles)
  - ***Reiter's disease***Q (compact, heaped up lesions resembling heads of nails = **keratoderma blenorrhagica** suggest dx)
  - ***Pityriasis rubra pilaris***Q (yellow hyperkeratosis with acute follicular eruption in adults and lesions on kees and elbows on children).
  - **Extensive hyperkeratotic eczema** (marked itching)
  - **Trichophytosis** (esp Trichophyton rubrum, is u/l and lack inflammatory sign)
  - **Crusted scabies**

- Striate (Brunauer-Fuhs-Siemens) keratoderma
- Hidrotic ectodermal dysplasia (Clouston's syndrome)
- Tylosis/Keratoderma with oesophageal cancer (Howel-Evan's syndrome)
- Cicatrizing K.with hearing impairment (Keratoma hereditarum mutilans/Vohwinkel's syndrome)
- Papillon Lefevre syndrome (K with peridontitis)
- Schopf- Schulz passarge syndrome (K With eyelid cyst/hypodontia and hypotrichosis)
- Oculocutaneous tyrosinaemia (tyrosinemia type II/ tyrosine-transaminase def/Richner-Hanhart syndrome)
- Punctate and porokeratotic (Brauer-Buschke-Fischer) K
- Filiform (Music box spine) K
- Marginal papular K/mosaic acral keratosis
- Aquagenic syringeal acrokertoderma
- Acro-osteolysis with K (Bureau-Barriere syndrome)

  - **Secondary syphilis**, hyperkeratotic late syphilides
  - **Late yaws** (crab like gait)
  - Viral warts (in immune compromised)/HPV
  - Lupus erythematosus
  - Immuno bullous disorder (with antidesmocollin 3 anti bodies)
  - Lichen planus and lichen nitidus
  - HIV associated keratoderma
  - Calluses and corns (clavi)
- Drug induced kertoderma
  - Hypersensitivity to iodine
  - Tegafur, glucan, lithium, and halogenated weed killers and dioxin intoxication.
  - Arsenic keratosis
- *Keratoderma climcterium (Haxthausen's disease)*
- PPK with myxoedema
- Lympoedematous keratoderma (e.g. in filaria)

DEFICIENCY DISEASES

Acrodermatitis Enteropathica (AE)

- A rare ***autosomal recessive (AR) disorder***[Q] characterized by abnormalities in zinc absorption d/t defect in intestinal zinc transporter, the human *ZIP- 4 protein* l/t ***zinc deficiency***[Q].
- Classically present during infancy on weaning from breast milk to formula or cereal which have lower zinc bioavailability than breast milk. Acquired AE may also dvelop if breast milk zinc levels is < 70 μ/dL (<12 μ mol/L). In such cases infant is symptomatic, while breast feeding & improve after weaning. Non breast fed infants develop AE during 4th- 10th week of life.
- Classical features of AE include: **Mn – "DEAL"**
  - Diarrhea[Q] , Depression
  - ***Eczematous erosive dermatitis***[Q] of *acute* onset, *symmetrical* distribution favoring **acral areas** – periorificial regions (perioral, periocular, perineal around nose genitals & anus), hands & feet. Over time vesicle *bullae & erosions with a characteristic peripheral crusted border develop.*
  - ***Alopecia (non scarring)***[Q], Apathetic look
  - Lethergy , irritability, whining & crying
- Acute hemorrhagic paronychia, Blepharitis, Conjunctivitis, Delayed wound healing (i.e. **ABCD**) and photophobia may also be observed.
- Subacute or chronic mild deficiency l/t growth retardation, hypogonadism, dysgeusia, poor appetite, poor wound healing, abnormal dark adaptation & impaired mentation.
- Normal plasma Zn levels is 70- 250 μg/dL. ***A low plasma zinc level is gold standard for diagnosis***[Q]. Serum AP – a zinc dependent enzyme is another useful indicator of zinc status.
- **Zn supplementation** with enteral (Zn sulfate) or parenteral (Zn- chloride) formula ***rapidly improves AE***[Q] in several days. In children 0.5-1.0 mg/kg of elemental zinc is given. Serum Zn is monitored during therapy d/t fear of Zn toxicity (i.e. *nausea, vomiting, lethargy, dizziness, dehydration, neuropathy & hypocupremia but no skin manifestations*). AE patients require *life long treatment*.

Miscellaneous

Lesion	Found In
Erythema Pernio (Chill blain) **Erythema marginatum** **Erythema migrans**	Cold ***Rheumatic fever***[Q] ***Lyme borreliosis***[Q]
Rose spots	***Systemic salmonella infection (enteric fever or typhoid)***[Q]
Lupus pernio & Epitheloid granuloma **Lupus profundus** Lupus Vulgaris	***Sarcoid***[Q] ***SLE***[Q] Skin TB
Phrynoderma **Sauroderma/Crocodile Skin**	***Vit. A def. /Essential fatty acid deficiency***[Q] ***Icthyosis Vulgaris***[Q]

Disease	Most Common Site
Morphea **Richl's melanosis**	***Forehead***[Q] ***Face & neck***[Q]
Fordyce Disease Peutz Jegher Syndrome (Pigmentation)	Lips Lips and Oral Mucosa
Acne, Impetigo, Herpes Simplex	Face Face
Herpes Zooster	Thorax

Weldt sores	*Desert areas*Q
Balck hairy tongue	Broad spectrum Antibiotics
Comadones	*Acne Vulgaris*Q
Koplik's spot, Coimpy's sign, Warthein fankeldy cell, Postauricular rash (1st)Q	*Measels*Q
Rhinophyma (glandular hyper trophy)	*Acne rosacae*Q
Darrier sign	*Uriticaria pigmentosa*Q
Pseudo Darrier Sign	Smooth Muscles Hypertrophy
Spongiosis	*Acute Eczema*Q
Xantheasma	Hypercholestemia
Oral Hairy Leukoplakia	*AIDS (not candidiasis)* Q
Rain drop pigmentation	*Chronic Arsenic Poisioning*Q
Pyoderma Gangrenosa	*Ulcerative Colitis*Q
Slapped Cheek appearance, Net like pattern erythema	*Erythema infectiosum*Q
Honey Crust	*Impetigo*Q
Angiod Streak	*Pseudoxanthoma Elasticum*Q
Axillary freckling & Lischnodule (Iris hamartoma)	*Neurofibromatosis*Q
Leonine face	Leprosy
Cardle cap appearance in	Seborrhoic Dermatitis (Pityriasis capitis)
Coyenne pepper stippling (d/t hemosidirin)	*Plasma cell balenitis of Zoom*Q

Herpes gestationales	Periumblical region
Shagreen Patch	*Lumbosacral*Q
Mongolian Spots	*Sacral > gluteal & lumbar*Q
Necrobiosis diabeticorum	Front of legs
Atopic dermatitis	*Antecubital & popletial fossa*Q

Questions

Xeroderma Pigmentosa

1. **Defective DNA repair is a/w** *(AIIMS Nov 09)*
   A. Albinism ☐
   B. Xeroderma pigmentosa ☐
   C. Vitiligo ☐
   D. Icthyosis ☐
2. **Genodermal disease that can cause skin malignancy are**
   A. Xeroderma pogmentosa *(DNB 98, PGI 03)* ☐
   B. Neurofibromatosis ☐
   C. Actinic keratosis ☐
   D. Porphyria cutanea tarda ☐
3. **Cells cultured from patients with this disorder exhibit low activity for the nucleotide excision repair process. This autosomal recessive genetic disease includes marked sensitivity to sunlight (Ultra voilet light) with subsequent formation of multiple skin cancers and premature death, the disorder is:**
   A. Acute intermittent Porphyria ☐
   B. Alkaptonuria *(Karnatak 98, TN 03, UP 02)* ☐
   C. Xeroderma Pigmentosa ☐
   D. Ataxia – Telangiectasa ☐

Incontinentia Pigmenti

4. **A girl child with verrucous lesions at an age of 2 weeks later on developed linear bands of hyperkeratotic papules and nodules followed by whorled pigmentation. Her mother had history of in utero child death and hypopigmented atrophic linear lesions. The diagnosis is**
   A. Neurofibromatosis *(AIIMS May 08)* ☐
   B. Xeroderma pirmentosa ☐
   C. Tuberous sclerosis ☐
   D. Incontinentia pigmenti ☐
5. **2-month-old girl present with verrucous plaque on the trunk. What is your most probable diagnosis?**
   A. Incontinentia pigmentosa *(AIIMS Nov 08, DNB 01)* ☐
   B. Darier disease ☐
   C. Congenital naevus ☐
   D. Icthyosis ☐
6. **The mode of inheritance of incontinentia pigment is :**
   A. Autosomal dominant *(Kerala 04, J&K 07, UP 06)* ☐
   B. Autosomal recessive ☐
   C. X- linked dominant ☐
   D. X- linked recessive ☐
7. **True about incontinenta pigmenti include the following except:** *(AI 09, CMC 08, AIIMS May 11)*
   A. X-linked dominant ☐
   B. Primary skin abnormality ☐
   C. Avascularity of peripheral retina ☐
   D. Ocular involvement is seen in almost 100% cases and is typically unilateral ☐

Neurofibromatosis

8. **Neurofibromatosis all are true except** *(AIIMS May 09)*
   A. Autosomal recessive ☐
   B. Scoliosis ☐
   C. Neurofibroma ☐
   D. Association with cataract ☐
9. **The pathognomonic sign of neurofibromatosis is :***(AI 89)*
   A. Cafe-au-lait macules ☐

B. Axillary frekling
C. Shagreen patch
D. None of the above

10. Lisch nodule is seen in : *(PGI 99)*
A. Von Reclinghausens disease
B. Lupus vulgaris
C. Leprosy
D. LGV

11. A patient had seven irregular hyperpigmented macules on the trunk and multiple small hyperpigmented macules in the axillae and groins since early childhood. There were no other skin lesions. Which is the most likely investigation to support the diagnosis?
A. Slit lamp examination of eye *(AI 06, DNB 02)*
B. Measurement of intraocular tension
C. Examination of fundus
D. Retinal artery angiography

12. Child with h/o hypopigmented macule on back, infantile spasm and delayed milestone has
A. NF *(AIIMS 02, CMC 05, DNB 07)*
B. Sturge weber syndrome
C. Tuberous sclerosis
D. Nevus anemicus.

13. All are seen in Tuberous sclerosis except *(AI 2K)*
A. Iris Nodule
B. Renal Cortical Cyst
C. Rhabdomyoma of heart and lung
D. Adenoma Sebaceum

14. Adenoma sebaceum is a feature of: *(AIIMS Nov 05)*
A. Neurofibromatosis *(UPSC 02)*
B. Tuberous sclerosis
C. Xanthomatosis
D. Incontinenetia pigmenti

15. Babloo a 4 year male presents with history of seizures. On examination there is hypopigmented patches on face & mental retardation. Most probable diagnosis is:
A. Neurofibromatosis *(AIIMS 2000)*
B. Tuberous sclerosis
C. Sturge Weber Syndrome
D. Incontinenta Pigmenti

16. Ash leaf maculae is found in :
A. Tuberous sclerosis *(Jharkhand 05)*
B. Neurofibromatosis
C. Lymphangioma
D. None

17. Koenen's periungual fibromas are seen in > 50% of cases with : *(JIPMER 02)*
A. Tuberous sclerosis
B. Sturge weber syndrome
C. Alaxia telangiectasia
D. Neurofibroatosis

18. All are true regarding tuberous sclerosis except
A. Autosomal dominant sporadic transmission
B. Vogt triad of epiloia *(PGI- June 08)*
C. Café au lait macules exclude the diagnosis
D. Fibrous facial plaque
E. Stippled confetti spots.

Icthyosis

19. Inheritence of ichthyosis vulgaris is : *(AI 93)*
A. X linked dominant
B. X linked recessive
C. Autosomal dominant
D. Autosomal recessive

20. Crocodile skin or sauroderma is seen in :
A. Toxic epidermal necrolysis *(AIIMS 96, DNB 97)*
B. Psoriasis
C. Darier's disease
D. Ichthyosis vulgaris

21. Granular layer is absent in: *(Orissa 98)*
A. Ichtyosis vugaris
B. X linked ichthyosis
C. Epidermolytic hyper keratosis
D. Lamellar ichthyosis

22. A male child with cryptorchidism presents with large black scales on body flexures. Skin biopsy showed hyper granulosis & steroid sulfatase deficiency. Probable diagnosis is: *(SGPGI 08)*
A. Icthysois vulgaris
B. Icthyosis –lamellar
C. X linked icthyosis nigra
D. Nonbullous icthyosiform erythroderma

23. Icthyosis is associated with: *(UP 06, CUPGEE 96)*
A. Hodgkins disease
B. AIDS
C. Hypothyroidism
D. All

24. Ichthysis is caused by: *(Bihar 06, Nimhans 01, DNB 99)*
A. Hemosiderosis
B. Refsum disease
C. Niacin deficiency
D. Steven johnson syndrome

25. Keratomdrma is/are seen in *(PGI May 11)*
A. Pemphigus
B. Pityriasis rosea
C. Pityriasis rubra pilaris
D. Dermatitis herpetiformis
E. Reiter's syndrome

Deficiency Diseases

26. Casal's paint necklace is caused by: *(PGI 97)*
A. Lichen planus
B. Pellagra
C. Pernicious anemia
D. SLE

27. Flaky paint appearence of skin is seen in *(AI 95)*
A. Dermatitis
B. Pellagra
C. Marasmus
D. Kwashiorkar

28. Reccurent oral ulcers with pain and erythematous halo around them, diagnosis is: *(AIIMS 96)*
A. Apthus ulcer
B. Herpes
C. Chicken pox
D. Measels

29. All are true about Achrodermatitis enteropathica except: *(AIIMS Nov 08, May 011)*
A. ↓Zn level (low serum zinc level)
B. Reverse with Zn supplement
C. Triad of acral dermatitis, dementia & diarrhea
D. AR

30. Dermatitis and alopecia are due to deficiency of:
A. Zinc *(SGPGI – 2001)*
B. Molybodenum
C. Magnesium
D. Calcium

31. Acrodermatitis entero pathica is d/t deficiency of:
A. Zn *(AIIMS 93, TN 97)*

B. Se ☐
C. Cu ☐
D. Cr ☐

Miscellaneous

32. The rash in measles occurs first in occurs first in the ..... region : *(Kerala 90)*
A. Forehead ☐
B. Post auricular ☐
C. Chest ☐
D. Neck ☐

33. Erythema marginatum is seen in : *(Bihar 05, Kerala 97)*
A. Drug reactions ☐
B. Typhoid fever ☐
C. Enteric fever ☐
D. Rheumatic fever ☐

34. Rose spot are seen in : (Kerala 98, *UP 06*)
A. Typhus fever ☐
B. Typhoid fever ☐
C. Enteric fever ☐
D. Rheumatic fever ☐

35. 'Slapped cheeks' appearance is seen in:
A. Roseloa infantum *(PGI 98, AIIMS 97)* ☐
B. Erythema subitum ☐
C. Erythema infectiosum ☐
D. Erythema multiforme ☐

36. Phrynoderma is a cutaneous manifest-ation of severe deficiency of vitamin :
A. A (Delhi 99, AMC 98) ☐
B. B ☐
C. C ☐
D. D ☐

37. Veldt sore is most common in -
A. Hilly areas *(JIPMER 98, AMU 99)* ☐
B. Tropical climate ☐
C. Rainy areas ☐
D. Deserts ☐

38. 'Cayenne pepper' stippling due to hemosiderin is found in : *(AI 96)*
A. Erythroplasia of Queyrat ☐
B. Pagets disease ☐
C. Plasma cell balantitis of zoon ☐
D. Metronidazole ☐

39. Common sites of mongolian spot are : *(PGI Dec 08)*
A. Face ☐
B. Neck ☐
C. Lumbo sacral area ☐
D. Leg ☐
E. Thigh ☐

40. Which of the following condition resolves spontaneously in an infant : *(PGI Dec 08)*
A. Erythema toxicum ☐
B. Mongolian spot ☐
C. Lymphoma ☐
D. Milia ☐
E. Port wine stain ☐

41. Erythema toxicum in a neonate indicates- *(PGI 96)*
A. Staphylococcal sepsis ☐
B. Pneumococcemia ☐
C. Drug hypersensitivity ☐
D. Is not of any significance ☐

42. Riehl's melanosis mainly invloves -
A. Face and Neck *(JIPMER 92, AIIMS 92)* ☐
B. Trunk ☐
C. Extremities ☐
D. Palms only ☐

43. M.C. site of Atopic dermatitis *(AIIMS 98)*
A. Scalp ☐
B. Elbow ☐
C. Antecubital fossa ☐
D. Trunk ☐

44. Monogolian spots is usually seen at region- *(AI 98)*
A. Cervicofacial ☐
B. Lumbosacral ☐
C. Deltoid ☐
D. Thoraco lumbar ☐

45. Shagreen patch is usually found in -
A. Face *(AI 98)* ☐
B. Cervical region ☐
C. Limbs ☐
D. Lumbosacral region ☐

46. Morphea occurs usually in: *(Jipmer 97, AIIMS 96)*
A. Forehead ☐
B. Sternum ☐
C. Limbs ☐
D. Back ☐

47. Fine reticular pigmentation with palmar pits are seen in : *(AIIMS May 2011)*
A. Dowling-Degos disease ☐
B. Rothmund Thomson syndrome ☐
C. Cockyane syndrome ☐
D. Bloom's syndrome ☐

Answers and Explanations:

Xeroderma Pigmentosa

1. **B i.e. Xeroderma pigmentosa**
2. **A i.e. Xeroderma pigmentosa** 3. **C i.e. Xeroderma pigmentosa**

[Ref: Rook's dermatology 7/e p-12.56 – 12.60; Roxburgh's 17/e P- 218; Harrison's 17/e p- 324, 327, 546-47, 387; Neena Khanna 3rd/e p- 34; Pasricha textbook of dermatology 3/e p- 14; Fitzpatrick 7/e p. 1315-19]

Xeroderma pigmentosa is an autosomal recessive ***genodermal disease in which DNA repair is defective d/t defective NER (nucleotide excision & repair) pathway***Q. This results in marked ***hypersensitivity to ultraviolet (sun) light, photosensitivity, dry pigmented skin, increased risk of skin malignancy and premature death***Q.

Incontinentia Pigmenti

4. **D. i.e. Incontinentia pigmenti** 5. **A i.e. Incontinentia pigmenti** 6. **C i.e. X linked dominant**
7. **D i.e. Ocular involvement is seen in almost 100% cases and is typically unilateral**

[Ref: Neena Khanna 5/e p- 36; Thomas Habif 4/e p. 580- 81; Fitzpatrick 7/e p. 79, 83, 631, 730, 1058; Harrison's 18/e p-413; Rook's 8/e p 58.15/17; IADVL Dermatology 2/e p- 634]

- **Incontinetia pigmenti (Bloch-Sulzberger Syndrome)** is ***X linked dominant disorder primarily affecting females as it is believed to be embryonically (in utero) lethal in males***Q.
- It is **primarily skin abnormality** presenting with 4 overlaping stages of ***linear or whorled cutaneous lesions along lines of Blaschko***Q. ***Linear streaks & plaques of erythematous vesicles & papules (stage 1, birth – few months); thickened verrucous warts & whorled plaques***Q (Stage 2, 2 weeks - months) both usually on extremities > trunk. Linear streaks, whorls, flacks & reticulated patches of ***hyperpigmentation mainly on trunk > extremities***Q (stage 3, first few months to adolescence) and anhidrotic, hairless, atrophic, hypopigmented linear patches or streaks usually on calves (stage 4, adolescence to adultohood).
- Dental/teeth (80-90%), bones (30-40%), CNS /neurological (30-40%) and ***ocular/ophthalmic (25-35%) involvement may be associated with skin involvement in few cases (but not in all cases)***Q. ***Retinal vaso-occlusive ischemia is primary mechanism***Q.
- **Icontinentia pigmenti** is an ***X-linked dominant disorder primarily affecting females***Q and belived to be embryonic lethal in males. It *primarily involves skin (in 100% cases)* and presents with typical skin lesions along the lines of Blaschko ***often at birth, usually before 1st week and rarely after the fist 2 months***Q. Four cutaneous stages, some times with some overlap are

1. Inflammatory macule, papule, vesicle and pustules **(vesicular stage)** from birth or shortly there after.
2. **Hyperkeratotic and verrucous** lesions (stage) between 2-8 weeks of age
3. Blue-Gray or slate to brown, bizarre **Chinese letter pattern hyperpigmentation** (several months of age into adolescence)
4. Atrophic **hypopigmented**, and depigmented, hariless, anthidrotic bands/streaks that fail to tan on sun exposure (from infancy through adulthood).

8. **A i.e. Autosomal recessive** 9. **B i.e. Axillary freckling**

[Ref: Thomas Habif Clinical Dermatology 4/e p. 905-08; Fitzpatrick 7/e p. 1331-39; Harrison's 17/e p- 326, 610, 2363, 2606-7; Neena Khanna 3/e p. 32-33]

Neurofibromatosis is ***autosomal dominant***Q disorder. **Axillary freckling (crowe sign)** is a ***pathognomic sign of von- Reckling hausen's type 1 neurofibromatosis***Q. Café – au – lait macules alone are not absolutely diagnostic of NF1, regardless of their size and number.

10. **A i.e. Von Recklinghausens disease** *[Ref: Roxburgh's-Common Skin disease 17/e p. 199, 257, 301]*

Features of **Von Recklinghausens ds. (neurofibromatosis)**

2. ***Café' au lait***Q (brown macules)
3. ***Axillary freckles***Q (diagnostic feature)
4. ***Lisch nodule (iris hamartoma)***Q
5. Skin coloured to pink mauve compressible soft tissue tumor.

11. **A i.e. Slit lamp examination** *[Ref: Roxburgh's 17/e p. 301, 199-200, 257; Fitzpatrick's 6/e p-1333; Harrison 16/e p – 306 – 02, 2457]*
Seven hyperpigmented macules on trunk with multiple hyperpigmented macules in axilla (freckling) point towards the diagnosis of neurofibromatosis. So for supporting the diagnosis we need to see iris hamartomas (lish nodules) by slit lamp examination.

Tuberous Sclerosis

12. **C i.e. Tuberous sclerosis**
13. **A i.e. Iris nodule** 14. **B i.e. Tuberous sclerosis**
15. **B i.e. Tuberous sclerosis** 16. **A i.e. Tuberous sclerosis**
17. **A i.e. Tuberous sclerosis** 18. **C i.e. Café au lait macules exclude the diagnosis.**
[Ref. Roxburgh's 17/e p. 201, 199; Fitzpatrick's 7/e p-1325-31; Harrison 17/e p 1798-1800; Thomas Habif 4/e p. 909-11; Neena Khanna 3/e p. 30; Pasricha 4/e p 167]

Tuberous sclerosis is *autosomal dominant disorder*[Q] presenting with classical **Vogt's triad** of **epilepsy, low intelligence/mental retardation / delayed mile stones and adenoma sebaceum** *(angiofibroma of face)*[Q] *and ashleaf (stippled or Confetti) hypomelanotic offwhite macules mostly on trunk & buttock*[Q]. (Acronym-**Epiloia**)

Icthyosis

19. **C i.e. Autosomal dominant** 20. **D i.e. Ichthyosis vulgaris** 21. **A i.e. Ichtyosis vugaris**
[Ref: Roxburgh's 17/e p. 246-47; Pasricha 3/e p. 5-10; Rooks 7/e p.34.5-34.25; Fitzpatric 7/e p. 401-423; Neena Khanna 3/e p. 20-28; Thomas Habif 4/e p. 115]

Icthyosis vulgaris

- **Icthyosis vulgaris** is *autosomal dominant disorder*[Q], occurring due to reduced or *absence of filaggrin protein and granular layer*[Q]. It presents with dry scaly skin resembling **fish (reptile or crocodile) skin K/a sauroderma.**
- AD means one parent should also manifest disease. It is a congenital condition which is not present at birth but develops during first year of life.
- Dirty looking large mosaic like scales most commonly *over anterior (extensor) surface of legs. Major flexors (axillae, groins, popliteal & cubital fossa) are always and face is usually spared;* though cheeks & forehead may be rarely involved.
- Condition improves in humid & summers and deteriorates in winter. It may be associated with *atopic diathesis, keratosis pilaris, hyper linear & exaggerated palm & sole creases,* and occasionally, keratoderma.

22. **C. i.e X- linked icthyosis nigra**

Icthyosis nigra is *X-linked recessive disease affecting only males and presenting with large, adherent, generalized, brown to black scales encroaching flexures along with cryptorchidism*[Q]. Skin biopsy shows *hyperkeratosis with hyper granulosis and steroid sulfatase deficiency*[Q].

23. **D. i.e. All** 24. **B. i.e. Refsum's disease**

Icthyosis is seen in ***Hypothyroidism, AIDS, Refsum disease and Lymphoma***[Q]. (Mn-"**HARLY** i.e. name of motor cycle Harly Davidson).

25. **C i.e. Pityriasis rubra pilaris; E i.e. Reiter's syndrome** *[Ref: Fitzpatrick 7/e p. 424-30; Rook's 8/e p. 19.117, 34.30]*

Keratoderma is seen in PRP, psoriasis, Reiter's syndrome (keratoderma blenorrhagica), arsenic and Haxthausen's disease[Q].

Deficiency Diseases

26. **B i.e. Pellagra** *[Ref: Nelson's 17/e P-183; Fitzpatrick's 6/e p-1405-07; OPG 5/e P-69]*
27. **D i.e. Kwashiorkar**

Pellagra

Pellagra is a deficiency disease caused by lack of ***niacin (nicotinic acid)***Q, occurs chiefly in countries where *corn (maize)- a poor source of trypthophan* is a basic food stuff. It's clinical presentations is **"3-D"**

- ***Dementia***Q
- ***Diarrhoea***Q
- ***Dermatitis***Q – most characteristic manifestation; occurs in form of pigmented, scaly, sharply demarcated & frequently changing cracked skin on parts exposed to sunlight. It may be of various types on location
  - *Pellagrous glove* ie lesion on hand
  - *Pellagrous boot* ie lesion on boot
  - ***Casal necklace***Q ie lesion around neck.

Kwashiorkor

Mn:		Essential Freatures	Other Imp Features
G	=	*Growth Retardation*Q	- *Flaky paint Dermatosis*Q
E	=	*Edema*	- *Flag Hair Sign*Q
M	=	*Mental Apathy*Q	- *Hepatomegaly*Q

28. **A i.e. Apthous ulcer**

Apthous Ulcers

- *Vitamine deficiency & Stress* are important etiological agents
- Charecterstically presents with ***reccurent painful oral ulcers with erythema & halo around it***Q.

29. **C i.e. Triad of acral dermatitis , dementia & diarrhea** **30.** **A i.e. Zinc** **31.** **A. i.e. Zn**

[Ref: Fitzpatrick's 7/e p-1215-17, 1456-57; Thomas Habif 4/e p. 469, 580-81; Pasricha 4/e p. 193; Harrison 17/e P448-49; Neena Khanna 3/e p. 334]

Autosomal recessiveQ disorder **acrodermatitis enteropathica** d/t ***deficiency of zinc***Q is characterized by ***diarrhea, depression, eczematous dermatitis, alopecia and lethargy.*** (Mn- **DEAL**). ***Zn supplementation rapidly improves condition***Q.

Miscellaneous

32. **B i.e. Post auricular** **33.** **D i.e. Rheumatic fever** **34.** **C i.e. Enteric fever**
35. **C i.e. Erythema infectiosum** **36.** **A i.e. A** **37.** **D i.e. Deserts**
38. **C i.e. Plasma cell balantitis of zoon** **39.** **C. i.e. Lumbosacral > E. i.e. Thigh D. i.e. leg.**
40. **A. i.e. Erythema tòxicum, B. i.e. Mongolian spot D. i.e. Milia** **41.** **D. i.e. Is not of any significance**
42. **A. i.e. Face & Neck** **43.** **C i.e. Antecubital fossae** **44.** **B i.e. Lumbosacral**
45. **D i.e. Lumbosacral** **46.** **A i.e. Forehead**

[Ref: Fitzpatrick 7/e p. 367, 1740-41, 633; Rooks 7/e p.18.1-18.30; Roxburgh's 17/e p. 107; Thomas Habif Clinical Dermatolofy 4/e p. 469, 582; Nelson 18/e p-2662-61; OP Ghai 6/e p-146, 47; Schaffer's disease of Newborn 5/e p-891]

- ***Mongolian spots, milia, miliaria, neonatal acne, transient neonatal pustular melanosis and erythema toxicum are benign, spontaneously self resolving conditions***Q. Whereas, **portwine stain** represents progressive *ectasia of superficial vascular plexus* mostly involving *face* and is best treated by 585 nm pulsed dry laser.
- **Mongolion spots** are blue / slate gray well demarcated macular lesions, ***most frequently involving buttock area (sacral > gluteal & lumbar trunk)***Q in 80% of black & Indians. Involvement of ***posterior thigh, legs, back & shoulders is not uncomon***Q. It is mis- nomer because it is not related to Down's syndrome & usually ***disappear before 1st birthday***Q.
- **Erythema toxicum neonatorum (toxic erythema of new born)** occurs in 20-50% of ***term infants – usually 2nd and later deliveries who are otherwise healthy***Q. It is rare in preterm & under weight (<2.5 kg) infants. Lesions are not present at birth and *mostly appear between 24-48 hours*, on face, trunk, buttocks & proximal extremities, or pressure sites, - in form of macule, papule, wheal & pustule. Palm & soles are not involved. Wright's stain of lesion show neumerous eosinophils without peripheral eosinophilia.

47. **A i.e. Dowling-Degos disease** *[Ref: Rook's 8/e p. 15.94-15.95, 58.21/22, 52.41, 15.76 – 15.82; Fitzpatrick 7/e p. 1324-19; IJD vol 62 p. 25-29]*

- **Dowling-Degos disease** presents *as* ***asymptomatic post-pubertal, symmetrical, progressive, reticular pigmentation involving flexural-areas (flexor folds) with scattered comedo like lesions (dark dot follicles) and pitted aceniform scars near angles of mouth***[Q].
- **Reticular acropimentation of kitamura** presents with **reticular freckle like pigmentation on dorsal hands, palmar pits**[Q] and breakage of epidermal ridge pattern.
- Cockayne's syndrome, Bloom's syndrome and Rothmund-Thomson syndrome are genodermatoses with defective DNA repairing, presenting as photo sensitivity.

Dowling-Degos disease

- **Dowling-Degos disease (reticular pigmented anomaly of flexures)** is a rare *autosomal dominant genodermatoses* usually presenting *post pubertally* with *multiple small, round pigmented macules* that resemble freckles. *Pigmentation is symmetrical and progressive;* and the lesions become progressively more numerous and *reticulate with time.* It characteristically ***involves flexurals areas***[Q] e.g: axillae, groins (mc sites), intergluteal/ infra-mammary folds, neck, scalp, trunk, arms and genitals. Except pigmentation, it is otherwise asymptomatic (rarely pruritic). ***Scattered comedo like lesions (dark dot follicles) pitted acneiform scars near angels of mouth***[Q] and hidradenitis suppurativa are other features.
- *Histology is diagnostic,* with a distinctive form of *acanthosis,* characterized by an *irregular elongation of rete ridges, with a concentration of melanin at the tips (filiform down growths in epidermis with hyperpigmentation of deepest areas);* the melanocyte count being normal. It involves follicular infundibulum with follicular plugging in some cases.

Reticulate acropigmentation of Kitamura

- **Reticulate acropigmentation of kitamura** is characterized by a *reticulate network of freckle like areas of pigmentation* which develop on *dorsa of hands* in first 2 decades, which may subsequently involve most parts of body. ***Palmar pits and breakages of epidermal ridge pattern are found***[Q]. Histologically, the pigmented macules show *epidermal atrophy and increased number of melanocytes.*
- **Hereditary symmetrical dyskeratosis of extremities (reticulate acropimentation of Dohi)** is AD disorder presenting in infancy or early childhood as mottled pigmentation with areas of depigmentation on dorsa of hands and feet or arms and legs.

Haber's syndrome

- **Haber's syndrome** is a familial condition characterized by *persistent/permanent rosacea like eruption* (i.e. facial flushing, erythema, telangiectasia, prominent follicles, comedones, small papules and tiny atrophic pitted areas) associated in some cases with *static, scaly/keratotic, flat, non-indurated plaques on trunk and limbs.*

Bloom's syndrome

- **Bloom's syndrome** (congenital telangiectatic erythema and stunted growth) is a AR disorder characterized by *photosensitive telagiestatic facial erythema* during infancy or early childhood (superficially resembling lupus erythematosus), *moderate and proportionate growth deficiency* both in utero and postnatally, *unusual facies* (narrow, slender, delicate face with a narrow, prominent nose, hypoplastic malar areas, receding chin and microcephaly and dolichocephaly i.e. long and narrow head).
- Patients are *predisposed to multiple infection (d/t immune dysfunction)* and *early cancers* (usually interanal) l/t early death (usually <30yr).
- Fertility is decreased although puberty and *neurological development is normal;* diabetes mellitus and testicular atrophy are common.

Cockayne's syndrome

- **Cockayne's syndrome** is AR degenerative disease with *cutaneous* (photosensitivity, premature skin aging), ocular (pigmentary retinal degeneration with salt-peper appearance of retina, optic atropy and cataract), *neurological* (sensorineural deafness, progressive neurological degeneration, extensive primary demyelination, peripheral neuropathy, normal pressure hydrocephalus, microcephaly, intellectual deterioration) and somatic abnormallties (postnatal growth failure, cachectic dwarfism with disproportionately long limbs with large hands and feet and ears). Child usually appears normal for the first year, when photosensitive butterfly facial erythema develop l/t mottled pigmentation, atrophic scars giving patient a *prematurely senile appearance* which is enhanced by marked loss of subcutaneous fat on face *(wizened appearance) and sunken eyes* with typical *bird headed facies* and *prominent Mickey mouse ear.*
- In contrast to xerodema pigmentosa, CS *don't have increased incidence of skin cancer and infection* and the CS patients have unusual facies, demyelination with delayed nerve conduction velocity and normal level of global NER.

Rothmund Thomson Syndrome

- **Rothmund Thomson syndrome** (congenital poikiloderma), an AR disorder is characterized by poikiloderma with variegated cutaneous pigmentation, atrophy and telangiectasia beginning in infancy (but not birth). Cheeks are fist and most severly involved but face, *buttock and extremities are also involved. Photosensitive erythema* and facial smelling may be accompanied by blister formation. Scalp hair, eyebrows, eyelashes, pubic and axillary *hair are often sparse or absent. Juvenile cataract (b/l), proportionate stunted growth* with slender delicate limb, small hands, feet and finger; *bird like small skull with a saddle nose, skeletel abnormalities* including radial ray defect (present as thumb hypoplasia, abnormal radial head or absence of radius) and a *predisposition for cancer* especially *osteosarcoma* (30%). Intelligence is normal and life expectancy depends on development of cancer; otherwise it appears to be normal.

14 MALIGNANT SKIN DISEASE

Cutaneous Markers of Internal Malignancy

Genodermatoses

Genetically determined syndrome with a cutaneous component & risk to develop neoplasm. On the basis of main organ affected or usual mode of presentation these may be

Skin

- Xeroderma pigmentosa
- Gorlin's (Naevoid basal cell carcinoma) syndrome
- Familial atypical naevi, melanoma, multiple mole &/or dysplastic naevus (B-K mole or familial melanoma syndrome)
- Melanoma astrocytoma syndrome (melanoma nervous system tumor syndrome).
- Incontinentia pigmenti
- Porphyria cutanea tarda
- Supernumerary nipples
- Tylosis/ Focal palmoplantar keratoderma/ Howel Evans syndrome
- Basex-Dupre Christol syndrome (Follicular atrophoderma)
- Sclerotylosis (Huriez syndrome)
- Familial leimyomas (cutaneous & uterine = Reed syndrome; hereditary leiomyomotosis and renal cell carcinoma)
- ***Muir-Torre/Torre syndrome (sebaceous tumor, keratocanthomas & visceral malignancy)***Q
- Brit-Hogg-Dube syndrome & Hornstein-Knickenberg syndrome

Endocrine

- Multiple endocrine neoplasia syndrome; multiple endocrine adenomatosis = MEA; MEN type I = Wermer; MEN type 2A = Sipple syndrome and MEN type 2B or 3

Neurological

- Neurofibromatosis type 1 (von Recklinghausen's disease) and type 2
- ***Tuberous sclerosis (Bournville disease)***Q
- Ataxia telangiectasia/ Louis-Bar syndrome (immunodeficiency also)

Immuno deficiency

- Wiskott-Aldrich syndrome
- Chediak-Higashi syndrome
- Fanconi's anaemia (usually present d/t congenital growth/ skeletal malformation)
- Dyskeratosis congenita (Zinsser-Cole Engman syndrome; haemopoietic involvement)

Gastrointestinal

- Gardner's syndrome
- Peutz Jeghers syndrome
- Bannayan-Riley-Ruvalcaba syndrome
- Turcot (mismatch repair cancer) syndrome

Growth/Skeletal

- Bloom's syndrome
- Rothmund – Thomson syndrome (poikiloderma congenitale)
- Werner's syndrome (adult progeria)
- Maffucci syndrome
- Goltz syndrome

Multisystem

- Cowden's (PTEN multiple hamartoma and neoplasia/tumor) syndrome
- **Carney complex (NAME syndrome** = naevi congenital melanocytic, atrial myxomas, myxoid neurofibromas, ephelides' **LAMB syndrome** = lentigines, atrial myxomas, mucocutaneous myxomas and blue naevi) or **myxoma syndrome**
- Von Hippel-Lindau disease
- Beckwith Wiedermann Syndrome (EMG syndrome)

Paraneoplastic Dermatoses Syndrome

Skin conditions that have an association with internal malignancy but are not themselves malignant. These may be of various type on the basis of **strength of correlation** with malignancy.

Strong

- **Acrokeratosis paraneoplastica or Bazex syndrome** (sq cell ca of upper respiratory or gastrointestinal tract)
- **Erythema gyratum repens** (wood grain appearance of skin + lung cancer esp)
- ***Necrolytic migratory erythema***Q (glucagonoma syndrome / α cell tumor of pancreas)
- **Acanthosis Palmaris (Tripe palm or pachydermatoglyphy)**
- Acquired (paraneoplastic) hypertrichosis lanuginose (aquisita)
- Trousseau's syndrome (recurrent migratory thrombophlebitis = Trousseau's sign)
- Carcinoid syndrome
- ***Paraneoplastic pemphigus***Q
- **POEMS** (polyneuropathy, organomegaly, endocrinopathy, **M** protein, skin changes) **syndrome**
- Scleromyxedema/ lichen myxoedematosus
- Necrobiotic xanthogranuloma
- Primary & myeloma associated systemic amyloidosis (AL protein deposition)

Moderate

- Sweet's syndrome
- Pyoderma gangrenosum
- *Dermatomyositis*
- Pityriasis rotunda
- Multicentric reticulohistio-cytosis (lipoid dermato-arthritis; reticuocytoma cutis)

Weak

- ***Acanthosis nigricans***Q
- Acquired icthyosis (unless widespread, deeply fissured, truncal pattern)
- Sign of Leser-Trelat (sudden numerous, eruptive seborrhoeic keratoses)
- Erythema annulare centrifugum
- Erythroderma & exfoliative dermatitis; Ofuji papuloerythroderma
- Erythromelalgia
- Prusitis
- Raynaud's phenomenon & digital ischemia (paraneoplastic acral vascular syndrome)
- Vasculitis
- Relapsing polychondritis
- ***Digital clubbing (unless with hypertrophic osteoarthropathy)***Q
- Cushing's syndrome
- Sclerederma
- Calcinosis cutis
- ***Bullous pemphigoid***Q
- Deep vein thrombosis, Mondor's disease

★ Genodermatoses that predispose to skin but not to internal cancers (such as albinism, epidermodysplasia verruciformis, dystrophic epidermolysis bullosa, prokeratosis of Mibelli and KID syndrome) are not included here.

Acanthosis Nigrican (AN)

- It is a cutaneous marker, ***most commonly of insulin resistance & obesity and less frequently of genetic disorder and malignancy***Q.
- **Clinical hallmark** is development of ***symmetrical grey- brown velvety plaques with feathered margins that may start as dirty appearance hyperpigmentation***Q. Later skin becomes *hypertrophied* with *increased markings* & papillomatosis and appears *rugose & mammilated.*
- The **most commonly** involved areas are ***neck, axilla, external genitalia, groin, face***Q, inner thighs, antecubital & popliteal fossa, umbilicus, perianal area & submammary folds. In some cases, **mucosa** (oral, oesophageal, pharyngeal, laryngeal, conjunctival, anogenital) may be invoved. However, the ***back of the neck is most consistently & severly affected area***Q. Florid cases may involve knuckles, or palms (rugated appearance is k/a **tripe palms** and is usually indicative of malignancy). Vulva is the common place to find AN in obese, hirsute, hyper androgenic, insulin resistant women.
- AN is considered a ***prognostic indicator for developing type 2 diabetes***Q, as it represents a ***cutaneous marker of tissue insulin resistane***Q and resultant hyperinsulinemia (a known risk factor for type 2 diabetes).
- **Benign** form presents at a *younger age* & has gradual progression on flexural surfaces. **Malignant** form is suspected when *a rapid appearance of lesion in older individual along with atypical sites such as oral mucosa* is seen. Tripe palsm, Leser- Trelat sign *severe itching* , Bazex syndrome & florid papillomatosis when associated with AN indicate a malignant (cause *mostly adenocarcinoma of stomach*).
- Etiological classification

Benign

D/t obesity & also k/a pseudo AN.

Malignant

D/t ***adenocarcinoma of stomach (most common)***Q & genitourinary tract

Drug induced

D/t *nicotinic acid, stillbestrol, corticosteroid, & oral contraceptives.*

Endocrinal & Syndromes

- **Type A** or **HAIR – AN syndrome** is hyper androgenemia (HA), *extreme insulin resistance (**IR**)*Q and acanthosis nigricans (AN). It is distinguished from type B insulin resistance by onset in infancy & childhood, lack of antibodies to insulin receptor or other evidence of autoimmune disease.
- Type B syndrome of insulin resistance
- ***Bloom syndrome***Q
- Acromegaly, Addison's disease, Alstrom sy, Bartter sy, Cushing's sy., Don houe sy., Laurence – Moon – Biedl sy., Werner sy., Stein- Leventhal sy. (polycystic ovarian ds.), MORFAN (mental retardation, over growth, remarkable facies and AN) etc.

Cutaneous Markers of Endocrine Disorders

Diabetes Mellitus

- Xanthomas (eruptive xanthomas)
- Infections (fungal, bacterial)/Ischemic changes (foot ulcers, protracted wound healing most common feature)
- **Necrobiosis lipoidica**Q/Neuropathic ulcers
- **Granuloma annulare**Q
- Acquired perforating disorders (Kyrle disease, reactive perforating collagenosis, perforating folliculitis, & elastosis perforans serpiginosa)
- **Bullosis diabeticorum**Q
- Acanthosis nigricans
- Diabetic dermopathy (pigmented peritibial papules or **Shin-spots**)Q
- Sclerederma diabeticorum and
- Scleroderma like skin & limited joint mobility syndrome
- Lipoatrophy, lipo hypertrophy (rare)

Mn – **"XING A BAD song"**. All of these **(except acanthosis nigricans) are not associated with malignancy.**

Hyper parathyroidism

- **Cutaneous (metastatic) calcinosis**
- Chronic urticaria
- **Calciphylaxis (calcific uremic arteriolopathy or CUA)** is

Hyperthyroidism (Grave's disease)

- Soft, velvety, infant like skin
- Soft, fine hair accompanied by **diffuse non scarring alopecia**
- Facial flushing, palmar erythema, hyperpigmentation, vitiligo
- Soft, shin, brittle nails with increased rate of growth
- **Plummer's nail** (concave nail with distal onycholysis) = not pathognomic
- Thyroid dermopathy (**pretibial myxedema**) = bilateral, painless, nonpitting nodules & plaques with variable colors & waxy induration, mostly on extensor surface of legs.
- **Thyroid acropachy** (digital clubbing, soft tissue swelling of hands & feet with periosteal reaction)

Hypothyroidism

- Cool & pale skin (d/t decreased core temperature & peripheral vasoconstriction)
- Doughy, dry, waxy, swollen skin with fine wrinkling but no pitting
- Yellow orange discoloration (β-carotenemia)
- Coarse, dry, brittle, and slowly growing hair and nail.
- **Myxedema** (d/t dermal accumulation of muco-polysaccharides: hyaluronic acid and chondroitin sulfate

non immunological, life threatening Ca^{++} deposition in walls of small/medium sized vessels resulting in skin necrosis; occurs mostly (not always) in CRF and secondary hyper parathyroidism.

★ Signs of hyperparathyroidism in a/w cutaneous skin tumor like angiofibromas, collagenomas, and lipomas indicates MEN 1.

Hypo parathyroidism

- Scaly, hyperkeratotic, edematous & puffy skin
- Patchy alopecia with hair thinning
- Brittle nails with transverse ridging

Acromegaly

- Enlargement of hands & feet with doughy texture
- Increasing ring, glove, shoe and hat size
- **Prognathism** (enlargement of jaw with separation of teeth), **Macroglossia**
- Cutis vertices gyri, acanthosis nigricans, hirsutism, hyperhidrosis and brittle thick nails.

there is doughy, swollen, waxy but without pitting skin. It may be generalized l/t broadened nose, thickened lips, puffy eyelids, and macroglossia with smooth & clumsy tongue or can appear more strikingly in extremities).

Cushing Syndrome (Excessive Cortisol)

- Increased central obesity (**moon facies, buffalo hump**) with thinning of extremities = Orange on sticks
- Skin thinning, easy bruisability and violaceous striae
- Acanthosis nigricans
- Increased dermatophyte & candidal skin & nail infections
- Hyper pigmentation (rare)

Addison Disease (loss of gluco/mineralo corticoid & adrenal androgens)

- ***Hyper pigmentation of skin & mucous membranes***Q
- Longitudinal pigmented bands in nails
- Calcification of auricular cartilage in men
- Vitiligo
- Decreased axillary/pubic hair in women

Mycosis Fungoides/Cutaneous T cell lymphoma

It is a multifocal, neoplastic disorder of T- lymphocytes that primarily affects the skin and may evolve into generalized lymphoma. It is ***most common primary cutaneous lymphoma***Q.

Pathology

- Histological hallmark is presence of ***Sezary – Lutzner cells***Q. These are ***T-helper cells (CD4 psitive)***Q that form band like aggregates within superficial dermis and invade epidermis as single cells and small clusters ***(Pautrier microabscess)***Q.
- **Epidermotropism** i.e. pronounced epidermal infiltration by sezary – lutzner cells. In more advanced nodular lesions, the malignant T cells *lose their epidermotropic tendency*, grow deeply into the dermis, and eventually ***seed lymphatic & peripheral circulation***Q.

Clinical Features

- It is an ***indolent lymphoma***Q with patients often having a several years of eczematous or dermatitis skin lesion before the diagnosis is finally established.
- The skin lesions progress from patch stage to plaque stage to cutaneous tumors.
- Lesions start off as a series of *red macules & scaly pathes over trunk and upper limbs*, which gradually extend & become more prolific. These eventually thicken & become *plaques*, &, later still *eroded tumor*.
- The ring worm like appearance of early patches & fungating plaques in late stage, were responsible for the term mycosis fungoides
- In advanced stage, lymph node enlargement, hepatospleenomegaly & infiltration of other viscera occur.
- A particular syndrome involve, ***erythroderma (diffus erythema & scaling) and circulating tumor cells with mycosis fungoides***Q. This is known as **Sezary's syndrome**

Treatment & Prognosis

- Early stage (rare) can be curved by radiotherapy, often ***total – skin electron beam irradiation***Q.
- Advanced disease has been treated with topical *glucocorticoids, topical nitrogen mustard, phototherapy, psoralen with UV-A (PUVA), electron beam radiation, interferon, antibodies fusion toxins, & systemic cytotoxic therapy.*
- ***Unfortunately these treatments are palliative***Q.
- The disorder is ***inevitably fatal***Q, although the rate of progression is quite variable, with survival ranging from 2-3 years in some patients to 20 years in others.

Langerhans Cell Histiocytosis (LCH) / Histiocytosis X

It is characterized by *proliferation (reactive or neoplastic,* is debatable) of ***antigen presenting immature dendritic cell (DC) called Langerhans cell (LH)***Q. In most instances proliferation is monoclonal, and dendritic cell show ***HLA DR, CD-1a, S 100, CD 207 (langerin), E-cadherin & Birbeck granules***Q (i.e. all positive); but ***CD14, CD68, CD163***Q, factor XIII **negative**.

- **Historical classification (4 types)**

1. **Litterer Siwe disease (LSD)** is ***acute, disseminated multifocal multisystem***Q fatal form that usually appears in *infants or newborn* and children <2years. It presents with *fever, diffuse eruption* like seborrheic dermatitis (esp on scalp, ear canal, front & back of trunk), repeated infections, *hepato spleenomegaly, lymphadenopathy, pulmonary lesions* & osteolytic bone lesions with bone marrow infiltration
2. **Hand – Schuller – Christian disease (HSC)** is *chronic progressive multifocal form,* commonly beginning in childhood & presenting

Clinical Features

- **Cutaneous lesions.**
- Are very common & may represent *earliest sign.*
- Typical lesion is 1 – 2 mm *small translucent, slightly raised, rose yellow papule* usually located on ***trunk, scalp and skin folds & frequently showing scaling***Q >> crusting &

with **HSC triad** i.e. ***calvarial defect in scalp, diabetes insipidus and exopthalmos***[Q].

3. **Eosinophilic granuoma (EG)** is *localized benign form presenting with **vertebra plana with no subperiosteal bone formation***[Q].
4. **Hashimto- Pritzker disease** (HPD) represent *benign self healing* variant, usually presenting *at birth or during first few days of life.*

- **Classification according to extent of diseae & treatment**

Restricted- Single System LCH Former EG & HPD

Skin lesions only

- **In children**

Only *observation* is the best option

persists ↓

N_2-mustard topically 20mg/dL daily for 5 days

↓

Systemic glucocorticoids or antimitotic drugs in resistant cases

- **In adults**

- Topical nitrogen mustard
- PUVA
- CO_2 laser in periorificial EG
- Thalidomide
- Isotretinoin

Bone lesions only

- **Monostotic lesions** with or without *diabetes insipidus, adjacent lymph-node involvement or rash*
- **Polyostatic lesions** (involving *several* bones or >2 lesions in one bone) with or without diabetes insipidus, (DI), adjacent lymph node involvement or rash.

- *Surgical excision or curetlage is treatment of choice* if lesions are accessible
- **Steroid injection**, in children to prevent injury to *growth plate of long bones* &developing teeth
- **Radiotherapy** is indicated for *involvement of vertebrae, sella turcica & weight bearing bones* with risk of spontaneous fracture, in adults but must be *reserved for resistant cases* that fail to respond to other measures in children
- **Monochemotherapy** in *multiple bone lesions.*

Extensive – Multi system (multiorgan) LCH Former LSD & HSC

Visceral organ **involvement**

- With or without signs of organ dysfunction or **lungs, liver or hematopoietic system.**
- With or without bone lesion, DI, adjacent lymph node involvement & /or rash

- **Monochemotherapy** with **vinblastin or etopaside** with or without *preceeding steroid* is most suitable.
- *Etopaside* may l/t *AML* (Cummulative doses > 4000 mg/m^2); so it is *not first choice in children* & should be reserved for *severe cases resistant to other drugs.*
- **Relapsed** or **Recurrent** (low risk organ involvement) disease
  - 60% respond to *same monotherapy reinduction* (usually vinblastin weakly & daily predinisolone), which can be canged to adding *methotrexate* – weekly & *merceptopurine* nightly & making vinblastin regimen 3 weekly.
- **Non responders** treated with **polychemotherapy** including
  - Vincristine, cytarabine (cytosine arabinoside) & prednisolone or
  - Vincristine, doxorubicine & prednisolone or
  - Salvage regimen including vincristine, cyclophosphamide, doxorubicin & chlorambucil
- **Refractory & advanced** (high risk involvement) **disease**
  - ***Cladribine (2- Chlor deoxy adenosine/2-CdA)***[Q] & cytosine arabinoside (cytarabine), cyclosporine, interferon - α2
  - **Hematopoietic stem cell transplantation** (HSCT) i.e. allogenic or auto (CD 1a depleted) bone marrow transplantation after reduced intensity conditioning, in patients refractory to chemotherapy.
- **Progressive disease** (i.e. progressive after 6 weeks or partial response after 12 weeks) is treated by 2- *CdA & 2 deoxycoformycin* salvage therapy (but is more effective in bone, lymph node, skin involvement)
- **Multiple reactivation** is treated with *continuous 2- CdA infusion for 3 days.*

ulceration.

- *Vesicle & pustules* are especially common during *neonatal period.*
- Appear more (LSD) or less (HSC) rapidly in *successive crops* and tend to merge on
  1. Folds (retroacuricular, axillary, genital) *mimicking intertrigo*
  2. Scalp (l/t alopecia) *mimicking seborrheic dermatitis* or folliculitis.
- *Purpura & nail changes* (eg. Fragile lamina, paronychia, sub ungal hyperkeratosis / pustules, nail fold destruction, onycholysis, and nail bed showing longitudinal – groving, pigmented & purpuric striae) are **poor prognostic signs.**
- Mucosal lesions are usually ulcerated nodules involving mainly gingival & perioral area, and esp. in EG, perigenital or perianal region. Although absence of mucousal lesion is a key feature of HPD,

- **Bone manifestations** are *most frequent* (80%) and present as *osteolytic lesion* involving:
  - *Temporo- parietal* region of *skull* forming ***map-lesions***[Q]
  - Lower maxillary bone l/t *floating teeth appearance* on x-ray
  - Retro ocular bone involvement l/t *exopthalmos*
  - Base of skull involvement l/t *growth retardation & diabetes insipidus* (d/t pituitary involvement)
  - Flat bones, vertebrae & long bones can be involved. At times significant periosteal reaction, adjacent tissue (eg. muscle) and bone marrow involvement may be present, making MRI advantageous.
  - *Isotope scan* is useful for multiple lesions & *fluoro-deoxy-glucose PET* for active osseous lesions. *Isolated bone lesion with bevelled margins & without sclerosis* has best prognosis.
- **Lymphadenopathy** (upto 75%) mostly involving cervical lymph-nodes, **hepatic & spleen involvement** (upto 50%) and **pulmonary involvement** (upto 25%) l/t *honey comb appearance or micronodular-pattern* are other features.
- ***Brain & gonadal involvements is rare***[Q]. Intercurrent candidial infections & malignancy are complications

Histopathological features & diagnostic markers

- A *dense infiltrate of histiocytes* with a *strong epidermotropism* and presence of **typical "LCH" cell** – i.e. a histiocyte approximately *4 – 5 times larger than small lymphocytes* with an *irregular, vesiculated an often reniform (kidney) shaped nucleus* containing linear grooves / folds and an *abundant slightly eosinophilic vacuolated cytoplasm* containing characteristic ***tennis racket shaped Birbeck granules***[Q].
- LCH cells test positive for ***S- 100 protein, CD1a and CD207 (langerin) diagnostic markers***[Q].

Epidermal Nevus

It is generalized term for *hamartomatous proliferation* of epidermis; which is subdivided according to *predominant histological cell type or distribution of lesion.*

Classification

Variant	Predominant structure	Morphology	Distribution
(Linear) Verrucous epidermal nevus • Localized • Systemized eg - Nevus unis lateris - Icthyosis hystrix • **Inflammatory linear verrucous epidermal nevus (ILVEN)**	***Keratinocyte (surface epidermis)***Q	***Verrucous plaques***Q Inflammed verrucous	 Localized Widespread Widespread unilateral Widespread bilateral Localized
Nevus sebaceous	*Sebaceous gland*	Yellow verrucous	Localized rarely diffuse
Nevus comedonicus	Pilosebaceous gland (hair follicle)	Comedones (grouped)	Localized rarely diffuse
Eccrine nevus **Apocrine nevus**	Eccrine sweat gland Apocrine gland	Papule (non-descript)	Localized
Becker's nevus	Surface epidermis hair follicles + smooth muscles, melanization	Pigmented hairy	Localized
White sponge nevus	Mucosal epithelium	Gray-white plaque	Localized or diffuse

Differential diagnosis

includes & on the basis of histology

Lichen Striatus

- *Lichenoid lymphocytic infiltrate involving 3-4 adjacent dermal papillae with* overlying epidermal aconthosis, dyskeratosis, hyperkeratosis & occasional parakeratosis
- Intraepidermal vesicle containing *Langerhans cells.*

Linear Darier disease

- *Hyperkeratosis, focal dyskeratosis* (abnomal & premature keratinization of single keratinocyte)
- ***Suprabasal acantholysis*** Q l/t clefs
- Rounded eosinophilic dyskeratotic cells are called ***corps rounds*** *in stratum spinosum &* ***grains*** *in upper epidermis.*

Linear porokeratosis

- **Hyper keratotic stratum corneum with** a thin column of poorly staining parakeratotic cells the **coronoid lamella** (arising from indentation of epidermis)
- Underlying the **coronoid lamella**, the *granular layer is either absent or markedly reduced* but is of normal thickness in other areas of lesion.
- Coronoid lamella is characteristic but not pathognomic & may also be seen in *viral warts, icthyosis, & nevoid hyperkeratosis.*
- Underlying keratinocytes are edematous with spongiosis & shrunken nuclei, and a dermal lymphocytic pattern.

Incontinentia pigment

- Dyskeratosis, pigment incontinence, eosinophilic exocytosis & ***basal layer vacuolization***Q & degeneration
- Extensive deposits of melanin (laden macrophages) in basal cell layer & dermis.

Linear & whorled nevoid hypermelanosis **(LWNH)**

Increased pigmentation of basal cell layer & prominence or ***vacuolization of melanocytes*** ± pigment incontinence

Clinical resentation

- Tend to appear ***between birth & adolescence***Q with majority of lesions appearing by age 14 years and ***80% of lesion appearing within 1st year of life***Q.
- **Linear verrucous epidermal nevus (LVEN) or linear epidermal nevus** is characterized by localized or diffuse, closely set, skin coloured (brown or gray- brown) ***verrucous plaques***Q that may coalesce to form *well demarcated papillomatous plaques,*
- ***Linear configuration (along Blaschko's relaxed skin tension) lines is common on limbs***Q ***and nevi take on transverse configuration on trunk***Q.
- ILVEN most commonly involve *buttocks & lower extremities* and show pruritis, erythema, & scaling
- Although congenital lesions do not expand significantly, the lesions that present after birth may expand in childhood, stabilize in size at or around puberty & remain quiescent after adolescence
- Rarely basal cell or squamous cell carcinoma or *offspring with epidermolytic hyperkeratosis (EHK)* may occur. In EHK a *mutation in one of two keratin- 10 (K-10) alleles* (i.e. *mosaicism* = presence of two genetically distinct cell lines) is demonstrated in parents & offspring.

Histology

- > 60% lesions display – *acanthosis, papillomatosis, & hyperkeratosis,* Rare features include – *thin elongated rate ridges,* compact orthokeratosis, ***vacuolization of keratinocytes in granular layer of epidermis***Q, and large keratohyline granules within or outside cells.
- ILVEN shows chronic dermal inflammatory infiltrate, psoriasiform epidermal hyperplasia, & alternating bands of ortho- & parakeratosis. ***In ILVEN granular layer is absent under lying the areas of parakeratosis***Q.

Cosmetic and Skin Care

Chemical Peel

- It is controlled application of 1 or more *exfoliating agents* to the skin resulting in *accelerated epidermal shedding* (by superficial peels) or *chemically destroying epidermis and* progressive layers of dermis by protein coagulation (indicated by white frost) and cell lysis (medium and deep peels). Skin damage is f/b release of cytokines and inflammatory mediators resulting in *thickened rejuvenated skin.*
- An area with *higher density of appendigeal structures (such as pilosebaceous glands)* i.e. *face* respond in a more predictable way than neck, chest and limb (i.e. areas with minimal sebanceous appendages. Medium depth peels can be used on face but care is required in using

them on other parts of body d/t risk of impaired healing, scarring and pigmantory changes in nonfacial areas. Superfacial peels should only be used in most areas other than face.

- Topical retinoids, tretnoin application prior to peel, enhances penetration and uniformity of peel. Because of risks of facial pigmentation, only skin phototypes III and above are treated with peels.

Chemical Peel type	Superficial	Medium	Deep
Depth of penetration (destruction)	**Epidermis** alone (± upper papillary dermis)	**Epidermis + Papillary dermis** (± upper reticular dermis)	**Reticular dermis** (mid)
Chemoexfoliants (see skin phototype table below)	- 10-25% ***TCA (tri chloroacetic acid)***[Q] - α hydorxy acids (glycolic acid 50-70%, lactic acid, malic acid, citric acid) - β hydroxyacid (salicylic acid) - α ketoacid (pyruvic acid) - ***Kojic acid***[Q] - Retinoic acid (tretinoin) - Solid CO_2 - Jessner's solution (lactic acid, salicylic acid and resorcinol 14g. each in ethanol 95% in quantity sufficient to yield 100ml). - Modified Unna's resorcinol paste.	- TCA 35-50% - 35% TCA and solid CO_2 - 35% TCA and Jessner's solution - 35% TCA and glycolic acid 70% - ***Phenol (carbolic acid) 88%***[Q] ★ Superficial peels remain valuable for treating **milder skin ageing problems, (photoaging, superficial pigmentation, wrinkling and scars and dilated pores)** and as an adjuvant treatment in acne ★ Medium and deeper peels are now replaced by laser skin rejuvenation ★ Cardiac, renal and hepatic toxicity is a/w phenol peels	- TCA 50%/Baker's phenol - **Baker-Gordon phenol peel (phenol** USP 88% 3ml + **croton oil** 3 dops + **hexachlorophene = septisol** liquid soap 8 drops + distilled water 2ml) - **Littons** fomula (replaces septisol with glycerine) and Belson – Mecollough formula (i.e. heaver application of Baker Gordon peel)

Skin Photo-type	Color	Reaction to skin (Burn)
I	**Very white or freckled**	**Always**
II	With	Usually
III	White to olive	Sometimes
IV	Brown	Rarely
V	Dark brown	Very rarely
VI	**Black**	**Never**

Clinical Condition	Type of laser and IPL (Intensed pulsed light)
Vascular lesions	Pulsed dye (585-595nm)
Telangiectasia	Copper bromide
Portwine statins/haemangiomas	KTP (Potassium titanyl phosphate)
Cambell de Morgan angiomas	IPL
Bengin pigmented lesions like photoageing, solar lentigo	Q switched, ruby (605nm), alexandrite (755nm), neodynium: YAG (532 and 1064 nm), Q switched KTP (532 nm)
Lentigo, melanosis, melasma (Photo damage)	IPL
Tattoos	Q switched, Ruby, alexandrite, Nd: YAG
Naevus of Ota	Q Switched pigment laser
Aging skin, rhytides, laxity	CO_2 Laser
Seborrhoea keratosis	Erbium YAG laser, Fractional lasers
Hirsutes (Pigmented hair)	Long pulsed ruby, alexadrite, Nd: YAG, IPL

Capillary Malformations

Present with *macular erythematous patch* and are of 2 types

Salmon patch (Stork bite/mark, Nuchal Stain, Angel's kiss or Nevus flammeus neonatorum)

- *Extremely common* vascular anomalies present clinically with irregular pink/red macular patches with or without fine telangiectasia.
- The commonly affected sites are *nape of neck* (most common) may be extending upto *occiput* (k/a **unna nevus**), and anteriority on forehead, glabella, upper eyelid or bridge of nose. Less common site include *sacral region.*
- ***Facial satins fade within 1st year of life***[Q] (or upto 4 years), whereas others sites may persist into adulthood.
- Sacral lesions may be a/w spinal dysraphism and warrant MRI if a/w lipoma, pit, dimple, hypertrichosis, cutis aplasia, hemangioma or sinus.

Port-Wine Stain (PWS)

- It is a *low-flow vascular malformation* defined as a red homogenous macular telangiectatic patch which is ***present at birth (congenital) and remains throughout life.***
- It is *often unilateral*, sometimes bilateral, but usually not median. Lesions are *flat and painless, don't bleed spontaneously*, and are *never warm* on palpation.
- Color varies from pink-red to deep purple with a geographic contour or a dermatomal distribution. Initial pale-pink lesions may mature into a violaceous/purple color (facial PWS), remain static or even lighten (trunk or limb).
- It involves skin, subcutis and sometimes mucosa. ***Most PWS are located on face***[Q] where they follow the distribution of **trigeminal nerve**; V_1 (front and upper eyelid); V_2 (lower eylid, cheek, upper lip); V_3 (lower lip chin, mandible)
- Facial stains evolve into thicker areas with vascular bleds, pyogenic granuloma and tissue hypertrophy (unilateral limb hypertrophy)
- It may be part of syndrome, such as ***Sturge-Weber syndrome (PWS, seizure and glucoma)***[Q], phakomatosis pigmento vascularis (PWS, epidermal naevus, Mongolian blue spots, nevus anaemicus, naevus spilus or naevus of ota); **Klippel-Trenaunay syndrome** (capillary-lympatico-venous malformation, hypertrophy of affected limb, lymphedema)

Sturge-Weber syndrome

It is *neuro-oculo-cutaneous syndrome* consisting of ***facial port-wine stain in association with ipsilateral vascular malformation of leptomeninges and eye***Q.

Cutaneous features

- ***Portwine stain (or macular telangiectatic patch) in the ophthalmic (V_1) and maxillary (V_2) branch of trigeminal nerve***Q is the commonest feature. V_1 branch (i.e. PWS extending to forehead and upper eyelid) must be involved in part or its entirety for true syndrome.
- Ocular and CNS involvement is only 9% in PWS affecting lower lid alone, but 90% if both upper and lower eye lids are involved.
- PWS can cross over the midline and is *bilateral* in 50% or additional macular patch may be on *trunk and limbs* in 40%. The oral and nasal mucosa may be affected l/t *gingival hypertrophy and accelerated dentition.*

Neurological features

- *Homolateral leptomeningeal capillary venous malformation* affecting the *occipto-parietal area* l/t *hypervascularity, calcification, atrophy and demyelination.*
- ***Epileptic seizures***Q is the most common neurological feature *usually starting within first 7months* of life, but may start later in adulthood.
- *Mental retardation, developmental delay, transient hemiplegia and homonymous hemianopia* later becoming permanent are other features.
- Plain X-ray shows **sinuous tramline opacification** typical of intra cranial corical calcification.
- **Gadolinium enhanced MRI** is superior for early detection, delineating extent, showing associated vascular abnormalities, parenchymal atrophy, ischmic damage and choroid plexus enlargement. PET can show areas of ischemia

Ocular Features

- Choroid angiomas l/t (overproducion) **glaucoma** (nearly always unilateral and is present at birth in 60%). **Buphthalmos** (enlarged eye) and **cloudy cornea** occurs when glaucoma is present at birth, whereas patients at later age present with *increasing myopia* and *retinal detachment.*
- Failure to treat early will l/t *optic nerve damage, field defects and ultimately blindness.*
- Management includes ***control of seizures (when present) with anticonvulsants, regular follow up for detection of glaucoma and treatment of PWS by tuneable dye laser (PDL)***Q

Questions

1. **Underlying internal malignancy is not shown by** *(AI 96)*
   A. Acanthosis nigricans & Annular erythema ☐
   B. Bullous pyoderma & migratory necrotizing erythema ☐
   C. Granuloma annulare ☐
   D. Erythema gyratum repens ☐
2. **Following are signs of internal malignancy except:** *(PGI 97)*
   A. Tuberous sclerosis ☐
   B. Acanthosis nigricans ☐
   C. Clubbing ☐
   D. Dermatomyositis ☐
   E. None ☐
3. **Skin markers of internal malignancy are/is** *(PGI Nov 11)*
   A. Acanthosis nigricans ☐
   B. Migratory necrolytic erythema ☐
   C. Necrobiosis lipodica ☐
   D. Bullous pemphigoid ☐
   E. Dermatomyositis ☐
4. **Which of the following is/are not the cutaneous manifestation of diabetes mellitus:** *(PGI May 13)*
   A. Necrobiosis lipodica ☐
   B. Diabetic bulla ☐
   C. Shin spots ☐
   D. Calcinosis cutis ☐
   E. Angiokeratoma ☐
5. **Multiple sebaceous tumors are seen in** *(AI 2011)*
   A. Gardner's syndrome ☐
   B. Cowden's syndrome ☐
   C. Carney complex ☐
   D. Muir- Torr syndrome ☐
6. **Predisposing factors for skin ca are :** *(PGI 02)*
   A. Lichen planus ☐
   B. Bowen's disease ☐
   C. Psoriasis ☐
   D. Behcet's disease ☐
   E. U Vrays ☐
7. **Changes of squamous cell carcinoma are seen in:** *(PGI 97)*
   A. Seborrhoeic keratosis ☐
   B. Bowen's disease ☐
   C. Lichen planus ☐
   D. DLE ☐
8. **Actinic keratosis is seen in :** *(AIIMS May 02)*
   A. Basal cell carcinoma ☐
   B. Squamous cell carcinoma ☐
   C. Malignant melanoma ☐
   D. Epithelial cell carcinoma ☐
9. **Which is related to sunlight exposure** *(AIIMS May 12)*
   A. Actinic keratosis ☐
   B. Molluscum contagiosum ☐
   C. Icthyosis ☐
   D. Basal cell carcinoma ☐
10. **Acanthosis nigricans is indicative of:** *(PGI 98, Kerala 97, DNB 99)*
    A. Internal malignancy ☐
    B. Endocrine disorder ☐
    C. Blooms syndrome ☐
    D. Pigmentation of face, neck etc. ☐
    E. All are correct ☐
11. **Acanthosis Nigricans in old patient usually indicate :** *(Jharkhand 04, DNB 06)*
    A. Skin Disorder ☐
    B. Malignancy ☐
    C. Senile Brain ☐
    D. Usually found in negro ☐
12. **False regarding acanthosis nigricans is** *(PGI – 07)*
    A. Prognostic indicator ☐
    B. Velvety plaques on dirty hyperpigmentation ☐
    C. Confirmatory sign of malignancy ☐
    D. Gastric adenocarcinma is commonest malignant association ☐
    E. Indicate hyper androgenic state ☐
13. **True about acanthosis nigricans** *(PGI 03)*
    A. Most commonly seen in obesity ☐
    B. Seen in axilla ☐
    C. It signifies internal malignancy ☐
    D. It is associated with insulin resistance ☐
    E. Seen inold age ☐
14. **Mycosis cells are altered :** *(AI 89, DNB 96)*
    A. T Lymphocytes ☐
    B. Monocytes ☐
    C. b lymphocytes ☐
    D. Eosinophils ☐
15. **Mycosis fungoides which is not true:** *(AIIMS Nov. 2006)*
    A. It is the most common form of cutaneous lymphoma ☐
    B. Pautriers microabscess ☐
    C. Indolent course and good prognosis, easily amenable to treatment ☐
    D. Erythroderma seen and spreads to peripheral circulation ☐
16. **Pautrier's micro-abcess is a histological feature of:** *(AIIMS Nov 05)*
    A. Sarcoidosis ☐
    B. TB ☐
    C. Mycosis fungoides ☐
    D. Ptyriasis lichenoides chronica ☐
17. **Which of the following statements about mycosis fungoides is not true?** *(AI 2007)*
    A. It is the most common skin lymphoma ☐
    B. Pautriers micro abscesses are common ☐
    C. It has a indolent course and good prognosis. ☐
    D. It presents with diffuse erythroderma. ☐
18. **TOC in mycosis fungoides** *(AIIMS 91)*
    A. 5 – FU ☐
    B. Radiotherapy ☐
    C. Full skin electron Threapy ☐
    D. I/V Adriamycin ☐
19. **Total skin electron irradiation is used for treatment of** *(AI 12)*
    A. Sezary syndrome ☐
    B. Mycoses fungoides ☐
    C. Psoriasis ☐
    D. Brain metastasis of skin cancer ☐
20. **Langerhans cells in skin are :** *(AI 96)*
    A. Antigen presenting cells ☐
    B. Pigment producing cells ☐
    C. Keratin synthesisng cells ☐
    D. Sensory neurons ☐
21. **All are true about Langerhans' histocytosis except?** *(AIIMS May 09)*
    A. Common before 3 years of age ☐
    B. Letterer Siwe disease is systemic manifestation ☐
    C. Radio sensitive ☐
    D. Testis is commonly involved ☐
22. **All are true regarding LCH except** *(PGI 07)*
    A. Papular trunk lesions with scaling & crusting ☐
    B. Ulcerative nodules on mucosa ☐
    C. Calvarial defect with map lesions & floating teeth ☐
    D. CD – 68 positive ☐

E. Polyostotis bone lesions t/t by polychemotherapy. ☐

23. Rx of refractory histiocytosis? *(AIIMS Nov 08)*
A. Cladarabine ☐
B. High dose MTX ☐
C. High dose cytosine arabinoside ☐
D. Fludarabine ☐

24. Child presents with linear verrucous plaques on the trunk with vacuolization of keratinocytes in s. spinosum and s. granulosum. Diagnosis is: *(AIIMS Nov 08, May 11)*
A. In continenta pigmenti ☐
B. Delayed hypersensitivity reaction ☐
C. Linear / Verrucous epidermal nevus ☐
D. Linear Darier's disease ☐

Cosmetics and Skin care

25. Chemical peeling is done by all except:*(AIIMS Nov, 2010)*
A. Trichloroaccetic acid ☐
B. Phosphoric acid ☐
C. Carbolic acid ☐
D. Kojic acid ☐

26. A mother brought her child which has got a vascular plaque like lesion over the lateral aspect of forehead mainly involving ophthalmic and maxillary division of trigeminal nerve. Mother says that the lesion remains unchanged since birth. Also mother gives a history that the child is on valproate for seizure disorder. The probable diagnosis is *(AIIMS May 12)*
A. Tuberous sclerosis ☐
B. Infantile hemangioma ☐
C. Sturage weber syndrome ☐
D. Incontinentia pigment ☐

27. Child with erythematous non blanching bosselated lesion on right side of face, Rx is: *(AIIMS May 2011)*
A. Erbium laser ☐
B. Nd-YAG laser ☐
C. Flash light pumped dye laser ☐
D. Q ruby laser ☐

Answers and Explanations:

1. C i.e. Granuloma annulare **2. E i.e. None**

3. A i.e. Acanthosis nigricans; B i.e. Migratory necrolytic erythema; D i.e. Bullous pemphigoid; E i.e. Dermatomyositis

4. D i.e. Calcinosis cutis; E i.e. Angiokeratoma
[Ref: Roxburgh 18/e p 293-97, 276-77; Neena Khanna 4/e p. 229, 233, 392-96; Rook's 8/e p 62.14-62.46; Fitzpatrick's 8/e p 1840-53; Harrison 18/e p. 2988]

- **Granuloma annulare, necrobiosis lipoidica, diabetic bulla (bullosis diabeticorum)** and **diabetic dermopathy (shin spots) are skin markers of diabetes mellitus** (and are **not associated with internal malignancy**).
- **Tuberous sclerosis** is AD condition of **angiokeratomas**, epilepsy, mental retardation which may be a/w multisystem tumors, mostly hamartomatous.
- **Calcinosis cutis (cutaneous calcinosis** or **metastatic calcinosis)** is seen in **hyperparathyroidism** (elevated Ca^{++} & phosphate), juvenile variant of dermatomyositis and in **scleroderma/systemic sclerosis** as a part of **CREST syndrome** (i.e. Calcinosis cutis, Raynaud's phenomenon, Esophageal dysmotality, Sclerodactyly, and Telangiectasia).

Skin Markers of Internal Malignancy

Mnemonic = "**BAD-MENS**"

- Bullous pemphigoid
- Acquired icthyosis
- ***Acanthosis nigricans***[Q]
- ***Annular erythema***[Q]
- Dermatomyositis
- ***Migratory Necrolytic erythema***[Q]
- ***Erythema gyratum repens***[Q] *(specific marker of C_A bronchus mostly)*
- ***Erythema multiforme***[Q]
- ***Necrolytic migratory erythema***[Q]
- Skin metastasis

★ Bullous pemphigoid, dermatomyositis, acanthosis nigricans, and figurate erythemas (i.e. annular erythema & erythema multiforme) are weakly / sometimes a/w underlying malignant disease whereas others have strong association.

★ **Clubbing** is seen in ***metastatic lung cancer & mesothelioma***[Q]

5. D i.e. Muir – Torre syndrome

Muir – Torre syndrome (i.e. *multiple seabecous tumors like adenoma, carcinoma or keratoacanthoma and visceral malignancy*) is a genodermatoses that is cutaneous marker of internal malignancy.

6. A i.e. Lichen planus; B i.e. Bowen's disease; E i.e. UV rays

7. B i.e. Bowen's disease, D i.e. DLE, C i.e. Lichen planus

8. B i.e. Squamous Cell Carcinoma **9. A i.e. Actinic Keratosis**
[Ref: Roxburgh's 17/e p. 209-13; Harrison 15/e P-554/558; Bailey & Love 23/e P-179-181; Fitzpatrick's 7/e p-1007-15; Rooks 8/e p. 52.30-32; CMDT (2002) p. 151]

Etiological Factors & Premalignant lesions for Squamous Cell CA

1. ***Actinic (Solar) Keratosis***Q, Arsenic (As) Keratosis
2. ***Bowen's disease***Q (Intra-epidermal epithelioma)
3. Chemical carcinogens eg. tar, pitch, Arsenic
4. ***DLE***Q, Dystrophic epidermolysis bullosa
5. Erythema ab igne (persistent heat injury)
   Erythroplasia of queyratQ (Bowen's ds. of glans penis)
   Epidermal naevus
   Epidermodysplasia verruciformis
6. Giant warty tumor of genitalia, ***Genodermal disease (i.e. Xeroderma)***Q
7. ***Hypertrophic lichen planus***Q
   Human Papilloma virus infection (more commonly in immunosuppressed renal transplant patients)
8. ***Xeroderma pigmentosa (Genodermal disease)***Q
9. ***UV radiation – UV-B***Q

Mnemonic = "**ABC D² E⁴ – G² H² - XU**"

Actinic/ Solar Keratosis (AK)

- These are hyperkeratotic lesions that ***develop in response to prolonged exposure to ultraviolet radiation (i.e. on chronically light exposed adult skin)***Q. Risk factors for development of AK include old age, male gender, fair skin that easily burns and freckles, blond/red hair, light colored eyes, immunosuppression, gentic syndromes (like XP, Bloom's and Rothmund-Thomoon syndromes), prior history of AK or other skin cancer and most importantly ***cumulative UV radiation exposure***Q.
- Historically being considered ***premalignant lesions***Q with focal areas of abnormal proliferation and differentiation that carry a ***low risk (0.2%) of progression to invasive sauqmous cell carcinoma***Q. However, now these are defined as malignant neoplasm with intra epithelial SCCs in evolution.
- It is raised, pink or grey, scaling or warty hyperkeratotic plaque or papule with *alternating parakeratoses & hyperkeratosis in histology.*

Premalignant lesion	Predisposed Cancer
*Actinic (Solar) Keratosis*Q	Squamous cell carcinoma
*Bowen's ds. (intra-epidermal-epithelioma)*Q	Squamous cell CA
*Erythroplasia*Q *of Queyrat*Q (bowen's ds. affecting glans penis)	Squamous cell CA
Lantigo maligna **(Hutchinson's freckle)**Q	Malignant Melanoma

- Also Know
  - **UV – radiation & Xeroderma pigmentosa** are risk factors for all 3 types of skin cancer (Basal, Squamous Cell, & Melanoma).
  - **Lentigo maligna (Hutchinson's freckle)** is premalignant lesion for ***malignant melanoma***Q.

10. **E i.e. All** 11. **B. i.e. Malignancy**
12. **C. i.e. Confirmatory sign of malignancy**
13. **A i.e. Most commonly seen in obesity; B i.e. Seen in axilla; C i.e. It signifies internal malignancy; D i.e. It is associated with insulin resistance** *[Ref: Thomas Habif 4/e p. 900 – 1; Neena Khanna 3rd/p 34-35; Fitzpatrick 7/e p. 635, 1448, 1462- 63, 1494-96; Roxburgh's 17/e p. 283; Davidson 19/e P-1099]*

14. **A. i.e. T lymphacytis** 15. **C i.e. It has indolent course and good prognosis easily amenable to treatment**
16. **C i.e. Mycosis Fungoides** 17. **C i.e. It has indolent course and good prognosis**
18. **C i.e. Full skin electron therapy** 19. **B i.e. Mycoses fungoides**

[Ref: Robbins 7/e 671, 685, 1249-50; Roxburgh's 17/e 224-5,131; Fitzpatrick's 6/e p- 1537-57, 719-35; Rook's 7/e p. 54.7-54.23; 36.26-36.42]

- **Mycosis fungoides** is an **indolent** ***cutaneous T – cell lymphoma***Q with patients often having several years of eczematous or dermatitis skin lesion before the diagnosis is finally established. But the disorder is ***inevitably fatal***Q, although the rate of progression is quite variable.
- ***Mycosis Fungoides and Sezary Syndrome are T-Cell neoplasm***Q. Mycosis fungoides (a T Cell malignancy) has skin manifestations like urticatia, erythema, eczema, itching & hard nodules which later on ulcerate containing fungating granulation. ***Pauterier's microabscess***Q is histological features of **mycosis fungoides.** *TOC is electron beam radiation*Q.

20. **A i.e Antigen presenting cells** 21. **D. i.e. Testis is commonly invoved**
22. **D i.e. CD – 68 positive; E. i.e. Polyostotis bone lesions t/t by polychemotherapy.** 23. **A. i.e. Cladarabine**

[Ref: National Cancer Institute www.cancer.gov; Fitzpatrick 7/e p. 1414- 24; CMDT 2009 p. 965; Neena Khanna 3rd p-323; Journal of Pediatric Onchology; Robbins 7/e p- 701-02, 199-200]

24. **C. i.e. Linear epidermal nevus**

[Ref: Fitzpatrick's 7/e p-1056-58, 631, 32, 443, 435; Thomas Habif 4/e p- 713-14; Department of DNYU, online journal 9(4)15]

Linear verrucous epidermal nervs presents with localized/diffuse, closely set, skin coloured ***verrucous plaques with liner configuration (along Blaschko's lines) on limbs and transverse configuration on trunk***Q. Histology shows acanthosis, papillomatosis, hyperkeratosis, compact orthokeratosis, alternating bands of ortho and ***parakeratosis, perinulclear vacuolization of keratinocytes in granular layer (stratum granulosum) and stratum spinosum***Q and irregular cellular boundaries peripheral to the vacuolization and increased number of *irregularly shaped large kerathinohyaline granules.*

Cosmetics and Skin care

25. **B i.e. Phosphoric acid** *[Ref: Fitzpatrick 7/e p. 2369-71; Roxburgh 18/e p. 347; Rook's 8/e p. 80.9 – 80.10; Neena Khanna 4/e p. 418; IAVDL 3/e p-1678]*

Chemical peeling is done by α hydroxy acids (glycolic acid, lactic acid, malic acid, citric acid), β hydroxy acid (salicyclic acid), ***trichloroacetic acid (TCA)***Q, α-ketoacid (pyruvic acid), ***phenol (carbolic acid), Kojic acid***Q, retinoic acid (tretinoin), resorcinol, solid carbon dixoxide, **Jessner's solution** (lactic acid + salicylic acid + resorcinol + 95% ethonol), **modified Unna's resorcinol paste** and **Baker –Gordon phenol peel** (phenol + croton oil + hexachlorophene/septisol+distilled water). ***But phosphoric acid is not used for chemical peeling***Q.

26. **C i.e. Sturge –Weber Syndrome** *[Ref: Rook's 8/e p. 18.6 – 18.65; Fitzpatrick 7/e p. 1651-53]*

Vascular plaque ***(capillary malformation) over lateral aspect of forehead mainly involving ophthalmic (V_1) and maxillary (V_2) division of trigeminal nerve and sezures***Q suggest diagnosis of **Sturge-Weber syndrome (encephalo-trigeminal angiomatosis).**

27. **C i.e. Flash light pumped dye laser** *[Ref: Rook's 8/e p. 78.5 -78.7, 18.63 – 18.64; Fitzpatrick's 7/e p. 2374-76; 1652-56]*

- ***Flash lamp pumped – pulsed tuneable dye lasers (PDL)***Q is the **intervention of choice for uncomplicated porwine stains (PWS) or capillary malformations (CM).**
- 1st generation PDLs operated at *577 or 585nm* and achieve lightening by reducing number and size of erythrocytes in vessels by *selective photothermolysis* (as oxyhemoglobin has absorption peak at 577/542/ and 418nm). **Flash lamp-pumped** PDL uses a high-power *Xenon flashlamp* to excite *rhodamine(organic) dye* to produce a *pulse of yellow light that* is absorbed by oxyhemoglobin. **Pulsed lasers** allowed for more precise targeting of oxyhemoglobin containing vessels with less thermal and mechanical injury of surrounding tissue. Because of emission of continuous thermal energy l/t scarring and pigmentary alteration, the use of early lasers such as argon laser (488/514nm), argon pumped tunable laser (488 to 638nm), copper and bromide laser (578nm), potassium –titanyl-phosphate (KTP) laser (532 nm) and krypton laser (568nm) is limited.
- **585nm short pulse PDL** is probably optimal for treating paediatric PWS because vessel diameters are relatively small. Success rate is 50-90%; the *size of vessels, its depth and density* will influence the response. Factors favoring a good response to PDL are presence of *more superficially located vessels, flat and red/scarlet* (as opposed to pink and purple) *PWS on head and neck* (a compared to other body sites), as well as *youth*. Although *peripheral facial lesions* respond better than midline-centrofacial or cheeks.
- Side effects of PDL are few and includes *bruising* (in all cases), *pain, swelling, crusting bleeding, pyogenic granuloma, both hypo and hyper-pigmentation, prtial re-emergence and redarkening*.
- 2nd generation PDLs, emit light with a longer *wave length of 595nm* (absorption of which by HbO_2 is 5 times lower), longer pulse width, higher fluences with addition of cooling system. This may be *suitable for deeper, bigger vessels* in **resistant or adult PWS.**
- In **PDL resistant** capillary malformations *KTP laser* may produce extra lightening. **Hypertrophic and PDL resistant** PWS are sometimes treated with near *infrared lasers* such as *alexandrite (755nm) and Nd: YAG (1064nm)* laser, multiple pass irradiation with *two PDL passes*: 1st at 590-600nm and 2nd at 585nm, and intense pulsed light (e.g. photoderm) or combined pulsed dye & Nd:YAG laser. Other possibilities under investigation include *electro-optical synergy and vaccum assisted laser treatment*. **Adult** patients in whom **progressive vascular ectasia** has resulted in very **exophytic lesions** are probably best treated with **CO_2 laser.**

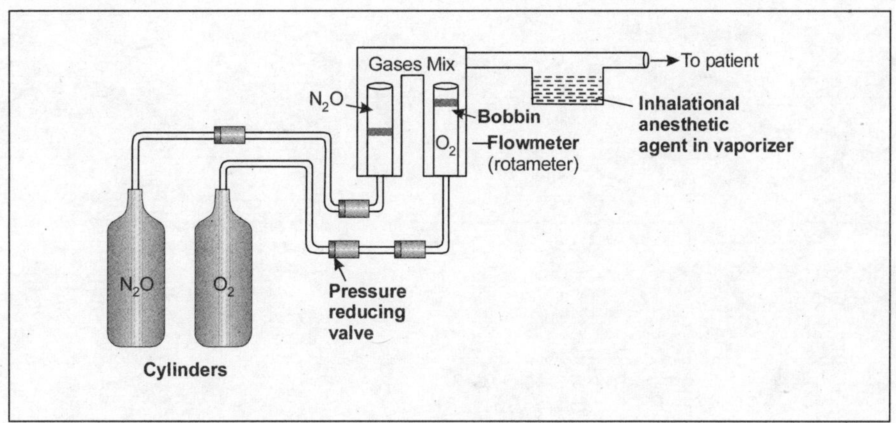

Anaesthesia

1 ANESTHESIA TROLLY, INSTRUMENTS, CIRCUITS, VENTILATION AND PREANAESTHETIC MEDICATION

Anaesthesia Machines & Cylinders

Anaesthesia Machine :Boyle's Apparatus

- Boyle's machine was first developed in *1917* by *Edmund Gaskin Boyle*. It operates on the ***continuous flow***Q principle, where gas flows all the time during the inspiratory and expiratory phase of patient respiration. During expiration, the gas flow is temporarily being stored in a reservoir bag.
- An anesthetic agent is delivered to the patient via flow controllers and mixture controllers. Normally a mixture of ***N_2O and O_2 would act as a carrier for the main agent eg halothane, which is in liquid form and thus provide anesthetic vapours***Q.
- Anesthetic machine has three parts according to pressure. *High pressure system* includes *cylinders* with pressure regulators yolk assembly, pressure reducing valve and oxygen flush. *Intermediate pressure system is from pressure reducing valve to flow control valve* and includes oxygen failure alarm & O_2-N_2O lock. And *low pressure system* is beyond flow control valve upto machine outlet and includes rotameter, vaporizer and high pressure valve.
- Gases in cylinder are at higher pressure 2000 psi (pound per square inch) for O_2 & ***760 psi for N_2O***Q, which is reduced to *50-60 psi* by first and *15-20 psi* by second pressure reducing valve. Now gases reach flow meters and mix at the top of flow meter from where they pass through a vaporizer containing inhalational agent, the vapours of which get incorporated in gaseous mixture which finally reaches the machine outlet at a pressure of *5-8 psi*.

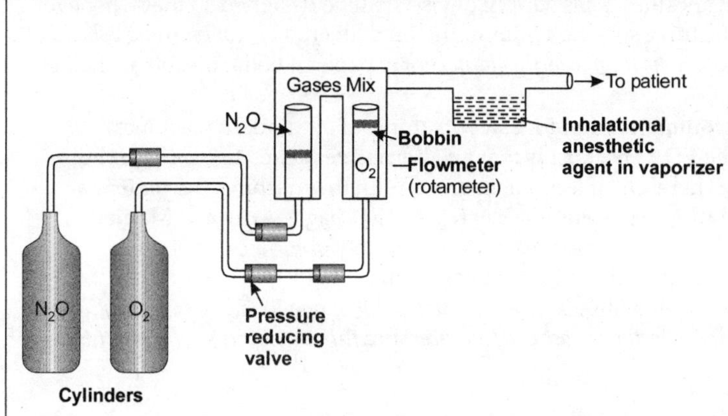

Rotameter

- ***It is a variable orifice, constant pressure flow meter.***Q
- It contains **bobbin or marker** to indicate the ***flow rate of gas***Q. *The height to which bobbin rises is increased with the flow rate.*
- Causes of inaccurate readings include- ***static electricity***Q, dirt, cracked and non-vertical flow meter tubes, a defect in the top sealing washer of a rotameter and back pressure.
- ***Static electricity & dirt can cause as much as 35% inaccuracy***Q due to sticking of bobbin, especially in low flows. To reduce effects of static electricity coating of tubes interior with a conductive substance is done.
- Dirt can also change the effective diameter of tube to cause inaccurate reading.

Respirometer (Spirometer / Ventilometer / Respiratory flow meter / Ventilation or respiratory meter or monitor / Volume measuring device)

- Respirometer is a device that *measures the volume of gas passing during a period of time* through a location in flow pathway.
- ***Monitoring respiratory volumes and flows*** can help in detecting breathing system obstruction, disconnections, leaks, apnea, ventilator failure, and high or low volumes in spontaneously breathing patients as well as in those whose ventilation is controlled. A discrepancy between expired & inspired tidal volume suggest a leak or incompetent unidirectional valve / reversed flow.
- ASA recommended *monitoring of volumes of expired gases*. So anesthesia workstation standard requires a device *to monitor*

Wright Respirometer (Vane Anemometer)

- It is an older, *mechanical respirometer* which employs a *rotating vane of low mass in expiratory limb* in front of the expiratory valve of breathing circuit of anesthesia machine.
- Gas entering through outer casing is *directed through a series of tangential slots* (enclosed in a cylindrical housing) and *strikes the vane in the center, causing it to rotate.* The vane is connected by a mechanical gear system to the hands on the dial (i.e. display indicator) so that a reading corresponding to the volume of gas passing through the device is registered.
- ***Because of inertia, Wright's respirometer over reads at high flows and under reads at low flows***Q. **Pulsatile flows** can also cause over-reading. It will give slightly higher readings with **N_2O & O_2 mixtures** than for air and will slightly over-read in presence of **xenon**.

the patient's exhaled tidal or minute volume or both.

- **Possible locations for spirometer** in the circle system may be 1) in ***exhalation limb*** upstream or downstream of unidirectional valve (most common); 2) ***between breathing system and patient*** (most desirable from the standpoint of accuracy); 3) ***downstream of CO_2 absorber*** (volume of gas measured is decreased d/t absorption); 4) ***on inspiratory limb*** (show high readings as the gas that does not inflate patient's lung will also pass; but disconnection may not be detected during controlled ventilation). *Pressure flow sensors are located at expiratory downstream & inspiratory positions.*
- Measurement of exhaled tidal volumes in expiratory limb includes gas that had been lost to the circuit (& not delivered to the patient).
- The difference b/w the volume of gas delivered to circuit & volume of gas actually reaching the patient becomes very significant with *long compliant breathing tubes, rapid respiratory rates & high airway pressures.* These problems (of position 4) are particularly overcome by measuring the tidal volume at Y connector to the patient's airway (position 2).
- Flow of gas across respirometer is measured *mechanically (Wright's R.),* electronically/ electro-magnetically (spiromed), photoelectrically, or by measuring *differential pressure* (flow sensor & D-lite gas sampler, novametrics side stream sensor), *thermal dissipation* (heated wire anemometer), and *discontinuities in gas flow* (ultrasonic flow sensor). A **pneumotachograph** is a fixed orifice flow meter that can function as spirometer.
- Advantages include small size, light weight, no power supply is needed and *low dead space* which makes it suitable b/w patient & breathing system.
- Disadvantages include **lack of alarms**, is difficult to read, expensive maintenance, needs to be cleaned & disinfected b/w patients and *inaccuracy* b/o poor mechanical condition or portability resulting in damage from being dropped or pocket dirt.
- ***It does not read bidirectional flow and does not give respiratory rate***Q. A clock is necessary to determine minute volume. ***Flow can be calculated by averaging recorded volumes over time***Q.

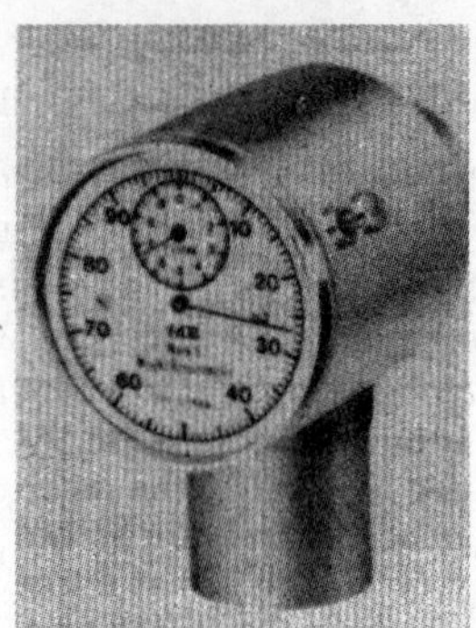

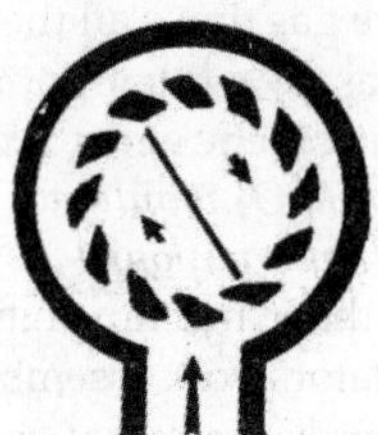

Wright Respirometer

Hypoxia Preventation Safety Devices

- **1998 ASTM F1850 – 00** (51.12.1/2) states that, "The anesthesia gas supply devise shall be designed so that whenever O_2 supply pressure is reduced to below the manufacturer specified minimum, the delivered *O_2 concentration shall not decrease below 19% at the common gas outlet*; and atleast *a medium priority alarm* (not capable of being disabled) shall be activated *within 5 sec.*
- In 1993, USFDA published **anesthesia checkout recommendation** for safety features of all modern machines/ workstations, by an educated user. **Item no. 1** on the FDA checklist is that an **alternative means to ventilate the patients lung should be present and functioning.** Therefore, if a problem arises with the machine, the **patient's lungs can be ventilated manually using a self inflating resuscitation bag (eg AMBU bag = Artificial Manual Breathing Unit).** If a machine problem arises and the cause/remedy is not immediately obvious, one should instinctively reach for the **resuscitation bag and start manual ventilation**Q and call for help.
- One of the most serious mishaps that occurred with early mahines, was *depletion of O_2 supply (usually from a cylinder) without the user's awareness resulting in delivery of 100% anesthetic gas.* ***Oxygen pressure failure devices****, to prevent this problem, include*

Oxygen Failure Safety Device (Valve)/ Low Pressure Guardian System/Oxygen Failure Protection Device/ Pressor Sensor Shut or Cut off Valve/N_2O Shut off System/Fail Safe Device or Valve.

- Oxygen can pass directly to its flow control valve , whereas, *N_2O, other gases & air (in some machine) must pass through a safety device – fail safe valve* before reaching their respective flow control valve. ***So fail safe valve is located down stream from N_2O supply source***Q.
- These valves permit the flow of other gases only if there is sufficient O_2 pressure in safety device. Safety devices sense O_2 pressure via a small piloting pressure line and *if pressure falls below a threshold eg* 20 psig, **shut off / cut off / fail safety** valve close, preventing the administration of any other gas. In datex –ohmeda machine, a pressure sensor shut off valve completely shut off the flow of all other gasses at 133 KPa (998mm Hg).
- **Fail Safe (Pressure Sensor) System shuts** off or proportionally decreases and ultimately interrupts the supply of N_2O if the O_2 supply pressure decreases; air supply may or may not be cut off.

Oxygen Supply Failure Alarm

- Acoording to standard specification, **whenever the O_2 supply pressure** (at inlet) **falls below a manufacture specified threshold** ~20-35 psig (usually 30 psig=205 KPa) **low pressure O_2 supply sensor, activate at least a medium priority alarm (gas whistle, electrical alarm) within 5 second.** It shall not be possible to disable this alarm.

Proportioning Safety Device

Most modern (Datex Ohmeda) machines use a *proportioning safety device* instead of threshold cutt off fail safe valve system.
These devices *proportionately reduce the pressure of N_2O & other gases except* air. Nitrous oxide & other gases are completely shut off only below a set minimum O_2 pressure (eg 0.5 psig for N_2O & 10 psig for other gases).

Balance regulator (Datex Ohmedamachine)

A **second stage O_2 regulator** down stream from O_2 supply source in intermediate pressure circuit ensuring a constant pressure of O_2 at the flow meter untill pressures fall below 80 –107 KPa (600 –802 mmHg | 14 psig)

Oxygen failure protection device (Draeger Narkomed)

A proportional system with complete shut off of N_2O occurring when O_2 pressure falls below 67 KPa (502 mmHg)

- **Both the O_2 failure safety device and alarm depends on pressure and not flow.** They **aid in preventing hypoxia caused by problems occurring upstream in the machine circuits (disconnected O_2 hose, low O_2 pressure in pipeline,** and **depletion of O_2 cylinders).** These devices **do not offer total protection against a hypoxic mixture being delivered,** because they do not prevent anesthetic gas from flowing **if there is no flow of oxygen.**

- **Flow control valve** seperate the intermediate pressure circuit from the low pressure circuit. ***High pressure* circuit** is confined to ***cylinders & cylinder's primary pressure regulators***Q. ***Intermediate pressure*** *circuit* includes ***pipeline (gasline) upto flow valves***Q and ***low pressure circuit*** is b/w ***flow valve & common gas outlet***Q. The operator regulates flow entering the *low pressure circuit* by turning flow – control. Valve. For safety, *O_2 knob is larger, fluted, protudes more than other knobs & situated furthest to the right.*

Link 25 proportion limiting control system (Datex ohmeda)

- Uses a chain to link O_2 & N_2O flow control knobs with 14- tooth sprocket attached to N_2O
- flow control valve & 28 tooth sprocket to O_2 valve
- Allows independent adjustment of either valve but automatically ***maintains a 25% O_2 concentration and a maximum N_2O- O_2 flow ratio of 3: 1***Q

Pneumatic interlock ORMC (oxygen ratio monitor controller) or **S – ORC (sensitive O_2 ratio controller)** Drager Narkomed machine

- Maintain fresh gas *O_2 concentration at 25 ± 3%* at O_2 flow rates of less than 1L/min
- Maintain O_2 conc. by limiting nitrous oxide flow, unlike that of link 25, which actively increases O_2 flow.

★ These safety device does not affect the flow of third gas (eg CO_2, air, helium)

- **Flow meter sequence** in a three gas machine: ***The safest configuration is when oxygen is located in down stream position (after both gases)***Q. However, a leak in O_2 flow tube can produce a hypoxic mixture even when it is located down stream.

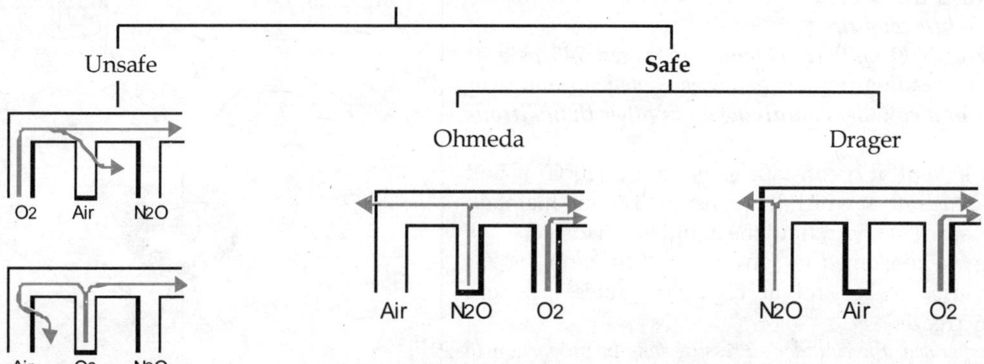

- **Oxygen flush valve** allows direct communication b/w the high & low pressure circuit; and ***delivers 100% O_2 at a rate of 35 –75 l/min on actuation (may l/t barotrauma)***Q.

Pin Index Safety System (PISS) & Coding of Gas Cylinder

- PISS consists of **7 hole positions on the cylinder valve** positioned in an arc (circumference of a circle) of 9/16 inch radius centered on the port. The **corresponding pins on the yoke or pressure regulator of anaesthesia machine** are positioned to fit into these holes. The pins are 4 mm in diameter and 6 mm long, except for pin 7 which is slightly thicker.
- PISS is a safety feature ***adopted to prevent incorrect gas cylinder attachment***Q. To prevent incorrect attachment or misconnection, each gas cylinder valve block have *holes drilled in 2 out of 6 positions* (a single hole in entonox). *The relative positioning of pins & holes is unique for each gas or gas mixture (k/a* ***pin index)*** and unless the pins & holes are aligned, the port will not seat.
- Each gas cylinder (A-E) has ***two holes in its cylinder valve that mate with corresponding pins in the yoke of anesthesia machine***Q. Each cylinder has a particular pin code and unless the correct cylinder valve is attached, the pins & holes will not coincide. Thus it is practically impossible to fit any cylinder to wrong yoke.
- It is possible for a yoke or a pressure regulator without pins to receive any cylinder valve, but ordinarily it is not possible for an undrilled cylinder valve to be placed in a yoke or pressure regulator containing pins.
- ***The pin index safety system is ineffective if yoke pins are damaged or cylinder is filled with wrong gas or using extra sealing washers (between cylinder and yolk).***
- There are *problems with PISS when specialized gas mixtures are used.* For example 5% CO_2 with O_2 has different pin index than 100% CO_2. But CO_2 mixture of 7% or greater CO_2 would be fitted with the pin index of 100% CO_2.

Pressure and Storage of Gases

- High pressure (H) gas cylinders are made up of ***steel alloy of molybdenum***Q **(molybdenum - steel) and gas pipes** are made of *seamless copper tubing.* **Height, size** and **volume** of cylinder increases from A onwards with **smallest available size AA and biggest H. So A<B<C<D<E<G<H<J.**
- E cylinders of O_2, N_2O and air attach, directly to anesthesia machine.
- ***Nitrous oxide (N_2O), carbondioxide (CO_2) and cyclopropane are stored in liquid form***Q in equilibrium with saturated vapours, whereas, oxygen, nitrogen, helium, air, xenon, nitric oxide & carbon monooxide are stored as gases.
- N_2O can be kept in liquid form without refrigeration system, because its *critical temperature 36.5°C* is above room temperature (in cold countries). Upto 80% of full N_2O cylinder volume contains liquid. *Filling ratio* of N_2O (i.e., ratio of weight of N_2O to weight of water that would fill the cylinder) is *0.67 in tropical & 0.75 in temperature countries.*
- ***Pressue gauge of N_2O cylinder should not exceed 745 psig at 20°C***Q. A higher reading implies gauge *malfunction,* tank over fill (liquid fill), ***or a cylinder containing a gas other than nitrous oxide***Q.
- If liquid N_2O is kept at a constant temperature (20°C) it will vaporize at a same rate at which it is consumed & will maintain a constant pressure (745 psig) until the liquid is exhausted.
- Because energy is consumed in conversion of *liquid to gas, the liquid nitrous oxide cools.* And at high flow rates, pressure regulators may freeze
- *As oxygen is expanded, the cylinder's pressure falls in proportion to its content.*
- N_2O is neither flammable nor explosive, but supports combustion even in absence of O_2, if high temperature (> 450°C) is provided to initiate decomposition into N_2 & O_2.

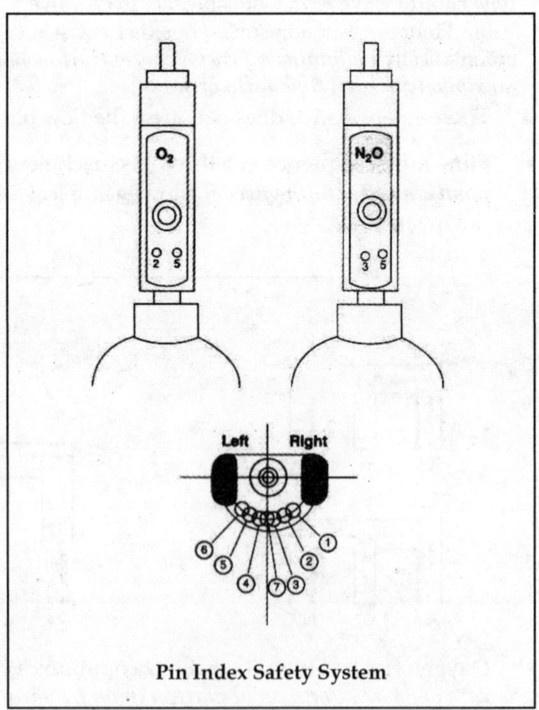

Pin Index Safety System

Coding of Gas Cylinders

Gas	UK Code / Australian Code		U S Code	Pin index position	Pressure at 15°C	
	Body	**Shoulder**			Ib in^{-2}	Bar
Oxygen	Black	White	Green	2, 5	1987	137
Nitrous oxide	Blue	Blue	Blue	3, 5	*638*Q	44
CO_2	Gray	Gray	Gray	1, 6	725	50
Helium	Brown	Brown	Brown	-	1987	137
Air	Grey	White / black quartered	Yellow	1, 5	1987	137
O_2/CO_2	Black	White / grey quartered	-	CO_2 < 7.5% = 2,6 CO_2 > 7.5%=1,6	1987	137
O_2/ Helium	Black	White /brown quartered	-	He > 80.5% = 4, 6 He < 80.5% = 2, 4	1987	137
N_2O/O_2 (Entonox)	Black	White / blue quartered	-	N_2O 47.5-52.5% = 7	1987	137
N_2	Black	Black	Black	1, 4		

Breathing System

- **Mapleson A / Magill system** *is most efficient for spontaneous ventilation*Q because fresh gas flow equals to minute volume is sufficient to prevent rebreathing of exhaled air. In Mapleson A circuit during spontaneous breathing, alveolar gas with CO_2 will be exhaled into B. tube or directly vented through an open pop off valve. Before inhalation occurs if the fresh gas flow exceeds alveolar minute volume, the inflow of fresh gas will force the remaining alveolar gas in B. tube to exit from valve and inspiration will only contain fresh gas.
- Flow rate of Mapleson A system is about *5 lit/ min*Q.
- **Mapleson D system** *is most efficient for controlled ventilation*Q since fresh gas flow forces alveolar air away from patient and towards pressure relief valve.

  Bain coaxial circuit is a popular modification of Mapleson D system that incorporates *fresh gas inlet tubing running coaxially* inside the corrugated breathing tube & ends at the point where the fresh gas would enter if the classic Mapelson D form were used. This modification *decreases the circuit bulk & retains heat and humidity better* than Mapleson D circuit as a result of partial warming of inspiratory gas by *counter current* exchange with the warmer expired gases. The possibility of kinking or disconnection of fresh gas inlet tubing l/t to re breathing of exhaled gases is the possible disadvantage.
- **Mapleson E system** is advocated primarly for use *in infants & young children*Q. The main advantage of -T- piece is absence of resistance to expiration, a factor of crucial importance to children.
- Efficiency of system with **spontaneous respiration**Q**: A** > D & E > C > B
- Efficiency of system with **IPPV**: **D & E**>B>C>A

Classification & Characteristics of Mapleson circuits

Mapleson Class	Other Name	**Spontaneous Fresh Gas Flow** Rate	**Controlled** FGFR
A	**Magill**Q	**Equal to minute ventilation (≈ 80 ml / kg / min)**Q	Very high & difficult to predict
B	–	2 x Minute ventilation (mv)	2-2½ x mv
C	Water's to and fro	2 x mv	2-2½ x mv
D	**Bain circuit**	2 – 3 x mv	1 – 2 x mv
E	**Ayre's -T- piece**Q	**2 – 3 x mv**Q	3 x mv
F	Jackson – Rees' modification	2 – 3 x mv	2 x mv

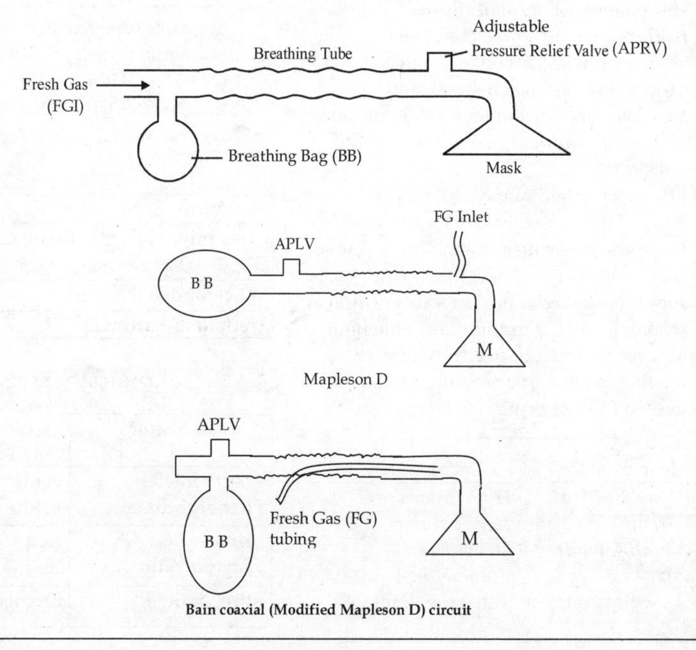

Bain coaxial (Modified Mapleson D) circuit

Rebreathing System

Rebreathing system are systems, in which some gas is rebreathed by the patient were designed originally to economize in the use of cyclopropane. In addition, they *reduce the risk of atmospheric pollution* and *increase the humidity of inspired gases*, there by *reducing heat loss from patient*. They may be used as close systems in which fresh gas is introduce only to replace oxygen & anesthetic agents absorbed by the patient. More commonly, the system is used with a small leak through a spill valve, and fresh gas supply exceeds basal oxygen requirements. Because rebreathing occurs these systems *must incorporate a means of obsorbing CO_2 from exhaled alveolar gas*. Examples are – ***To and fro (Waters's / Mapleson C) system***Q ***and Circle system***Q.

2

ANAESTHESIA

CO_2 Absorption

- Heat & humidity conserving rebreathing systems eliminate exhaled CO_2 by using CO_2 absorbent (eg. Soda / bara line).
- *Hydroxide salts* of sodalime are *irritating to mucosa* & skin; thats why *adding silica increases hardness and minimizes the risk* of inhaling sodium hydroxide dust. As barium hydroxide (in baraline) incorporates water of crystalization in its structure, its sufficiently hard & safe without silica.
- Water is essential, as the chemical reaction only takes place in presence of water. So water is aded to both soda & bara line to provide optional condition for carbonic acid formation
- Delayed induction or emergence may occur as dry *absorbent granules* can absorb & latter release large amounts of volatile anesthetics
- The generated heat inside the sodaline can break ***trichloroethylene to dichloroacetylene, which is potent neurotoxin***Q. Sodalime may also decompose **sevoflurane**, so it is *not used for periods > 3 hours* in a closed system without flushing the system. If soda lime is allowed to dry (by leaving fresh gas flowing through canister), then its subsequent use ***with desflurane, isoflurane & enflurane***Q has been associated with carbon monoxide production (Clinical insignifcant). However ***dry barium hydroxide can cause clinically significant carbon monoxide poisoning***Q
- Efficiency of sodialime depends on its *physical structure* such as granule size. Too large granules cause channeling of gas so that it fails to come in contact with sodalime and results in less absorption whereas, smaller granules provide high absorptive area but pack too tightly leading to excessive resistance to flow of gas. So CO_2 absorption is:

Increased by	Decreased by
- ***Resistance in circuit***Q - ***Small granule size***Q - Low flow rate	- ***High flow rate & tidal volume***Q - *Dead space* - ***Channeling***Q - Too large granule size

Composition of CO_2 Absorbers in Rebreathing Systems

Soda Lime

Ca $(OH)_2$	94 %
NaOH	5 %
KOH	< 1% or nil
Silica	0.2 %
Moisture	14 – 19%

- ***94% $Ca(OH)_2$ + 5% NaOH as catalyst + 1% KOH***Q
- Granule size is ***4-8 mesh***Q
- Absorbs upto ***23L of CO_2/100 g***Q (20% of its own weight)
- It can absorb & later release significant amount of volatile anesthetic (eg. Fluranes). This property is responsible for delayed induction & emergence.
- The drier the sodalime more likely that it will absorb & degrade volatile anesthetics.
- **With trilene, sodalime forms neurotoxin phosgene gas**Q, so it is contraindicated with trilene.
- **Sevoflurane** reacts **with sodalime** & produces **compound-A i.e. Pentafluoro isopropenyl-fluro-methyl ether.**
- **Sodalime should not be used with**Q

C	-	Chloroform
T	-	Trilene (form neurotoxin
	-	dichloracetylene)
Scan		Sevoflurane

Amsorb

- $Ca(OH)_2$
- Ca Cl_2
- $CaSO_4$ & polyvinylpyrro-lidone added to increase hardness
- Cause less degradation of volatile anesthetics (eg sevoflurane into compound A or desflurane into carbon mono oxide)

Baralime

$Ca(OH)_2$	80%
Ba $(OH)_2$	20%
KOH	< 1% or
Moisture	nil

- ***80% $Ca(OH)_2$ + 20% $Ba(OH)_2$***Q
- Granule size 4-8 mesh
- Absorb upto 18L CO_2/100 g
- **Desflurane can be broken down to CO**Q **by** dry barium hydroxide lime.

★ It is exothermic reaction resulting in drop of pH (d/t $CaCO_3$) and water formation. If sodalime canister is not felt warm it is not functioning)

$CO_2 + 2NaOH \rightarrow Na_2CO_3 + H_2O$ (fast)

$Na_2CO_3 + Ca(OH)_2 \rightarrow 2NaOH + CaCO_3$ (slow)

★ Note that initially required H_2O & NaOH are regenerated.

	Soda Lime	Barium Hydroxide Lime
Mesh Size	4 – 8	4 – 8
Absorptive capacity (liters) of CO_2 / 100 g granules	14- 23	9 – 18
Indicator dye (Ususal)	Ethyl violet	Ethyl voilet
Method of hardness	**Silica**	***Water of crystallization***Q

Indicator Dye changes signaling absorbent exhaustion

Indicator	Color When Fresh	Colour when exhausted
Ethyl violet	White	Purple
Phenolphthalein	White	Pink
Mimosa 2	Red	White
Clayton yellow	Red	Yellow
Ethyl orange	Orange	Yellow

★ Absorbent should be changed when 50–70% has changed colour. Although if rested, granules may revert to their original colour but absorptive capacity is not significantly recovered

Airway Management

Total dead space (Physiological dead space) = Anatomical dead space + Alveolar dead space

Anatomical Dead Space is increased by

- Old age
- ***Standing (upright) posture***Q
- Neck extension
- Jaw protrusion
- ***Bronchodilators anticholinergic e.g. (Atropine), halothane***Q
- *Increase lung volume*
- Anasthesia mask & Circuits
- IPPV (Intermittent positive pressure ventilation)
- PEEP (Positive end expiratory pressure)
- Pulmonary embolism, hypotension, emphysema

Anatomical Dead Space is decreased by

- ***Supine position***Q
- ***Neck flexion***Q
- ***Artificial airways eg intubation***Q
- ***Tracheostomy***Q
- Hyperventilation
- ***Bronchoconstrictors***Q
- ***Massive pleural effusion***Q

Alveolar Dead Space is increased by

- IPPV
- PEEP
- General anesthesia
- Hypotension
- Lung pathologies affecting diffusion membrane like interstitial lung disease, pulmonary embolism, pulmonary edema, ARDS.

Dead Space

- **Anatomical**: Area in the tracheobronchial tree where the gaseous exchange between the lung and capillaries is not possible. It starts from nasal cavity, includes larynx trachea, bronchi and end of terminal bronchiole
- **Physiological**: Space where gaseous exchange is occurring (alveoli)

Factors affecting Dead Space

Factor	Effect
Posture	
*Upright*Q	↑
*Supine*Q	↓
Position of airway	
*Neck extension*Q	↑
*Neck flexion*Q	↓
Age	↑
Artificial airway	↓
Positive pressure ventilationQ	↑
Drug-anticholinergicQ	↑
Pulmonary perfusion	
Pulmonary embolism	↑
Hypotension	↑
Pulmonary vascular disease	
EmphysemaQ	↑

O_2 Delivery Equipment (Devices)

High flow/fixed performance equipments

- *Provide complete source of inspired O_2*
- O_2 is supplied at *predetermined rate* & at *fixed concentration*, inspite of patients respiratory, pattern (i.e. flow rate is not affected by respiratory pattern). This is achieved by delivering O_2 at a flow rate greater than the peak inspiratory flow rate. A flow of more than 20l/min. is adequate because a normal inspiratory flow rate is 20-30l/min for an adult. Because of high flow rate expired gases are rapidly flushed out and thus, there is no rebreatning & no increase in dead space.
- ***Venturi mask***Q is ***colour coded*** and marked with *recommended oxygen flow rate.* It uses Bernoulli's principle to deliver fixed & predetermined O_2 concentration.
- Indications of ventimask (fixed performance device) are
  - Consistent FiO_2 & /or
  - Large inspiratory flow of gas (>40l/min)
- ***Maximum O_2 that can be delivered by venturimask is 60%***Q

Low flow or variable performance equipments

- Provides a fraction of inspired O_2. Here the FiO_2, the patient is getting is uncertain.
- It is only used when it is not critical to deliver a fixed oxygen concentration. Patient whose ventilation is dependent on a hypoxic drive must not receive O_2 from variable performance mask.
- The final conc. of inspired O_2 depends upon.
  - *O_2 supply flow rate*
  - How *tight the mask* fits on the face.
  - The *pattern of ventilation* i.e. if there is a pause between expiration & inspiration, the mask fills with O_2 and a high concentration is available at the start of inspiration.
  - Patients *inspiratory flow rate* – during inspiration O_2 is diluted by the air drawn in through the holes. If the inspiratory flow rate exceeds the flow of O_2 supply.
- Low flow devices are:
  - ***Nasal cannula (maximum O_2 delivered is 44%)***Q
  - ***Oxygen tents***Q
  - Simple mask
  - Mary carterall mask
  - Non breathing masks
  - Rebreathing masks
  - ***Polymasks***Q

Laryngeal Mask Airway (LMA)

Laryngeal Mask Airway (LMA)

1. It's a reusable (upto 40 times) *supra glottic airway device* providing ***an airway intermediate between the face- mask and tracheal tube in terms of anatomical position, invasiveness, security to protect the airway***Q, and facilitate gas exchange.
2. Also known as **Brain mask** (after the name of its inventor **Archies Brain**). It consists of 3 components: an inflatable mask, mask inflation line and airway tube. Mask is placed blindly in oropharynx and cuff is inflated until no air leak is detected. It is important to ensure that the *maximum inflation volume is not exceeded*. Cuffed mask is designated to fit closely over laryngeal aperture forming a *low pressure seal* around it. An ideally positioned cuff is boardered by the base of tongue (superiorly), pyriform sinus (laterally) and upper esophageal sphincter (inferiorly).
3. It is very effective in maintaining a patent airway in spontaneously breathing patient. Positive pressure ventilation may be applied if necessary. It is used ***in place of a face mask or ETT during administration of an anesthetic to facilitate ventilation & passage of ETT in a patient with difficult airway***Q and to aid in ventilation during fiberoptic bronchoscopy (FOB) as well as placement of bronchoscope.
4. LMA partially protects the larynx from pharyngeal secretions but not gastric regurgitation .The mask is **not suitable** for patients who are at *risk from regurgitation of gastric content (emergency surgery, hiatus hernia, or h/o reflux, and obesity)*.
5. It is avoided in bronchospasm or high airway resistance (but not C/I)
6. It is available in ***7 different sizes***Q (i.e. 1, 1.5, 2, 2.5, 3, 4, 5). The **flexible LMA** differs from standard LMA in that it has a flexible wire reinforced tube available in sizes 2, 2.5, 3, 4, and 5. The size of the cuff is similar but the *tube is longer and narrower*; and therefore offering *more resistance* to breathing. Because of wire, it is unsuitable for MRI.
7. **Intubating LMA** is an advanced form with a *shorter tube* and a *metal handle* permitting *single handed insertion* without moving the head and neck and without placing fingers in the mouth. It is available in sizes *3, 4 and 5*; and may be passed through an interdental gap as narrow as *20 mm*. ***It allows a tracheal tube to be passed in order to intubate trachea***Q.
8. **LMA PRO-SEAL** is another advanced form of classic LMA that has a *double lumen*. The airway tube is wire reinforced to prevent collapse and has *built in bite block* (to reduce airway obstruction d/t bitting). The *drainage tube* passes lateral to the airway tube and allows passage of orogastric tube, drainage of gastric content and prevents gastric insufflation. The cuff allows a higher seal than classical LMA.

Characteristics of LMAs:

Size	Length	Volume of cuff (mL) upto	Largest size tracheal tube that fits into LMA	Size of patient
1	8	4	3.5	***Neonates & infants upto 6.5 kg***Q
1.5	10	7	4	Infants 5 – 10 kg
2	11	10	4.5	Infants & children 10-20 kg
2.5	12.5	14	5	Children 20 – 30 kg
3	16	20	6	***Children & small adults 30 – 50 kg***Q
4	16	30	6	Normal adults 50 – 70 kg
5	18	40	7	Large adult > 70 kg

Indications

- ***To facilitate ventilation & passage of ETT in patient with a difficult airway***Q & to aid in ventilation during fiberoptic bronchoscopy as well as placement of bronchoscope
- ***Difficult airway management during cardiopulmonary resuscitation.*** Q
- ***Difficult intubation*** Q is anticipated
- In emergency where intubation & mask ventilation is not possible
- For minor surgeries, where anaesthetist wants to avoid intubation
- As a conduit for bronchoscopes, small size tubes, gum elastic bougies.
- For extra & intra-ocular surgeries including retinopathy surgery in ex-premature infants (better access the surgical field and does not affect the IOT)
- LMA have little effect on intraocular pressure. Therefore they may be useful for airway management of patient undergoing examination of eye under anesthesia : ***the absence of face mask may facilitate eye examination.*** Q
- Mouth opening < 1.5 cm

Contraindications

- ***Oropharyngeal abscess or mass*** Q
- **Conditions with high risk of aspiration**
  - Hiatus hernia
  - Pregnancy
- ***Full stomach patients who are vulnerable to go in bronchospasm***Q
- Pharyngeal pathology (eg. abscess)
- Pharyngeal obstruction
- **Full stomach (eg pregnancy, hiatus** hernia) as it ***partially protects larynx from pharyngeal secretions but not gastric regurgitation***Q
- Low pulmonary compliance (eg. obesity)
- Peak inspiratory pressure > 20 cm of H_2O.

Advantage

- Easy to insert
- ***Does not require any laryngoscope, visualization, & muscle relaxants***Q
- Does not require any specific position of cervical spine so *can be used in cervical injuries*

Disadvantage

- Does not prevent aspiration so should not be used for full stomach patients.
- High incidence of laryngospasm and bronchospasm.

Endotracheal Intubation

Process of Endotracheal Intubation

- Moderate head elevation and ***extension of atlanto occipital joint***[Q] places the patient in desired sniffing position. The ***lower portion of cervical spine is flexed***[Q] by resting the head on pillow.
- *Preoxygenation with 100%* O_2 provides extra safety in difficult airways.
- The blade is intorduced into right side of oropharynx & tongue is swept to left
- ***The tip of curved blade is usually inserted into the vallecula while the straight blade tip covers the epiglottis***[Q]
- ***Trapping lip between teeth & blade and leverage on the teeth are avoided***[Q]
- The ETT *cuff* should lie in *upper tranchea but beyond the larynx.* The cuff is inflated with the *least amount of air necessary to create a seal* during positive pressure ventilation.

Indications of Endotracheal Intubation

- ***To deliver positive pressure ventilation***[Q]
- Protection of the respiratory tract from aspiration of gastric contents
- Surgical procedures involving the head and neck or in non-supine positions that preclude manual airway support
- Almost all situations involving neuromuscular paralysis
- Surgical procedures involving the cranium, thorax, or abdomen
- Procedures that may involve intracranial hypertension
- ***To maintain patent airway***[Q]
- Profound disturbance in consciousness with the inability to protect the airway.
- ***Tracheobronchial toilet***[Q]
- Severe pulmonary or multisystem injury associated with respiratory failure, such as sepsis, airway obstruction, hypoxemia and hypercarbia.

Oral Tracheal Tube Size Guidelines

Age	Internal Diameter (mm)	Cut Length (cm)
Full term infant	3.5	12
Child	$4+\frac{Age}{4}$	$14+\frac{Age}{2}$
Adult		
Female	7.0 – 7.5	24
Male	7.5 – 9.0	24

Internal Diameter (mm) of Endotracheal Tube

- **< 6 years** → $\frac{\text{Age in years} + 3.5}{3.5}$
- **> 6 years** → $\frac{\text{Age in years} + 4.5}{4.5}$

Difficult Airway

It means difficulty in tracheal intubation solely or problems with mask ventilation. Number of signs, scale & tests have been proposed and these are-

- ***Mallampati oropharyngeal Scale***[Q]
- **Patil Thyromental Distance Test**
  If it is < *7 cm* there is an increased likelihood of a difficult intubation.

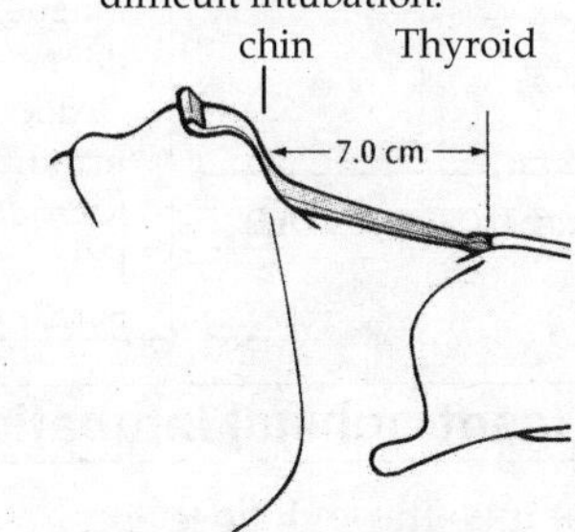

✶ The ***cricoid cartilage***[Q] is the narrowest point of airway in **children younger than 5 years of age**; in **adults**, the narrowest point is the ***glottis***[Q].

Signs Of Difficult Laryngoscopy

Sign	Score
- **Micrognathia with acute mandibular angle**	5
- **Glossoptosis or Basal macroglossia**	4
- Difficulty with prior laryngoscopy	3
- Long, high arched palate with long, narrow dental arch	2
- **Temporomandibular joint limitation**	4
- Short muscular neck with full dentition	2
- Protuding maxillary dentition with premaxillary over growth	2
- Increased alveolomental depth	1
- **Limited extension of upper cervical vertebrae**	2
- **Limited motion of lower cervical vertebrae**	3
- Pathological signs of airway obstruction	3
- Decreased distance between hyoid & thyroid	2
- Decreased distance of epiglottis from posterior wall of pharynx	3
- **Miller sign**	3
- Skill of anesthesiologist, planning for endoscopy	1-5

Mallampati Oropharyngeal Scale

The view of posterior wall of pharynx, obtained after asking patient to open mouth widely and protuding the tongue, may be divided into *four grades of increasing difficulty in tracheal intubation.*

- **Class I**
  - ***Soft palate, uvula, faucial pillars & posterior pharngeal wall are visible***[Q]
- **Class II**
  - Lower part of faucial pillar & uvula masked by base of tongue
  - Upper part of faucial pillars & soft palate are visible
- **Class III**
  - ***Only soft palate is visible***[Q]
- **Class IV**
  - All of these structures masked
  - ***Only hard palate visible***[Q]

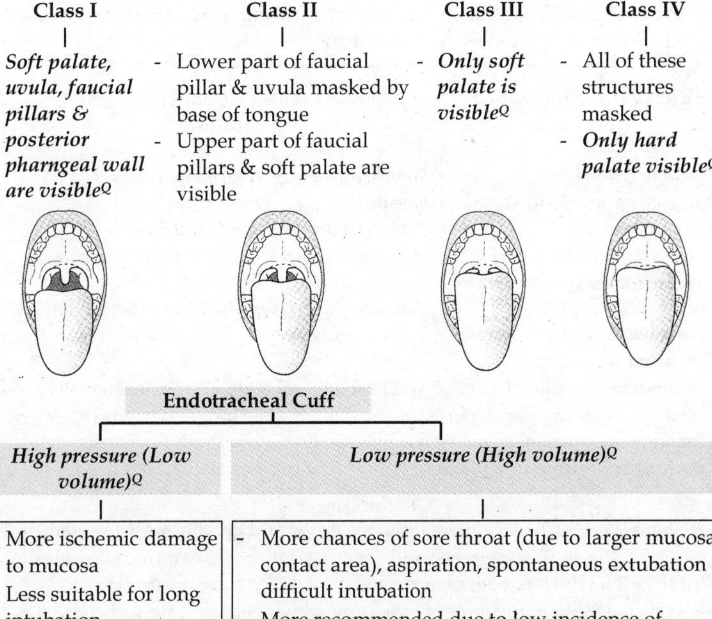

Endotracheal Cuff

High pressure (Low volume)[Q]	*Low pressure (High volume)*[Q]
- More ischemic damage to mucosa - Less suitable for long intubation	- More chances of sore throat (due to larger mucosal contact area), aspiration, spontaneous extubation & difficult intubation - More recommended due to low incidence of mucosal damage

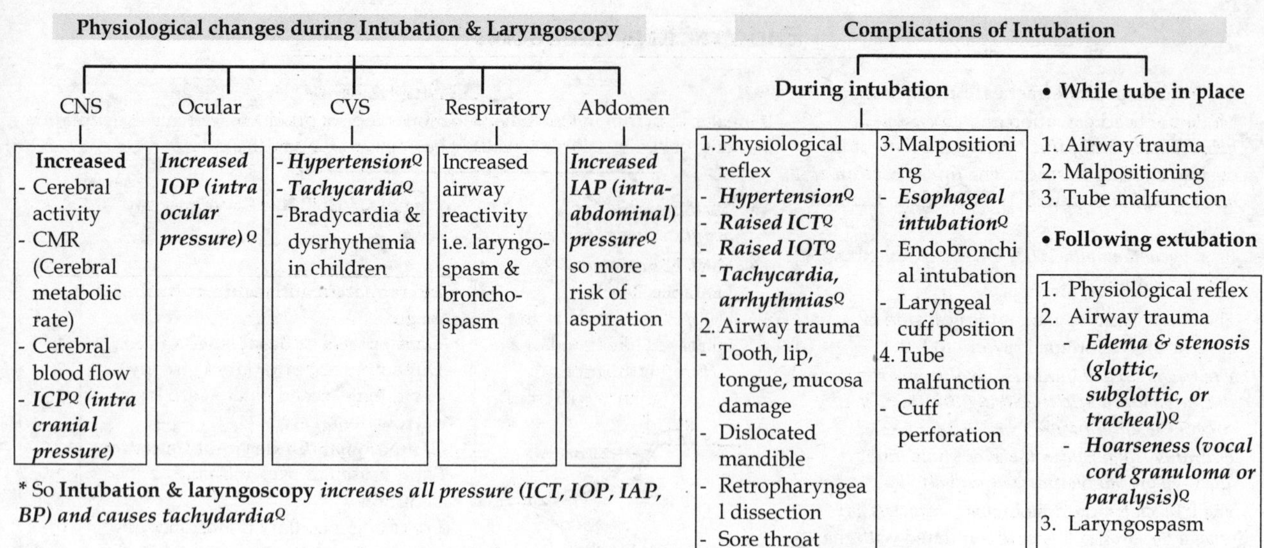

Physiological changes during Intubation & Laryngoscopy
CNS
Increased
- Cerebral activity
- CMR (Cerebral metabolic rate)
- Cerebral blood flow
- ICP^Q (intra cranial pressure)
Ocular
Increased IOP (intra ocular pressure)^Q
CVS
- Hypertension^Q
- Tachycardia^Q
- Bradycardia & dysrhythemia in children
Respiratory
Increased airway reactivity i.e. laryngo-spasm & broncho-spasm
Abdomen
Increased IAP (intra-abdominal) pressure^Q so more risk of aspiration
* So Intubation & laryngoscopy increases all pressure (ICT, IOP, IAP, BP) and causes tachydardia^Q
Complications of Intubation
During intubation
1. Physiological reflex
- Hypertension^Q
- Raised ICT^Q
- Raised IOT^Q
- Tachycardia, arrhythmias^Q
2. Airway trauma
- Tooth, lip, tongue, mucosa damage
- Dislocated mandible
- Retropharyngeal dissection
- Sore throat
3. Malpositioning
- Esophageal intubation^Q
- Endobronchial intubation
- Laryngeal cuff position
4. Tube malfunction
- Cuff perforation
• While tube in place
1. Airway trauma
2. Malpositioning
3. Tube malfunction
• Following extubation
1. Physiological reflex
2. Airway trauma
- Edema & stenosis (glottic, subglottic, or tracheal)^Q
- Hoarseness (vocal cord granuloma or paralysis)^Q
3. Laryngospasm

Nasal (Nasotracheal) Intubation (NTI)

Nasal intubation (ie placement of endotracheal tube through nose and nosopharynx) is necessary when oral route is not possible (eg limited mouth opening) or would impede surgical access (eg intraoral surgery). NTI was formely considered the **technique of choice for resuscitation**, but **orotracheal intubation using the rapid sequence technique** is now usually the first choice. **Rapid sequence induction (RSI)** is indicated when there is significant *risk of airway soiling from gastro-oesophageal* contents (eg pregnancy, intestinal obstruction, oesophageal dilatation, inadequate starvation, trauma, emergency). RSI involves *preoxygenation (at least 3 min or E_TO_2 > 90%), intravenous induction (thiopental and suxamethonium) and cricoid pressure.*

Advantages and Disadvantages

- NTI tubes are longer and narrower than oral tracheal or tracheostomy tubes so the *airway resistance is greater and therapeutic aspiration of pulmonary secretions is more difficult.*
- NTI has been used in critical care as an alternative to tracheostomy because it is *better tolerated than oral intubation* (Miller 1586). NTI is less popular then formerly in ICU b/o increased recognition of the risk of sepsis from sinusitis (Aitkenhead 739).
- Both nasal & oral (translaryngeal) tracheal intubation are safe at least for 2-3 weeks. When compared with oral intubation;

Benifits of nasal intubation are

- ***Good oral hygiene***^Q
- More comfortable for patient
- ***More secure (less extubation/displacement incidences)***^Q
- *Less* likely to cause laryngeal damage

Adverse events associated with nasal intubation

- ***Significant mucosal damage & nasal bleeding***^Q
- ***Transient bacteremia (infection)***^Q
- Submucosal dissection of nasopharynx and oropharynx
- ***Sinusitis & otitis media***^Q (d/t obstruction of auditory tubes)

- When used for more than 2 –3 weeks, both oral & nasal translaryngeal-tracheal tubes predispose to *subglottic stenosis*. So if longer periods (> 1 week for some institution) of mechanical ventilation is required, tracheostomy is performed (within first few days) and *cuffed tracheostomy* tube is used.

Technique

After phenylephrine (vasoconstrictor) nose drops and good lubrication slightly smaller tube (7 mm ID for women and 7.5 mm ID for men) is introduced into nostril through which patient breathes most easily (or right nostril) and advanced gently along the floor of nose preferably over a soft tip catheters as a guide.

Indications

- Obstructing mass in oral cavity
- Abscess in oral cavity
- Oral surgery
- Fracture mandible (no mouth opening)
- TM joint dysfunction (inadequate mouth opening)
- Cervical spine injury
- Awake intubation
- Tube is to be kept for long periods

Contraindications

- ***Old or new base of skull (eg cribiform plate) fracture and surgery and severe mid facial trauma b/o risk of intracranial tube placement***^Q.
- ***CSF rihnorrhea***^Q may l/t cerebral infection
- Nasal trauma & abnormalities like polyp, abscess, foreign body.
- Adenoids
- Coagulopathy of bleeding disorder
- Previous nasal surgery is relative contraindication

Blind Nasal Intubation

Nasal intubation may be accomplished under vision to guide the tube into larynx or by **blind technique** (BNI). Distance b/w nares and crania in adult men is 32 cm and women is 27 cm. It is done in

- Where laryngoscopy is not possible due to inadequate mouth opening, like in:
- ***Temporomandibular joint ankylosis***^Q
- Trismus (d/t , tetanus, quinsy)
- Neck contracture

Indications of Tracheostomy

Respiratory obstruction

1. Infection - ***Diptheria***[Q], ***Ludwig's angina***[Q], laryngo-tracheo-bronchitis, epiglottis, retro/parapharyngeal abscess
2. Neoplasm of larynx, pharynx, trachea, tongue, thyroid
3. ***Foreign body larynx***[Q]
4. ***B/L abductor paralysis***[Q]
5. Congenital anomalies
   - Laryngeal web, cyst
   - Tracheo-esophageal fistula
   - B/L choanal atresia
6. Laryngeal edema

Retained Secretion

1. Painful cough
   - Chest trauma
   - ***Multiple rib fracture (flail chest)***[Q]
2. Inability to cough due to:
   - ***Coma (eg. head injury)***[Q]
   - Paralysis of respiratory muscle eg. Spinal injury, G. B. Syndrome, polio, myasthenia gravis
3. Respiratory muscle spasm eg. ***Tetanus***[Q], ecclampsia, strychnine poisoning

Respiratory insufficiency

Chronic lung ds. ex- atelectasis, COPD, Bronchiectasis

Hazards of O_2 therapy / Hyperoxia / Oxygen Toxicity

Mechanism

- Enzymes containing *sulfhydryl group* are inactivated by O_2 derived *free radicles.*
- Neutrophil recruitment & inflammatory mediators accelerate ***endothelial & epithelial damage***[Q] & impairment of surfactant system.
- *Super oxide dismutase & catlase* provide protection against free radicles (reactive O_2 metabolites) such as , *superoxide, activated hydroxyl ions, singlet O_2 & H_2O_2*
- Additional protection is provided by antioxidants & free radicle scavangers eg. ***glutathione peroxidase, vit C (ascorbic acid), vit-E (α -tocopherol), acetyl cysteine & probably mannitol.***

Dose-time toxicity relationship

- The risk & expected degree of toxicity are directly related to duration, inspired O_2 partial pressure (P_IO_2) & individual susceptibility. Alveolar rather arterial O_2 tension is important.
- Clark & Lambertsen equation

$$\text{UPTD} = tx\ ^{m}\sqrt{0.5/(P-0.5)}$$

UPTD = Unit pulmonary toxic dose of O_2, t = exposure time (min), P= inspired P_IO_2 in ATA, M = Slope constant

- Between 0.21 – 0.50 atmospheres absolute (ATA), anatomical, physiological & biochemical changes are adaptive rather than pathological.
- Maximum nontoxic PIO_2 is 0.5 ATA. Pulmonary function & blood gas exchange has no measurable changes during exposure to<*50% O_2*
- 60% oxygen should not be administered for more than 36 hrs., 80% O_2 for not > 24hrs and 100% O_2 for not more than 12 hours.
- The degree to which O_2 is toxic is related to PO_2 of inspired gas. At 1ATA, 100% O_2 is as toxic as 16.7% O_2 at 6ATA or 2% O_2 at 50 ATA.
- ***Lungs are first to demonstrate toxicity with normobaric (1ATA) exposures***[Q]. CNS toxicity is not observed below inhaled O_2 partial pressure of 2ATA. However it may occur before pulmonary toxicity at pressures above 3ATA.

Organ system involvement

Lung

- Pulmonary toxicity
- Dominant symptom is *substernal distress* begining as mild irritation in area of carnia & occasional coughing
- *Burning chest pain, urge to cough & to deep breathe* becomes more intense.
- Severe dyspnea, paroxysmal coughing, & ***decreased vital capacity***[Q] (In F_IO_2 1 for > 12 hrs).
- ***Pulmonary function test as compliance & blood gases deteriorate***[Q].
- Alveolar – capillary membrane injury l/t *ARDS* (type 1 alveolar cell decrease & type 2 cells proliferate)
- *Pulmonary interstitial edema* (exposure for few days – 1 week) & *Pulmonary fibrosis* (exposure > 1 week)
- **Hypoventilation *(Ventilatory depression)***[Q] in COPD patients who have been ventilating in response to a hypoxic drive resulting in hypercapnia but not necessarily hypoxia (b/o increased FIO_2)
- ***Absorption atelectasis***[Q] in areas of low V/Q ratios.
- Brochopulmonary dysplasia in new born

Central nervous system

- O_2 at 2ATA or more may l/t nonfocal *tonic – clonic seizure* with or without warning symptoms (eg. behaviour changes, nausea, vertigo, facial numbness, twitching, olfactory / gustatory / acoustic symptoms).
- Probability of convulsions is greater at *higher P_IO_2* & in acute indications such as *CO poisoning*
- Metabolic factors such as *high dose penicillin* (for clostridial infection), sepsis & hypoglycemia reduce seizure threshold.
- T/t is immediately decreasing inspired O_2 concentration.

Eye : Retinopathy of prematurity

- Premature infants (*i.e., < 1kg birth weight & 28 weeks gestation)* are most susceptible to retrolental fibroplasia
- In contrast to pulmonary toxicity, RoP ***corelates better with arterial than with alveolar O_2 tension***[Q].
- Whenever fraction of inspired O_2 (F_IO_2) causes PaO2 to be > *80 mm Hg for > 3hrs in infants whom combined gestational age + life age < 44 weeks;* the risk of ROP exists
- *50 – 80 mmHg* (6.6 –10.6 KPa) is the recommended arterial conc. for premature infants receiving O_2.
- In cardiopulmonary patients fear of causing worse ROP is not a reason to withhold O_2

- Insignificantly decreased heart rate, cardiac output & pulmonary artery pressure
- Fire hazard

Helium (He) and Heliox (He – O_2) Therapy

- **Helium (He)** isolated by Sir W. Ramsey is an ***inert (nobel), colorless, odourless gas with high diffusibility and low mass, density, solubility and density to viscosity ratio***[Q]. Helium cylinders are *brown* & heliox cylinders are *brown with brown-white shoulder* quadrants. The pressure in full cylinder is 137 bar.
- *Low solubility* of He enables it to be used in *measurement of lung volumes by gas dilution*. Whereas, *combination of high diffusibility and low solubility* make (He) *less* likely than nitrogen to be *responsible for decompression sickness*. Its high thermal capacity encourages loss of body heat.
- *Helium has a significantly lower density but a similar viscosity to air*. So He has *low Reynold's number* (b/o low density) and *significantly lower density /viscosity ratio*.
- Low Reynold's number (< 1000) is associated with laminar flow whereas high value (>1500) produces turbulent flow. Laminar flow normally occurs distal to small bronchioles (< 1mm). Flow in upper air way is usually turbulent. During **turbulent flow (i.e. in upper large airways)** airway resistance depends on **gas density** whereas, during **laminar flow** (i.e. in ***small distal airways***) resistance depends on **gas viscosity**. So a **gas (He)** or a **gas mixture (Heliox)** with **low density** leads to a *dramatic decrease in airway resistance and turbulent in upper large airways; lower Reynold's number will encourage laminar flow in larger airways*; but because its *viscosity is very similar to air (He)/O_2 (heliox)* it will make *no difference to laminar flow in small airways*.
- **Heliox** is a ***mixture of helium with oxygen***[Q] in several blends (80-20% He to 20-80% O_2). However, most popular mixtures are *80%/20% and 70%/30% helium-oxygen*, which have densities that are 1.805 and 1.586 times less dense, respectively, compared to pure oxygen. *Lower density greatly increase flow for any given pressure gradient or allows the same flow for a smaller pressure gradient*. However, the higher the concentration of helium in mixture, the *lower the F_{IO2} (oxygenation)*. So heliox can be used in
  1) Patients with *acute distress (& stridor) from upper airway obstruction* such as subglottic edema, foreign bodies, tracheal tumors, epiglottitis, laryngo-tracheo-bronchitis, tracheitis, angioneurotic edema and bilateral vocal cord palsies etc. to obtain relief until more definitive care can be delivered/effective.
  2) *Pressure needed to ventilate patients with small diameter endo-tracheal tubes is substantially reduced* (halved with 80/20 He-O_2) in anesthesia.
  3) ***Inspiratory driving pressure and work of breathing can be reduced***[Q] when heliox is delivered via the mechanical ventilator (non invasive - non intubated via mask or invasive via an artificial airway)
  4) May also be used as a *driving gas for small volume nebulizers* for bronchodilator therapy in asthma. However, the 80/20 heliox flow needs to be increased to 11 lit/min versus the usual 6-8 L/min with O_2.
  5) It has less convincing evidence in treating lower airway obstruction in COPD & asthma.
  6) *For deep sea diving (> 50 meters)*, nitrogen (air) should be avoided and replaced with a helium - oxygen mixture to reduce chances of decompression sickness. Whereas *risk of high pressure nervous syndrome (HPNS)*, at depths of > 500 m (very high pressure > 70 atmospheric) or during rapid compression (> 1m/min) is reduced by adding *low concentrations (5%) of nitrogen to heliox (trimixes)*.
- *At higher partial pressure* (produced by hyperbaric exposure *eg during hyperbaric O_2 therapy or underwater diving)* most inert gases *produce CNS depression (anesthetic potency)* which approximately follows their *lipid solubility*. **Increasing order of lipid solubility, anesthetic/narcotic potency and CNS depression** and **decreasing order of MAC** is: **He < Ne < H2 < N2 < Ar < Kr < Xe.** MAC is in reverse order except Kr > Ar. *At high partial pressures, the blood and tissue content of dissolved inert gas is also increased*, the magnitude of which depends upon the pressure, duration and solubility of gas. So less soluble gas like helium are less likely to produce decompression sickness. And similarly b/o very low solubility, He has such a low anesthetic potency (chances of CNS depression) that the pressure required to produce CNS depression exceeds those required to produce HPNS (i.e. CNS depression has not been observed).

Ventilation

Positive Airway Pressure Therapy (PEEP & CPAP)

Positive airway pressure therapy can be used in patients breathing spontaneously as well as those mechanically ventilated. The principal indication for PAPT is a **symptomatic decrease in FRC**, resulting in *absolute or relative hypoxemia*. By increasing transpulmonary distending perrssure, PAPT can *increase FRC and lung compliance*, and reverse V/P mismatching (reflected as decreased venous admixture & improved arterial O_2 tension).

Continuous Positive Airway Pressure (CPAP)

A constant level of positive pressure applied to a spontaneous breathing cycle is named CPAP. It is **indicated** in.

Clinical Presentation	Conditions responsive to CPAP (with ≥1clinical presentations)
- On **examination** – the presence of increased work of breathing (i.e. respiratory distress) as indicated by increase in respiratory rate >30% of normal, grunting,	- ***Very preterm infants***[Q] (born at < 28 weeks gestation age, weight

When *positive pressure* is applied *during expiration* as an adjunct to a mechanically delivered breath (that allows expiratory flow to occur only when airway pressure exceeds or equals the PEEP level), the therapy is referred to as **positive end-expiratory pressure** & while, *positive pressure* is applied *during both inspiration & expiration* during spontaneous breathing therapy is k/a **continuous positive airway pressure.**

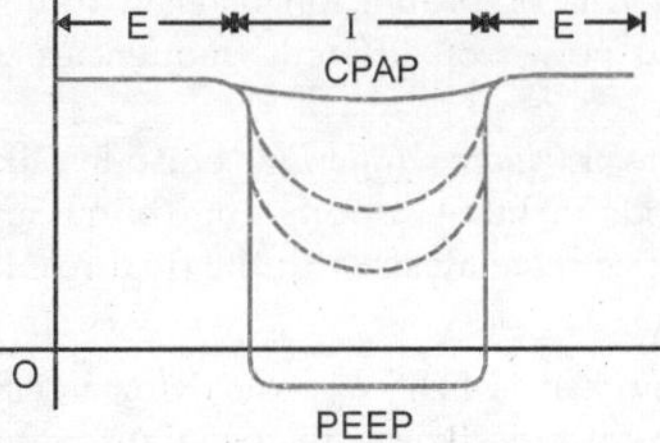

So pure PEEP is a ventilator cycled breath, while CPAP provides only sufficient continuous or on demand gas flows (60-90 L/min) to prevent inspiratory pressure from falling below the expiratory level during spontaneous breaths. ***By increasing inspiratory gas flow, PEEP progressively becomes CPAP.***Q

Pulmonary Effects

- ***Useful in situations where PO_2 is low***Q
  - ***Increase FRC, tidal ventilation, compliance***Q
  - Correct ventilation-perfusion abnormalities
  - ***Improve arterial oxygenation***Q by decreasing intrapulmonary shunting, reexpanding functionally collapsed alveoli, redistributing lung water, & thereby reducing V/Q mismatch
- Side effects due to excessive PEEP/CPAP l/t over distension of alveoli & bronchi
  - Increase dead space
  - *Decrease lung compliance*Q
  - Increase in pulmonary vascular resistance & right ventricular after load
  - ***Barotrauma (Pneumothorax, Pneumopericardium, Pneumoperitoneum, Subcutaneous emphysema)***Q

Extra pulmonary effects

- ***Decrease cardiac output***Q (due to rise in mean airway pressure & intrathoracic pressure
- ***Decrease in hepatic & renal blood flow***Q (due to decrease in CO & increase in central venous pressure)
- ***GFR, urinary output, free water clearance decreases & ADH and angiotensin levels are increased (i.e. renal functions are impaired***Q.
- ***Raised ICT***Q

E = Expiration &
I = Inspiration

nasal flaring, and suprasternal & substernal retractions; the presence of pale or cyanotic skin colour, and agitation

- **On chest x-ray** presence of poorly expanded &/or infiltrated lung fields.
- Inadequate **arterial blood** gas values i.e **inability to maintain PaO_2 >50 mmHg** with

1. $FiO_2 \leq 0.60$ (provided V_E is adequate as indicated by a $PaCO_2$ 50 mmHg & a pH $\geq$ 7.25) i.e. patient is breathing 60% of oxygen in moderate to severe respiratory distress or recurrent apnea
2. FiO_2 of 0.40 in newborns with RDS

Guidelines for CPAP use

Start at pressure of 5 cm of H_2O and FiO_2 of 40-50%

↓ No improvement / Worsening

Pressure is increased by 1 – 2 cm H_2O to maximum of 8-12 cm of water.

↓ Still impaired oxygenation

Increase FiO_2 by 5% to maximum of 80%

<1kg) = nasal CPAP + surfactant therapy.

- Apnea of prematurity (prolonged & recurrent attacks)
- ***Respiratory distress syndrome***Q (in both term and preterm infants)
- Weaning of chronically ventilator dependent infants.
- Recent extubation (following mechanical ventilation)
- Post operative thoracotomy care
- Conditions associated with atelactasis, decreased functional residual capacity, right to left shunts, V/Q mismatch, alveolar edema and airway instability
- Atelactasis & one lung ventilation
- Pulmonary edema
- Tracheal malacia or other similar abnormalities of lower airway
- *Sleep apnea*
- For administration of NO in spontaneously breathing infants

Devices providing CPAP

Nasal prong (6 – 15mm)

Nasopharyngeal CPAP (40-90 mm)

Endotracheal tube CPAP

Monitoring of Patient

BIS/Bispectral Index

- ***Bispectral imaging analyses EEG*** **date and quantitates anesthetic effects on the brain, specifically the** ***hypnotic component.*** It is a *composite numerical index,* which represents a dimensionless numerical value that has been correlated with the patient's current hypnotic state or depth of anaesthesia and provides some assurance that paralyzed (anesthetized) patient is also asleep (unaware).
- BIS analysis may *reduce chances of patient awareness during anesthesia.* It may *also reduce resource utilization* because less drug is required to ensure amnesia, facilitating a faster wake up time and a shorter stay in recovery room. The **BIS number** decreases with increasing hypnosis.
- To perform BIS, data measured by EEG are taken through a number of steps. BIS estimates *phase coupling* between different frequency components in EEF signal. The BIS is derived from complex EEG analysis

Assessing Consciousness Intraoperative

1. **Bispectral index (BIS) analysis**
2. **Narcotrend monitor** (Monitor Technik)
3. **Patient state index (PSI, Physiometrix)** is based on

ANAESTHESIA 2

incorporating weighted information derived from the **degree of burst suppression, spectral (β band) power and the bispectrum coherance**. To make the EEG signals easier to interpret it uses 2 principles which are, which are, **spectral analysis (power)** (ie any complex wave may broken down into a series of sine waves) and **fast fourier analysis** (ie an analysis in terms of proportion of each frequency that contributes to total signal). BIS analysis uses the phase and power of different frequencies within the original signal.

- BIS identifies EEG patterns with 30 second periods, by first *excluding (filtering)* episodes likely to be produced by *artifact (diathermy or muscle activity)* and periods of burst suppression (burst suppression ratio and QUAZI). The remaining activity is subjected to bispectral analysis with the final result adjusted to take account of the proportion of suppressed EEG.

BIS	Awareness level and Depth of anesthesia
100	**Awake** (memory intact, respond to verbal command)
85-65	**Sedation**
65-40	**General anesthesia** (no awareness, deep hypnosis, memory function lost)
<40	Cortical suppression becomes discernible, increasing burst suppression
0	**Cortical silence (isoelectric), deeply anesthetised**

- Although it is FDA approved for assessing the depth of anesthesia in paediatric and adult patients, it has not yet become a standard monitor *b/o high cost and inaccuracy*. BIS values had *better response with hypnotic drugs (eg isoflurane, propofol) than with opiates*. BIS values *decrease in patients receiving NM blocker*, while fully conscious. BIS value remains *unchanged or even elevated during N_2O anesthesia*, and elevated during IV ketamine (both acting through NMDA glutamate receptor).

quantitative EEG signal relationship b/w frontal and occipital brain regions

4. **Entropy monitors** measure *state entropy* (response over the rangeof 0.8 - 32 Hz, reflecting EEG dominant spectrum and *response entropy* (response over range of 0.8 - 47 Hz, reflecting both EEG and EMG spectra)
5. **Stimulus - response technique of auditory evoked potential.**

Neurophysiological Monitoring

Electroencephalography (EEG)

- EEG are most useful for **assessing the adequacy of *cerebral perfusion* during *carotid endarterectomy (CEA) & controlled hypoventilation* and for *assessing anesthetic depth*[Q].**
- EEG activation (i.e. predominantly *high frequency & low voltage* activity) is seen with *light anesthesia*, and surgical stimulation, whereas EEG depression (i.e. predominantly *low frequency & high voltage activity*) occurs with *deep anesthesia or cerebral compromise*. Most anesthetics produce a **biphasic pattern** consisting of an *initial activation* (at subanesthetic low doses) *f/b dose dependent depression*.
- IV agents: Opioids produce monophasic, dose dependent depression whereas ketamine produces unusual activation consisting of rhythmic high amplitude theta activity f/b very high amplitude gamma and low amplitude beta activity. **Benzodiazepines, barbiturates, etomidate & propofol** produce typical **biphasic pattern** (last three produce *burst suppression* & electrical silence at high dose).
- Inhalational anesthetics: halothane produces biphasic pattern; **isoflurane** can produce **isoelectric EEG** at high doses (1-2 MAC); **desflurane & sevoflurane** produce a **burst suppression pattern** at high doses (1.2 & > 1.5 MAC respectively) but not electrical silence; and **N_2O** increases both frequency & amplitude **(high amplitude activation)**.

Activation (high n, low v)	**Depression** (low n, high v)
- Light anesthesia & surgical stimulation	- Deep anesthesia or cerebral compromise
- Hypoxia (early) - Mild hypercapnia - Barbiturates (small dose) - Benzodiazepines (small dose) - Etomidate (small dose) - Inhalational agent (sub anesthetic)	- Hypoxia (late), Ischemia - Marked hypercapnia - Barbiturates - Benzodiazepines - Etomidate - Inhalational agents (1-2 MAC)
- **N_2O** - **Ketamine** - Sensory stimulation	- **Propofol** - **Opioids** - ***Hypothermia***[Q] - Hypocapnia

Evoked Potentials (EP)

- **Somatosensory evoked potentials (SSEPs)** test the integrity of *dorsal spinal column & sensory cortex* and may be useful during spinal tumor resection, spine instrumentation, CEA & aortic surgery. Adequacy of spinal cord perfusion is better assessed by *motor evoked potential.*
- **Brain stem auditory evoked potential or response (BAER)** test the integrity of 8th cranial nerve and auditory pathways above pons & are used for surgery in posterior fossa. **Visual evoked response (VER)** monitor optic nerve & upper brain stem during resections of large pituitary tumors. ***VER are most, whereas BAER are least affected by anesthetics***[Q].
- Short latency of EP arise from nerve stimulation or brain stem. Long & intermediate latency EP are of cortical origin. So *short latency EP are least whereas long latency EP are most affected* (by even sub-anesthetic levels of most anesthetics).

Agent	**SSEP**		**VER**		**BAER**	
	Amp	Lat	Amp	Lat	Amp	Lat
N_2O	↓	±	↓	↑	±	±
Halothane	↓	↑	±	↑	±	↑
Isoflurane	↓	↑	↓	↑	±	↑
Barbiturates	±	±	↓	↑	±	±
Opioids	±	±	±	±	±	±
Etomidate	(↑)	↑				
Propofol	↓	↑			↓	↑
Benzodiazepines	↓	±				
Ketamine	±	↑				

Ability of **anesthetic drugs** to produce a change in **sensory and motor EPs (evoked potentials)** that could be mistaken for surgically induced change.

Drugs	Visual EP		Trans cranial motor EP		Somoto Sensory EP		Brain stem Auditory EP	
	Lat	Amp	Lat	Amp	Lat	Amp	Lat	Amp
Inhalation: **Isoflurane, Enflurane, Halothane, N_2O**	Yes	Yes	Yes	Yes	Yes	Yes	**No**	**No**
Barbitrates, Propofol, Diazepam, Midazolam	Yes	Yes	Yes	Yes	**Yes**	**Yes**	**No**	**No**
Droperidol	-	-	Yes	Yes	No	No	No	No
Etomidate, Ketamine	Yes	Yes	No	No	No	No	No	No
Opiates	No	No	No	No	No	No	No	No
Dexmedeto-midine	No	ND	ND	No	No	No	No	No

Guidelines for choosing anesthetic technique during procedure in which sensory evoked responses are monitored

- *Intravenous agents have significantly less effect* than equipotent doses of inhaled anesthetics.
- Combinations of drugs generally produce *additive effects*
- ***Subcortical (spinal or brain stem) sensory evoked potentials (responses) are very resistant to the effects of aesthetic drugs***Q. If subcortical responses provide sufficient information for surgical procedure, anesthetic technique is not important, and effects on cortically recorded responses may be ignored.
- In general, *balanced anesthetic techniques (N_2O, NM relaxant, and opioids) cause minimal changes, whereas volatile agents* (halothane, sevoflurane, desflurane and isoflurane are best avoided or used at a constant low dose.
- *Early occurring (specific) EPs are less affected by anesthetics* than the late occurring (nonspecific) responses. ***Most sensitive to anesthesia is VEP >>Transcranial motor EP> SSEP> BAER (least sensitive/most resistant)***Q. Changes in BAERs may provide a measure of the depth of anesthesia.

Characteristics and Uses of EPs

Type	Stimulus	Delivering method	Used in
Auditory (BEAR)	Click, tones	Ear transducer	Cerebello pontine tumor resection, acoustic neuroma, cranial nerve V and VII decompression, infratentorial mass
Somato-sensory (SEP/SSEP)	Electric current	Electrodes	**Spinal or thoraco abdominal aortic aneurysm surgery,** supra/infratentorial mass lesion, intracranial aneurysm clipping, carotid endarterectomy
Motor (MEPs)	Electric current, magnetic current	Electrodes	**Spinal** or **thoraco abdominal aortic** aneurysm surgery

- **Indications for intraoperative monitoring of EPs** (evoked potentials) include surgical procedures *a/w possible neurological injury* eg. intracranial, spinal and thoracoabdominal aortic aneurysm repair etc. *Persistent obliteration of EPs is predictive of postoperative neurological defecit.* Although *SSEPs identify spinal cord damage* because of their different anatomic pathways, sensory (dorsal spinal cord) EP preservation does not guarantee normal motor (ventral spinal cord) function (false negative). Furthermore, *SSEPs elicited from posterior tibial nerve stimulation cannot distinguish between peripheral and central ischemia (false positive).* The advantage of using motor EPS as apposed to SSEPs for spinal cord monitoring is that *MEPs monitor the ventral spinal cord*, and if sensitive and specific enough, can be used to *indicate which patient might develop a postoperative motor deficit.*
- Motor evoked potentials (MEP) monitoring require monitoring of level of *neuromuscular blockade and hypothermia* (<32°C). MEPs are contraindicated in patients with *retained intracranial metal, after seizure, with a skull defect and after any major cerebral insult.*

Situation	Effect On EEG
- Hypothermia (<35°C) - **Profound hypothermia** (7- 20°C)	***Progressive slowing of EEG***Q Complete electrical silent
CO_2 level - Hypocarbia - Hypercarbia (5-20%) - Hypercarbia (>30% above normal) - Hyper carbia (>50% above normal)	- Slowing of EEG - Decreased cerebral excitability & increased electroshock seizure threshold - Increased cerebral excitability & epileptiform discharge - *EEG depression.*
O_2 levels - Hyperoxia - **Early Hypoxia** - **Persistent Hypoxia** - **Late Hypoxia approching anoxia**	- Cerebral excitation l/t low amplitude fast frequency EEG - Cerebral excitability (d/t peripheral cemoreceptor stimulation) l/t. ***acute increase in amplitude of EEG***Q - ***Diffuse slowing of EEG***Q ***l/t marked reduction in amplitude with appearance of slow waves***Q - EEG silence
Sensory stimulation (in awake)	Desynchronization of EEG patterns, increased amplitude, & increased frequency.

Situation	Effect On EEG
Narcotic Analgesics - Low dose - High dose	 - Increase amplitude of both α & β bands. - Theta & delta frequencies develop heralding the onset of sedation
Enflurane	Dose dependent *depression of EEG activity*, but at moderate high concentration (>3%), it produces ***epileptiform paroxymal spike activity and burst suppression***Q. ***It should be avoided in epileptic patients***Q.
Isoflurane, Desflurane and Sevoflurane	- No seizure activity on EEG & excitatory effects (as seen in enflurane) - Dose dependent depression of EEG activity - Does not cause seizure activity at any level of anesthesia with or without hypocapnia.
Propofol	- EEG frequency decreases & amplitude increase
Ketamine	- Unlike those seen with other IV. anesthetics, and consists of ***loss of alpha rhythm and predominant theta activity***Q.

2

ANAESTHESIA

Neuromuscular Monitoring by Peripheral Nerve Stimulation

- **Monitoring of neuromuscular function** (or **depth of neuromuscular block during anesthesia)** is accomplished by delivering an electrical stimulus near a peripheral motor nerve and evaluating the evoked reponse of the muscles innervated by that nerve. Methods for evaluating evoked responses include **visual assessment, tactile evaluation, mechanomyography/MMG, (gold standard** for scientific measurement of neuromulscular response but rarely used clinically), **accelero myography** (ACG, AMG is better than visual or tactile methods), **Kinemyography** (KMG: can measure TOF, duble burst & single twitch), **piezoelectric film, electromyography (EMG)** and **phonomyography (acoustic myography= PMG/AMG)**. Neuromuscular block (NMB) should be monitored when muscle relaxants are used to avoid drug overdosage or under dosage and residual NMB during recovery.
- Because it is inhibnition of neuromulscular receptor that needs to be monitored, **direct stimulation of muscle should be avoided** by placing the electrodes over the course of nerve and not over the muscle itself.
- Neuromuscular function is monitored by evaluating the muscular response to *supramaximal stimulation of peripheral motor nerve*. Neuromuscular blocking drugs decrease the muscle response in parallel with the number of fibers blocked. So the reduction in response, reflects the degree of blockade.
- For monitoring, the stimulus must be truely maximal throughout the period; therefore the applied electrical stimulation is usually atleast 20- 25% above that is necessary for response, which is k/a supramaximal stimulus.
- *Electrical stimulation* is the most commonly used method, and *single twitch, train of four, tetanic, post – tetanic count (PTC), & double burst stimulation* are the most commonly used patterns.
- ***Ulnar nerve is most popular site***Q followed by facial, median, posterior tibial & common peroneal. Stimulation of ulnar nerve causes contraction of *adductor pollicis* & stimulation of facial nerve l/t contraction of *orbicularis oculi*. ***The diaphragm, rectus abdominis, laryngeal adductors, and orbicularis oculi muscles recover from neuromuscular blockade earlier than adductor pollicis***Q.
- Best site for stimulation of ulnar nerve is *volar side of wrist*, with distal electrode placed about 1cm proximal to the point at which *proximal wrist flexion crease crosses the lateral side of FCU* (flexor carpi ulnaris) tendon.
- *Peripheral nerve stimulation cannot replace direct observation* of the muscles (eg. diaphragm) because different muscles have different sensitivity to n-m blocking agents. And further more adductor pollicis recovery does not exactly indicate recovery of muscles required to maintain airway.
- *Sustained (≥ 5sec) head lift, forceful hand grip, & ability to generate an inspiratory pressure of atleast (-) 25cm H_2O* are other indicators of adequate recovery.
- All stimuli are *200 μs (0.2ms)* in duration, of equal current intensity & of square wave pattern.

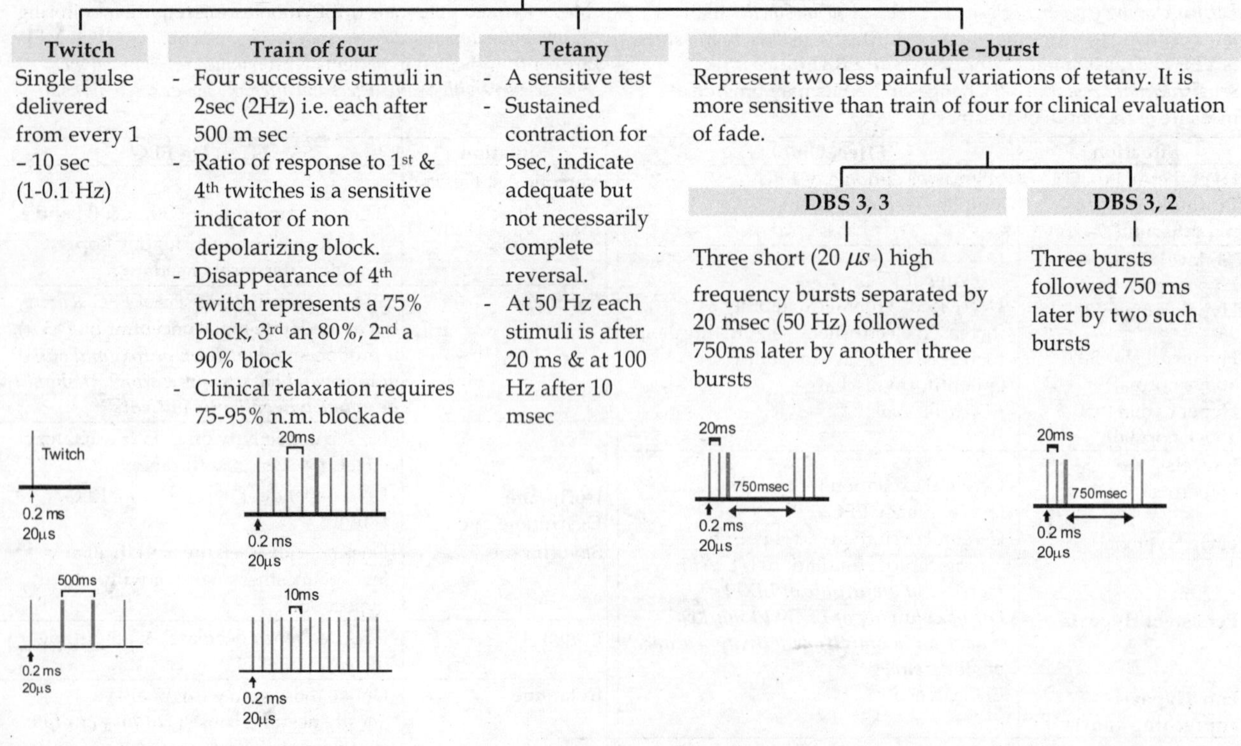

Twitch	Train of four	Tetany	Double -burst
Single pulse delivered from every 1 - 10 sec (1-0.1 Hz)	- Four successive stimuli in 2sec (2Hz) i.e. each after 500 m sec - Ratio of response to 1st & 4th twitches is a sensitive indicator of non depolarizing block. - Disappearance of 4th twitch represents a 75% block, 3rd an 80%, 2nd a 90% block - Clinical relaxation requires 75-95% n.m. blockade	- A sensitive test - Sustained contraction for 5sec, indicate adequate but not necessarily complete reversal. - At 50 Hz each stimuli is after 20 ms & at 100 Hz after 10 msec	Represent two less painful variations of tetany. It is more sensitive than train of four for clinical evaluation of fade. **DBS 3, 3**: Three short (20 μs) high frequency bursts separated by 20 msec (50 Hz) followed 750ms later by another three bursts **DBS 3, 2**: Three bursts followed 750 ms later by two such bursts

Capnography

Capnography is the study of *shape or design in the analog (waveform) format* of the changing *concentration of CO_2* in respired gas.

Capnometer is an instrument that measures CO_2 concentration numerically. A device that continuously records and displays CO_2 concentration in form of a tracing or wave form is called a **capnograph** and the tracing on recording paper is called capnogram. *Capnograph or capnogram, is vastly to be preferred to a capnometer or even a fast digital display.* Indeed the last two are useless in anesthetic practice, in which the breath by breath wave form needs to be displayed to permit continuous monitoring and analysis.

Principle

Luft developed the principle of capnography from the fact that *CO_2 absorbs infrared* (IR) radiation of a particular *(43 μm) wavelength*, producing absorption band on IR electromagnetic spectrum. A beam of IR radiation is passed across the gas sample to fall on a sensor. The intensity of IR radiation, passing through CO_2 is diminished by absorption, which allows CO_2 absorption band to be identified, and is *proportional to the amount of CO_2 in mixture*

Erroneous Readings

IR rays are given off by all warm objects and absorbed by non elementary gases (i.e. those composed of dissimilar atoms). There is some overlap in absorption bands of other gases eg. *N_2O distorts the absorption band of CO_2* and produce **collision pressure broadening effect.**

Two way radios and new digital telephones using global positioning satellite (GPS), when used within 2 m of medical device cause disruptions of IR capnogram because the electric field can exceed the immunity record of *7Vm* recommended by USFDA.

Contamination of IR cell by liquids or particu-late matter causes erroneous high readings because of their high IR absorbance.

Types of analyzer

- **Sidestream analyzer** capnography draw a fixed volume of sample gas continuously at rate b/w *50 and 500*

Normal Capnogram

Most commonly used type of capnograph *plots PCO_2 (partial pressure or concentration of CO_2) on Y axis versus time* on x axis. It is divided into an *inspiratory and 3 (sometimes 4) expiratory phases.*

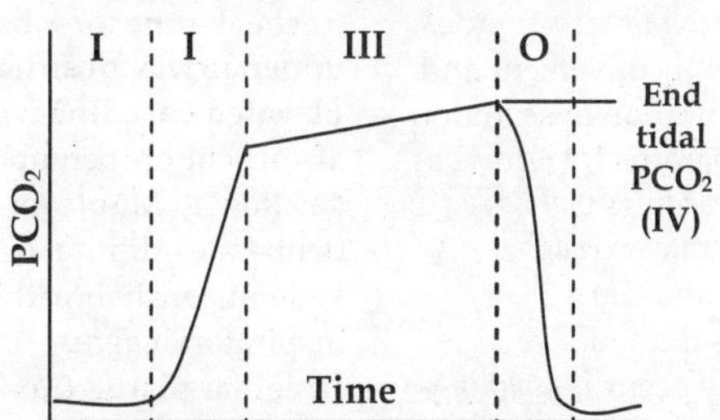

Phase	Feature
I	It represents **beginning of expiration**. The first part of the gas passing out of patent's mouth comes from **mechanical and anatomical dead spaces** (large airways) and contain **no CO_2.** So capnograph register **zero**. This is the **base line**
II	It is a sharply rising **expiratory upstroke** front, which represents *mixing of dead space gas with alveolar gas.* (**Airway + alveolar gas**).
III	It is **end expiratory slowly rising platue** representing **mostly alveolar gas exhalation**. It is not isocapnic; as it shows a very slight & steady increase in CO_2 concentration. PCO_2 value at the end of exhalation is referred to as end **tidal PCO_2 (P_{ET} CO_2)**
IV	Sometimes, there is a *sharp rise in PCO_2* at the terminal end of phase III platue and it is k/a phase IV. It is thought to occur b/o **sudden closure of small airways** abruptly releasing CO_2 rich gases. Bhavani shankar's explanation: well ventilated open lung units have *upsloping increase* in PCO_2 whereas poorly ventilated closure prone lung units have *linear increase* When poorly ventilated units close, the pattern from well ventilated units predominates and slope of platue rise suddenly.
O	**Inspiratory phase**. It is a *sharp downward return* of traces towards zero at the *onset of inspiration.*

Abnormal Capnograms

- Good alveoler plateau with (graph 1) a **low end tidal CO_2** may be seen in **hyperventilation** or an increase **in dead space ventilation** (distinguished by comparision of P_{ETCO2} and Pa_{CO2}) and (graph 2) with **elevated E_{TCO2}** may be caused by **hypoventilation** or **increased CO_2 delivery to lungs.**

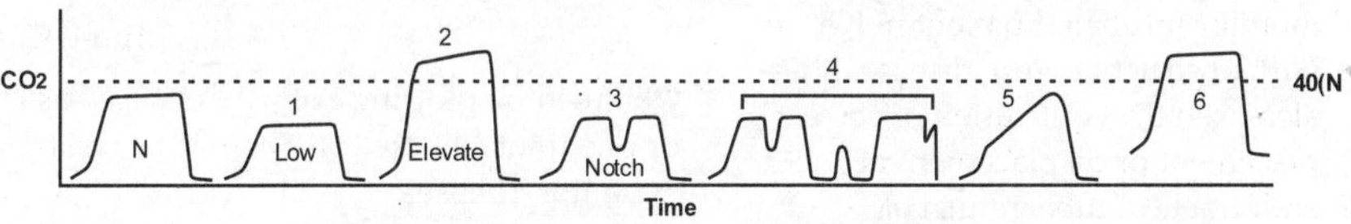

- **Curare cleft or notch** (3) seen during **spontaneous ventilation**[Q] is caused by *lack of synchronous action between the intercostal muscles and diaphragm* most commonly d/t *inadequate muscle relaxant reversal.* The depth of notch is *proportional to the degree of muscle paralysis. The postion of cleft is fairly constant* in same patient but is not *necessarily present in every breath.* Notch (cleft) can also be seen in **cervical transverse lesions, flail chest, hiccups, pneumothorax** and when a patient tries to breath during mechanical ventilation.
- Spontaneous respiratory efforts during mechanical ventilation causes **small breaths at various places during expiration and inspiration** on capnogram (graph 4). Causes include *maladjusted ventilator (hypoventilation), inadequate muscle paralysis, severe hypoxia, patient waking up, pressure on the patient's chest or ventilator malfunction.*

2

ANAESTHESIA

mL/min through nylon or Teflon tubing (as halogenated hydrocarbons react with PVC). Sampling should take place as close to the patient as possible. But usually *proximal end of endo tracheal* tube is preferred over just above the carine site for taking samples as though the latter provides better sample but is inconvenient and has high risk of aspiration of secretion and water into apparatus l/t *erroneous reading. Erroneous readings will be obtained if sampling rate exceeds expiratory flow* rate and causes inspired gas to be sampled. *Hypoventilation* may occur *if sampling flow* exceeds fresh gas flow especially in children in which expired and fresh gas flow are quiet low.

- **Mainstream analyzer capnography** incorporate IR sensors into the circuit very close to ET tube thus eliminating many problems of siestreaming. This is more expansive, *more preferable (in clinical practice), no loss, very fast response system.* The risk of condensation of water vapour is minimized by heating measurement chamber to 40°C but there remains the possibility of contamination from secretion.

Clinical Use

- In cardiovascular stability, the end tidal CO_2 concentration (P_{ET} CO_2) bears a constant relation to arterial CO_2 conc. ($PaCO_2$); and **normal $P_{ET}CO_2$ – P_aCO_2 = 0.7 kPa (5 mmHg),** because of presence of small amount of alveolar dead space. If all alveoli of lung empty synchronously, P_{ET} CO_2 will be synonymous with $PaCO_2$. Normal P_{ET} CO_2 is **32 – 42 mmHg** (1 – 5 mmHg less than $PaCO_2$)
- Capnography ($P_{ET}CO_2$) is used to monitor intubated patient in ICU, or with obstructive lung disease. It is also used for verification of correct placement or displacement of endotracheal tube, return of spontaneous circulation, adequacy of CPR and predict survivability. (i.e. without a return of P_{ET} CO_2 levels of ≥10mmHg after 20 minutes of CPR, the mortality rate is 100%)

E_{TCO2} may slightly rise b/o increasing metabolism of contracting respiratory muscles. Small **indentations** or **dips** in **final (later third) portion** of alveolar platue may represent gas movement d/t someone leaning on chest or patient making very small movements of diaphragm as a **muscle relaxant** is wearing off (**curare cleft**).

- **Prolonged and progressive slanting expiratory upstroke** (5) is caused by start of inspiration before prolonge expiration is complete, so that P_{ETCO2} reading is decreased. It is seen in obstruction to gas flow caused by **partially obstructed tracheal tube or obstruction in patientis airway eg COPD, bronchospasm** or **upper airway obstruction.**
- **Elevated base line** with normal wave form shape (6) may be caused by **exhausted absorbent or incompetent expiratory valve in a circle system**[Q]; insufficient fresh gas flow to **Maplesm system**; problems with the inner tube of the Bain system; deliberate addition of CO_2 to the fresh gas; rebreathing under drapes in a spontaneously breathing patient who is not intubected or an incompetent inspiratory valve.
- **Irregular platue &/or baseline** (7) may result from displacement of tracheal tube into the upper larynx or lower pharynx with intermittent ventilation of stomach and lungs or from pressure on chest, which causes small volumes of gas to move in & out of lungs.

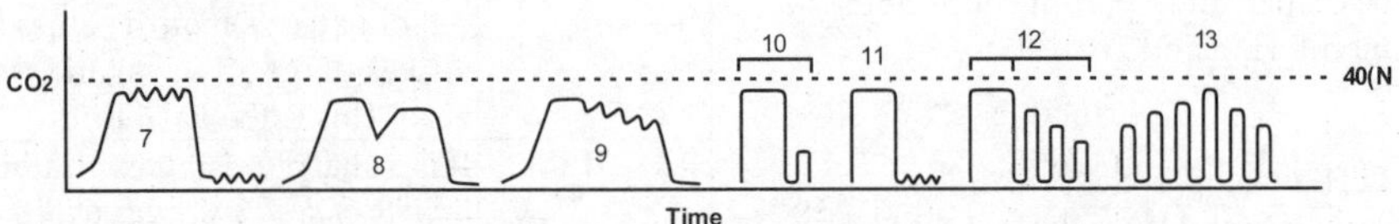

- **Biphasic expiratory platues** (8) is seen in patient with *servere kyphoscoliosis and following single lung transplantation* or in conditions when compliance, airway resistence or V-P ratios in one lung differ substantially from the other lung. **Camel capnogram** (i.e. a second alveolar platue superimposed on the first) represents *one lung emptying slightly before the other* (usually seen in lateral position).
- **Cardiogenic oscillations (small regular tooth like humps** at the end of expiratory phase) caused by heart beating against the lungs is seen in **pediatric patients** as a rule (b/o relative size of infant's heart and thorax). Negative intrathoracic pressure, low respiratory rate, diminution in vital capacity; heart size ratio, low inspiratory: expiratory ratio, low tidal volume and muscular relaxation contribute to cardiogenic ossilation.
- **Sudden drop of E_{TCO2} to a low but nonzero** (graph 10) value include a *poorly fitting tracheal tube or mask, partial obstruction of a tracheal tube and a leak or partial disconnection* in breathing system. **Sudden drop of E_{TCO2} to zero** (11) is caused by acute events relating to the airway, such as *extubation, esophageal intubation, complete breathing system disconnect, ventilator malfunction, totally obstructed tracheal tube or plugged gas sampling tube.* **Exponential decrease in E_{TCO2}** (12) is caused by ***sudden hypotension owing to massive blood loss, or obstruction of major blood vessel, circulatory arrest with continued pulmonary ventilation and pulmonary (air, clot, thrombus, marrow) embolism***[Q]. Sudden increase in E_{TCO2} that gradually returns to normal (13) is seen in *tourniquet release or unclamping of major vessel.*

Volume Capnography

Obtained by plotting *expired PCO_2 versus exhaled gas volume* (measured by spirometer or pneumotachometer). There is *no inspiratory phase* & the curve is divided into 3 expiratory phases

Total **area under** the **PCO_2 curve** is *total volume of CO_2 (Vco_2) exhaled* for that single breath. It measures partition of dead space components (i.e. total physiological dead space, alveolar dead space), fraction of expired CO2 (F_ECO_2), and value of mixed expired PCO_2 (P_ECO_2).

Incompetent inspiratory valve and rebreathing during mechanical ventilation may require volume capnography to be detected reliably. It is also better (than time capnography) for diagnosis of pulmonary embolism and titration of PEEP settings.

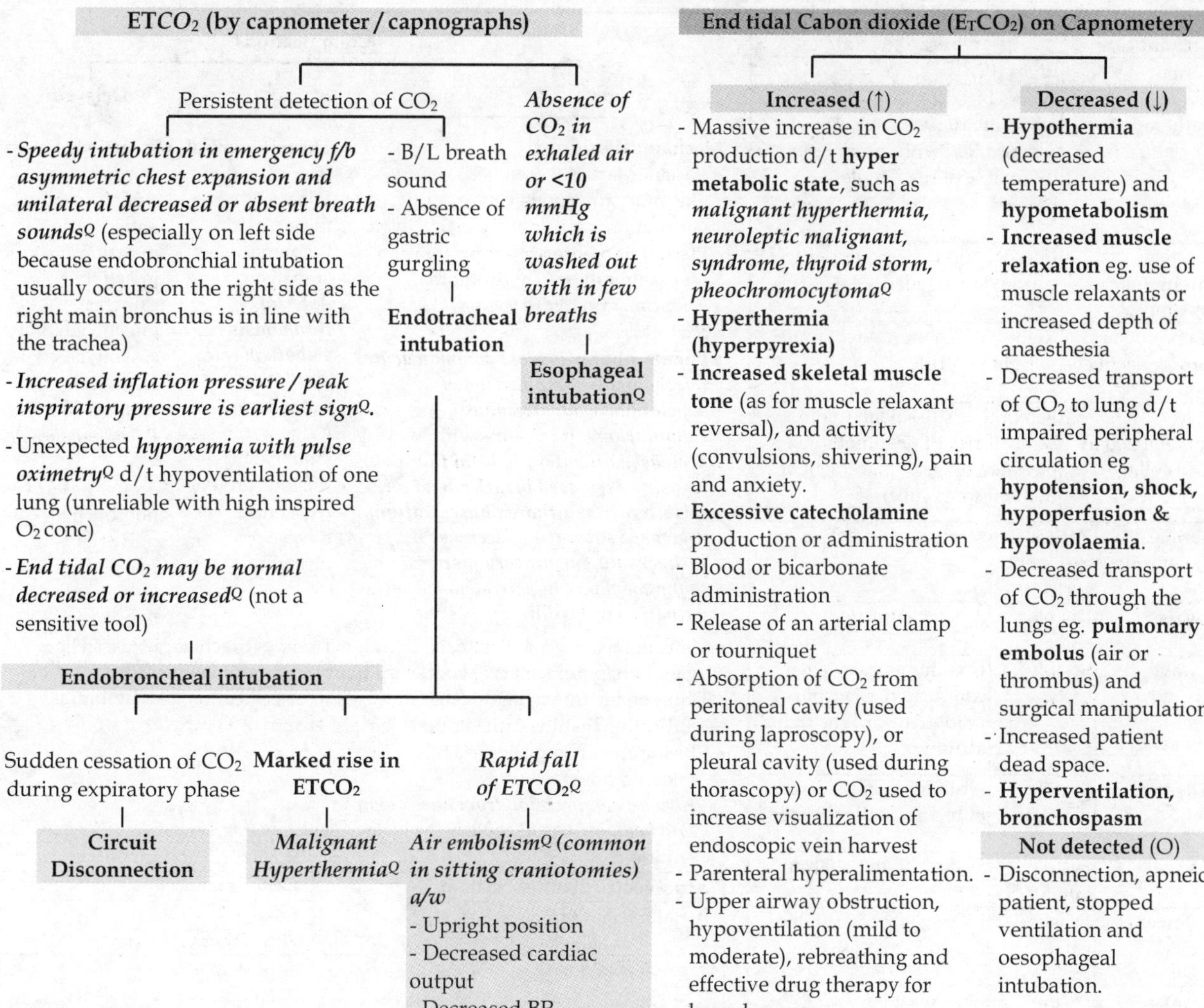

ETCO2 (by capnometer / capnographs)
Persistent detection of CO2
Absence of CO2 in exhaled air or <10 mmHg which is washed out with in few breaths
Esophageal intubationQ
- Speedy intubation in emergency f/b asymmetric chest expansion and unilateral decreased or absent breath soundsQ (especially on left side because endobronchial intubation usually occurs on the right side as the right main bronchus is in line with the trachea)
- Increased inflation pressure / peak inspiratory pressure is earliest signQ.
- Unexpected hypoxemia with pulse oximetryQ d/t hypoventilation of one lung (unreliable with high inspired O2 conc)
- End tidal CO2 may be normal decreased or increasedQ (not a sensitive tool)
- B/L breath sound
- Absence of gastric gurgling
Endotracheal intubation
Endobronchial intubation
Sudden cessation of CO2 during expiratory phase
Circuit Disconnection
Marked rise in ETCO2
Malignant HyperthermiaQ
Rapid fall of ETCO2Q
Air embolismQ (common in sitting craniotomies) a/w
- Upright position
- Decreased cardiac output
- Decreased BP
End tidal Cabon dioxide (ETCO2) on Capnometery
Increased (↑)
- Massive increase in CO2 production d/t hyper metabolic state, such as malignant hyperthermia, neuroleptic malignant, syndrome, thyroid storm, pheochromocytomaQ
- Hyperthermia (hyperpyrexia)
- Increased skeletal muscle tone (as for muscle relaxant reversal), and activity (convulsions, shivering), pain and anxiety.
- Excessive catecholamine production or administration
- Blood or bicarbonate administration
- Release of an arterial clamp or tourniquet
- Absorption of CO2 from peritoneal cavity (used during laproscopy), or pleural cavity (used during thorascopy) or CO2 used to increase visualization of endoscopic vein harvest
- Parenteral hyperalimentation.
- Upper airway obstruction, hypoventilation (mild to moderate), rebreathing and effective drug therapy for bronchospasm.
Decreased (↓)
- Hypothermia (decreased temperature) and hypometabolism
- Increased muscle relaxation eg. use of muscle relaxants or increased depth of anaesthesia
- Decreased transport of CO2 to lung d/t impaired peripheral circulation eg hypotension, shock, hypoperfusion & hypovolaemia.
- Decreased transport of CO2 through the lungs eg. pulmonary embolus (air or thrombus) and surgical manipulation.
- Increased patient dead space.
- Hyperventilation, bronchospasm
Not detected (O)
- Disconnection, apneic patient, stopped ventilation and oesophageal intubation.

★ Inspiratory CO_2 is zero in all except rebreathing (↑); All show normal wave form on capnograph except all causes of E_TCO_2=O, showing absent waveform, rebreathing showing elevated baseline, use of muscle relaxant showing curare cleft and upper airway obstruction showing abnormal wave form. E_T to arterial gradient is normal in all except rebreathing, increased dead space and pulmonany embolism (in which it is elevated).

Central Venous Pressure (CVP) Monitoring

- 7 Fr (French), 20 cm multiport chatheter that allows monitoring of CVP & infusion of drugs and fluid simultaneously are the most common type used. It should be noted that because of smaller diameter of each individual lumen and the overall catheter length, increases resistance to flow significantly. So the rapid fluid resuscitation is more efficient with short length, large bore catheter inserted peripherally.
- **Right internal jugular vein** (Daily method) is the most popular & preferred site b/o consistent, predictable, readily identifiable & palpable anatomical location, and a short, straight course to superior vena cava. Alternative CV cannulation sites are left internal jugular vein, subclavian vein, external jugular vein, femoral vein, axillary and other peripheral veins. Ultrasound guided CV catheter placement (one look technique) is preferred.
- **Confirmation of intravenous catheter position** is done intraoperatively by aspiration of blood and postoperatively by radiography. Ideally the catheter tip should lie within the superior venacava, parallel to vessel walls, & be positioned below the inferior border of clavicles and above the level of *3rd rib/T_4-T_5 interspace / azygous vein / tracheal carina/ or the take off of the right main bronchus.* Catheter tips located with in the heart or below the pericardial reflection of superior vena cava increase the risk of cardiac perforation & fatal cardiac tamponade.

Condition	Preferred site
Normal	Right IJV
Severe bleeding diatheses	Where bleeding from vein or adjacent artery is easily detected & controlled with compression Internal/external jugular is preferred & subclavian avoided
Severe emphysema or pneumothorax	Internal jugular is preferred & subclavian avoided
Transvenous cardiac pacing is required	Right IJV b/o most direct route to right ventride
Neck immobilized in hard collar	Femoral or subclavian (more safely if risk of pneumothorax is obviated by prior placement of thoracostomy tube)

Normal waveform	Phase of cardiac cycle	Mechanical event
a wave	Distole end	Atrial contraction
C wave	Systole early	Isovolumic ventricular contraction, tricuspid motion toward the right atrium
X descent	Systole mid	Atrial relaxation, descent of base, systolic collapse
V wave	Systole late	Systolic filling of atrium
Y descent	Diastole early	Early ventricular filling, diastolic collapse
h wave	Diastole mid-late	Diastolic plateau

Contraindications

- ***Renal cell tumor extension into the right atrium or fungating tricuspid valve vegetations***Q.
- IJV cannulation is relatively contraindicated in patients who are *receiving anticoagulants* or who have *had an ipsilateral carotid endarterectomy*, b/o the possibility of unintentional carotid artery puncture.

Complications

Acute

Mechanical Injury

- Vascular (arterial or venous) injury like injury to venous valves, aortic perforation, avulsion of facial vein etc.
- **Pleural or mediastinum perforation** l/t pneumothorax, hydrothorax, ***hemothorax***Q, hydro/hemo/ chylothorax.
- **Pneumothorax** is ***most common acute (mechanical) complication of subclavian central venous cannulation***Q. It presents with ***decreased air entery in hemi thorax (causing decreased breath sound on ipsilateral hemithorax auscultation), decreased saturation, decrease BP, tachycardia, respiratory distress (dypnoea) and hyperresonance on palpation of ipsilateral chest***Q

- **Thromboembolism**
  - Venous thrombosis
  - Pulmonary embolism
  - ***Arterial thrombosis & embolism (air, clot)***Q
  - Catheter or guide wire embolism
- Misinterpretation of data & misuse of instrument

Delayed

- **Infection** is most common late complication and include insertion site infection, catheter infection, blood stream infection ***(septicemia)***Q & endocarditis
- ***Pseudoaneurysm***Q & aortoarterial/venobronchial/carotid artery-internal jugular vein **fistula** are *uncommon*

- Subcutaneous / mediastinal emphysema, nerve (brachial plexus, stellate ganglion, phrenic nerve) vocal cord injury, arrhythmias & cardiac tamponade (most life threatening vascular complication). **Arrhythmias** indicating that the catheter tip is in right atrium or ventricle.
- Respiratory compromise d/t:
  - Pneumothorax
  - ***Airway compression from hematoma***Q
  - ***Tracheal, laryngeal injury***Q

Condition	Waveform abnormalities
Atrio-ventricular dissociation	***Cannon a wave***Q
Atrial fibrillation	Loss of a wave Prominent C wave
Tricuspid stenosis	Tall a wave Attenuation of y descent
Tricuspid regurgitation	Tall systolic C-V wave Loss of x descent
Right ventricular ischemia / pericardial constriction	Tall a and v waves Steep x and y descents M or W configuration
Cardiac tamponade	Dominant x decent Attenuated y descent
Respiratory variation during spontaneous or positive pressure ventilation	Measure pressures at end expiration

Swan-Ganz Pulmonary Artery Catheter

It is the mainstay for *cardiac function assessment* in *critically ill patient* especially in *perioperative setting*. It can help to distinguish neuronal pulmonary edema from other causes of edema, and can be used to direct fluid and catecholamine therapy, if necessary, and to exclude cardiogenic causes, such as pericardial temponade and MI. It is used to measure

- ***direct pressure in pulmonary artery (PAWP), right atrium & right ventricle***Q.
- right ventricle ejection fraction
- indirect pressure in left atrium
- ***cardiac out-put by indicator dilution.***Q
- ***mixed venous oxygen saturation***Q } by addition of thermistors, pressure transducers and fiberoptics
- measurement of pulmonary flow }

Complications

- Resulting from catheter placement (catheterization)
  - Arrhythmias, ventricular fibrillation
  - Right bundle branch block, complete heart block
- Associated with in vivo presence / catheter residence
  - Mechanical, catheter knots
  - Thromboembolism
  - Pulmonary infarction
  - Endocarditis, infection
  - Endocardial damage, cardiac valve injury
  - Pulmonary artery rupture
  - Pulmonary artery pseudoaneurysm
- Misinterpretation of data & misuse of equipment

Pulmonary Artery Catheterization

Location	Pressure tracing	
Catheter passes via SVC to right atrium **(Right atrial pressure)**	Low pressure waves	3-8 mm Hg
Catheter enters right ventricle through tricuspid valve **(Right ventricle pressure)**	Tall pressure waves	15-25 mm Hg systolic and 0-10 mm Hg diastolic
Entery in pulmonary artery through pulmonary valve is heralded by **Pulmonary artery pressure**	***Sudden increase in diastolic pressure***Q (10-20 mm Hg). Systolic pressure remains same ***Dicrotic notch caused by closure of pulmonary valve***Q	10-20 mm Hg diastolic pressure
Catheter advances into a branch of pulmonary artery (where it wedges) **Pulmonary capillary wedge pressure.** This reflects left atrial pressure	Dampened pressure wave form	4-12 mm Hg

Allen's Test

- Allen's test is used to check the adequacy of *blood supply to hand by assessing integrity of palmar arch, patency of radial and ulnar arteries.*
- It is a simple but not reliable, method for assessing the safety of (radial) artery cannulation or AVF ligation. If the arteries are not patent or arch is incomplete, these procedures are risky as the blood supply of hand may be compromised.
- In this test, patient exsanguinates his hand by elevating and making a fist several times. While **operator occludes the radial & ulnar arteries with fingertip pressure** at wrist, the patient relaxes the blanched hand. The tip of the finger should go pale. In this test return of colour is observed with release of each (ulnar & radial) artery in turn.
- Collateral flow through palmar arterial arch is confirmed by flushing of thumb (little finger) within **5 seconds** after pressure on the ulnar (radial) artery is realeased. Delayed return of normal color (5-10s) indicates an equivocal test or insufficient collateral circulation (> 10s)
- It is of questionable utility and require patient cooperation. Alternatively blood flow distal to arterial occlusion and adequacy of collateral circulation can be detected by *palpation, doppler, plethysmography or pulse oximetry* (patient cooperation is not required).

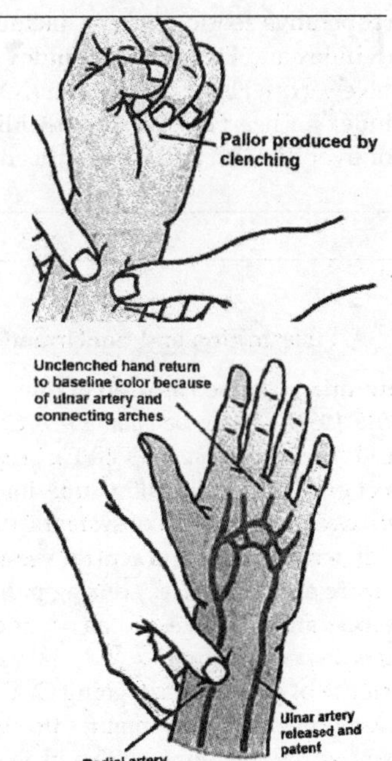

American Society of Anesthesiologists (ASA) Physical Status Classification

- **American Society of Anesthesiologists (ASA) Physical Status Classification** of patient is a **scoring system to assess physical status (main) and help quantify relative risk**Q.
- ASA risk classification system developed in 1941 by **Meyer Saklad**, was the first attempt to quantify the risk associated with anesthesia and surgery. Neither the type of anesthesia, nor the location of procedure or operation was considered in the development or as a component of this risk classification. Thus it attempts to **give a subjective and relative risk based only on patients preoperative medical history or physical status** (ie no consideration of diagnostic studies). ASA Physical Status (ASAPS) 2 patients are

Class	Definition of Patients's Physical Condition (Status)
ASA 1	***Normal healthy patient*** *without organic, physiological, biochemical or psychiatric disease/* disturbance. The pathological process for which surgery is to be performed is localized and does not entail a systemic disturbance.
ASA 2	A patient with **mild systemic disease** caused by the condition to be treated surgically or other pathophysiology **eg mild asthma, well controlled hypertension (even by drugs)** mild heart disease, anemia, obesity, mild chronic bronchitis, **stable diabetes mellitus and old age** (patients aged > 80 yrs are automatically placed in class II). Disease does not limit patient's activity in any way (**no functional limitation & no significant impact on daily activity).** Unlikely to have an impact on anesthesia & surgery.

ANAESTHESIA

2

at higher risk than ASAPS 1 patients, but only if undergoing the same operation.

- **ASA-PS classification defines relative risk** prior to conscious sedation and surgical anesthesia. Its advantages includes: it is time honored, simple, reproducible and most importantly it has been shown to be strongly a/w perioperative risk (Morgan). However, most importantly, there is **no attempt to quantify the risk**, which hampers the ability to use this risk assessment tool for **communicating meaningful expectations** to patients and other care givers (Miller).
- **ASA classification which ranks physical status** is most widely used system for **describing patients physical condition**. However, it does not accommodate the asymptomatic patients who, for example may have severe coronary artery disease. It also **ignores risks incurred by the proposed operation. Therefore, it is not synonymous with the risk of morbidity and mortality.**[Q]
- Other preoperative scoring systems include **Goldman index** and **Fleischer risk index** (for cardiac disease); New York Heart Association (NYHA) scoring index for heart disease**; Pugh-Childs Scoring index (**for liver disease) and GCS for head injury.

ASA 3	- Patient with **severe (significant) systemic disease** from any cause which causes some **functional limitations** (ie limits normal activity or have significant impact on daily activity in form of **limited life style**) eg *renal failure on dialysis or classic congestive heart faillur*. It may not be possible to define the degree of disability with any precision eg *angina, cardiac failure and **severe (uncontrolled) diabetes mellitus.*** - Probable impact on anesthesia & surgery.
ASA 4	- A patient with **severe systemic disease that is a constant threat to life (ie already life threatening)** or **requires intensive therapy** and not always correctible by operation eg *acute MI, respiratory failure requiring mechanical ventilation, marked cardiac insufficiency, persistent angina (unstable),* severe respiratory, renal or hepatic insufficiency. - Severe limitations of daily activity **(functionally incapacitated).** - Major impact on anesthesia & surgery.
ASA 5	**Moribund patient** who is **equally likely to die in the next 24 hours** without or even with surgery. **Little chance of survival,** but submitted for operation in desperation.
ASA 6	**Brain dead organ donar.**
E	E added to classification indicates **emergency surgery**; and the patient is considered to be in poorer physical condition. eg 2E is poorer condition than 2

Hypothermia

Definition and Confirmation

- **Hypothermia** is defined as drop of *core body temperature below 35ºC (95º F)*. It can be *mild (35-28ºC), moderate* (27-21°C) **and** *severe or profound* (< 20ºC); *primary (accidental)* d/t direct exposure of a healthy individual to cold or *secondary* as a complication of systemic disorder.
- Core body temperature and **central venous blood temperature** are same except during periods of relatively rapid temperature changes as can occur during *extracorporeal perfusion*.
- Temperature of patient undergoing G.A. should be monitored (except for < 15 minutes procedure) by thermistor or thermocouple with a probe placed over tympanic membrane, rectum, nasopharynx, esophagus, bladder & skin. Hypothermia is confirmed by measuring core temperature preferably at 2 sites such as *15 cm deep rectal probes* (not adjacent to cold feces) and *esophageal probe* (placed 24 cm bellow larynx); relying solely on *infrared tymapanic thermography* is not advisible.

Mechanism & Thermoregulation

- Heat loss occurs through 5 mechanisms: **radiation** (body **looses 55-65% of heat**; most important mechanism), **conduction (10-15%** of heat loss but becomes greater in cold water immersion), **convection** (increased in wind**), respiration** and **evaporation** (affected by ambient temperature and relative humidity).
- **Preoptic anterior hypothalamus** normally orchestrates thermoregulation. Immediate defence of thermoneutrality is via *autonomic nervous system* (include release of epinephrine, increased muscle tone, and shivering l/t thermogenesis and increased BMR); whereas, delayed

Benefits/Advantages and Uses

- ***Hypothermia*** (ie body temperature <36° C) reduces metabolic oxygen requirements, is proved to **be *protective during times of cerebral or cardiac ischemia***[Q]. Hypothermia causes a *greater reduction in cerebral metabolic rate* for glucose & O_2 than the level attained at EEG silence because its reduction of metabolism is caused by a *reduction in both neuronal electrical activity* and enzyme activity related to maintenance of cellular function. **Unlike anesthetic agents, *hypothermia decreases both basal & electrical metabolic requirements throughout the brain***; which continues to decrease even after complete electrical silence.
- Hypothermia also ***reduces release of excitatory neurothransmitters, reduces free radicals and other mediators of ischemic injury. It is an effective method for protecting the brain during focal and global ischemia.***[Q] Induced hypothermia has shown ***benefit following cardiac arrest and is a routine part of most post arrest protocols for comatose patients***[Q]. Profound hypothermia is used for *upto 1 hour of total circulatory arrest.*
- Hypothermia provides ***protection against ischemia & hypoxia***[Q] **by *reducing metabolic rate about 8 %/°C***[Q]**. It reduces metabolic rate/oxygen requirements** and can be **protective during cerebral or cardiac ischemia.**
- ***1-3°C*** **hypothermia (core temperature ≈ 34°C)** is indicated in

1. ***Neurosurgery***[Q]
2. Carotid artery surgery
3. ***Cardiac surgery***[Q]
4. Traumatic brain injury
5. ***ARDS***[Q] ***(Neonatal asphyxia)***
6. ***Malignant hyperthermia***[Q]
7. Procedure where tissue ischemia is anticipated
8. ***Prolonged surgeries***[Q]
9. ***Recovery after cardiac arrest and for asphyxiated neonates***[Q]

control is mediated by *endocrine system (eg thyroid axis).*

- Normally in unanesthetized patients **the hypothalamus maintains core body temperature** with a very narrow range **(interthreshold range)** with the threshold for sweating and vasodilation at one extreme and the threshold for vasoconstriction and shivering at the other. Raising body temperature induces vasodialation & sweating while hypothermia triggers vasoconstriction & shivering as compensatory mechanism.
- During anesthesia body cannot compensate for hypothermia because ***anesthetics inhibit central thermoregulation by interfering with hypothalamic function***Q. Eg isoflurane produces a dose dependent decrease in threshold temperature that triggers vasoconstriction (3° ↓ for each % of isoflurane).
- **Both general and regional anesthetics** increase the threshold range, although by different mechanism. Like general anesthetics, *spinal & epidural anesthesia* also lead to hypothermia by vasodialation & internal redistribution of heat. The accompanying thermoregulatory impairment from regional anesthesia is due to an *altered perception of temperature in blocked dermatomes by hypothalmus as opposed to central effect of G.A.*
- Unintentional **perioperative hypothermia occurs in nearly every patient during anesthesia & surgery** (especially in extremes of age, abdominal surgery, long procedure, cold operating room temperature, prolonged exposure of large wound, use of large amount of room temperature IV fluids or high flows of unhumidified gases) unless steps are taken to prevent this complication.

Phases

- When there is no attempt to actively warm an anesthesized patients core temperature usually decreases in 3 phases.

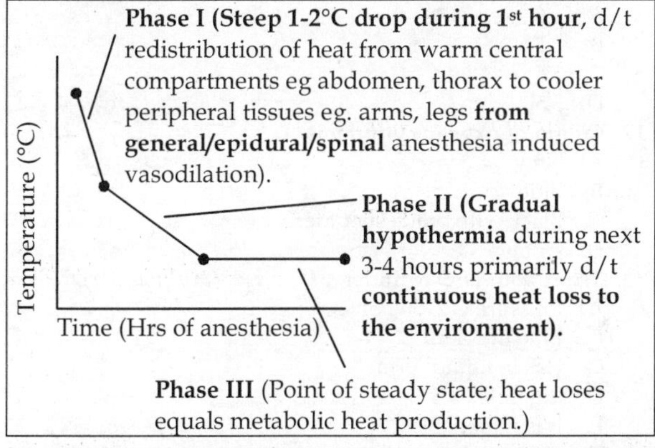

Phase I (Steep 1-2°C drop during 1st hour, d/t redistribution of heat from warm central compartments eg abdomen, thorax to cooler peripheral tissues eg. arms, legs from general/epidural/spinal anesthesia induced vasodilation).
Phase II (Gradual hypothermia during next 3-4 hours primarily d/t continuous heat loss to the environment).
Temperature (°C)
Time (Hrs of anesthesia)
Phase III (Point of steady state; heat loses equals metabolic heat production.)

Deleterious Effects & Complication

Nevertheless, hypothermia has **multiple deleterious physiological effects. Complications** of unintentional perioperative hypothermila include.

1. **Cardiac arrhythmias and ischemia.**Q
2. **Reversible coagulopathy** (d/t platelet dysfluntion related to local>> core temperature; routine coagulation screening done at 37°C cannot recognized it) causing increased blood loss & transfusion requirements
3. Impaired wound healing and **increased risk of wound infection** (most common serious complilcation)
4. Impaired renal functions**, increased urinary nitrogen excretion**
5. Decreased /delayed drug metabolism.
6. Increased postoperative protein catabolism and stress response (increased BP, heart rate and catecholamine concentration)
7. Increased morbid myocardial outcomes (3 times; d/t stress) and increased mortality rate.
8. Markedlly impaired thermal comfort (feeling extremely cold).
9. Altered mental status
10. Increases peripheral vascular resistance; hyperglycemia
11. Left shift of hemoglobin oxygen saturation curve.

Management

- Prewarming the patient for ½ an hour with **convective forced air warming blankets** prevents phase 1 hypothermia by eliminating the central peripheral temperature gradient.
- Methods to minimize phase 2 hypothermia include ***use of forced air warming blankets, warm water blankets (cutaneous warming), increasing ambient room temperature, heat humidification of inspired gases and warming of intravenous fluid***Q. Passive insulators such as heated cotton blankets (space blankets) are of limited utility unless the entire body is covered (Morgan).
- **Patients cannot be warmed by administering heated fluids because the fluids cannot (much) exceed body temperature**. On the other hand, heat loss from cold IV fluids *becomes substantial when large amounts of* crystalloid soluition or blood are administered. 1 unit of refrigerated blood or 1L of crystalloid administered at room temperature each decreases mean body temperature ~0.25°C. Fluid warmers minimize these losses and should be used when large amounts of IV fluids or blood are administered.
- Post operative **shivering (shaking)** is a protective mechanism to hypothermila. Its likelihood can be reduced by maintaining normothermia. Post operative shivering can be effectively treated with small doses of **meperidine** (12-25 mg), **pethidine (doc), tramadol (2nd choice** i.e. opioids but not morphine), clonidine, ketanserin, physostigmine, nefopam, dexmedetomidine, and magnesium sulfate.

Brain Death

- It is defined as ***irreversible cessation of all brain function. Spinal cord function below C_1 may still be present***Q**.** Brain death criteria can be applied only in absence of ***hypothermia, hypotension, drug depressing brain function, neuromuscular blocking agent, endocrinal & metabolic abnormalities***Q, *(Clinical criteria are:*
  - ***Coma***Q
  - ***Absence of brain stem (i.e., pupillary, gag, corneal, oropharangeal, respiratory, vestibuloocular (caloric) & or cough) reflexes***Q.
  - Absence of motor activity including decrebate & decorticate posturing.
  - Absence of ventilatory effort with the arterial CO_2 tension 60 mm Hg or 20 mmHg above pretest level
- ***Spinal cord reflexes may be preserved in coma & re- examination (not < 2hour apart) is optional.***Q *Apnea test* should be done at last because of its harmful effects on intracranial pressure. ***Isoelectric EEG, absent brain stem auditory evoked potentials & absence of cerebral perfusion***Q (on angiography, radioisotope scan or transcranial Doppler) are confirmatory but not required tests.

QUESTIONS

ANAESTHESIA MACHINES & CYLINDERS

1. **Acronym AMBU stands for:** *(AIIMS May 13)*
   A. Automated manual breathing unit
   B. Artificial manual breathing unit
   C. Artificial mechanical breathing unit
   D. Artificial mechanical balloon unit
2. **A 4 year old child was intubated while posted for craniotomy. Suddenly anesthetic machine started showing bellowing (alarming). Next management is:**
   A. Start manual ventilation *(AIIMS Nov 12)*
   B. Do nothing
   C. Larger size of endotracheal tube
   D. Increase flow rate
3. **Which of the following is true about anesthesia machine**
   A. Desflurane vapourizer is heated to 39°C *(AI 12)*
   B. Halothane vaporizers at 39°C
   C. Rotameter is a variable pressure flow meter & variable orifice device for gases only.
   D. O_2 sensor is attached to inspiratory limb at the machine end.
4. **True about Boyle's apparatus:** *(PGI Dec 06)*
   A. Continuous flow machine
   B. Liquid anesthetic vapours not used
   C. Resistance very high
   D. Resistance low
5. **True about Rotameter:** *(DNB 09, MP 06)*
   A. Rotameter reading may not get affected by dirt inside the tube
   B. Rotameter reading may not get affected by static electricity
   C. The height to which bobbin rises indicates the flow rate
   D. A rotameter is a variable pressure flowmeter
6. **True about Wright's Spirometer is/are** *(PGI Nov 11)*
   A. Flow rates can be calculated *(DNB 10)*
   B. Gives false high values at low flow rates
   C. Gives false low values at high flow rates
   D. Used for calculation of expired volume
   E. Read bidirectional flow
7. **True about anaesthesia breathing circuit is:** *(PGI June 08)*
   A. Cylinder is a part of high pressure system
   B. O_2 flush delivers < 35 lts.
   C. O_2 flush delivers > 35.00 lts
   D. Pipelines is a part low pressure system
8. **All of the following are safety measures to prevent the delivery of hypoxic gas mixture to the patient except:** *(AIIMS May 08)*
   A. Location of oxygen valve after the N_2O Valve
   B. Presence of a PIN index system to prevent wrong attachment of the N_2O and oxygen cylnders
   C. Location of a fail-safe valve downstream from the nitrous oxide supply source
9. **Pin index system is a safety feature adopted in anaesthesia machines to prevent:** *(AIIMS 03, DNB 08)*
   A. Incorrect attachment of anaesthesia machines.
   B. Incorrect attachment of anaesthesia face masks.
   C. Incorrect inhalation agent delivery
   D. Incorrect gas cylinder attachment.
10. **The Pin index code of Nitrous oxide is :**
    A. 2, 5. *(AIIMS 03, CMC 02)*
    B. 1, 5.
    C. 3, 5.
    D. 2, 6.
11. **True statement regarding pin index:** *(PGI May 10)*
    A. Pin is present on cylinder *(DNB 08)*
    B. Pin is present on machine
    C. Not effective if wrong gas is filled in cylinder
    D. Pin index of air is 2, 5
    E. Hole positions on cylinder valves
12. **Gas is filled as liquid in cylinder in:**
    A. O_2 *(PGI Dec 07)*
    B. CO_2
    C. N_2O
    D. Cyclopropane
    E. Halothane
13. **Colour of O_2 cylinder** *(AIIMS 92)*
    A. Gray
    B. Orange
    C. Blue
    D. Black & White
14. **An anaesthetist orders a new attendant to bring the oxygen cylinder. He will ask the attendant to identify the correct cylinder by following color code:** *(AI 03, DNB 98)*
    A. Black cylinders with white shoulders
    B. Black cylinders with grey shoulders
    C. White cylinders with black shoulders
    D. Grey cylinder with white shoulders
15. **For high pressure storage of compressed gases cylinders are made up of.** *(DNB 99, CMC 04)*
    A. Molybdenum steel
    B. Iron + Mo
    C. Steel + Cu
    D. Cast iron
16. **Pin Code index of N_2O is** *(AI 97)*
    A. 1,6
    B. 2,5
    C. 2,6
    D. 3,5
17. **Colour of oxygen cylinder is** *(AI 97)*
    A. Grey
    B. Blue
    C. Black with white shoulder
    D. Orange
18. **True about N_2O cylinder** *(PGI June 04, DNB 05)*
    A. Pressure is 2200 PSI
    B. Blue in colour
    C. Gas in liquid form
    D. Pin index 3.5
    E. It is flammable
19. **True about N_2O:** *(PGI June 08)*
    A. Pin index 3,5
    B. Blue in colour
    C. Stored as liquid
    D. MAC 105
20. **True about N_2O cylinder is/are A/E:**
    A. Blue color *(PGI 2000)*
    B. N_2O in liquid form in cylinder
    C. 2220 PSP is the pressure in cylinder
    D. Pin index 3,5
21. **All statements are true about gas cylinders except**
    A. Pressure of N_2O is 745 psig at 20°C *(MAHE 04)*
    B. Higher pressure indicates impurity in N_2O *(DNB 01)*
    C. N_2O is in liquid form *(Jipmer 02)*

D. Emergency oxygen 'E' cylinder has more gas than 'H' cylinder ☐

22. Regarding critical temperature which of following is true: *(PGI Dec 08)*
A. TC of O_2 is – 119°C ☐
B. TC of N_2 is – 119°C ☐
C. TC of N_2 is 36.5°C ☐
D. TC of N_2O is 36.5°C ☐
E. TC of air is - 140.6°C ☐

23. Most commonly used cylinder in anaesthesia machine is: *(PGI May 12)*
A. A ☐
B. B ☐
C. D ☐
D. E ☐
E. F ☐

BREATHING SYSTEM

24. All of the following are suitable anaesthetic circuits for both controlled and assisted ventilation except *(AIIMS 2003)*
A. Mapleson A ☐
B. Mapleson B & C ☐
C. Mapleson D ☐
D. Mapleson E ☐

25. Not true for magills circuit *(AIIMS 93, CMC 99)*
A. Ideal for adults ☐
B. Ideal for infant ☐
C. Semiclosed ☐
D. Spontaneous breathing is a must ☐

26. A 25 year old male is undergoing incision and drainage of abscess under general anaesthesia with spontaneous respiration. The most efficient anaesthetic circuiit is:
A. Maplelson A ☐
B. Mapleson B ☐
C. Mapleson C ☐
D. Mapleson D ☐

27. True about Bain circuit : *(PGI May 10, 09, DNB 06)*
A. Mapleson type B ☐
B. Mapleson type D ☐
C. Can be used for spontaneous respiration ☐
D. Can be used for controlled ventilation ☐
E. Coaxial ☐

28. In magil circuit airflow is *(AI 2K, 98, WB 05)*
A. 1/2 of minute volume ☐
B. equal to M.V. ☐
C. 2 x m.v. ☐
D. 3 x m.v. ☐

29. The most appropriate circuit for ventilating a spontaneously breathing infant during anaesthesia is:
A. Jackson Rees' modification of Ayres' T Piece. ☐
B. Mapleson A or Magill's circuit. *(AI 2005)* ☐
C. Mapleson C or Waters' to and fro canister. ☐
D. Bains circuit. ☐

30. True about oxygen concentrator: *(PGI June 2005)*
A. Zeolite activation ☐
B. Delivers O_2 ☐
C. Requires power supply ☐
D. Gives O_2 at 100% ☐

REBREATHING SYSTEM

31. For rebreathing prevention valve incorrect is
A. Should be as far as possible from the patient ☐
B. Should be light *(AIIMS 1994)* ☐
C. Well designed ☐
D. Used at expiratory end of tube ☐

32. All ↓CO_2 absorption in circuit except: *(PGI Dec 07)*
A. Resistance in circuit ☐
B. High flow ☐
C. Small granule size ☐
D. Medium granule size ☐
E. Chanelling ☐

33. All decrease CO_2 absorption in circuit except *(AIIMS 1993)*
A. Resistance in circuit ☐
B. Flow ☐
C. Dead Space ☐
D. Tidal Volume ☐

34. Reacts with soadaline *(AI 1993)*
A. Methoxyfluene ☐
B. Ketamine ☐
C. Trilene ☐
D. SO_2 ☐

35. Which is the main component of sodalime in closed circuit *(AIIMS May 12)*
A. Sodium hydroxide ☐
B. Barium hydroxide ☐
C. Calcium hydroxide ☐
D. Potassium hydroxide ☐

36. All are constituents of soda lime except *(PGI 96, Jipmer 2K, DNB 03)*
A. $Ca(OH)_2$ ☐
B. $Ba(OH)_2$ ☐
C. Silica ☐
D. Moisture ☐

37. Water is used for hardening in *(PGI 96, AI 92, DNB 02)*
A. Sodalime ☐
B. Baralime ☐
C. Both ☐
D. None ☐

38. Clayton is used in a close breathing system for the purpose of *(PGI 96, AMU 98)*
A. As a hardner ☐
B. As an absorbent ☐
C. As a softner ☐
D. As an indicator ☐

39. Rebreathing systems are A/E *(PGI 95, SGPGI 2K, DNB 99)*
A. To & fro system ☐
B. Circle system ☐
C. Water's system ☐
D. Mapleson F ☐

AIRWAY MANAGEMENT

40. **Which of the following are used to protect airways:** *(PGI Nov 2009)*
A. LMA ☐
B. Endotracheal tube ☐
C. Ryles tube ☐
D. Combitube ☐
E. Sengstaken Blackmore tube ☐
F. Bag & Mask ☐

41. Dead space is increased by all except *(AIIMS May 09)*
A. Anticholinergic drugs ☐
B. Standing ☐
C. Hyperextension of neck ☐
D. Endotracheal intubation ☐

42. Seen after tracheostomy is *(AIIMS May 09)*
A. Inversion of V/P ratio ☐
B. Increased V/P ratio ☐
C. Decrease in dead space ☐
D. Increased resistance to air flow ☐

43. The physiological dead space is decreased by: *(AIIMS May 2005)*
A. Upright position ☐
B. Positive pressure ventilation ☐
C. Neck flexion ☐
D. Emphysema ☐

44. Anatomical dead space is increased by all /except *(AI 1999)*
A. Atropine ☐
B. Halothane ☐

C. Massive pleural effusion ☐
D. Inspiration ☐

45. True about endotracheal intubation is: *(AI 1999)*
A. It reduces normal anatomical dead space ☐
B. It produces decrease in resistance to respiration ☐
C. Subglottic edema is most common complication ☐
D. All of the above ☐

46. Which one of the following device provides fixed performance oxygen therapy:
A. Nasal Cannula *(AIIMS May 2005)* ☐
B. Venturi mask ☐
C. O_2 by T-piece ☐
D. Edinburg mask ☐

47. O_2 delivery is regulated by A/E *(AIIMS 94)*
A. O_2 tent ☐
B. Venti mask ☐
C. Poly mask ☐
D. Noval Catheter ☐

48. All of the following are examples of definite airways, except: *(AI 11)*
A. Nasotracheal tube ☐
B. Orotracheal tube ☐
C. Laryngeal Mask airway ☐
D. Cricothyroidotomy ☐

49. Trendelenberg position produces decrease in all of the following except- *(AIIMS Nov 04, DNB 05)*
A. Vital capacity ☐
B. Functional residual capacity ☐
C. Compliance ☐
D. Respiratory rate ☐

50. Maximum vital capacity decreased in
A. Prone *(AIIMS 1992)* ☐
B. Supine ☐
C. Trendelenberg ☐
D. Left lateral ☐

51. Which of the following does not represent a significant anaesthetic problem in the morbidly obese patient?
A. Difficulties in endotracheal intubation ☐
B. Suboptimal arterial oxygen tension *(AIIMS Nov 2004)*☐
C. Increased metabolism of volatile agents ☐
D. Decreased cardiac output relative to total body mass ☐

52. True about Laryngeal mask airway: *(PGI May 10, June 09)*
A. More reliable than face mask ☐
B. Prevent aspiration ☐
C. Alternative to Endotracheal tube (E.T.T) ☐
D. Does not require laryngoscope & visualization ☐
E. Can be used in full stomach ☐

53. Laryngeal mask Airway (LMA) is used for;
A. Maintenance of the airway *(AIIMS 03)* ☐
B. Facilitating laryngeal surgery ☐
C. Prevention of aspiration ☐
D. Removing oral secretions ☐

54. The laryngeal mask airway used for securing the airway of a patient in all of the following conditions except:
A. In a difficult intubation *(AI 05)* ☐
B. In cardiopulmonary resuscitation ☐
C. In a child undergoing an elective/routine eye surgery. ☐
D. In a patient with a large tumour in the oral cavity. ☐

55. Laryngeal mask airway is indicated in :
A. To prevent aspiration of stomach contents*(PGI 2001)* ☐
B. Short surgical procedure ☐
C. Where endotracheal intubation is contra-indicated ☐
D. Difficult airway ☐
E. Facilitate endotracheal intubation ☐

56. True about LMA (Laryngea Mast Airway): *(PGI June 08)*
A. Available in 8 sizes ☐
B. Intubation can be done ☐
C. Size 1 for neonates ☐
D. Size 3 for adults ☐
E. Full protection from aspiration ☐

57. High air way resistance is seen in *(DNB 08)*
A. Respiratory bronchiole ☐
B. Terminal bronchiole ☐
C. Intermediate bronchiole ☐
D. Main bronchus ☐

58. During laryngoscopy and endo-tracheal intubation which of the maneuver is not performed: *(AIIMS 2003)*
A. Flexion of the neck. ☐
B. Extension of Head at the atlanto-occipital joint. ☐
C. The laryngoscope is lifted upwards levering over the upper incisors. ☐
D. In a straight blade laryngoscope, the epiglottis is lifted by the tip. ☐

59. Which of the following is not an indication for endotracheal intubation?
A. Maintenance of a patent airway *(AI06)* ☐
B. To provide positive pressure ventilation ☐
C. Pulmonary toilet ☐
D. Pneumothorax ☐

60. Malampatti grading is for *(AI 2K, DNB 03)*
A. Mobility of cervical spine ☐
B. Mobility of atlanto axial joint ☐
C. Assessment of free rotation of neck before intubation ☐
D. Inspection of oral cavity before intubation ☐

61. True about endotracheal cuff: *(PGI June 04)*
A. Low-volume, high pressure ☐
B. Low-volume, low pressure ☐
C. High-volume, low pressure ☐
D. High-volume, high pressure ☐
E. Equal-volume, pressure ☐

62. All are features of difficult airway except
A. Miller's sign *(PGI 99)* ☐
B. Micrognathia with macroglossia ☐
C. TMJ ankylosis ☐
D. Increased thyromental distance ☐

63. Plan C of anesthetic airway management is
A. Standard laryngoscopy & intubation *(DNB 05)* ☐
B. Intubation catheter guided intubation ☐
C. Insertion of laryngeal mask airway & fiberoptic bronchoscopy ☐
D. Cancel the surgery or perform tracheostony ☐

64. Sellick manouever is used to prevent: *(PGI Nov 09)*
A. Alveolar collapse ☐
B. Hypertension ☐
C. Aspiration of Gastric content ☐
D. Bradycardia ☐
E. Glaucoma ☐

65. Sallick's manouvere is used for *(AIIMS 97)*
A. To prevent gastric aspiration ☐
B. To facilitate Respiration ☐
C. To reduce dead space ☐
D. To prevent alveolar collapse ☐

66. Size in < 6 years old child, of endotracheal tube is
A. Age +3.5/3.5 *(DNB 02, AI 04)* ☐
B. Age +2.5/2.5 ☐
C. Age + 4.5/4.5 ☐
D. Age –4.5/4.5 ☐

67. In infant (full term) diameter (mm) length (cm) of ETT used are *(DNB 02, AIIMS 03)*
A. 3.5, 16 ☐
B. 7, 12 ☐

C. 3.5, 12
D. 7, 10

68. Merits of nasotracheal intubation is
A. Good oral hygiene *(AIIMS May 07)*
B. Less infection
C. Less muscosal damage and bleeding
D. More movement or displacement of endotracheal tube

69. Nasal intubation is contra indicated in
A. CSF Rhinorrhea *(AIIMS 1995)*
B. Fracture cervical spine
C. Fracture mandible
D. Short neck

70. A 40 year old man who met with a motor vehicle catastrophe came to the casualty hospital in an hour with severe maxillofacial trauma. His Pulse rate was 120/min, BP was 100/70 mm Hg, SpO_2 - 80% with oxygen. What would be the immediate management – *(AIIMS Nov 10)*
A. Nasotracheal intubation
B. Orotracheal intubation
C. Intravenous fluid
D. Tracheostomy

71. Both Oral and Nasal intubation are C/I
A. Laryngeal endema *(AIIMS 1995)*
B. CSF – Rhinorrhoea
C. Comastose patient
D. Acute Tracheo - Laryngo - bronchitis

72. Mendelson's syndrome is *(AIIMS 1994)*
A. Air leak
B. Tracheal rupture during intubation
C. Oesophageal rupture
D. Aspiration of gastric content

73. Position with least vital capacity in G.A.
A. Trendelenburg *(AI 91)*
B. Lithotomy
C. Prone
D. Lateral

74. True about Laryngoscopy & intubation
A. Hypertension *(PGI June 2004)*
B. Tachycardia
C. ↑ ICT
D. ↑ Intra ocular pressure
E. ↓ Lower oesophageal sphincter tone

75. True about endotracheal intubation (during the process) is all except: *(PGI 2001)*
A. Hypertension & tachycardia
B. Raised IOT
C. Raised ICT
D. Arrhythmias
E. Increased oesophageal peristalsis

76. In venturi mask maximum O_2 concentration attained is :
A. 90% *(BIHAR - 2005)*
B. 100%
C. 60%
D. 80%

77. Indications of tracheostomy are
A. Flail chest *(PGI 2003)*
B. Head injury
C. Tetanus
D. Cardiac tamponade
E. Foreign body

78. Side effects of oxygen therapy are all except:
A. Absorption atelactasis *(AIIMS May 07)*
B. Increased pulmonary compliance
C. Decreased vital capacity
D. Endothelial damage

79. In a patient with fixed respiratory obstruction Helium is used along with Oxygen instead of plain oxygen because
A. It increases the absorption of oxygen
B. It decreases turbulence *(AI 02)*
C. It decreases the dead space
D. For analgesia

80. True about Heliox: *(PGI Nov 2010)*
A. Helium is a inert gas
B. Less viscous than air
C. Higher density than air
D. Reduces work of breathing
E. Mixture of He & O_2

81. Properties of Helium *(PGI June 07)*
A. Atomic no 2
B. Vscosity is zero
C. Used in COPD
D. All

VENTILATORS

82. Which of the following produces the least damage to blood elements *(AIIMS Nov 04)*
A. Disc oxygenator
B. Membrane oxygenator
C. Bubble oxygenator
D. Screen oxygenator

83. In volume-cycled ventilation the inspiratory flow rate is set at: *(AIIMS 2002)*
A. 140-160 L/min
B. 110-130 L/min
C. 60-100 L/min
D. 30-50 L/min

84. Not seen with controlled ventilation
A. Barotrauma *(AIIMS 1993)*
B. Alkalosis
C. Pulmonary embolism
D. Cardiac Temponade

85. The following modes of ventilation may be used for weaning off patients from mechanical ventilation except:
A. Controlled Mechanical ventilation (CMV) *(AI 05)*
B. Synchronized intermittent mandatory ventilation (SIMV).
C. Pressure support ventilation(PSV)
D. Assist-control ventilation (ACV)

86. All are true about PEEP except: *(PGI 1999)*
A. Useful in situations where P02 is low
B. ↓ CO
C. Impaired renal function
D. ↓ ICT

87. About CPAP all are true except: *(AIIMS May 09)*
A. Given prophylactically in all preterm with respiratory distress
B. Started with FiO2 50 to 60 percent
C. Given in infants less than 28 weeks and less than 1 kg weight
D. Improves oxygenation and improves lung compliance

MONITORING OF PATIENTS

88. EEG in anesthesia is useful in: *(AIIMS Nov 12)*
A. Depth of general anesthesia
B. Depth of local anesthesia
C. Depth of neuromuscular block
D. Depth of analgesia

89. A 40 year old female underwent surgery. Postoperatively she told the anesthetist that she was aware of preoperative events. Individual intraoperative awareness is evaluated by: *(AI 11, 12; AIIMS May 12)*
A. Cerebral pulse oximetry ☐
B. Colour Doppler ☐
C. Bispectral imaging ☐
D. End tidal CO_2 ☐

90. Which of the following in anesthesia will produce decreased EEG activities *(AIIMS 06; DNB 08)*
A. Hypothermia ☐
B. Early Hypoxia ☐
C. Ketamine ☐
D. N_2O ☐

91. Which of the following can lower EEG amplitude
A. N_2O *(AIIMS Nov 11)* ☐
B. Ketamine ☐
C. Hypothermia ☐
D. Early hypoxia ☐

92. During anesthesia, which is least affected *(AI 12)*
A. Visual evoked response ☐
B. Somatosensory evoked potential ☐
C. Brainstem auditory evoked potential ☐
D. Motor evoked potential ☐

93. Kinemyography is used for: *(AIIMS Nov 12)*
A. Monitoring of neuromuscular function ☐
B. Monitoring of muscle spindle activity ☐
C. Monitoring of exercise capacity ☐
D. Monitoring of depth of anesthesia ☐

94. M.C. nerve used for monitoring during anaesthesia
A. Ulnar nerve *(AIIMS May 2007)* ☐
B. Facial nerve ☐
C. Radial nerve ☐
D. Median nerve ☐

95. Which of the following is not a cardiovas-cular monitoring technique: *(AIIMS Nov 05)*
A. Transesophageal echocardio- graphy ☐
B. Central venous pressure monitoring ☐
C. Pulmonary artery catheterization ☐
D. Capnography ☐

96. All are true statement about capnography except:
A. E_{TCO2} in pulmonary embolism *(PGI May 12)* ☐
B. Elevated baseline represent exhausted absorbent in the circle system ☐
C. To check confirmation of ETT ☐
D. Curare cleft or notch represent start of spontaneous ventilation ☐
E. In malignant hyperthermia E_{TCO2} decreases ☐

97. Flat capnogram found in A/E *(AIIMS May 09)*
A. Disconnection of anesthetic tubing ☐
B. Accidental extubation ☐
C. Mechanical ventilation failure ☐
D. Bronchospasm ☐

98. Placement of a double lumen tube (DLT) is best confirmed by: *(PGI Dec 08)*
A. Clinically by Auscultation ☐
B. Fibreoptic bronchoscopy ☐
C. Capnography ☐
D. Chest radiography ☐
E. Chest inflation on positive pressure ☐

99. Placement of double lumen tube for lung surgery is best confirmed by: *(AIIMS Nov 05, DNB 06)*
A. $EtCO_2$ ☐
B. Airway pressure measurement ☐
C. Clinically by auscultation ☐
D. Bronchoscopy ☐

100. A 27 year old female was brought to emergency department for acute abdominal pain following which she was shifted to the operation theatre for Laparotomy. A speedy intubation was performed but after the intubation, breath sounds were observed to be decreased on the left side and a high end tidal CO_2 was recorded. The likely diagnosis is: *(AI 10)*
A. Endotracheal tube blockage ☐
B. Bronchospasm ☐
C. Esophageal intubation ☐
D. Endobronchial intubation ☐

101. End-tidal CO_2 is increased to maximum level in :
A. Pul. embolism *(PGI 2K, DNB 05)* ☐
B. Malignant hyperthermia ☐
C. Extubation ☐
D. Blockage of secretion ☐

102. Rise in end tidal CO_2 during thyroid surgery can be due to all except: *(AI 11)*
A. Anaphylaxis ☐
B. Malignant hyperthermia ☐
C. Thyroid storm ☐
D. Neuroleptic malignant syndrome ☐

103. Best to monitor intraoperative myocardial ischemia (infarction) is *(AI 11)*
A. ECG ☐
B. CVP monitoring ☐
C. Transesophageal echocardiography ☐
D. Invasive intracarotid arterial pressure ☐

104. The most sensitive and practical technique for detection of myocardial ischemia in the perioperative period is: *(AIIMS Nov 2005)*
A. Magnetic Resonance Spectroscopy ☐
B. Radio labeled lactate determination ☐
C. Direct measurement of end diastolic pressure ☐
D. Regional wall motion abnormality detected with the help of 2D transoesophageal echocardio-graphy ☐

105. The most common cause of hypoxia during one lung ventilation is: *(AIIMS Nov 2005)*
A. Malposition of the double lumen tube ☐
B. Increased shunt fraction ☐
C. Collapse of one lung ☐
D. Soiling of lung by secretions ☐

106. Most common complication of central venous catheter
A. Local bleeding *(AI 12)* ☐
B. Thrombosis ☐
C. Catheter related infection ☐
D. Pneumotherax ☐

107. In an ICU, following righ subclavian rein cannulation for putting CV line, patient developed respiratory distress, dyspnoea, hypotension (BP 100/55) and tachycardia (140/min HR), chest examination revealed diminished air entery and decreased breath sounds on auscultation and hyper resonance on percussion towards right side of chest. Left sided breath sounds were minimally reduced. The probable diagnosis is *(AI 12)*
A. Tension pneumothorar ☐
B. Acute MI ☐
C. Air embolism ☐
D. Pulmonary edema ☐

108. All are the Complication of CVP line except: *(PGI June 09)*
A. Airway injury ☐
B. Haemothroax ☐
C. Septicemia ☐
D. Air embolism ☐
E. Pseudoaneurysm ☐

109. Swan Ganz catheter measure

A. PCWP (PGI Dec 06) ☐
B. C.O. ☐
C. Mixed venous O_2 saturation ☐
D. Right atrial pressure ☐

110. While introducing the Swan-ganz catheter, its placement in the pulmonary artery can be identified by the following pressure tracing: (AIIMS Nov 2005)
A. Diastolic pressure is lower in PA than in RV ☐
B. Diatolic pressure is higher in PA than in RV ☐
C. PA pressure tracing has diacrotic notch from closure of pulmonary valve ☐
D. RV pressure tracing for plateau and sharp drop in early diastole ☐

111. Pulse oxymetry detects inaccurately in presence of:
A. Hyperbilirubinemia (PGI June 2005) ☐
B. Nail polish ☐
C. Methemoglobinemia ☐
D. Skin pigmentation ☐

112. The gas used to create pneumoperitoneum is
A. CO_2 (PGI 2001) ☐
B. N_2 ☐
C. O_2 ☐
D. Room air ☐
E. N_2O ☐

113. Incubator heat is delivered by except :
A. Conduction (PGI 1998) ☐
B. Convection ☐
C. Radiation ☐
D. Evaporation ☐

114. Which of following is used to monitor respiration in neonate (not intubated) –
A. Capnography (AI 2007) ☐
B. Impedence pulmonometry ☐
C. Chest movements ☐
D. Infrared End Tidal CO_2 ☐

PREOPERATIVE ASSESSMENT & MEDICATION

115. A 45 year old male with h/o smoking is scheduled for elective surgery. All are true except (AIIMS May 12)
A. Effect of nicotine on aortic and carotid bodies can increase sympathetic tone ☐
B. Carbon monoxide shift O_2-Hb dissociation curve to right ☐
C. Muscle relaxant dose requirements are increased ☐
D. Smoking dereases surfactant levels ☐

116. A patient is on regular medication for medical illness. Which of the following drugs can be safely stopped with least adverse effects before an abdominal surgery
A. Stains (AIIMS May 12) ☐
B. Steroids ☐
C. Beta blockers ☐
D. ARB ☐

117. A patient who was on aspirin for long period was selected for an elective surgery. What should be done (AIIMS 2001)
A. Stop aspirin for 7 days ☐
B. Infusion of fresh frozen plasma ☐
C. Infusion of platelett concentration ☐
D. Go ahead with surgery maintaining adequate hemostasis ☐

118. Most potent antiemitic agent used in preoperative period
A. Glycopyrolate (AIIMS 1996) ☐
B. Hyoscine ☐
C. Atropine ☐
D. Metochlorpromide ☐

119. Atropine as preanesthesia has all effects except (AI 1996)
A. Decrease secretion ☐
B. Bronchoconstriction ☐
C. Prevent bradycardia ☐
D. Prevent hypotension ☐

120. Preanesthethetic Medication is for A/E
A. Secretion decrease (AI 1992) ☐
B. ↓Anxiety ☐
C. ↓dose of inducing agent ☐
D. Allay Anxiety ☐

121. During G.A. shivering is abolished by suppression of
A. Hypothalmus (AI 1991) ☐
B. Thalmus ☐
C. Cerebral Cortex ☐
D. Medulla ☐

122. Hypothermia is used in all except : (PGI 98, DNB 01)
A. Neonatal asphyxia ☐
B. Cardiac surgery ☐
C. Hyperthermia ☐
D. Arrythmia ☐

123. Which of the following is true about hypothermila during anesthesia? (AIIMS May 13)
A. Beneficial to patients ☐
B. Prevented by giving warm fluids ☐
C. Body looses heat mainly by conduction ☐
D. Occur irrespetive of the type of anesthesia ☐

124. Drugs commonly used in pre-anaesthetic medication-
A. Diazepam (PGI Dec 2004) ☐
B. Scopolamine ☐
C. Morphine ☐
D. Succinylcholine ☐
E. Atracurium ☐

125. Preanesthetic medication is used for A/E :
A. Decrease of anesthetic dose ☐
B. Decrease BP (PGI 2002) ☐
C. Prevent aspiration ☐
D. Produce amnesia for peri-operative events ☐
E. Relieve anxiety ☐

126. A patient with hypertension, under control by medication falls under which grade? (AIIMS Nov 12)
A. ASA 1 ☐
B. ASA 2 ☐
C. ASA 3 ☐
D. ASA 4 ☐

127. ASA classification is done for:
A. Status of patient (Rajasthan 2001) ☐
B. Risk ☐
C. Pain ☐
D. Lung disease ☐

128. Modified Allen's test is for checking the proper arterial supply at the: (AIIMS Nov 12)
A. Wrist ☐
B. Arm ☐
C. Elbow ☐
D. Forearm ☐

129. Criteria for brain death A/E (PGI Dec 2007)
A. ECG ☐
B. EEG ☐
C. Brain stem reflex ☐
D. ↓ body temperature ☐
E. Pupillary dilatation ☐

130. Clinical criteria of brain death is all except
A. Coma (JIPMER – 2005) ☐
B. Absent brain stem reflex ☐
C. Absent spinal cord reflex ☐
D. Absent motor activity ☐

ANSWERS AND EXPLANATIONS

Anaesthesia Machnes & Cylinders

1. **B i.e. Artificial manual breathing unit** *[Ref: Drosch 5/e p 495; Ajay Yadav 5/e p 40-41]*

Acronym "**AMBU**" stands for **Artificial Manual Breathing Unit."**

2. **A i.e. Start manual ventilation** *[Ref: Dorsch 5/e 99-100, 828-30; Morgan 5/e 43, 52, 58; Miller 7/e p. 667-81; Wylie 7/e p. 473-72; Yao 7/e p 1280-81]*

Oxygen supply failure alarm starts bellowing in anesthesia machine whenever O_2 supply pressure (not flow) falls below a manufacture specified threshold (~20-35 psig). USFDA 1993 guidelines rcommend immediately starting manual ventilation (eg by AMBU bay)Q in this situation.

3. **A i.e. Desflurane vapourizer is heated to 39°C** *[Ref: Dorsch 5/e p. 131-33]*

- **Rotameter** *is constant pressure, variable orifice (area) flow meter for gases and liquid both*Q.
- Halothane vaporizes at 50.2°C (ie boiling point)
- **O_2 sensor** *can be attached both on expiratory and inspiratory limb of circle system's breathing circuit but not into the fresh gas line of machine*Q.
- **Desflurane's vaporizer are externally heated to 39°C** to compensate for significant heat loss a/w desflurane vaporization. It also increases the vapour pressure (to 1300 mmHg), preventing the possibility of boiling in warm rooms.
- **Tech 6 vaporizer** is used only with desflurane. Desflurane is heated to ***39°C (102°F)***Q**,** which is well above its boiling point (22.8°C), by two heaters in the base. An external *heating is needed, because the potency of desflurane requires that large amount be vaporized.* And also because the boiling point of desflurane is near room temperature and depending on ambient temperature *would make the output unpredictable.* These factors make thermo compensation using the usual mechanical devices impossible.

4. **A i.e. Continuous flow machine; D i.e. Resistance low**
5. **C i.e. The height to which bobbin rises indicates the flow rate**
[Ref. Wiley & Davidson 7/e p-466-475; Machintosh 2/e p. 277; Ajay Yadav 2/e p. 19-23; Lee's Anaesthesia 12/e p. 86-87]

6. **D i.e. Used for calculation of expired volume >> A i.e. Flow rates can be calculated**
[Ref: Morgan 4/e p. 71-73; Drosch 5/e p. 732-33, 239, 740-41]

Wright's Respirometers (spirometers) are used to ***measure expiratory (exhaled) tidal volumes***Q in breathing circuit of anesthesia machine. A clock is necessary to determine minute volume. It ***overreads at high flows and under reads at low flows***Q.

7. **A. i.e. Cylinder is a part of high pressure system C.i.e. O_2 flush delivers > 35 lts**
8. **B i.e., Presence of a PIN index system to prevent wrong attachment of the N_2O and oxygen cylnders**
9. **D i.e. Incorrect gas cylinder, attachement** 10. **C i.e. 3, 5**
11. **B i.e. Pin is present on machine, C i.e. Not effective if wrong gas is filled in cylinder, E i.e. Hole positions on cylinder valves** *[Ref: Wylie 7/e p- 472, Miller's 6/e p. 275-78; Barash 4/e p-188; Lee's 13/e ,p – 86; Morgan 4/e p –50- 59, Dorsch: 5/e p- 108 – 11, 5-8]*

- **Pin Index safety system (PISS)** consists of *2* ***holes on the cylinder valve that mate with corresponding pins on the yolke or pressure regulator of anesthesia machine***Q. PISS is a safety feature adopted in anaesthesia machine to prevent incorrect gas cylinder attachment. But this becomes ineffective if the cylinder is filled with wrong gas, yolk pins are damaged or extrasealing washers are used.
- Pin Index of entonox is (7); N_2 (1,4); **air (1, 5)**; CO > 7.5% (1, 6); He < 80.5% (2, 4); **O_2 (2, 5)**; CO_2 < 7.5% (2, 6); **N_2O (3, 5)**; cyclopropane (3, 6); and He > 80.5% is (4, 6).

12. **B i.e. CO_2; C i.e. N_2O; D i.e. Cyclopropane**
13. **D i.e. Black & White** 14. **A i.e. Black Cylinder with white shoulder** 15. **A i.e. Molybdenum Steel**
16. **D i.e. 3, 5** 17. **C i.e. Black with white shoulder**

Gases	Pin Code Index
Entonox	Single central hole (7)
Air	1, 5
CO_2 >7.5 %	1, 6
O_2	2, 5
CO_2 <7.5 %	2, 6
N_2O	3, 5
N2	1,4
Cyclopropane	3,6
He > 80.5%	4, 6
He < 80.5%	2, 4

Cylinder	Colour
Cyclopropane	**Orange**[Q] (liquid form) In pronanciating this cyclo there come O (orange)
N_2O	**Blue**[Q] (liquid form) 'N' for Neela (Blue)
Thiopentone	**Yellow**[Q] Peela (Yellow)
CO_2	Grey (liquid form)
Halothane	Amber (Purple - Red)
Entonox (O_2 & N_2O in equal volumes)	Blue body with Blue and white shoulders
O_2	**Black body with white shoulders**[Q] (UK) or Green (US)
N_2	Black
Air	Grey body with black & white shoulder

18. **B i.e. Blue in colour; C i.e. Gas in liquid form; D i.e. Pin Index 3, 5**
19. **A. i.e. Pin index 3, 5 B. i.e. Blue in colour, C. i.e. Stored as liquid, D. i.e. MAC 105**
20. **C i.e. 2220 PSP is the pressure in cylinder** *[Ref: Dorsch 4/e p.13;Lee 12/e p. 104; Aitkenhead 4/e, P- 374-376; Morgan's 4/e p. 19-21; Wiley & Davidson 7/e p-471-472; Paul's 4/e p. 67]*

Gas	Colour of cylinder	Pin Index	State in cylinder	Pressure	Volume
N_2O	*Blue*[Q]	*3.5*[Q]	*Liquid gas*[Q]	745 psig	1590 L
O_2	*Black with white shoulder*[Q]	*2.5*[Q]	Gas	1900 psig	660 L

N_2O **cylinder is** ***blue in colour***[Q] ***with pin index 3, 5***[Q] contain gas in ***liquid form***[Q] at a pressure of ***750 lb/sq inch (psi)*** [Q] at 20° C. Its MCA is 104[Q].

21. **D i.e. Emergency oxygen 'E' cylinder has more gas than 'H' cylinder** *[Ref: Morgan's 4/e p-19; Wikepedia]*
22. **A.i.e. Tc of O_2 is - 119°C, D. i.e. Tc of of N_2O is 36.5°C , E. i.e. Tc of air is – 140.6°C**
23. **D i.e. E** *[Ref: Miller 7/e p 675; Morgan 5/e p 49-52; Ajay Yadav 5/e p 25-26]*

- **Most commonly used cylinder, in anesthesia** work station (machine) is **E (>>H)**, when a pipeline supply source is not avaible.
- **For high pressure storage of compressed gases, cylinders are made up of molybdenum steel**[Q].
- **Height, size** and **volume** of cylinder increases from A onwards with **smallest available size AA and biggest H. So A<B<C<D<E<G<H<J.**

Critical Temperature (Tc)

Tc of a substance is the temperature *at and above which vapour of the substance can not be liquefied, no matter how much pressure* is applied (i.e. critical point is reached).

Critical point (Vapor- liquid)

A point reached at Tc above which distinct liquid & gas phases do not exist. As the Tc is approached, the properties of gas and liquid phases approach one another, resulting in only one phase **(a homogenous supercritical fluid)** at Tc.

Critical Pressure (Pc)

It is the vapor pressure at critical temperature

Critical Molar Mass (Vc)

It is the volume of one mole of material at Tc & Pc

Substance	Tc(°C)	Pc (atm)
Oxygen (O_2)	*- 119*[Q]	49.8
Argon	- 122.4	48.1
Air	- 140.6	39
Nitrogen (N_2)	***- 146.9***[Q]	33.5
Hydrogen (H_2)	- 242	12.8
Helium	- 267.96	2.24
Xenon	16.6	57.6
Carbondioxide	31.04	72.8
Nitrous oxide (N_2O)	*36.5*[Q]	1072 (Ps°)
Water (H_2O)	374	217.7

Liquid O_2 must be stored well below its critical temperature (-119°C), because gases can be liquefied by pressure only if stored below their critical tempderature[Q]. A liquid O_2 storage system is more economical for large hospital.

Breathing System

24. **A i.e. Mapleson A** 25. **B i.e. Ideal for infants** *[Ref. Morgon's 4/e p-32-34, Lee's 12/e p-1168, 117, Paul's 5/e p89, 90, 91]*

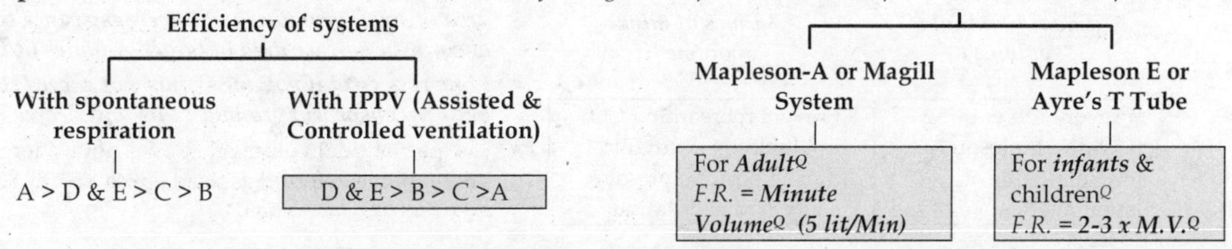

26. A ie Mapleson A

27. B, D, E, C i.e. Mapleson type D; Can be used for controlled ventilation; Can be used for spontaneous respiration; Coaxial

28. B i.e. Equal to minute volume

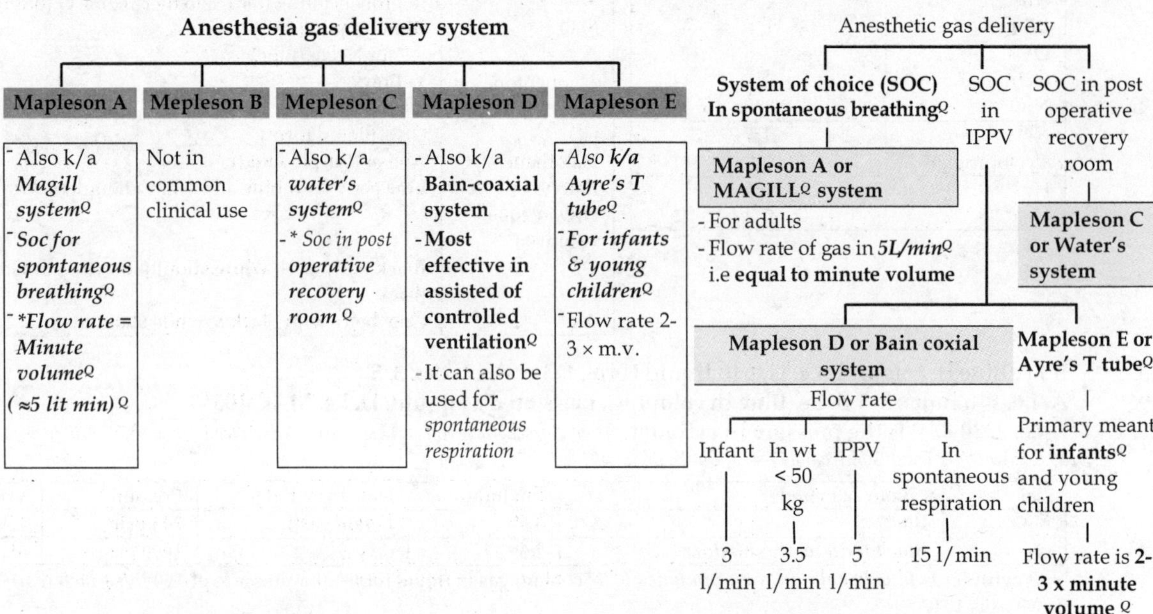

29. **A i.e. Jackson Rees modification of Ayre's T Piece** *[Ref: Lee 12/e p117; Ajay Yadav 2/e p27]*

Mapelson E system (i.e. Ayre's T Piece) is advocated primary for use in ***infants and young children***Q. The main advantage of T-piece is *absence of resistance to expiration,* a factor of crucial importance to children. Type E is basically a circuit for spontaneous respiration, as it does not contain a breathing bag. Jackson's Rees *modified* it and *added a bag for monitoring and IPPV (mapleson F).* **Jakson's Rees modification of Ayre's T piece (Mapleson F. system)** has thus become the ***most appropriate circuit for ventilating a spontaneous breathing infant.*** Q

30. **A i.e. Zeolite activation; B i.e. Delivers O_2; C i.e. Requires power supply** *[Ref: Dorsch & Dorsch 4th/68]*

Oxygen concentrators ***extract O_2 from atmospheric air***Q for which a ***Zeolite molecular sieve***Q is used. The atmospheric air is exposed to the Zeolite sieve at a certain pressure which selectively retains N_2 & other constituents of air and thus giving about *95% O_2*Q

Rebreathing Sysytem

31. **A i.e. Should be as far as possible from patient.** *[Ref: Aitkenhead 4/e P- 388; Morghan's 4/e p. 38; Wiley & Davidson 7/e p- 474]*

Rebreathing Prevention Valve

- ***Installed at expiratory end***Q
- prevents rebreathing of expired air
- ***Should be as near as possible from the patient,***Q to serve it's purpose because more distance from patient will l/t more tube length (in which there will be larger amount of expired air) prior to valve which will be taken in by patient with each inspiration.

32. **A i.e. Resistance in circuit; C i.e. Small size granule**

33. **A i.e. Resistance in circuit** *[Ref: Aitkenhead 4/e P- 388; Morghan's 4/e p. 38; Wiley & Davidson 7/e p- 474, 480]*

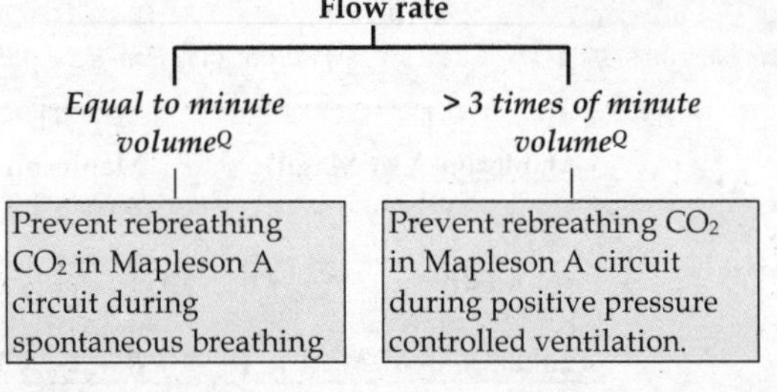

- ***CO_2 absorbers increase circuit resistance***Q. **Granule size** is a compromise between ***high resistance & high absorptive surface area of small granules and lower resistance to gas & lesser absorptive surface area of larger granules (d/t channeling)***Q
- ***Flow rate &tidal volume should not exceed the air space between absorbent granules; this will decrease CO_2 absorption.***Q
- The part of tidal volume that does not undergo alveolar ventilation is referred as dead space; so any *increase in dead space decreases CO_2 absorption.*

34. **C i.e. Trilene** **35.** **C i.e. Calcium hydroxide** **36.** **B i.e. $Ba(OH)_2$**
37. **B i.e. Baralime** **38.** **D i.e. As an indicator** **39.** **D i.e. Mapleson F**

- **Calcium hydroxide [$Ca(OH)_2$]** is the ***main component of both sodalime (94%) and baralime*** Q ***(80%).***
- ***$Ba(OH)_2$ is not a constituent of soda lime, it is used in baralime. Water (of crystalization) is used to produce hardening in baralime*** Q.
- ***Clayton, mimosa*** Q, ethyl violet, phenolphthalein & ethyl orange are **indicators.**

Airway Management

40. **A, B, D i.e. LMA, Endotracheal tube, Combitube**
[Ref: Morgan 4/e p-94-99; Harrison 17/e 1977; Ajay yadav 3/e p-32-35; Wylie 7/e p-445-48; Paul 6/e p-249-59]

- **Laryngeal mask airway & endotracheal tubes** (eg **combi/double lumen tubes**, coles tube, endotrol tube, microlaryngeal tube, RAE preformed tubes) are used for airway protection (i.e. maintenance of patency of upper airways for maintaining ventilatory function.
- **Ryles tube** is used for feeding and aspiration of gastric contents. **Sengstaken- Blakemore (Minnesota) tube** is used for balloon tamponade of variceal haemorrhage in portal hypertension.
- Different type of tubes to protect airways include
  - **Endotracheal tubes** may be *orotracheal /oral* (short & curved with radius of curvature of *14 cm*, bevel angle $\geq 45^0$ and passed through oral cavity to the trachea) or *nasotracheal /nasal* (long & curved with radius of curvature of *25 cm*, bevel angle $\geq 30^0$ and passed through nose)
  - **Latex armoured (spiral embedded / flexometallic) tube** are *non kinkable, non collapsible* rubber/ latex/ plastic / or silicon spiral tubes with a metal wire or nylon filament embedded into the wall of tube. These are useful in cases where *acute flexion of the neck* is expected as in *posterior craniotomy.* It is not possible to cut this tube to desired length, thus incrasing the risk of bronchial intubation.
  - **Oxford nonkinking endotracheal tube** is made of red rubber & moduled to *form 90^0 bend inside the mouth.* It is useful when the patient is *prone or sitting position* & sometimes in *cleft palate* surgery. But the tube is longer, thus increasing the risk of bronchial intubation.
  - **Cole orotracheal tube** with *narrow distal (or patient) end* for subglottic vocal cord to trachea region is used in *pediatric patients.*
  - **RAE (Ring, Adair & Elwyn) preformed tubes** has a bend at the mouth to prevent kinking & a connector at chin to allow good access for surgery on head & neck. North facing RAE tubes are used for lower lip surgery & south facing for upper (cleft) lip & palate surgery.
  - **Endotrol tube** with a built in stylet system & a ring pull on its inner curvature that helps bending the tip. So it is excellent for oral & nasal intubation, particularly when good visualization of cords is difficult.
  - **Combitube** is a **double lumen tube** with two cuffs. It is placed with its tip in the oesophagus & the lower small cuff is inflated. The upper larger cuff is then inflated behind the base of tongue. One tube lumen passes through the lower cuff & provides a route for regurgitation. The other lumen ends blindly above the lower cuff, but has side holes between the 2 cuffs that permit ventilation through the 2nd lumen by virtue of the cuff sels above & below the hypopharynx.
  - **Microlaryngeal** & laryngotracheal surgery **tubes** (MLT, LTST) are available in 4/5/6 mm internal diameter with standard length & cuff size *f* for microlaryneal surgeries.

41. **D. i.e. Endotracheal intubation** **42.** **C. i.e. Decrease in dead space** **43.** **C i.e. Neck flexion**
[Ref: Morgan 4/e 553; Ajay Yadav 3/e p. 4]

Physiological dead space is decreased in – ***supine posture, neck flexion*** Q and use of ***bronchoconstrictors*** and ***artificial airway* (eg. *intubation, tracheostomy*).**

44. **C i.e. Massive Pleural effusion** *[Ref: Lee & Morgan 3/e, P-139; KDT 349]*
- Pleural effusion normally tends to decrease physiological dead space initially. However when massive it also decreases anatomical dead space.
- *Atropine, halothane are bronchodialators,* so ↑ anatomical dead space. *Inspiration* may also streatch airways to ↑ anatomical dead space.

45. **A i.e. It reduces the normal anatomical dead space** *[Ref: Mikhail, Murray 3/e P-80, Snow old edition - 139]*
- Endotracheal tube decreases the anatomical dead space (150 ml) to as less as 25 ml.
- Endotracheal intubation increases the resistance to respiration; obstruction from kinking, foreign body or secretions further increase resistance.
- Subglottic edema, though a complication, is not the most common one.

46. **B i.e. Ventimask** *[Ref: Stakey's Essentials of anaesthesia 2/e p. 76-77]*

Ventimask or venturimasks are *high flow or fixed performance* (performance not affected by changes in patient's tidal volume and respiratory rate) ***oxygen delivery devices*** Q delivering accurate oxygen concentration.

47. D i.e. Noval Catheter *[Ref. Paul Essentials of Anethesiology 6/e p. 41]*

- Nasal catheter is used for O_2 delivery not novel catheter.
- O_2 is delivered through various devices. The common used methods are.

1. *Oxygen tent*Q
2. *Oxygen apparatus*Q
3. *Polymask*Q
4. *Ventimask*Q
5. *Nasal catheter*Q
6. BLB mask

48. C i.e. Laryngeal Mask airway
[Ref. Dorsch 5/e p. 450-500; Clinical Surgery-Cushieri, Darzi, Rowley 2/e p. 37; Miller 7/e p. 1580-90]

Airways

Non-definitive Airways

- **Oropharyngeal (oral) airway** eg. Gudel airway, Berman airway, Patil-Syracus endoscopic airway, William airway intubator, Ovassapian fiber optic intubating airway and Berman intubating/pharyngeal airway.
- **Nasopharyngeal (nasal) airway or nasal trumpet** eg Linder nasopharyngeal (bubble tip) airway, cuffed nasopharyngeal airway and binasal airway
- **Laryngeal mask airway (LMA)** is a *supraglotlic airway device-periglottic type* that forms a seal around larynx with an inflatable cuff.

Definitive- Airway

- **Tracheal tubes (endotracheal tubes)**ie
  - *Oral (oro-tracheal) tubes*Q
  - *Nasal (naso-tracheal) tubes*Q
  - *Tracheostomy tubes*Q
  - Cuffed murphy tracheat tubes, Cole uncuffed pediatric TT, Spiral embedded tubes, Hunsaker Mon-Jet ventilation tube, **laryngectomy tube**, microlaryngeal tracheal surgery tube, endotrol (trigger) tube, endoflex tube, Parker flex tip tube, **LITA** (*laryngotracheal instillation of topical anesthesia*) etc.
- **Percutaneous (transcutaneous) airway**
  - Tracheostomy
  - *Cricothyrotomy*Q (surgical, needle/cannula, Seldinger). **Perilaryngeal airway** is used for percutaneous dilatation cricothyroidotomy in *difficult to intubate/difficult to ventilate* scenario.

49. D i.e. Respiratory rate **50. C i.e. Trendelenberg** *[Ref: Morgan's Anaesthesia 3/e p. 522, 899]*

- **Trendelenburg (head down) position** causes cephalad shift of abdominal viscera and diaphragm leading to marked *decrease in lung capacities (i.e. vital capacity, functional residual capacity, total lung volume, lung compliance)* Q
- *Respiratory rate is not affected in any position.*Q

Physiological effects of patient position

Trendelenburg	Horizontal	Lithotomy	Prone	Lateral decubitus
• Cardiac : Activation of baroreceptors produce decrease in - Cardiac output - Heart output - B.P. - Peripheral vascular resistance • Respiratory : Cephalad shift of abdominal viscera produces - ***Marked decrease in lung capacities (VC, FRC, Total lung volume, lung compliance)***Q - Atelactasis - Increase ventilation perfusion mismatch - Increase likelihood of regurgitation • Others - Increase intraocular pressure in glaucoma - Increase in intracranial pressure & decrease in cerebral blood flow.	• Cardiac - Decreased heart rate - Decreased peripheral resistance - Equalization of pressure through out the arterial system - Increased right sided filling & cardiac output. • Respiratory - Diaphragm is displaced cephalad by abdominal viscus - Increase perfusion of dependent (posterior) segment - Functional residual capacity decreases	• Cardiac - Increase in circulating blood volume and preload. - Effect on blood pressure and cardiac output depends on volume status. • Respiratory - Decreased vital capacity. - Increase likelihood of aspiration	• Cardiac - Decrease preload, cardiac output, blood pressure due to peripheral pooling of blood. • Respiratory - Decreases total lung compliance and increases work of breathing.	• Cardiac - Cardiac output unchanged unless venous return obstructed. - Arterial blood pressure may fall as a result of decreased vascular resistance. • Respiratory - Decreased volume of dependent lung. - Increased perfusion of dependent lung. - Increased ventilation of dependent lung in awake patient (No v/q mismatch) - Decreased ventilation of dependent lung in anaesthetized patient (v/q mismatch) - Further decrease in dependent lung ventilation with paralysis and open chest.

51. **D i.e. Decreased cardiac out put relative to total body mass.** *[Ref: Lee 12/e p9; Morgan's 3/e p748-9]*

Obesity related changes

Cardiovascular	Respiratory	Gastrointestinal	Problems during anesthesia
- ↑ Blood volume - ↑ ***Cardiac output***[Q] - ↑ B.P. - ↑ Stroke volume - ↑ Cardiac workload - ↑ Cardiomegaly	- ↓ Compliance - ↓ Respiratory drive - ↓ Vital capacity & FRC - ↓ ***Blood O_2 (Hypoxemia)*** [Q] - These patients require high FiO_2 to achieve adequate oxygenation, the ratio of N_2O/O_2 is kept 2/3	- Hiatus hernia - Gastroesophageal reflux poor gastric emptying Hyper acidic gastric fluid.	- ***Difficult intubation*** [Q] - Increased risk of aspiration pneumonia - ***Volatile agents are metabolized rapidly while the action of nonvolatile agents are prolonged.*** [Q] - Difficulties in regional anesthesia - ***Respiratory failure is the major post operative problem*** [Q]

52. **A i.e. More reliable than face mask; C i.e. Alternative to Endotracheal tube (E.N.T); D i.e. Does not require laryngoscope & visualization**

53. **A i.e. Maintenance of airway** 54. **D i.e. In a patient with large tumor of the oral cavity**

55. **D i.e. Difficult airway); E i.e. Facilitates endotracheal intubation**

56. **B. i.e. Intubation can be done; C i.e. Size 1 for neonates; D i.e. Size 3 for adults**
[Ref: Aitkenhead 5/e p 258-60; Wylie's Anesthesia 7/e p-445, 46, 701, 832; Ajay yadav 4/e p 40 ; Miller's aneshthesia 7/e p- 1581-84; Morgan 3/e p 63-66; Lee's 12/e p248, 249; Paul's anethesia 5/e p-93, Pediatric anesthesia: Gregory 4/e p210, 701, 339]

- **Laryngeal mask airway (LMA)** or **Brain mask** is an ***alternative airway intermediate between the face mask and endotracheal tube***[Q] in terms of anatomical position, invasiveness, *reliability & security to protect airway &* facilitate gas exchange.
- LMA ***does not require any laryngoscope, visualization-muscle relaxants or specific position of cervical spine***[Q].
- It is used if ***difficult intubation***[Q] is indicated, for ***difficult airway management***[Q] during CPR, in emergency and to ***facilitate ventilation & passage of ETT in patient with difficult airway***[Q]. **Size 1** LMA is used in ***neonates***[Q] and **size 3** in ***children & small adults (30-50 kg)*** [Q].
- ***Oropharyngeal abscess or mass and risk of gastric regurgitation & aspiration is a contraindication to the use of laryngeal mask airway.***[Q]

57. **D i.e. Main bronchus**
Medium size airways like main bronchus has maximum resistance[Q]

58. **C i.e. The laryngoscope is lifted upward levering over the upper incisiors**

59. **D. i.e. Pneumothorax** *[Ref: Sabiston 17/e p. 425; Lee's anesthesia 12/e p-236; Morgan's clinical anesthesiology 3/e p-71, 72, 73]*

This Q is based on this fact that during intubation & laryngoscopy ***trapping of lip between teeth & blade and leverage on the teeth are avoided.***[Q]

60. **D i.e. Inspection of oral cavity before intubation**

Malampatti grading** is for **assessment of difficult air way (inspection of oral cavity for intubation)[Q].

61. **A i.e. Low volume, high pressure; C i.e. High volume, low pressure**

62. **D i.e. Increased thyromental distance** *[Ref: Lee 12/e P-233; Wiley &Davidson 7/e p-450; Morgan's 4/e p104-05, 924]*

63. **C i.e. Insertion of laryngeal mask airway& fibrotic bronchoscopy**

American Society of Anesthsiologist (ASA) developed practice guidelines & an algorithm that involves four plans: *Plans A, B, C, and D, which go in sequence.*

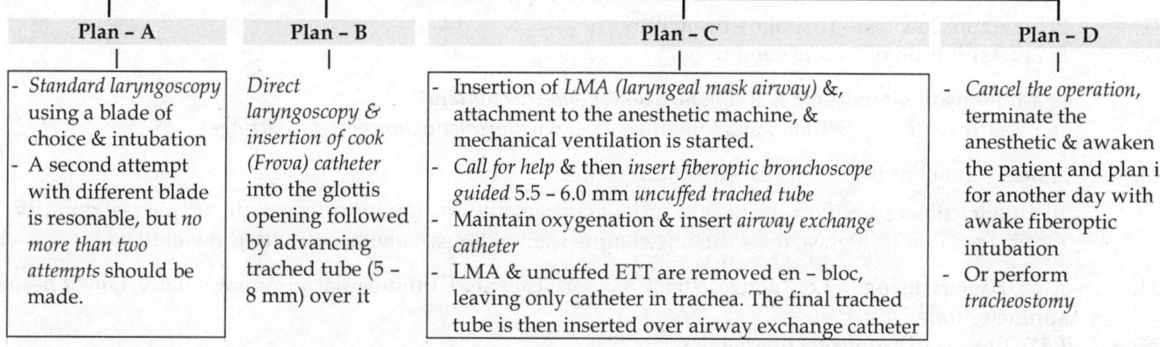

Plan – A
- Standard laryngoscopy using a blade of choice & intubation
- A second attempt with different blade is resonable, but no more than two attempts should be made.
Plan – B
Direct laryngoscopy & insertion of cook (Frova) catheter into the glottis opening followed by advancing trached tube (5 – 8 mm) over it
Plan – C
- Insertion of LMA (laryngeal mask airway) &, attachment to the anesthetic machine, & mechanical ventilation is started.
- Call for help & then insert fiberoptic bronchoscope guided 5.5 – 6.0 mm uncuffed trached tube
- Maintain oxygenation & insert airway exchange catheter
- LMA & uncuffed ETT are removed en – bloc, leaving only catheter in trachea. The final trached tube is then inserted over airway exchange catheter
Plan – D
- Cancel the operation, terminate the anesthetic & awaken the patient and plan it for another day with awake fiberoptic intubation
- Or perform tracheostomy

64. C i.e. Aspiration of Gastric content **65. A i.e. To prevent gastric aspiration**

Sellick's manuvere is application of *backward pressure on cricoid cartilage to prevent gastric aspiration (Mandelson's syndrome).*[Q]

66. A i.e. Age +3.5/3.5 **67. C i.e. 3.5 mm, 12 cm** *[Ref: Lee's 13/e p-208-9; Morgan's 4/eP-103-106,110-17]*

Endotracheal Intubation

- Endotracheal tube is sterilized by ***boiling***[Q] and cuffed E.T. tube is inflated at pressure *15-22 mmHg*
- **In neurosurgical** operations ***Armoured Endotracheal tube***[Q] is used.
- *For quick intubation, DOC is **Suxamethonium.***[Q]

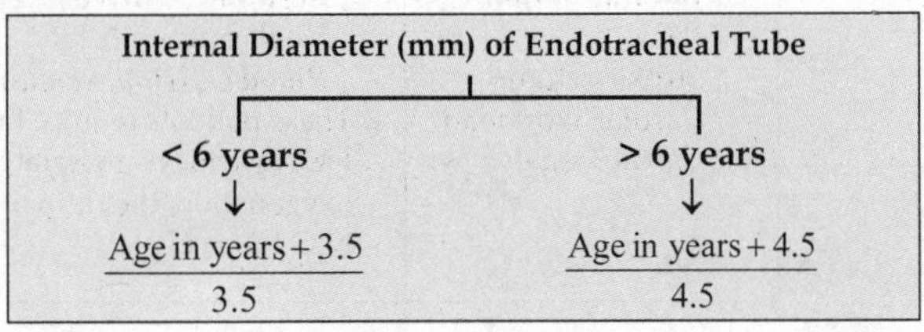

68. A i.e. Good Oral hygiene

69. A i.e. CSF Rhinorrhea *[Ref: Miller's 6/e p-1628-46; Aitkenhead 4/e, p- 464-67; Wiley & Davidson 7/e p- 447-48; Lee's 13/e p-208-9; Morgan's 4/e, p. 103-06, 111, 1035]*

Nasal (naso-tracheal) intubation is required when oral (orotracheal) tube will interfere with surgery (eg intraoral surgery) and may be indicated when oral intubation is difficult (eg inability to open month). It ***provides good oral hygiene and more secure fixation with less chances of displacement and extubation. But it is more commonly a/w significant nasal/mucosal bleeding, submucosal placement, transient bacteremia (infection), sinusitis and otitis media***[Q]. These side effects make nasotracheal intubation **contraindicated** in *base of skull fracture, CSF rhinorrhea*[Q], nasal abnormalities and trauma and coagulopathy.

70. B i.e. Orotracheal intubation

[Ref. Milley 7/e, p. 1580-1603, 2378, 2859, 2666; Aitkenhead 5/e, p. 306, 601, 739; Wylie 7/e, p. 446-48, Stoelting 5/e, p 212-18, Morgan 4/e, p 103-7, 111; Lee 13/e p. 698, 212-13]

- **ABCDE** of trauma care includes Airway maintenance and cervical spine protection, Breathing and ventilation, Circulation with haemorrhage control, Disability and neurological assessment and Exposure (undress) to assess for other injures. So option C is excluded. And decreased O_2 saturation (80%) with oxygen (most probably through mask or nasal tube) indicate that patient needs tracheal intubation. The tube in trachea can be put via nose (nasotracheal), via oral cavity (orotracheal) or trachea itself (tracheostomy).
- *Ideally tracheostomy should be performed under GA.* And technically tracheostomy with an awake local anesthetic in a patient with severe airway compromise is difficult because the ideal positioning with an extended head and supine is often not tolerated by patient, and the procedure is to be undertaken in a semi upright sitting position. ***Because tracheostomy is a relatively time taking procedure in comparison to intubation, it does not have much role in emergency airway management***[Q]***. Tracheostomy is usually done when immediate O_2 requirements are taken care of by rapid intubation and prolonged intubation is planned***[Q] (>1 to 2-3 weeks). However, if intubation is impossible, **cricothyroidotomy** is an emergency procedure. So option D is excluded.
- ***Orotracheal intubation using rapid sequence induction is the technique of choice for resuscitation***[Q]. *And nasotracheal intubation is preferred in awake patients.* But it is important to understand that in case of maxillary fracture, awake intubation is not possible. ***Nasotrached intubation is contraindica in severe mid facial injury***[Q]. So for maxillary fracture, orotracheal intubation is method of choice for immediate management of hypoxia.

71. D i.e. Acute Tracheo - Laryngo - bronchitis

72. D i.e. Aspiration of gastric content

- **Mendelson's syndrome** is d/t ***aspiration of gastric content***[Q]
- It is prevented by **Sellick's maneuver** i.e. backward ***pressure on cricoid cartilage***[Q].

73. A i.e. Trendelenburg *[Ref: Morgan's 3/e, P-693]*

In trendelenburg position, head end is lowered so due to gravity and weight of intra-abdominal viscera, diaphragm is at its highest level causing compression of lungs; so vital capacity is lowered.

74. A i.e. Hypertension; B i.e. Tachycardia; C i.e. ↑ ICT; D i.e. ↑ Intra ocular pressure; E i.e. ↓ Lower oesophageal sphincter tone

75. E i.e. Increased esophageal peristalsis

76. **C i.e. 60%** *[Ref: Stakey's Essentials of Anaesthesia 2/e p. 76-77; Ajay Yadav 2/e p. 35-39]*

Equipment	Maximum Oxygen Concentration Delivered
Nasal Canula	44% Q
Venturi mask/Oxygen mask	60%Q
Ventilators	100% Q

77. **A i.e. Flail chest; B i.e. Head injury; C i.e. Tetanus; E i.e. Foreign body** *[Ref: P. L. Dhingra 3/e P-382]*

78. **B i.e., Increased pulmonary compliance** *[Ref: Yao & Artusios Anesthesiology 6/e p- 67; Morgan 4/e p –1028-29; Wylie 7/e p- 1177, 1168-69, Miller 6/e p. 716-17, 2676-78,711]*

Hyperoxia (oxygen toxicity) may lead to ***hypoventilation, hypercapnia (but not necessarily hypoxia), absorption atelectasis,*** **decreaed vital capacity,** ***deterioration of pulmonary compliance & blood gases***Q, interstitial edema, pulmonary fibrosis, tonic clonic seizure & retinopathy of prematurity d/t free radicle induced damage of sulfhydryl group enzymes, ***endothelium***Q, epithelium and surfactant systems

79. **B i.e. It decreases turbulence**

80. **A i.e. Helium is a inert gas, D i.e. Reduces work of breathing, E i.e. Mixture of He & O_2**
[Ref: Morgan 4/e p. 1028; Lee's 13/e p. 85, 147, 738, 787-88; Wylie 7/e p. 1169; Miller 7/e p. 2360]

- **Helium (He)** is a colorless, odourless, ***inert nobel gas***Q, with high diffusibility, low solubility, ***low density***Q and low density to viscosity ratio.
- **Heliox** is a ***mixture of helium & oxygen***Q, which ***decreases large airway resistance and turbulence and therefore reduces patients work of breathing***Q.

81. **D i.e. All**

- **Helium (He)** has ***no freezing point, approximately zero (0) viscosity, atomic number 2 and atomic weight 4.006***Q. It is *second most lightest* gas (after hydrogen) *and 2nd most abundant* element in universe, *after hydrogen.* However, it is rare on earth.
- It solidifies at – 272. 20°C at pressure above 26 atm; & boils at – 268.9°C. Its density is 0.1664 g/lit at 20°c & 1 atm.
- ***It is used with O_2 as HELIOX in COPD & bronchial asthma***Q. Inhaled helium is used in MRI to produce high contrast images. And beams of He from synchrocyclotron are used in eye tumors for shrinking it and for vascular malformation.

Ventilators

82. **B i.e. Membrane Oxygenator** *[Ref: Morghan's 3/e p. 436]*

Membranous (pump) oxygenators produce ***least damage to blood elements (RBCs, WBCs, platelets)***Q and *cause least denaturation of proteins.* They have improved the efficiency of gas exchange while minimizing the trauma to blood elements. Due to these advantages membrane oxygenators have largely replaced bubble oxygenators.

Oxygenators are devices used in cardiopulmonary bypass surgeries. Currently only two types of oxygenators - *Membranous & bubble* oxygenators are in use.

- Membranous oxygenators imitate the natural lung by interspersing a thin membrane between gas and blood phases. This *eliminates gaseous micro emboli formation & minimizes blood element trauma.*
- Hematological advantages of membranous oxygenator (vs bubble oxygenators) are – less trauma to RBC, WBC, platelet & less protein denaturation. Due to these advantages membranous oxygenators have largely replaced bubble oxygenators.
- Disc oxygenators & vertical screen oxygenators were used in past.

83. **C i.e. 60-100L/min** *[Ref: Evita 2 Dura : A book on ventilators; Harrison 15/e P-1528]*

- The ventilators *serve as energy source only during inspiration* replacing the muscles of chest wall & diaphragm; expiration is passive driven by the recoil of the lung & chest wall
- In volume cycled ventilation inspiratory flow rate is *usually maintained at **60L/min***Q

Intensive Care Ventilatory Manual

Adult Ventilation	Paediatric Ventilation
Tidal Volume = 100 ml to 2000 ml	Tidal Volume 20 ml to 300 ml
Inspiratory Flow Rate = ***6 lit/min to 120 L/min***Q	Inspiratory Flow Rate = ***6 L/min to 30 L/min***Q

84. **D i.e. Cardiac Temponade** *[Ref: Morgan's 3/e P-960]*

Prolonged controlled ventilation may cause ***barotrauma*** & ***pulmonary embolism***[Q]. And CO_2 wash out causes ***alkalosis***[Q] in controlled ventilation.

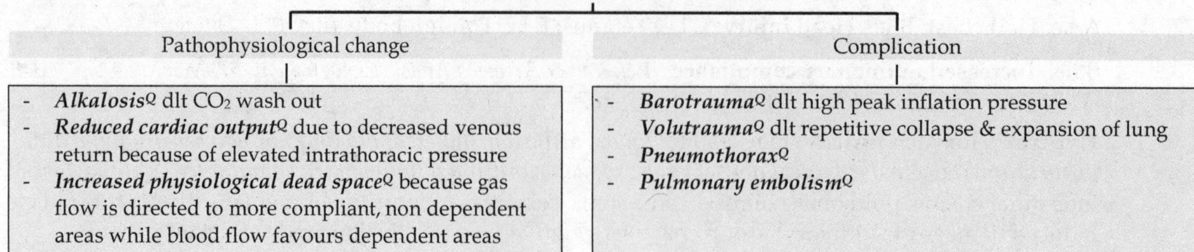

Intermittent Positive Pressure Ventilation (IPPV)
Pathophysiological change
Complication
- Alkalosis[Q] dlt CO2 wash out
- Reduced cardiac output[Q] due to decreased venous return because of elevated intrathoracic pressure
- Increased physiological dead space[Q] because gas flow is directed to more compliant, non dependent areas while blood flow favours dependent areas
- Barotrauma[Q] dlt high peak inflation pressure
- Volutrauma[Q] dlt repetitive collapse & expansion of lung
- Pneumothorax[Q]
- Pulmonary embolism[Q]

85. **A i.e. Controlled mechanical ventilation** *[Ref: Morgan 4/e p1030-40; Ajay Yadav 2/e p182-83]*

Controlled mechanical ventilation (CMV) is *best reserved for patients capable of little or no ventilatory effort.* In this mode, V_T and ventilatory rate are fixed (minute ventilation) regardless of patient effort, because patient can not breathe spontaneously. So this mode will pay no role in weaning a patient from mechanical ventilation, setling to limit inspiratory pressure ***guard against pulmonary barotrauma***[Q].

In Assist control ventilation (ACV) by incorporating a pressure sensor in breathing circuit, the *patients inspiratory effort can be used to trigger inspiration.* The ventilator can be set for a fixed ventilatory rate, but each patient effort of sufficient magnitude will trigger the set V_T (tidal volume). And if the spontaneous inspiratory efforts are not detected the machine functions as if in the control mode.

Criteria for Discontinuing (weaning) of Mechanical Ventilation

Mechanical Criteria		**Weaning Modes**
- Inspiratory pressure	< 25cmH_2O	- ***Synchronized Intermittent mandatory ventilation (SIMV)***[Q]
- Tidal volume	> 5ml/kg	- ***Intermittent mandatory ventilation (IMV)***
- Vital Capacity	> 10ml/kg	- ***Pressure support ventilation(PSV)***[Q]
- Minute ventilation	< 10ml	- Weaning with a T-piece or CPAP (continuous positive airway pressure)
- Rapid shallow breathing index	< 100	- ***Assist control ventilation (ACV)***[Q±]

86. **D i.e. ↓ICT** *[Ref: Morgan's anaesthesia 4/e p. 1038-40]*

87. **B. i.e. Started with $FiO_2$50-60%**

[Ref: Miller's aneshthesia 7/e p-2882-84, 2666-67, 2716, 1851-52; www.guideline.gov.; Wylie's & Davidson Anesthesia 7/e p-476-77, 1085; Clinical anesthesia: Barash, Cullen stoelting 6/e p- 237, 1240; American association for respiratory care: clinical practical guide.]

(Nasal CPAP or intubation at birth for very preterm infants. The new England journal of medicine Feb 08 vol 358: 700 – 708 nuber 07)

Bronchopulmonary dysplasia is associated with ventilation (intubation) & O_2 treatment. Infants who were born at 25 – 28 weeks gestation and were breathing spontaneously were treated with nasal **continuous positive airway pressure (CPAP)** shortly (at 5 minutes) after birth. 50% were subsequently intubated. Infants in CPAP group had a better outcome at 28th day than did those in intubated group (i.e. required significantly lower rate of O_2 treatment and underwent fewer days of ventilation) even though the rate of pneumothorae was higher in CPAP group.

A CPAP of 8 – 12 cm of water was used to maintain functional residual capacity and for improving lung compliance and oxygenation.

The study suggests that starting respiratory support with CPAP does not adversely affect, infants even if upto 50% of them subsequently undergo ventilation (intubation), some because of pneumothorax. Ammar et al also showed that 76% of infants < 1.251 kg and 50% of those weighing < 0.751 kg did not need to undergo ventilation (intubation).

[Nasal CPAP in preterm infants – does it works & how? J-Hammer]

Previous research suggest that **CPAP (nasal) application in preterm infants** is associated with *benefits in terms of reduced respiratory failure and reduced duration and invasiveness of respiratory support; without worsening of other standard measures of neonatal outcome* (bronchopulmonary dysplasia & death).

Among spontaneously breathing **very premature infants, surfactant therapy** administered within 1st hour of life along with **nasal CPAP** decreases the oxygen requirement, need for mechanical ventilation and may prevent chronic lung disease.

Monitoring of Patient

88. **A i.e. Depth of general anesthesia**
89. **C i.e. Bispectral imaging** *[Ref. Miller 7/e, p 35-36, 254-55; Morgan 5/e p. 129-135; Lee 13/e p. 117-18; Aitkenhead 5/e, p 199, 359]*

- During anesthesia, **electroencephalography (EEG) is most useful** for assessing the **adequacy of cerebral perfusion during carotid endarterectomy (CEA) & controlled hypoventilation and for assessing depth of general anesthesia.**[Q]
- **Bispectral index (BIS) can assess intraoperative awareness and consciousness**[Q] and has been approved by FDA for **evaluating the depth of general anesthesia in adult & pediatric patients.**

90. **A i.e. Hypothermia** *[Ref: Aitkenhead 4/e, P-147-48; 157-62,175; Wiley & Davidson 7/e p-515- 16; http ://www. Pubmedcentral. Nih. Gov / article render fcgi artid – 28985; Harrison 16/e p. 123]*

Hypothermia causes *progressive slowing of brain activity* at core temperatures below 35°C. Severe hypothermia (<28°C) results in loss of cerebrovascular auto regulation, decrease in cerebral blod flow, coma, loss of ocular reflex, and ***progressive decrease in EEG***[Q].

91. **C i.e. Hypothermia** *[Ref: Morgan 4/e p. 624-26; Aitkenhead 5/e p. 358-59]*

- **EEG activation** (i.e. high frequency & low voltage activity) is seen in (Mn-**"Small BBC In English Stimulates No Hypoxic Keets"**) i.e. Barbiturates *(small dose)*, Benzodiazepines *(small dose)*, *Mild* hypercapnia (↑CO_2), **In**halational agents *(subanesthetic)*, Etomidate *(small doses)*, sensory **stimulation**, **N_2O**, **Hypoxia** *(early)*, **ket**amine. Here small = small, mild, early or subanesthetic dose.
- EEG depression is caused by (Mn- **Marked Hypo**) i.e. **hypo**thermia, **hypo**capnia, Propofol and Opioids and all marked (i.e. marked hypoxia (late), marked hypercapnia, large dose of barbiturates, etomidate & inhalational agents (1-2 MAC).

92. **C i.e. Brainstem auditory evoked potential** *[Ref. Miller 7/e, p 1488, Morgen 4/e p, 147]*

Brain stem auditory evoked potential (BAEP) is ***most resistant (i.e. least affected) during anesthesia***[Q].

93. **A i.e. Monitoring of neuromuscular function** *[Ref: Dorsch 5/e p. 805-17; Morgan 5/e p. 138-40; Miller 7/e p. 1488]*
94. **A i.e. Ulnar nerve**

- **Kinemyography** (KMG), **acceleromyography** (ACG/AMG), **piezoelectric film, electromyographyh** (EMG), **phono/acoustic-myography (PMG/AMG), mechanomyography** (MMG; gold standard) and tactile or visual assessment methods are used for evaluating evoked responses during **monitoring of neuromuscular function (block).**
- **Ulnar nerve stimulation of adductor pollicis** (most common) and **facial nerve stimulation of orbicularis oculi are most commonly used monitoring sites during anesthesia.**

95. **D i.e. Capnography** *[Ref: Morgan's 3/e p. 110-11]*

- **Capnography** is a *respiratory monitoring system (not cardiovascular)*. It is the determination of end tidal CO_2 (Et CO_2) concentration to confirm adequate ventilation.
- Cardiovascular monitoring techniques are – ECG, Echocardiography, BP, CVP, pulmonary artery catheterization.

96. **E i.e. In malignant hyperthermia E_{TCO2} decreases**
97. **D. i.e. Bronchospasm** *[Ref: Dorsh 5/e p 705-19; Miller 7/e p. 1213-14, 1425-29; Ajay Yadav 5/e p 61; Wylie 7/e p- 432-36; Capnography: Clinical aspectis by J.S. Gravenstein; Capnography.com]*

- **Capnography (E_{TCO2} = end tidal CO_2) is the best method to confirm endotracheal tube (ETT) placement**[Q].
- **Malignant hyperthermia** shows **a marked rise and pulmonary** (air) **embolism** shows a **rapid fall of E_{TCO2} on capnography.**
- **Elevated baseline** (and normal waveform shape) may be caused by **exhausted absorbent in the circle system**[Q]. And **curure notch or cleft** on copnogram is seen during **spontaneous ventilative**[Q].
- **Flat line on capnogram (Flat capnogram)** instead of normal square step shaped wave form is indicative of absence of CO_2 in expired air. It is seen in – ***accidental extubation, dissociation (disconnection) of anesthetic tube, equipment failure, total occlusion, mechanical ventilation failure and complete severe bronchospasm***[Q].
- In **partial bronchospasm** *steep platue (not flat)* capnogram is seen. And *end tidal CO_2 (ET CO_2) is increased* in **inadequate ventilation.**

98. **B. i.e. Fiber optic bronchoscopy**

99. **D i.e. Bronchoscopy**

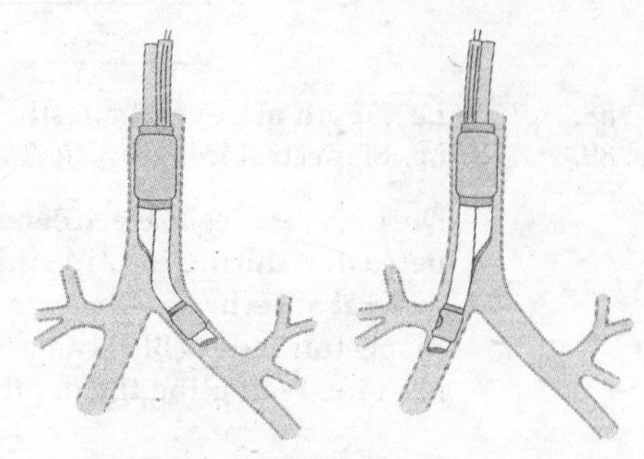

- During thoracic surgery there may be a need for one lung to be deflated offering surgeon easier and better access. This is achieved by **double lumen endotracheal tubes** that allows anesthetist to selectively deflate one lung while maintaining standard ventilation of other.
- The position of the tube should be checked by auscultation immediately after intubation but the ***confirmation of correct placement of the tube should be done by flexible fiberoptic bronchoscopy***Q
- $EtCO_2$ (Persistent detection of CO_2 by capnography) is best confirmation of tracheal placement endotracheal tube. Capnography *can detect whether the tube is in trachea or oesophagus but cannot differentiate between tracheal intubation /endobronchial intubation.*

Double lumen endotracheal tube

Best confirmation of tracheal placement (i.e. detection whether tube is in trachea or oesophagus)	**Best confirmation of placement** (Whether tube is in trachea or bronchus)
*Capnography ($EtCO_2$)*Q	*Flexible fibreoptic Bronchoscopy* Q

100. **D i.e. Endobronchial intubation** *[Ref: Miller 7/e p-1600; Benumof 2/e p-1/95 2008/101; Morgan's 3/e, P-59, 73, 110]*

101. **B i.e. Malignant hyperthermia**

- ***Unilateral absence (or decrease) of breath sounds over one lung (especially left) after a speedy intubation suggests a diagnosis of inadvertent endobronchial intubation. End tidal CO_2 may be low, normal or raised after an endotracheal intubation.*** *The presence of high end tidal CO_2 however excludes a diagnosis of esophageal intubation which is associated with reduced or absent end tidal CO_2.*
- ***Malignant hyperthermia show marked rise in E_TCO_2.***

102. **A i.e. Anaphylaxis** *[Ref. Drosch 5/e p. 705-8; Shaikh-Simon 2/e p. 119; Mller 7/e p. 1213, 1425-29, 1088]*

- **Thyroid storm, malignant hyperthermia, neuroleptic malignant syndrome** and **pheochromocytoma are hypermetabolic states with a massive increase in CO_2 production**, characterized by hyperpyrexia, tachycardia striking alteration in consciousness and ***rise in E_T CO_2 (end tidal CO_2 on capnometery)***Q.
- **Anaphylaxis** l/t hypotension and shock results in hypoperfusion of lungs and ***deceased E_T CO_2***Q.

103. **C i.e. Transesophageal echocardiography** *[Ref. Aitkenhead 5/e 353, 722-24, 749]*

- **Tranoesophageal echocardiography** provides a real time picture of all 4 cardiac chambers and valves. It can identify any malfunctioning valves in addition to any wall motion abnormalities related to myocardia ischemia. **It is very useful during anesthesia. Abnormal motion of ventricular wall detected in this way is a reliable index of myocardial ischemia** and may guide drug therapy, can identify if therapy has successfully treated the ischemia or indicate the need for further surgical revascularization
- **CVP** (catherter in central vein) measures right sided filling pressure whereas **pulmonary artery catheter** measures/monitors left heart filling pressure.
- **Arterial cannulation** measures direct systemic arterial pressure and facilitate sampling of arterial blood for analysis.

104. **D i.e. Regional wall motion abnormality detected with the help of 2D transoesophageal echocardiography** *[Ref: Morgan's Anesthesia 4/e p. 460-462, 502-503]*

Intraoperative Monitoring of Ischemic heart disease

For detection of ischemia	**Hemodynamic monitoring (m.c. are hypertension & tachycardia)**
Trans-oesophageal echocardiographyQ - Detection of new regional wall motion abnormalities is a rapid & more sensitive indicator of myocardial ischemia (than ECG) - Decreased systolic wall thickening may be more reliable index for ischemia than endocardial wall motion alone	Pulmonary artery pressure monitoring

105. **A i.e. Malposition of the double lumen tube** *[Ref: Morgan's Anesthesia 4/e p. 591-593]*

- Malposition of a double lumen tube is usually indicated by poor lung compliance and low exhaled tidal volume
- ***Most common cause of hypoxemia during one lung ventilation is malposition of double lumen tube.*** Q
- Hypoxemia can also occur due to occlusion of tube & increased shunt fraction.

106. **C i.e. Catheter related infection** **107.** **A i.e. Tension pneumothorar**

108. **None** *[Ref: Miller 7/e p-1290-97; Morgan 4/e, p 131-32; Silberzweig et al vascular interventional radiology]*

- ***Infection is most common (5-26%) late complication*** Q f/b thromboembolism (2-26%) and mechanical (5-19%) of CVP catheter placement.
- **Pneumothorax** is ***most common acute (mechanical) complication of subclavian central venous cannulation*** Q. It presents with ***decreased air entery in hemi thorax (causing decreased breath sound on ipislateral hemithorax auscultation), decreased saturation, decreased BP, tachycardia, respiratory distress (dynpnoea) and hyperresonance on palpation of ipsilateral chest*** Q.

109. **A i.e. PCWP; B i.e. CO; C i.e. Mixed venous O_2 saturation; D i.e. Right atrial pressure**

110. **C i.e. PA pressure tracing has diacrotic notch from closure of pulmonary valve**

111. **B i.e. Nail polish; C i.e. Methemoglobinemia; D i.e. Skin pigmentation**

112. **A i.e. CO_2; C i.e. O_2; D i.e. Room air; E i.e. N_2O**

113. **A i.e. Conduction** *[Ref: Morgan 4/e p. 134-136; Dorsch 4/e p. 827; Forfar & Arneil's textbook of pediatrics 4/e P-167, 168]*

Following factors may lead to inaccurate reading in pulse oxymeter:

- ***Methemoglobin*** Q
- Carboxyhemoglobin (over read d/t HbCO)
- Fetal hemoglobin (at very high levels only)
- Hemoglobin S (?)
- Severe hyperbilirubinemia does not affect readings
- Malpositioning of sensor
- Poor peripheral pulsation
- ***Skin pigmentation*** Q
- Dyes-methylene blue, indocyanine green
- Optical interference
- Electrical interference
- ***Nail polish & covering*** Q

Gas used to create pneumoperitoneum

1. *CO_2* Q
2. *O_2* Q
3. ***Room air*** Q
4. *N_2O* Q *(not N_2)* Q

- In incubator heat is delivered by-
  1. ***Radiation*** Q
  2. ***Convection*** Q]— mainly
  3. ***Evaporation*** Q
- In infants, heat loss (& also heat delivery) through conduction is very small as infants are not usually in direct contact with structure of high thermal capacity.
- In infants, heat loss (& also heat delivery) through evaporation is also very small if incubator have humidifiers.

114. **B i.e. Impedence pulmonometry** *[Ref: Lee's 13/e p-622- 23; Miller's 6/e p-1435-75, 2394- 95; Morgan's 4/e p. 932- 33; Aitkenhead 4/e, P- 371, 476- 77; Wiley & Davidson 7/e p- 437- 40, 975]*

Monitoring Respiration

Require Intubation
- ***Capnography*** Q
- ***Infrared End Tidal CO_2 measurement*** Q

Don't require Intubation
- ***Impedence pulmonometry*** Q
- Pulse oximetry
- Transcutaneous gas analysis. (only effective in infants d/t thin skin)

Preoperative Assessment & Medication

115. **B i.e. Carbon monoxide shift O_2-Hb dissociation curve to right** *[Ref. Yao and Artusio's 7th p 32, 33; Lee's 13/e p41, 43; Miller 7th p 1103-4, 1022; Stoelting 5/e p 412-14; Goodman and Gilman 12/e p 271, 657, 657-58]*

- Smoking increases airway irritability & secretions, decreases surfactant mucopulmonary transport and increases the incidence of postoperative pulmonary complications.
- ***Cessation of smoking for 12 to 24 hrs before operation decreases the level of carbon monoxide and carboxyhemoglobin, which shift oxy-hemoglobin dissociation curve to the right*** Q and increases the O_2 available to tissue. (CO shift oxyHb dissociation curve to left).
- Improvement in mucociliary transport and small airway function and decrease in sputum production require prolonged abstinence (8–12 weeks) from smoking. So the incidence of postoperative pulmonary

complications decrease with abstinence from cigarette smoking for **> 8 weeks in patients undergoing cardiac (coronary artery bypass) surgery and > 4 weeks** in patients underging pulmonary surgery.

- Smoking shortly before surgery may be a/w an increased incidence ST segment depression on ECG.
- Major action of nicotine consists **initially of transient stimulation** (at small doses) and subsequently of a more persistent ***depression of all autonomic*** **(sympathetic and parasympathetic) ganglia** (at larger doses). Nicotine also possess *a biphasic action on adrenal medulla* i.e. small doses evoke whereas larger doses prevent the discharge of *catecholamines* in response to splanchnic nerve stimulation. The effect of nicotine on **neuromuscular junction** are similar to those on ganglia i.e. initial stimulant phase (contractions) f/b blockade by receptor desensitization (l/t rapidly developing paralysis). Nicotine, like Ach, *stimulates* number of *sensory receptors* such as *mechanoreceptors* (to stretch or pressure) of skin, mesentry, tongue, lung and stomach; ***chemoreceptors of carotid and aortic body***, *thermal receptors* of skin and tongue; *pain receptors;* and *emetic chemorecepto trigger zone (CTZ) in the area postrema of medulle oblongata* (causing vomiting). Nicotine markedly stimulates *CNS* i.e. weak analgesia at low doses; tremors and convulsion at higher doses followed by CNS depression and death from respiratory failure. So it can be assumed for the above description that **smoking (low nicotine) can stimulate aortic and carotid body, increase sympathetic tone and stimulate NMJ thereby increasing the muscle relaxant dose requirements.**

116. **D i.e. ARB** *[Ref. Miller 7/e, p (2)-2268]*

- ***β blockers (antihypertensive), steroids and stains are continued (ie taken) on the day of operation***Q. Whereas ***angiotensin receptor blockers (ARB) are stopped preoperatively***Q.
- **ACE inhibitors** (capto/enala /lisino/rami-pril, enalaprilat) and ***angiotension II receptor blockers*** *(valsartan)* are increasingly used as 1st line antihypertensive drugs and appear to improve quality of life of patients taking antihypertensive drugs. However, **ACE inhibitor, angiotensin II receptor blockers and ACE receptor blocking agents** may be a/w *more peripheral vasodilation and hypotension on induction of anesthesia* (than sympatholytic drugs are). These last 2 classes of drugs are a/w ***such severe hypotension with standard anesthetic induction that these are either discontinued or at least considered discontinuing preoperatively***Q.

117. **A i.e. Stop Aspirin for 7 days**

- Mode of action of aspirin

Aspirin in even small doses inhibit
TxA2 synthesis by platelets (irreversibly)
↓
Platelet aggregation is interfered and
Bleeding time prolonged nearly to twice
↓
Effect lasts for about *one week (turn over time of platelets)*

- So if aspirin is stopped for a week before surgery all platelet will change and Bleeding time will become normal. Other measure will not help as - ***Aspirin is irreversible inhibitorof*** T_xA_2Q

118. **D i.e. Metochlopromide** *[Ref: Morgan's 3/e, P-210, 245]*

- Metochlopramide increases lower esophageal sphinter tone, speeds gastric emptying & lowers gastric fluid volume & decreases risk for aspiration pneumonia due to antiemetic effect
- Antiemetics
  - Metoclopramide = Preoperative
  - $5HT_3$ antagonist (ondansteron) = Postoperative
  - Hyoscine = Out of use

119. **B i.e. Bronchoconstrictor** *[Ref: KDT 5/e P-105]*

Atropine is a **bronchodialator**Q

120. **C i.e. ↓ dose of inducing agent** *[Ref: KDT 5/e]*
Preanesthetic medication is for the **Amnesia, Antiemesis, Analgesia; Decreasing Anxiety, Seretions & Acidity.** It has nothing to do with induction.

121. **A i.e. Hypothalmus** 122. **D i.e. Arrythmia**
123. **D i.e. Occur irrespective of the type of anesthesia**
[Ref: Yao 7/e p 567; Miller 7/e p 1538-48; Pardo 6/e p 330, 377, 725-27; Ajay Yadav 5/e p 132-33; Harrison 18/e p 165-69, 1868; Wylie 7/e p 547; Morgan 5/e p 1183-85, 587]

- **During GA shivering is abolished by suppression of hypothalamus.**Q
- **Hypothermia is protective during cerebral or cardiac ischemia** and it is *used in neurosurgery, cardiac surgery,* carotid artery surgery/prolonged surgeries, where tissue ischemia is anticipated, in **recovery after cardiac**

arrest and for neonatal asphyxiaQ. Dysarrhythmia occurs at temperature below 30°C, spontaneous ventricular fibrillation may be seen but is not likely above 20°C. As ***hypothermia is arrythmogenic so hypothermia is C/I in arrythmia***Q

- **Hypothermia during anesthesia occur in nearly every patient during both general & regional (spinal/epidural) anesthesia**, unless steps are taken to prevent this complication. ***Body looses heat mainly by internal re-distribution and radiation***Q. It is **beneficial (in ischemia)** as well as **deleterious**Q (coagulopathy, cardiac arrhythmia, wound infection etc) to patients. It can **be prevented by giving warm fluids only if large amounts of IV fluids are to be administered** (which is mostly not the case.) However, **patients cannot be warmed by using heated fluids** because the fluid cannot (much) exceed body temperature.

124. A i.e. Diazepam; B i.e. Scopolamine; C i.e. Morphine
125. B i.e. Decrease BP *[Ref: Lee 12th/13-18; KDT 5/e P-345]*

Main drugs used in preanaesthetic medication are-

- Opioids- Morphine
- Anxiolytics- Diazepam
- Hypnotics- Barbiturate
- Anticholinergics- Atropine, Hyoscine(Scopolamine)
- Neuroleptic- Chlorpromazine
- H_2 blocker- Ranitidine
- Antiemetics- Metoclopramide, Ondansetron

Aims of preanesthetic medication

1. ***Allay anxiety & apprehension***Q
2. ***Amnesia***Q for pre & postoperative events
3. ***To decrease dose of anesthetic***Q
4. ***To prevent aspiration***Q by antiemetics & decreasing secretions
5. ***To decrease acidity***Q so that it is less damaging if aspirated

126. B i.e. ASA 2 **127. A i.e. Status of patient**
[Ref: Lee's 13/e p 6-7; Morgan 5/e p 297; Wiley 7/e p- 415, 478; Miller 7/e p. 1002, 1297-99]

- **American Society of Anesthesiologists (ASA) Physical status classification** of patient is a **scoring system to assess physical status** (main) **and help quantify relative risk**Q.
- A patient with **mild systemic desease with no functional limitations eg mild asthma or well controlled hypertension (by medication)** falls under **ASA grade 2**.

128. A i.e. Wrist *[Ref: Morgan 5/ep 92-93]*

Modified Allen's test is for checking the proper **arterial supply at the wrist**Q. It is a simple (but not very reliable) method for assessing the *integrity (patency) of palmar arterial arch, radial and ulnar arteries.*

129. A i.e. ECG; D i.e. Body temperature decrease
130. C i.e. Absent spinal cord reflex *[Ref: Morgan 4/e p – 1022]*

2

NEUROMUSCULAR BLOCKERS

Classification of Muscle Relaxants (according to)

Duration of Action of Neuromuscular Blockers

	Long Acting (>50 min)	**Intermediate Acting** (20-50min)	**Short Acting** (10-20 min)	**Ultra short Acting** (<10 min)
Others	Glallamine Allocuronium			- *Succinyl choline*Q - GW280430 A - TAAC3
Steroidal compound	*Pancuronium*Q Pipecuronium	*Vecuronium*Q Rocuronium	*Rapacuronium*Q	
Benzylisoquinolinium compound	d- Tubocurarine Metocurine Doxacurium	Atracurium Cisatracurium	*Mivacurium*Q	

* **Onset time** is time to 95% depression of twitch height following an intubating dose
* **Clinical duration** is time to 25% recovery of twitch height

Onset time

Drug (In order of fastest to slowest onset time)	**Onset time In Seconds**	**Clinical Duration In Minutes**
*Succinyl choline*Q	60 (*most rapid onset*Q)	10
RapacuroniumQ	< 75	15
RocuroniumQ	75	33
Atracurium	110	43
Cisatracurium	150	45
Mivacurium	170	16
Vecuronium	180	33
Pancuronium	220	75
D- tubocurarine	220	80
Doxacurium	250	83
Gallamine	300	80
Pipecuronium	300	95
Alcuronium	420	70

Action

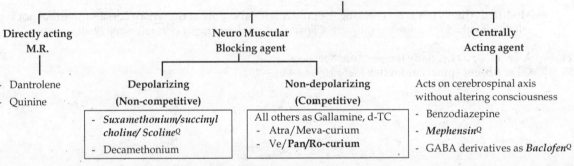

Directly acting M.R.
- Dantrolene
- Quinine

Neuro Muscular Blocking agent

Depolarizing (Non-competitive)
- *Suxamethonium/succinyl choline/ Scoline*Q
- Decamethonium

Non-depolarizing (Competitive)

All others as Gallamine, d-TC
- Atra/Meva-curium
- Ve/**Pan/Ro-curium**

Centrally Acting agent

Acts on cerebrospinal axis without altering consciousness
- Benzodiazepine
- ***Mephensin***Q
- GABA derivatives as *Baclofen*Q

Reversal of Muscle Relaxation

- **Anticholinesterase** act by inhibiting acetylcholinesterase enzyme (a type B carboxylesterase) at neuromuscular junction. **Antagonism of nondepolarizing blockade** is time dependent and recovery rate primarily depends on 5 factors
  1) *Depth of blockade & type of neuromuscular blocking agent* (i.e. long, intermediate or short duration of action).
  2) *Type of anticholinesterase administered:* at moderate depth of blockade (i.e. 2-3 palpable twitches by TOF monitoring) the order of rapidity of antagonism of residual blockade is *edrophonium* > *neostigmine* > *pyridostigmine*. But ***edrophonium becomes less potent relative to neostigmine as the depth of blockade becomes more intense.***
  3) *Dose of anticholinesterase: larger doses* (upto the point of maximum effective dose) *antagonize NM blockade more rapidly and more completely than smaller doses.* Maximum effective dose for neostigmine is **60-80 μg/kg,** pyridostigmine is **350 μg/kg** and for edrophonium **1- 1.5 mg/kg**. Mixing or combining do not potentiate and is not advisible. If maximal dose fail to antagonize the residual blockade, it is *not advisible to administer additional anticholinesterase* because giving too much may actually render patient weaker.
  4) *Rate of spontaneous recovery* which depends on duration of action of NM blocker.

5) *Concentration of inhaled anesthetic:* recovery is slow & reversal is prolonged by inhalational agents (sevoflurane > desflurane > isoflurane).
6) **Hypokalemia & calcium channel blocker verapamil** potentiate nondepolarizing blockers and decrease the ability of drugs to antagonize the block. Both *metabolic & respiratory respiratory acidosis* may augment the nondepolarizing block but only respiratory acidosis (CO_2 arterial partial pressure > 50 mmHg d/t hypoventilation caused by narcotics) prevents antagonism. *Metabolic alkalosis* not metabolic acidosis, prevents neostigmine antagonism of dTC & pancuronium, suggesting that **extracellular pH is not as important as intracellular pH & electrolyte concentration.** *Mild hypothermia* (i.e. 34° - 35°C), which commonly occurs intraoperatively decreases clearance and delays onset on peak effect of neostigmine.

- A *modified γ-cyclodextrin,* **sugammadex** (su=sugar, & gammadex = gamma cyclodextrin structural molecule) or **ORG – 25969** is the first selective muscle relaxant binding (reversal) agent. Its 3 dimensional structure resembles a *doughnut or hollow truncated cone with a hydrophobic cavity & a hydrophilic exterior.* Hydrophobic interactions trap the drug in *doughnut hole (cyclodextrin cavity)* thereby forming very tight water soluble guest-host complexes in *1:1 ratio* with steroidal neuromuscular blocking agents **(rocuronium > vecuronium >> pancuronium)**. The **combination of rocuronium & sugammadex** could replace succinylcholine for rapid sequence induction of anesthesia & completely eliminate residual paralysis in postanesthetic recovery room.
- **Cysteine:** Gantacurium undergoes rapid degradation in plasma by chemical hydrolysis and inactivation by *cysteine adduction.* So exogenous administration of cysteine can accelerate the antagonism of gantacurium induced NM blockade.

Choice of Anticholinesterase

TOF visible twitches	TOF fade (estimated)	Anticholinesterase drug & dose (mg/kg IV)	Anticholinergic drug & dose (μg/kg IV)
None	-	Not recommended	Not recommended
≤ 2	++++	**Neostigmine** (0.07)	Glycopyrrolate (7) or atropine (15)
3 – 4	+++	Neostigmine (0.04)	Glycopyrrolate (7) or atropine (15)
4	++	**Edrophonium** (0.5)	Atropine (7)
4	0	Edrophonium (0.25)	Atropine (7)

1. ***Depolarizing (Non Competitive) M.R. are not antagonized.*** Q
2. *Non-D (compatitive) M.R. are antagonized by Acetyl choline or* ***Anti Choline Esterase – Neostigmine, Pyridostigmine, Edrophonium*** Q

In order *to prevent muscarinic effects* ***Glycopyrrolate/Atropine*** *is given in combination* Q

Features of Neuromuscular Blocking Drugs

Depolarising (Non competitive)

- Depolarizing NM blocker succinyl choline is composed of *2 molecules of acetylcholine linked back to back* through acetate methyl group. It is a long, thin, flexible molecule *which stimulates (like Ach) cholinergic receptors* at NM junction at nicotinic (ganglionic) and muscarinic autonomic sites, thereby *opening the ionic channels in Ach receptors.* So Sch produces *prolonged depolarization resulting in decreased sensitivity of postsynaptic nicotininc acetylcholine receptor & inactivation of sodium channels* so that propagation of action potential across the muscle membrane is inhibited.
- Na^+ channel are blocked open, the muscle is unresponsive to other mechanical or electrical

Non depolarizing (Competitive)

- ***They are mostly hydrophilic,*** mono or bisquaternary salts with interonium distances of 0.7 – 1.4 nm or steroidal non depolarizing muscle relaxants produce neuromuscular blockade by *competing with acetylcholine for post synaptic α-subunits.*
- Relativey slow onset (1-5 min) and relatively slow dissociation at receptors. ***Time of onset of neuromuscular block is dose dependent*** Q.
- *Speed of onset is inversely proportional to the potency* of nondepolarizing agent. With the exception of atracurium, *molar potency is highly predictive of drug's rate of onset of effect.* Molar-potency (ED_{95}) of rocuronium is 13% of vecuronium & 9% that of cisatracurium; so its onset of

Differences

Characteristic	**Depolarizing Block (Phase I Block)**	**Nondepolarizing Block (Phase II Block of Sch)**
Effect on single twitch height	Depression	Depression
Train of four fade	Absent	***Present*** Q ***(marked)***
Tetanic stimulation fade	Absent	***Present*** Q
Post tetanic facilitation	Absent	***Present*** Q
Effect of anticholinesterase agent eg endorphium	***Potentiation of block*** Q	***Reversal of block*** Q
Effect of nondepolarising drugs	Less blockade	More blockade
Train of four ratio	***> 0.7*** Q	***< 0.4*** Q
Recovery	Rapid	Increasingly prolonged
Tachyphylaxis	Absent	Present
Dose of Sch (mg/kg)	2-3	>6

stimuli and repolarization does not happen until phase 2 block develops, when the resting membrne potential returns to – 80 mv.
- ***Rapid onset of effect & ultrashort duration of action***[Q] b/o its rapid hydrolysis by *butyryl cholinesterase.*
- Fast dissociation at receptors.
- Causes ***muscle fasciculation***[Q] (but not in myasthenic humans), and extraocular muscles exhibit a tonic response.
- In partial paralysis, there is depression of muscle twitch, ***no 'fade' and no post tetanic facilitation***[Q].
- ***Block is not reversed by neostigmine or other anticholinesterases***[Q].
- They are potentiated by ***isoflurane***[Q], *respiratory alkalosis, hypothermia & magnesium.*
- Antagonised by *acidosis* and nondepolarising relaxants
- Repeated or continuous leads to phase 2 block.

action is more rapid than that of either agents. Dose of drug required to produce an effect (50%, 90% or 95% depression of twitch height) is taken as a measure of potency.
- ***No muscle fasciculation***
- Relaxed muscle remains responsive to other mechanical & electrical stimuli
- In partial paralysis, there is depression of muscle twitch, 'fade', and posttetanic facilitation, followed by exhaustion.
- ***Reversed by anticholinesterases***[Q] *(neostigmine, pyridostigmine & edrophonium)*, sugammadex & cysteine (for gantacurium).
- Effects are reduced by suxamethonium (but not in mysthenics)
- ***Potentiated by volatile agents, acidosis, magnesium and hypokalemia***[Q], verapamil.
- ***Mild cooling antagonises but further cooling below 33°C potentiates them***[Q].

Effect of nondepolarizing neuromuscular blocking agent

Muscle	Onset	Maximum blockade	Duration
Resistant muscles			
Diaphragm[Q], Laryngeal adductors, corrugator supercilli (eye brow muscle)	Fast	Shallow	Short
Abdominalis, Intercostals	Fast	Intermediate	Intermediate
Ms. of hypothenar eminence	Slow	Intermediate	Long
Sensitive muscles			
Adductor pollicis, flexor hallucis, first dorsal interosseous (hand)	Slow	Deep	Long
Geinohyoid, upper airway ms; orbicularis oculi	Fast	Very Deep	Long

Evoked responses during depolarizing (phase I and phase II) and non depolarizing block

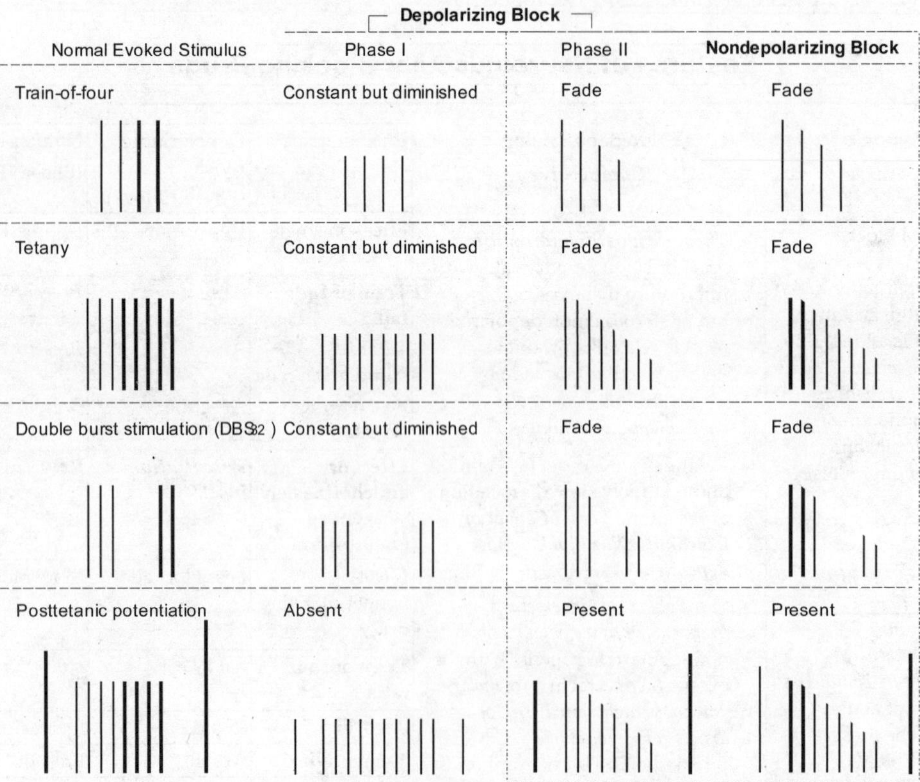

Succinylcholine (Scoline, Suxamethonium or Diacetylcholine)

Suxamethonium chloride, a dicholine ester of acetyl choline, is a **clear, colourless aqueous solution of ph 3.0-5.0 with a shelf life of 2 years** Q and stored at 4°C. Spontaneous hydrolysis occurs in alkaline or warm conditions.

Metabolism

- Sch is the ***only depolarizing (non-competitive) muscle relaxant***Q in clinical use. It is a *long, thin, flexible* molecule composed of 2 *acetylcholine (Ach) molecules* linked back to back through acetate-methyl group. Because of similar (copycat) structure, Sch (like ACh) *stimulates cholinergic receptors at NM junction & at nicotinic (ganglionic) and muscarinic autonomic sites*, thereby opening the ion channels in Ach receptor and depolarize the post synaptic membrane. Although its *effect is more persistent than Ach*, which is metabolized much more rapidly by Ach-esterase (acetylcholinesterase).
- It is the only neuromuscular blocker with a **rapid onset of action (30-60 seconds)** and **ultrashort (shortest) duration of action (3-5 min; typically < 10 min)**. Its rapid onset effect is *mainly d/t its low lipid solubility* (all MRs are highly charged & water soluble) and *relatively overdose that is administered*. The short duration of action is d/t rapid hydrolysis by **butyrylcholinesterase** (also k/a ***plasma cholinesterase or pseudocholinesterase***Q).
- Butyrylcholinesterase hydrolyzes Sch into succinylmonocholine & choline so efficiently that *only a small fraction (10%) of injected drug ever reaches the neuromuscular junction*. The initial metabolite, succinylmonocholine, is a much weaker neuromuscular blocking agent (than Sch) & is slowly metabolized to *succinic acid & choline*. As there is no or little pseudocholinesterase at NMJ, the blockade of Sch is *terminated by its diffusion away from the NMJ back into circulation* when drug serum level falls. Therefore pseudocholinesterase, influences the onset & duration of action of Sch by controlling the rate at which the drug is hydrolyzed before it reaches & after it leaves NMJ. The duration of action is prolonged by *abnormal metabolism (d/t hypothermia, low pseudocholinesterase levels or genetically aberrant enzyme*) and *high doses*; although increasing the dose does not result in prolongation of effect of the same magnitude as with nondepolarizing MR.

Pseudocholinesterase & Dibucaine Number

- Butyrylcholinesterase is *synthesized by liver and found in plasma*. Normal serum level is 800ml & is not found in CSF, RBC & nerves. Sch block is prolonged by decreased concentration or activity of enzyme. ***Factors lowering pseudocholinesterase activity*** *are liver disease, renal failure, pregnancy, advanced age, burn, malnutrition* and drug therapies like *Oral contraceptive pills*, phenelzine *(MAO inhibitor), ecothiophate* (organophosphate used ofr glucoma), *neostigmine & pyridostigmine (cholinesterase inhibitors or anticholinesterase drugs), pancuronium* (NDMR), esmolol (β blocker), cyclophosphamide (antineoplastic), tetrahydroaminacrine, hexafluorenium & metoclopramide (antiemetic or prokinetic) and bambuterol (prodrug of terbutaline). Whereas, histamine type 2 receptor antagonist have no effect. However, this is of **little concern in clinical practice** because *even large decreases in pseudocholinesterase activity results in only moderate increase in the duration of action of Sch (2-20 minutes).*
- **Dibucaine,** a local anesthetic, **inhibits normal butyrylcholinesterase to a far greater extent (80%) than it inhibits the abnormal enzyme (20%).** Succinylcholine induced neuromuscular blockade is significantly prolonged if the patient has an abnormal genetic variant of butrylcholinesterase (pseudocholinesterase). **Dibucaine number** indicates the *percentage of inhibition of pseudocholinesterase (butyrylcholinesterase) enzyme activity by local anesthetic dibucaine* and it is a measure of **qualitative** activity of pseudocholinesterase. The dibucaine number indicates the genetic make up of an individual with respect to butyrylcholinesterase, it ***does not measure the concentration of enzyme in plasma, nor does it indicate the efficiency of enzyme in hydrolyzing substrate succinylcholine or mivacurium***Q. Both are determined by measuring butyrylcholinesterase activity, which may be influenced by genotype. ***So dibucaine number is proportional to enzyme function (quality) and independent of amount of enzyme (i.e. quantity)***Q. In other words adequacy of pseudocholinesterase enzyme can be determined qualitatively by dibucaine number (major factor) and quantitatively in units per liter (minor factor).

Potentiation (+) & Resistance (-) of NM Blocking Drugs

Drugs	Depolarizing Block	Nondeplarizing Block
Magnesium sulfate (used to treat preeclampsia & eclampsia), **local anesthetics** (high dose), **volatile inhalational anesthetics** (sp. isoflurane), antiarrhythmics **(quinidine, CCB)** & antibiotics (streptomycin, aminoglycoside, kanamycin, neomycin, clindamycin, lincomycin, tetracycline, polymyxin, colistin)	+	-
Lithium	+	?
Ketamine, Dantrolene	?	+
Anticonvulsants (phenytoin, valproate, carbamazepine, primidone)	?	-
Cholinesterase inhibitor	+	-

Side Effects

- Sch is a relatively safe drug but *b/o risk of hyperkalemia, rhabdomyolysis and cardiac arrest (profound bradycardia) in children with undiagnosed myopathies*, Sch is considered contraindicated in routine management of children & adolescent.
- Side effects of sch include an increase in (Mn– "**Music KIT**")

- ***Muscle tone (masseter spasm)***Q
- ***Muscle fasciculations (signal onset of paralysis)*** Q
- ***Muscle pains (ache or soreness) or myalgig (most common complication)***Q
- K+ i.e. ***hyperkalamia l/t diastolic cardiac arrest refractory to CPR***Q
- Introcular, intracranial, intra abdominal, intragastric pressure and opening pressure of lower oesophageal sphincter (all increased)
- Temperature (ie l/t ***malignant hyperthermia*** Q)

Dibucaine number and fluoride no indicates the percentage of enzyme function inhibited.

- **Plasma cholinesterase level** is a quantitative measure of this enzyme. Plasma cholinesterase should not be confused with *cholinesterase activity which is the assessment of RBC or erythrocyte cholinesterase*. The combination of plasma cholinesterase level and dibucaine number can differentiate genetic from non genetic causes of prolonge apnea after Sch use.
- **Normal individuals** are **homozygous** for **wild type (more normal enzyme)** and have **80 dibucaine number because their plasma cholinesterase is 80% inhibited by dibucaine. Homozygous for atypical genes (ie more quantity of atypical pseudocholinesterase) have a dibucaine number of 20 because of 20% inhibition.** These patients have **prolonged Sch induced NM blockade.** Hetrozygous have 60 DN because of 60% inhibition.

Pseudocholin-esterase type	Genotype	Incidence	Dibucaine number	Response to substrate Sch or Mivacurium
Homozygous typical	$E_1^U E_1^U$	Normal	**70-80**	***Nomral***Q
Heterozygous atypical	$E_1^U E_1^a$	1/500	50-60	Lengthened by 50-100%
Homozygous atypical	$E_1^a E_1^a$	1/3200	20-30	***Prolonged for 4-8 hours***Q

Mn:
- **High dibucaine number (80)** means **high quantity normal and low quantity atypical pseudocholinesterase = normal response to Sch/mivacurium.**
- **Low dibucaine number (<30) means low quantity normal & high quantity atypical pseudocholinesterase = prolonged Sch/mivacurium block.**

- Of the recognized abnormal pseudocholinesterose genes, *dibucaine resistant (1/100 activity), fluoride resistant and silent (no activity)* are common. ***Prolonged paralysis from succinylcholine caused by atypical (abnormal) pseudocholinesterase should be treated with continued mechanical ventilation until muscle fasciculation returns to normal***Q. ***Anticholinesterases neostigmine & pyridostigmine are avoided***Q, as these may prolong the effect of Sch.

Dual/Biphasic Block

- Usual adult dose of Sch is ***1-1.5 mg/kg intravenously***Q. Because of *nonlipid solubility*, Sch distribution is limited to the *extracellular space*. Therefore *dosage for pediatric patients (neonates & infants) are often greater (in mg/kg) than for adults* as they have a larger extra cellular space (per kg) than adults. Sch produces a characteristic *depolarizing (phase I) block at usual dosage* that is a/w ***absence of fade in response to train of four and tetanic stimulation, absence of post tetanic facilitation and increased block in presence of anticholinesterase drugs***Q. It is important to note that although anticholinesterase drugs reverse nondepolarizing paralysis, they markedly prolong a phase I depolarizing block. And *small doses of non-depolarizing relaxants antagonize the effect of Sch (phase I block)*. The transition from phase I depolarizing block to phase II nondepolarizing block is gradual and usually occurs after ***administration of large doses (7-10mg/kg)***Q or *prolonged exposure (30-60 minutes)* of Sch. The recovery from phase II block is much slower. So Sch causes ***dual or biphasic block***Q.

Features	Phase I	Transition	Phase II
Tetanic stimulation (fade)	No	Slight	Fade
Train four fade	No	Moderate	Marked
Post tetanic facilitation	No	Slight	Yes
Train of 4 ratio	>0.7	0.4-0.7	< 0.4
Tachyphylaxis	No	Yes	Yes
Dose required (mg/kg)	2-3	4-5	>6Q
Edrophonium	Augments	Little effect	Antagonizes
Recovery	Rapid	Rapid-slow	***Increasingly prolonged***Q

- Sch can increase or decrease BP and heart rate. At low doses it produces *negative chrono and ino-tropic effects* but higher doses usually *increase heart rate and contractility* and elevate circulating *catecholomine* levels. ***Sinus bradycardias, nodal (junctional rhythms and ventricular dysrhythmias***Q also occur. Children are particularly susceptible to **profound bradycardia,** which may occur in adults only if a 2nd bolus of sch is given in ~3-8 min after first dose (because sucuinylmonocholine sensitizes muscarinic cholinergic receptors in SA node to 2nd dose of Sch). **Intravenous atropine** is prophylactically, given to children prior to first dose and always before a 2nd dose
- Side effects esp **myalgia and fasciculation** can be prevented by precurarization, self taming with iv scoline, iv lignocaine and faster infusion. But pretreatment **with small doses of nondeplarizing relaxant** (eg. rocuronium) ***remain the most commonly used method***Q
- Sch may increase serum K^+ by 0.5 mEq/L normally which can be **life threatening in** patients with *pre-existing hyperkalemia, renal failure, extensive burn, massive trauma (7-10 days after injury); skeletal muscle disease, neurological disorders, (GB syndrome, stroke, severe Parkinson's ds, ruptured cerebral aneurysm, closed head injury, polyneuropathy, spinal cord injury, myopathy (Duchenne's), encephalitis, tetanus, severe intraabdominal infections, hemorrhagic shock with metabolic acidosis and prolonged total body immobilization*. Subsequent **cardiac arrest** may be refractory to routine CPR requiring calcium, insulin, glucose, bicarbonate, epinephrine, cation – exchange resin, dantrolene, & even cardiopulmonary bypass to reduce metabolic acidosis & serum K^+ levels.
- *Malignant Hyperpyrexia* is autosomal dominant condition precipitated specially in Muscular dystrophies as Duchene, *causing persistant muscle contraction and heat production d/t intra cellular release of Ca^{++} from sarcoplasmic reticulum.*Q Predisposing conditions for M.H. are - *Muscle disorder Ex.* ***Duchene ms dystrophy***Q, ***Halothane***Q and ***Succinyl choline***Q Treatment of Malignant Hyperpyrexia is - ***Dantrolene***Q, Bromocriptene and External Cooling
- S/E of scoline (esp. myalgia) can be prevented by – Precurarization, Self taming with IV Scoline, IV lignocaine, Faster infusion. ***Small dose of non depolarizing relaxant remain the most commonly used method.***Q

Mivacurium

- *As with other non depolarizing blockers, increase in dose increases the rapidity of onset of neuromuscular block*[Q].
- It is the *shortest acting non depolirizing muscle relaxant*[Q]. The increase in the duration of action with increasing dose is not as marked as with other non depolarizing blockers. As in the case of other non depolarizing relaxants, spontaneous recovery is slower in the presence of isoflurane (potent volatile anesthetic)
- Repeat infusion or bolus dose not significantly change recovery profile, suggesting *minimal cumulation*
- *Mivacurium has tendency for histamine release thus reducing arterial (blood) pressure & systemic vascular resistannce*[Q], even in clinically useful doses. And causing *tachycardia, bronchospasm & flushing*[Q].
- Duration of action is increased in *elderly & marked hepatic & renal disease* d/t reduction in plasma cholinesterase activity. The prolongation is significantly marked in individuals with homozygous silent or atypical gene or atypical plasma cholinesterase variants.

It is a mixture of 3 stercoisomers :

- *2- Short acting cis – trans & trans-transisomer*
  - constitute 94% of mixture, have half lives of 2min, almost entirely broken down by plasma cholinesterase with a high rate of clearance & short duration of action
- *1-long acting cis- cis isomer*
  - Has about one – tenth the (N- M blocking) potency of the other two isomers.
  - Under goes *some renal excretion* & also being broken down by *plasma cholinesterase* with a half life of about *50 min.*

2

ANAESTHESIA

Atracurium/Cisatracurium

Metabolism

- Only 45% atracurium is eliminated by Hofmann degradation, 10% by ester hydrolysis and remaining by metabolism or excretion by liver & / or kidney. ***Like atracurium, cisatracurium undergoes Hoffmann elimination (77%) but produces lesser amount of laudanosine.***[Q] But ***nonspecific ester hydrolysis do not appear to be involved in metabolism of cisatracurium***[Q].
- **Organ independent spontaneous degradation (or Hofmann elimination)** is purely a *chemical process* that results in *loss of positive (+) charges by molecular fragmentation* producing **laudanosine** (a tertiary amine) and a monoquarternary **acrylate** at physiological pH & temperature. These breakdown products may actually be used to synthesize the parent compound under proper chemical conditions.
- **Ester hydrolysis** of atracurium by *non specific esterases* (not acetylcholine esterase or pseudocholinesterase) produces a *monoquarternary alcohol,* which also undergoes *hofmann degradation* to laudanosise.
- *2 molecules of laudanosise* are produced from break down of one molecule of atracurium – *1 mol. from Hofmann degradation* & *1 mol. from ester hydrolysis.*
- Cisatracurium is 4 times more potent stereoisomer of atracurium. Atracurium contains ~15% cisatracurium. ***Because of 4-5 times greater potency & so 4-5 times lesser amount of used drug***[Q]***. Laudanoside levels are much less when cisatracurium, rather than atracurium is given by continuous infusion to critically ill patients with renal dysfunction in ICU. So ciatracurium is neuromuscular blocking agent of choice for critically ill patients needing infusion of relaxant for several days***[Q].
- At *physiological PH & temperature,* atracurium is eliminated by *spontaneous nonenzymatic organ independent degradation* through **Hofmann elimination** and **ester hydrolysis**. Hofmann degradation is considered as' ***safety net in the sick patient with imparied liver or renal function , as atracurium will still be cleared from the body***[Q].
- The unique metabolism of atracurium makes it ***suitable for use in the critically ill patient as it is associated with a rapid recovery***[Q]. This is even true in ***renal failure & liver failure (cirrhosis)***[Q].
- ***Spontaneous recovery occurs reliably from an atracurium neuromuscular block***[Q]. Repeated administration of atracurium does not l/t an increase in the duration of action

Difference

Atracurium	Cisatracurium
Atracurium besylate is a synthetic bisquaternary benzylisoquinolinium nondepolarizing neuromuscular blocking drug (ND-NMBD). It is a mixture of *10 optical isomers.*	Cisatracurium is benzylisoquinolinium ND-NMBD. It is *one of the 10 isomers of atracurium.* Cisatracurium is **1R cis-1′ R cis isomer** of atracurium. Atracurium contains **~15%** cisatracurium.
ED_{95} = 0.22 mg/kg is ~4 times greater than ED_{95} of cisatracurium, which means 4 times more atracurium is required to produce same effect (i.e. atracurium is **less potent**).	ED_{95} = 0.05 mg/kg or 50 µg/kg, making it abut **4 times more potent** than atracurium. Being more potent, the drug has slightly *longer onset & duration of action* (i.e. **slower onset & longer duration**)
Metabolized by organ-independent spontaneous degradation by **Hofmann elimination** (45%) and **ester-hydrolysis** (by non specific esterases not acetylcholinesterase or pseudocholinesterase). Both accounting for 60-90% metabolism. So 10-40% (a/t Fischer 60%) of total clearance occur via other pathways, presumably by *metabolism or excretion by kidney (<10 - 40%) or liver.*	More cisatracurium is metabolized by **Hofmann degradation (~77%)**. In contrast, however there is **no ester hydrolysis**. 23% of drug is eliminated through organ dependent means with renal elimination accounting for 16%
4-5 times more laudanosine is produced[Q].	Because of 4-5 times greater potency (& so 4-5 times lesser drug being administered); *4-5 times lesser metabolites (laudanosine & mono quaternary acrylate)* are produced.
Atracurium triggers **dose dependent histamine release** that becomes significant at doses > 0.5 mg/kg giving transient hypotension & tachycardia a/w facial & truncal flushing. Atracurium may also cause a *transient drop in systemic vascular*	Cisatracurium is ***devoid of histamine releasing effects***[Q], therefore is a/w ***greater cardiovascular stability***[Q]. It does not affect heart rate or BP, nor does it produce autonomic effects even at rapid & large IV doses (>8 times of ED_{95}).

- The reversal of an atracurium block can be easily accompalished by neostigmine or endrophonium; however the later is not reliable if the block is relatively deep.
- Possible adverse effect of atracurium are –

resistance & an increase in cardiac index independent of any histamine release, which can be minimized by slow rate of injection.	

Laudanosine related seizure activity & toxicity

- Laudanosine is *more lipid soluble* than atracurium; it is metabolized in liver and also excreted unchanged in urine. Unlike atracurium, laudanosine *is dependent on liver (bile) & kidney for its elimination* and has a long elimination half life. Laudanosine *freely crosses the blood brain barrier,* has *CNS stimulating property* resulting in *elevation of MAC and even seizures.* It enhances the stimulation evoked release of norepinephrine (partly accounting for CNS excitation). Laudanosine concentrations are elevated in patients with *liver disease & those who have received atracurium for many hours in ICU.*
- At concentrations *above 17 μgML^{-1}*, it produces ***epileptiform fits,*** (in animals) as it has slow renal elimination & crosses blood brain barrier. Although this complication ***has never been reported in humans***[Q].
- Laudinosine may have cardiovascular effect (sever hypotension & bradycardia) at higher concentration (only one case reported).

Histamine Release

- Observed in upto 40% giving transient *hypotension and tachycardia associated with facial & truncal flushing.*
- Local wheal or flare around the injection site especially if a small vein is used.
- Atracurium has minimal cardio vascular effects except for some histamine liberation, if the drug is *given rapidly or in high doses.*
- This can be prevented by injecting the drug slowly over 75 seconds, reducing the dose, or prior treatment with chlorpheniramine & cimetidine intravenously.

Anaphylaxis

- ***Neuromuscular blocking drugs are the commonest***[Q] cause of anaphylactic reaction. ***Succinyl choline is the most common culprit***[Q]
- Common drugs l/t anaphylaxis are – Sch, alcuronium, ***atracurium***[Q], thiopental, alfathesin, d- TC, gallamine, pancuronium vecuronium, hemexccel, & cephazolin etc
- It presents with *cardiovascular collapse (eg. no pulse), bronchospasm (cough, asthma), cutaneous manifestations (eg. erythema, angioedema, rash, urticaria),* generalized edema, pulmonary edema & gastrointestinal disturbance.

Others

- Atracurium should be *avoided in asthmatic patients* b/o risk of *severe bronchospasm.* Atracurium's duration of action may be prolonged by hypothermia & to lesser extent by *acidosis.* Atracurium will *precipitate as free acid* if it is mixed into IV line containing alkaline solutions *(as thiopental).* Except for bronchospasm, cisatracurium also shares same sensitivity for pH, temperature & chemical incompatibility.

QUESTIONS

1. **Which of the following is the neuromuscular blocking agent with the shortest onset of action?** *(AIIMS May 06)* *(DNB 01)*
   A. Mivocurium ☐
   B. Vecuronium ☐
   C. Rapacuronium ☐
   D. Succinylcholine ☐
2. **Site of action of vecuronium is** *(AIIMS 06, AI 12)*
   A. Cerebrum ☐
   B. RAS ☐
   C. Motor neuron (ganglion) or motor end plate ☐
   D. Myo-neural junction ☐
3. **Which ones are Non-Depolaring Muscle Relaxants:**
   A. Mivacurium *(PGI Nov 09, DNB 03)* ☐
   B. Halothane ☐
   C. Desflurane ☐
   D. Isoflurane ☐
   E. Ether ☐
4. **Neostigmine is used for reversing the adverse effect of:**
   A. dTC + pancuronium *(PGI 1997)* ☐
   B. d TC only ☐
   C. Alcuronium only ☐
   D. Ketamine complication ☐
5. **All of the following statements about neuromuscular blockage produced by succinylcholine are true, Except**
   A. No fade on Train of four stimulation *(AI 2010)* ☐
   B. Fade on titanic stimulation ☐
   C. No post titanic facilitation ☐
   D. Train of four ratio >0.4 ☐
6. **Features of depolarising neuromuscular blocking agents are all / except** *(PGI 2K, JIPMER 99, DNB 02)*
   A. Cause muscle fascicutation ☐
   B. No fade ☐
   C. No post tetanic facilitation ☐
   D. Isoflurane potentiates ☐
   E. Reversed by neostigmine ☐
7. **For non depolarization block which of the following statement is correct** *(AIIMS 93, PGI 99)*
   A. Post tetanic potentiation is seen ☐
   B. Tetanic fade is absent ☐
   C. Train of four is absent ☐
   D. Anticholinergic drugs potentiation of block ☐
8. **Train of four' is characteristically used in concern with**
   A. Malignat hyperthermia *(AI 08)* ☐
   B. Non-depolarizing neuromuscular blockers ☐
   C. Mechanical ventilation ☐
   D. To check hemodynamic parameters ☐
9. **Muscle most resistant to non depolarizing block is**
   A. Intercostal *(Jipmer 03, DNB 05)* ☐
   B. Abdominal ☐
   C. Diaphragm ☐
   D. Adductors. ☐
10. **True about non-depolarizing muscle relaxants :**
    A. Competitive inhibitor of acetylcholine ☐
    B. Metabolised by pseudocholinesterase ☐
    C. Mg^{2+} predisposes the block *(PGI 05, DNB 06)* ☐
    D. Ca^{2+} antagonizes the block ☐
    E. Hypothermia prolongs the block ☐

SUCCINYLCHOLINE

11. **Suxamethonium is available as a clear, colourless aqueous solutions. The shelf-life of suxamethonium is:**
    A. 6 months *(AIIMS May 13)* ☐
    B. 1 year ☐
    C. 2 years ☐
    D. 3 years ☐
12. **Shortest acting muscle relaxant** *(AI 1992)*
    A. Succinyl choline ☐
    B. d-TC ☐
    C. Gallamine ☐
    D. Ketamine ☐
13. **Phase II blocker is seen in:** *(PGI 98, AIIMS 99)*
    A. D-TC ☐
    B. Cocaine ☐
    C. Scoline ☐
    D. Vencuronium, ether, N_2O ☐
14. **Which muscle relaxant increases intracranial pressure?**
    A. Mivacurium *(AIIMS 2002)* ☐
    B. Atracurium ☐
    C. Suxamethonium ☐
    D. Vecuronium ☐
15. **Muscle pain after anaesthesia is caused by:**
    A. Vecuronium *(PGI 1999)* ☐
    B. D-tubocurare ☐
    C. Suxamethonium ☐
    D. All ☐
16. **Post anesthetic mucsle soreness is caused by**
    A. Gallamine *(AIIMS 1994)* ☐
    B. d-TC ☐
    C. Suxamethonium ☐
    D. Dantrolene ☐
17. **Post operative muscle ache is caused by**
    A. D-Tubocurarine *(AI 1991)* ☐
    B. Suxamethonium ☐
    C. Gallamine ☐
    D. Poncuronium ☐
18. **True about scoline are following except:**
    A. Fasciculations *(PGI 1997)* ☐
    B. ICT increases ☐
    C. Non depolarising neuro muscular blocker ☐
    D. Short acting muscle relaxant ☐
19. **Fasciculation are caused by** *(AI 1997)*
    A. Suxamethonium ☐
    B. Pancuronium ☐
    C. d-TC ☐
    D. Vecuronium ☐
20. **Bradycardia is common after injection of:**
    A. Midazolam *(AIIMS NOV 05, DNB 07)* ☐
    B. Succinyl choline ☐
    C. Dopamine ☐
    D. Isoprenaline ☐
21. **Drugs metabolized by cholinesterase-**
    A. Succinylcholine *(PGI Dec 04)* ☐
    B. Mivacurium ☐
    C. Esmolol ☐
    D. Remifentanyl ☐
    E. Ketamine ☐
22. **All of the following statements are incorrect about the treatment of prolonged suxamethonium apnoea due to plasma cholinesterase deficiency (after a single dose of suxamethonium) except-** *(AIIMS NOV 2004)*
    A. Reversal with incremental doses of neostigmine ☐
    B. Continue anaesthesia and mechanical ventilation till recovery ☐
    C. Transfussion of fresh frozen plasma ☐

D. Plasmapheresis ☐

23. A 70 kg old athlete was posted for surgery, Patient was administered succinylcholine due to unavailability of vecuronium. It was administered in intermittent dosing (total 640 mg). During recovery patient was not able to respire spontaneously & move limbs. What is the explanation –
A. Pseudocholinesterase deficiency increasing action of syccinylcholine (AIIMS Nov 2010) ☐
B. Phase 2 blockade produced by succinylcholine ☐
C. Undiagnosed muscular dystrophy and muscular weakness ☐
D. Muscular weakness due to fasciculation produced by succinylcholine ☐

24. Myasthenics are resistant to following muscle relaxant : (PGI 2000)
A. Suxamethonium ☐
B. Pancurium ☐
C. Atracuronium ☐
D. Vecuronium ☐

25. Regarding Mysthenia true about senstivity to curare and Scoline is (AIIMS 1994)

	Curare	Scoline	
A.	↓	↑	☐
B.	↓	Normal	☐
C.	↑	Normal	☐
D.	↑	↓	☐

26. Regarding **scoline** apnoea all are true except
A. Caused by suxamethonium (AIIMS May 12) ☐
B. Cab be inherited ☐
C. Deficiency of cholinesterase ☐
D. Mortality is very low in recent times with proper management ☐

MIVACURIUM

27. Shortest acting non depolarizing muscle relaxant
A. Mevacurium (AI 03, AIIMS 98) ☐
B. Vercuronium ☐
C. Atracurium ☐
D. Succynil Choline ☐

28. Mivacurium when given in high doses, all are true except
A. Bronchospasm (AIIMS Nov 07) ☐
B. Hypertension ☐
C. Flushing ☐
D. Increase in dose increases the rapididity of onset ☐

ATRACURIUM

29. Dose of which of the following muscle relaxant has to be calculated on the basis of total body weight of an obese person rather than its ideal weight? (AIIMS Nov 12)
A. Atracurium ☐
B. Vecuronium ☐
C. Pancuronium ☐
D. Rocuronium ☐

30. All of the following drugs are eliminated by kidney except- (AIIMS Nov 2004)
A. Pancuronium bromide ☐
B. Atracurium besylate ☐
C. Vecuronium bromide ☐
D. Pipecuronium ☐

31. Which of the following skeletal muscle relaxants undergo Hoffman's elimination?
A. Atracurium (PGI June 07, 99, 98) ☐
B. Cis-atracurium ☐
C. Mivacurium ☐
D. Vecuronium ☐

32. A patient with bilirubin value of 8mg/dl and serum creatinine of 1.9 mg/dl is planned for surgery. What is the muscle relaxant of choice in this patient:
A. Vecuronium (AI 2010) ☐
B. Pancuronium ☐
C. Atracurium ☐
D. Rocuronium ☐

33. Muscle relaxant of choice in hepatic and renal failure
A. Cisatracurium (AIIMS May 07) ☐
B. Rocuronium ☐
C. Vecuronium ☐
D. Rapacuronium ☐

34. Muscle relaxant used in renal failure :
A. Ketamine (PGI 1999, 97) ☐
B. Atracurium ☐
C. Pancuronium ☐
D. Fentanyl ☐

35. An ICU patient on atracurium infusion develops seizures after 2 days. The most probable cause is: (AI 2006)
A. Accumulation of landonosine ☐
B. Allergy to drug ☐
C. Due to prolong infusion ☐

36. Cis atracurium is prefferd over atracurium due to advantage of - (AIIMS May 2011)
A. Rapid onset ☐
B. Short duration of action ☐
C. No histamine release ☐
D. Less cardiodepressant ☐

37. Laudanosine is metabolite of - (AIIMS May 2011)
A. Cisatracurium ☐
B. Atracurium ☐
C. Pancuronium ☐
D. Gallamine ☐

38. A 21 year old lady with a history of hypersensitivity to neostigmine is posted for an elective caesarean section under general anesthesia. The best muscle relaxant of choice in this patient should be: (AIIMS May 2004)
A. Pancuronium ☐
B. Atracurium ☐
C. Rocuronium ☐
D. Vecuronium ☐

39. The ideal muscle relaxant used for a neonate undergoing porto-enterostomy for biliary atresia is: (AIIMS 2003)
A. Atracurium. ☐
B. Vecuronium ☐
C. Pancuronium. ☐
D. Rocuronium. ☐

40. At the end of a balanced anaesthesia technique with non-depolarizing muscle relaxant, a patient recovered spontaneously from the effect of muscle relaxant without any reversal. Which is the most probable relaxant the patient had received. (AI 2003)
A. Pancuronium ☐
B. Gallamine ☐
C. Atracurium ☐
D. Vecuronium ☐

d-TC

41. True about d-TC is all except: (PGI 1998)
A. Excreted unchaged by kidney ☐
B. Causes hypotension by ganglion blocking action ☐
C. Vagolytic action ☐
D. Effects lasts for 2-3 hours. ☐

42. The drug used for d-Tc reversal is
A. Atropine (AI 1991) ☐

B. Atracurium
C. Diazepalm
D. Neostigmine

PANCURONIUM

43. Intubation dose of pancuronium *(AIIMS 1993)*
A. 0.02 mg/Kg
B. 0.04 mg/Kg
C. 0.06 mg/Kg
D. 0.08 mg/Kg

44. A 25 year old overweight female was given fentanyl-pancuronium anesthesia for surgery. After surgery and extubation she was observed to have limited movement of the upper body and chest wall in the recovery room. She was conscious and alert but voluntary respiratory effort was limited. Her blood pressure and heart rate were normal. The likely diagnosis is: *(AI 2010)*
A. Incomplete reversal of pancuronium
B. Pulmonary embolism
C. Fentanyl induced chest wall rigidity
D. Respiratory depression

VECURONIUM

45. Which of the following statement is not correct for vencuronium *(AIIMS 2002)*
A. It has high incidence of cardiovascular side effects
B. It has short duration of neuromuscular block
C. In usual doses the dose adjustment is not required in kidney disease
D. It has high liphophilic property.

46. Cardiovascular side effects are minimal with: *(PGI Dec 06, 02)*
A. Pancuronium
B. Rocuronium
C. Doxacurium
D. Vecuronium
E. Mivacurium

47. Which of the following muscle relaxant can cause pain on IV injection Site *(AI 12)*
A. Succinyl choline
B. Vecuronium
C. Rocuronium
D. Pancuronium

GALLAMINE

48. Muscle Relaxant excreted exclusively by Kidney *(AIIMS 1998)*
A. Gallamine
B. Atracurium
C. Vercuronium
D. Sch

49. Muscle relaxant contra indicated in Renal faliure is *(AI 99, 95, 91)*
A. Gallamine
B. d-TC
C. Vecuronium
D. Atracurium

50. Muscle Relaxant most sensitive to patient of mysthenia gravis (M.G.) *(AI 1993)*
A. Scoline
B. Neostigmine
C. Gallamine
D. Decamethonium

51. Muscle relaxant with ganglion blocker action are A/E *(AIIMS 1993)*
A. Pancuronium
B. Trimethaphan
C. Curare
D. Halothane

ALCURONIUM

52. Drug causing anaphylactoid reaction : *(PGI 1998)*
A. Propofol
B. Alcuronium
C. Thiopentone
D. Glycopyrrolate

2

ANAESTHESIA

Answers and Explanations:

1. **D i.e. Succinylcholine** *[Ref: Lee's 13/e p-188; Aitkenhead 4/e, P- 225- 30; Wiley & Davidson 7/e p-583- 94; Morgan's 4/e p. 218; Miller's 7/e p-876]*

Succinyl choline has ***most rapid onset of action*** and ***shortest duration of course***Q

2. **D i.e. Myo-neural junction** 3. **A i.e. Mivacurium** 4. **A i.e. dTC + Pancuronium**

As d-TC & Panduronium, both are non-depolarizing muscle relaxant, so neostigmine is used to reverse the drugs.

5. **B i.e. Fade on titanic stimulation** 6. **E i.e. Reversed by neostigmine**
7. **A i.e. Post titanic potentiation is seen** 8. **B i.e., Nondepolarizing neuromuscular blockers**

[Ref: Miller 7/e p. 867; Lee's Anesthesia 13/e p-182-84; Wiley & Davidson 7/e p-282-86; 583 -94; Aitkenhead 4/e, P- 227-33; Morgan's 4/e p. 206–15]

Post titanic stimulation, and fade on titanic stimulation & train of fourQ is a characteristic feature present in **non depolarizing block** or **phase II block**.

Succinyl choline is typically a **depolarizing neuromuscular blocker** that classically presents with features of depolarizing or **phase I block**. However, when administered at high doses (>500 mg) or over a long period, it causes **dual** or **biphasic block** i.e. phase I followed by phase II (or non depolarizing) block. This transition occurs from desensitization of receptors to acetylcholine. During transition from phase I to phase II dose is 4-5 mg/kg and train of four ratio is 0.4-0.7.

9. **C i.e. Diaphragm**
10. **A i.e. Competitive inhibitor of acetylcholine; C i.e. Mg^{2+} predisposes the block; D i.e. Ca^{2+} antagonizes the block; E i.e. Hypothermia prolongs the block**

Non-Depolarizing Neuromuscular Block

- Non-depolariszing muscle relaxants are ***competitive blockers of ACh receptors on NMJ***Q. They don't cause depolarization.
- Among non-depolarizing blockers only, ***mivacuronium is metabolized by pseudocholineaterase***Q.
- Block is reversed by neostigmine and other anticholinesterases.
- Block is ***potentiated by hypokalemia and Mg^{+2}*** Q
- ***Ca^{+2} increases the release of ACh from nerve endings;thus partially antagonizes the block*** Q
- Acodosis increases the duration and degree of block.
- ***Mild cooling antagonize the block but greater cooling (<33°C) potentiates block.*** Q

Succinylcholine

11. **C ie 2 years**
12. **A i.e. Succinylcholine** 13. **C i.e. Scoline** 14. **C i.e. Suxamethonium**
15. **C i.e. Suxamethonium** 16. **C i.e. Suxamethonium** 17. **B i.e. Suxamethonium**
18. **C i.e. Nondepolarizing neuromuscular blocker** 19. **A i.e. Suxamethonium** 20. **B i.e. Succinylcholine**
21. **A, B i.e. Succinylcholine, Mivacurium** 22. **B i.e. Continue anesthesia & mechanical ventilation till recovery**
23. **B i.e. Phase 2 blockade produced by succinylcholine** *[Ref: Miller 7/e p. 862-67; Morgan's 4/e p 210-15; Wylie 7/e p. 584-86; Lee 13/e p 181-91; Stoelting 5/e p. 136-50; Aitkenhead 5/e p. 82-86]*

Suxamethonium chloride, a dicholine ester of acetyl choline, is a **clear, colourless aqueous solution of ph 3.0-5.0 with a shelf life of 2 years** Q and stored at 4°C. Spontaneous hydrolysis occurs in alkaline or warm conditions.

- Sch is ***depolarizing/ non competitive***Q M.R. with ***shortest duration of action***Q (3-5 min) d/t rapid hydrolysis by ***pseudo cholinesterase***Q. It causes **dual/ biphasic block**Q. It *increases K^+ (ie **hyperkalemia**Q l/t* diastolic cardiac arrest), *intraocular & intragastric pressure* and temperature *(l/t)* ***malignant Hyperthermia)***Q
- ***Depolarizing block (phase I & II)*** caused by ***Succinyl***

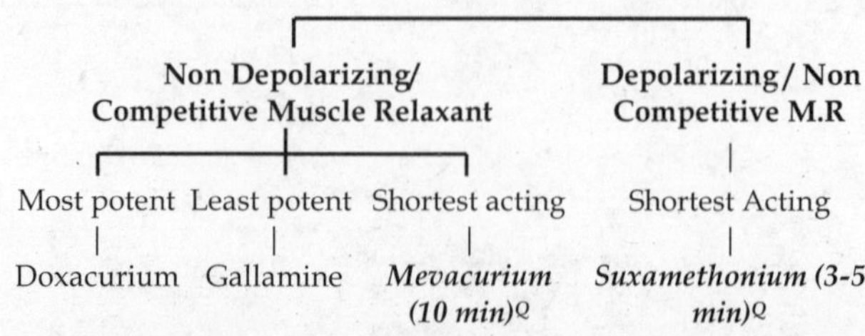

*choline*Q is also called **Dual or Biphasic Block**. In contrast to phase II depolarization block & Non depolarizing block, phase I depolarization block does not exhibit fade during tetanus or train-of-four, neither does it demonstrate post tetanic potentiation. Phase I block is potentiated by isoflurane, Mg, Li & Anticholine-esterase while phase II block is potentiated by enflurane.

- **The onset of paralysis by succinylcholine is signaled by visible motor unit contractions called fasciculation.**Q Patients who have received suxamethonium have an increased incidence of ***postoperative myalgia***Q. This is more common in *healthy female outpatients. Pregnancy & extremes of age* seem to be *protective*.
- **Succinylcholine** releases a metabolite **succinylmonocholine**, causing excitation of the cholinergic receptors in the sinoatrial node resulting in ***bradycardia.*** Q **Intravenous atropine** is given prophylactically (particularly in children, who are more susceptible) in *children* and always before a *second dose of sch.*

Succinylcholine (Suxamethonium) causes increase in
(a) ***Intracranial Pressure***Q
(b) ***Intraocular Pressure***Q
(c) ***Intra gastric pressure***Q

Rise in ICT dlt Sch use can be prevented by
(a) Good airway control & insulating hyperventilation
(b) Pretreatment with nondepolarizing muscle relaxant
(d) IV lidocaine 2-3 minutes prior to intubation

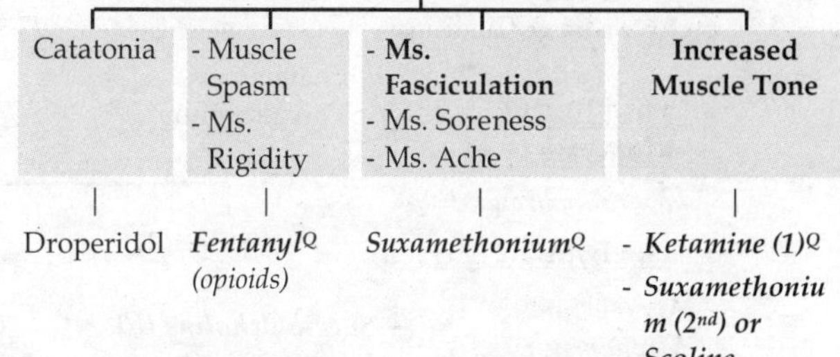

- Prolonged apnea after suxamethonium is best managed by providing ***mechanical ventilation, maintaining anesthesia and continuous monitoring until muscle function returns to normal.***Q Transfusion of fresh frozen plasma is beneficial (as it provides pseudocholinesterase) its infectious risks outweigh its potential benefits –*Morgan*
  Administration of purified pseudocholinesterase, blood or plasma may antagonize the block. However because of the risk associated with their use, infusion of banked blood or fresh frozen plasma cannot be recommended – *Churchill.*
- ***Succinylcholine & mivacurium are metabolized by pseudocholinesterase, while esmolol and remifentanyl are metabolized by RBC esterase.***Q
- **Pseudo cholinesterase deficiency** causes prolonged residual paralysis at ***normal Sch dose (1-2 mg/kg)***Q whereas, **phase 2 non-depolarization blockade** occurs after administration of **higher doses >6 (7-10) mg/kg**Q
- Despite large decrease in pseudo cholinesterase activity (level) there is only moderate increase in duration of action of Sch. In contrast to the doubling or tripling of blockade duration seen in patients with low pseudo cholinesterase enzyme levels or hetozygous atypical enzyme, patients with homozygous atypical enzyme will have a very blockade (4-8 hrs) following Sch administration.

24. **A i.e. Suxamethonium** **25.** **D i.e. ↑for curare & ↓ for Sch** *[Ref: Morgan's 3/e, P-747]*

In **Myasthenia gravis** response to

Succinyl choline (Depolarizing M.R.)	**Non depolarizing M.R. (ex d-TC)**
Unpredictable ie patients may manifest a *relative resistance*Q, prolonged effect or unusual response (phase II block)	***Increased sensitivity***Q (even a defasciculating dose can result in complete paralysis)

Mnemonic: "**R.D.** (Radio diagnosis) **No Seat**" i.e.
Resistance for Depolarising M.R.
Non depolarising M.R. has increased Sensitivity.

26. **C i.e. Deficiency of cholinesterase** *[Ref. Morgan 4/e, p 225]*

Scoline apnoea is prolonged residual paraysis after administration of succinyl choline (suxamethonium) l/t apnoca. It can be seen in patients with ***hereditary (inherited) atypical pseudochdinesterase enzyme (homozygous >>> heterozygous)***Q and ***phase II (non depolerizing) block***Q. ***Decreased level of normal pseudocholinestrerase (not choline esterase) enzyme***Q would usually not result in prolonged apnea unless the surgery was very short. In other words, in contrast to doubling or tripling of blockade duration seen in patients with heterozygous atypical enzyme or patients with low (normal/typical) enzyme levels, patients with homozygous atypical enzyme will have a very prolonged blockade (4-8 hrs) following Sch administration. ***Prolonged paralysis (apnoea) should be treated with continued mechanical ventilation until muscle function returns to normal which has reduced mortality to very low levels***Q.

Mivacurium

27. **A i.e. Mivacurium** **28.** **B i.e. Hypertension**
[Ref: Wylie – Anesthesia 7/e p- 590- 91; Miller 7/e p. 882; Morgan 4/e p – 221-22; Lee's 13/e ,p – 186, 190, 192]

- Shortest acting non-depolarizing muscle relaxant = *Mivacurium*[Q] (12-20 minutes)
- Shortest acting depolarising muscle relaxant = *Sch*[Q] (3-6 minutes)
- Overall shortest acting muscle relaxant = *Sch.*[Q]
- Shortest acting local anaesthetic = *Chlorprocaine*[Q]

- *Speed of onset is inversely proportional to the molar potency (ED_{95}) of nondepolarizing MR* (with the exception of atracurium). In other words, ***increase in dose of nondepolarizing blocker (like mivacurium), increases the rapidity of onset***[Q].
- Mivacurium has tendency for **histamine release** thus ***reducing systemic vascular resistance and BP (i.e. causes hypo-tension not hypertension)***[Q], increasing heart rate (tachycardia) and causing ***bronchospasm & flushing***[Q] (usually at higher doses).

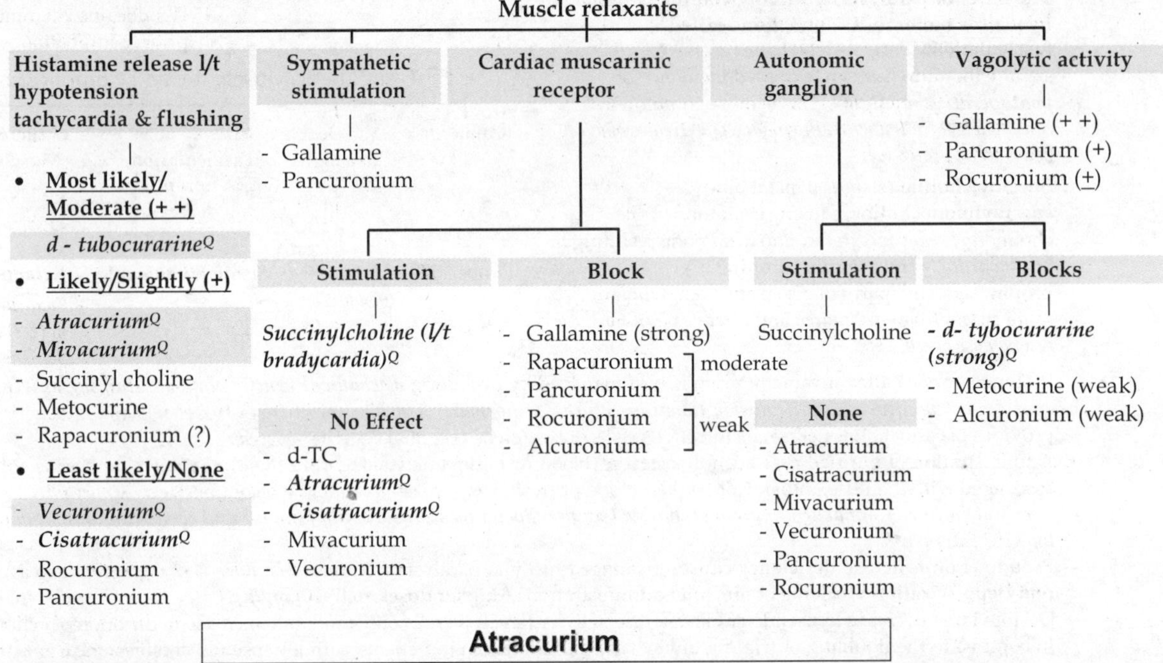

Atracurium

29. **A i.e. Atracurium** *[Ref: Goodman 12/e p. 263-65; http://ceaccp.oxfordjournals.org/4/5/152/T1.expansion.html; Oxford Journals Medicine BJA: CEACCP Volume 4 Article]*

In morbidly obese persons, doses of **atracurium, cisatracurium, succinyl choline, mivacurium,** *neostigmine, midazolam (intiation dose) and propofol (maintenance dose)* are calculated on the basis of ***total body weight (TBW)***; *dose of featanyl, alfentanyl or sufentanil* are calculated on the basis of total body weight *(TBW) or corrected weight (ie IBW + 0.4 × excess weight;) and* ***pancuronim, vecuronium, rocuronium***, remifentanil, morphine, paracetamol, propofol (induction dose) and midazolan (continuous dose) are calculated on the basis of **ideal body weight (IBW).**

30. **B i.e. Atracurium besylate** 31. **A i.e. Atracurium; B i.e. Cisatracurium** 32. **C i.e. Atracurium**
33. **A i.e. Cisatracurium** 34. **B i.e. Atracurium** 35. **A i.e. Accumulation of laudanosine**
36. **C i.e. No histamine release > D i.e. Less cardiodepressant**
37. **B i.e. Atracurium** *[Ref: Stoelting-Miller 5/e p. 144, 148, 149; Miller 7/e p. 881; Wylie 7/e p. 404-40, 590-89, 868-69; Irwin & Lee's 13/e p. 191-92; Morgan 4/e p. 220-21; Ripp's IC Medicine 6/e p. 226; Aitkenhead 5/e p. 87-88]*

- ***Laudanosine is mainly a metabolite of atracurium***[Q]. Because of 4-5 times greater potency its 4-5 times lower dose is needed to produce same effect. And therefore cisatracurium produces 4-5 times less plasma concentration of metabolites (eg. laudanosine) than equipment dose of atracurium.
- ***Being more potent, the cisatracurium has slightly longer onset & duration of action (i.e. slower onset and longer duration) than atracurium***[Q].

Drug	Duration	Hydrolysis in plasma	Hepatic degradation	Bilary excretion	Renal excretion (% unchanged)
Mivacurium	Short	Enzymatic (pseudocholinestarase)	NS	NS	NS (<10%)
Atracurium	Intermediate	Enzymatic (ester-hydrolysis) spontaneous (Hoffman's)	NS	NS	NS (10%)
Cisatracurium	Intermediate	Spontaneous (Hoff man's)	NS	NS	NS (15%)
Vacuronium	Intermediate	No	20-30%	40-75%	15-30%
Rocuronium	Intermediate	No	10-20%	50-70%	10-33%
Pancuronium	Long	No	10%	5-10%	80%

- Unlike atracurium, ***cisatracurium is devoid of dose dependent histamine releasing effects***[Q] and therefore is associated with greater cardiovascular stability.
- **Atracurium** and **Cisatracurium** undergoes ***spontaneous degredation by Hoffmann elimination*** [Q]. So its ***pharmacokinetics are independent of renal and hepatic functions***[Q]. ***Spontaneous recovery occurs reliably from atracurium/cisatracurium neuromuscular block***[Q].
- ***Atracurium/Cisatracurium > mivacurium are muscle relaxant of choice in patients with liver and renal disease (or failure)***[Q].
- Laudanosine concentration are elevated in ***patients with liver disease & those who received atracurium for hours***[Q] (in Q it is given for 2 days). At concentrations > 17µg/ml; it produces ***epileptiform fits (seizures)***[Q] in animals. Although it has never been reported in humans.

38. **B i.e. Atracurium**

You might be thinking that this Q has never been asked, but think a while and try to understand that around which concept the Q is based. In other words, they are trying to ask that which muscle relaxant will not require reversal? I think now you need no explanation

- In pancuronium reversal is often required d/t its longer duration of action
- Ve/Ro-curonium seldom require reversal unless repeated doses have been given
- **In atracurium & cis-atracurium** reversal is mostly not required due to its unique feature of ***spontaneous non eyzmatic degradation (Hoffmann elimination)*** [Q].

39. **A i.e. Atracurium**

In this case a muscle relaxant is required whose metabolism has nothing to do with liver (preferabely) & it should not be excreted through bile. The straight forward answer is *atracurium/cisatracurium* as these are inactivated in plasma by *spontaneous non enzymatic degradation (Hoffman elimination)* independant of hepatic or renal function and biliary or urinary exceretion.

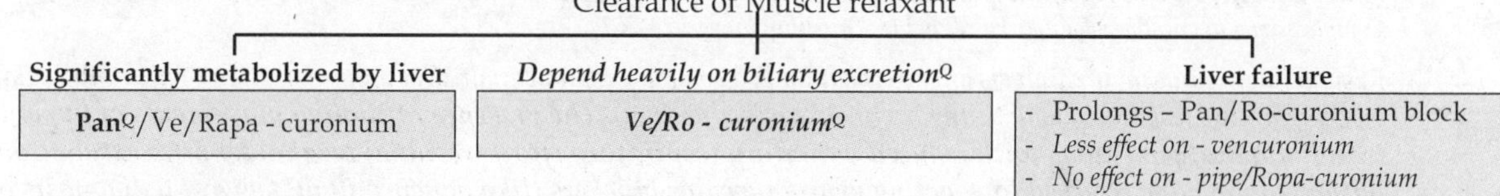

40. **C i.e. Atracurium**

- *Atracurium gets inactivated in plasma by spontanous non-enzymatic Hoffman's elimination. So reversal is mostly not required.*
- The concept of **Balanced anaesthesia** was introduced by **Lundy** and evolved to consist of-

Thiopental	for	Induction
N$_2$O	for	Amnesia
Mepiridine (or other opioid)	for	Analgesia
Curare	for	Muscle relaxation

- *Pancuronium & Gallamine oftenly need reversal*
- In *vecuronium, recovery is generally spontaneous not needing neostigmine reversal,* unless repeated doses are given. Longterm administration of vecuronium to patients in ICU has resulted in prolonged neuro muscular blakade (upto several days) d/t accumulation of 3-Hydroxy metabolite, or development of polyneuropathy.
- Best answers, are **Mivacurium and Rapacuronium** as they are short acting (Vecuronium & Atracurium are intermediate acting)

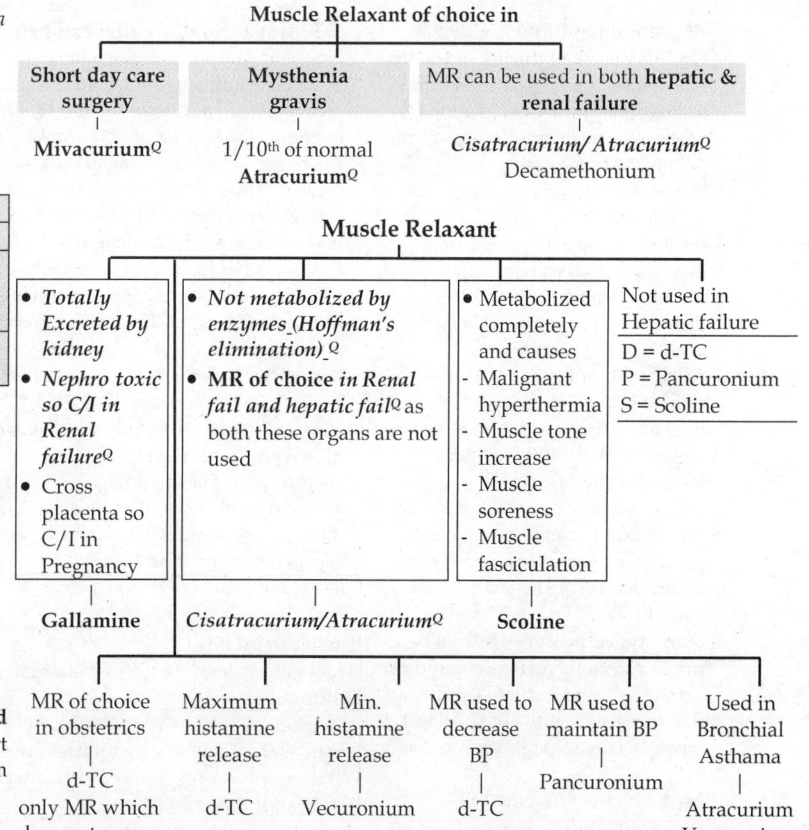

d-TC

41. **D i.e. Effect lasts for 2-3 hours** *[Ref: KDT 5/e P-313]*
42. **D i.e. Neostigmine**

d-tubocurarine

- d-TC produce significant **hypotension** by
  1- ***Ganglion block***Q
  2- Histamine release
  3- ↓ed venous return
- d-TC produce **tachycardia** d/t ***vagolytic action***Q
- d-TC is partly metabolized; the ***unchanged drug is excreted in urine as well as in bile***Q duration of action is ***30-60 minutes***Q.

- d-tubocurarine (d-TC) is *nondepolarizing* (competitive) M.R. with *maximum histamine release* (so L/t bronchospasm & *C/I in asthma)* and *maximum ganglion block*. It is only MR which does *not cross placenta (So MR of choice in obstetrics)*.
- Nondepolarizing muscle relaxants are antagonized by *Acetyl choline or* ***Anticholine esterase (Neostigmine,***Q *pyridostigmine,*Q *Edrophonium, physostigmine)*. In order to prevent muscarinic S/E ***anticholinergic agent*** *(ex glycopyrolate or* ***atropine****)*Q is given in combination.
- ***Cholinesterase inhibitors prolong depolarization blockade***Q***; inspite of antagonizing it.***

Pancuronium

43. **D i.e. 0.08 mg/Kg** *[Ref: Morgan's 3/e P-195]*
    - Pancuronium is *commonly used MR.* d/t lack of S/E like flushing, bronchospasm as it causes less histamine release. It causes hypertension by releasing Noradrenaline and is safe in malignant hyperpyrexia.
    - *Dose for intubation is* ***0.08-0.12 mg/kg***Q

44. **A i.e. Incomplete reversal of pancuronium** *[Ref: Wylie 7/e p-550, 592; Miller 7/e p-781-82, 887-89, 1525-26, 1601; Complications in anesthesiology-kirby 3/e p-114; Stroetling 6/e p-524-25]*

Residual neuromuscular paralysis after extubation is a common complication after administration of neuromuscular blocking agents (especially long acting agents like pancuronium). ***The presence of limited movements of upper body (residual paralysis) along with reduced voluntary respiratory effort (residual weakness) after extubation in patients who have received long acting neuromuscular blockers (like pancuronium) suggest a diagnosis of incomplete reversal of the muscle relaxation effect of the anesthetic drug.***

Opioid induced Rigidity	Residual paralysis after extubation (incomplete reversal of muscle relaxant)
- Usually observed **during induction** of anesthesia; however rarely may occur either immediately upon emergence from anesthesia, or upto 3-5 hrs.Postoperatively. - Occurs with *larger doses* of opioids (eg. alfentanil) - It is often associated in the first instance with the **chest wall muscles** ***frequently preventing ventilation of lungs with a bag & mask***Q. - Affects virtually all the major muscle groups in the body, beginning first in upper body (sternocleidomastoid, deltoid, biceps, forearm) - Often *sudden in onset* and could be provoked by stimulation such as passive movement of an extremity, manipulation of anesthesia mask, or a loud sound - **Stereotyped postures:** flexion of upper extremity, extension of lower extremity, rigid immobility of head, flexion of neck with chin on chest, & *severe rigidity of the abdomen & chest wall.* - Mediated by μ *receptors* in brainstem midline nuclei. *Naloxone*	- Frequent complication ***seen in recovery room after extubation following surgery***Q - The maximum antagonist effect of neostigmine occurs in **< 10 minutes.** ***If adequqte recovery does not occur within this time, subsequent recovery is slow & requires ongoing elimination of NM blocker from plasma***Q. So subsequent recovery occurs at the same rate as spontaneous recovery and is caused by decrease in plasma concentration of NM blocker drug as it is eliminated. And now the time at which full recovery of NM function will occur depends on inherent duration of action of NM blocker. With the drug that have a **long duration of action (eg. pancuronium)**, this period of inadequate neuromuscular function can be **30-60 minutes** or even longer, whereas with drugs that have an **intermediate duration of action**, it will be much shorter eg **15-30 minutes**. It occurs if the blockade at the time of neostigmine administration is sufficiently deep. Administration of second dose of neostigmine has no further effect on recovery if acetylcholinesterase is already maximally inhibited by maximum dose (70μg/kg). - ***Risk is highest with long acting muscle relaxants like pancuronium. (42%)***Q. It has also been seen with intermediate duration drugs like atracurium, vecuronium, or rocuronium. The advantage of using intermediate or short acting agent is that any residual paralysis will be of short duration. - Anticholinesterases (neostigmine) are used to reverse the effect of neuromuscular blocker. The *incidence is high if reversal of block is not routinely carried out.*

Sign & symptoms of reversal	Train of four ratio
Unable to lift head or arm Tidal volume may be normal but vital capacity & inspiratory force reduced.	≤0.4
Lift head for 3 seconds Open eyes widely & stick out their tongue Vital capacity & inspiratory force are often still reduced	0.6
Lift head for 5 seconds Normally cough sufficiently but grip strength 60% of normal	0.7-0.75

<table>
<tr><td rowspan="3">relieved rigidity implicating an opioid mechanism
- Currently only reliable treatment is administration of neuro muscular blocker, in doses large enough to facilitate intubation.
- Drugs that act on GABA-ergic, serotonergic or adrenergic pathway affect rigidity. Ketanserin (serotonin receptor antagonist), dexmedetomidine (α2- adrenergic agonist) prevent (in rats) and benzodiazepines & thiopentone (GABA ergic) attenuate rigidity in humans & rats.</td><td>Diplopia & visual disturbance
Inability to maintain apposition of incisor teeth
Tongue depressor test negative
Inability to sit up without assistance
Severe facial weakness, speaking a major effort
Over all weakness & tiredness</td><td></td></tr>
<tr><td>Diplopia & visual disturbances Generalized fatigue</td><td>0.85-0.90</td></tr>
<tr><td colspan="2">• Residual blockade (TOF<0.9) decrease chemoreceptor sensitivity to hypoxia & thereby l/t insufficient response to a decrease in O_2 tension in blood. Moreover it is a/w function impairment of pharyngeal & upper oesophageal muscles, which most probably predisposes to regurgitation & aspiration of gastric content. Even without sedation or impaired consciousness, a TOF ratio ≤0.9 may impair the ability to maintain the airwayQ.
• It is therefore imperative that all patients satisfy extubation criteria (Sustained head lift of more than 5 seconds or a strong hand grip) before removal of the tracheal tube. The patient in question has limited movements of the upper body and hence is not satisfying the extubation criteria due to incomplete reversal/residual paralysis</td></tr>
</table>

Vecuronium / Rocuronium

45. **A i.e. It has high incidence of cvs side effects** *[Ref: Miller's 5/e P-427; Morgan's 4/e p 207-223; Lee P-215]*

Vecuronium

- *Even at high doses, **vecuronium is devoid of significant cardiovascular side effects.***Q
- The ***lipophilic***Q effect of single quaternary nitrogen enhances rapid uptake into hepatocytes.
- *Duration of action is 10-20 min and is **not influenced by renal failure.***Q

46. **B i.e. Rocuronium; C i.e. Doxcurium; D i.e. Vecuronium** *[Ref: Lee 12/e P-212-16]*

- ***Rox/Ve-curonium & Dox-curium***Q have no CVS side effects.

47. **C i.e. Rocuronium** *[Ref. Pharmacology for Nurse Anesthesiology 2/e, p. 111; Wylie 7/e p. 589; Lee's 13/e p. 188; Miller 7/e p. 728-50]*

- **Rocuronium** is *desacetoxy analog of vecuronium* with a low potency (1/6 - 1/8 of vecuronium) and so *rapid onset of action* (because potency and speed of onset are inversely related). It is the ***fastest (most rapid) acting nondepolarizing muscle relaxant***Q (75 sec), which is slightly **slower than depolarizing muscle relaxant succinylcholine only.**
- ***Rocuronium injection can cause pain on injection site***Q, which may be decreased by alkalinizing the solution. Other painful injections include ***etomidate, propofol, methohexital and thiopental***Q.

Gallamine

48. **A i.e. Gallamine** *[Ref: Morgan's 4/e, P-207-223]*

GallamineQ (M.R.) and ***Methoxyflurane***Q (G.A.) are C/I in renal failure.

Metabolization of Muscle Relaxant

Metabolized by organ independent Hofmann elimination into acryulate & laudanosine	Least potent	Only Pan / Ve / Rapa – curonium metabolized by liver	Metabolized by pseudocholine esterase	Maximum histamine release	Minimum histamine release
*Metabolized by organ independent **Hofmann elimination***Q into acryulate & laudanosine It *can be used **in both hepatic & renal failure***Q	*Least potent*Q Totally excreted by kidney, so ***C/I in Renal failure***Q	Only **Pan / Ve / Rapa – curonium** are metabolized to significant degree by **liver** but clinically, liver failure prolongs *pancuronium &* *rocuronium* blockade with less effect on *vecuronium & no* effect on *pipecuronium or Rapacuronium.*	Metabolized by ***pseudocholine esterase***Q	*Maximum histamine*Q realease so ***C/I in Asthma***Q	Minimum histamine release so used in asthma
- **Atracurium** - **Cisatracurium**	- **Gallamine** - Metocurine		- **Succinylcholine *(shortest acting M.R.)***Q - **Mivacurium *(shortest acting nondepolarizing M.R)***Q	**d-TC**	Vecuronium

- **Rapacuronium** would clearly be the best choice of nondepolarizing M.R. for rapid sequence induction, because of its rapid onset of action, short duration of action, minimal cardiovascular S/E.
- **Rocuronium** is also suitable for rapid sequence induction but at cost of much longer duration of action.

ANAESTHESIA 2

49. **A i.e. Gallamine** *[Ref: Lee 12/e P-215 Morgan 3/e P-188]*

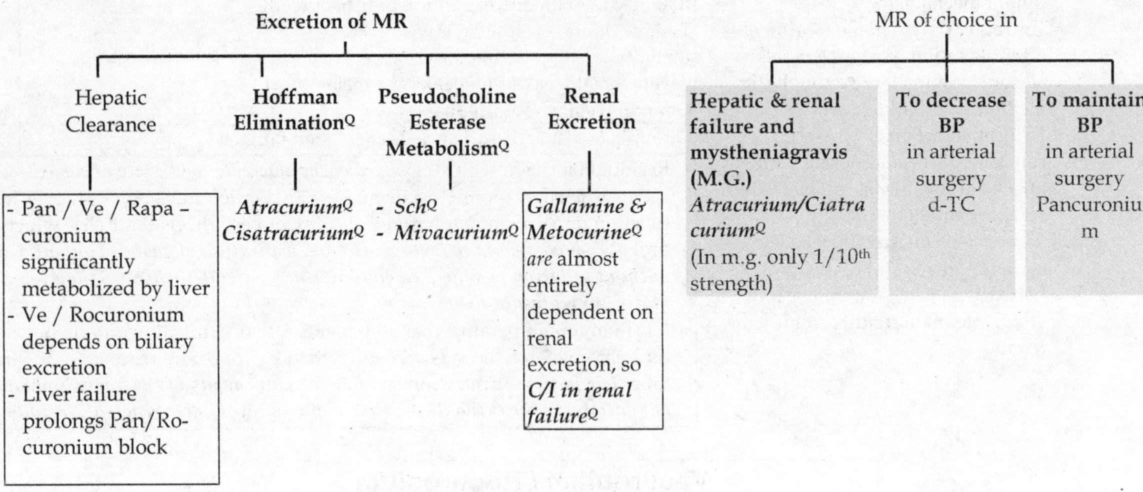

50. **C i.e. Gallamine** *[Ref: Morgan's 3/e P-752]*

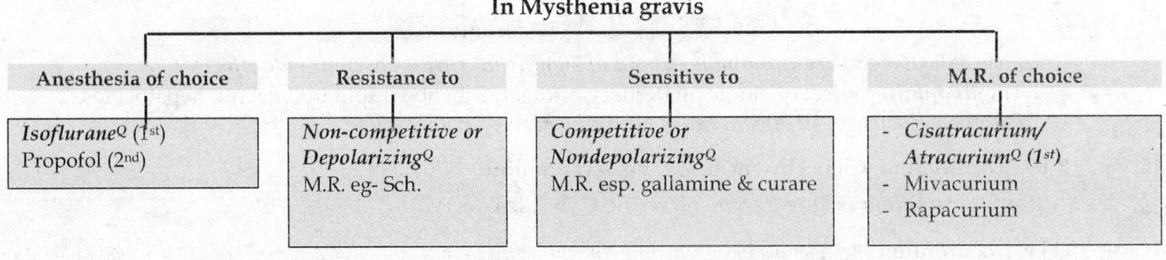

Mnemonic = **No Seat** of **R.D.** i.e.
Mysthenics are **S**ensitive to **No**n-Depolarising M.R. & Resistant to Depolarising M.R.

51. **D i.e. Halothane** *[Ref: Clinical Anesthesiology 3/e P-392]*

- **M.R. with ganglion block :**

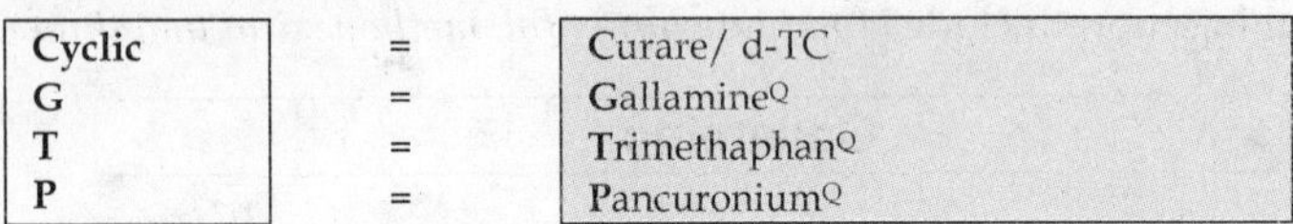

Cyclic	=	Curare/ d-TC
G	=	Gallamine^Q
T	=	Trimethaphan^Q
P	=	Pancuronium^Q

- ***Nicotine, Anticholinesterase, Acetyl Choline are ganglion stimulant.***^Q

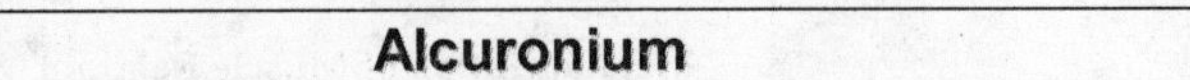

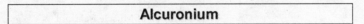

Alcuronium

52. **B i.e. Alcuronium** *[Ref: Lee 12/e P–210]*

Exposure to any **nondepolarizing muscle relaxant** (i.e. *alcuronium*^Q) may lead to development of ***true allergy or antibody formation & tachyphylaxis***^Q

3 INTRAVENOUS ANAESTHETICS

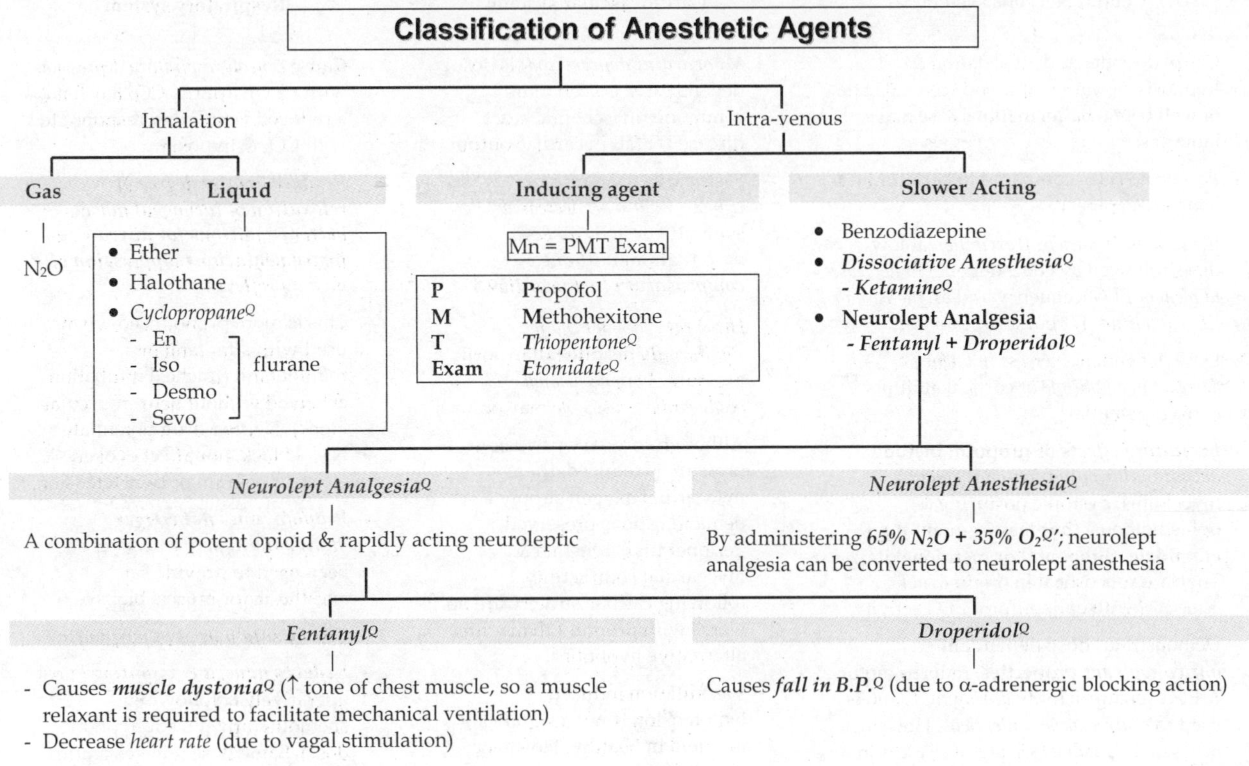

Propofol

- It is an alkylphenol, **2, 6-Disopropylphenol**^Q. It is highly *soluble in lipid but not water* and formulated as an *aqueous emulsion* with intralipid, specifically an isotonic 1% solution with *10% soyabean oil, 2.25% glycerol, and 1.2% **purified egg phosphatide***^Q. The addition of *disodium acetate* 0.005% *supresses bacterial growth.*
- **Propofol** is ***2,6-disopropylphenol (an alkyl phenol not barbiturate)***^Q nonbarbiturate intravenous anesthetic agent. It is formulated as an aquous emulsion with ***soyabean oil, glycerol and purified egg phosphatide***^Q. So it can ***provoke allergic reactions in individuals having allergy to egg lecithin***^Q. Propofol and other intravenous anesthesia should not be used in **airway obstruction** (i.e. absolutely contraindicated if there is anticipated difficulty in maintaining an adequate airway eg epiglottis, oral or pharyngeal tumors). Propofol should not be used **for long term sedation of children** (<17 years old) in ICU.
- Propofol is ***safe in porphyric patients and patients prone to malignant hyperthermia***^Q. Because of early induction and smooth recovery propofol is ***intravenous induction agent of choice for day care (out patient) anesthesia***^Q. *Because of suppression of laryngeal reflexes* (resulting in reduced coughing & laryngospasm), propofol is regarded by most anesthetists as *drug of choice for induction of anesthesia when laryngeal mask airway (LMA) is to be used.*
- **Propofol** causes ***respiratory & cardiovascular depression***^Q and CNS excitement.
- Propofol is most commonly used induction agent & hypnotic component of a balanced anesthetic technique. ***Smooth and rapid induction***^Q, easy titration to effect, short clinical duration of action and a demonstrable antiemetic effect represent the most (near to ideal) balanced clinical profile of available intravenous hypnotic.
- Following IV bolus, plasma levels initially decline rapidly, d/t redistribution of propofol from highly perfused low capacity tissues (eg brain) to high capacity sites with lower perfusion. ***The rapid distribution and high hepatic clearance accounts for rapid recovery, after a bolus dose***^Q. Hepatic metabolism is by glucuronidation (40%) to OH group and oxidation (60%) to 4–OH- propofol, a quinol derivative responsible for *green colour of urine.*
- It has *no anelgesic effect* and *injection in small veins cause pain* (*no thrombophlebitis* and less chances in large veins),

- Dilution or addition of drug, to reduce the pain or provide systemic analgesia, can destabilize the emulsion. It can only be mixed with *preservative free lidocaine,* 0.5% or 1% (20 : 1 ratio) and immediate administration; and with *alfentanil,* 500 mg ML- for use with in 6 hours.
- **Effects on**

Central Nervous system

- Cause dose dependent sedation & hypnosis, elevation of mood, general state of well being, hallucinations & sexual fantasies.
- *Poor amnesia* (as compared to barbiturate & benzodiazepines)
- EEG shows *transient β excitation* at low dose, followed by conc. dependent *decrease in median EEG* frequency and an *increase in EEG amplitude* l/t burst suppression.
- Dose dependent *increase in latency & decrease in amplitude* of cortical auditory evoked potentials.
- ***Excitatory effects* of propofol include *occasional involuantry movements,*** myoclonus, dystonic posturing & ophisthotonus. **(but less frequent than etomidate, thiopental or methiohexital).** They are subcortical in origin & *not associated* with epileptiform EEG activity.
- Demonstrates **dose dependent *anticonvulsant* properties**, reduces motor & EEG seizure activity *during ECT,* and is used to *control status epilepticus.* However, occasional *grandmal seizures may occur* in patients with past h/o seizures. (relative not absolute C/I)
- It *reduces cerebral oxygen consumption (CMRO2), cerebral blood flow (CBF), & intra cranial pressure (ICP).* However great fall in mean arterial pressure can *reduce cerebral perfusion pressure* (CPP)

Cardiovascular system

- ***Myocardial depression***Q is dose dependent & is seen more commonly in ischemic heart disease l/t fall in cardiac output
- *Systemic vascular resistance is reduced (~30% d/t decreased* sympathetic activity & vasodilation) ***without compensatory tachycardia***Q.
- *Heart rate does not change significantly* despite fall in aortic pressure. *Very occasional bradycardia & asystole* may occur.
- Although coronary perfusion pressure is reduced, the myocardial oxygen supply – demand ratio is preserved. Perioperative ischemia & myocardial contractility following cardiac surgery are no worse with propofol than with alternative hypnotics
- Vasodilation induced hypotension is not a significant problem in healthy. However *patient with limited cardiovascular reserve may demonstrate exaggerated hypotension.*

Respiratory system

- Cause *central respiratory depression* with rise in arterial CO_2 tension & a reduced ventilatory response to both CO_2 & hypoxia.
- ***Produce greater degree of relaxation of laryngeal muscle & better conditions for airway instrumentation (suppression of airway reflexes)*** Q
- This is more pronounced when used with alfentanil or remifentanil (tracheal intubation acheived without neuromuscular block). Neither drug potentiate NM – block, nor affect evoked electromyogram or twitch tension.
- ***Propofol does not trigger malignant hyperpyrexia***Q & has been used to provide safe anesthesia for muscle biopsy.
- ***Can be safely used in porphyria***Q
- ***Reduces nausea & vomiting***Q post operatively & following chemotherapy (on subhypnotic dose). Same dose relieves *praritis* in choleastasis & spinal opiates.

Ketamine

- **Ketamine (phencyclidine)** is a ***noncompetitive inhibitor at the NMDA (N-methyl D-aspartate) receptor (a subtype of glutamate receptor)***Q. Its ***NMDA receptor antagonist***Q action may mediate the general anesthetic & some analgesic actions. It is also a *ligand at opioid receptors, both μ & κ,* where *S(+) ketamine* is more potent and fewer side effects than R(-) ketamine. The primary site of CNS action of ketamine seems to be *thalamo-neocortical projection system.* The drug selectively *depresses* neuronal functions in parts of *cortex (esp association areas) and thalamus,* while stimulating parts of limbic system. This process creates *functional disorganization* of nonspecific pathways in midbrain & thalamic area. In contrast to *depression of RAS* induced by barbiturates, *ketamine dissociates thalamus* (which relays sensory impulses from RAS to cerebral cortex) *from the limbic cortex* (which is involved with the awareness of sensation). Clinically this state of **dissociative anesthesia** causes the patient to appear conscious (eg eye opening, swallowing, muscle contraction) but unable to process or respond to sensory input.
- *Psychic emergence reactions* of ketamine include vivid dreaming *extracorporeal experiences* (sense of floating out of body) & *illusions* often a/w confusion, excitement, euphoria & fear. They occur in 1st hour & occur secondary to ketamine induced *depression of auditory & visual relay nuclei* l/t misinterpretation or misperception of auditory & visual stimuli.

Disadvantages	Advantages & Indication
- ***Unlike – propofol and thiopental, ketamine increases cerebral blood flow, oxygen consumptoin, metabolism, and intracranial pressure, making it unsuitable for neuroanesthesia***[Q]. Rise in ICT is particularly marked in the presence of *intracranial pathology*, and may exceed sympathetically mediated increase in mean arterial pressure, with a reduction in cerebral perfusion pressure. ***so ketamine is contraindicated in raised intracranial pressure***[Q] or ***intracranial pathology with a mass effect***[Q]. - Cerebrovascular responsiveness to ketamine is preserved, and *reducing the arterial CO2 tension by hyper ventilation attenuates the ketamine induced rise in intracranial tension.* - A parallel increase in intraocular pressure may be detrimental in patients with *open eye injuries*, or *glucoma*, or during *vitro- retinal surgeries.* - The propensity to *tachycardia and hypertension* means that ketamine must be used extremely carefully in patients with ***ischemic heart disease or vascular aneurysm***[Q]. - Ketamine sensitizes heart to small doses of epinephrine (d/t sympathomimetic effect) and can *precipitate arrythmias* in anxious patients. - Its *indirect sympathomimetic effect predominate over direct negative ionotropic & vasodilatory effects.* Thus the net effect is increase in heart rate, blood pressure, cardiac output, and myocardial oxygen consumption. So resistance to sympathetic effect of ketamine, in critically ill & shocked patients can unmask direct *myocardial depression and peripheral vasodilation.* - Increased laryngeal spasm, tracheobronchial and salivary secretion and airway obstruction can be troublesome, particularly in children. *Inhalation agents should be used for induction if airway obstruction is anticipated.* - ***Unpleasant & troublesome psychomimetic emergence reactions characterized by vivid dreams, surreal experiences and illusions during first hour of recovery***[Q].	- War & civilian disasters often coexist with limited medical resources for anesthesia & post operative are. ***Ketamine may be anesthetic agent of choice when supplies of oxygen and monitoring & disposable equipment are limited and anesthesia is administered by inexperienced anesthesiologists or paramedical personnel.*** - ***Profound analgesia***[Q] & sesation of subanesthetic dose has been used during minor painful procedures eg. dressing; patient positioning - It produces minimal respiratory depression & an unaltered response to CO_2. FRC, MV, & tidal volume and contribution of intercostal muscle function to inspiration are maintained. It is ***potent bronchodilator***[Q] owing to sympthominetic effect. It has been used in ***life threatening and unresponsive status asthmaticus***[Q], during one lung anesthesia in patients with severe pulmonary disease. - It *increases uterine tone and intensity of uterine contraction.* Sympathetic stimulation & maintenance of cardiovascular tone makes ketamine a potentially ***life saving anesthetic for parturients with exsanguinating obstetric hemorrhage and a flaccid uterus***[Q]. - There is no widespread or consistent clinical indications but is promoted by enthusiasts for patients with *severe shock* or who are *cardiovascularly compromised.*

Effects

Cardiovascular	CNS	Respiratory System
- ***Directly causes cardiodepression by inhibiting calcium channels*** [Q] but this is masked by cardiotonic action of sympathetic system. Once the sympathetic system is blocked the cardiodepressant action gets unmasked. - It increases – HR, CO, BP, pulmonary artery pressure, myocardial work & dysrhythmia d/t stimulation of sympathetic system & increase in NA (noradrenaline) - So it is ***contraindicated in – coronary artery disease, hypertension, CHF & arterial aneurysm***[Q] - Because of cardiotonic action it is the ***anesthesia of choice for shock***[Q].	- ***It increases cerebral metabolism & O_2 consumption, cerebral blood flow & intracranial pressure so it is C/I in patients with space occupying lesion of CNS***[Q] - Hallucination (most common S.E.), illusions, delusions & disturbing dreams are seen at emergence. ***More likely if pretreated with anticholinergics and reduced when pretreated with benzodiazepene*** [Q]	- Potent bronchodilator (can be used in asthma) - Upper airway reflexes are maintained (decreased risk of aspiration) - Tracheobronchial & salivary secretions are increased (may l/t aspiration) ★ Ketamine increases intraocular, intragastric- pressure and muscle tone.

Barbiturates

Three processes are involved in termination of action of barbiturates :

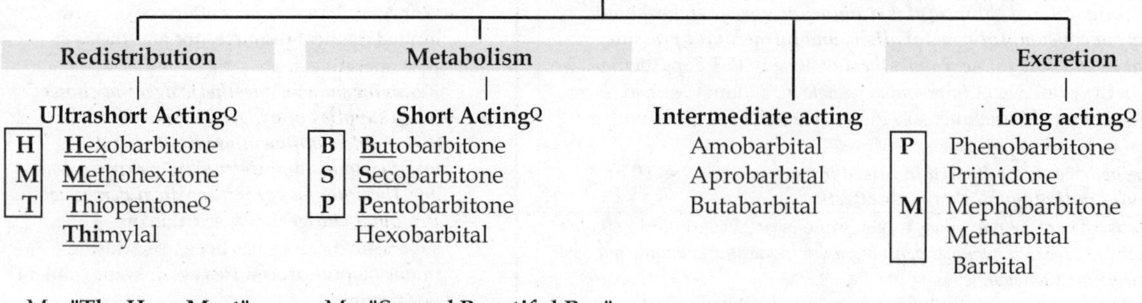

Barbiturates: Thiopentone & Methohexital

Thiopental, methohexital & thiamylal are the only barbiturates in common use as *intravenous hypnotic agent*

Formulation

- ***6% anhydrous sodium carbonate***[Q] (by wt) is mixed for formulation of barbiturate as sodium salt, and then water or normal saline is mixed to produce a **2.5% *solution of thiopental***[Q], 2% solution of thiomylal, & 1% solution of methohexitol.
- Thiopental is *prepared & stored under nitrogen*, which prevents release of free thio barbituric acid in presence of atmospheric CO_2.
- If refrigerated after reconstitution, thiobarbiturates (i.e., thiopental & thiamylal) are stable for 1 week & methohexital for 6 weeks. The solutions are bacteriostatic, although freshly prepared solutions should be used within 24 hours.
- Are highly lipid soluble weak acids dissolved in a strongly alkaline aqueous solution (PH >10). So *intra arterial or subcutaneous injection can cause serious*
- Cannot *be reconstituted with Ringer lactate or other acidic solution as decrease in alkalinity of solution can precipitate barbiturates as free acids*
- Precipitates & can block iv-line, when mixed with

Dose

Dose of thiopental & thiamylal *(2.5 – 4.5 mg/kg)*[Q] is about twice that of methoxhexital (1-2mg/kg).

Chemistry

- Barbiturates are barbituric acid (formed by malonic acid & urea) derivative. At position 2, *oxybarbiturates have O_2 and thiobarbiturates have sulfur (S)*
- *Tautomerization* (at position 2) *to enol* form allows formation of *water solubile salts* in alkaline solution
- *Substitution of hydrogen at C5* position with *aryl or alkyl* group produces *hypnotic or sedative effects*. And increase in length of alkyl chain at C5 increases hypnotic potency.
- Phenyl group substitution at C5 produces *anticonvulsant activity*
- *Sulfur at position 2* produces *a more rapid onset of action*
- Addition of *ethyl or methyl group at position 1* also produce a more rapid onset of action but with excitatory side effects including *tremors, hyper tonus & involuantry movements.*
- Short duration of action is d/t thio substitution & a branched group on C5. Larger unbranched group of prolong duration of action & increase convulsant activity.
- Evidence of stereoselective differences b/w the

Mechanism of action

- Barbiturates preferentially *affects of function of nerve synapses* rather than axon
- Transmission of ***excitatory neurotransmitters (eg glutamate & acetyl choline) is suppressed and inhibitory neurotransmitters (eg. gamma amino butyric acid = GABA) are enhanced***[Q]
- *$GaBA_A$ receptor is a chloride ion channel* with specific site of action for GABA, barbiturates & benzodiazepines. Barbiturates are *positive allosteric modulators* at $GABA_A$ & glycine receptor. At low conc. it enhances the effect of GABA (by decreasing its rate of dissociation), and is responsible for hypnosis & sedation. At higher conc. barbiturates have agonist (mimetic) action and directly activate chloride channel. Mimetic effect is responsible for barbiturate anesthesia

Metabolism

- Barbiturates (*except phenobarbi-tone) are hepatically metabolized by* (1) oxidation of aryl, alkyl or phenyl at C5 most common) (2) N- dealkylation (3) desulfuration of thiobarbiturates at C2, and (4) destruction of barbituric acid ring.
- Renal excretion of phenobarbital is enhanced by alkalinization of urine with bicarbonate.

Contraindications

- ***In porphyria***[Q], as barbiturates induce hepatic enzymes can precipitate attack by stimulating γ *-aminolevulinic acid synthetase*, the enzyme responsible for production of porphyrins.
- Patient with respiratory obstruction or inadequate airway
- Status asthmaticus

Clinical Uses

- Preop. sedation
- Sole anaesthetic agent for short operational procedure
- ***Induction and maintenance of anesthesia***[Q]
- ***Rapid control of seizure(status epilepticus)***[Q]
- Treatment of ***raised ICT***[Q]
- ***As cerebral protector by reducing cerebral metabolism***[Q]
- Modified ECT
- To facilitate verbal communication in psychiatric patient, known as **narcoanalysis, narcotherapy** or ***truth spells***[Q]

2

ANAESTHESIA

acidic solutions of muscle relaxants. So pancuronium, ***vecuronium, atracurium, alfentanil, sufentanil & midazole are not mixed***[Q] in solution

enantiomers, *S (l) isomer is twice as potent as R (d) isomer,* despite their similar access to CNS. This suggests presence of chirally active centers on stereoselective receptor.

- ***Severe cardiovascular instability, pericardial temponade uncompensated mycardial disease & shock***[Q].
- Without proper equipment for administration & airway equipment (artificial ventilation)

Thiopentone

Thiopentone is an ultrashort acting barbiturate used for induction of anesthesia. Its effects on various organs are as follows-

CNS

- **Barbiturates (thiopental)** *are* **cerebro protective (neuroprotective)** ***primarily b/o depression of cerebral electrical activity and cerebral metabolism***[Q]. *It may protect the brain from transient effect of focal ischemia (eg cerebral embolism) but probably not from global ischemia (eg cardiac arrest)*
- Barbiturates (like other CNS depressants) ***decrease cerebral metabolism resulting in depression of cerebral metabolic oxygen consumption rate (CMRO₂) and ATP consumption rate***[Q] and protecting from incomplete cerebral ischemia.
- Alterations in cerebral (metabolic) activity and O_2 requirements are reflected by *progressive slowing of EEG.* The *awake α* pattern progress to *low voltage-fast activity* with small doses *to high amplitude (voltage) slow frequency (activity) δ and θ waves* until burst suppression (silence precedes a flat EEG at very large doses.
- With reduced $CMRO_2$, cerebral vascular resistance increases. ***Reduce $CMRO_2$ causes cerebral vasoconstriction, there by reducing cerebral blood flow (cerebral perfusion) and intracranial pressure (↓ ICT)***[Q]
- The drop in ICP exceeds the drop in arterial BP, so the ***cerebral perfusion pressure/CPP is usually increased (CPP=MAP-ICP).*** Cerebral perfusion pressure equals cerebral artery pressure minus the greater of cerebral venous pressure or ICP. The decrease in *CBF is also not detrimental, as barbiturates induce even greater decline in cerebral O_2 consumption.*
- ***Thiopental is a potent anticonvulsant***[Q]. However methohexital, has proconvulsant properties and increases incidence of post operative seizures in undiagnosed epileptics and following neurosurgery.
- ***Antianalgesic effect***[Q]
- ***Pain***[Q] is felt some times due to lowering of pain thresold
- CNS depression from sedation to unconsciousness
- Feel a *taste of garlic or onion,* during induction
- Some barbiturates ***induce involuntary muscle contraction (eg methoxital) but small dose of Thiopentone rapidly controls most grandmal seizures.***[Q]

Cardiovascular

- Peripheral *vasodilatation* l/t pooling of venous blood
- ***Decreased contractility*** d/t less availability of Ca^{++}
- *Decreased cardiac output* & negative ionotropic effect
- *Increased heart rate* & myocardial O_2 consumption.
- In conditions where *baroreceptor response* is *inadequate* eg. *congestive heart failure, hypovolemia & β-adrenergic blockade* the cardiac output & BP may fall dramatically d/t uncompensated peripheral blood pooling & unmasked direct cardiac depression. So it is ***contraindicated in shock***[Q].
- In *coronary artery disease* increased heart rate & myocardial O_2 consumption is potentially deleterious.

Respiratory

- ***Dose dependent central respiratory depression & apnea. Response to hypoxia & hypercapnia are also depressed***[Q]
- Upper ***airway*** obstruction d/t ***laryngo/broncho spasm***[Q]. Although laryngeal & tracheal reflexes are depressed to lesser degree than propofol.

Musculoskeletal

Mild ***muscular excitatory movements***[Q] such as tremor, twitching & respiratory excitatory effects including cough & hiccup.

Eye

- Pupils I[st] dilate then constrict
- ↓IOP
- *Loss of eyelash reflex is excellent sign of adequate induction*

Immunological

Rash[Q], angioedema & photosensitivity rarely

CNS Physiology and Anesthesia

- Under normal circumstances **global cerebral blood flow (CBF)** is maintained at *~50 mL/100gm/min* (75-80 for cortical, mostly gray matter and ~20 ml/100gm/min for subcortical, mostly white matter). There is substantial reserve below normal CBF levels, and it is not until CBF has *fallen to 20 mL/100gm/min, the EEG evidence of ischemia begins to appear.* At *15ml/100gm/min,* the cortical EEG is *isoelectric.* CBF range between 6 to *15 ml/100gm/min* l/t *neuronal dysfunction* which is *temporarily reversible* but neuronal death will occur if flow is not restored. As CBF reduces to about **6ml/100 gm/min potentially irreversible membrane failure (*ie elevated extracellular k^+ and loss of direct cortical response*)** is rapidly evident.
- **Severe reduction in CBF (<10mL/100gm/min)** l/t *rapid ischemic neuronal death,* characterized by early excitotoxicity and delayed apoptosis.
- **60%** of brains energy consumption is used to *support electro-physiological functions* and remainder *40%* energy consumed by brain is involved in *house-keeping (cellular hemostatic)* activities. Glial cells make up most of brains volume and require less energy than neurons do.

- In general, anesthetic drugs suppress cerebral metabolic rate (CMR). With **ketamine and N_2O** being notable **exception**. With several anesthetics including ***barbiturates, iso/sevo/des-flurane, propofol and etomidate,*** increasing plasma conc. cause progressive suppression of electrophysiological (EEG) activity and a concomitant reduction in CMR. However, increasing the plasma level beyond what is required to first achieve suppression of EEG results in no further depression of CMR, because IV anesthetics reduce only neuronal (not house keeping) function.
- **Hypothermia** decreases CMR by 6 to 7% /°C and causes complete suppression of EEG at 18° to 20°C (like anesthetis). However, in contrast with anesthetic drugs, hypothermia beyond this level produce a further decrease in CMR. This occurs *because hypothermia decreases both electrophysiological and basal house keeping energy consumption.* **Hyperthermia** has an opposite influence and between 37 *to* 42°C, CBF and CMR increase. However, above 42°C cerebral O_2 consumption decreases dramatically b/o protein denaturation.
- ***Hypercarbia is most potent cerebral vasodilator***[Q]. CBF varies directly with $Paco_2$. The effect is *greatest within the physiological range* of Pa_{CO2} variation. CBF changes 1-2 mL/100gm/min for each lmmHg change in Pa_{CO2} around normal Pa_{CO2} values. This respose is attenuated below a Pa_{CO2} value 25 mmHg.
- Changes **in Pa_{O2}** from 60 to >300 mmHg have a little influence on CBF. Below a Pa_{O2} 60 mmHg. CBF increases rapidly.
- ***Barbiturates (thiopental), etomidate, and propofol decrease*** *cerebral metabolic rate (CMR)* and can produce burst suppression of EEG. CMR is reduced by abut 60% and because flow and metabolism coupling is preserved cerebral blood flow (CBF) is also decreased. **Opiates and benzodiazepines** cause minor decrease in CBF and CMR whereas **Ketamine and N_2O** can *increase CMR, CBF and ICP.* Ketamine is best avoided as sole agent in patients with impaired intracranial compliance.
- **Barbiturates, propofol, ketamine (?), volatile anesthetics and xenon** have ***neuroprotective efficacy and can reduce ischemic cerebral injury***[Q]. Anesthetic neuroprotection is sustained only when the severity of ischemia is mild; with moderate to severe injury *long term protection is not achieved.*
- Administration of **etomidate** is a/w regional reduction in blood flow and this can ***exacerbate ischemic brain injury***[Q]. Etomidate was proposed as a potential neuroprotective anesthetics in setting of aneurysm surgery. However, administration of etomidate result in exacerbation of *brain tissue hypoxia and acidosis* in patients with temporary intracranial vessel occlusion. Additional concerns of *adrenocortical suppression and renal injury* caused by propylene glycol vehicle will preclude more than episodic use
- Order of **vasodilation potency (increase in CBF, CB volume and ICP)** of volatile anesthetics is *halothane* >> *enflurane* > *desflurane* ~ *isoflurane>sevoflurane.*
- **Epileptogenesis** can be seen with ***volatile anesthetics (enflurane >>>> sevoflurane)***[Q], methohexital (barbiturate), ketamine, rarely etomidate, propofol, narcotics and ***atracurium (laudanosine)***[Q].
- With the exception of *tissue plasminogen activator (t PA) for thrombolysis, and calcium channel blockers nimodipine and nicardipine for management of subarachnoid haemorrhage,* pharmacological neuroprotective anesthetics are not available for the treatment of patients with cerebral ischemia.

Recommendations for use of Anesthetic Drugs in Acute Porphyria

	IV induction agents	Analgesic	Local anesthetic	Inhalation agent	Neuro muscular blocker	N M block reversing agent	Sedative & antiemetic	Cardiovascular drugs
Avoid/ Contraindi-cation	- *Barbiturates eg thiopentone, methohexitone*[Q] - *Etomidate*[Q]	*Pentazocine*[Q]	Ropivacaine (no data)					
Use with extreme caution only		Diclofenac Ketorolac Phenacetin Tilidine					Chlordiazepoxide Nitrazepam	Hydralazine Nifediapine Phenoxybenzamine
Use with caution	Ketamine		Cocaine Mepivacine	Enflurane Isoflurane Sevoflurane Desflurane	Alcuronium Atracurium Rocuronium Mivacurium Vecuronium		Benzodiazepines (others) Diazepam Lorazepam Midazolam Oxazepam Cimetidine Metoclopramide Ondansteron	Diltiazem Disopyramide Sodium nitroprusside Verapamil
Use	Propofol	Paracetamol (acetaminophen) Aspirin Alfentanil Fentanyl Sufentanil Buprenorphine Codeine Pethidine Morphine Nalozone	Bupivicaine Lidocaine Prilocaine Procaine Tetracaine	Nitrous oxide Halothane Cyclopropane	Tubocurarine Pancuronium Suxamethonium	Atropine Glycopyrrolate Neostigmine	Droperidol Phenothiazines Temazepam Triazolam	Epinephrine Magnesium Phentolamine Procainamide α- agonists β- blocker β- agonists

Opioid: Remifentanyl

- It is newest fentanyl analog, deliberately developed by *incorporating ester moiety*, to have *ultra short duration* of action, as this makes drug susceptible to ester hydrolysis (other example is *esmolol*)
- It is ***rapidly metabolised by non specific esterase present in tissue (significantly) and RBC***[Q]. Remifentanil is not metabolised by pseudo cholinesterase, plasma cholinesterase, acetyl cholinsteras or carbonic anhydrase. So the patients with pseudocholinesterase deficiency have a normal response to drug.
- *The very large clearance (3-5L/min)* is several times greater than that of normal hepatic blood flow which *indicates wide spread extahepatic* metabolism and results' in rapid decrement of blood levels of drug following discontinuation of continuous infusion. So there is ***absence of metabolic toxicity in patients with hepatic dysfunction***[Q].

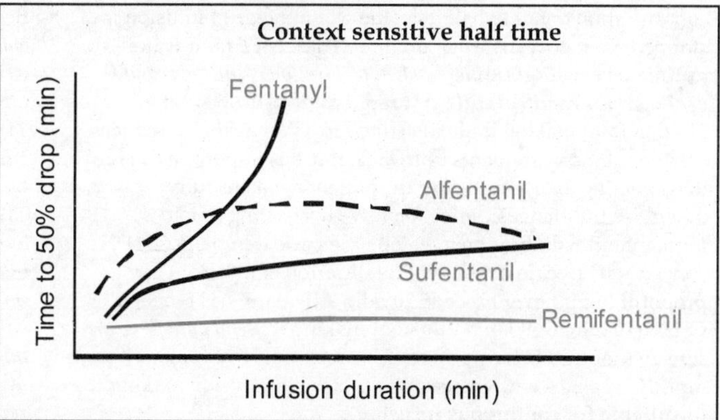

- Remifentanil is a ***μ receptor agonist with analgesic potency (& pharmacological profile) similar to that of fentanyl (15-20 times more potent than alfentanyl)***[Q]. It has low lipid solubility and the drug is not significantly metabolized or sequestred in lung, whereas significant amount of very highly lipid soluble opioids (fentanyl, sufentanil > alfentanil) can be retained by lungs (in first pass uptake) and latter diffuse back into system circulation. *Very low lipid solubility* of *morphine* l/t slow passage across BBB and resulting in *slow onset & prolonged duration* of action. Similarly very high lipid solubility of sufentanil & fentanyl allows rapid onset and short duration of action. However, alfentanyl has more rapid onset & shorter duration of action than fentanyl even though it has less lipid solubility than fentanyl. This is d/t very high (90%) nonionized fraction of drug available for diffusion.
- Remifentanil is de- esterified to form a carboxylic acid metabolite G 190291 which is 0.001 – 0.003 times as potent as or *4600 times less potent than remifentanil*. Its low potency is explained by a low affinity to μ receptor with poor brain penetration. Its excretion is dependent on renal clearance. So in renal failure patient, G1902 91 is accumulated but the substantial clinical effect is not clinically significant. ***So the pharmacokinetics or pharmacodynamics of remifentanil is not appreciably influenced by renal or hepatic failure***[Q].
- The elimination half life of remifentanil is < 10 min and context sensitivity half time (time required to decline plasma drug concentration 50% after termination of continuous infusion) is ~ 3 min regardless of duration of infusion.

Opioid	Lipid solubility	Non ionized fraction	Protein binding	Potency (mg relative to morphine, 10mg)
Morphine	Very low (+)	Low (++)	Low (++)	10
Meperidine	Low (++)	Very low (+)	High (+++)	75
Remifentanil	Low (++)	High (+++)	High (+++)	0.10
Alfentanil	High (+++)	Very high (++++)	Very high (++++)	1.0
Sufentanil	Very high (++++)	Low (++)	Very high (++++)	0.01
Fentanyl	Very high (++++)	Very low (+)	High (+++)	0.10

Total Intravenous Anaesthesia (TIVA)

TIVA is *induction and maintenance of anesthesia using the intravenous route*. Today, b/o availability of favourable drugs and more appropriate means of delivering them has markedly promoted TIVA.

Ideal drug profile and suitable drugs

- Ideal profile includes rapid onset and offset of action, with short effect compartment half life (t ½ Keo), constant context sensitive half life, rapid non organ dependent elimination (metabolism), slow redistribution and non-accumulation
- The concentration at effect site – the **biosphere concentration** – and not the plasma concentration governs the drug effect (*effect*

Problems with inhalation anesthesia

- Adverse effect on cardiac output, respiratory rate, total volume and respiratory dead space
- Environmental damage i.e. depletion of ozone layer and green house effect
- Diffusion hypoxia, distension of gas filled spaces and production of fluoride ions.

compartment model). Mathematical constant (Keo) determines the time delay b/w changes in blood conc. of drug and drug effect (on/off rates). So short effect compartment half life (t½ Keo) **means rapid equilibrium b/w blood and brain.**

The equilibrium b/w plasma and effect site is **rapid** for ***thiopental, propofol, alfentanil, and ramifentanil***Q; **intermediate**, *for fentanyl, sufentanil and nondepolarizing muscle relaxants; and* **slow** *for morphine and ketorolac.*

- **Context sensitive half time (CSHT)** is the time taken for plasma concentration to fall to half its value when the drug infusion is stopped. So it governs wake up time. The **CSHT (and wake uptime) is** ***constant*** *(ie independent of duration of infusion) and very short* ***for ramifentanil*** (d/t rapid ester hydrolysis at > 3L/min rate) making it ideally suited to TIVA as it also reduces the propofol requirements upto 50%. But it is important to give longer acting analgesic before the patient awakens fully otherwise the analgesic effect of very short acting opioid remifentanil will disappear leaving the patient in pain. CSHT is context sensitive (ie dependent on duration of infusion) for **propofol** but it never exceeds **20 min**. Alfentanil has longer CSHT (40 min for 90 min infusion) making it *useful only for short surgery* (not suitable for prolonged cases). CSHT of **fentanyl** rapidly escalates with increasing duration of infusion making it **unsuitable for continuous infusion.**
- **Propofol and opioid combination** (± midazolam) is commonly used resulting *in synergism* where *propofol provides hypnosis, amnesia, antiemesis and opioid provides analgesia, hemodynamic stability, while blunting responses to noxious stimuli.* **Propofol and remifentanil** ***(forgiving drug) is idealy suited to TIVA***Q
- For infusion durations of 15-600 min, the CSHT of the opioids decrease in following order: **fentanyl >alfentanil > sufentanil >> remifentanil (FASR)**. So the *optimal propofol concentration* (for propofol-opioid TIVA) also decreases in the same order. A shorter CSHT *allows the administration of greater amounts of opioids (and less propofol)* during anesthesia without creating **prolonged opioid effects.**

Methods of drug delivery

- Manually controlled infusion eg Bristol infusion regimen
- **Target controlled infusion (TCI)** devices eg ***Diprifusor*** TCI pumps for propofol. TCI devices enable the (theoretical) drug concentration in plasma to be controlled continuously and administered without the need for complex calculations by the anaesthetist. The computer program in TCI devices continuously calculates the distribution and elimination of drug (based on pharmacokinetic data of drug (and automatically adjust the infusion rate to maintain predicted plasma drug concentration. However, Diprofusor system does not determine how much anesthesia a patient needs. It is not a monitor of the depth of anesthesia, & control still rests with anesthesiologist, who should be using *clinical signs or BIS to monitor the depth of anesthesia.*

Advantages of TIVA

- Provides truly *balanced anesthesia* by selecting a pure hypnotic propofol and an opioid together with muscle relaxant. By independently titrating each of these different drugs to *provide the desired level of hyponosis, analgesis, relaxation and suppression of autonomic and somatic responses*, it is possible to *adjust anesthesia to the needs of individual patient* a/t surgical situation.
- TIVA has potential to provide anesthesia with equal or *greater flexibility and control* than with the use of inhalational agents.
- Because the onset and offset times of drugs a known, TIVA *obtains a specific desired effect* (eg quick induction, rapid response to increased analgesia or hypnosis, convenient and stress for emergence) *with in a specific time frame.*
- TIVA is especially useful when delivery of inhaled agents is compromised or anesthetised patient needs to be transferred eg between radiology and theatres.
- TIVA (with propofol) provides extremely clear-headed awakening (which is useful after neurosurgery for patient evaluation) *and* ***reduced incidence of post operative nausea and vomiting (PONV)***Q compared to volatile anesthesia. ***It can be safely used in patient susceptible to malignant hyperpyrexia***Q and reduces release of scavenged anesthetic gases into the atmosphere. ***The paralysis is not always required, avoiding reversal agents and emergence is rapid***Q (especially when propofol TIVA is used with remifentanil)
- TIVA avoids all disadvantages of inhalation anesthesia. Broadly ***TIVA provides rapid-smooth induction with minimal coughing and hiccups, rapid-easier-flexible control of anesthetic depth; and rapid-stress free-more predictable emergence with lower incidence of POVN***Q. *It* **decreases organ toxicity** ***(eg nephrotoxicity), atmospheric pollution and side effects of inhalation agents (eg expansion of closed air spaces and bone marrow suppresses related to*** N_2O***)***Q. ***It allows ideal operating conditions for neurosurgical operation with reduced cerebral metabolic rate (CMR) and cerebral blood flow (CBF)***Q.

Disadvantages of TIVA

- Propofol is more expansive then volatile agents in low flow systems
- It needs electrical power, infusion devices and requires experience to run smoothly
- *There is risk of awareness* if iv access is not maintained (eg disconnection, dislodgement and blockade) – so the infusion site must be visible at all times
- *There is no direct monitoring of plasma concentration, unlike end tidal concentrations of volatile agents.* BIS may be desirable to reduce the possibility of awareness. The actual plasma concentration may be desirable of agent is subjected to biological variability and may not match model's predictive value. Therefore predicted plasma conc. must be adjusted to control the depth of anesthesia assessed clinically, in the same way as end expired partial pressure would be adjusted when using inhalational technique.

Etomidate

- **Etomidate** is a *carboxylated imidazole* compound, that is a *selective positive allosteric modulator at GABA A receptor* and, unlike thiopental does not appear to affect other pentameric ion channels. It is *structurally unrelated* to other agents.
- It is rapidly acting general anesthetic agent with a *short duration of action* (2-3 min), resulting predominantly from *redistribution,* although it is also eliminated rapidly from body. It is characterized by ***hemodynamic stability, minimal respiratory depression & cerebroprotective effect***Q.
- It is a ***sedative hypnotic but lacks analgesic properties***Q
- As with thiopental, ***cerebral blood flow and metabolism, intracranial & intraocular pressure all fall with etomidate***Q

- As with methohexital, *excitatory phenomenon* (on induction) may be seen which can be prevented by benzodiazepine premedication or concomitant use of opioid.
- *Central sympathetic out flow is stimulated*, which maintains hemodynamics. Because of minimal cardiovascular effect, *CPP is well maintained.*
- *It enhances somatosensory evoked potentials* on EEG.
- It causes ***adreno – cortical suppression***[Q] by *inhibiting enzymes 11β hydroxylase (mainly) & 17 α hydroxylase* ***involved in cortisol and aldosterone (mineralocorticoid) production***[Q]. Vit C supplimentation restores cortisol level.
- *Excitatory phenomenon* causing myoclonus, hiccups & other involuantry movements (40%); *emergence phenomenon* causing restlessness & delirium during recovery; high incidence of *nausea and vomiting (highest among all IV anesthetics i.e. ~40%)*; and *pain on injection, vitamin C deficiency*, & thrombophlebitis are other adverse effects of etomidate.

2

Induced / Deliberate / Controlled – Hypotensive Anesthesia

Indications: When hypotension is used to reduce blood loss the BP is deliberately reduced (to 1/3rd of preoperative value, reducing the systolic BP to 80-90 mm Hg or mean arterial pressure to 50-65 mm Hg) to achieve desired response. In contrast when hypotension is used to facilitate vessel surgery or to enhance myocardial performance, the goal is to control BP so as to prevent an unwanted rise or to maintain a slightly hypotensive state. A reliable IV line & accurate BP monitoring is mandatory.

I. Reduction of surgical blood loss
- To produce dry operative field & improve visualization for intracranial neuro surgery
- When blood is not available or cannot be given d/t religious reasons (Jehovah's convention)
- Large blood loss is expected eg. malignancy

II. Facilitation of vascular surgery

By keeping large vessels soft & preventing progressive stretching of their walls, hypotension makes suturing or clipping easier. Applications include:
- *Clipping of intracranial aneurysm or arteriovenous malformations.*
- Cardiovascular surgeries like coarctectomy, aortic surgery, coarctation of aorta & patent ductus arteriosus repair.
- ***Excision of vascular tumors (like nasopharyngeal angiofibroma)***[Q]
- Operations for portal hypertension
- Hypertension after cardiopulmonary by pass/ in pheochromocytoma

III. Improvement of myocardial performance by reducing the preload & afterload.

Contraindications (relative)
1) Infants
2) Pregnancy
3) Significant decrease in O_2 delivery
4) Systemic disease compromising major organ function
5) Renal, cerebral, or coronary artery disease
6) Children with cardiac shunt
7) Patient with sickle cell disease
8) Un corrected polycythemia
9) Ganglionic blocking drugs in patient with narrow angle glaucoma
10) Inexperience

Techniques and drugs used
- **Ganglionic blocking** drugs eg pentolinium, trimethaphan
- **Direct acting vasodilators** eg ***SNP (sodium nitroprusside), nitroglycerine/glycerol trinitrate***[Q], hydralazine, adenosine, prostaglandin E_1.
- **α-adrenergic blocking drugs** eg ***phenotolamine***[Q], urapidil, nicergoline
- **β-adrenergic blocking drugs** eg propranolol (both β1 & $β_2$ blocker), practolol, metoprolol and esmolol (cardioselective) β blockers)
- **Both α & β blocker** eg labetalol
- **Calcium channel blocker** eg nicardipine, verapamil
- **Fenoldopam**, a pure dopamine (D_1) receptor antagonist with selective coronary, renal, mesenteric & peripheral arteriolar vasodilator action.
- Tilting patient (head up or foot down) decreases arterial pressure as a result of peripheral pooling. Patient should not be tilted too quickly as cerebral auto regualion requires several minutes.
- High spinal /epidural
- ***Inhalation anesthetics eg isoflurane (inhalation agent of choice), halothane***[Q], enflurane, savoflurane, desflurane. However, the use of these drugs as sole means of inducing hypotension is not recommended because they cause:

- *Impairment of myocardial contractile function*
- With increasing inhalation anesthetics concentration, cerebral autoregulation is impaired & cerebral blood flow (CBF) and intracranial pressure may increase.
  Dose related depression of cardiovascular function by inhalation agents, with some differences, is well documented
- In healthy people, both halothane & enflurane have minimal (no) effects on systemic vascular resistance (SVR) & hypotension is 2^0 to dose dependent decrease in left ventricular function
- Halothane has little (no) effect on heart rate, (H R) whereas isoflurane & enflurane increase HR
- Isoflurane causes hypotension by decreasing SVR whereas cardiac output is preserred b/o associated decrease in after load.
- Isoflurane (up to 1 MAC) produce a conc. related depression of cerebral metabolism, influence the global cerebral oxygen supply-demand ratio favourably & may afford cerebral protection. But with higher conc. CBF & ICP increases.

Prevention of tachyphylaxis (i.e. diminished response) to hypotensive drugs
- Halothane & other inhalation agents (inactivates baro-receptor response)
- Avoid or decrease fluid overload/belladonna drugs
- Preoperative sedation/IV opioids/β blockers
- Premedication with clonidine/ACE inhibitor/angiotensin II competitive antagonist
- Combining hypotensive drugs

Sodium Nitroprusside

- It is an effective *antihypertensive* agent which *dilates both arteries and veins.* Short term side effects are d/t excessive vasodilation with *hypotension* and its consequences.
- Pharmacokinetics : SNP is accumulated in RBC, receive electron from iron of hemoglobin and gets converted to methaemoglobin and unstable radical yielding nitric oxide and ***cyanide (main toxic)***[Q]. There are 4 pathways for disposal of this free CN-
  - Conversion to cyanomethemoglobin (1/5)
  - Most of the cyanide remains localized in RBC, binding to mitochondrial cytochrome oxidase, inhibiting oxidative phosphorylation. The subsequent anaerobic metabolism l/t lactic acidosis (metabolic acidosis).
  - Cyanide in plasma is *converted to thiocyanate* in *liver and kidney,* catalyzed by *enzyme rhodenase & cofactor* B_{12a}. It is *major metabolic pathway* for CN- in humans. Added *thiosulfate* speeds the reaction by providing sulfur atom. Thiocyanate is a relatively nontoxic compound & is excreted in urine.
  - In presence of hydroxocobalamin, CN- becomes cyanocobalamin (not important pathway in humans)
- The limiting factor in the metabolism of cyanide is availability of sulfur containing substrate thiosulfate in the body. Cyanide accumulates in the RBC & thiocyanate diffuses out in the plasma, hence ***monitoring plasma thiocyanate concentrations during prolonged nitroprusside infusion is a useful marker of impending cyanide toxicity.***[Q]

Detection of cyanide toxicity

- In children, 3 abnormal responses suggesting impending CN- intoxication are
1. *requirement of high dose* of SNP (>10 μg kg^{-1} min^{-1})
2. *tachyphylaxis* which is apparent 30-60 min after the start of infusion
3. *resistance* apparent within 5-10 min after the start of infusion.
- **Clinical manifestations** of CN- toxicity are
  - Metabolic acidosis
  - Increased requirements for SNP
  - Progressive hypotension with narrow pulse pressure
  - Refractory hypotension unresponsive to fluids & vasopressors but responsive to thiosulfate
  - Cardiovascular collapse
  - Bright venous blood
  - Increased SvO_2 & PvO_2
- Most sensitive metaolic indicators (in dogs) are blood pH, blood lactate (or lactate /pyruvate) levels, Pvo_2 or Svo_2, sagittal sinus O_2 tension (reflecting ↓ cerebral O_2 uptake), cerebral metabolic rate for O_2 and brain lactate (or lactate/pyruvate).
- In humans lethal levels of *blood CN-* is ~500μg/dl & thiocyanate can be as low as *~340μg/dl.* However this varies with rate of CN- release as well as with the total dose. Measurements of blood CN- release as well as with the total dose. ***Measurements of blood CN- or thiocyanate levels does not reflect the magnitude of CN- released***[Q]. So nonspecific lab tests are relied upon as indicator of CN- toxicity.

Prevention of CN- toxicity

- Total dose should not exceed 1.5 mg/kg/hr for short exposures or 0.5 mg/kg/hr for prolonged exposures. Infusion rates exceeding 10μg/kg/min are contraindicated.
- *Initial rate* of SNP infusion should be *0.5-1μg/kg/min* and response is *monitored during first 30 min.* If either a constant requirement of high doses of SNP or tachycardia is noted a *β-blocker* should be administered & *inhaled anesthetic concentration increased.* A rapid response is usually seen & SNP dose can be decreased. If resistance is still detected (within 5-10 min), the SNP is stopped & *a different hyptensive drug given.*

Treatment of cyanide toxicity

- **Sodium thiosulfate** (STS) can afford complete protection against CN^- & complete detoxification if *three times more* thiosulfate than CN^- is present by ensuring plentiful supply of sulfhydryl radicals needed to form thiocyanate from CN^-.
- STS bolus injection of 30 mg/kg f/b 60mg /kg /hr continuous infusion is most effective antidote against CN- toxicity.
- **Hydroxocobalamin (vitamin B12a)** prevents an increase CN- conc. in RBC when given prophylactically with large doses of SNP. Dose is 50 mg/kg bolus f/b 100 mg/kg/h
- *Correction of acidosis, fluid replacement & blood transfusion,* if patient is bleeding.

QUESTIONS

CLASSIFICATION

1. **Not intravenous Anasthetic agent**
   A. Ketamine (AI 1995) ☐
   B. Thiopantone ☐
   C. Etomidate ☐
   D. Cyclopropane ☐

PROPOFOL

2. **A 20 yr old patient presented with early pregnancy for Medical Termination of Preg-nancy (MTP) in day care facility. What will be the anesthetic induction agent of choice?**
   A. Thiopentone (AIIMS May 2006) ☐
   B. Ketamine ☐
   C. Propofol ☐
   D. Diazepam ☐
3. **Regarding features of propofol, which of the following statement is correct:** (PGI Dec 05)
   A. It suppresses adrenocortical hormone secretion ☐
   B. I.M.inj. is painful ☐
   C. Undergoes hepatic metabolism ☐
   D. Chemically it is derivative of D-isopropyl phenol ☐
   E. Cerebral protector action ☐
4. **All are true about propofol except** (PGI 99, 02, DNB 02)
   A. Plesant sedation & recovery ☐
   B. Safe in porphyria ☐
   C. Antiemetic effect ☐
   D. Suppression of airway reflexes ☐
   E. Cardiac stimulant ☐
5. **Which of the following is NOT TRUE regarding PROPOFOL?** (AI 08)
   A. It is used in day care anesthesia ☐
   B. It is contraindcated in porphyria ☐
   C. Commercial preparation contains egg extract ☐
   D. It does not cause airway irritation ☐
6. **True about propofol:** (PGI May 2010)
   A. Indicated in egg allergy ☐
   B. Can be used in porphyria ☐
   C. It is of barbiturate group ☐
   D. Used in day care surgery ☐
7. **A severely ill patient was maintained on an infusional anaesthetic agent. On the 2nd day he started detiorating. The probable culprit may be** (PGI 99, Jipmer 04, DNB 05)
   A. Etiomidate ☐
   B. Propofol ☐
   C. Opioid ☐
   D. Barbiturate ☐
8. **The following anaesthetic drug causes pain on intravenous adminstration:**
   A. Midazolam (DNB 07, AIIMS May 06) ☐
   B. Propofol ☐
   C. Ketamine ☐
   D. Thiopentone sodium ☐
9. **Bradycardia during anaesthesia seen in**
   A. Pancuronium (PGI June 2004) ☐
   B. Vecuronium ☐
   C. Atracurium ☐
   D. Propofol ☐
   E. Succinylcholine ☐

KETAMINE

10. **Dose of Ketamine is** (AIIMS 1993)
    A. 0.5 mg/Kg I/m ☐
    B. 2 mg/kg I/v ☐
    C. 5mg/kg I/v ☐
    D. 10mg / kg I/m ☐
11. **Which of the following anesthetic agents is contraindicated in a 32 yr old patient with hypertension planned for elective cholecystectomy?** (AI 2011)
    A. Ketamine ☐
    B. Propofol ☐
    C. Etomidate ☐
    D. Diazepam ☐
12. **Which of the following drugs produces dissociative anesthesia** (AIIMS Nov 2006, AI 96)
    A. Ketamine ☐
    B. Propofol ☐
    C. Thiopentone ☐
    D. Enflurane ☐
13. **Which drug of anesthetics causes delirium & hallucination** (AI 98, 93)
    A. Ketamine ☐
    B. Trilene ☐
    C. Halothane ☐
    D. Trichloroethylenev ☐
14. **Increased Cardiac Oxygen demand is caused by**
    A. Halothane (AIIMS 1993) ☐
    B. Thiopentone ☐
    C. N_2O ☐
    D. Ketamine ☐
15. **Intraocular Pressure is lowered by A/E (or increased by)**
    A. Ketamine (DNB 99, AI 91, 93) ☐
    B. Morphine ☐
    C. Halothane ☐
    D. Thiopentane ☐
16. **ICT is raised due to:** (AI 02, PGI 97)
    A. Ketamine ☐
    B. Scoline ☐
    C. Halothane ☐
    D. Ether ☐
17. **Which of the following anaeshetic agents have good (maximum) analgesic property?**
    A. Ketamine (PGI June 06, AI 97) ☐
    B. Nitrous oxide ☐
    C. Thiopentone ☐
    D. Propofol ☐
    E. Midazolam ☐
18. **Cerebral metabolism and O_2 consumption are increased by:** (AIIMS Nov 2007)
    A. Propofol ☐
    B. Ketamine ☐
    C. Atracurium ☐
    D. Fentanyl ☐
19. **With regard to Ketamine, all of the following are true except:** (AIIMS Nov 05)

A. It is a direct myocardial depressant ☐
B. Emergence phenomenon are more likely if anticholinergic premedication is used ☐
C. It may induce cardiac dysarythmias in patients receiving tricyclic antidepressants ☐
D. Has no effect on intracranial pressure ☐

20. **All statements regarding ketamine are true except**
A. May be arrythmogenic *(PGI 04, 02)* ☐
B. Raised ICT do not respond to CO_2 level ☐
C. Vasodialator and negative ionotropic effect ☐
D. Psychomimetic emergence
E. Indirectly sympathetic action ☐

21. **Ketamine is safe in** *(AIIMS 91, 02)*
A. Raised ICT ☐
B. Open eye injury ☐
C. Ischemic heart disease ☐
D. Severe shock ☐

22. **Ketamine can be used in all of the situations except**
A. Status asthamaticus *(AI 92, 2K)* ☐
B. For analgesia & sedation ☐
C. Obstetric hemorrhage ☐
D. Ischemic heart disease ☐
E. Aortic aneurysm ☐

23. **An unconcious patient of head injury comes in casualty. On examination shows raised intracranial pressure. Which anesthetic agent is contraindicated:**
A. Thiopentone *(AIIMS 98, 99; AI 06)* ☐
B. Propofol ☐
C. Ketamine ☐
D. Etomidate ☐

THIOPENTANE (BARBITURATE)

24. **Total cerebral metabolic failure occurs at blood flow of**
A. 10 ml/100 gm/min *(AIIMS May 12)* ☐
B. 20 ml/100 gm/ml ☐
C. 30 ml/100 gm/min ☐
D. 40 ml/100 gm/ml ☐

25. **Most potent cerebral vasodilator is** *(AIIMS May 12)*
A. B blocker ☐
B. Nitro-glycerine ☐
C. Hyper carbia ☐
D. Nitroprusside ☐

26. **Anesthetic agent (s) safe to use in ↑ICP** *(PGI Nov 2009)*
A. Halothane ☐
B. Thiopentone ☐
C. Ketamine ☐
D. Ether ☐

27. **Sodium Thiopentone is ultra short acting d/t**
A. Rapid absorption *(AI 1996)* ☐
B. Rapid metabolism ☐
C. Rapid redistribution ☐
D. Rapid excretion ☐

28. **Commonly used in narcoanalysis** *(AI 2010)*
A. Atropine ☐
B. Scopolamine ☐
C. Opium ☐
D. Thiopentone ☐

29. **% of thiopentone used in induction**
A 0.5% *(AIIMS 1995)* ☐
B. 1.5% ☐
C. 2.5% ☐
D. 4.5% ☐

30. **Use of Thiopentone-** *(PGI Dec 2004)*
A. Seizure ☐
B. Truth spell ☐
C. Reduction of ICP ☐
D. Cerebral protection ☐
E. Maintenance of an anesthesia ☐

31. **Dose of Thiopentone used for induction is**
A. 1 mg/kg *(JIPMER 96)* ☐
B. 2 mg/kg ☐
C. 5 mg/kg ☐
D. 10 mg/kg ☐
E. 15 mg/kg ☐

32. **All are true about Thiopentone except:** *(AIIMS Nov 07)*
A. $NaHCO_3$ is a preservative ☐
B. Contraindicated in Porphyria ☐
C. Agent of choice in shock ☐
D. Has cerebroprotective action ☐

33. **Drugs contraindicated in acute intermittent porphyria-**
A. Thiopentone *(PGI Nov 09, Dec 2004)* ☐
B. Etomidate ☐
C. Ketamine ☐
D. Propofol ☐
E. Midazolam ☐

34. **Thiopentone is C/I in:** *(AIIMS 1997)*
A. Acute intermittent porphyria ☐
B. Bronchial Asthma ☐
C. Both ☐
D. None ☐

35. **Intravenous thiopentone pentox, produces**
A. Rash *(PGI 2003)* ☐
B. Pain ☐
C. Spasm ☐
D. Hypotension ☐
E. Muscular excitation (locally) ☐

36. **Intra artireal injection of thiopentone causes:**
A. Vasospasm *(AIIMS 1995)* ☐
B. Vasodialation ☐
C. Necrosis of vessel wall ☐
D. Hypotension ☐

37. **If thiopentone is injected accidently into an artery the first symptom is** *(AI 1997)*
A. Analgesia ☐
B. Paralysis ☐
C. Skin ulceration ☐
D. Pain ☐

38. **Which of the following anaesthetic agent lacks analgesic effect:** *(PGI Dec 2005)*
A. N_2O ☐
B. Thiopentone ☐
C. Methohexitone ☐
D. Ketamine ☐
E. Fentanyl ☐

39. **Primary mechanism responsible for cerebral protection effect of thiopentone is** *(AI 12)*
A. GABA action, calcium channel block and free radicle removal ☐
B. Increased cerebral blood flow ☐
C. Decreased (lowered) cerebn metabolism ☐
D. Reduces cerebral O_2 demand by limiting CBF ☐

NEUROLEPTIC ANAESTHESIA

40. Neurolept analgesia all are true except :
A. Can be used along with O_2 & N_2O ☐
B. Causes focal dystonia *(PGI 1998)* ☐
C. Fentanyl- droperidol ☐
D. Causes hypotension ☐
E. None ☐

41. Characteristics of Remifentanyl:
A. Metabolised by plasma esterase ☐
B. Short half life *(PGI Dec 07)* ☐
C. More potent than Alfentanyl ☐
D. Dose reduced in hepatic and renal disease ☐
E. Duration of action more than Alfentanyl ☐

42. Which one of the common side effects is seen with fentanyl? *(AIIMS May 2006)*
A. Chest wall rigidly ☐
B. Tachycardia ☐
C. Pain in abdomen ☐
D. Hypertension ☐

43. Drug contraindicated in renal failure is *(AI 12)*
A. Morphine ☐
B. Pethidine ☐
C. Fentanyl ☐
D. Alfentanil ☐

44. Muscle Rigidity is caused by which agent
A. Fentanyl *(AI 1991)* ☐
B. Halothane ☐
C. Ketamine ☐
D. Droperidol ☐

45. Least sedative narcotic? *(AIIMS Nov 09)*
A. Morphine ☐
B. Codeine ☐
C. Papaverine ☐
D. Noscapine ☐

Total Intravenous Anaesthesia (TIVA)

46. There have been many recent advances in TIVA compared to inhalational anesthesia. Which of the following is true about TIVA *(AIIMS May 12)*
A. Reduces cerebral metabolism (CMR) and CBF ☐
B. Smooth induction with high incidence of post operative nausea and vomiting ☐
C. Propofol inhibits pulmonary vasoconstriction d/t hypoxia, and is a/w increased pulmonary toxicity, malignant hyperthermia and enhanced N_2O effects ☐
D. Higher chances of nephrotoxity ☐

ETOMIDATE

47. Which anaethetic induction agent that may cause adrenal cortex suppression is: *(AIIMS 10, AI 03, PGI June 06)*
A. Ketamine ☐
B. Etomidate ☐
C. Propofol ☐
D. Thiopentone ☐
E. Fentanyl ☐

48. A intravenous anesthetic agent that is associated with hemodynamic stability , maintenence of CPP with post operative nausea, vomiting and myoclonus
A. Ketamine *(PGI 2002, SGPGI 2004)* ☐
B. Etomidate ☐
C. Propofol ☐
D. Opioids. ☐

49. Which anesthetic induction agent produces cardiac stability. In other words cardiostable anesthesia is.
A. Ketamine *(AIIMS May 09)* ☐
B. Propofol ☐
C. Thiopental ☐
D. Etomidate ☐

50. All of the following cause myocardial depression except:
A. Halothane *(PGI June 09)* ☐
B. Etomidate ☐
C. Thiopentone ☐
D. Ketamine ☐
E. Propofol ☐

HYPOTENSIVE ANAESTHESIA

51. Hypotensive Anesthesia in nasopharyngeal angiofibroma is/are given by: *(PGI Nov 2009)*
A. Propofol ☐
B. Ketamine ☐
C. Phentolamine ☐
D. Halothane ☐
E. Na Nitroprusside ☐

52. Sodium nitroprusside infusion may result in:
A. Hypertension *(AIIMS May 2005)* ☐
B. Pulmonary oedema ☐
C. Cyanide toxicity ☐
D. Heart block ☐

Answers and Explanations:

1. **D i.e. Cyclopropane**
2. **C i.e. Propofol**
3. **C i.e. Undergoes hepatic metabolism; D i.e. Chemically it is derivative of D-isopropyl phenol; E i.e. Cerebral protector action**
4. **E i.e. Cardiac stimulant**
5. **B i.e. It is contraindicated in porphyria**
6. **B i.e. Can be used in porphyria, D i.e. Used in day care surgery**
[Ref: Aitkenhead 5/e, P- 41-45, 616–17; Miller's 6/e p-318–26, 2590- 2610; Lee's 13/e p- 158-60, 586- 88; Morgan's 4/e p. 200–202; Wiley & Davidson 7/e p-570-72, 1024-33, 571]

Propofol

- ***Smooth induction, rapid onset of action, easy titration to effect, short clinical duration of action and demonstrable antiemetic effect*** – make ***propofol an induction agent of choice for day care (out patient) anesthesia***Q.
- It is **extremely useful in** situations in which volatile anesthetic agents are not available or applicable and intravenous anesthetic technique must be employed, for example ***rigid laryngoscopy or bronchoscopy, tracheobronchial surgery with apneic oxygenation or ventilation, transfer of anesthelized patients, high risk of post operative nausea & vomiting, and susceptibility to malignant hyperpyrexia***Q.
- Its advantages are particularly evident in –*day case anesthesia, neuroanesthesia, cardiac anesthesia especially during cardiopulmonary bypass, sedation for intensive care, or comfort during radiological intervertions, endoscopy or minor surgery with local anesthesia.*
- Its role in pediatric anesthesia is controversial. It is ***not approved for anesthesia in children less than 3 years old***Q or for sedation for intensive care, or surgical and diagnostic procedure.
- Metabolism – *Lung* play an important role in first pass elimination and responsible for approximately 30% of removal of drug after a bolus dose. Drug is metabolized in *liver* by glucoronide conjugation to produce water soluble compound which are excreted by *kidney.*

Effect on organ system						
CVS		Respiratory		CNS		
HR	**MAP**	**Vent.**	**Bronchiodilation**	**CBF**	**Cerebral Oxygen consumption**	**ICP**
- -/↓Q	↓↓↓	↓↓↓	- -	↓↓↓	↓↓↓	↓

- ***Propofol and thiopental provides similar degree of cerebral protection*** Q.
- Unless the propofol is given very slowly or by infusion, ***severe dose dependent myocardial depression***Q is seen following a bolus dose of propofol and is likely to cause **hypotension** in *hypovolaemic or untreated hypertensive* and those with *cardiovascular/ischemic heart disease* more commonly. CVS depression is modest if drug is administered slowly or by infusion.

7. **A i.e. Etomidate; B i.e. Propofol**

- ***Increased infection and mortality in a group of patients sedated with etomidate infusion in an ICU was associated with low cortisol levels***Q and is attributed to ***etomidate induced supression of adrenal cortisal synthesis***Q.
- Etomidate is a dose dependent but *reversible inhibitor of 11 - β hydroxylase* in the adrenal cortex and is more potent than **metyrapone.** This enzyme is required for both mineralocorticoid and corticosteroid production. Minor adrenocortical supressive effects (i.e. impaired response to ACTH) follow induction doses or short infusion doses.
- Propofol is not recommended for sedation of *critically ill pediatric patients in ICU*. The drug has been associated with higher mortality d/t ***propofol infusion syndrome***. Its essential features are *metabolic acidosis, multiple organ failure, hemodynamic instability, hepatomegaly, and rhabdomyolysis*. Very rarely, it may occur in adults, and in patients undergoing long term propofol infusion (> 48 hours) for sedation at high doses (>5 mg/kg/hr).

8. **B i.e. Propofol** *[Ref: Wiley & Davidson 7/e p-570–71; Miller's 6/e p-318- 20; Morgan's 4/e p. 200–202; Aitkenhead 4/e, P- 170-76; Lee's 13/e p-158-60]*

ANAESTHESIA 2

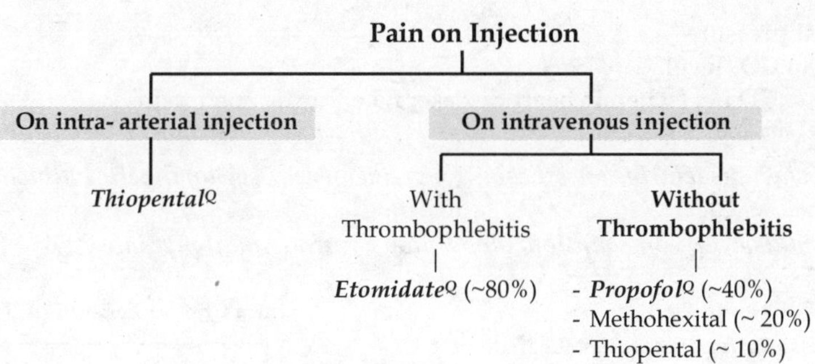

- Incidence of pain on injection after intravenous administration of drug in small vein (eg. dorsum of wrist or hand) is 80% for **etomidate**, 40% for **propofol**, 20% for **methohexital** 1% and 10% for **thiopental 2.5%** anesthetic agents
- This incidence is greatly reduced if a *large vein* is used, if a *small dose of lidocaine* (10mg) is injected shortly before.
- Thiopental 2.5% also causes pain on IV administration but the incidence is much higher for propofol.

9. **C i.e. Atracurium; D i.e. Propofol; E i.e. Succinylcholine**
[Ref: Lee's Anesthesia 13/e p-156-162; Miller's anesthesia 5/e p. 443; KDT 5/e p. 343, 313, 312]

- **Propofol** causes ***bradycardia***Q (d/t central vagal activity) & ***hypotension***Q (d/t vasodilation)
- **d-TC, Pancuronium, Vecuronium** Q **& Rocuronium** Q causes ***bradycardia & fall in BP.*** Q
- **Succinylcholine** causes bradycardia initially d/t stimulation of vagal ganglia followed by tachycardia & hypertension d/t stimulation of sympathetic ganglion
- Other nondepolarizing M.R. have negligible effect on BP & heart rate.
- **Atracurium** may cause ***bradycardia.*** Q

Ketamine

10. **B i.e. 2mg/Kg IV**

Ketamine
- IM - 6 mg/kg (3-6 mg/Kg)
- IV - 2 mg/kg (1-2 mg/Kg)

Ketotifen
- 2 mg/Kg

Ketorolac
- 2 mg/Kg/IV
- 10 mg/Kg/IM

11. **A i.e. Ketamine**
[Ref. Morgan 4/e, p 197-99]

In sharp contrast to most other anesthetic agents (propofol, etomidate, opioids except meperidine and most benzodiazepines), ***ketamine increases arterial blood pressure (BP), heart rate (HR) and cardiac output***Q. These *indirect effects* are d/t central stimulation of sympathetic nervous system and inhibition of reuptake of norepinephrine. *Increase in pulmonary artery pressure and myocardial work* accompany these changes. Hence **ketamine should be avoided** in patients with ***ischemic heart (coronary artery) disease, uncontrolled hypertension, congestive heart failure and arterial aneurysm***Q. On the the other hand it's ***indirect stimulatory effects are beneficial to patients with acute hypovolemic shock***Q.

Cardiovascular effects

	Ketamine	Barbiturates (thiopental, thiamylal methohexital)	Droperidol	Benzodiazepines (diazepam, lorazepam, Midazolam*)	Etomidate	Propofol	Opioids		
							Fentanyl Sufentanyl Al/Remi-fentanil*	Morphine	Meperidine
HR	↑↑	↑↑	↑	O/↑	O	O	↓↓	↓	↑
MAP (BP)	↑↑	↓↓	↓↓	↓	↓	↓↓↓	↓/↓↓*	H	H

H means depends on extent of histamine release; * Midazolam and droperidol have same effects

12. **A i.e. Ketamine** 13. **A i.e. Ketamine** 14. **D i.e. Ketamine** 15. **A i.e. Ketamine**
16. **A i.e. Ketamine** 17. **A i.e. Ketamine; B i.e. Nitrous oxide** 18. **B i.e. Ketamine**

19. D i.e. Has no effect on intracranial pressure
20. B i.e. Raised ICT do not respond to CO_2 level
21. D i.e. Severe Shock **22. D i.e. Ischemic heart disease; E i.e. Aortic aneurysm**
[Ref: Aitkenhead 4/e, P- 178-79; Wiley & Davidson 7/e p-576-75; Miller's 6/e p-345- 50; Morgan's 4/e p. 197- 99; Lee's 13/e p-162- 65]

Ketamine causes ***profound analgesia***Q, ***disociative anesthesia***Q, and ***emergence psychomimetic hallucinations and delirium*** Q.
Ketamine increases ***cerebral metabolism, O_2 consumption, blood flow & intracranial pressure.***Q

Ketamine

- It causes ***profound analgesia***Q and ***dissociative anesthesia***Q (i.e. patient appears conscious e.g. eye opening, swallowing but unable to process or respond to sensory input). Ketamine causes ***Dissociative Anesthesia***Q by acting on **cortex and subcortical areas (not on RAS)** l/t feeling of dissociation from ones own body and surroundings. *Post Operative Delirium and Hallucination*Q is part of this Dissociative phenomenon. **Drug of choice for post op. delirium & hallucination is Lorazepam.**Q
- It is *closest to being a complete anesthetic* since it induces analgesia, amnesia & unconsciousness.
- It is associated with ***emergence psychotomimetic side effects (delirium, illusions, hallucination)***Q. It is less common in children and pretreatment with ***lorazepam (drug of choice)***Q.
- It is a *sympathetic stimulant,* so it causes:

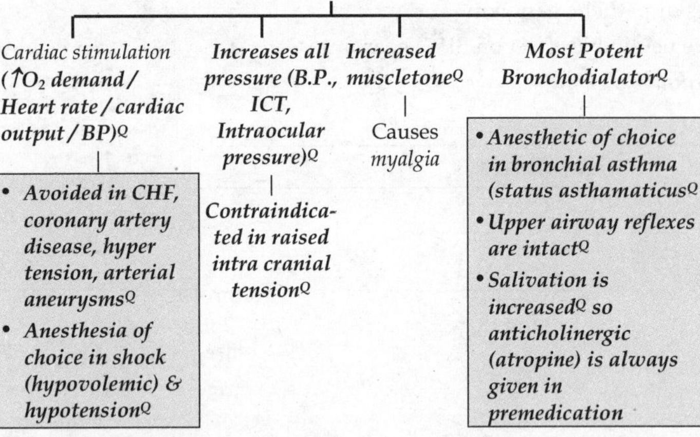

Cardiac stimulation (↑O_2 demand / Heart rate / cardiac output / BP)Q
Avoided in CHF, coronary artery disease, hyper tension, arterial aneurysmsQ
Anesthesia of choice in shock (hypovolemic) & hypotensionQ
Increases all pressure (B.P., ICT, Intraocular pressure)Q
Contraindicated in raised intra cranial tensionQ
Increased muscletoneQ
Causes myalgia
Most Potent BronchodialatorQ
Anesthetic of choice in bronchial asthma (status asthamaticusQ
Upper airway reflexes are intactQ
Salivation is increasedQ so anticholinergic (atropine) is always given in premedication

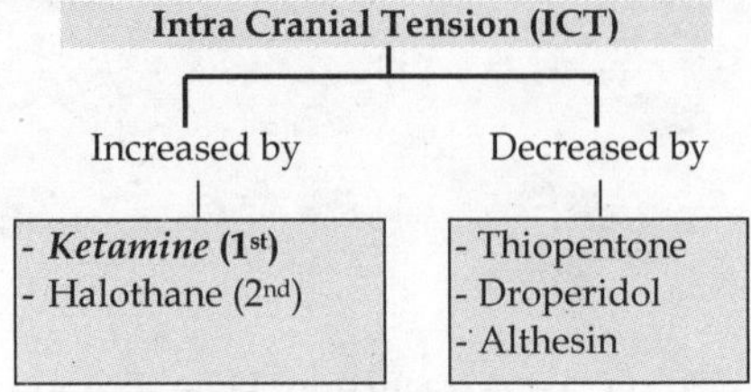

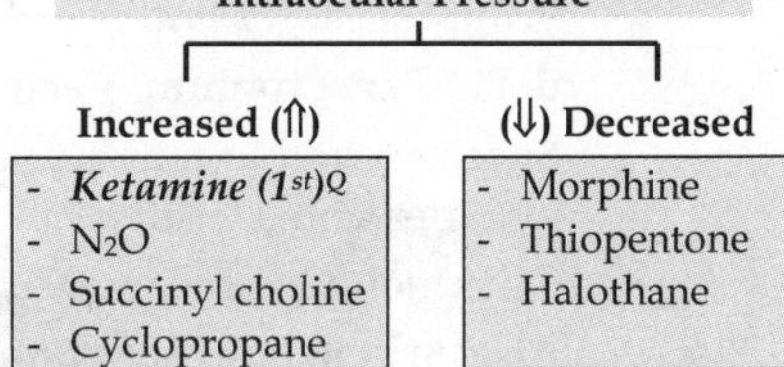

Intraocular Pressure
Increased (⇑)
(⇓) Decreased
- Ketamine (1st)Q
- N_2O
- Succinyl choline
- Cyclopropane
- Morphine
- Thiopentone
- Halothane

Maximum i.e. very good) analgesic agents are
- *Ketamine*Q
- Buprenorphine
- Trilene
- Sufentanyl

23. C i.e. Ketamine

Ketamine causes increase in all pressure i.e. *intracranial, intraocular, intragastric and intravascular (Blood) pressure.* So it is not used in raised ICT/IOT & Hypertension as it may increase the pressure to morbid levels.

Preferable **anesthetic agents of choice in head injury are** :
- ***Thiopentone***Q ***(cerebro protective)***Q
- *Propofol*
- *Etomidate* (protection against circulatory depression)
- *Isoflurane*
- M.R. = Ro/Ve/Pipe-curonium, Doxocurium, Sch (although ↑ ICT but given in difficult airway)

Barbiturate (Thiopentone)

24. A i.e. 10 ml/100 gm/min **25. C i.e. Hyper carbia** *[Ref. Miller 7/e, p 305]*

Severe reduction in CBF (< 10 mL/100 gm/min) l/t rapid ischemic neuronal death, characterized by early excitotoxicity and delayed apoptosis. ***Hypercarbia is most potent cerebral vasodilator***Q.

26. B i.e. Thiopentone *[Ref: Morgan 4/e p-167, 200]*

Anesthetic agents safe to use in raised intracranial pressure (ICP) are ***thiopentone, propofol & etomidate***Q

CNS effects of anesthetic agents

Inhalational agents						Nonvolatile agents							
Ether	N_2O	Halothane	Isoflurane	Desflurane	Sevoflurene	Barbiturates eg thiopental	Benzodiazepines eg diazepam, lorazepam, midazolam	Opioids eg morphine, meperidine, su/al/remi-fentanyl	Ketamine	Etomidate	Propofol	Droperidol	
↑	↑	↑↑	↑	↑	↑	↓↓↓	↓↓	↓	↑↑↑	↓↓↓	↓↓↓	↓	Cerebral blood flow **(CBF) & ICP**
↑	↑	↓	↓↓	↓↓	↓↓	↓↓↓	↓↓	↓	↑	↓↓↓	↓↓↓	O	Cerebral **metabolic rate/oxygen consumption**
↑	↓	↓	↓	↓	↓	↑/↓	↓		↑	↑/↓	↑/↓		**Seizures**

27. **C i.e. Rapid redistribution** **28.** **D i.e. Thiopentone** **29.** **C i.e. 2.5%**
30. **All** **31.** **C i.e. 5 mg/kg** **32.** **C i.e. Agent of choice in shock**

[Ref: Good man & Gillman 10/e – 415, 419, Wylie 7/e p- 572-73; Morgan 4/e p – 184- 87; Lee's 13/e ,p – 150- 56; Miller 6/e , p- 326-34 –Aitkinhead 4/e P- 171- 75; Stoeling 4/e P- 457]

- ***Thiopentone, a pale yellow powder, is ultrashort acting smooth inducing agent because of rapid redistribution***Q***. It is used in 2.5% conc. at 2.5 – 4.5 mg/kg mixed with 6% anhydrous*** Na_2CO_3 ***as perservative***Q
- **Thiopentone** is **contraindicated** in ***porphyria, status asthmaticus, severe shock, pericardial temponade and uncompensated myocardial disease***Q

33. **A, B i.e. Thiopentone, Etomidate** **34.** **A i.e. Acute intermittent porphyria**

- In **porphyria** ***(AIP), barbiturates (eg thiopentone, methohexital & thiamylal), etomidate, pentazocine and ropivacaine are avoided/ contraindicated***Q whereas diclofenac, ketorolac, phenacetin, tilidine, chlordiazepoxide, nitrazepam, hydralazine, nifedipine, and phenoxybenzamine are used with extreme caution only.
- **Barbiturate (Thiopentone)** induces *aminolevulenic acid synthetase & formation of porphyrin* which may precipitate ***actue intermittent or variegate prophyria***Q***. ; so it is contraindicated in porphyria.***Q
- Due to cholinergic nerve stimulation, histamine release or direct bronchial smooth muscle stimulation, barbiturates may *cause bronchospasm;* which would *be preventable by pretreatment with atropine,* so it is *not C/I in asthma.*

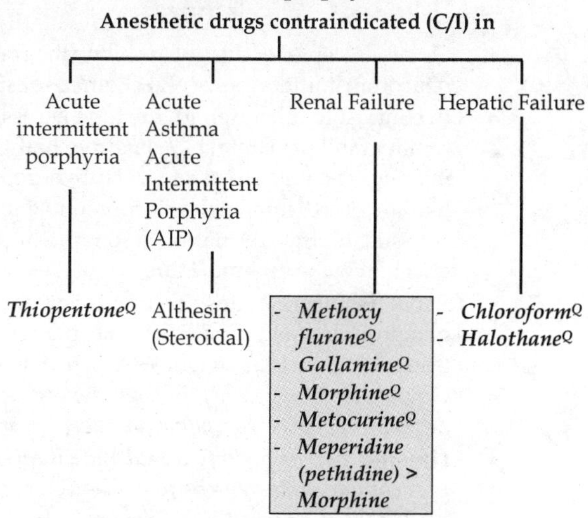

35. **A i.e. Rash; B i.e. Pain; C i.e. Spasm; D i.e. Hypotension; E i.e. Muscular excitation**
36. **A i.e. Vasospasm** **37.** **D i.e. Pain** *[Ref. Aitkenhead 5/e, p 37-38, Miller 7/e, p 307-8, 728-32]*
38. **B & C i.e. Thiopentone, Methohexitone** **39.** **C i.e. Decreased (lowered) cerebn metabolism**

Barbiturates (thiopental), primarily decreases cerebral metabolismQ resulting in a dose related *depression of cevebral metabolic oxygen consumption* ($CMRO_2$).
Reduced $CMRO_2$ causes progressive slowing of ***EEG, a reduction in rate of ATP consumption, cerebral vasoconstriction (reducing cerebral blood flow and intracranial tension) and protection from incomplete cerebral ischemia***Q.

Thiopentone Sodium

- Thiopentone is a *yellow coloured* powder used as 2.5 % solution at *5 mg/kg* dose for *smooth induction.* It is ***ultrashort acting***Q ***due to rapid redistribution***Q. It is **contraindicated in porphyria.**Q.

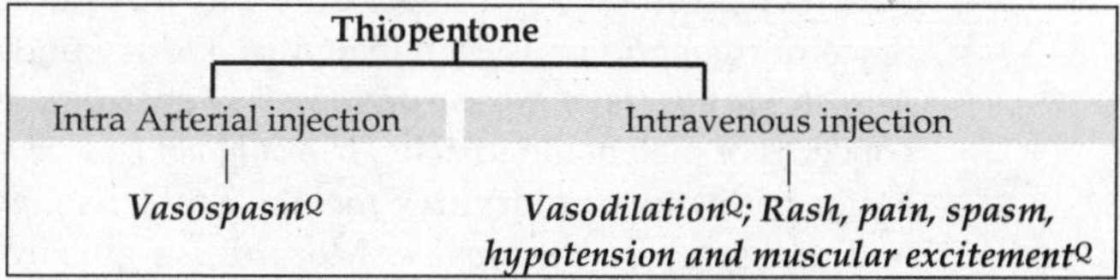

- On ***intravenous injection.*** Thiopentone causes ***vasodialation***Q *and* on ***intra-arterial*** injection, it causes, ***vasoconstriction***Q.
- To prevent intrarterial injection it is preferably given in veins of *outer aspect of forearm* in adults; *anterior to wrist* in chubby babies and on *scalp vein* in infants, not in cubital fossae.
- On intrarterial injection
  - ***1st symptom is pain***Q
  - ***1st sign is white hand with cynosis***Q of nail d/t arterial spasm.
- **Treatment**Q - ***Leave canula into the artery***Q
  - Immediate heparinisation
  - Inject ***papaverine / prosta cyclin***Q
  - ***Stellate ganglion or Brachial plexus block***Q to remove vasoconstrictor impulse.
- ***Intra-arterial injection of thiopentone l/t arterial spasm***Q. So in question if option spasm means arterial spasm, it is excluded from answer & if spasm means Laryngospasm it is included in answer.
- **Methohexitone and thiopentone belong to barbiturates and lack analgesic effect.** Infact thiopentone *decreases pain threshold* or show *antianalgesic effect.*
- *N_2O* is the only inhalational agent which shows analgesic effect.
- **Other inducing agents which have analgesic effect are:**
  - ***Ketamine***Q
  - ***Opoids e.g. fentanyl***Q
  - *Trielene* was anaesthetic agent that shows maximum analgesia but it is toxic to trigeminal nerve and abducens nerve, so, has been withdrawn.
- Features which shows that anaesthetized patient is in pain are-
  - Tearing
  - Unexplained tachycardia
- ***Pain is measured by visual analogue scale (VAS) and Mc Gill pain Questionnaire (MPQ).***Q

Neurolept Anaesthesia

40. **E i.e. None** **41.** **B i.e. Short half life; C i.e. More potent than alfentanyl**
[Ref: Wylie 7/e p- 556; Morgan 4/e p – 192- 97; Miller's 6/e p. 411- 12, 403]

Remifentanil is 1st *ultrashort acting opioid, metabolized by RBC & tissue esterase that is not appreciably influenced by hepatic & renal failure*Q*. It is 10 times more potent than alfentanil and 100 times more potent than morphine & methadone.*

42. **A i.e. Chest wall rigidity** *[Ref: Aitkenhead 4/e, P- 211- 219; Morgan's 4/e p. 192–96]*

Nonvolatile Anesthetic Agents: Opioids

- Opiate- receptor activation, inhibits the presynaptic release and post synaptic response to excitatory neurotransmitters (eg. acetyl cholne , substance P) from nociceptive neurons.
- In contrast to other opioid, the time necessary to achieve a 50% decrease in the plasma concentration of remifentanil (**its context - / sensitive half time**) is very short (~ 3 min) and *is not influenced by the duration of infusion.* The unique easter structure of remifentanil, an ultrashort acting opioid with a terminal elimination half life of <10 min, makes it susceptible to rapid ester hydrolysis by non specific esterases in blood (RBC) & tissue. Biotransformation is so rapid and so complete, that duration of remifentanil infusion has little effect on wake up time. Patient with *pseudo cholinesterase deficiency has a normal response to remifentanil.*
- Renal dysfunction cause accumulation of normeperidine (end product of meperidine) & morphine 3/6 – glucuronides (end products of morphine). **Toxic effects** of **normeperidine** cause excitatory effect on CNS, leading to *myoclonic activity & seizure* that are *not reversed by naloxone.*
- Opioids *elevated apneic threshold* (the highest $PaCO_2$ at which a patient remains apneic) and *decrease hypoxic drive. Morphine & mepiridine can cause histamine induced bronchospasm.*
- ***Opioids (particularly fentanyl, sufentanil and alfentanil) can induce chest wall rigidity, severe enough to prevent adequate ventilation***Q. This centrally mediated muscle contraction is most frequent after large drug boluses & effectively treated with neuromuscular blocking agent.
- *IV meperidine* (25mg) has been found most effective opioid for *decreasing shivering.*

43. **B i.e. Pethidine** *[Ref. Wylic 7/e, p 315, Goodman and gilmann 13/e, p. 499-504]*

- **Meperidine (pethidine, demerol)**, a *phenylpiperidine* is metabolized chiefly in liver to **nonmeperidine**, which is *eliminated by the kidney and liver.* In patients or addicts who are tolerant to the depressant effects of meperidine, large doses repeated at short interval may produce an **excitatory syndrome** including hallncination, tremors, muscle twitches, dilated pupils, hyperactive reflexes and convulsions. These excitatory symptoms are d/t accumulation of normeperidine, which has a *half life of 15-20 hours, compared to 3 hours for meperidine.* In patients with cirrhosis, the bioavailability of meperidine is ~80% increased and t½ of both meperidine and normeperidine are prolonged.
- Since normeperidine is eleminated by kidney and liver, ***decreased renal or hepatic function predispose to neurotoxic effects of nor-meperidine***Q. Meperidine is also *not recommended for the treatment of chronic pain* b/o concerns of metabolite toxicity. *It should not be used for longer than 48 hours or in doses > 600 mg/day.*
- Major pathway for **morphine** metabolism is *conjugation with glucuronic acid* forming *morphine -6- glucuronide* and *morphine -3- glucuronide.* **Morphine-6-glucuronide** is **twice as potent as morphine with somewhat**

longer t½. (t½ of morphine is 2 hours) and pharmacological actions indistinguishable from those of morphine. With chronic morphine administration, the 6-glucuronide accounts for most of analgesia and its blood levels exceed those of morphine. **Morphine-6-glucuronide is excreted by kidney,** so its levels increase in renal failure, perhaps *explaining morphine's potency and long action* in compromised renal function. So in patients with renal failure decreased protein binding of morphine (resulting in higher plasma free drug level) and accumulation of morphine -6- glucuronide predispose them to **respiratory depression**. So morphine is given cautiously in low doses in renal failure.

- Respiratory depression is also reported in patients with CRF receiving **sufentanyl.** Except for slightly decreased protein binding, the free drug volume of distribution and clearance of **alfentanil** *appears to be unaffected by renal failure.* **Fentanyl,** has short half life and its metabolites are inactive. Therefore, it ***is a good choice in patients with renal disease***[Q].
- In **renal disease (renal failure) remifentanil > fentanyl > alfentanil > sufentanil** are safe. Whereas **morphine** (d/t morphine 6 glucoronide) l/t **respiratory depression** is used very cautiously in low dose and **meperidine (pethidine)** is contraindicated d/t very long acting metabolite **nor-meperidine** causing **neurotoxic excitatory syndrome.**

44. A i.e. Fentanyl

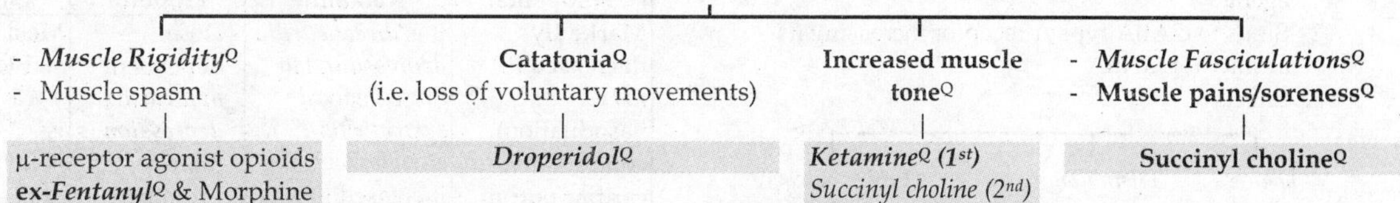

Opioid receptors are of four variety – mu (μ), Kappa (κ), delta (δ) & sigma (σ)

Receptor	Clinical effect	Agonist
Mu (μ) [(μ1), (μ2)]	*Muscle rigidity*[Q] Physical dependence Supraspinal analgesia (μ1) Respiratory depression (μ2)	Morphine *Fentanyl*[Q] Met- Enkephalin β- Endorphin
Kappa (κ)	Sedation Spinal analgesia	Morphine Nalbuphine Dynorphin (endogenous opioid) Butorphanol Oxycodone
Delta (δ)	Analgesia Behavioral Epileptogenic	Leu – Enkephalin β- Endorphin
Sigma (σ)	Dysphoria *Hallucination*[Q] Respiratory stimulation	Pentazocine Nalorphine *Ketamine*[Q]

45. C i.e. Papaverine *[Ref: Lee's 13/e p-318-20]*

Papaverine is an opioid alkaloid ***with almost no central effects***[Q] (i.e. analgesia, sedation, euphoria, anxiolytic, addictive, respiratory depression). *It does not suppress intestinal peristalsis, and relieves spasm in arteries.*
It is used to *treat visceral (GI tract, bile duct, ureter) spasm, vasopasm of coronary & cerebral vessels and erectile dysfunction.* It can also be used as smooth muscle relaxant in microsurgery, & cryopreservation of blood vessels and as a topical growth factor.

Total Intravenous Anaesthesia (TIVA)

46. A i.e. Reduces cerebral metabolism (CMR) and CBF
[Ref. Miller 7/e p1176, 802-3; Lee 13/e, p.164-72; Morgan 4/e, p.509, Aitkenhead 5/e p.311-13, 47, 48; Wylie 7/e p.637-41]

- TIVA (with propofol) provides extremely clear-headed awakening (which is useful after neurosurgery for patient evaluation) *and **reduced incidence of post operative nausea and vomiting** (PONV)*[Q] compared to volatile anesthesia. ***It can be safely used in patient susceptible to malignant hyperpyrexia***[Q] and reduces release of scavenged anesthetic gases into the atmosphere. ***The paralysis is not always required, avoiding reversal agents and emergence is rapid***[Q] (especially when propofol TIVA is used with remifentanil).

Etomidate

47. **B i.e. Etomidate** **48.** **B i.e. Etomidate** **49.** **D. i.e. Etomidate** **50.** **B i.e. Etomidate**
[Ref: Lee's 13/e p-157-58; Morgan's 4/e p. 199-201; Miller's 6/e p-350-53; Aitkenhead 4/e, P-176-78; Wiley & Davidson 7/e p-573-75]

- Etomidate causes ***adreno – cortical suppression***[Q] by *inhibiting enzymes 11β hydroxylase (mainly) & 17 α hydroxylase* ***involved in cortisol and aldosterone (mineralocorticoid) production***[Q]. Vit C supplimentation restores cortisol level.
- **Etomidate** and **midazolam** ***provide cardiovascular stability***[Q]. But ***etomidate is most cardiostable agent***[Q] that causes the least hemodynamic disturbance of any of the ***intravenous anesthetic agents. So it is intravenous anesthetic agent of choice for patients with cardiac disease and aneurysm surgery***[Q].
- **Direct myocardial depression** is caused by ***halothane (severe), nitrous oxide (moderate), iso/sevo/des-flurane (mild), thiopental (marked), propofol (dose dependent) and ketamine***[Q] (but this is masked by cardiotonic sympathetic stimulatory action). ***Etomidate > midazolem are most cardiostable agents***[Q].

Etomidate

1. It is a *carboxylated imidazole* ***(steroidal)***[Q] anesthetic agent
2. Binds to GABA type A receptor increasing its affinity for GABA.
3. Effects

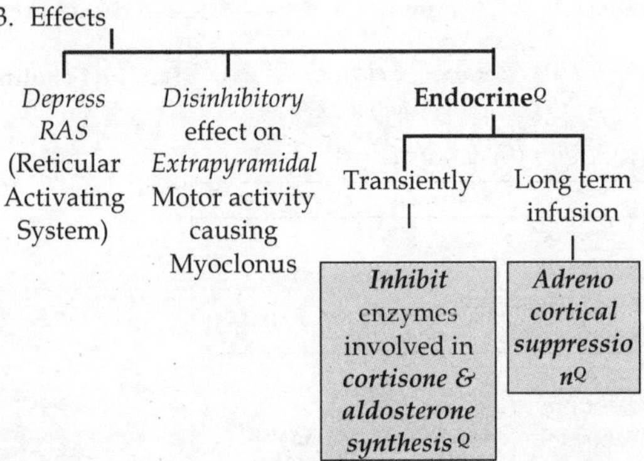

4. Opioids decrease the myoclonus characteristic but increase the chances of apnea.
5. Contraindicated in ***Porphyria***[Q] ***& Adrenal insufficiency***[Q]

Cardiovascular Effects of

Thiopental	Ketamine	Propofol	Etomidate
Markedly decreased BP (d/t vasodilation), contractility, cardiac output (CO) and **increased** heart rate (HR), and myocardial O_2 consumption (MOC). So it is **contraindicated or avoided** in - ***Shock***[Q] (hypovolemia, CHF, β adrenergic blockade) - Coronary artery disease	It is ***direct cardio depressant***, *but causes marked sympathetic stimulation* l/t increased BP, CO, HR, pulmonary artery pressure, and MOC. So it is - ***Contraindicated in coronary artery disease, CHF, hypertension and arterial aneurysm***[Q] but - ***Anesthesia of choice for shock***[Q]	- Dose dependent ***myocardiac depression*** is more prominent in *ischemic heart disease* (l/t ↓CO) - *Exaggerated hypotension* (d/t vasodilation) in patients with limited *cardio vascular reserve.*	**Most cardio stable agent** in a way that there is - No histamine release - Unchanged cardiac contractility - No or minimal decrease in CO, systemic vascular resistance & BP - No or minimal increase in HR - Maintained coronary perfusion
Ultrashort acting smooth inducing agent	Moderately rapid onset and recovery	Smooth & rapid induction	Rapid onset & moderately fast recovery

★ **Midazolam** is *slow onset cardiostable agent* used in balanced anesthesia & conscious sedation. It produces marked amnesia and its reversal is available (i.e. *Flumazenil*).

Hypotensive Anaesthesia

51. **C, D, E i.e. Phentolamine, Halothane, Na Nitroprusside** *[Ref: Wylie 7/e p-204-9; Miller 7/e p-2065; Ajay yadav 4/e p-132-33]*

Hypotensive anesthesia used to facilitate vessel surgery such as ***clipping of intracranial aneurysm, excision of highly vascular tumor (eg nasopharyngeal angiofibroma)***[Q] is given by variable combinations of ***vasodialators (sodium nitroprusside, nitroglycrine), ganglion blocker (phentolamine, trimethaphan), inhalation agent (isoflurane, halothane) and β-blockers***[Q].

52. **C i.e. Cyanide toxicity** *[Ref: Aietkenhead 4/e p. 686; Miller 7/e p. 211-13Lawrence 9/e p470; KDT 5/e p. 513]*

Sodium nitropruside has five cyanide groups within its structure and ***cyanide toxicity***[Q] is a problem if it is used is high doses. Its formula is $Na_2[Fe(CN)_5NO]X_2H_2O$

4 INHALATIONAL ANAESTHETICS

Minimal Alveolar Concentration (MAC)

It is alveolar vapour phase concentration of an inhaled anesthetic that prevents movement in 50% of patient in response to a standard noxious stimulus surgical incision[Q].

1. It is the ***best measure of anesthetic potency***[Q] as it *mirror brain partial pressure* (better than oil gas partition coefficient)
2. Surprisingly the absence of response to noxious stimuli is primarily mediated by *anesthetic action in spinal cord.*
3. Best unit for expressing potency is chemical potential (% saturation) > vapour phase concentration (% by volume or fraction of 1 atm) >aqueous concentration units (molar).
4. Alveolar partial pressure rather than alveolar vapour concentration is important because the latter alters with change in altitude. High altitude requires higher inspired conc of anesthetic to achieve same partial pressure, so *MAC is expressed as a % of 1atm.*
5. MAC is *unaffected by species, sex or duration of anesthesia.* And regardless of volatile anesthetic, it ***decreases 6% per decade***[Q]
6. MAC values of different anesthetics are *additive for CNS depression but not for myocardial depression.*
7. **MAC - awake** is value at which 50% subjects fail to respond to command (i.e. value required to prevent awareness) during induction . *0.3 –0.4 MAC* is associated with awakening from anesthesia (MAC awake)
8. 0.3 MAC is required to suppress learning & memory of auditory or verbal information during nonsurgical conditions. And lack of response to intubation (MAC- intubation) needs higher anesthetic conc, than required to prevent movement to surgical incision.
9. **MAC - BAR** is blockade of adrenergic response (i.e., ↑ heart rat & BP) in 50% subjects on surgical incision.
10. **ED/AD 95** is dose to prevent movement in 95% of subjects & is more useful. It is roughly 1.3 –1.5 MAC
11. **Decreasing value of MAC = Increasing Order of Potency**:
    N_2O (104) > Xenon (71) > Ethylene (67) > Cyclopropane (9.2) > Desflurane (6) > Fluroxene (3.4) > **Sevoflurane** (2.1) > **Diethyl ether** (1.92) > **Enflurane** (1.68) > **Isoflurane** (1.15) > **Halothane** (0.74) > Methoxyflurane (0.16).
12. Physical property that best correlates with anesthetic potency is *lipid solubility* (**Meyer – overton rule**). There is direct relationship between MAC and lipid solubility (*oil – gas partition coefficient*)

Factor affecting MAC

Variable	Effect on MAC	Comments
Temperature		
Hypothermia	↓	
Hyperthermia	↓	↑ if > 42°C
Age		
Young	(↑)	
Elderly	↓	
Alcohol		
Acute intoxication	↓	
Chronic abuse	(↑)	
Anemia		
Hematocrit < 10%	↓	
PaO_2		
< 40 mm Hg	↓	
$PaCO_2$		
> 95 mm Hg	↓	Caused by < pH in CSF
Thyroid		
Hyperthyroid	No change	
Hypothyroid	No change	
Blood pressure		
MAP < 40 mm Hg	↓	
Electrolyte		
Hypercalcemia	↓	Caused by altered CSF
Hypernatremia	(↑)	Caused by altered CSF
Hyponatremia	↓	
Pregnancy	↓	MAC decreased by 1/3 at 8 wks gestation; normal by 72 hours postpartum
Drugs		
Local anethetics	↓	
Opioids	↓	
Ketamine	↓	
Barbiturates	↓	
Benzodiazepines	↓	
Verapamil	↓	
Lithium	↓	
Sympatholytics		
Methyldopa	↓	
Reserpine	↓	
Clonidine	↓	
Dexmedetomidine	↓	
Sympathomimetics		
Amphetamine		
Chronic	↓	
Acute	(↑)	
Cocaine	(↑)	
Ephedrine	(↑)	

Meyer Overton Hypothesis : Hydrophobic State

Ease with which an anesthetic dissolve in olive oil, octanol & other membrane like substance such as lecithin & amphipathic phospholipid with hydrophobic & polar components, is correlated with its potency. In other words, *potency correlates best with lipid solubility*; and anesthesia starts when anesthetics reached a conc of *50 mmol /mol of lipid membrane.*

Evidences for

- Capacity of anesthetics to strongly *change phase transition* (from fluid to gel) *temperature*
- *Decreased lateral phase separation* in mixture of phospholipids (Area of solid phase phospholipid surrounded by fluid phase lipid in membrane is k/a lateral phase seperation)
- ***Hydrophobic site***[Q]

Evidences against (i.e., Exception)

- Hydrophilic site
- ***Nonanesthetics or non immobilizers (do affect learning & recall) provide most striking deviation***[Q], as their lipid solubilities are such that they should be anesthetics according to meyer- overton correlation (MOC)
- **Transitional compound** produce anesthesia but at a much higher concentration than predicted by MOC. The potencies of nonimmobilizers & transitiional compounds correlate poorly with theri oil –gas partition coefficient. The extent of halogenation & % of fluorine increase in this order : anesthetic > transitional > non immobilizer.
- **Cut off effect** i.e., decreased potency in higher members of homologus series. Eg. perfluromethane (CF_4) is anesthetic, whereas longer chain perfluroethane is not (true cut off). Similarly less lipid soluble paraffin – n- pentane causes anesthesia whereas highly lipid soluble n decane is not anesthetic.
- **Convulsant gases**: Complete halogenation of end methyl gp of alkanes & ethers decrease their anesthetic potency and increase convulsant activity. Compound 485 is isomer of en & isoflurane.
- **Isomers**
- **Critical volume hypothesis**

Metabolism and Toxicity of Inhalational Anesthetics

- Nitrous oxide and xenon are both non-halogenated inhalation anesthetics. And halothane, iso/en/sevo/des-fluranes are halogenated inhalation anesthetics
- The propensity of **liver injury** appears to parallel metabolism of parent drug to produce *trifluoroacetylated hepatic protein adducts*, thus, **halothane (20%) >>>>enflurane (2.5%) >>>>isoflurane (0.2%) >desflurane (0.02%)**. Sevoflurane does not produce acetylated protein adducts (ie not hepatotoxic) . Liver toxicity and injury show *cross-sensitization phenomenon* ie reported after repeat exposure on subsequent occasions to different fluorinated anesthetics.
- **Methoxyflurane** is no longer used because of **polyuric renal failure (nephrotoxicity) caused by high levels of inorganic fluorides** > (50-80= moderate injury, 80-120 = severe renal injury, >120 μmol/L = death). Sevoflurane defluorination rate in vitro (lab) is approximately same as that of methoxyflurane, howere, serum F^- conc. after sevoflurane are significantly less than those after methoxyflurane because of sevofluranes *low blood gas solubility* (B/G partition coefficient 0.69 versus 10.2 for methoxyflurane) and its rapid elimination. **Serum fluoride concentration** is **elevated** by **methoxyflurane>>sevoflurane>enflurane>>isoflurane>desflurane**. Although peak fluoride levels may be higher to those with enflurane, *sevoflurane has less nephrotoxic potential,* as measured by maximum urine concentrating ability and NAG (N-acetyl-β-glucosaminidase), an indicator of renal tubular damage
- Sevofluorane is metabolized to hexafluoroisopropanol, formaldehyde, inorganic fluoride and CO_2. The major base-catalyzed breakdown product of sevoflurane (with soda and bara-lime) is **nephrotoxic vinyl ether (compound A)** that induces both *dose and time dependent renal injury.* The toxic threshold reaches only on prolonged sevoflurane anesthesia showing *glucosuria and enzymeuria but unchanged BUN and creatinine levels.* To date, no significant clinical renal toxicity has been a/w the use of sevoflurane. New **calcium hydroxide-based CO_2 absorbents**, such as Amsorb and Drager Sorb Free, contain neither NaOH or KOH and thus are chemically inert and donot degrade inhaled anesthetics to carbon monoxide or degrade sevoflurane to compound A
- Inhaled anesthetic and desiccated CO_2 absorbent interactions can l/t **production of CO** in anesthetic circuit: **Desflurane>>>enflurane>isoflurane**. Negligible amounts of carbon monoxide are formed from halothane and sevoflurane.
- *The interaction* of inhaled anesthetics with CO_2 absorbents is an exothermic reaction resulting in production of heat (CO_2 canister temperature 25-45°C), *hydrogen, fire* and toxic gas. *Decreased fresh gas flow and sevoflurane are a/w greatest production of heat.*
- Fluorinated inhaled anesthetics containing bromine and chlorine **deplete ozone (halothane >>>enflurane>isoflurane)** and contribute to **green house effect** and **global warming**. N_2O does not deplete ozone but cause green house effect and global warming.
- **Enflurane** shows *maximum epileptiform activity (Spikes) on EEG and frank seizures (convulsions)* especially with hypocapnia (hyperventilation) and high doses (>1.5 MAC). **Epileptiform activity and seizure activity on EEG has been induced by administration of sevoflurane** in patients without epilepsy but no clinical seizure activity has been reported in pediatric patients with h/o epilepsy during induction with sevoflurane . However, seveflurane, similar to

other inhalation agents, is not suitable for use during electrocardiography for localization of seizure foci. **Isoflurane** use can show *isolated epilepliform patterns on EEG* (at 1.5-2 MAC) and halothane at 3-4 MAC (a dose that l/t prolonged cardiovascular toxicity). There is ***no evidence of epileptic form activity with desflurane***Q (despite hyperventilation and MAC 1.6 doses) and it has been used as *a treatment of refractory status epilepticus*.

So epileptiform activity on EEG and seizures may occur with: ***enflurane***Q **>>>>** ***sevoflurane***Q **> Isoflurane > halothane**. ***Desflurane has no epileptiform activity and is used in treatment of refractory status epilepticus***Q.

XENON - ANESTHESIA

- Xenon was isolated by William Ramsay (Nobel prize for chemistry) in 1904 and 1st used as anesthetic in 1950. It is one of the noble gases. It is ***colourless, odurless, nonirritating, non flammable and does not support combustion*** and ***non explosive***Q gas that is ***heavier than air (4 times) and more viscous than N_2 & N_2O***Q.
- Being *extremely unreactive*, it does not interact with soda lime, but will *diffuse readily through rubber*.
- The main factor limiting the use of xenon is *availability*. Although it is an atmospheric gas, it only constitutes *0.0000087%* of atmosphere (0.086ppm), and produced by *fractional distillation* of air often as a *byproduct* of oxygen production.
- Xenon cannot be manufactured but is recovered in the process of *fractional distillation of liquefied air* and a purity of > 99.99% can be obtained after several separation steps. The process makes it costly. Unlike all other inhaled anesthetics, it is *not an environmental pollutant*.
- Except for cost, ***xenon would be the most ideal inhaled anesthetic agent because Xenon (MAC of 71%) is more potent than nitrous oxide, can provide anesthesia in 30% O_2, is very insoluble (blood-gas partition coefficienct of 0.14) and has positive medical & environmental effects***Q. Xenon exhibits minimal cardiovascular & hemodynamic side effects, is *not* known to be *metabolized in liver or kidney*, is *not teratogenic* and does *not trigger malignant hyperthermia* (in susceptible swine). It is *neuroprotective* and cardioprotective. The unique combination of *analgesia, hypnosis and lack of cardiovascular depression* in single agent makes xenon a very attaractive choice for patients with limited cardiovascular reserve. Environmental positives are that it *does not deplete stratospheric ozone, or contribute to green house effect & global warming*.
- Xenon provides favourable cardiovascular stability & left ventricle contractility (not reduced) both in patients with or without cardiac disease. *Emergence from xenon anesthesia is faster*.
- During Xenon anesthesia, N_2 released from the patient's body accumulates in the anesthesia circuit. So it is necessary to perform *prolonged denitrogenation* before starting xenon administration *to reduce the risk of hypoxia*. Transition from denitrogenation to *closed circuit xenon anesthesia* (most economical technique for clinical use) is a technical challenge. Xenon must be given with a *rebreathing system, low fresh gas flow or a closed circuit system*. Xenon, krypton and argon are all chemically inert & have anesthetic properties.
- ***Xenon is more potent than nitrous oxide with MAC 71% (but even than is a weak anesthetic agent)***Q. ***It is a good analgesic***Q. Although it has a ***blood – gas solubility coefficient of less than one third of N_2O***Q, there is still the *potential of diffusion hypoxia during recovery* (although less then N_2O), and it should also offer the benefit of the *concentration effect and second gas effect during induction* (as for N_2O). Similar considerations would apply as with N_2O regarding *diffusion into gas filled cavities*. However, the lower blood gas coefficient of Xenon results in ***rapid induction and recovery***Q.
- Its a *noble gas*, which implies that it is *extremely unlikely* to be involved in any *biochemical reactions*. It does not undergo biotransformation & is *harmless to the ozone layer*. The elimination is mainly through lung, has low toxicity & devoid of teratogenicity.
- Produces highest regional blood flow in brain, liver, kidney, and intestine; thus greatly reducing the dangers of tissue hypoxia and providing an interesting *alternative for transplant surgery*. It should be used *with caution in patients at risk for raised intra cranial pressure* (as it causes increase in cerebral blood flow and intra cranial pressure). And for the same region it has ***neuroprotective effect*** (protect neural cell against ischemia) during cardiopulmonary surgery.
- It is *radiodense* and inhaled Xe – 133 is used to *inhance CT images of brain* and to *measure cerebral blood flow* and its regional distribution in severe head injury. It is *not used for neurosurgery*.
- It has *higher density and viscosity than N_2 and N_2O*, leading to *higher airway resistance and increased work of breathing*. It probably should not *not be used or used with caution* in cases of *narrowing or obstruction of airways (moderate to severe COPD), morbidly obese, premature infants & in other patients in whom increase in work of breathing might have adverse effects*.
- It provides ***good hemodynamic stability with little change in blood pressure***Q. Causes slight reduction in heart rate, otherwise ***it has no effect on heart***Q (no cardiac depresion / stimulation and does not sensitise to catecholamines.)
- It ***inhibits – calcium pump in plasma membrane***Q & NMDA receptor in dorsal horn neuron.
- In common with N_2O, it appears to be associated with post operative *nausea' & vomiting*.
- Xenon has many properties of an ideal anesthetic (eg. echo friendly). The reason that it is not commonly used are its *unavailability, very high cost*, its concentration *can not be measured with conventional anesthetic gas analysers* and new anesthetic system need to be developed to provide for recycling of xenon.

2

ANAESTHESIA

Nitric Oxide (NO)

Synthesis

- NO is ***naturally occurring* potent *vasodialator***Q released by *endothelial cells*Q **(Endothelium derived relaxing factor)**Q with ultra short duration of action (6 sec half life). NO ***activates guanylyl cyclase***Q enzyme, which forms *C-GMP*Q
- **Endothelium derived relaxing factor (EDRF),** also k/a ***nitric oxide*** is synthesized ***from L-arginine by nitric oxide synthase (NOS) enzyme***Q in endothelium of blood vessels
- NOS is *NADPH diaphorase (NDP)* and *requires NADPH*. Three forms of NOS are
  - **NOS 1,** found in nervous system
  - **NOS 2,** in macrophage & other immune cells.
  - **NOS3,** found in *endothelium*
- 1 & 3 isoforms of NOS are induced by agents that increase *intracellular* Ca^{++}, such as *vasodilators, acetyl choline & bradykinin, or shear stress.* NOS_2 is induced by cytokines (not Ca^{++})
- Unlike other transmitters it is gas, which diffuses to *smooth muscle cell* where it ***activates guanylyl cyclase producing C- GMP***Q
- ***NO binds rapidly to hemoglobin & gets inactivated***Q
- **Endothelial independent vasodilation** is caused by adenosine, ANP & histamine via H2 receptors; whereas **endothelium dependent** vasodilation is due to *acetyl choline , bradykinin, histamine via H1 receptor , VIP, substance P, NO* & prostaglandin I_2 (a prostacyclin).
- ***Endogenous NO causes vasodilation throughout the body***Q, *whereas* **inhaled NO** (NO;) a colourless, odourless gas is a ***selective pulmonary vasodilator***Q.
- **Prodrugs**: These drugs form NO (exogenous) and do not need intact endothelium to cause vasodilatation. Hence effective in hypertension, atherosclerosis & vasospastic disorder where endothelium function is impaired
  1. ***Sodium Nitroprusside***Q (both arteriolar & venous dialator)
  2. ***Nitroglycerine***Q (venous dialation >arterial d.)
  3. *Hydralazine* (arteriolar dialator)
  4. Nitrosothiols
  5. Molsidomine

Physiological role

1. Cause ***vasodilation & decrease vascular resistance throughout the body***Q
   - in kidney this l/t *increased GFR*
   - vasodilation of corpora cavernosa l/t ***penile erection***Q
   - in lung ***decrease pulmonary artery pressure & pulmonary hypertension***Q
   - tonic release of NO is necessary to *maintain normal blood pressure*
2. Involved in vascular remodeling, angiogenesis & pathogenesis of atherosclerosis. As vessels with damaged endothelium rapidly develop atherosclerosis.
3. *Platelet aggregation* (in intact endothelium)& *sudden increase of flow* to a tissue cause release of NO & vasodilation (later is k/a flow induced dilation).
4. NO inhibits *adhesion , activation & aggregation of platelets.*
5. In GI tract its a major *dilator of smooth muscle*
6. Necessary for *cytotoxic ability of macrophages* & also for their cancer cell killing ability
7. Secreted by nerve terminals in brain responsible for *long term behaviour & memory*. It differs from other transmitters in that it is *not preformed & stored* in vesicle in presynaptic terminals. Instead, it is *synthesized instantly as needed* and diffuses out rather than being released in vesicular packets.

- Because NO binds rapidly with hemoglobin, ***inhaled NO exerts its effects on pulmonary but not systemic vasculature***Q.
- ***Inhaled NO is selective pulmonary vasodialator & decreases pulmonary artery pressure in infants & adults***Q, so used in ***treatment of pulmonary artery hypertension***Q.
- ***Improves perfusion (dilates vessels) only in ventilated areas***Q, so used in ARDS or one lung ventilation, after mitral valve surgery in patients known to have long standing pulmonary hypertension & after cardiac transplantation.
- During **one lung ventilation**, *inhaled NO (NOi) to ventilated lung* and almitrine (potent *pulmonary vaso constrictor) to lung undergoing surgery* (to decrease perfusion) markedly improve oxygenation (esp in) *supine position*. The effect of NOi is directly ***proportional to the degree of pulmonary vascular resistance present in ventilated lung before NO administration***Q. So, most patients undergoing pulmonary resection & usually having normal or slightly elevated pulmonary artery pressure have disappointing result (improvement in oxygenation) esp in *lateral position.*
- Direct infusion of *prostaglandin* E_1*, (Vasodilator)* into pulmonary artery of *ventilated lung* and prostaglandin F2 α (*Vaso constrictor*) into pulmonary artery of *non- ventilated lung* during one lung ventilation improve arterial oxygenation (PaO_2) & decrease shunt.

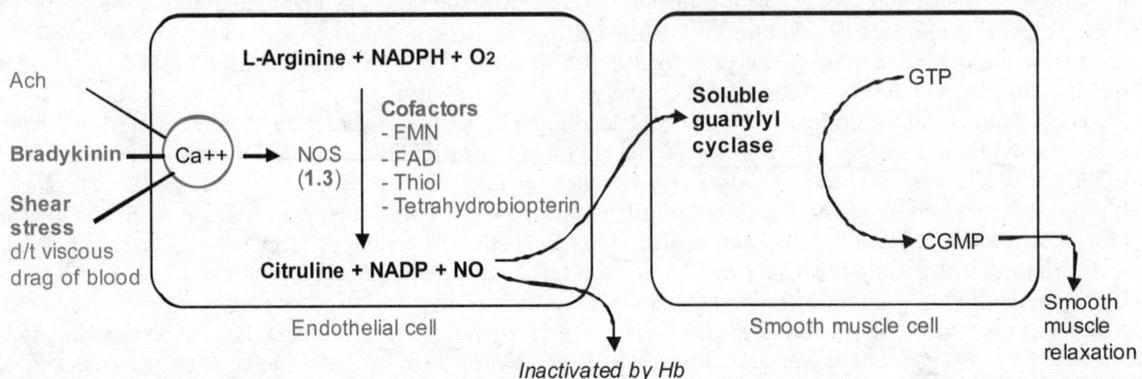

Nitrous Oxide (N_2O)

- N_2O has two important effects as it is given at 70-80% concentration. **N_2O has second gas effect** during ***induction***[Q] & **diffusion hypoxia** after discontinuation of anesthesia in ***recovery phase***[Q]

Diffusion Hypoxia

- It occurs during ***recovery phase***[Q] after discontinuation of prolonged anesthesia. N_2O having low blood solubility rapidly diffuse into alveoli & dilutes the alveolar air – PP of O_2 in alveoli is reduced i.e. ***diffusion hypoxia***[Q]
- N_2O has *low blood solubility,* so after discontinuation it rapidly *diffuses to alveoli* (from blood) and dilutes the alveolar air. This causes excess of N_2O in alveoli so partial pressure of O_2 in alveoli is reduced, *resulting in hypoxia.* It is not of much consequence if cardio pulmonary reserve is normal but may be dangerous if it is low.
- It can *be **prevented by continuing 100% O_2 inhalation for a few minutes after discontinuing N_2O***[Q]

Second Gas Effect

- It occurs in initial part of ***induction of anesthesia***[Q] as N_2O is used in high concentration (70-80%); this high concentration l/t entery of N_2O in blood at a rate higher than minute (1lit/min) volume. If another potent anesthetic eg. halothane is added, it also will be delivered to the blood at a rate higher than Minute volume & the induction will be faster.
- Due to high conc. of inhaled N_2O it ***enters blood at rate of 1 lit/min, which is higher than minute volume*** if another potent anesthetic eg halothane (1-2%) is being given at same time it also will be delivered to blood at same rate (1 lit/min) ***& induction will be faster.***[Q]

- N_2O is a *sweet smelling, nonflammable gas of low potency (MAC = 104%)* that is *relatively insoluble in blood.* It is most commonly used as *an anesthetic adjuvant* or carrier in combination with opioids or volatile anesthetics. A mixture of 70% N_2O +25-30% O_2 + 0.2 – 2% another potent anesthetic is applied to reduce the concentration of other agent to 1/3 for same level of anesthesia. **Unlike potent volatile anesthetics, N_2O *does not produce significant muscle relaxation;* but it is a *good analgesic.***
- **Nitrous oxide** is a **good analgesic** and **a very weak anesthetic (ie mainly or only analgesia).** N_2O produces analgesia that is in part mediated by release of **proenkephalin derived family of endogenous opioid peptides.**
- O_2 is used to **correct hypoxia; NO** inhalation **dilates pulmonary vasculature** and **CO_2** is used for **insufflations during endoscopic procedures.** The implies that combining N_2O with an opioid may not take best advantage of drug interaction synergism as this combination is **neither synergistic or additive.** Although amnesia and intraoperative conditions may improve, N_2O does not produce any effect that is not produced by either opioid or a sedative hypnotic.
- **N_2O is a good analgesic** and **50:50 N_2O – O_2 mixture** is used to alleviate pain in labour and minor surgical procedures. N_2O is a very weak anesthetic, inadequated as as sole anesthetic agent and generally used in combination with a second agent. *It reduces MAC & and the amount required for the effect of second agent* and it also ***increases the uptake and elimination of other agent by second gas effect, increasing the rate of induction and recovery***[Q]**.**

- Although not flammable, ***nitrous oxide will support combustion***[Q] (Barash)
- **Microlaryngoscopy tubes** (long length, small (4-5 mm) internal and external diameter with high volume low pressure cuff) are *not suitable for laser surgery*. Two main hazards of laser surgery (of larynx) are ***laser induced airway fire***[Q] and risk to operating room staff & patient from diverted laser. (Miller)
- The *transient flaring of fat deposits* occasionally seen in the airway during laser surgery is self terminating and would not produce a blow torch airway fire regardless of ambient O_2 concentration. For a blow torch airway fire to occur, a *non metal foreign material, has to be present.*

- N_2O **expands air filled closed spaces and bubbles** because of its greater solubility in blood compared to N_2
- Several closed gas spaces, such as *middle ear and bowel,* exist in body and other spuces may occur as a result of disease or surgery such as pneumothorax, ***pneumoperitonium, pneumocephalus, COPD, emphysema, intestinal obstruction and tympanic membrane grafting***[Q]**.**
- N_2O diffuses from blood to air space; the amount depends on concentration of N_2O and duration of anesthesia. As N_2O diffuses into middle ear cavity its pressure is increased resulting in *overlay graft displacement*. Many ENT surgeons now use *underlay grafts* (which are hold in position by increased middle ear pressure) and many ***anesthesiologist do not use N_2O in ear surgery***[Q]**)**, and instead use a mixture of air and O_2 or limit N_2O concentration to 50%.
- After discontinuation of N_2O, the gas is rapidly reabsorbed (or rapid Eustachian tube opening allowing gas to escape) creates negative pressure in cavity l/t *serous otitis media, disarticulation of stapes & impaired hearing*. Accumulation of N_2O in middle ear can diminish post operative hearing and is ***relatively contraindicated in tympanoplasty***[Q]**.**
- In **fluid-gas exchange technique** of **vitreoretinal surgery**, the surgeon injects intravitreal air bubble to tamponade the retina against the wall of the

- To minimize these risks, inspired O_2 ***concentration should be lowest that maintains adequate O_2 saturation, and air (N_2) or helium should be used in preference to N_2O***[Q]. The potential fuel source should be removed (supra glotlic jet ventilation technique) or should have laser resistant properties. (Only non inflammable laser proof tube is all metal **Nortan tube** which has no cuff).

globe. **Sulfur hexafluoride or perfluoropropane** (C3 F8, never agent) are poorly soluble gases used to prolong the resorption of intravitreal air bubbles. Nitrous oxide diffuses and causes bubble expansion, with the potential increase in IOP. N_2O should be shut off for **15 minutes before** placing the sulfur hexafluoride bubble and should be avoided **7-10 days (SCL6 use)** / for **at least a month (C3F8 use)** thereafter. So it is important to ask for recent retinal procedure.

- Air filled *cuffs of pulmonary artery catheters and endotracheal tubes* also expand with the use of N_2O, possibly causing tissue damage via in pulmonary artery and trachea respectively.

- N_2O has 5'P'

- **Priestely** was discoverer
- In Practice safest anaesthesia
- Poor muscle relaxant i.e. only relieves pain
- **Poynting Effect** Entonox (50% N_2O + 50% O_2) and mixture of gases (N_2O & O_2) keeps them in gaseous form
- ***Not used in Pneumoconditions***[Q] as Pneumothorax, Pneumoperitonium, pneumocephalus & other conditions where air containing cavities are found as COPD, Emphysema, tympanic membrane grafting Intestinal obstruction etc. especially **for 7 days** as N_2O leads to **expansion of air filled cavities**

- N_2O is **laughing gas** which is **lighter than air** with **high insolubility in blood** (but more soluble than N_2 and of course less than solubility of CO)
- S/E mainly are:
  - ***Bone marrow suppression***[Q] or Agranulocytosis
  - Megaloblastic anemia
  - ***Second gas effect or Diffusion hypoxia***[Q]

Ether

- B/G co. of ether is 12 i.e. ***slow induction & slow recovery.***[Q]
- *Irritant vapour,* which can readily induce laryngeal spasm and make induction even slower and ***stimulates salivary and bronchial secretions***[Q]. So atropine pre medication is required.
- Ether is ***highly inflammable and causes explosion with cautery***[Q]***. It should not be used when diathermy is needed in the airways because of risk of fire or explosion***[Q]***. Muscle relaxants need not to be used as ether itself produces excellent relaxation.***
- ***Ether liberates catecholamines and tends to maintain blood pressure. Cardiac arrythmias occur rarely with ether and there is no sensitization of myocardium to circulating catecholamines***[Q]. BP and respiration are well maintained due to reflex sympathetic stimulation and does not ***sensitise heart to adrenaline***[Q].
- ***Adrenaline is relatively safe with ether***[Q]. Bronchial smooth muscle is relaxed. The products of its metabolism (alcohol, acetaldehyde and acetic acid) are relatively non toxic.
- **Guedel's staging** of anesthesia was given for **ether**

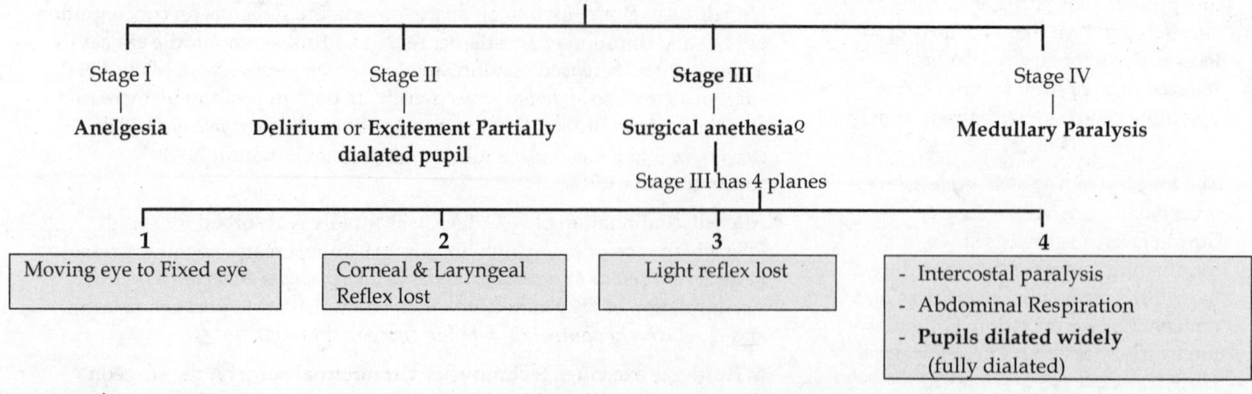

Halothane

- ***Least expansive, least pungent (non-irritant), potent anesthesia without analgesia***Q
- **Mn-D**[3] i.e. *Dissolve rubber*Q and ***corrodes metals***Q; Drager narko Test is done for halothane and Dilates bronchi, uterus & vessels
- *Best uterine relaxant is Halothane followed by ether. Best Muscle relaxant is ether followed by Halothane.*
- Halothane contains ***0.01%***Q **thymol** for stability and is decomposed by light but is stable when in *amber coloured bottles*. **15-20%**Q of absorbed halothane is metabolized. Halothane may persist in the liver for as long as 12 days after administration & is usually ***not given in same patient within 3 months***Q. Tissue : Blood ratio is maximum *in fat*. ***Trichloracetic acid is found in urine***Q

Dialator

- **Best Bronchodialator**Q, it's action is not reversed by B Blocker and it reverses asthma induced bronchospasm
- **Best uterine relaxant**Q,
  - ***It is not used in pregnancy as it increases postpartum haemorrage***Q
  - Anesthesia of choice for uterine titanic contraction and version
- **Vasodialator (peripheral)**
  - *Hypotension (so used in hypotensive anesthesia)*
  - *Chills & shivering due to cutaneous vasodialation*
- **Coronary Artery Vasodialator**
  But the coronary artery blood flow decreases, owing to systemic hypotension caused by peripheral vasodialation

Side Effects (HAM)

- **Hepatitis (Centrilobular necrosis)**Q
  -Primarily involves ***post puberty age group***Q, *more common in middle age, obese female*
  -More chances after hypoxia & phenobarbitone exposure)
  - ***Chloroform is more hepatotoxic than halothane so both are C/I in liver disease***Q
- **Arrythmogenic**Q
  -It ***sensitizes heart to arrythmogenic action of epinephrine***Q, so doses of epinephrine above 1.5 μg/kg should be avoided.
- **Malignant Hyperthermia**Q
- **Raised Intra Cranial Tension**
  but of lesser degree in comparison to Ketamine

Contra indications

1. ***Liver dysfunction***Q
2. ***Halothane use with in 3 months***Q

] ***due to S/E of halothane hepatitis***

3. *Hypovolemia & severe cardiac disease (aortic stenosis);* due to negative inotropic effect.
4. *Pheochromocytoma & exogenous catecholamines administration* as it sensitize heart to catecholamines.

Anesthesia with

No Analgesia	=	**Halothane**
Only Analgesia	=	**N_2O**
Profound Analgesia	=	**Ketamine**
Best / Maximum Analgesa	=	**Trilene**

Fluranes

Isoflurane

- *Barbiturate* induction followed by ***Isoflurane in*** ***O_2 or N_2O – O_2*** **mixture (+** ***cisatracurium***Q as neuro-muscular blocking agent) is method of *choice in patients of liver disease (cirrhosis),* for employing general anesthesia.
- Isoflurane is *AOC for* ***neurosurgical procedure***Q as it does not increase cerebral blood flow & CSF pressure.

Desflurane

- Desflurane's structure is ***very similar to that of isoflurane. The only difference is substitution of a fluride atom for isofluranes chlorine atom.*** Q
- It is recently developed ***fluorinated congener of isoflurane.*** Q
- Its special properties are – highly volatile, extremely low oil – gas partition coefficient and very low solubility in blood and tissues i.e. ***very low blood and tissue – gas partition coefficients*** Q. Because of these properties its ***induction and recovery are very fast*** Q. Due to its short action it is ***commonly used as***

Sevoflurane

- Sevoflurane is ***fluorinated methyl propyl ether.***Q
- It is volatile anesthetic, which is ***well tolerated in children & elderly.*** Q
- Minimum alveolar conc. (MAC) for sevoflurane is 2 Q.
- Blood gas partition coefficient of sevoflurane is lesser than halothane and isoflurane.(halothane-2.3, isoflurane-1.4, sevoflurane-0.69, desflurane 0.42)

Enflurane

- ***C/I in Epilepsy***Q because it causes raised ICT & tonic-clonic seizure.
- Epileptiform activity of Enflurane is increased by hypocapnea (↓ CO_2) so ***hyperventilation is not recommended to attenuate enflurane induced ↑ ICT.***

2

ANAESTHESIA

- Isoflurane cause *coronary steal syndrome*Q.
- Isoflurane is used in *daycare anesthesia*Q.
- Isoflurane is a preferred anesthetic agent for ***neurosurgical procedure***Q, *in renal failure*Q and *myasthenia gravis*Q.
- Isoflurane presents no unique C/I other than controversy concerning possibility of *coronary steal and severe hypovolemia*Q.

anesthesia for out patient departments.

- It under goes *minimal metabolism in humans* Q therefore serum and urine inorganic fluoride levels following anaesthesia are essentially unchanged from pre anaesthetic levels.
- It causes *minimal cardiac depression like isoflurane* Q. It causes Blood pressure – decrease; Systemic vascular resistance – decrease; Heart rate – No change or increase; Cardiac output – No change or increase.
- **Desflurane** is pungent but a *safe anesthetic agent for geriatric age group* as *its cardiovascular effects are similar to isoflurane but without coronary steal phenomenon*Q.

- *Sodalime & baralyme,both,absorb sevoflurane and form compound A.*
- *Sevoflurane is not recommended in closed circuit because there is chance of production of a toxic metabolic product compound A,* Q *(an olefin) in closed circuit.*
- *Sevoflurane is inhalational agent of choice for inductioin of anesthesia in pediatric patients and adults, because of rapid onset of action & nonpengency* Q

Methoxyflurane

- High boiling point (104° C)
- Highest fluride content
- Highly *Nephrotoxic*Q
- *High output renal failure*Q
- *High risk of oxalate stone*Q

Cardiovascular Side Effects

	N_2O	Halothane	Isoflurane	Desflurane	Sevoflurane
Heart rate	No change (nc)	↓	↑	↑ /nc	Nc
Cardiac output	nc	↓	nc d/t tachycardia	nc or ↓	↓ d/t no (or little) tachycardia
Systemic vascular resistance	nc	nc	↓ ↓	↓ ↓	↓
Blood pressure	nc	↓ ↓ (d/t dose dependent direct myocardial depression) BP & CO decrease	↓ ↓	↓ ↓	↓
Normal coronary artery dilation & coronary blood flow		Coronary artery vasodilator but coronary blood flow decrease d/t drop in BP	Dilates but not is potent as nitroglycerine or adenosine	dose not increase	does not occur
Coronary steal syndrome		No	May be present (±) d/t diversion of blood away from fixed stenotic lesion	Absent	Absent
Rapid increase in drug concentration	Sympathetic hyperactivity l/t unchanged or slightly elevated BP, CO, HR despite direct myocardial depression		Transient rise in HR, BP, & plasma nor epinephrine level	Transient but worrisome elevation of heart rate BP & catecholamines Attenuated by fentanyl, esmolol or clonidine	
Direct myocardial depression	+ +	+ + +	Minimal (+)	Minimal (+)	Mild (+)
	- Vasoconstriction of cutaneous & pulmonary vasculature - ↑ed pulmonary vasculature resistance & rt ventricular end diastolic pressure				Prolong QT interval
Sensitized to cate cholamines	↑endogenous catecholamines & higher incidence of epinephrine induced arrythmia	Sensitize heart to arrythmogenic effect of epinephrine so its dose >1.5 µkg/kg avoided	no	no	no

QUESTIONS

GENERAL

1. Lowest concentration of anesthetic agent in aveoli needed to produce immobility in response to painful stimulus in 50% of individual is termed as *(AIIMS 98)*
A. Minimum alveolar concentration ☐
B. Minimal analgesic concentration ☐
C. Minimal anaesthetic concentration ☐
D. Maximum alveolar concentration ☐

2. All of the following factors decrease the Minimum Alveolar Concentration (MAC) of an inhalation anaesthetic agent except. *(AIIMS 03, DNB 05)*
A. Hypothermia ☐
B. Hyponatremia ☐
C. Hypocalcemia ☐
D. Anemia ☐

3. Index of potency of general anaesthesia *(PGI 1997)*
A. Minimum alveolar concentration ☐
B. Diffusion coefficient ☐
C. Dead space concentration ☐
D. Alveolar blood concentration ☐

4. Partition coefficient of gas *(PGI 98, DNB 97)*
A. Measure of potency ☐
B. Directly proportional to potency ☐
C. Measures solubility ☐
D. All of the above ☐

5. The potency of an inhalational anesthetic depends on:
A. Blood gas partition co-efficient *(PGI 99, DNB 03)* ☐
B. Oil-gas partition co-efficient ☐
C. Gas pressure ☐
D. Blood pressure ☐

6. Characteristic of an ideal gas is
A. Volume is directly proportional to change in pressure *(PGI 98)* ☐
B. Volume is inversely proportional to change in temperature ☐
C. At absolute temp. volume of gas is 1 ☐
D. Obeys Carles, Byles and Avagadro' laws ☐

7. Exception of Meyer overton rule are A/E
A. Nonanaesthetics *(Jipmer 03, J&K 04)* ☐
B. Nonimmobilizer ☐
C. Cut off effect ☐
D. Hydrophobic site ☐

8. Least soluble anesthetic agent is:
A. Desflurane *(DNB 06, TN 05)* ☐
B. Sevoflurane ☐
C. Halothane ☐
D. Methoxyflurane ☐

9. Least blood gas partition coeficient anesthetic agent:
A. Desflurane *(DNB 05, WB 06)* ☐
B. Nitrous oxide ☐
C. Halothane ☐
D. Ether ☐

10. Fastest acting agent: *(DNB 04, J&K 06)*
A. Sefoflurane ☐
B. Desflurane ☐
C. Isoflurane ☐
D. None ☐

11. Least diffusion coefficient is for:
A. Isoflurane *(JIPMER 04, AMU 05)* ☐
B. Enflurane ☐
C. Halothane ☐
D. N_2O ☐

12. Which one of the following is the fastest acting inhalational agent? *(AI 05)*
A. Halothane ☐
B. Isoflurane. ☐
C. Ether. ☐
D. Sevoflurane. ☐

13. Pungent volatile anesthetic agents are: *(PGI Nov 09)*
A. Halthane ☐
B. Isoflurane ☐
C. Sevoflurane ☐
D. Desflurane ☐
E. Nitrous oxide ☐

14. Which of the following inhalational agents has the minimum blood gas solubility coefficient?
A. Isoflurane *(AIIMS May 06)* ☐
B. Sevoflurane ☐
C. Desflurane ☐
D. Nitrous oxide ☐

15. Which of the following anesthetic does not depress ciliary function: *(PGI Nov 12)*
A. Ketamine ☐
B. Enflurane ☐
C. Ether ☐
D. Sevoflurane ☐
E. Desflurane ☐

XENON

16. Which of the following is not true about xenon anesthesia
A. Non explosive *(AIIMS Nov 11, 06)* ☐
B. Minimal cardiovascular side effects ☐
C. Slow induction and slow recovery ☐
D. Inhibits Ca^{++} pump and low blood gas solubility ☐

17. True about xenon anaesthesia: *(PGI Nov 2010)*
A. Rapid induction and recovery ☐
B. Low potency ☐
C. High blood solubility ☐
D. Non-explosive ☐
E. Heavier than air ☐

18. True about Xenon: *(PGI Nov 12)*
A. Blood: gas partition coefficient is 0.14 ☐
B. Minimum alveolar concentration is high ☐
C. Minimal hemodynamic effect ☐
D. Heavier than air ☐
E. High blood solubility ☐

NO

19. True about nitric oxide *(PGI June 2007)*
A. Formed from L-Arginine by NO synthase ☐
B. Causes vasodilation in all vessels ☐
C. Used in portal hypertension ☐
D. Interacts with Hb ☐
E. Used in erectile dysfunction ☐

20. Which of the following statements is true regarding Nitric oxide: *(PGI 01)*
A. Used in pulmonary hypertension ☐
B. Decreases the dose of anaesthetics ☐
C. Sympathomimetic action ☐
D. Causes systemic hypotension ☐
E. Used as a vasoconstrictor ☐

21. True about inhaled nitric oxide *(PGI June 07, 09, Nov 10)*
A. Causes generalized (systemic) vasodilation ☐

B. Dilates pulmonary arteries ☐
C. Causes hypotension, increase pulmonary artery pressure ☐
D. Least systemic effects ☐
E. Better (improves) ventilation perfusion match ☐

22. Which of the following inhaled gas is used to decrease pulmonary artery pressure in adults and infants?
A. Nitrous oxide *(AIIMS 2002)* ☐
B. Nitrogen dioxide ☐
C. Nitric oxide ☐
D. Nitrogen ☐

N_2O

23. Diffusion hypoxia is seen during: *(PGI 1998)*
A. Induction of anaesthesia ☐
B. Recovering anaesthesia ☐
C. Preoperatively ☐
D. Postoperatively ☐

24. At the end of anaesthesia after discontinuation of nitrous oxide and removal of endotracheal tube, 100% oxygen is administered to the patient to prevent: *(AIIMS 2003)*
A. Diffusion Hypoxia ☐
B. Second gas effect ☐
C. Hyperoxia ☐
D. Bronchospasm ☐

25. Bone marrow depression is seen with.
A. Halothene *(AIIMS 1996)* ☐
B. N_2O ☐
C. Ether ☐
D. Isoflurane ☐

26. Use of nitrous oxide is contraindicated in all of the following surgeries except: *(AIIMS Nov 08)*
A. Cochlear implant ☐
B. Microlaryngeal surgery ☐
C. Vitrioretinal surgery ☐
D. Exentration operation ☐

27. Most potent analgesic agent among following:
A. Nitrous oxide *(AIIMS Nov 12)* ☐
B. Nitric oxide ☐
C. CO_2 ☐
D. Oxygen ☐

TRILENE

28. Not compatible with soda lime
A. Ether *(AIIMS 1997)* ☐
B. Halothene ☐
C. Trilene ☐
D. N_2O ☐

29. Sodalime circuit is not used with
A. Enflurane *(AIIMS 1993)* ☐
B. Isoflurane ☐
C. Methoxyflurane ☐
D. Trilene ☐

30. Inhalation agent incompatable with sodaline
A. Isoflurane *(AIIMS 1992)* ☐
B. Trichloro Ethylene ☐
C. Methoxy flurane ☐
D. Enflurane ☐

ETHER

31. Stages of anesthesia were established by
A. Ether *(AIIMS 1997)* ☐
B. N_2O ☐
C. Halothane ☐
D. Chloroform ☐

32. No effect on heart *(AIIMS 1992)*
A. Chloroform ☐
B. Ether ☐
C. Methoxyflurane ☐
D. Halothane ☐

33. All of the following are the disadvantages of anesthetic ether, except: *(AI 2005)*
A. Induction is slow ☐
B. Irritant nature of ether increases salivary and bronchial secretions ☐
C. Cautery cannot be used. ☐
D. Affects blood pressure and is liable to produce arrhythmias. ☐

HALOTHANE

34. True about halothane *(PGI 2003)*
A. 1% Thymol is used as preservative ☐
B. It senitizes heart to catecholamines at 1 MAC ☐
C. 20% metabolized ☐
D. It is not usually given in same patient within 3 months ☐
E. It forms compound -A with sodalime ☐

35. True about Halothane *(PGI Dec 06)*
A. Non irritant ☐
B. Antiarrhythmic ☐
C. It antagonizes bronchospasm ☐
D. Vasodilator ☐

36. True about halothane: *(PGI 2002)*
A. Causes bronchodilation ☐
B. Anti-arrhthmic ☐
C. Can be used in hepatitis ☐
D. Uterine contraction occurs ☐
E. Causes hepatitis ☐

37. Which of the are the following contraindication for halothane used:
A. Male sex *(PGI 2001)* ☐
B. Middle age ☐
C. Recent halothane use ☐
D. Associated liver pathology ☐
E. Obesity ☐

38. Post operative jaundice is because of use of: *(PGI 1999)*
A. Isoflurane ☐
B. NO ☐
C. Methoxyflurane ☐
D. Halothane ☐

39. Hepatitis is caused by: *(PGI 1997)*
A. Cyclopropane ☐
B. Halothane ☐
C. Isoflurane ☐
D. Enflurane ☐

40. Repeated use of halothane causes
A. Hepatitis *(AI 1999)* ☐
B. Pancreatitis ☐
C. Encephalitis ☐
D. Meningitis ☐

41. Anesthesia agent with least analgesic property
A. N_2O *(AI 1994)* ☐
B. Halothane ☐
C. Ether ☐
D. Propane ☐

42. Hepatotoxic agent is *(AIIMS 1997)*
A. Ketamine ☐
B. Ether ☐
C. N_2O ☐
D. Halothane ☐

43. Agent which dissolves rubber

2

ANAESTHESIA

A. Halothane (AIIMS 1993) ☐
B. Enflurane ☐
C. Cyclopropane ☐
D. Ether ☐

44. Maximum uterine relaxation (AIIMS 1992)
A. Ether ☐
B. N_2O ☐
C. Halothane ☐
D. Chloroform ☐

45. All are true except (AI 2001)
A. Halothane is good analgesic agent ☐
B. Halothane sensitize heart to catacholamines ☐
C. Halothane relaxes bronchi. ☐
D. Halothane causes hepatitis and liver cell necrosis ☐

46. Bronchospasm is not caused by (AIIMS 1994)
A. Regurgitation ☐
B. Aspiration ☐
C. Intubation ☐
D. Halothane ☐

47. Which of the following fluorinated anaesthetics corrodes metal in vaporizers and breathing systems?
A. Sevoflurane (AIIMS May 2006) ☐
B. Enflurane ☐
C. Isoflurane ☐
D. Halothane ☐

FLURANES

48. Nephrotoxic agent is (AI 98, AIIMS 1997)
A. Methoxy flurone ☐
B. Isoflurone ☐
C. Halothane ☐
D. N_2O ☐

49. Fluoride content is least: (PGI 1997)
A. Methoxyflurane ☐
B. Enflurane ☐
C. Isoflurane ☐
D. Sevoflurane ☐

50. Which of the following inhalational agent is contraindicated in a patient with history of epilepsy;
A. Isoflurance (AIIMS 03, 94) ☐
B. Enflurane ☐
C. Halothane ☐
D. Sevoflurane ☐

51. A patent has to undergo neurosurgery for intracranial space occupying lesion, inhalatonal agent of choice is:
A. Enflurane (AIIMS May 13) ☐
B. Sevoflurane ☐
C. Isoflurane ☐
D. Desflurane ☐

52. In increased ICT, agent used for anesthesia
A. N_2O (AIIMS 1994) ☐
B. Trilene ☐
C. Ether ☐
D. Isoflurane ☐

53. Least effect on myocardial contractility
A. Ether (AIIMS 1993) ☐
B. Halothane ☐
C. Trilene ☐
D. Isoflurane ☐

54. Coronary steal is caused by (AIIMS 1993)
A. Halothane ☐
B. Isoflurane ☐
C. Enflurane ☐
D. Ether ☐

55. Least Cardiotoxic anaesthetic agent (AI 2K, 98, 96)
A. Enflurane ☐
B. Isoflurane ☐
C. Sevoflurane ☐
D. Halothane, Trilene, ketamine ☐

56. Which of the following statements regard-ing desflurane is correct? (AIIMS Nov 04)
A. It causes severe myocardial depression ☐
B. It is a structural analogue of isoflurane ☐
C. It has vary high blood and tissue gas partition coefficients ☐
D. It is metabolically unstable ☐

57. A seventy year old patient is posted for a surgery which is likely to last 4-6 hours. The best inhalational agent of choice for maintenance of anesthesia in such a case is:
A. Methoxyflurane (AIIMS May 2004) ☐
B. Ether ☐
C. Trichlorethylene ☐
D. Desflurane ☐

58. Rapid induction of anesthesia occurs with which of the following inhalation anesthetics? (AIIMS 02)
A. Isoflurane ☐
B. Halothane ☐
C. Desflurane ☐
D. Sevoflurane ☐

59. Anesthetic agents associated with epilepsy: (PGI Nov 12)
A. Enflurane ☐
B. Desflurane ☐
C. Propofol ☐
D. Sevoflurane ☐
E. Thiopentone ☐

60. Which of the following is an epileptogenic anesthetic agent (AI 11)
A. Isoflurane ☐
B. Sevoflurane ☐
C. Methoxyflurane ☐
D. Halothane ☐

61. A six year old child is posted for elective urology surgery under general anesthesia. He refuses to allow the anaesthesiologist an I.V. access. The best inhalational agent of choice for induction of anesthesia is:
A. Sevoflurane (AIIMS May 04, DNB 06) ☐
B. Methoxyflurane ☐
C. Desflurane ☐
D. Isoflurane ☐

62. Which is C/I in closed system anesthesiology :
A. Methoxyflurane (Bihar 05, DNB 05, UP 06) ☐
B. Isoflurane ☐
C. Sevoflurane ☐
D. Desflurane ☐

63. True about Sevoflurane- (PGI Dec 04)
A. Isopropyl ether ☐
B. MAC is 2% ☐
C. Good to use in old age ☐
D. Blood gas partition coefficient is more than halothane ☐
E. Formation of compound A with baralyme ☐

64. NOT TRUE regarding sevoflurane (AI 08)
A. MAC is higher than isoflurane ☐
B. Blood gas coefficient is higher than desflurane ☐
C. Potency more than cardio depressant than isoflurane ☐
D. Sevoflurane is less cardio depressant than isoflurane ☐

65. Which of following is/are false: (PGI Nov 2010)
A. Enflurane interacts with sodalime ☐
B. Sevoflurane causes seizures ☐
C. Rapid recovery from propofol ☐
D. Ketamine acts through GABA-A receptors ☐
E. MAC indicates potency of inhalational agents ☐

GENERAL

1. **A i.e. Minimum alveolar concentration**
2. **C i.e. Hypocalcemia**
3. **A i.e. Minimum alveolar concentration**
4. **C i.e. Measures solubility**
5. **B i.e. Oil gas partition Co-efficient**

[Ref: Morgan 4/e p – 163- 65; Lee's 13/e ,p – 125' Miller 6/e , p- 107-9, 115; Wylie 7/e p- 260- 61, 988 – 89]

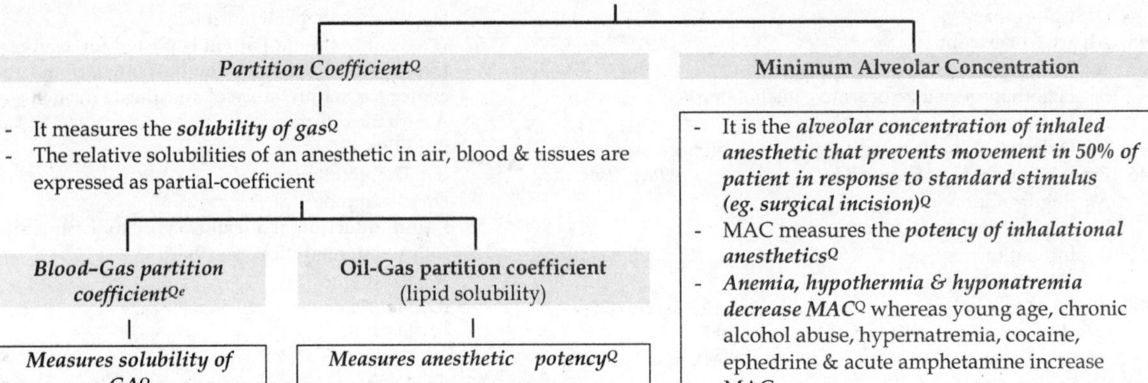

Partition CoefficientQ
- It measures the solubility of gasQ
- The relative solubilities of an anesthetic in air, blood & tissues are expressed as partial-coefficient
Blood-Gas partition coefficientQe
Measures solubility of GAQ
Oil-Gas partition coefficient (lipid solubility)
Measures anesthetic potencyQ
Minimum Alveolar Concentration
- It is the alveolar concentration of inhaled anesthetic that prevents movement in 50% of patient in response to standard stimulus (eg. surgical incision)Q
- MAC measures the potency of inhalational anestheticsQ
- Anemia, hypothermia & hyponatremia decrease MACQ whereas young age, chronic alcohol abuse, hypernatremia, cocaine, ephedrine & acute amphetamine increase MAC.

6. **D i.e. Obeys Charles, boyle's & avogadro's laws**

- An *ideal gas obeys charle's, boyle's & avogadro's law*Q
  - Boyle's law: at constant temperature $V \propto \frac{1}{P}$
  - Charle's law: at constant pressure $V \propto T$ (absolute temperature)
  - Avogrados law: Equal volumes of gas at same temperature & pressure contains same no. of molecules
- At STP (Standard temperature i.e. 37 C) the volume of a mole of gas is 22.4 liters.
- For ideal gas – PV = nRT

7. **D i.e. Hydrophobic site** *[Ref: Wylie 7/e p 259-60; Miller's 6/e p- 116-117]*

***Non anesthetics / nonimmobilizers, cut off effect convulsant gases, isomers, hydrophilic site and critical volume expanism hypothesis provide exceptions to the meyer – overton rule*Q.**

8. **A i.e. Desflurane**
9. **A i.e. Desflurane**
10. **B i.e. Desflurane**
11. **D i.e N_2O** *[Ref: Miller's 6/e p. 115, Lee's 13/e p –124- 29]*

Inhalation Anesthetic

- **Increasing order of**
  - **Blood gas coefficient**
  - **Diffusion coefficient**
  - **Solubility**
- **Decreasing order of induction & recovery**

***Xe (minimum B/G coefficient /solubility and maximum i.e., fastest induction & recovery)*Q → *Desflurane* → Cyclopropane → N_2O → *Sevoflurane* → *Isoflurane* → *Enflurane* → *Halothane* → *Halothane* → Chloroform → Trielene → Ether → *Methoxy flurane* (maximum B/G coefficient /solubility & solowest induction & recovery)*Q.

Mn : for fluranes – "**D S I E M**"

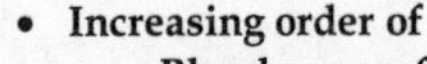

N_2O (b/w 1st two) - Halothane - Ether (b/w last 2)

Decreasing value of MAC = Increasing Order of Potency

N_2OQ > Xenon > Ethylene > Cyclopropane > *Desflurane* > Fluroxene > *Sevoflurane* > Diethyl ether > *Enflurane* > Isoflurane > Halothane > Methoxyflurane.

Mn: for flurane – "**D S E I M**"

N_2O — Halothane (b/w last 2) — Ether (before Enflurane)

Lesser MAC = Higher Potency

12. **D i.e. Sevoflurane**
[Ref: Morgan 4/e p155, 157-60, Lee's 13/e p. 123-24]

i. The greater the uptake of anesthetic agent, the greater the difference between inspired and alveolar concentrations, and the slower the rate of induction.
ii. Three factors affects anesthetic uptake: Solubility in the blood, alveolar blood flow and difference in partial pressure between alveolar gas and venous blood.
iii. Many of the **factors that speed induction** also speed **recovery:** elimination of rebreathing, high fresh gas flows, low anesthetic circuit volume, low absorption by the anesthetic circuit, *decreased solubility*, high cerebral flow, and increased ventilation.
iv. Because the concentration of a gas is directly proportional to its partial pressure, the alveolar partial pressure will also be slow to rise. The alveolar partial pressure is important because it determines the partial pressure of anesthetic in blood and, ultimately, in the brain. Similarly the partial pressure of anesthetic in brain is directly proportional to its brain tissue concentration, which determines clinical effect.
v. Blood gas partition coefficient (B/G Coff.) is most important factor in determining the uptake of agent and so the speed of induction and recovery. The **higher** the **B/G coefficienct** of an anesthetic, the **greater its solubility in blood** and its **uptake in pulmonary circulation.** As a result of this alveolar *partial pressure rises* much slowly & **induction is prolonged.** Agents with low blood gas partition coefficient will have high alveolar concentration. So the ***induction & recovery will be fast with agent with less B/G Coff.; and induction and recovery will be slower with agents with high, B/G partition coefficients.*** Q
vi. **Agents in increasing order of B/G coefficients (or decreasing order of induction & recovery)**

Xe (0.14) → **Desflurane** (0.42) > Cyclopropane (0.44) > N_2O (0.47) > ***Sevoflurane*** (0.69) > **Isoflurane** (1.38) > Enflurane (1.8) > Halothane (2.4) > Chloroform (8) > Trielene (9) > Ether (12) > Methoxyflurane (15)

13. **B, D i.e. Isoflurane, Desflurane** 14. **C i.e. Desflurane**
[Ref: Wiley 7/e p- 524; Miller's 6/e p-240-38; Lee's 13/e p129; Morgan's 4/e p.158; Aitkenhead 4/e,p152-64; KDT 5/e P-338]

Pungent volatile anesthetic agents **are** *desflurane, isoflurane, enflurane and ether*Q. **(Mn-"DIE')**

Volatile Anesthetic Agent	Physical property	Blood / Gas partition coefficient	
Xenon	Colourless, odourless, **nonirritating** (i.e. **non pungent**)	0.115	**Low B/G Coeffiecient = Low solubitity** in blood i.e. ***fast induction & rapid recovery***Q
Desflurane	**Pungent** (irritating / unpleasant to inhale)	0.42	
Nitrous oxide (N_2O)	Colourless, sweet smelling, non irritant (i.e. **non pungent**)	0.47	
Sevoflurane	Colourless, **non pungent**	0.69	
Isoflurane	**Pungent** ethereal odor (i.e. moderately irritating)	1.4	Mn-**"Xena- Dislikes No Save" "IE HEAT"**
Enflurane	**Pungent**	1.9	
Halothane	Colourless, **non irritating (non pungent/pleasant)** odor	2.5	**High B/G** coefficient = **High solubility** in blood i.e. ***Slow induction & slow recovery***Q
Ether	Extremely irritating **(pungent)**	12	

★ Because of lack of chlorine / bromine ions; sevoflurane & desflurane have no effect on ozone layer.
Pungent = Unpleasant= Causing Cough = Irritant

15. **C i.e. Ether >>> A i.e. Ketamine** *[Ref: Miller 7/e p. 567-68; Ajay Yadav 5/e p. 74]*

- **All inhalational agents except ether inhibit ciliary activity. Volatile anesthetics and nitrous oxide** may diminish rate of mucus clearance (Tantalum powder clearance) by decreasing ciliary beat frequency, disrupting metachronism or altering the physical characteristics or quantity of mucus. **Halothane, enflurane, isoflurane and sevoflurane, in contrast to many intravenous anesthetics, reduced ciliary movement and beat frequency**Q. Among the volatile anesthetics, *sevoflurane exhibited the weakest cilia-inhibitory effects* in vitro (but still more inhibition than total intravenous anesthesia consisting propofol & remifentanil). = Miller/Yadav.
- Some intravenous sedating agents such as *benzodiazepines, barbiturates,* ***opioid and ketamine*** *may impair ciliary motility* (unboundmedicine. com). However, this statement is not supported by all anesthesia text books, which consider intravenous agents to be not affecting ciliary function.

XENON

16. **C i.e. Slow induction and recovery**
17. **A i.e. Rapid induction and recovery, D i.e. Non-explosive, E i.e. Heavier than air**
18. **A i.e. B/G Partition coefficient 0.14; B i.e. MAC is high; C i.e. Minimum hemodynamic effect; D i.e. Heavier than air** *[Ref: Wiley & Davidson 7/e p-536; Morgan's 4/e p. 155-59; Aitkenhead 4/e, P- 168; Miller's 7/e p-640, 567, 626, 317-18, 2137-38; Lee's Anesthesia 13/e p-143]*

- **Xenon** is inert/nobel, colourless, odorless, nonirritating, ***nonflammable and non explosive gas that is heavier than air (4 times), more dense/viscous than N_2 & N_2O, more potent than N_2O, is very blood insoluble***Q **(B/G partition coefficienct 0.14)** ***most ideal inhaled anesthetic agent with very rapid induction & recovery***Q. It is neuro & cardioprotective, non teratogenic, and safe (to liver & kidney) anesthetic which is environmental friendly.
- At 0.115, **Xenons'** B/G partition coefficient is the lowest coefficient of all available agents, resulting in ***rapid induction and recovery***Q.
- ***Xenon is more potent than nitrous oxide with MAC 71% (but even than is a weak anesthetic agent)***Q. ***It is a good analgesic***Q. It is **neuroprotective, and provides favourable cardiovascular stability (ie has minimum hemodynamic effects)**Q.

NO

19. **A i.e. Formed from L-arginine by NO Synthetase; B i.e. Causes vasodilation of all vessels; C i.e. Used in portal hypertension; D i.e. Interacts with Hb; E i.e. Used in erectile dysfunction**
20. **A i.e. Used in pulmonary hypertension; D i.e. Causes systemic hypotension**
21. **B i.e, Dilates pulmonary arteries D i.e., Least systemic effects E i.e., Better ventilation perfusion mismatch**
22. **C i.e. Nitric oxide**
[Ref: Wylie 7/e p- 158, 186, 207, 797, 1099, Miller's 7/e p. 949; Guyton 11/e p-564, 199- 200, 322; Ganong 22/e p- 115, 598-99, 427-28]

- **Nitric oxide (NO)** or **endothelium derived relaxing factor (EDRF)** is ***synthesized from L-arginine by nitric oxide synthase (NOS) enzyme in endothelium of blood vessels***Q. Physiologically it causes ***vasodilation & decreases vascular resistance throughout the body***Q. It activates guanylyl cyclase producing C-GMP and ***binds rapidly to Hb & gets inactivated***Q.
- Whereas **inhaled NO** is a **selective pulmonary-vasodilator** ***decreases pulmonary artery pressure in infants & adults and improves V/P ratio***Q. So it is used in ***treatment of pulmonary artery hypertension***Q. ***It has no systemic vasodilatory effect***Q. Systemic effects of breathing NO includes platelet & leukocyte inhibition and oxidation of extraerythrocytic hemoglobin.
- Inhaled NO decreases vascular smooth muscle cell hyperplasia & increases alveolarization in the injured developing limb. This *pulmonary vascular & alveolar developmental effect of NO* is used to prevent or ameliorate pulmonary hypertension in infants with congenital heart disease and chronic lung disease in premature infants.

N_2O

23. **B i.e. Recovering anesthesia** 24. **A i.e. Diffusion Hypoxia**
25. **B i.e. N_2O** 26. **D.i.e. Excentration operation**
[Ref: CDTP 2000 p-423-24; Miller's 7/e p-2373,2383;KDT 6/e p.370-71; Aitkenhead 5/e p .575-76, 257, 28-31, 581-95]

- **Diffusion hypoxia** is seen during **recovery phase** after discontinuation of prolonged **N_2O anesthesia**. It ***can be prevented by continuing 100% O_2 inhalation for a few minutes after discontinuing N_2O***Q.
- **Second gas effect** occurs in initial part of **induction** of N_2O anesthesia. N_2O also shows ***bone marrow suppression***Q.
- **Excentration** is enucleation + wide dissection of periorbital tissue. In it there is no closed space formation so N_2O can be used. In **microlaryngeal lesser surgery, *N_2O is contraindicated d/t risk of airway fire***Q

27. **A i.e. Nitrous oxide** *[Ref: Wiley 7th /536; Goodman & Gilman 12/e p 558-60; Miller7th/813]*

- **Nitrous oxide** is a **good analgesic** and **a very weak anesthetic (ie mainly or only analgesia).** N_2O produces analgesia that is in part mediated by release of **proenkephalin derived family of endogenous opioid peptides.**
- **O_2 is used to correct hypoxia; NO** inhalation **dilates pulmonary vasculature** and **CO_2 is used for insufflations during endoscopic procedures.**

TRILENE

28. **C i.e. Trielene** [Ref: Morgan's 4/e, P-38] 29. **D i.e. Trilene** 30. **B i.e. Trichloro ethylene**

Sodalime with trilene forms phosgene (neurotoxic) gas.Q So this combination is contraindicated.

Sodalime is a mixture of ***94% ($Ca(OH)_2$ + 5% NaOH as catalyst + 1% KOH***Q; with granule size of **4-8 *mesh***Q. **It should not be used with :**

C	-	Chloroform
T	-	*Trilene*Q
Scan	-	*Sevoflurane*Q

The drier the sodalime, the more likely it will degrade & absorb volatile anesthetics. It produces ***compound A with sevoflurane***Q (clinically significant) and *carbon monoxide with desflurane, isoflurane & enflurane (clinically insignificant)*. However, desflurane can be broken down to CO by dry barium hydroxide lime to such an extent that it is capable of causing clinically significant CO poisoning.

ETHER

31. **A i.e. Ether** 32. **B i.e. Ether**
33. **D i.e. Affects blood pressure & is liable to produce arrythmias.** *[Ref: Morgan's anaesthesia 4/e p. 166-69]*

Staging of anesthesia (Guedel's) were established for *ether*Q. Ether is **highly inflammable** (so ***cautery can't be used***Q), irritant (stimulates laryngospasm & bronchial secretion) has ***slow induction & slow recovery***Q but ***maintains BP & respiration, cardiac arrhythmias are rare and does not sensitize heart to circulating catecholamines***Q (i.e. relatively safe).

HALOTHANE

34. **B i.e. It sensitizes heart to catecholamines at 1 MAC; C i.e. 20% metabolized; D i.e. It is not usually given in same patient within 3 months**
35. **A i.e. Non irritant; C i.e. It antagonizes bronchospasm; D i.e. Vasodilator**
36. **A i.e. Causes bronchodialation; E i.e. Causes hepatitis**
37. **C i.e. Recent halothane use; D i.e. Associated liver pathology** 38. **D i.e. Halothane**
39. **B i.e. Halothane** 40. **A i.e. Hepatitis** 41. **B i.e. Halothane**
42. **D i.e. Halothane** 43. **A i.e. Halothane** 44. **C i.e. Halothane**
45. **A i.e. Halothane is a good analgesic** 46. **D i.e. Halothane** 47. **D i.e. Halothane**

[Ref: Lee's 13/e p-140- 43; Aitkenhead 4/e, P-153- 65; Wiley & Davidson 7/e p-524-26; Miller's 6/e p-237- 38; Morgan's 4/e p. 166- 69]

- **Halothane** (2- bromo – 2- chloro – 1, 1, 1 trifluoroethane) is a *potent, non inflammable, non toxic* (relatively), *colourless* liquid with relatively ***non pungent (pleasant)*** vapour. It is *decomposed by light* and stabilised by ***0.01% thymol***Q, but is stable when stored in *amber coloured bottles.* Although it is decomposed by soda lime, it may be used safely with this mixture. ***The vapour is absorbed by rubber***Q (rubber/gas partition cofficient is 120). ***It corrodes metals in vaporizers and breathing systems***Q. ***In the presence of moisture, it corrodes aluminium, tin, lead, magnesium and alloys***Q. It should be stored in a closed container away from light and heat. It is ***soluble in rubber, and plastics***Q commonly found in ansethetic circuits. This has obvious implications for patients with halothane sensitivity, or who are at risk for malignant hyperthermia, in whom anesthetic free circuit should be used.
- ***Halothane, Ketamine & Atropine***Q **are *bronchodialators.*** These agents decrease airway resistance and increase anatomical dead space.
- ***Aspiration, regurgitation & intubation leads to reflex bronchospasm.***

FLURANE

48. **A i.e. Methoxy flurane** [Ref: Lee 12/e P-328, Morgan 3/e P-672 & 143] 49. **C i.e. Isoflurane**

Isoflurane has least & methoxyflurane has highest fluride contentQ. Methoxyflurane causes ***vasopressin resistant high output renal failure.***Q

Nephrotoxicity of anesthetic agents

Methoxyflurane	Enflurane & Sevoflurane	Isoflurane, Desflurane, Halothane
Has **5 Highs** 1. High Boiling point (104 c)Q 2. High *nephrotoxicity*Q 3. ***Highest fluride content***Q 4. ***Causes High output (Polyuric) renal failure***Q which is vasopressin resistant 5. *High risk of* **Oxalate stones**Q	Prolonged use l/t significant fluoride production & nephrotoxicity.	- Fluride production is negligible - **Can be used in Renal failure**Q - Halothane & Isoflurane decrease renal blood flow, GFR & urinary output but desflurane does not. - **Desflurane** has high vapour pressure (boils at room temp. in high altitude), ***ultrashort duration of action (wake up time is less)***Q

50. **B i.e. Enflurane** *[Ref. KDT 5th/e p 340; Morgan's 3/e p-142]*

Enflurane is ***contraindicated in epilepsy***Q.
Mn- **E** is contraindicated in **E**

- Enflurane increases cerebral blood flow, secretion of CSF, resistance to CSF flow & intra cranial pressure
- During deep enflurance anesthesia *high voltage high frequency EEG* changes can progress *to spike & wave pattern* that culminates in *frank tonic clonic seizures*Q.
- This epileptiform activity is exacerbated by high anesthetic concentrations & hypocapnia, so ***hyperventilation is not recommended to attenuate enflurane intracranial hypertension.***

Isoflurane	Enflurance
- **Coronary Steal Syndrome**Q - **Least affect myocardial contractivity**Q - **AOC in neurosurgery like increased ICT**Q	- ***C/I in Epilepsy***Q because it causes raised ICT & tonic-clonic seizure. - Epileptiform activity of Enflurane is increased by hypocapnea (↓ CO_2) so ***hyperventilation is not recommended to attenuate enflurane induced ↑ ICT.***

51. **C i.e. Isoflurane** *[Ref: Yao 7/e p. 524; Pardo 6/e p 477-81; Morgan 5/e p 169, 581-83; Miller 7/e p 307-21; 2048-50, 2069]*
52. **D i.e. Isoflurane** **53.** **D i.e. Isoflurane**
54. **B i.e. Isoflurane** **55.** **B i.e. Isoflurane** *[Ref: Morgan's 3/e P-142]*

- A patient undergoing **neurosurgery for intracranial space occupying lesion, inhatational agent of choice is isoflurane**Q.
- Isoflurane increases ICT but less than halothane & enflurane; which can be reversed by hyperventilation. So isoflurane is a preferable agent in raised ICT. Isoflurane is anaesthesia of choice *(AOC) for* ***neurosurgical procedure***Q as it does not increase cerebral blood flow & CSF pressure.
- *Of various inhalation agents available,* ***isoflurane has the advantage of providing stability of cardiac rhythm & lack of sensitizention of the heart to exogenous & endogenous adrenaline***Q.
- In coronary artery disease ***isoflurane should be avoided d/t coronary steel phenomenon***Q.
- In ischemia of cardiac muscle selective vasodialation of vessels of Ischemic zone and maintained tone of non ischemic zone l/t selective increase of blood supply to ischemic areas.
- But in ***coronary steal phenomenon (Isoflurane & Dipyridomole) there is dialation of vessels of non ischemic zone also so there is decrease of flow in ischemic zone.***Q That is why **isoflurane is avoided in ischemic heart disease.**

★ In *Myocardial Infarction* operation should be ***with held for 6 months***Q.
★ **Goldman Index** is for cardiac risk factor and when it is > 13 it is associated with poor prognosis.
★ In **hypertension, halothane** is AOC (for hypotensive surgery)
★ In **hypovolumia, Light G.A.** (preferably Ether and Cyclopropane) with **IPPV is method of choice**

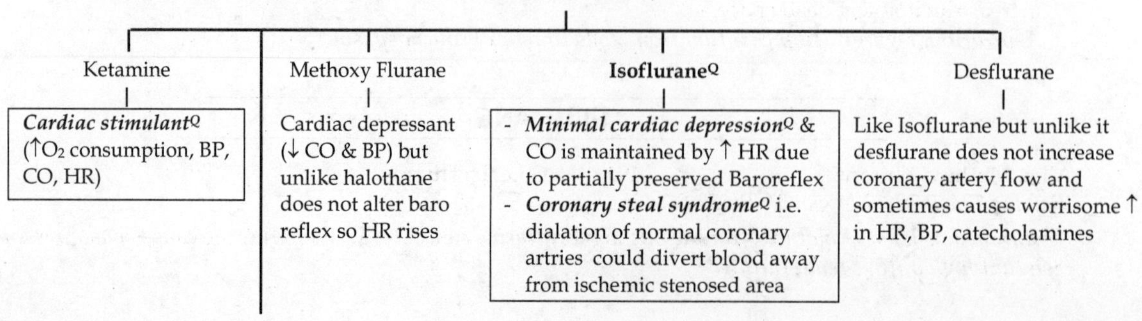

Cardiovascular S/E
Ketamine
Cardiac stimulantQ (↑O2 consumption, BP, CO, HR)
Methoxy Flurane
Cardiac depressant (↓ CO & BP) but unlike halothane does not alter baro reflex so HR rises
IsofluraneQ
- Minimal cardiac depressionQ & CO is maintained by ↑ HR due to partially preserved Baroreflex
- Coronary steal syndromeQ i.e. dialation of normal coronary artries could divert blood away from ischemic stenosed area
Desflurane
Like Isoflurane but unlike it desflurane does not increase coronary artery flow and sometimes causes worrisome ↑ in HR, BP, catecholamines

Halothane	Enflurane	Sevoflurane
- *Arrythmogenic*Q - Cardiac depressant leading to ↓ CO & BP - Blunts baroreception of aortic arch & carotid body leading to ↓ HR (inspite of decreased Blood Pressure) - Coronary artery dilator but coronary artery blood flow decreases d/t hypotension	- Cardiac depressant (↓ CO, BP & O_2 consumption) due to baro reflex HR ↑ - Sensitize heart to arrythmogenic action of epinephrine	- Cardiac depressant - HR does not increase so CO is not maintained

56. **B i.e. It is a structural analogue of isoflurane**
[Ref: KDT 5/e p341; Morgan's 3/e p144]

Desflurane's structure is ***very similar to that of isoflurane. The only difference is substitution of a fluride atom for isofluranes chlorine atom.*** Q

57. **D i.e. Desflurane** *[Ref. KDT 4/e p-349; Morgan's 3/e p-144 145 & 874]*

This is a long surgery (4-6 hours) so a safe anesthetic agent should be used as in many cases diminshed cardiac reserve in many elderly patient may be manifested as exaggerated drop in BP during inductioin of G.A.

- A prolonged circulation time delays the onset of intravenous drug but speeds induction with inhalational agent.
- Methoxy flurane, Trichloroethylene & Cyclopropane are no longer used.
- Ether is a safe anesthetic agent but is highly volatile, irritating, inflamable and explosive, induction is prolonged, unpleasant with struggling, breath holding, salivation & marked respiratory secretion so ether is not a preferred agent
- **Desflurane** is pungent but a ***safe anesthetic agent for geriatric age group* as its *cardiovascular effects are similar to isoflurane but without coronary steal phenomenon*Q.**

58. **C i.e. Desflurane** *[Ref: Clinical Anesthesology 3/e, P-145, 884; Goodman Gilman 10/e P-349]*

- You should know that *rate of induction of inhalational anesthetic agent is inversely proportional to its blood gas partition coefficient (i.e. the solubility of agent in blood & tissue)*. The *speed of induction* by inhalational anesthetics *in descending order* is

	Mn:
- **Des**flurane	**Disco**
- **Sevo**flurane	**Serves**
- **I**soflurane	**Ice**
- **Hal**othane	**Hall**

- **Non pungency & rapid increase in alveolar anesthetic concentration, makes sevoflurane an excellent choice for smooth & rapid inhalational induction in pediatrics & adult population.**
- ***Induction and recovery are very fast in desflurane*Q**. Due to its short action it is commonly used as *anesthesia for OPD*.

59. **A i.e. Enflurane >>>> D i.e. Sevoflurane**
60. **B i.e. Sevoflurane** *[Ref. Morgan 4/e, p, 167-73, Aitken head 5/e, p 24-23, Lee 13/e, 135-36, Miller's 7/e, p 1500-2, 642]*

Epileptiform activity on EEG and seizures may occur with: ***enflurane*Q >>>> *sevoflurane*Q > Isoflurane > halothane**. ***Desflurane has no epileptiform activity and is used in treatment of refractory status epilepticus*Q**

61. **A i.e. Sevoflurane**
62. **C i.e. Sevoflurane**
63. **A, B, C, E i.e. (Isopropyl ether), (MAC is 2%), (Good to use in old age) (Formation of compound A with baralyme)** *[Ref: Morgan 4/e p – 167, 169 –74; Lee's 13/e p. 135; Wylie 7/e p. 532]*
64. **D i.e., Sevoflurane is less cardiodepressant than isoflurane**

- ***Sevoflurane is inhalational agent of choice for inductioin of anesthesia in pediatric patients and adults, because of rapid onset of action & nonpengency*** Q
- ***Desflurane & isoflurane are more pungent and are associated with more coughing, breath holding & laryngeal spasm during inhalational inudction, so not used as first choice*Q.**
- Methoryflurane is highly nephrotoxic, so not preferred.
- ***Sevoflurane is not recommended in closed circuit because there is chance of production of a toxic metabolic product compound A,*** Q ***(an olefin) in closed circuit.***
- Unlike isoflurane & desflurane, both of which lead to tachycaridia, sevoflurane has minimal effect on heart rate.
- Sevoflurane can cause direct myocardial depression (via calcium channels) and produce dose dependent depression of cardiac output, & reduction in systemic vascular resistance similar to that seen in isoflurane

65. **B i.e. Sevoflurane causes seizures, C i.e. Rapid recovery from propofol >> A i.e. Enflurane interacts with sodalime** *[Lee's 13/e p. 136-39, 162; Morgan 4/e p. 38, 197; Miller 7/e p. 743]*

- ***MAC (minimal alveolar concentration) is the best measure of anesthetic potency*Q.**
- **Sevoflurane** has ***anticonvulsant properties*Q** with no excitatory phenomenon, no increase in CBF or intracranial pressure. Muscle tone is reduced, potentiating nondepolarizing muscle relaxants. Cerebral O_2 demand is decreased.
- ***Sevoflurane, isoflurane & desflurane have anticonvulsant properties*Q.** Whereas, the main disadvantage of enflurane is that it often causes ***epileptiform EEG changes*Q** (more commonly during hypocapnia) that may persist for several weeks. *Cerebral blood flow* is doubled at MAC 1 and ***convulsions*Q** occur at MAC2, so it should be used with extreme caution (or avoided) in patients with h/o epilepsy. Muscle relaxation is greater with enflurane than with halothane or isoflurane, enhancing the action of nondepolarizing relaxants.
- Enflurane interacts with sodalime but produce clinically insignificant amount of carbonmonooxide.
- ***Propofol has smooth & rapid induction and rapid recovery*Q.**
- **Ketamine** is a ***noncompetitive NMDA (glutamate) receptor antagonist*Q** and does not act on GABA-A receptor.

5 CLINICAL ANESTHESIA

DAY CARE (OUT PATIENT) ANESTHESIA

In day care surgery, patient is discharged on the same day, so anesthetic agents with short duration of actions are used.

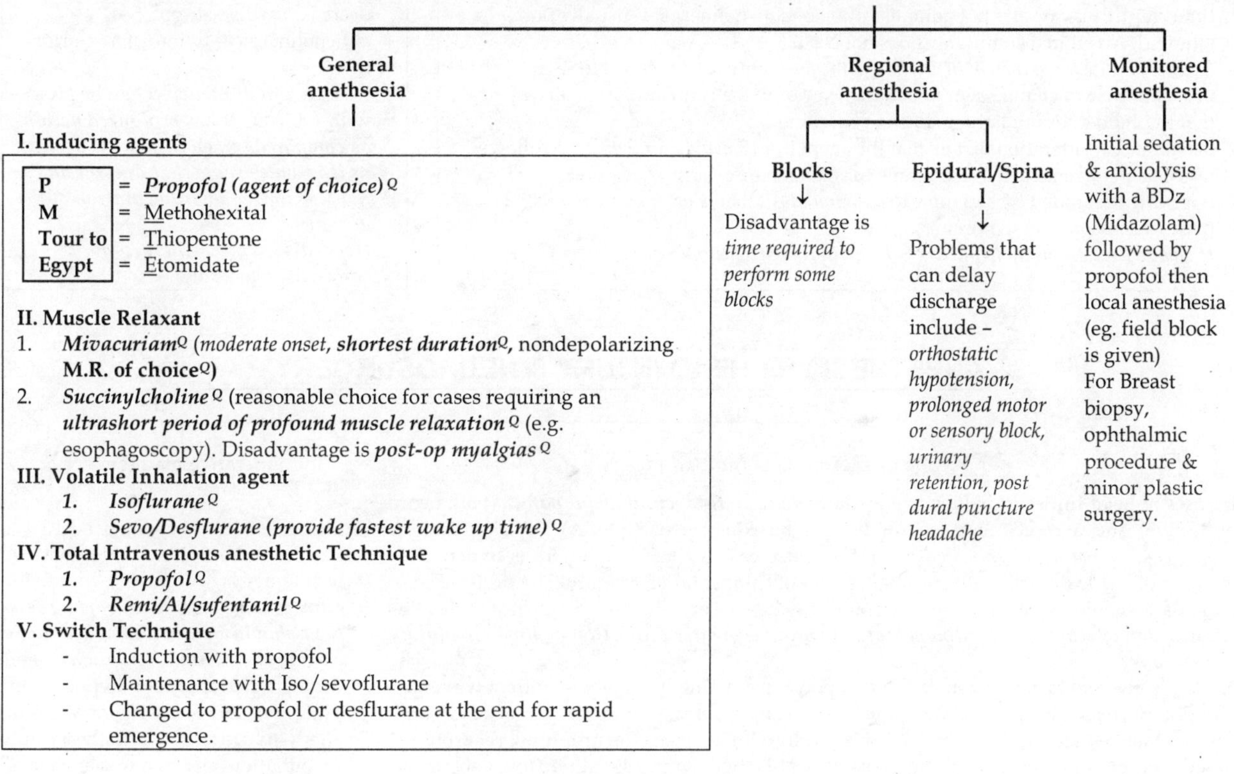

General anethsesia
I. Inducing agents
P = Propofol (agent of choice)Q
M = Methohexital
Tour to = Thiopentone
Egypt = Etomidate
II. Muscle Relaxant
1. MivacuriamQ (moderate onset, shortest durationQ, nondepolarizing M.R. of choiceQ)
2. Succinylcholine Q (reasonable choice for cases requiring an ultrashort period of profound muscle relaxation Q (e.g. esophagoscopy). Disadvantage is post-op myalgias Q
III. Volatile Inhalation agent
1. Isoflurane Q
2. Sevo/Desflurane (provide fastest wake up time) Q
IV. Total Intravenous anesthetic Technique
1. Propofol Q
2. Remi/Al/sufentanil Q
V. Switch Technique
- Induction with propofol
- Maintenance with Iso/sevoflurane
- Changed to propofol or desflurane at the end for rapid emergence.
Regional anesthesia
Blocks
Disadvantage is time required to perform some blocks
Epidural/Spinal
Problems that can delay discharge include – orthostatic hypotension, prolonged motor or sensory block, urinary retention, post dural puncture headache
Monitored anesthesia
Initial sedation & anxiolysis with a BDz (Midazolam) followed by propofol then local anesthesia (eg. field block is given)
For Breast biopsy, ophthalmic procedure & minor plastic surgery.

PAEDIATRIC ANESTHESIA

- ***Intravenous route is most preferred method for induction in children***Q because it provides overall better control of anesthesia & less chances of aspiration. The only problem is that it is difficult to put IV line.
- Neonates, infants & young children have relatively high alveolar ventilation and lower FRC compared with adults. This higher minute ventilation to FRC ratio relatively higher blood flow to vessel rich organs contributes to a rapid rise in alveolar anesthetic concentration. These factors result in ***rapid induction & recovery from G.A.***Q,
- ***In children for tracheal intubation muscle relaxant is used.***Q
- Mivacurium, atracurium & cisatracurium are preferred M.R. in neonates.
- ***Avoidance of needles is considered a major advantage of inhalational induction in young children***Q, while older children and adolescents often prefer an intravenous induction.

Inhalational induction	Intravenous – induction
- Avoidance of needles is considered a major advantage of inhalation induction in younger children, - MAC value changes with age. From birth, it increases to a peak at the age of 6 months and then gradually declines until the adult value is reacehed - N_2O is used as carrier for most inhalational agents - All volatile anesthetic agent potentiates the duration of	- Older children & adolscent often prefer an intravenous induction. - The main advantage of barbiturate (thiopental) that injection into a small vein is pain free. - It is more commonly used method - ***Propofol is useful*** in ***child with porphyria***Q - Ketamine is used in ***status asthamaticus***Q - Opioids may be used in large dose as sole agent to provide stable

neuromuscular blocking drugs, and may also l/t *malignant hyperthermia.*

hemodynamic condition for *children with heart disease.*

Sevoflurane

- It is now the ***drug of choice for inhalation induction***Q because of its *low pungency* & relatively *low blood solubility*, which allows rapid induction of anesthesia
- 8% exposure can be given experiencing significant problems of coughing, breath holding, or laryngeal spasm.
- There is little to be gained by including N_2O during induction as MAC sparing effect is not great.
- Bradycardia may occurs but administration of anticholinergic is usually not required. Arrythmia commonly does not occur.
- *Excellent choice for induction in children with upper airway obstruction* but it is probably wise to change over to halothane prior to instrumentation of airway so that the child does not lighten during procedure.
- Economic consideration dictate that the agent is *used mainly for induction*, followed by a cheaper agent such as isoflurane for maintenance.
- It is partly degraded by sodalime to ***compound A***Q that is *nephrotoxic in rats.* (hazard is theoretical in humans).
- ***It can be used safely in hepatitis & intestinal obstruction***Q.

Halothane

- This agent has been the *gold standard for induction of anesthesia* in children because, until recently its smell was one of the ***least pungent (non irritant)***Q.
- Depress myocardium, slows heartrate, decrease cardiac output. So anticholinergic is administered prior to it.
- Has smooth induction & can be given with 100% O_2. It has ***prolonged action as compared to newer volatile agents, as it is undesirable that anesthesia lightens during instrumentation of the airway***Q.
- ***Hepatitis is extremely rare***Q in comparison to adults.

ANESTHESIA for HEAD INJURY & NEUROSURGERY

Induction of anesthesia & Intubation

- In cases of **head injury** induction is ***preferably done by thiopental or propofol***Q (both neuro protective) and a rapid onset neuromuscular blocking agent (NMBA) *following adequate preoxygenation and hyperventilation* by mask (to decrease ICP). If the patient is **hypotensive** (systolic BP < 100 mmHg), either a smaller dose of **thiopental or propofol** should be used or **etomidate** should be substituted. Propofol provides a very short recovery time where as ***substitution of etomidate for thiopental may provide greater protection against circulatory depression***Q.
- NMBA is given to facilitate ventilation and prevent straining or coughing both of which can abruptly increase ICP. So *NMBA can lower ICP*, resulting in lowering of *CVP* with concomitant reduction in cerebral venous outflow impedance. **Rocuronium, vecuronium, pipecuronium and doxacurium** provide greatest hemodynamic stability. Doses should be limited to ranges not a/w hypotension *for metocurium, mivacurium and atracurium, and hypertension (and ↑ ICP) for pancuronium.*
- The use of **succinylcholine** in closed head injury is controversial (and best avoided) b/o ***potential for increasing ICP***Q and causing hyperkalaemia (although rarely). **Rocuronium or mivacurium** is a suitable alternative. However, Sch may be the agent of choice in patients at increased *risk for aspiration* or with a potentially difficult airway because *hypoxemia and hypercarbia are even move detrimental.* Significant muscle wasting is a relative contraindication to sch b/o, risk of hyperkalemia.
- If a difficult intubation is anticipated, awake intubation, fiberoptic technique or tracheostomy may be necessary. ***Blind nasal intubation is contraindicated*** *in presence of* ***basilar skull fracture***Q, which is suggested by **CSF rhinorrhoea, or otorrhea hemotympanum, or ecchymosis into periorbital tissue (raccoon sign) or 'behind the ear' (Battle's sign)**.

Hypotension, Monitoring & Diagnostic Studies

- Hypotension in cases of head injury is nearly always related to other associated injuries (usually abdominal) or scalp laceration in children. **Correction of hypotension take precedence** over radiographic diagnostic studies and definitive neurosurgical treatment because *systolic arterial BP <80 mmHg correlates with poor outcome.*
- **Colloid solutions and blood** should generally be used to restore intravascular volume deficit as it may be more advantageous than crystalloid solutions in preventing brain edema. *Glucose free isotonic crystalloid (normal saline) solutions* can be used for maintainance fluid requirements. Hyperglycemia is common in neurosurgical patients (corticosteroid effect)

Intraoperative maintenance of anesthesia

- Like mass lesion a/w raised ICT, a **barbiturate-opioid- N_2O-NMBA** technique is commonly used for *intraoperative maintenance anesthesia.* ***N_2O should be avoided when air is entrapped within cranium***Q and during periods of hypotension. Transient hypotension may occur after induction of anesthesia d/t vasodilation and hypovolemia and should be treated with α **adrenergic agonist vaspressors (ephedrine or phenylephrine)**-preferred and volume infusion (if necessary).
- **Hypertension** (d/t surgery or d/t/ acutely raised ICP which is also a/w bradrcardia k/a Cushing phenomenon) can be treated by *deepening the anesthesia with additional dose of induction agents (thiopental or propofol), or with increased dose of inhalation anesthetics (<1 MAC isoflurane), or with antihypertensives.* β adrennergic blockade (eg esmolol) is usually effective in controlling hypertension a/w tachycardia. *Vasodilators (eg nitroprusside, nitroglycerine, CCB and hydralazine should be avoided until dura is opened.* Hyperventilation to $Paco_2$<30 should be avoided in head injury patients to avoid excessive decrease in CBF. Excessive vagal tone should be treated with atropine or

and has been implicated in increasing ischemic brain injury. ***Glucose containing or hypotonic solutions should not used***[Q]***;*** large amounts of hypotonic crystalloids can worsen brain edem. Temporary infusion of vasopressor is often necessary for severe hypotension.

- Hematocrit should be maintained above 30%. Invasive monitoring of intra arterial pressure, CVP, or pulmonary artery pressure and ICP is extremely valuble but should not delay diagnosis and treatment. *Arrhythmias and ECG abnormalities in T wave, U wave, ST segment & QT interval* are common and not necessarily indicate cardiac injury: they likely represent *altered autonomic function.*
- Patient should be stabilized prior to diagnostic CT or angiography. *Sedation without airway control should generally be avoided* b/o the risk of further increase in ICT from hypercapnia and hypoxemia.

glycopyrrolate.

- DIC (d/t brain thromboplastin released in head injury) may l/t ARDS. DIC should be diagnosed by coagulation profile and treated with *platelets, fresh frozen plasma and cryoprecipitates,* wereas ARDS require *mechanical ventilation. PEEP* should only be applied on ventilator if ICP is monitored or when the dura is opened.

2

ANAESTHESIA

ANESTHESIA for TRAUMA PATIENTS

- Regional anesthesia (neuraxial and other blocks) is usually inappropriate and impractical in hemodynamically unstable patients with life threatening injuries, as these are time consuming. Airway management (intubation) and fluid resuscitation is done.
- **Ketamine and etomidate** are ***most commonly used induction agents for non head injury trauma patients***[Q]. Ketamine is beneficial in patients with *acute hypovolemic shock* (d/t indirect sympathetic stimulatory effects) whereas etomidate provides *greater cardiovascular stability* (ie no or minimal effects on myocardial contractility, cardiac output and cardiovascular system; mild reduction in peripheral vascular resistance and BP; and no histamine release).
- Even after adequate fluid resuscitation, the induction doses for propofol are greatly (80-90%) reduced in patients with major trauma. Even drugs such as *ketamine and N_2O that normally indirectly stimulate cardiac function can display cardiodepressant properties in patients who are in shock & already have maximal sympathetic stimulation.* Hypotension may also occur following etomidate administration.
- Maintenance of anesthesia in unstable patients may consist primarily the use of *muscle relaxants (NMBD) with general anesthetic agents* titrated as tolerated (mean arterial pressure >50-60 mm Hg) in an effort to provide amnesia. Small doses of ***ketamine, low concentrations of volatile agents (<0.5 MAC), midazolam or scopalomine***[Q] are well tolerated and prevent recall of events.
- *N_2O can be avoided* b/o possibility of pneumothorax and because it limits inspired oxygen concentration. ***Histamine releasing drugs (eg atracurium and mivacurim) that tend to lower blood pressure should be avoided in hypovolemic shock***[Q]***.***
- Effects of iv anesthetics are exaggerated as they are injected into a smaller intravascular volume. And similarly b/o ↓CO and ↑ ventilation, the rate of rise of alveolar concentration of inhalation anesthetics is greater in shock. Higher alveolar anesthetic partial pressure l/t higher arterial partial pressure and greater effects (myocardial depression). *So the key to safe anesthetic management of shock patients is to administer small incremental doses of selected agent.*

OBSTETRICS ANESTHESIA

Physiological Changes during Pregnancy

Central Nervous System (CNS)

- *MAC of inhaled anesthesia decreases progressively during pregnancy*-at term, by as much as 40% for all general anesthetics. Changes in maternal hormones, endogenous opioids, β endorphin and progesterone levels have been implicated. MAC returns to normal by the 3rd day after delivery.
- *Obstruction of IVC* by gravid uterus *distends epidural venous plexus* and *increases epidural blood* volume resulting in
  1. ***Decreased potential volume of epidural space and subarachnoid space (ie spinal CSF volume) resulting in enhanced cephalad spread of LA solution during epidural and spinal (intrathecal) anesthesia***[Q]
  2. *Increased epidural (space) pressure* makes identification of epidural space without dural puncture difficult thus predisposing to *higher incidence of dural puncture* with epidural anesthesia.

Parameter	Change
Neurological	
MAC	- 40%
LA dose	- 30%
Respiratory	
O_2 consumption	+ 20 – 50%
Minute ventilation	+ 50%
Tidal volume	+ 40%
Respiratory rate	+ 15%
P_aO_2	+ 10%
Airway resistance	- 35%
FRC	- 20%
P_aCO_2, HCO_3	- 15%
Cardiovascular (CVS)	
Plasma volume	+ 45%
Blood volume	+ 35%
RBC volume	+ 20%

- Bearing down during labor further accentuates all these effects (1 & 2). *Engorgement of epidural veins increase the chances of inadvertent intravascular injection.*
- **Decreased dose requirements** (~30%) d/t ***enhanced sensitivity to LA***Q during regional anesthesia appears to be mediated by ***hormonal factors and engorgement of epidural venous plexus (l/t decreased epidural and subarachnoid space volume and enhanced cephalad spread of LA)***Q. However, pregnancy does not increase susceptibility to LA toxicity.
- **MLAC (Minimal Local Analgesic Concentration)** is median effective analgesic concentration (EC_{50}) in a 20 mL volume for epidural analgesia in 1st stage of labor. MLAC is used in obstetric anesthesia to compare relative potencies of LA and the effects of additives.

★ Decreased FRC and increased O_2 consumption promotes rapid O_2 desaturation during periods of apnea.

★ Regardless of the time interval since the ingestion of food, women in labour must be treated as having a full stomach and an increased risk for pulmonary aspiration of gastric content.

Cardiac output	+ 40%
Stroke volume	+ 30%
Heart rate	+ 20%
Pulmonary resistance	– 30%
Peripheral resistance	– 15%
Diastolic BP	– 15%
Systolic BP	– 5%
Hematological	
Hemoglobin	– 20%
Platelets	– 10%
Clotting factors	+ 30 to 250%
Renal	
GFR	+ 50%
Gastrointestinal	
GI motility, volume of GI secretion, lower esophageal tone	Decreased
Risk of regurgitation and aspiration, gastric acidity, gastric emptying time	Increased

Analgesia in Labor for Vaginal Delivery

Epidural (Neuraxial) Analgesia

- **Epidural (neuraxial) analgesia** is the ***most effective and least depressant method of intrapartum pain relief and is often viewed as technique choice for relief of labor pain***Q. It blunts the hemodynamic effects of contractions and associated pain response, which is *desirable for patients with hypertensive disorders, asthma, diabetes, and cardiac and intracardiac neurovascular disease.*
- Pregnant women remains awake and alert without sedative side effects, hyper ventilation is avoided and the ability of mother to cooperate and participate actively during labor is facilitated
- Further advantage of lumbar epidural analgesia include its

1. ability to achieve *segmental bands of analgesia* (T_{10}-L_1) during first stage of labor when total anesthesia is not required
2. ability to extend the *block to include S_2-S_4* segments during the second stage of labor and
3. *extension of sensory anesthesia to T_4* for cesarian delivery if necessary

- Effective epidural analgesia *reduces maternal catecholamine levels, increasing intervillous blood flow* resulting in *improved uteroplacental perfusion.* A greater effect is seen in patients with pre-eclampsia.
- Epidural analgesia is specifically indicated if *when tracheal intubation is excepted to be difficult or impossible.*
- Obstetric indications include *prolonged labour, primigravida, small pelvis, oxytocin augmentation of labor,* and any factors that place the parturient at *high risk for cesarian* section. Fetal indications include *prematurity, large baby, mal (breech) presentation and multiple*

Systemic Inhalational Analgesia

- Entonox (50% N_2O in O_2) provides safe and satisfactory analgesia in some, while the mother remain awake with intact protective laryngeal reflexes.
- ***Maternal cardiovascular and respiratory depression is minimal, uterine contractility is not affected and neonatal depression does not occur***Q regardless of duration of (subanesthetic) N_2O administration.
- Overall, 50% N_2O is a weak analgesic, and is delivered via a demand valve through a low resistant breathing system and fully trained personnel are essential to ensure safety.
- As it *takes 45 sec for the analgesic effect* to be achieved, the parturient should start breathing. Entonox at the start of contractions, so that an adequate brain concentration can be achieved at the contraction peak.
- *Deep, slow breathing and abstinence b/w contractions,* is encouraged. The female may *breathe entonox prior to expulsion efforts* during 2nd stage.
- All apparatus must be checked regularly to avoid inhalation of 100% O_2 first, f/b N_2O resulting from gas mixture becoming separated, as may occur at low temperatures.

Systemic Parenteral (IM/IV) Analgesia

- Opioids are most commonly used systemic medication for pain relief. However, *excessive maternal sedation, loss of maternal protective airway reflexes, maternal respiratory depression and risk of neonatal depression* limit the safe amount of opioids.
- It is recommended that systemic opioids be administered in smallest possible doses while minimizing repeated dosing to reduce accumulation of drug and metabolite in fetus. The amount of analgesia is less in comparision to epidural. So it is *used in multipara with relatively short, predictable labor with minimal pain* and in primiparas in early labor as adjuncts to major regional anesthasia.
- **Meperidine (pethidine), fentanyl, and mixed agonist/antagonist nalbuphine and butorphenol** (both showing respiratory depression but exhibit a **ceiling effect** with increasing dose) are most commonly used opioid for PCA. **Morphine** is a/w higher incidence of neonatal respiratory depression than other opioids and is not a popular agent for obstetric patient.
- Promethazine (mild respirator stimulant), ketamine, rarely phenothiazine (anxiolytic and **antiemetic) are added** also

gestation, as greater control of delivery is possible and the depressant effects of systemic opioids are avoided.
- Contraindications are similar to those of neuraxial block in general population. Complications include hypotension (l/t fetal hypoxemia and acidosis), accidental subarachnoid or intravenous injection and inadequate analgesia.
- Usually very dilute LA *(bupivacaine, ropivacaine) and an opioid (eg fentanil, nalbuphine) are used.*

Spinal Analgesia

- Single shot injection is not suitable for 1st stage of labor in most cases b/o limited duration of action and multiple injections increase the risk of PDPH. Occasionally, it may be employed to provide analgesia in *multiparous women presenting at advanced stage of cervical dilation*, when only one injection is anticipated.
- Continuous spinal analgesia (intrathecal catheter) can be used for patients *in whom epidural catheter placement is problematic (morbid obesity, abnormal vertebral anatomy).*
- **Paracervical block** (3 and 9 o'clock position injection; a/w fetal bradycardia) **lumbar sympathetic block** are beneficial only in 1st stage of labor. **Pudenda nerve block with perineal infiltration** provide analgesia in 2nd stage of labour and are of value in situations in which epidural/spinal are unavailable or contraindicated.

ANESTHESIA FOR LIVER DISEASE

Effects of Anesthesia on Hepatic blood Flow (HBF)

Hepatic Blood flow is usually *decreased during regional (i.e. spinal & epidural) and general anesthesia.* Regional anesthesia decreases HBF by lowering arterial BP, whereas general anesthesia decreases it through decrease in BP, and cardiac out put (+sympathetic stimulation). Decrease in CO l/t reflex sympathetic stimulation → vasoconstriction of both arterial & venous splanchnic vasculature → reduced hepatic blood flow. Various factors are responsible including:

Anesthetic agents & drugs

- All anesthetic agents indirectly decrease hepatic blood flow in proportion to decrease in mean arterial blood pressure or cardiac output.
- **All volatile anesthetic agents reduce portal hepatic blood flow.** This decrease is ***greatest with halothane and least with isoflurane***Q.
- **Isoflurane** is only volatile agent causing significant *direct arterial vasodilation* that can *increase hepatic arterial blood flow*. None theless, even with isoflurane total hepatic blood flow (i.e. = portal hepatic blood flow+hepatic artery blood flow) decrease because the decrease in portal blood flow usually offsets any increase in hepatic artery flow.
- β adrenergic blockers, H2-receptor blocker's α1-adrenergic agonists and vasopressin reduce hepatic blood flow
- **Low dose dopamine** infusions may increase hepatic blood flow.

	Halothane	Isoflurane	N_2O	Desflurane	Sevoflurane
Hepatic Blood flow	↓↓	↓/-	↓	↓	↓
Renal Blood flow, GFR, urinary output	↓↓	↓↓	↓↓	↓	↓

Surgical procedures

Surgery *near liver* can reduce hepatic blood flow upto 60% by sympathetic activation, local reflexes & direct compression

Type of ventilation

- **Spontaneous ventilation** is *advantageous in maintaining HBF*, which may decrease in controlled positive pressure ventilation **(CPPV)** and positive end expiratory pressure **(PEEP)**.
- CPPV with high mean airway pressures reduces venous return to heart (so increasing hepatic venous pressure) and decreases cardiac output (increasing sympathetic tone of splanchnic vessels). Both mechanism compromise HBF.
- **Hypoxemia** decreases hepatic blood flow via sympathetic activation.
- Direct effects of **hypercapnia** and ***acidosis*** *increase* and **hypocapnia and alkalosis** *decrease HBF*. However, indirect secondary effects of sympathetic activation with hypercapnia & acidosis l/t variable effects.

Anesthesia for Patient with Liver Disease

Biliary Tract Obstruction

Opioid induced **sphincter of oddi spasm** may result in false positive intraoperative cholangiogram & increased biliary pressure (fentanyl = alfentanyl > morphine > mepiridine > butorphanol > nalbuphine). So ***opioids are better avoided or given after intra-operative cholangiography***Q

- Treament of sphincter spasm is *Naloxone* or *glucagons*
- *Halothane* & to lesser extent *enflurane* may blunt the increase in biliary pressure following opioid administration.

Cirrhosis (alcoholic, biliary, cardiac etc)

- *Regional anesthesia* with more care to avoid hypotension is preferable in patients without coagulopathy.
- ***Barbiturate induction followed by isoflurane in O_2 or O_2 – N_2O mixture is most common employed G.A.***Q
- ***Cisatracurium is neuromuscular blocking agent of choice***Q

Hepatitis (viral, alcohol, drugs)

- *Alcoholic* patients require *close cardio vascular monitoring*, because cardiac depressant effect of alcohol are additive to those of anesthetics.
- *Inhalation anesthetics are preferable* to intravenous agents because latter are dependent on liver for metabolism or elimination
- Standard induction dose of I.V. induction agents can be used because their action are terminated by redistribution, rather than metabolism or excretion.
- Halogenated anesthetics may lead to hepatitis. Halothane has maximum incidence > methoxyflurane > enflurane > ***isoflurane (rare) > desflurane & sevoflurane (not described)***Q

ANESTHESIA FOR RENAL DISEASE

Anesthetic Drugs in patients with Reduced Renal Function

Most anesthetics are ***weak electrolytes & lipid soluble in unionized state.*** Termination of their action depends on metabolism & redistribution (not on renal excretion). After biotransformation, these drugs are excreted in urine as water – soluble, polar, and *pharmacologically inactive* compounds; and their retention is *harmless.* Most drugs with prominent central & peripheral nervous system activity, including *most narcotics, barbiturates, phenothiazines, butyrophenone derivatives, benzodiazepines, ketamine and local anesthetics,* fall into this category.

Several drugs are **lipid insoluble** or are *highly ionized* in physiological pH & are *eliminated unchanged in urine.* Their *duration of action is extended* in patients with impaired renal function. Drugs in this category include *muscle relaxants, cholinesterase inhibitors, thiazide diuretics,digoxin, & many antibiotics.*

Inhaled Anesthetics

- Because of the greater ease of reversibility, ***inhaled anesthetics offer some advantages (over intravenous drugs) for induction***[Q] of general anesthesia in uremic patients.
- All are biotransformed (to some extent) and nonvolatile products are eliminated entirely by kidney. However, *CNS effect of inhaled anesthetics depends on pulmonary excretion.* So impaired kidney function would not alter the response to these drugs.
- Inhaled anesthetics cause a transient reversible depression in renal functions (GFR, RBF, urine output, & urinary excretion of sodium). **Renal blood flow** is ***maintained with halothane, isoflurane, and desflurane***[Q] but it is decreased with enflurane and sevoflurane.
- For the viewpoint of selecting an anesthetic, its biotransformation to *inorganic fluoride level determines nephrotoxicity* (nephrotoxic threshold is *50μM)*

Anesthetic	Fluoride level
Desflurane	< 1μmol/L
Halothane	1-2 μM
Isoflurane	3 - 5μM
Enflurane	19 μM
Sevoflurane (prolonged use)	50 μM
Methoxyflurane	50μM

So ***desflurane, isoflurane and halothane have no nephrotoxic potential***[Q].

- Desflurane is highly stable, resists degradation by soda lime and liver. Whereas, sevoflurane is not stable, decomposed by sodalime (to **toxic compound A**) and is biotransformed by liver.

Intravenous Anesthetics

- **Ultrashort acting barbiturates** such as **thiopental & methohexital** are safe to be used in uremia. However, *the dose to produce and maintain anesthesia should be reduced* because, the metabolison is unaffected and the proportion of unbound drug increases.
- **Propofol** does not adversely affect renal function. However, prolonged infusion may result in innocuous *green discolouration* of urine d/t presence of phenol. *Urate excretion* is also increased and may result in *cloudy urine.*
- When combined with 30-50% N_2O, narcotics and tranquilizers, should not have a particularly prolonged effect. Benzodiazepines esp diazepam, have a long life, so they tend to accumulate.

Opioids

- Neither the pharmacodynamics nor kinetics of **remifentanil** are altered by impaired renal function.
- ***Remifentanil > fentanyl > alfentanil > sufentanil are safe***[Q] to be used in renal failure
- **Morphine** is *not a good choice* (i.e. unsafe), as its 40% is metabolized in kidney (60% liver). And *water soluble glucuronide metabolites (morphine 3/6 glucuronide)* are excreted by kidney. Accumulation of *morphine 6 glucuronide* may l/t **life threatening repiratory depression**.
- Normeperidine, the chief metabolite of **meperidine**, has analgesic & CNS excitatory effects and is excreted through kidney. So its accumulation in renal failure l/t CNS toxicity.
- **Hydromorphone**, does not but its metabolite H-3-glucuronide does accumulate between dialysis treatment, which is effectively removed during hemodialysis. So it *may be used safely in dialysis patients.* However, it should be used with caution in patients with *GFR <30 mL/min who have yet to start dialysis or who have withdrawn from dialysis.*

Muscle Relaxants

- **Atracurium** is degradated by ***enzymatic ester hydrolysis & nonenzymatic alkaline degradation (Hofman elimination)***[Q], to inactive products that are not dependent on renal excretion for *terminal action. So its* ***terminal elimination half life and neuro muscular blockade indices (onset, duration, & recovery) are the same in patients with normal and absent renal function***[Q].
- Renal failure has only very little impact on **cisatracurium** because only 16% elimination occurs through kidney (77% through organ independent Hoffman elimination)
- Short acting **mivacurium** is metabolized by plasma pseudocholinesterase, which has decreased activity in uremia & hemodialysis. So its effects are prolonged (by 10-15 minutes) and requirement is decreased in anephric (end stage renal disease) patient.
- **Rocuronium** has longer duration of action in anephric patients b/o increase in volume of distribution with no change in clearance.
- Pancuronium, (50%), vecuronium (30%), pipercuronium, d-tubocurarine, and doxacurim are either not used or used very cautiously (with smaller maintenance doses at longer intervals).
- **Succinyl choline** has been used without difficulty in patients with decreased or absent renal function. It is metabolized by pseudocholinesterase into nontoxic succinic acid & choline. Sch is excreted by kidney, so large doses are avoided in renal failure. It causes a *rapid transient increase of 0.5m Eq/L* in serum K^+, which could be particularly dangerous in uremic patient with hyperkalemia (l/t CV collapse); so it is *inadvisable, unless the patient has undergone dialysis within 24 hours before surgery.* It is safe if the ***patient has undergone recent dialysis or has normal serum potassium level***[Q].

Cholinesterase inhibitors & Anticholinergics

- Renal excretion is of major importance, with ~ 50% of neostigmine and 70% of pyridostigmine & edrophonium excreted in urine. So excretion of all cholinesterase inhibitors is delayed in patients with impaired renal function
- Anticholinergics – atropine & glycopyrorolate are also partially dependent on kidney for excretion.

ANESTHESIA FOR LUNG DISEASE

Rapid Sequence Induction / Crash Induction

This is induction technique used in patient with risk of **aspiration pneumonia (mendelson's syndrome)** eg. hiatus hernia or any emergency operation with full stomach. ***Characteristic features are-***

- ***Patient is always preoxygenated prior to induction*** Q
- ***Prior Curarization*** with nondepolarization MR to prevent increase in intraabdominal pressure that accompanies use of succinyl choline
- *Endotracheal tube, one-half size smaller* than usual to maximize the chances of easy intubation
- Firm ***pressure over cricoid cartilage*** prior to inductipn **(*Sellick's maneuver*)**Q, applied to make oesophagus collapsed and prevent regurgitation
- ***Thiopental*** is given in induction dose as bolus.
- ***Succinylcholine or Rocuronium*** is immediately admistered
- The patient is ***not artificially ventilated*** to avoid filling of stomach with gas and thereby increasing the risk of emesis
- If intubation fails, spontaneous ventilation should be allowed to return and *awake intubation* performed
- After surgery, patient should *remain intubated* until airway reflexes and consciousness has been regained.

Anesthesia for Patient with Mitral Stenosis

Hemodynamic Goals

The principal objectives in MS are to

- ***Maintain a sinus rhythm***Q (if present preoperatively) *and to* ***avoid tachycardia***Q or rapid ventricular response rate during atrial fibrillation.
- *Avoid marked increases in central blood volume* (a/w over transfusion or head down position) and *cardiac output*. Avoid both hypovolemia and fluid overload by judicious fluid therapy.
- Avoid drug induced ***decrease in systemic vascular resistance (vasodilation)***Q
- Avoid events that may exacerbate *pulmonary hypertension* and evoke right ventricular failure, such as *arterial hypoxemia and hypoventilation*

Hemodynamic goals of other valvular lesions

Lesion	HR and Rhythm	Preload	Afterload	Contractility
AS	60-70, sinus	Full	Maintain	-
AR/AI	80-90	Maintain	Lower	May need support
MS	60-70	Full	-	-
MR	80-90, sinus	Maintain	Lower	May need support

Choice of Anesthesia

- Patients may be very sensitive to **vasodilating effects of spinal and epidural anesthesia** (so better avoided). Epidural is preferable to spinal b/o more gradual onset of sympathetic blockade.
- **Induction** is achieved with **intravenous** drug with possible *exception of ketamine,* which may be *avoided* b/o its sympathetic stimulation (l/t tachycardia)
- Tracheal intubation is facilitated by **hemodynamically neutral MRs** suchas ***vecuronium, rocuronium and cisatracurium***Q. And *pancuronium induced tachycardia* is to be *avoided.*
- So **general anesthesiawith endotracheal intubation** is the obvious choice. Goals can be achieved with combinations using *smaller total narcotic (opioid) doses, low concentrations of volatile inhalation anesthetics and short acting intravenous anesthetis (as propofol) with or without N_2O. Opioid may be a better choice than volatile agent because latter can produce undesirable vasodilation or precipitate junctional rhythm with loss of an effective atrial kick.* **Halothane** is the most suitable volatile agent because it decreases heart rate and is least vasodilating, but other volatile agents have also been used safely. Rapid increase in desflurane concentration may cause sympathetic stimulation with accompanying tachycardia and pulmonary hypertension. *N_2O should be used cautiously*, as it can acutely increase pulmonary vascular resistance (esp in severe coexisting pulmonary hypertension). ***Because of no effect on heart, little change in BP and good hemodynamic stability, xenon may be inhalation agent of choice***Q.
- **Intraoperative tachycardia** may be controlled by ***deepening anesthesia with an opioid (excluding meperidine) or β blocker (esmolol or propranolol)***Q. In presence of atrial fibrillation, ventricular rate may be controlled with *diltiazem, or digoxin.* Verapamil is less preferred b/o associated vasodilation. Sudden supraventricular tachycardia causing marked hemodynamic deterioration necessitates *cardioversion.* ***Phenylephrine*** is preferred over ephedrine as a vasopressor because the former lacks β adrenergic agonist activity.

Anesthesia for Patients with Aortic Stenosis (AS)

Pathophysiology

- **In critical AS,** with aortic valve orifice reduced to **0.5-0.7** cm^2 (normal is 2.5-3.5 cm^2), patients have a transvalvular gradient of ~50mm Hg *at rest (with a normal cardiac output)* and are **unable to increase cardiac output in response to exerction.** Moreover, further increase in transvalvular gradient do no significantly increase stroke

Monitoring

- Close monitoring of ECG (for ischemia) and intraarterial pressure is desirable as many patient **do not tolerate even brief episodes of mild hypotension** (b/o an already precarious myocardial oxygen demand supply balance). **Higher than normal pulmonary capillary wedge pressure** is often required to maintain adequate LV end diastolic volume & cardiac output. Pumonary artery wedge pressure often show prominent **a waves.**

Choice of Anesthesia

- **Spinal and epidural anesthesia are relatively contraindicated is patients with severe AS.** However, generally asymptomatic patients with mild to moderate AS may tolerate cautiously employed epidural (preferable b/o slower onset hypotension is easy to manage) or spinal anesthesia.

2

ANAESTHESIA

volume because with chronic AS, myocardial contractility progressively deteriorates & compromises left ventricular function.

- Advanced AS patients **have classical triad of dyspnea on excretion, orthostatic or exertional syncope** (b/o vasodilation in muscle tissue) and **angina** in absence of of coronary artery disease (because ventricular hypertrophy increases myocardial O_2 demand whereas high (upto 300 mmHg) intracavitary systolic pressure decreases myocardial O_2 supply by compressing intramyocardial coronary vessels.

- In sereve AS, the choice of general anesthetic agent is less important than managing their hemodynamic effects, as most GA agents can produce vasodilation and hypotension (in volatile agents this is done by controlling concentration).

Severe hypertension & significant tachycardia can precipitate ischemia	Most patients tolerate moderate hypertension and **are sensitive to vasodilators** they **tolerate even episodes of mild hypotension poorly.**	Intraoperative **supraventricular tachycardias with hemodynamic compromise**.	**Frequent ventricular ectopy** (reflecting ischemia).
Mx immediately **by increasing anesthetic depth** or administration **of β adrenergic blocking agent.**	Hypotension promptly treated with **escalating doses (25-100 mcg) of phenylephrine.**	**Immediate synchronized cardioversion.**	**Amiodarone** is effects for both supraventrical and ventricular arrhythmias.

ANAESTHESIA

Anaesthesia in Ischemic Heart Disease

Induction agents

- Propofol, barbiturate, etomidate, benzodiazepines, opioids & combinations are used
- Ketamine is relatively contraindicated because its indirect sympathominetic effect can adversely affect the myocardial oxygen demand-supply balance. When combined with a benzodiazepine or propofol, however, ketamine does not appreciably increase sympathetic activity and results in relatively stable hemodynamics with minimal myocardial depression. The *combination of benzodiazepine and ketamine* may be *most useful in patient with poor ventricular function (ejection fraction <30%)* and in frail patient with hemodynamic compromise.
- ***High dose opioid anesthesia had previously been used widely for patients with significant ventricular dysfunction***Q. With the exception of meperidine (in large doses), opioids alone are generally associated with minimal or no cardiac depression. Apparent cardiac depression may also occur wth pure high dose opioid inductions : this likely represents withdraw of an elevated baseline sympathetic tone. Patients with poor ventricular function often rely on an elevated sympathetic tone to maintain their cardiac output & may decompensate even with pure high dose opioid anaesthesia. (That's why now mixed I.V & inhalation anaesthesia is used)

Maintenance agents

- Patients are generally managed with an *opioid-volatile anaesthetic technique*
- Patients with ejection fraction < 40% may be very sensitive to the depressant effects of potent volatile agents or large bolus of opioids
- *N_2O, Particularly in presence of opioids, can also produce significant cardiac depression*
- All volatile agents generally have favorable effect on myocardial oxygen balance, reducing demand more than supply. Isoflurane dilates intramyocardial arteries more than the larger epicardial vessels but there is little evidence that isoflurane causes an intracoronary steal phenomenon in clinical practice.

Evolution of Anaesthesia for Ischemic Heart Disease

High dose opioid anaesthesia
Was developed to circumvent the myocardial depression associated with older volatile anesthetics such as halothane & enfleurane. But it produces prolonged post op. respiratory depression, patient awareness & often fails to control the hypertensive response to stimulation in many patients with good left ventricular function

→

Total Intravenous Anesthesia / Fast track anaesthesia
It is associated with decreased ICU stays and early hospital discharge. It employs infusion of propofol & remifentanil. Because short half life of remifentail, I.V morphine has to be given at end of surgery to provide post operative analgesia.

↓

Mixed Intravenous / Inhalation Anesthesia

- Renewed interest in volatile agents came about following studies demonstrating the protective effects of volatile agents on ischemic myocardium, and the availability of volatile inhalation anesthetics that produce less myocardial depression than older agents & that are rapidly eliminated (e.g. desflurane & sevoflurane) and an emphesis on fast track management.
- *Propofol or etomidate* is most commonly used for induction. Atlernate induction agents include *thiopentone & midazolam*
- *Opioids* are given in small dose together *with volatile agent for maintenance anesthesia.* To facilitate fast track management, total dose of fentanyl and sufentanil should generally not exceed 15 & 5 μg/kg respectively. The major advantage of volatile agent & I.V. infusion of remifentanil (or propofol) is the ability to change the anaesthetic concentration and depth rapidly. *Isoflurane, sevoflurane & desflurane are most commonly used volatile anesthetics*. Early reports of isoflurane inducing intracoronary steal have not been substantiated and it remains a commonly used volatile agent.
- N_2O is generally not used because its tendency to expand any intravascular air bubbles that may form during CPB.
- Muscle relaxants : *Vecuronium* is not used with opioids as it enhances opioid induced bradycardia. *Pancuronium* may be a good choice in patients with marked bradycardia because of its vagolytic effects.

Anesthesia for Endoscopic Surgeries of Airway

- Endoscopy includes laryngoscopy, *microlaryngoscopy (i.e. aided by an operating microscope)*, bronchoscopy & oesophagoscopy. These procedures may be accompanied by *laser surgery*.
- **Microlaryngoscopic surgeries** include biopsy / surgery of laryngeal malignancy, vocal cord polyps etc. It is associated with some specific problems as – common field for anesthetist & surgeon, already reduced glottic opening d/t growth, *laryngospasm* (mediated by superior laryngeal nerve) d/t laryngeal stimulation, *very high chances of aspiration and myocardial ischemia* (~ 4% due to sympethetic stimulation).

Preoperative Considerations

- ***Sedative premedication is contraindicated in any patient with any significant degree of upper airway obstruction***Q, d/t fear of aspiration. *Glycopyrrolate*, 1 hour before surgery minimize secretions, thereby facilitate ventilation.
- Pethidine & promethazine are only given if there is no airway obstruction.

Laser Precautions

- General laser precautions include *wearing protective spectacles* to prevent retinal damage and *evacuation of toxic fumes (laser plume) from tissue vaporization* which may have potential to transmit microbacterial diseases.
- Greatest fear during laser airway surgery is **a tracheal tube fire**. This can be avoided by using a technique of ventilation that does not involve a flammable tube or catheter (eg *intermittent apnea or jet ventilation through the laryngoscope side port*). *The potential fuel source should have laser resistant properties* (laser tubes or wrapping a tracheal tube with metallic tape) or be removed (supraglottic jet ventilation technique). The only non inflammable, laser proof tube is the *all metal Norton tube, which has no cuff.* Most laser tubes have laser resistant properties around the shaft, but the cuff is not protected and can ignite. So there are double cuffs to seal the airway- if upper cuff is struck by laser and saline escapes, the lower cuff will continue to seal the airway.
- No cuffed tracheal tube, or any currently available tube protection is completely laser proof. Therefore, whenever laser airway surgery is being performed with a tracheal tube in place, the following precaution should be observed.
  - Inspired O_2 conc. should be as low as possible may be upto 21%
  - ***N_2O support combustion & should be replaced with air (N_2) or helium***Q
  - Tracheal tube cuffs should be filled with saline dyed with methylene blue to dessipate heat & signal cuff rupture
  - A cuffed tube will minimize O_2 conc. in the parynx. The addition of 2% lidocaine jelly (1:2 mixture with saline) can seal small laser induced cuff leaks, potentially preventing combustion
  - Laser intensity & duration should be limited as much as possible.
  - Saline soaked pledgets (completely saturated) should be placed in the airway to limit risk of ignition.
  - A source of water (60 ml) should be immediately available in case of fire.

Muscle Relaxation

- Profound muscle relaxation is the aim to provide masseter muscle relaxation for introduction of suspension laryngoscope & an immobile surgical field.
- Anesthesia is induced with IV induction agent followed by a *non depolarizing muscle relaxant*; the vocal cords are ***sprayed with 3 ml lidocaine 4% to assist smooth anesthesia & to minimize the possibility of postextubation laryngospasm***Q
- Alternatively the cords

Oxygentation & Ventilation

- **Microlaryngoscopy tubes** are *long, have a small internal and external diameter*, and are designed specifically for endoscopic procedures (but not suitable for laser surgery). Typically **4 to 5 mm** internal diameter tubes with *high volume, low pressure cuffs are used in nasal or oral versions*. The most popular anesthetic technique use a **Coplan's microlaryngoscopy tube** (5mm ID, 31cm long, 10ml cuff volume and constructed from soft plastic). It is designed for micro laryngeal surgery or for patient whose airway has been narrowed to such an extent that a normal sized tracheal tube cannot be inserted. The small tube diameter provides better visibility and access to surgical field but may l/t incomplete exhalation and occlusion.
- Most commonly the patients are ***intubated with small diameter (4 – 6 mm) tracheal tubes***Q;
- *Standandard tracheal tubes* of this size, however, are designed *for pediatric patients*. They tend ***to be too short for adult trachea (in length)***Q with a low volume cuff that will exert high pressure against it
- *A 4 – 6 mm microlaryngea tracheal (MLT) tubes* (Mallinckrodt critical Care) is the same length as the adult tube, has disproportionately *large high volume low pressure cuff*, and is stiffer and less prone to compression than a regular tracheal tube.
- **The advantages of intubation** include – protection against aspiration, and the ability to administer inhalational anesthetics and ***enable monitoring of ventilation by capnography and spirometry, by measuring end tidal CO_2***Q
- In some cases (eg those involving posterior commissure), intubation may interfere with surgeon's visualization and then alternatives are:

may be painted with *3% cocaine* at the end of procedure, which has the added advantage of reducing bleeding from operative site.

1. *Insufflation of high flows of oxygen* through small catheter placed in the trachea
2. *Intermittent apnea technique.*
3. Jet ventilation through laryngoscope
4. High frequency positive pressure ventilation (HFPPV)

Cadriovascular Stability

- Short acting anesthetics (eg propofol, remifentanil) or sympathetic antagonists (eg esmolol) as per needed
- *Regional nerve blocks of glossopharyngeal & superior laryngeal nerve would minimized intraoperative swing in BP*[Q].

Airway Fire Protocol

If airway fire or explosion occurs, the surgeon and anaesthesiologist must act quickly, decisively and in co-ordinated manner following this emergency protocol. A surgeon who detects an endotracheal or other source of airway fire should remove the source as quickly as possible and simultaneously inform anaesthesiologist who should-

1. ***Immediately stop ventilation and remove tracheal tube***[Q]
2. Turn off oxygen and temporarily disconnect the breathing circuit from anesthesia machine
3. ***Flaming material (eg tracheal tube) should be extinguished (submerged) in a bucket of water or by pouring sterile water***[Q]
4. Ventilation with 100% O_2 should be provided by face mask and anesthesia should be continued and patient reintubated
5. Assess airway damage with direct laryngoscopy, rigid (venture-ventilating)/fiberoptic bronchoscopy, serial chest x-rays and arterial blood gases
6. Consider **bronchial lavage** (for interior blowtorch fire to remove debrise), **reintubation** (if air way damage is apparent), **low tracheostomy** (for severe damage), **prolonged intubation and mechanical ventilation** (in pulmonary damage d/t heat or smoke) and a **brief course of high dose steroids.**

Disadvantages of metallic tape wrapping (of tracheal tube)
- Adds thickness to tube and rough edges may damage mucosal surface - No cuff protection, adhesive backing may ignite - May reflect laser onto nontargated tissue, not approved by FDA

Type of tube	Advantage	Disadvantage
Polyvinyl chloride	Inexpensive, **non reflective**	Low melting point, highly **combustible**
Red rubber	**Non reflective**, puncture resistant, maintains structure	Highly **combutible**
Silicon rubber	**Nonreflective**	Combustible, turns to toxic ash
Metal	**Combustion-resistant**, kink resistant	Transfers heat, reflects laser flammable cuff, thick walled, cumbersome

QUESTIONS

ANESTHESIA FOR OUT PATIENT/DAY CARE SURGERY

1. **The following combination of agents are the most preferred for short day care surgeries** *(AIIMS 03, DNB 08)*
   A. Propofol, fentanyl, isoflurane ☐
   B. Thiopentone sodium, morphine, halothane ☐
   C. Ketamine, pethidine, halothane ☐
   D. Propofol, morphine, halothane ☐
2. **Which of the following intravenous induction agent is the most suitable for day care surgery?**
   E. Morphine *(AI 06, AIIMS 98)* ☐
   F. Ketamine ☐
   G. Propofol ☐
   H. Diazepam ☐
3. **Which of the following is the best indication for propofol as an intravenous induction agent?**
   A. Neurosurgery *(AI 04)* ☐
   B. Day care surgery ☐
   C. Patients with coronary artery disease ☐
   D. In neonatesq ☐
4. **A 38 year old man is posted for extraction of last molar tooth under general anaesthesia as a day care case. He wishes to resume his work after 6 hours. Which one of the following induction agents is preferred:** *(AI 03, 02)*
   A. Thiopentone sodium ☐
   B. Ketamine ☐
   C. Diazepam ☐
   D. Propofol ☐
5. **Best anaesthetic agent for out patient anasthesia is**
   A. Fentanyl *(AIIMS 94, DNB 02)* ☐
   B. Morphine ☐
   C. Alfentanyl ☐
   D. Penthidine ☐

PAEDIATRIC ANAESTHESIA

6. **Method of choice for induction in children is by**
   A. I.M. *(AIIMS 1993)* ☐
   B. Inhalation ☐
   C. I.V. ☐
   D. O_2 tent ☐
7. **Inhalational agent of choice in children:**
   A. Sevoflurane *(AI 06;AIIMS 04, 02;PGI 08,05; DNB 02)* ☐
   B. Isofurane ☐
   C. Desflurane ☐
   D. Halothane ☐
   E. N_2O ☐
8. **A six year old child is posted for elective urology surgery under general anesthesia. He refuses to allow the anaesthesiologist an I.V. access. The best inhalational agent of choice for induction of anesthesia is**
   A. Sevoflurane *(AIIMS 04)* ☐
   B. Methoxyflurane ☐
   C. Desflurane ☐
   D. Isoflurane ☐
9. **In a child with intestinal obstruction with deranged liver function test, the anesthetic of choice is :** *(PGI June 2006)*
   A. Enflurane ☐
   B. Isoflurane ☐
   C. Halothane ☐
   D. Sevoflurane ☐
   E. Ether ☐
10. **All agents can be given for induction of anesthesia in children except:** *(AI 01)*
    A. Halothane ☐
    B. Sevoflurane ☐
    C. Morphine ☐
    D. N_2O ☐
11. **In a 2 months old infant undergoing surgery for biliary atresia, you would avoid one of the following anaesthetic**
    A. Thiopentone *(AIIMS 03; DNB 05)* ☐
    B. Halothane. ☐
    C. Propofol. ☐
    D. Sevoflurane. ☐
12. **The narrowest part of larynx in infants is at the cricoid level. In administering anesthesia this may lead to all except.** *(AIIMS 2003)*
    A. Choosing a smaller size endotracheal tube ☐
    B. Trauma to the subglottic region ☐
    C. Post operative stridor ☐
    D. Laryngeal oedema ☐
13. **Regarding neonatal circumcision, which one of the following is true:** *(AIIMS 03; WB 05)*
    A. It should be done without anaesthesia, as it is hazardous to give anaesthesia. ☐
    B. It should be done without anesthesia, as neonates do not perceive pain as adults. ☐
    C. It should be done under local anaesthesia only. ☐
    D. General anaesthesia should be given to neonate for circumcision as they also feel pain as adults. ☐
14. **A two month old infant has undergone a major surgical procedure. Regarding postoperative pain relief which one of the following is recommended:** *(AI 06; DNB 07)*
    A. No mediaction is needed as infant does not feel pain after surgery due to immaturity of nervous system ☐
    B. Only paracetamol suppository is adequate ☐
    C. Spinal narcotics via intrathecal route ☐
    D. Intravenous narcotic infusion in lower dosage ☐
15. **A five-year old child is scheduled for strabismus (squint) correction. Induction of anesthesia is uneventful. After conjunctival incision as the surgeon grasps the medial rectus, the anaesthesiologist looks at the cardiac monitor. Why do you think he did that?** *(AIIMS 02; DNB 03)*
    A. He wanted to check the depth of anaesthesia ☐
    B. He wanted to be sure that the blood pressure did not fall ☐
    C. He wanted to see if there was an oculocardiac reflex ☐
    D. He wanted to make sure there were no ventricular dysarhythmias which normally accompany incision. ☐
16. **A six-year old boy is schedules for examination of the eye under anaesthesia. The father informed that for the past six months the child is developing progressive weakness of both legs. His elder sibling had died at the age of 14 years. Which drug would you definitely avoid during the anaeshetic management?**
    A. Succinylcholine *(AIIMS 02; CMC 05)* ☐
    B. Thiopentone ☐
    C. Nitrous oxide ☐
    D. Vecuronium ☐
17. **A 5 year old boy suffering from Duchenne Muscular dystrophy and polymyositis has been fasting for 8 hrs and has to undergo tendon lengthening. Which anaesthesia should be used.** *(AIIMS 2000)*
    A. Induction by IV Thiopentone & maintenance by N_2O & halothene ☐

2

ANAESTHESIA

B. Induction by IV Propofol and maintenance by N_2O & O_2 ☐
C. Induction by IV scoline and Maintenance by N_2O & Halothene ☐
D. Inhalation N_2O, O_2 & halothene ☐

18. A 5 year old boy suffering from Duchenne muscular dystrophy has to undergo tendon lengthening procedure. The most approp-riate anaesthetic would be: *(AI 2003)*
A. Induction with intravenous thiopentone and N_2O; and halothane for maintenance ☐
B. Induction with intravenous suxamethonim and N_2O; and oxygen for maintenance ☐
C. Induction with intravenous suxamethonium and N_2O; and halothane for maintenance ☐
D. Inhalation induction with inhalation halothane and N_2O; oxygen for maintenance ☐

19. A 5-year old patient is schedules for tonsillectomy. On the day of surgery he had running nose, temperature 37.5°C and dry cough. Which of the following should be the most appropriate decision for surgery. *(AI 06; DNB 09)*
A. Surgery should be cancelled ☐
B. Can proceed for surgery if chest is clear and there is no history of asthma ☐
C. Should get X-ray chest before proceeding for surgery ☐
D. Cancel surgery for 3 weeks and patient to be on antibiotic ☐

20. The following are used for treatment of postoperative nausea and vomiting following squint surgery in children except: *(AI 05)*
A. Ketamine. ☐
B. Ondansetron. ☐
C. Propofol. ☐
D. Dexamethasone. ☐

21. A child is posted for operative repair of exostrophy of bladder with renal failure. Which anesthetic should be preferred? *(AIIMS Nov 09)*
A. Pancuronium ☐
B. Vecuronium ☐
C. Ataracurium ☐
D. Rocuronium ☐

ANESTHESIA for HEAD INJURY & NEUROSURGERY

22. Blood brain barrier is permeable to all except *(AIIMs Nov 10)*
A. Water ☐
B. Gas ☐
C. Lipophilic drug ☐
D. Protein ☐

23. A case of road traffic accident (RTA) came with head injury, BP is 90/60, pulse is 150/min. Which anesthetic agent should be used for induction. *(AIIMS May 12)*
A. Thiopentone ☐
B. Ketamine ☐
C. Halothane ☐
D. Succinylcholine ☐

24. Which of the following is contraindicated in an epileptic patient? *(AIIMS May 13)*
A. Propofol
B. Thiopentone
C. Ketamine
D. Midazolan

ANESTHESIA for TRAUMA PATIENTS

25. Following RTA, a patient suffered splenic ruture. His BP is 90/60 mmHg, PR 126/min and SpO_2 92%. Induction agent of choice is *(AIIMS May 12)*
A. Remifentanyl ☐
B. Halothane ☐
C. Midazolam ☐
D. Etomidate ☐

26. Amount of K^+ (mEq/l) in ringer lactate (RL) *(AIIMS Nov 10)*
A. 2 ☐
B. 4 ☐
C. 5 ☐
D. 6 ☐

ANESTHESIA for CARDIOVASCULAR SURGERY

27. A 30 year old woman with coarctation of aorta ia admitted to the labour room for elective caesarean section. Which of the following is the anaesthesia technique of choice: *(AIIMS Nov 05)*
A. Spinal anaesthesia ☐
B. Epidural anaesthesia ☐
C. General anaesthesia ☐
D. Local anaesthesia with nerve block ☐

28. A 5 year old child is suffering from cyanotic heart disease. He is planned for corrective surgery. The induction agent of the choice would by: *(DNB 07, AIIMS 05)*
A. Thiopentone ☐
B. Ketamine ☐
C. Halothane ☐
D. Midazolam ☐

29. A 6 month old child is suffering from patent ductus arteriosus (PDA) with congestive cardiac failure. Ligation of ductus arteriosus was decided for surgical management. The most appropriate inhalational anaesthetic agent of choice with minimal haemodynamic alteration for induction of anaesthesia is: *(DNB 08, AIIMS 05)*
A. Sevoflurane ☐
B. Isoflurane ☐
C. Enflurane ☐
D. Halothane ☐

30. The most common cause of morbidity and mortality in patients undergoing major vascular surgery is: *(AIIMS May 05)*
A. Renal complications ☐
B. Thrombo embolic phenomenon ☐
C. Coagulopathies ☐
D. Cardiac complications ☐

31. A 52 year old male diagnosed as triple vessel coronary artery disease with poor left ventricular function. Coronary artery bypass grafting surgery was decided. During maintenance of anaesthesia which one of the following agents should be preferred? *(AIIMS Nov 04)*
A. IV Opioids ☐
B. Isoflurane ☐
C. Halothane ☐
D. Nitrous oxide ☐

32. During surgery for aortic arch aneurysm under deep hypothermic circulatory arrest, which of the following anesthetic agent administered prior to circulatory arrest that also provides cerebral protection? *(AIIMS 2002)*
A. Etomidate ☐
B. Thiopental sodium ☐
C. Propofol ☐
D. Ketamine ☐

33. Patient with mitral stenosis is having surgery tomorrow. There is some liver compromise. Which of the following inhalational agent is preferred *(AIIMS Nov 10; DNB 11)*
A. Halothane ☐
B. Enflurane ☐
C. Xenon ☐
D. Sevoflurane ☐

34. Which of the following is not used in controlling heart rate intraoperatively. *(AI 07; DNB 08)*
- A. Propanolol/Metoprolol ☐
- B. Verapamil ☐
- C. Esmolol ☐
- D. Procainamide ☐

35. Vasopressor of choice in anesithesia for a patient of aortic stenosis developing hypotension during surgery:
- A. Ephedrine *(AIIMS May 13)* ☐
- B. Dopamine ☐
- C. Dobutamine ☐
- D. Phenylephrine ☐

ANESTHESIA for ENT & DENTAL SURGERY

36. Following will be the choice of anaesthesia in an infected tooth posted for extraction: *(MP 2006)*
- A. Local block with lignocaine ☐
- B. Local block with lignocaine and adrenaline ☐
- C. Isoflurane ☐
- D. Enflurane ☐

37. Fire breaks out during laser vocal cord surgery. What is not to be done? *(AI 2011)*
- A. Pouring sterile water ☐
- B. Removing endotracheal tube ☐
- C. 100% oxygen after discontinuing anesthetic gases ☐
- D. Treatment with steroid and antibiotics ☐

38. Anaesthesia used in microlaryngoscopy is *(AIIMS 1996)*
- A. Pollarad tube of 10 mm diameter with heavy sedation ☐
- B. Pollarad tube of 15 mm diameter with topical xylocaine ☐
- C. Pollarad tube with infiltration block ☐
- D. Heavy sedation on and Endotracheal intubation. ☐

OBSTETRICS ANAESTHESIA

39. Important factor(s) deciding reduced dose of anesthetic drug in pregnancy: *(PGI May 13)*
- A. Mechanical factor of gravid uterus ☐
- B. Hormonal factors ☐
- C. Altered pharmacokinetic of drugs ☐
- D. Alteration in CSF PH ☐

40. In pregnancy, there is decreased requirement of anesthetic agent b/o all except reasons *(AIIMS May 12)*
- A. Higher sensitivity of nerves to LA ☐
- B. Engorged spinal veins ☐
- C. Decreased subarachnoid space ☐
- D. Increased lumbar lardosis ☐

41. A 25 year old primigravide with mitral stenosis and mitral regurgitation is under labor. She wants normal delivery which would be the best way to provide analgesia in this lady *(AIIMS May 12)*
- A. Inhalational analgesia ☐
- B. Intravenous opioids ☐
- C. Spinal anesthesia ☐
- D. Neuraxialblockde analgesia ☐

42. Anaesthesia of choice for manual removal of placenta
- A. GA *(AIIMS 1993)* ☐
- B. Spinal ☐
- C. Epidural ☐
- D. Para Cervical ☐

ANESTHESIA FOR LIVER DISEASE

43. A patient of alcohlic liver faliure requires general anesthesia AOC is *(AI 01)*
- A. Ether ☐
- B. Halothane ☐
- C. Isoflurane ☐
- D. Methoxyflurane ☐

44. All anesthetic agent decrease portal vein flow. Portal flow is maximally reduced by: *(AIIMS 10; DNB 11)*
- A. Ether ☐
- B. Halothane ☐
- C. Isoflurane ☐
- D. Enflurane ☐

ANESTHESIA FOR RENAL DISEASE

45. Anaesthesia of choice in renal disease: *(PGI June 08, 09)*
- A. Atracurium ☐
- B. Cisatracurium ☐
- C. Vecuronium ☐
- D. Rocuronium ☐
- E. Mivacuronium ☐

46. Anesthesia of choice in renal failure *(AI 01, DNB 06)*
- A. Methoxy flurane ☐
- B. Isoflurane ☐
- C. Enflurane ☐
- D. None ☐

ANESTHESIA FOR LUNG DISEASE

47. After hyperventilation for some time holding the breath is dangerous since *(AIIMS 2000)*
- A. It can lead to CO_2 narcosis ☐
- B. due to lack of stimulation by CO_2, anoxia can go into dangerous level ☐
- C. $\downarrow CO_2$ shift O dissociation curve to left. ☐
- D. Alkalosis can lead to tetany. ☐

48. Best anaesthesia for status asthamaticus
- A. Thiopentone *(AIIMS 1997)* ☐
- B. Ketamine ☐
- C. Ether ☐
- D. N_2O ☐

49. Inducing agent contraindicated in asthma is
- A. Ketamine *(AIIMS 1993)* ☐
- B. Thiopentone ☐
- C. Propofol ☐
- D. Althesin ☐

50. During rapid sequence induction of anaesthesia: *(AI 03)*
- A. Sellick's maneuver is not required ☐
- B. Pre-oxygenation is mandatory ☐
- C. Suxamethonium is contraindicated ☐
- D. Patient is mechanically ventilated before endotracheal intubation ☐

51. Which is safest to be used in asthmatic patients:
- A. Nitrazepam *(PGI 2001)* ☐
- B. Phenobarbitone ☐
- C. Chloral hydrate ☐
- D. All hypnotics are safe ☐
- E. Morphine ☐

Answers and Explanations:

ANESTHESIA FOR OUT PATIENT / DAY CARE SURGERY

1. **A i.e. Propofol, Fentanyl, isoflurane** 2. **C i.e. Propofol** 3. **B i.e. Day care surgery**
4. **D i.e. Propofol** 5. **C i.e. Alfentanyl**

[Ref: Morgan's 3/e, P-173, 884; Lee 12/e P-417; Aitkenhead 4/e, P-617]

Propofol is the most suitable intravenous induction agent for day care surgery because of its tendency to provide a rapid, clear headed wake up with low incidence of nausea and vomitting.

Preferable agents in Day Care Anesthesia

Manmohan	- Mivacurium (muscle relaxant of choice)
Singh	- *Succinyl choline (for Ultrashort period of muscle relaxation as esophagoscopy*
Is	- *Isoflurane (volatile inhalational agent)*[Q]*/ sevo or desflurane*
A	- *Alfentanyl*[Q] (remi or sufentanyl)
Prime	- *Propofol* (as inducing agent)[Q]
Minister	- Midazolam (for initial anxiolysis & sedation)

★ N_2O is also used in day care surgeries

Preferred induction agents in other situations

Neonates	Preferred induction agent *Sevoflurane (inhalation)*[Q]
Neurosurgery	*Isoflurane*[Q] with thiopentone/propofol/etomidate with hyper ventilation to maintain Pa CO_2 between 25-30 mm Hg
Coronary artery disease & hypertension	Barbiturate, Benzodiazepines, Propofol & Etomidate are equally safe
Day care surgery	*Propofol (best choice)*[Q]

PAEDIATRIC ANAESTHESIA

6. **B i.e. Inhalational > C i.e. Intravenous** 7. **A. i.e. Sevoflurane**
8. **A i.e. Seroflurane** 9. **D i.e. Sevoflurance** 10. **C i.e. Morphine**

[Ref: Morgan's 4/e p. 922-38; Lee's 13/e p. 628–35; Miller's 6/e p. 2395-98; Wiley 7/e p. 968–75; Aitkenhead 4/e p. 654–61]

- ***Intravenous route is most preferred method for induction in children***[Q] because it provides overall better control of anesthesia & less chances of aspiration. The only problem is that it is difficult to put IV line.
- ***Sevoflurane is inhalational agent of choice for inductioin of anesthesia in pediatric (and adult) patients, because of rapid onset of action & nonpengency***[Q]. It can be used safely in ***hepatitis & intestinal obstruction***[Q].
- Desflurane & isoflurane are more pungent and are associated with more coughing, breath holding & laryngeal spasm during inhalational inudction, so not used as first choice.
- Methoryflurane is highly nephrotoxic so not preferred
- ***Infants and elderly are more susceptible to respiratory depressant action of morphine*** (KDT). In infants this is d/t poorly developed respiratory centre.

Induction of Anesthesia in Pediatric Patient

Inhalation	Intravenous	Intra-muscular
• Single Breath Induction - *Sevoflurane in N_2O*[Q] for rapid induction • Classical method - *N_2O & O_2* and *Sevoflurane/ halothane*[Q] is added	*Rapid acting barbiturate (eg thiopental) or Propofol*[Q] f/b nondepolarizing muscle relaxant (eg. rocuronium, atracurium, mivacurium) or Succinyl choline	**I.M. Ketamine** reserved for combative children

11. **B i.e. Halothane** *[Ref. Lee's anesthesia 12/e p-167; Morgan's anesthesia 3/e p-159, 140*

Among all these options only *halothane is hepatotoxic* so it should be avoided

Lets revise some important facts.

- All coagulation factors with ***exception of factor VIII (8) & von wille brand factor*** **are produced by *liver***[Q]
- ***Vit K* is necessary for synthesis of *prothrombin (factor II) and factor VII, IX and X***[Q].
- *PT* is normally ***11-14 seconds***, mesures the activity of ***fibrinogen, prothrombin and factors, V, VII, and X***[Q]
- All opioids cause spasm of sphincter of oddi & increase biliary pressure
- **Halothane hepatitis** is more common in middle age, obese, female sex, and a repeated exposure (esp with in 28 days)

12. **A i.e. Choosing a smaller size endotracheal tube** *[Ref. Morgan's 3/e p-861, Paul's p-281, BDC 3/e p-208, 3rd vol.]*

- Endotracheal tube that passes through the glottis may still impinge upon the cricoid cartilage; ***the cricoid cartilage is the narrowest point of the airway in children younger than 5 years of age***[Q]
- Mucosal trama can cause ***post operative edema, stridor, croup & airway obstruction***[Q] in subglottic & glotic region
- The appropiate size of tube is estimated by an age based formula, which provides only a rough guide line however. Exceptions include premature neonates (2.5 to 3 mm tube) and full term neonates (3-3.5 mm tube)

Pediatric Endotracheal Tube

Inside diameter	Length
↓	↓
Tube dia (mm) = (4 + Age)/4	Tube length (in cm) = (12 + Age)/2

- Correct tube size is confirmed by *easy passage into the larynx* and the *development of gas leak at 15-20 cm H_2O pressure.*
- So the size of ETT depends on age, easy passage & gasleak at 15-20 cm H_2O pressure.

13. **D i.e. G.A. Should be given to neonate for circumcision as they also feel pain as adults**

14. **D. i.e. Intravenous narcotic infusion in lower dosage**

[Ref: Miller 7/e pg-2593; Wylie 7/e p-975; Practical Procedures:Issue7(1997) Article 2: p. 6; Lee's 12/e p 480, 518]

- ***Though neonates have immature brain, they nevertheless feel pain***Q and analgesia is needed.
- During circumcision of babies, standard techniques of G.A. are suitable. They are given a normal intravenous or inhalational induction and spontaneous respiration is maintained using O_2 N_2O & volatile agent.
- ***Morphine is the drug of choice for children who are inpatients. The preferred route of injection is intravenous***Q but other routes can be used. Intrathecal route is not the first choice.
- **Following minor surgical procedures,** *oral acetaminophen (paracetamol), codeine phosphate and ibuprofen* may be givn either alone or in combination. After more **major surgery** ***continuous infusion of a potent opioid analgesic such as morphine may be required***Q.
- **Regional nerve blocks & direct local infiltration of surgical wounds with long acting local anesthetics** are simple yet very effective methods of providing pain relief for all children.
- Supplementing the analgesia of ether opioid or regional technique with 40 mg/kg **acetaminophen rectally** at the beginning of procedure is also recommended (generally in children still in diapers).

15. **C i.e. Wanted to see if there was an oculocardial reflex.** *[Ref: Millar 5/e P-2181; Morgan's 3/e, P-763]*

- **Traction on extraocular muscles or pressure on eye ball** can elicit cardiac dysrhythmias, ranging from bradycardia to sinus arrest. This reflex consists of **trigeminal afferent** and **vagal efferent** pathway. **It is most common in pediatrics undergoing strabismus surgery.**
- It can be evoked in cataract extraction, enucleation and retinal detachment repair also.
- It is treated by temporary cessation of surgery until heart rate increases intravenous atropine 10mg/kg.

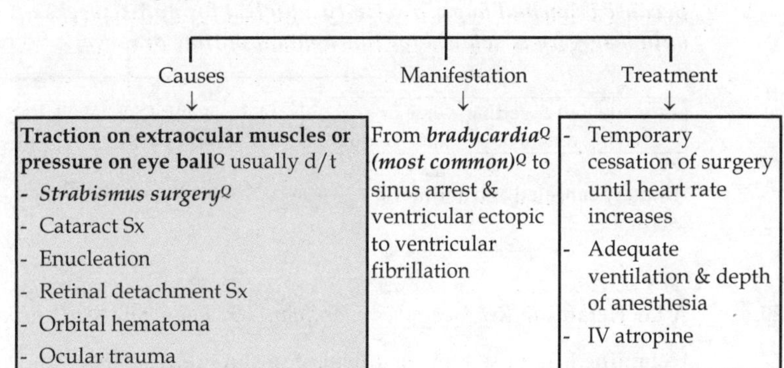

16. **A i.e. Succinylcholine** *[Ref: Morgan's 3/e, P-186]*

Boy is having some myopathy (probably duchenne's). So Sch may lead to life threatening hyperkalemia.

17. **B i.e. Induction by Propofol & maintenance by N_2O & O_2**

The boy is suffering from duchene muscular dystrophy. So anesthetic considerations would be about three things that are more probable in these patients and these are-***malignant hyperthermia, marked hyperkalemia & aspiration.***

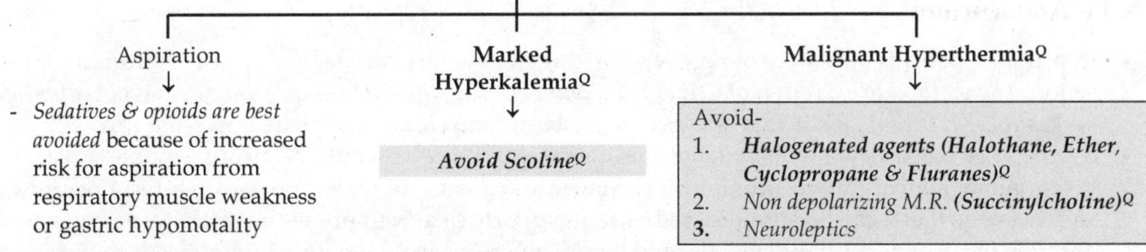

- ***Propofol***Q is anesthetic ***agent of choice*** in malignant hyperpyreria.
- *By avoiding scoline & halothane, we are left with only one option – (B)*

18. **A i.e. Induction with intravenous thiopentone and N_2O; and halothane for maintenance**

In this boy with duchene muscular dystrophy, there is high risk of malignant hyperthermia. **The earliest signs of malignant hyperthermia are masseter muscle rigidity (MMR), tachycardia, and hypercarbia** due to increased CO_2 production.

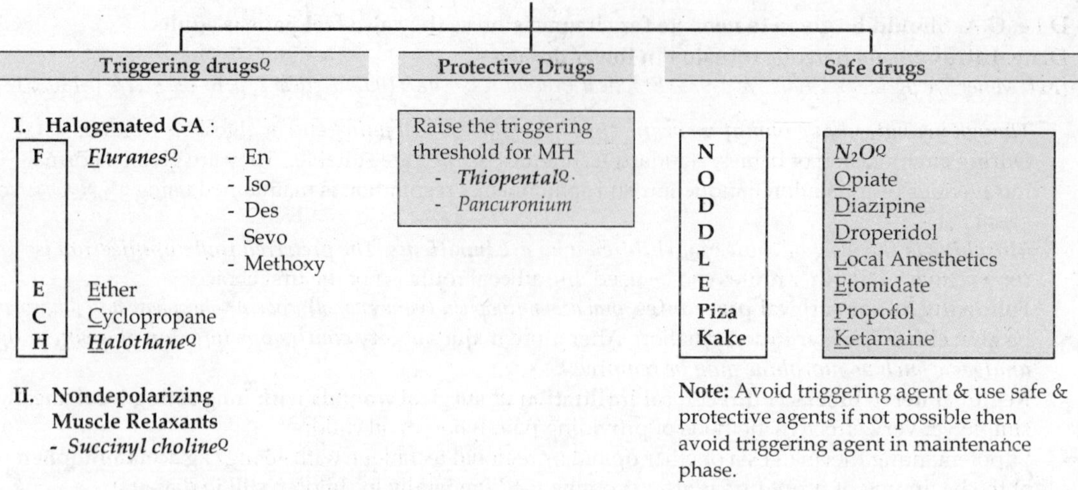

19. **D i.e. Cancel surgery for 3 weeks and patient to be on antibiotic** *[Ref: Miller 7/e p-2575; Morgan 4/e p-944]*

Surgery should be postponed if there is evidence of acute infection or suspicion of a clotting dysfunction (eg. recent aspirin ingestion)Q.

Child with an upper respiratory tract infection (URI) has an irritable airway and is at increased risk for laryngospasm, bronchospasm, post intubation croup, atelectasis, pneumonia & episodes of desaturation. ***Because bronchial hyper reactivity may last for upto 6 weeks after a URI, cancellation will make a difference only if surgery is delayed for this amount of time or longerQ.*** So patients who are

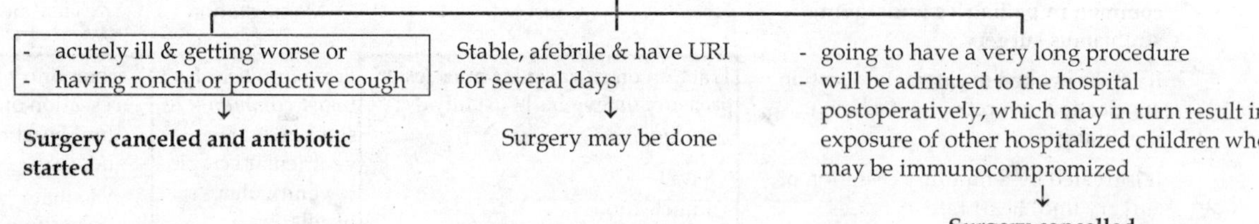

- acutely ill & getting worse or
- having ronchi or productive cough
Surgery canceled and antibiotic started
Stable, afebrile & have URI for several days
Surgery may be done
- going to have a very long procedure
- will be admitted to the hospital postoperatively, which may in turn result in exposure of other hospitalized children who may be immunocompromized
Surgery cancelled

20. **A i.e. Ketamine** *[Ref: An aesthesia for infants & children by Smith 6/e p.645; Lee 12/e p.192; Aitkinhead 4/e p244-49, 179]*

Ketamine is not used for treatment of postoperative nausea and vomiting. In fact ketamine use is ***itself associated with nausea & vomiting (d/t increase in intragastric pressure)*** and requires prophylaxis.

Antiemetics used for post operative nausea & vomiting (PONV)

Anticholinergics	$5HT_3$-Antagonists	Dopaminergic-Antagonists	Others
- Cyclizine	- ***Ondansterone***Q - Granesiterone	- Metoclopramide - Droperidol - Phenothiazines - Prochlorperazine - Butyrophenones	- ***Dexamethasone***Q - ***Propofol infusion plus nitrous oxide***Q - Transdermal scopolamine

21. **C i.e. Ataracurium** *[Ref: Miller 7/e p-2572; Wylie 7/e p 968-69]*

- In pediatric patients the choice of non depolarizing muscle relaxant depends on side effects and duration of action. ***The method of excretion of atracurium and cisatracurium (Hofman elimination and ester hydrolysis) makes these relaxants particularly useful in newborns and children with liver or renal diseaseQ.***
- If *tachycardia is desired* (eg with fentanyl anesthesia), *pancuronium* would be an appropriate choice. Vecuronium, atracurium, rocuronium & cisatracurium are useful for shorter procedures. **Rocuronium** offers an advantage that it can be administered intramuscularly (like Sch) preferably in deltoid however, the duration of action is ~ 1 hour, which could be a distinct disadvantage for a brief procedure. Vecuronium is valuable because no histamine is released; however, its duration of action is prolonged in newborns, which makes it similar to pancuronium
- The *potential for rhabdomyolysis & hyperkalemia* (particularly in boys < 8 yrs who may have unrecognized muscular dystrophy), as well as for *masseter spasm (jaws of steel), malignant hyperthermia, cardiac arrhythmias, and myoglobinemia* after administration of succinyl choline suggests that **Sch should not be used routinely in children.** Unlike adult patients *profound bradycardia & sinus node arrest* can develop in pediatric patients following 1st dose of Sch *without atropine pretreatment.* If a child unexpectedly experiences cardiac arrest

following Sch administration, *immediate treatment for hyperkalemia* should be instituted. However, it is the only available ultrashort acting muscle relaxant that provides a dependable, rapid onset of action. IV use of Sch should be limited to children who have full stomach or to treat laryngospasm. *Intramuscular, intralingual (Submental)* use is indicated for children with difficult intravenous access when control of airway is deemed essential.

- Mivacurium is an alternative to Sch when profound neuromuscular block of short duration is required but rapid onset of action is unnecessary.
- Antagonism of neuromuscular blockade in all neonates & small infants, is recommended, even if they have recovered clinically, because any increase in work of breathing may cause fatigue and respiratory failure.
- **Sugammadex**, a cyclodextrin whose endoskeleton forms a water soluble complex with exoskeleton of rocuronium, is designed to antagonize the effects of rocuronium. As it is made of sugars and antagonize by covalent bonding the *side effects are minimal*. Antagonism is *more rapid* than neostigmine/atropine. It also reverse the *other steroidal relaxants vecuronium & pancuronium to a lesser extent.* The mechanism of reversal is lowering of plasma conentation & thus reversing the concentration gradient and pulling the rocuronium off the myoneural junction.

ANESTHESIA for HEAD INJURY & NEUROSURGERY

22. **D i.e. Protein** *[Ref. Morgan 4/e, p 615-17, Miller 7/e, p 306, 322]*

- In the brain, with the *exception of choroid plexus, pituitary and the area postrema*, cerebral blood vessels are unique in that the junctions between vascular endothelial cells are nearly fused (8 Å pore size in comparison to 65 Å of body's capillary). The **paucity of pores is responsible for blood brain barrier (BBB).**
- The movement across BBB is influenced by the ***size, charge, lipid solubility and degree of protein binding* (in blood) of substance. So *carbondioxide (CO_2), oxygen (O_2), lipid soluble substances (as most anesthetics) and water freely enter brain (via BBB) whereas most ions (even small), protein and large substance such as mannitor penetrate poorly*[Q].**

23. **A i.e. Thiopentone** *[Ref. Miller 7/e, p 322-13, Morgan 4/e, p 866, 640-9; Stoelting 5/e, p 610-13]*

- In **head injury, induction** is preferably done by ***thiopental or propofol (both neuroprotective)***[Q] and a *rapid onset NMBD (usually rocuronium or mivacurium) following adequate preoxygenation hyperventilation* by mask. A **barbiturate (thiopentone) – opioid – N_2O-NMBA technique** is commonly used or intraoperative maintenance anesthesia.
- ***Ketamine, halothane, succinylcholine can increase ICP and are better avoided***[Q], however, Sch can be used in difficult intubation. Glucose containing or hypotonic crystalloid solutions, sedation without airway control and vasodilators (CCB, hydralazine, nitro-glycerine, nitroprusside) and PEEP are also avoided (or used very cautiously) in head injury.

24. **C i.e. Ketamine** *[Ref: Morgan 5/e p 618-17]*

- In patients with **seizure disorders,** in selecting anesthetic agents, **drugs with epileptogenic potential** should be avoided, most notably **enflurane**, theoretically **ketamine**[Q] and **methohexital** (in small doses) and hypothetically **large doses of atracurium, cisatracurium** or **meperidine** (relatively contraindicated b/o epileptogenic potential of their respective **metabolites, laudanosine and normeperidine).**
- In seizure patients, chronic antiseizure therapy **induces hepatic microsomal enzymes** and *increases the dose requirement and frequency of anesthetics and nondepolarizing neuromuscular blockers* and may increase the risk for **hepatotoxicity from halothane**.

ANESTHESIA for TRAUMA PATIENTS

25. **D i.e. Etomidate** *[Ref. Morgan 4/e, p 866-67, 199, 197, Miller 7/e, p 2285]*

Ketamine and etomidate are ***most commonly used induction agents for (non head injury) trauma patients***[Q]. Ketamine is beneficial in patients with *acute hypovolemic shock* (d/t indirect sympathetic stimulatory effects). Whereas etomidate provides *greater cardiovascular stability* (ie no or minimal effects on myocardial contractility, cardiac output and cardiovascular system, mild reduction in peripheral vascular resistance and BP, and no histamine release).

26. **B i.e. 4** *[Ref. Morgan 4/e, p 693]*

RL Contains 130 mEq/L Na^+, 109 mEq/L Cl^-, **4 mEq/L K^+**[Q], 3 meq/L Ca^{++} and 28 meq/L lactate.

Solution	**Tonicity** (mOsm/L)	**Na^+** (mEq/L)	**Cl^-** (mEq/L)	**Glucose** (g/L)
5% Dextrose in water (D_5W)	Hypo (253)	-	-	50
Normal saline (NS)	Iso (308)	154	154	
½ NS	Hypo (154)	77	77	
D_5 NS	Hyper (586)	154	154	50
D5 ½ NS	Hyper (432)	77	77	50
D5 ¼ NS	Iso (308)	38.5	38.5	50
3% Saline (S)	Hyper (1026)	513	513	
5% S	Hyper (1710)	855	855	

Solution	**Ringer lactate (RL)**	**D_5RL**	$NaHCO_3$ (7.5%)	**Plasmalyte**
Tonicity	Iso (273)	Hyper (525)	Hyper (1786)	Iso (294)
Na^+	130	130	893	140
Cl^-	109	109		98
K^+	4[Q]	4		5
Ca^{++}	3	3		
Mg^{++}				3
Lactate	28	28		
HCO_3^-			893	
Acetate				27
Gluconate				23
Glucose		50		

ANESTHESIA for CARDIOVASCULAR SURGERY

27. **C i.e. General anesthesia**

- In **coarctation of aorta** any decrease in cardiac output or cardiac return is deleterious to the fetus because the placental circulation is already comprised on account of coarctation. So any anesthetic procedure/drug which causes hypotension should be avoided.
- ***Regional anaesthic procedure such as spinal anesthesia and epidural anesthesia should be avoided***[Q] in these patients because hypotension is the most common side effect of these procedure.
- ***General anesthesia is technique of choice***[Q] for performing cesarian section in a patient with **coarctation of aorta,** as it has advantage of – rapid induction, better airway & ventilation and less hypotension.

28. **B i.e. Ketamine** *[Ref: Morgan's Anesthesia 4/e p. 478-82]*

- **Ketamine (intramuscular or intravenous)** is a commonly used *induction agent because it maintains or increases systemic vascular resistance* and it does not appear to increase pulmonary vascular resistance and *therefore does not aggravate the right to left shunting (in cyanotic heart disease)*
- Patients with milder degree of right to left shunting can also tolerate inhalational induction with halothane, because it tends to maintain systemic vascular resistance (due to minimal systemic arterial vasodilatation).
- Halothane is not used in very young patients due to its pungent nature & slow action.
- Halothane is also not preferred for patients with low cardiac output.
- Important facts about cyanotic heart disease are-
  - Cyanotic heart disease has predominantly right to left shunt i.e. blood flows directly from right ventricle to left ventricle by-passing the pulmonary circulation
  - Anaesthetic drugs and procedures which increase systemic vascular resistance & decrease pulmonary vascular resistance should be preferred.
  - R→L shunting tends to slow the uptake of inhalational anaesthetics. In contrast, it may accelerate the onset of intravenous agents.
  - N_2O is usually used with inhalational induction (does not ↑ PVR).

29. **A i.e. Sevoflurane** *[Ref: Morgan's Anesthesia 4/e p. 935; 480-1]*

Sevoflurane is the agent of choice for inhalational induction in pediatric patient[Q]. Desflurane & isoflurane are not used for induction because theyr are more pungent & are associated with more coughing, breath holding & laryngospasm during an inhalational induction.

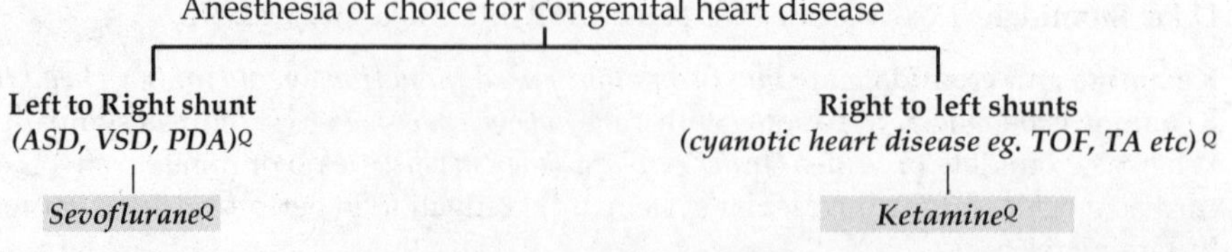

30. **D i.e. Cardiac Complication** *[Ref: Miller's Anaesthesia 6/e p. 2053; Clinical anesthesia by Gold Stone & Pollard p. 444; Clinical anaesthesia practice by Kirby, Gravenstein, Lobuto 2/e p. 1353]*

- ***Myocardial performance***Q is the single most important determinant outcome following a major vascular operation.
- ***Non fatal and fatal MIs***Q are the most important & specific outcomes that determine per operative cardiac morbidity in a patient undergoing vascular surgery.
- The **dominant risk factor for perioperative morbidity & mortatity in patients scheduled for abdominal aortic aneurysmectomy is** found to be – ***cardiac (47%) > pulmonary (31%)***Q > age older than 85 years (17%) > Renal failure (2%) > Retroperitoneal fibrosis (2%) > Cirhosis with ascites (1%)

31. **A i.e. Opioids > B i.e. Isoflurane** *[Ref: Morgan, Mikhail, Murray 4/e p507-10, 523-; 462-63]*

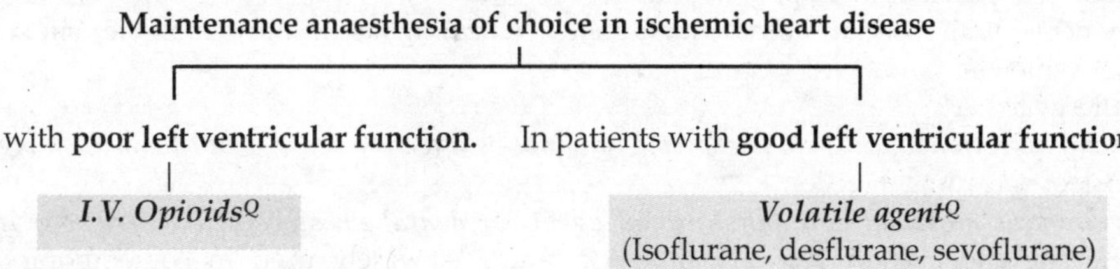

32. **B i.e. Thiopentone Sodium** *[Ref: Morgan's clinical anesthesiology 3/e, P-562]*

- Surgery from aortic arch aneurysm carries a great risk for hypoxic injury of brain; so surgery is performed using ***deep hypothermia***Q ***& circulatory arrest method*** (based on principle that brain can tolerate circulatory arrest for periods of upto 45 minutes if temperature is lowered to 15-17° C during surgery.
- During this process a **cerebroprotective agent**Q is needed which lowers the metabolic demands of brain by eliminating metabolic cost of electrical activity and protect brain from hypoxia by reducing cerebral edema & free radicle formation.
- ***Thiopentone (Barbiturate)***Q is definitely a **cerebroprotective drug**Q
- Other probable drugs are *Etomidate, Propofol, Isoflurane, Ketamine*

33. **C i.e. Xenon** *[Ref. Morgan 4/e, p 469; Yao 7/e, p-205-7, Miller 7/e, p 1929-30; Stoelting 5/e p. 373]*

Xenon provides ***good hemodynamic stability with little change in blood pressure***Q. It causes slight reduction in heart rate, otherwise it ***has no effect on heart (ie no cardiac depression*** **or** ***stimulation and does not sensitize to catecholamines) and systemic vascular resistance***Q. It has ***no hepatic and renal toxicity***Q. So it can be used safely in surgery of mitral stenosis with some liver compromise. Halothane cannot be used in this case b/o liver compromise.

34. **B i.e. Verapamil** *[Ref: Stoelting 5/e p. 377-79]*

- **Intraoperative administration** of **intravenous β blockers** ***(atenolol, metoprolol, propranolol or esmolol)***Q is done to *avoid tachycardia* during induction of anesthesia.
- The onset of paroxysmal atrial tachycardia or fibrillation in perioperative period can be treated by the iv administration of drug that abruptly prolong the refractory period of AV node (**adenosine**) or lengthen the refractory period of accessory pathways ***(procainamide)***Q Digitalis and verapamil may decrease refractory period of accessory pathways (in pre-excitation syndromes like Wolff-Parkinson-White syndrome) responsible for atrial fibrillation and thereby result in an increase in ventricular response rate during this dysrhythmia and thus should be avoided.
- **Ventricular tachycardia** not a/w hypotension is initially treated by iv administration of **lidocaine, amiodarone** or **lidocaine, amiodarone** or **procainamide**. Symptomatic VT is **best treated** by external electrical cardioversion.

35. **D i.e. Phenylephrine** *[Ref: Yao 7/e p 205; Lee 13/e p. 39; Morgan 5/e p 414-16]*

Phenylephrine (α-agonist) is **vasopressor agent of choice** in anesthesia for a **patient of aortic stenosis developing hypotension during surgery**. It is preferred over ephedrine becacause *it lacks β adrenergic agonist activity and restores coronary perfusion.* Patients with aortic stenosis experiencing angina may require administration of α agonist such as phenylephrine rather than nitroglycerine to increase coronary perfusion pressure.

ANAESTHESIA 2

ANESTHESIA for ENT & DENTAL SURGERY

36. **D i.e. Enflurane** *[Ref: Lee's 13th/e p. 695]*

*"General anaesthesia is indicated in case of acute infection when LA may not be effective because of the local change in pH and there is a risk of spreading infecton".*Q

Anaesthesia in Dental Extraction

- Local anesthesia would be adequate except in few situations as –
  - inability to tolerate dental treatment using LA (especially children).
  - failure of previous attempt to treat under LA.
  - patients with special needs or disability which make it impossible to sit still (e.g. uncontrolled movements).
  - allergy to LA
  - *acute infection when local anesthesia may not be affective because of the local change in pH*Q and there is risk of spreading infection.
- *Enflurane is most suitable inhalational agent for dental anesthesia with fewer irritant properties*Q than isoflurane and a short recovery time. Isoflurane is widely used in contemporary practice, but is not recommended for dental surgery in spontaneously breathing patients as it is irritant and is associated with coughing, salivation, and desaturation.

37. **C i.e. 100% oxygen after discontinuing anesthetic gases** **38. C i.e. Pollarad tube with infiltration block**
[Ref: Aitkenhead 5/e, p. 575-76; Morgan's 4/e p. 438-40; Wylie 7/e p. 840-41; Miller 7/e p. 2373, 2416; Dorsch 5/e p. 568-67]

When fire breaks out during laser vocal cord surgery, oxygen should be turned off, ventilation stopped, tracheal tube removed and submerged in water and the patient should be ventilated with facemaskQ. Airway damage is assessed with bronchoscopy and bronchial lavage, steroids, can be used for treatment.

OBSTETRICS ANAESTHESIA

39. **A, B, C i.e. Mechanical factor of gravid uterus; Hormonal factors; Altered pharmacokinetic**
40. **D i.e. Increased lumbar lardosis** *[Ref. Morgan's 4/e, p 875, Yao and Artusio's 7/e, p 78]*
[Ref: Miller 7th/e p. 2203-10); Pardo 6/e p. 515-31; Ajay Yadav 5/e p. 201-205; Lee 13/e p. 657-665]

- **Pregnant** patients *display enhanced sensitivity to LA during regional anesthesia because of hormonal factors and engorgement of epidural venous plexus resulting in decreased epidural space and subarachnoid space (CSF fluid) volume*Q. This enhances the cephalad spread of LA solution during spinal and epidural anesthesia.
- **Lower doses of local anesthetic agents and pain relief drugs are use in pregnant than in nonpregnant women because of altered pharmacokinetics and pharmacodynamics during partuition**Q as a result of hormonal and cardiovascular effects. For example lignocaine (Lidocaine) is less protein bound and **nerves are more sensitive to LA agents.**

41. **D i.e. Neuraxialblockde analgesia** *[Ref. Yao & Artusios7/e p 788, Morgan 4/e p 883-84, Stoelting 5/e p 490-484, Wylie 7/e p 926]*

Epidural (neuraxial) analgesia is the *most effective and least depressant method of intrapartum pain relief and is often viewed as technique choice for relief of labor pain*Q. It blunts the hemodynamic effects of contractions and associated pain response, which is *desirable for patients with* ***hypertensive disorders, asthma, diabetes, and cardiac and intracardiac neurovascular disease***Q.

42. **A i.e. GA** *[Ref: Morgan's 3/e P-828]*

Obstetric Anesthesia

- **Indications of GA during vaginal delivery**

- Fetal distress during 2nd stage
- Tetanic uterine contractions.
- Breech extraction
- Version & extraction
- ***Manual removal of a retained placenta***[Q]
- Replacement of an inverted uterus
- Uncontrollable psychiatric patients

- N_2O can be given in Early pregnancy
- Anesthesia is dangerous in all three trimesters but **comparatively 2nd *trimester is safest***[Q].
- **Supine Hypotensive Syndrome** : In late pregnancy (IIIrd Trim) circulatory depression occurs due to diminished venous return because of ***pressure of gravid uterus over inferior venacava in supine position.***[Q]
- ***Best uterine relaxant is halothane,*** *so uterine tetanic contractions are most rapidly treated by halothane.*[Q]
- ***M.C. cause of death during G.A. in obstetrics is Mendelson's syndrome***[Q] ***i.e. Aspiration of gastric content during anesthesia.*** On X-Ray, butterfly motteling in hilar area is seen.
  This is prevented by:
  - Empty stomach and H_2 blockers
  - Esophageal Intubation
  - ***Secillik's maneuver i.e. backward pressure on cartilage.***[Q]
- Contraindications
  - Gallimanie is C/I as it crosses placenta.
  - Morphine is C/I until delivery as it causes respiratory depression in mother and baby. For respiratory depression of morphine or pathidine. **Naloxane 0.01 mg/Kg** is given through **umbilical vein.**

ANESTHESIA FOR LIVER DISEASE

43. **C i.e. Isoflurane** *[Ref: Lee's 12/e, P-331,332; Morgan's 4/e, P-781-82]*

- ***Isoflurane***[Q] is volatile ***anesthetic agent of choice***[Q] in patients with liver disease because it has the least effect on hepatic blood flow.
- ***Cisatracurium***[Q] is ***neuromuscular blocking agent of choice***[Q] owing to its unique non hepatic metabolism.

44. **B i.e. Halothane** *[Ref: Morgan 4/e p-781, 167]*

All volatile anesthetic agents reduce portal hepatic blood flow. This decrease is greatest with halothane and least with isoflurane[Q].

ANESTHESIA FOR RENAL DISEASE

45. **A. i.e. Atracurium > B. i.e. Cisatracurium > D. i.e. Rocuronium E. i.e. Mivacuronium**
[Ref: Miller's 7/e p-2112-16; Morgan's 4/e p-219]

Anesthetics which can be used safely in (uremic/anephric) patients with renal disease include –

- **Inhalation anesthetics**: *desflurane, halothan, isoflurane*[Q], and enflurane (with caution).
- **Intravenous anesthetics**: *ultrashort acting barbiturates such as thiopental & methohexital, propofol*[Q], and narcotics combined with 30-50% N_2O
- **Opioids**: *Remifentanil, fentanyl, sufentanil*[Q], and hydromorphone (with caution).
- **Muscle relaxants** : ***Atracurium (best)***[Q], ***cisatracurium, mivacurium and rocuronium***[Q].

Pancuronium (~50%), vecuronium (30%), pipercuronium and doxacurium are partially excreted through kidney, & their action is prolonged in patients with renal failure. So these are either not used or administered very cautiously.

46. **B i.e. Isoflurane** *[Ref: Lee's 12/e p. 328, Morgan's 3/e, P-672, 143]*

Nephrotoxicity of anesthetic agents

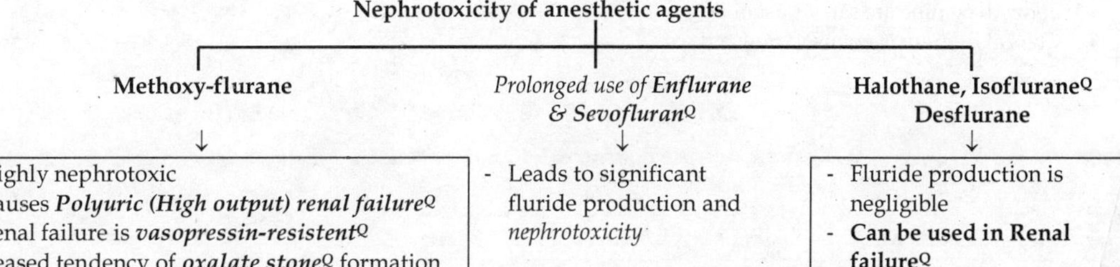

- Halothane & Isoflurane decrease renal blood flow, GFR & urinary output but desflurane does not.

ANESTHESIA FOR LUNG DISEASE

47. B i.e. Due to lack of stimulation by CO_2, anoxia can go into dangerous level

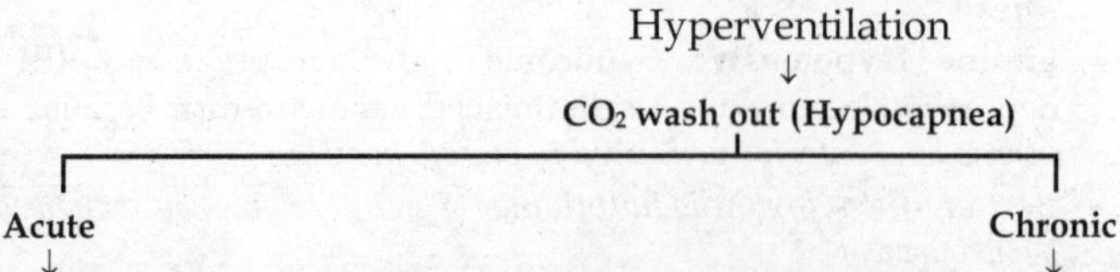

Acute	Chronic
Decrease respiratory drive[Q] ↓ Breath Holding may produce total lack of respiratory drive	- *Cerebral ischemia d/t vasoconstrictor effect of hypocapnea l/t* light headedness, dizziness - Increased cardiac output d/t peripheral vasoconstriction - Respiratory alkalosis *l/t* fall in plasma Ca^{++} level (Total P.Ca^{++} level does not change) and individual develops **carpopedal spasm, positive chove stek sign & other signs of tetany**

48. B i.e. Ketamine *[Ref: Morgan's 3/e, P-515]*

Anesthetic agent of choice in status asthamaticus

In children → ***Halothane***[Q]	In adults → ***Ketamine***[Q]
• It can sensitize the heart to aminophylline & β-adrenergic agonist administered during anesthesia; for that reason together with concern over hepatotoxicity – halothane is generally avoided in adults.	• Should not be used in patients with high theophylline levels, as the combined actions of the two drugs can precipitate seizure

- *Propofol & Etomidate, Isoflurane & desflurane are suitable alternatives and infact preferred by some clinicians.*

49. D i.e. Althesin *[Ref: Morgan's 3/e P-515]*

Contraindications

- Steroidal agent (Althesin) is contraindicated in *Porphyria and Asthama*[Q]
- *Adernaline is C/I with Halothane and Ring block is C/I in finger*
- **Ether** and **Cylopropane** are C/I with cauery
- ***Trilene*** is C/I with ***sodalime***
- In pregnancy — **Gallamine** and **Morphine**
- In Diabetics — **Ether** (better answer) & **Chloroform** as both causes hyperglycemia
- In liver damage **Choloroform (1st) & Halothane**
- In renal damage **Methoxyflurane** & **Morphine** as both leads to **High Output renal failure.** **Gallamine** is also C/I
- Thiopentone is C/I in acute intermittent porphyria

50. B i.e. Preoxygenation is mandatory *[Ref. Morgan 3/e p. 252; Lee's 12/e p. 233, 238]*

51. C i.e. Chloral hydrate *[Ref: KDT 5/e P-361; Harrison 15/e P-1462]*

In **Asthamatic**

Contraindicated	**Absolutely avoided** in acutely ill asthamatic
- ***β-Blockers***[Q] - Parasympathetic agonist	- ***Opiates***[Q] - ***Sedative & Tranquilizers***[Q] eg Barbiturate, BDZ's - Thiopentone

- Benzodiazepine are safe at usual dose.
- Chloral hydrate is not used now a days.

6 ANAESTHETIC COMPLICATION & MANAGEMENT

Venous Air (Gas) Embolism (VAE)

Etiology

- Gas usually enters the circulation *through a surgical wound.*
- *Subatmospheric venous pressure* greatly encourages air entrapment in venous system. So ***sitting, headup, park-bench, knee-chest positions that place operative site above the right atrium* carry an increased risk.**
- *Vascular catheters*, particularly during insertion are potential route for air entry
- ***Air (usually CO_2) embolism may occur during laproscopy & thoracoscopy***[Q].
- Highest incidence is seen in *sitting craniotomies (20-40%)*

Pathophysiology

- Clinical presentation varies with the volume as well as rate of air entery and whether patient has probe patent foramen ovale (10-25% incidence). An entery rate 0.5mL/kg / min produce clinical signs
- Patient foramen ovale can facilitate passage of air into the arterial circulation (**paradoxical air embolism**).
- Air entering venous system usually lodge in *pulmonary* circulation, diffuse into alveoli & ultimately exhaled. So small amounts are well tolerated in most.
- When the amount entrained exceeds the rate of *pulmonary clearance, pulmonary artery pressure (i.e. right ventricular after load) increases eventually decreasing cardiac output*
- Preexisting cardiac or pulmonary disease and *nitrous oxide* accentuate the effects

Clinical Presentation

- Sudden decrease in right ventricular output results in a ***rapid decrease in end-tidal carbon dioxide concentration***[Q]
- A decrease in end-tidal CO_2 or arterial O_2 saturation might be noticed prior to hemodynamic changes
- Only *slight increase* in (arterial) $PaCO_2$ as a result of increased pulmonary dead space (areas with normal ventilation but decrease perfusion)
- ***Sudden hypotension***[Q] followed by hypoxemia, tachycardia, ECG changes (arrhythmias) and an *increase in pulmonary artery pressure* are seen
- **Millwheel murmur**[Q] heard via precordial or oesophageal stethoscope is a late sign & occurs with very large emboli.
- ***Sudden circulatory arrest***[Q]
- Paradoxical gas embolism can result in *myocardial (coronary) or cerebral ischemia & infarction,* particularly when the normal transarterial (left > right) pressure gradient is reversed (d/t hypovolemia & PEEP)

Monitoring for VAE

- Most sensitive (intra operative) monitors are **transesophageal echocardiography (TEE)** and **pre cordial Doppler ultrasonography**. Both can detect air bubbles as small as *0.25 ml*
- TEE has added advantage of detecting the amount & any transatrial passage of bubble as well as evaluating cardiac function.
- **Interruption of regular swishing sound by sporadic roaring sounds on Doppler** indicates
- **Sudden decrease in end-tidal CO_2 tension & increase in pulmonary artery pressure** are less sensitive but important monitors that can detect VAE before overt clinical signs are present.
- Reappearance (or increase) of N_2 in expired gases
- ***BP changes & mill wheel murmur***[Q] are late manifestations.

Management

- Further AE is prevented by *flooding* the operative site *with saline* or applying the *bone wax* to skull edges and packing the wound.
- Venous pressure at the surgical site may be increased by compressing the jugular veins (in head & neck surgery) or by lowering the operative site relative to right atrium or by PEEP application.
- N_2O should be discontinued to avoid expansion of gas bubbles & lungs ventilated with 100% oxygen.
- Central venous catheter aspirated in an attempt to retrieve entrained air (only worth if a catheter is already in place)
- *Intravascular volume infusion* to increase CVP, *vasopressors* to treat hypotension
- Placing the patient in a head down left lateral position may help by allowing gas escape from right ventricle into atrium & vena cava.
- *Resuscitation*, external & internal cardiac massage for persistent cardiac arrest.

Anaesthetic Drug in Acute Porphyria

Class	Safe (Use)	Use with caution	Use with extreme caution	Avoid
Inhalation agents	N_2O, Halothane, Cyclopropane	Enflurane, Isoflurane Sevoflurane, Desflurane	-	-
Intravenous agents	***Propofol***[Q]	***Ketamine***[Q]	-	- ***Barbiturates***[Q] - ***Etomidate***[Q]
Analgesics	Paracetamol, aspirin, alfentanil, fentanyl, buprenorphine, morphine, codeine, pathedine, naloxone		- Diclofenac - Ketorolac - Phenacetin - Tilidine	- ***Pentazocine***[Q]

ANAESTHESIA 2

Neuromuscular blocking agents	Tubocurarine, Suxamethonium, Pancuronium	Alcuronium, Atracurium, vecuronium, rocuronium, mivacurium	-	-
N-M block reversing drugs	Atropine, glycopyrrolate, neostigmine	-		
Local anesthetics	Bupivacaine, lidocaine, prilocaine, procaine , tetracaine	Cocaine, mepivacaine	-	- *Ropivacaine*[Q]
Sedative and Antiemetics	Droperidol, phenothiazine, triazolam, timazepam	Other benzodiaze pines, diazepam, Lorazepam, midazolam, oxazepam, Cimetidine, metoclopramide,ondanst eron, Ranitidine	- Chlordiazepoxide - Nitrazepam	
Cardiovascualr drugs	α - agonists, β-agonists, β-blocker, epinephrine, Mg, procainamide, phentolamine	Diltiazem , Disopy ramide, Verapamil, sodium nitroprusside	- Hydralazine - Nifedipine - *Phenoxybenzamine*	

Anaesthetics Causing

Increased ICT	**Decreased ICT**	**↑IOT**	**↓IOT**	**Increased BP**	Bronchodilation (preferred in asthamatics)	Bronchospasmodics (contraindicated in asthamatics)
- ***Sevoflur-ane***[Q] - Desflura-ne - Isoflurane - Enflurane - Methoxyflur ane - **Halothane** - ***Ketamine***[Q] - Nitrous Oxide (N_2O) - Althesin	- Barbiturates *(e.g. **thiopentone sodium)*** [Q] - Benzodiaze-pines - Cyclopropane - Droperidol - Etomidate - ***Lidocaine***[Q] - ***Propofol***[Q] - Succinylch-oline	- **Barbiturates (e.g thiopentone Na)** - Cyclopropane - Etomidate - Succinyl Choline - ***Ketamine***[Q] - N_2O	- Morphine - Halothane - Hexameth-onium - Trimetha-phan	- Ketamine - Pentazocin - Pancuro-nium	- ***Ketamine (most potent)*** - ***Halothane*** - ***Morphine*** - ***Promethazine*** - ***d-TC***	- Ether - *N_2O* - ***Thiopentone***

Causes & Classification of Hyperthermia Syndromes

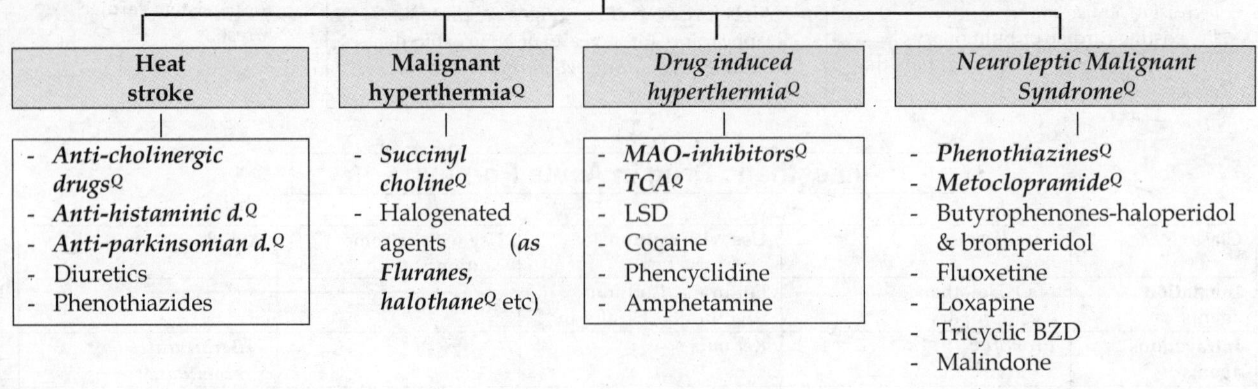

Malignant Hyperthermia

M. H is autosomal dominant genetic disorder of skeletal muscle that occurs in susceptible individuals due to exposure to some triggering agents, *typically suxamethonium or volatile agents* which cause an abnormal rise in intracellular calcium. It is caused by dysregulation of excitation - contraction coupling in skeletal muscles.

Mechanism

- Defect in *ryanodine receptor in sarcoplasmic retinaculum* (SR) that permits sudden outporing of calcium into cytoplasma from SR. Unchecked MH ultimately damages *mitochondria & sarcolemma.*
- Sch causes a *brief marked* rise in intracellular Ca^{++} & predominantly l/t *muscle damage (i.e., myoglobnuria & renal failure)*
- *Inhalation* agents cause a *sustained* rise & their effects are mainly *metabolic* due to the effect of Ca^{++} on *glycolysis enzymes;* with hyper capnia, hypoxia, hyperkalaemia & acidosis.
- *Previous uneventful exposure with Sch & inhalating agent do not exclude MH,* as it is not necessary to occur on every exposure.

MH associated Syndrome

- **Masseter spasm (thiopental - succinylcholine or halothane -succinylcholine rigidity)** *is defined as jaw muscle rigidity in association with limb muscle flaccidity* after administration of succinylcholine. This *tight/rigid/very rigid - jaw or jaw of steel (increase tone of jaw muscle)* occurs with Sch because the masseter and lateral pterygoid muscles contain slow tonic fibers that can respond to depolarizing NM blocker even after pretreatment with defasciulating dose of nondepolorizing relaxant.
- **If there is rigidity of other muscles in addition to trismus,** the association with **MH is absolute,** and anesthesis should be halted as soon as possible and treatment started. However in *>80% of patients with trismus but no rigidity of other muscles,* it is a variant found in *normal* patients. However, if trismus occurs, proper monitoring should include E_TCO_2, pigmenturia, acid base status, arterial-venous CK, electrolyte esp K^+.

Classical Clinical Manifestation Scenario

1. Rigidity after thiopental and Sch induction but successful intubation followed rapidly by the symptoms listed after scenario 2
2. Normal response to induction and uneventful anesthetic course until onset of these symptoms

- ***Unexplained ventricular arrhythmias or sinustrachycardia***Q, or both
- ***Tachypnea***Q if spontaneous ventilation is present
- Unexplained decrease in O_2saturation(b/o decease in venous O_2 saturation)
- ***Increased end tidal Pco₂ with adequate ventilation***Q (in most cases unchanged ventilation)
- ***Unexpected metabolic and respiratory acidosis***Q
- Central venous desaturation
- ***Unexplained increased in body temperature (> 38.8°c)***Q

Susceptible individual

- Patient with ***muscular dystrophy eg. Duchene***Q
- ***Pediatric age***Q (more chance)

Evaluation of Susceptibility

- A genealogy about anesthetic exposure & agent
- **Blood CK (creatine kinase)** in resting, fasting state without recent trauma reflects muscle membrane stability. If *CK is elevated in close relative of known MH person, he may be considered to have MH without contracture testing.*
- **Muscle Biopsy - Contracture studies (definite diagnostic procedure)** *if CK is normal on several occasions.* The patient *must travel to test center* for biopsy to ensure viability & accurate results. It involves exposure to *halothane, caffeine, & ryanodine. 4-chloro-m- cresol* may add to precision. Dantrolene must be avoided prior to biopsy because it masks the response to contracture producing drugs. Pseudo positive results may be seen in myopathies that bear no relation to MH & therefore may not indicate susceptibility.
- After a patient is diagnosed as being MH susceptible, **DNA testing for mutation** should follow. Other *relatives of patient with same mutation should be considered MH susceptible* without the need for invasive contracture test.

Anesthesia for Susceptible Patients

- **Safe Anesthetics** consist of

Mn - "**NOTE B**lood **P**ressure **AND Re**flex"

N	- *Nitrous oxide (N_2O)*Q
	- Non depolarizing muscle relaxant
O	- Opiates
T	- Tranquilizers
E	- Etomidate
B	- Barbiturates
P	- *Propofol*Q

AND - *Atropine, Neostigmine, Droperidol*

Reflex - **Regional anesthesia** (even with amide such as lidocaine which was once considered dangerous) is safe & may be preferred.

- Before use for MH-sensitive patients, **anesthetic machines cleansed** of potant volatile agents by removal or sealing of the vaporizers, changing the soda lime, replacing the fresh outlet hose, and using a disposable circle with a flow of 10L/min for 5 minutes
- ***Potent volatile anesthetics & succinyl choline must be avoided***Q, even in presence of dantrolene
- A minimum recovery room stay of 4 hours has been recommended for patients who are susceptible to MH.

Acute Treatment for an Episode

- Treatment is directed at terminating the episode and treating complications such as acidosis and hyperkalaemia. ***The triggering agent (anesthesia) must be stopped and dantrolene must be given immediately***Q. Even trace amounts of anesthetics absorbed by sodaline, breathing tubes and bags may be detrimental. So *anesthetic tubing and soda lime are changed.* The patient should be *aggressively ventilated with 100% O_2 to minimize* the side effects of hypercapnia, metabolic acidosis and increased O_2 consumption. Nonetheless, *the* ***mainstay of therapy for MH crisis is immediate administration of IV dentrolene***Q. Calcium channel blockers should not be used with

Triggering Agents

- **Depolarizing muscle relaxant: Succinyl choline (most common)**Q
- ***Halogenated inhaled general anesthetics***
  - **Halothane**Q
  - Ether
  - Chloroform
  - **Fluranes(methoxy, en, iso, des and sevo-fluranes)**

Drugs that are Probably safe

- Cyclopropane
- MAO inhibitors
- Tricyclic antidepressants
- Haloperidol
- Phenothiazines

Drugs safe in MH

- ***Benzodiazepines***Q
- Barbiturates: thiopental
- ***Ketamine***Q
- ***Propofol***Q
- Opioids
- Nondepolarizing neuromuscular blocking drugs
- **Nitrous oxide (N_2O)**Q
- All local anesthetics
- Atropine
- Neostigmine
- Droperidol
- Metoclopramide

Clinical Features

- ***Rise in end tidal CO_2 (Ist sign)***Q, ***Masseter muscle rigidity (MMR) and tachycardia are earliest sign***Q
- **Hypermetabolic features**
  - Increased CO_2 production & O_2 consumption; so blood gas analysis shows increasing hypoxemia & rising PCO_2
  - Low mixed venous O_2 tension
  - Fall in O_2 saturation, cyanosis, and mottling
  - ***Metabolic acidosis***Q
  - Tachypnaea (in spontaneously breathing)
- **Hyperthermic features**
  - Fever, hyperthermia (late), sweating
- **Sympathetic overactivity features**
  - ***Tachycardia***Q & arrhythmias
  - ***Unstable blood pressure, initial hypertension***Q
  - Mortality, most commonly d/t ventricular fibrillation.
- **Muscle Damage**
  - ***Masseter muscle spasm***Q, ***generalized rigidity***
  - ***Hyperkalemia***Q, *hypernatremia, hyperphosphatemia, myoglobinemia & myoglobinuria*
  - Increased creatine kinase levels
- DIC

dentrolene d/t risk of hyperkalemia

- ***Discontinue all anesthetic agents and hyperventilate with 100% oxygen***Q at high flow (to remove additional CO_2 produced) may be adequate t/t for slow onset brief exposure MH.
- Administer ***dantrolene***Q (2.5 mg/kg IV to a total dose of 10 mg/kg IV) every 5-10 minutes until symptoms subside
- Administer **bicarbonate ($NaHCO_3$),** 2-4 MEq/kg IV to correct the metabolic acidosis with frequent *monitoring of blood gases and pH.*
- Control fever by **cooling measures** (eg cooling body surface & cavities with ice fluids, cooling blanket, cold IV solution, cold dialysis, and if necessary using a heat exachanger with a pump oxygenater). Cooling is halted at 38°C to 39°C to prevent inadvertent hypothermia.
- **Monitor urinary output** & establish diuresis to protect kidney from *myoglobinuria* by mannitol infusion (0.5 g/kg) and/or furosemide.
- Consider invasive monitoring of CVP and arterial blood pressure.
- Further therapy is guided by blood gases electrolytes, temperature, arrhythmia, muscle tone, and urinary output.
- Treatment of hyperkalemia with *glucose and insulin* should be slow; and the most effective way to decrease serum K^+ is reversal of MH by *dantrolene*
- Analyze **coagulation studies** eg INR, PT, platelet count, fibrinogen, fibrin split or degradation products.

Dantrolene

- It is packed in 20mg bottles with *NaOH* (for a pH of 9-10, otherwise it would not dissolve) and with mannitol (converts hypotonic solution to isotonic).
- It is reconstituted in *sterile water* (not in salt solution or it will precipitate)
- Has a half life of atleast *10 hours* (so repeate at 10-15 hours)
- *Cholestasis* during long term (> 3 weeks) therapy is the only side effect.
- ***Only drug to be effective in reversing the symptoms and preventing the episode***Q.

Preoperative (procedure) Medication Instruction Guidelines

Drugs continued on the day of operation/procedure with a small sip of water even if otherwise NPO (nothing by mouth)

- Antihypertensive medications (like catecholamine/ sympathetic receptor blockers eg α adrenergic receptor blocking drugs, **β blockers**; arteriolar dilators and ***calcium channel blockers***Q.)
- Antidepressant, antianxiety & psychiatry (eg dopamine receptor antagonists), antiseizure and asthma medications.
- Birth control pills, cardiac medication (eg digoxin), diuretics, eye drops
- Narcotic pain medication, heart burn/reflux medication, steroids (oral & inhaled), statins (eg zocor, Lipitor) and thyroid medication.
- COX-2 inhibitors (unless surgeon concerned about bone healing).

Usually continue; but discontinued before plastic & retinal surgery

- NSAIDS (48 hrs before)
- Aspirin (7 days before)

Discontinue on the day of operation

- Topical creams & ointments, *oral hypoglycemic drugs*
- Vitamins, iron, premarin
- **Insulin** (Type 2 diabetic should discontinue all inssulins of any type). Type I should take small (1/3rd) amount of morning long acting insulin (Lente or NPH) only. Patient with insulin pump should take their basal rate only.

Discontinue days before surgery

- Viagra, levitra, cialis or similar drugs (discontinue 36 hours before)
- **Warfarin** (4 days before except in cataract surgery without bulbar block).
- **Clopidogrel** (7 days before except for vascular patients or those undergoing cataract surgery).
- Herbal & non vitamin supplements (7 days before)
- MAO inhibitors – antidepressant need anesthesia consultation 3 weeks before surgery.

- **Lithium should be stopped 2 days before major surgery because it potentiates nondepolarising relaxants**. So in emergency, suxamethonium (ie depolarizing relaxant) and regional blocks should be considered as an alternative. It **is** *usually safe to continue lithium therapy before minor surgery if proper attention* is paid to fluid and electrolyte balance *(Lee's)*.
- Lithium inhibits neuromuscular transmission presynaptically and muscular contraction postsynaptically by activation of K^+ channels. The combination of *Li and pipecuronium* results *in synergistic inhibition* of NM transmission, whereas combination of *Li and succinylcholine results in additive inhibition. Prolongation of NM blockade is reported in patients taking Li and both depolarizing and nondepolarizing blockers*. So in patients who are stabilized on Li therapy and undergoing surgery, NM blockers should be *administered in incremental and reduced doses* to the degree of blockade required (Miller).
- Although Li is reported to decrease minimum alveolar concentration and prolongs the duration of some NMBs, clinically these effects seem to be minor. *Sodium depletion (secondary to thiazide or loop diuretics) decrease renal excretion of Li and can cause lithium toxicity*. Fluid restriction & over diuresis should be avoided. Lithium dilution cardiac output measurements are contraindicated in patients on Li therapy. (Morgan)
- **Antihypertensive drugs** are normally continued upto the time of surgery to maintain normal blood volume and minimize the risk of dangerous hypotension at induction. However, some prefer to omit **ACE & angiotensin II receptor blockers**, which both may nevertheless cause significant hypotension.
- **Anti anginal drugs (calcium channel blockers or nitrates)** either orally or transdermally, should be continued to the time of suergery to prevent angina. **Levodopa** is continued upto the time of surgery to prevent Parkinsonism.
- **Lithium** should be stopped **2 days** before, & **non selective MAO inhibitor** (Phenelzine, isocarboxazid & especially tranylcypramine) should be discontinued **2 weeks** before elective major surgery. Reversible specific **MAO-A inhibitors (Moclobemide) and MAO-B inhibitors** (selegiline) may be *continued upto the day before surgery*.
- **Oestrogen containing combined OCP** increase the risk of *DVT* and *reduce the activity of antithrombin III*. The risk is maximum following *major pelvic, cancer and orthopaedic surgery* and in patients with *factor V laden mutation*. Combined OCP should be **discontinued 4 weeks before** major elective surgery or leg surgery (eg varicose vein stripping or ligation) and started again at first menstrual period following an interval of 2 weeks after surgery providing the patient is fully mobile. *Because of urgency, if this is not possible, prophylactic heparin should be considered.*
- **Low dose corticosteroid therapy** (<10 mg prednisolone/day) has assumed to have little effect. For **higher dose** therapy it is safe to give **extra hydrocortisone over the period of suergery** (eg hydrocortisone 25 mg at induction, followed by 25 mg 6 hourly for 24 hours for intermediate or 48 hours for major surgery; preferably by intramuscular route which provides more sustained plasma levels.

Cardio-Pulmonary Resuscitation (CPR) = CP and Cereberal Resuscitation (CPCR): Emergency Cardiac Care (ECC): BLS, ACLS/PALS

- **Cardiac arrest** (ie inability of heart to maintain effective cardiac output impairing tissue perfusion) is mostly of **cardiac origin (mostly d/t VT or VF secondary to myocardial ischemia) in adult** and usually of **respiratory origin (arterial hypoxemia & respiratory compromise**; or asystole) in ***children***. *Thus, airway management and breathing are critical to successful pediatric resuscitation, whereas defibrillation is an early important intervention in adults. However, **pediatric BLS or CPR follows the same algorithm as for adults: C-A-B***
- CPR is performed until return of spontaneous circulation, the patient is declared dead or placed on ECMO (extracorporeal membrane oxygenation).
- CPR and emergency cardiac care (ECC) should be considered **any time in an individual who cannot adequately oxygenate or perfuse vital organs-and not only following respiratory or cardiac arrest**.
- Now a days, CPR would be considered **basic life support (BLS)** ie life support without the use of special equipement, whereas **advanced cardiac life support (ACLS) and pediatric advanced cardiovascular life support (PALS)** include the use of pharmacotherapy **(drugs) and other definitive special equipement & techniques**.
- BLS and ECC in suspected, impending or confirmed cardiac arrest involves (1) **early recognition of medical emergencies**, (2) **activation of emergency response system** (eg dialing 911 in USA) and retreaving an automated external defibrillator (AED), (3) **CPR or BLS** intended to maintain organ perfusion until definitive intervention can be instituted. Order of priorty is **CAB ie compression,**
- ICC-2005 recommendations for CPR is "**push hard and push fast"** chest compression performed at **a rate of 100/min** and **with enough force to generate a palpable carotid or femoral pulse** are considered ideal. There is increased emphasis on **limiting interruptions in chest compressions, even for other resuscitative measures** (ie rescue breaths, attempts at defibrillations, tracheal intubation, IV line). **Guidline 2005 recommend compression-ventilation ratio of 30:2 in both single and 2 person CPR scenario with minimal interruption in chest compressions for rescue breaths.**
- **AHA & ILCOR-2010 recommendations for CPR-ECC include**
  - (To lay persons) that the **pulse should not be checked** and the **chest compression without ventilation may be as effective as compression with ventilation for first several minutes** (b/o enough O_2 already present in blood). If rescuer is unwilling to perform mouth to mouth ventilation, **chest compressions alone are preferred to doing nothing.**
  - (For health care provider) **defibrillation using biphasic electric current works best and tracheal tube (TT) placement should be confirmed with a quantitative capnographic wave form analysis.**Q
  - The sequence of steps in CPR has been **changed from ABC** (airway & breathing first before comprssion) to **CAB (compression first, with airway and breathing treated later)**
  - Emphasis has been placed on quality & adequacy of comprssions, minimizing interruption time of compressions and the preshock pause (time taken from last compressions to the delivery of shock); on physiological monitoring methods to optimize CPR quality and return of

airway and breathing. If the patient has no pulse, no signs of life or the rescuer is unsure, **chest compression should be started immediately. During pulseless cardiac arrest** (ie VF, rapid VT, pulseless electrical activity = PEA, and asystole) the **primary goal is to provide effective chest compressions** and **early defibrillation** if the rhythm is VF or VT. After initaiting CPR and defibrillation rescuers can then establish intravenous access, obtain a more definitive airway, all while providing continued chest comprssion and ventilation, (4) interventions made in response to sudden cardiac arrest (SCA), heart attack, stroke and airway obstruction by foreign body.

- Airway, breathing, circulation are BLS assessments. Rescue breathing, Heimlich maneurer, CPR and automated external defibrillater (AED) are BLS interventions
- CPR or CPCR is a most important part of BLS (or primary ABCD survey), ECC, and ACLS (Secondary ABCD surrey).

spontaneous circulation (ROSC).

- **Rule of tens and multiples ie < 10s to** check for **pulse**; < 10s for placing & securing **airway**; target chest compression adequacy to maintain end tidal pressure CO_2 **($PETco_2$) > 10, arterial diastolic BP > 20 and central venous oxygen saturation ($Scvo_2$)>30.**
- **Atropine use is excluded** in settings *of pulseless electrical activity (PEA) and asystole*; use of **chronotropic drug infusions** as an alternative to pacing in *ustable/symptomatic bradycardia* and recommended use of **adenosine** in management *of wide complex monomorphic tachycardia.*

- **ABCD** of CPR are- Airway, Breathing, Circulation and Defibrillation. Although A of mnemonic stands for airway, it should also stand for the initial **Assement** of patient. **Before CPR is initiated, unresponsive is established and the emergency response system activated.**

Airway

- Most common cause of airway obstruction in unconscious patient is **posterior displacement (fall) of tongue or epiglottis**. It can be managed by **head tilt (neck extension) and chin lift** (in patients without evidence of cervical spine instability) or **jaw thurst (ie mandible pulled forward)** in patients with cervical spine fracture. However, 2010 guidelines recommend use of head tilt-chin lift for cervical spine injury patients to save life; if it is not possible to maintain airway only by jaw thurst.
- Any foreign body, vomitus visible in mouth should be removed. If the patient is conscious or foreign body cannot be removed by finger sweep, the **Heimlich (subdiaphragmatic abdominal thurst) maneuver**, expelling a blast of air form lungs that displaces foreign body is recommended. A combination of **back blows and chest thursts** is recommended to clear foreign body obstruction in infants. **Rib fracture, trauma to internal viscera** and regurgitation are complications of Heimlich maneuver.
- The old **ABCD** (airway, breathing, circulation, & defibrillation) with look, listen and feel sequence has been changed to **CAB (compression, airway, breathing). So airway maneuvers should occur quickly, efficiently and**

Breathing (Ventilation)

- Chest compressions and ventilation should not be delayed for intubation if a patent airway is established by jaw thurst maneuver. **In apneic patients, initially 2 breaths** are slowly administered (2s per breath in adults, 1-1½ s in infant and children). If these breaths cannot be delivered, airway obstruction must be removed.
- Mouth to mouth or mouth to mask (barriers device) rescue breathing should be instituted in apneic patients, even in hospital settings when the crash cart is on its way.
- Successful rescue breathing (**V_T 700-1000mL**, 8-10 times per minute in an adult with a secured airway and a **ratio of 30 compression to 2 ventilations** if the airway is unsecured) is confirmed by observing the chest rising and falling with each breath and hearing and feeling the escape of air during expiration.

Circulation

- Circulation takes precedence over airway and breathing in cardiac arrest situation and **chest compression should begin even prior to initial breaths** in this scenario.
- Lay men should assume that an unresponsive man is in cardiac arrest and need not check pulse. Health care provider should assess for presence or absence of pulse and should take no more than 10 seconds to check for a definitive pulse.
- After successful delivery of 2 initial breaths (each 2s in duration), **circulation is rapidly assessed**. If the patient has/is

Adequate pulse or BP → Breathing is continued at 10-12 breaths/min for > 8 yrs old child & adult and 20 breath/min for < 8yr old child and infant.

Pulseless or **severly hypotensive,** no signs of lilfe or rescuer is unsure → Chest compression started immediately

- During short duration chest compression (CPR) the blood flow is created more by **cardiac pump mechanism** (ie directly compressing heart); but as CPR continues, the heart becomes less compliant and **thoracic pump mechanism** (ie by increasing intra thoracic pressure) becomes more

Defibrillation

- Time from collapes to defibrillation is the most important determinant of survival, which declines at a rate of **7-10% every minute** without defibrillation. **So cardia arrest patients should be defibrillated at the earliest possible moment** (especially in VF/VT). Shock should be delivered **within 3 min (±1) of cardiac arrest.**
- No definite relationship exists between the body size and energy requirement for successful defibrillation. A shock with too low energy may be unsuccessful and too high energy may cause functioned and morphological injury.
- **Biphasic waveforms are recommended for cardioversion** as they deliver an in series *bidirectional energy charge and achieve the same degree of success but with less energy (120-200 joule) and theoretically less myocardial damage* (in comparison to 200-300 J monophasic damped sine MDS wave form shocks).
- **Decreasing preshock pause** (time delay between last compression and delivery of shock) is important (a/t 2010 guidellines). **Stacking shocks** increase the time to next compression and thus should be **replaced by single shock** (~ 90% efficacy) **followed by immediate resumption of chest compression.**
- **Cardioversion should be synchronized with QRS complex** and is recommended for *homodynamically stable, wide complex tachycardia requiring cardioversion, PSVT, atrial fibrillation and atrial flutter. Polymorphic VT should be treated as VF with unsynchronized shocks.*

Indications	Energy of Biphasic shocks (Joules) using biphasic truncated

minimize interruptions in chest compressions.

- If there is no evidence of adequate breathing, even after opening the airway, the rescuer, should initiate **assisted ventilation** by inflating victims lungs with each breath using *mouth- to mouth/ nose/stoma/barrier device/face shield/ mask rescue breathing or using a bag mask device.* **Breaths are dlivered showly (inspiration lime ½-1s) with smaller tidal volumes** (V_T) [~700-1000 mL, smaller (400-600 mL) if supplemental O_2 is used] than was recommended in past.
- Because of riskof regurgitation & aspiration (esp with positive pressure ventilation) the **airway should be secured with TT (method of choice)** or an alternative airway (eg esophageal tracheal combitube (ETC), LMA, pharyngotracheal lumen airway, king laryngeal tube and cuffed oropharyngeal airway. Artificial airway **must be carefully secured with a tie or tape. However chest compression should not be interrupted for> 10 second to place any airway**.
- **The 2010 CPR-ECC guidelines** recommend a **TT (tracheal tube) as the airway adjunct of choice** (if persons skilled in placing it are available). And rescuers must **confirm TT placement with a P_{ETCO_2} detector**-**an indicator** a **capnograph** or a **capnometric device**. The **best choice for confirmation of TT placement is continuous capnographic waveform analysis**[Q]. All confirmation devices are considered adjuncts to clinical confirmation techniques eg auscultation.
- **Cricothyrotomy** (ie placing 12-14 gauge intravenous catheter through CT membrane) **or tracheotomy** may be necessary in case where TT intubation may be impossible (eg severe facial trauma) or unwise (cervical spine trauma). 0Cricothyrotomy is not generally recommended in children younger than 10 years age.
- Because exhaled air has 16-17% O_2 concentration only with significant CO_2, **the supplemental oxygen (preferrably 100%)** should always be used if available. In such a case, a smaller **V_T of 400-700ml** is recommended.
- **Cricoid pressure** to prevent regurgitation during cardiac arrest resuscitation is considered but not routinely recommended (in 2010 guidelines).
- **Tracheal intubation** should be attempted as soon as practicle. However, **intubation attempts should not interrupt ventication for more than 10s.**
- In neonatal resuscitation, indications for **positive pressure ventilation** include (1) apnea, (2) gasping respirations, (3) persistant central cyanosis with 100% O_2, and (4) a persistant heart rate <100 beats/min. Assisted ventilation (by bag & mask) should be at a rate of **30-60 breaths/min with 100% O_2**. Initial breaths may have 40 cm H_2O peak pressure but it should not exceed **30 cm H_2O** thereafter. Indications for endotracheal intubation include ineffective or prolonged mask ventilation and need to administer medication.

important.

- **Whether, adult resuscitation is performed by a single rescuer or by 2 rescuers, 2 breaths are administered every 30 compression (30:2)**, allowing 3 to 4s for 2 breaths. The cardiac compression should be **100/min regardless of numbers of rescuers**. Compression and relaxation times should be equal. High quality CPR includes push fast (100/min), push hard (2 inches), allow full chest recoil, minimize interruptions in chest compressions (of > 10s)and avoid excessive ventilation (or large tidal volume, breath rate > 10-12 and 1 breath duration > 1 second).
- Compression rate of > 100/min with 2 breath delivered every 30 compressions in infants; and > 120/min compression rate and 3:1 compression ventilation ratio is rercommended in neonates. Indication for chest comprssions (in neonate are a heart rate < 60/min or 60-80/min and not rising after 30s of adequate ventilation with 100% oxygen.
- **Adequacy of chest compressions** can be assessed (a/t 2010 guidelines) by monitoring **end tidal CO_2 ($PETco_2$), $Scvo_2$ (in jugular vein) and arterial diastolic pressure (in radial brachial or femoral artery). Coronary perfusion pressure** (CPP) is difference between aortic diastolic pressure and right atrial diaslolic pressure. **$PETCO_2$ > 10mmHg, arterial diastolic pressure> 20 mmHg and $Scvo_2$ > 30%** indicate good quality chest compression. $PETCO_2$ <10mm Hg is predictor of poor outcome and decreased chances of ROSC (recovery of spontaneous circulation). In $PETCO_2$ a transient increase is seen with **sodium bicarbonate administration** and an abrupt & sustained rise of $PETCO_2$ indicates ROSC. Arterial pulsations **during resuscitation are not a good measure of adequate chest compression**; however, spontaneous arterial pulsations indicate ROSC.

	exponential (BTE) or rectilinear (RBW) morphology
Unstable atrial fibrillation	120-200 (with further escalation if needed)
Unstable atrial flutler/ tachycardia (PSVT)	50-100
Monomorphic ventricular tachycardia	100
Polymorphic ventricular tachycardia or ventricular fibrillation	120-200

ACLS: Drugs and Routes of Administration

- The preferred route of administration of all drugs during CPR is **intravenous**. *The most rapid and highest drug levels occur with administration into a central vein.* Therefore, **when available central (internal jugular or subclavian) venous line is ideal** and should be used in CPR. If there is no central line access, then one should attempt to establish *peripheral venous line* either in antecubital or external jugular vein, *because placement of central line usually necessitates stoping CPR.* **Sites of upper extremity or neck are preferred over lower extremity because paucity of blood flow below diaphragm during CPR may cause extreme delay.**
- If intravenous cannulation is difficult, an ***intraosseous infusion*** can provide emergency vascular access in children or even in adults (upper tibia, distal radius, ulna).
- Some drugs are well absorbed following administration through an *endotracheal tube. They do not injure the lungs and can be absorbed for tracheal mucosa (eg. epinephrine*[Q], atrophine, vasopressin, lidocaine, naloxone but not sodium bicarbonate).
- **Epinephrine (adrenaline)** in CPR is given in dose of **1mg (10 ml of a 1:10000 solution) repeated every 3-5 minutes through central or peripheral venous line, intra tracheal route** (dosage 2-2.5 times higher) or **intraosseous route** (in children). Contrary to general belief that **epinephrine increases the amplitude of ventricular fibrillation (β adrenergic effect) and makes defibrillation easier,** clinical studies have shown no effect on defibrillation success (Wylie). **Adrenatline converts fine fibrillations to coarse** ones.

Basic Life Support – Summary

Features	Neonates	Infant (1-12 months)	Child (>1 yr to adolescence)	Adult
Breathing rate	**30-60/min** with 100% O_2 by bag & mask	20 breaths/min	20 breaths/min	10-12 breaths/min 8-10 breath/min if airway secured with TT
Compression rate	**120/min**	>100/min	100/min	100/min
Compression method push hard & fast and allow complete recoil	**Two thumb/Encircling technique** (preferred b/o higher peak systolic & coronary perfusion pressure) or **two finger technique**	*Two-Three fingers*Q or two thumbs encircling hands	Heel of one hand	***Hands interlaced***Q
Compression-ventilation ratio	**3 : 1**	**30:2** *new; 5:1*Q *old*	**30:2** *new; 5:1*Q *old*	**30:2** new; *15 : 2*Q, 5 : 1 if tracheal tube is used Old
Compresison depth	**1/3rd of AP diameter** of chest & enough to generate a palpable pulse	½ - 1 inch (1½ - 2½ cm)	1 - 1.5 inch (2 - 4 cm)	1.5 - 2 inch (4 - 5cm)
Pulse check		Brachial/Femoral	Carotid	Carotid
Foreign body obstruction		Back blows & Chest thursts	Hemlich maneuver	***Hemlich maneuver***Q

★ ***CPR in newborn should deliver 90 compressions and 30 ventilation (3:1) per minute.***Q

If after 30s, heart rate is

- **< 60/min** or **60-80/min without an increase** in response to resuscitation → **neonate intubuted & chest compression started**
- **60-80/min & increasing** → **assisted ventilation is continued and neonate observed**
- **>100/min** and spontaneous ventilation become adequate → **Assisted ventilation is no longer necessary**

Hydroxyethyl Starch (HES, Hespan)

- **Hydroxyethyl starches (HES)** are *modified natural polysaccharides similar to glycogen* and are mainly **amylopectin esterified with hydroxyethyl group**Q. They are derived from highly branched corn or potato starch amylopectin. *Substitution with hydroxyethyl group (at C_2, C_3 and C_6 carbon position) delays* **α-amylase break down with subsequent elimination from blood**, of HES.
- Most important physiochemical characteristics of HES are **molar substitution (MS)**, **C_2/C_6** ratio and **molecular weight**. MS is defined as the mol hydroxyethyl residues per mol glucose subunits. According to MS, HES can be classified into solutions with **high (hetastarch, hexastarch**; 0.7 & 0.6 ie 7 & 6 HE groups for every 10 glucose units respectively), **medium (pentastarch**; 0.5), and **low substitution (tetrastarch ; 0.4).** Tetrastarch, pentastarch, and hexastarch are 40%, 50% and 60% etherified (ie 40/50/60 hydroxyethyl group for every 100 glucose unit) respectively. **High MS prolonges degradation.**
- **C_2/C_6 ratio** refers to pattern of hydroxyethylation at the carbon atoms of glucose rings and is considered **high (>8)** or **low (< 8).** HE groups at C_2 *position are being cleared more slowly, than at position 6; therefore* ***high $C_2/C6$ ratio solutions are being slowly degraded and have longer plasma life.***
- ***Plasma half life*** of HES solution **increases with increasing molecular weight** because low MW fraction (< 60 - 70KD) is rapidly excreted by kidneys, whereas larger molecules have to be hydrolysed by serum α-amylase before elimination.
- **HES (Hespan** = 6% solution in 0.9 NaCl) is **stored in reticuloendothelial system** for several hours. The **plasma expanding (volume) effect** primarily depends on *concentration* of HES. They are considered longer lasting (**4 hours**) as plasma expanders than **dextrans and gelatins/haemaccel (~ 2 hours)**
- HES **reduce whole blood viscosity**, thereby decreasing vascular resistance, enhancing vonous return and cardiac output (indirectly). Improved blow fluidity **improve microcirculation, tissue perfusion and oxygenation.**
- HES (esp 1st generation high MS-hetastarches) cause **coagulation abnormalities by decreasing the levels of Von Willebrand factor (VWF) and associated factor VIII activity** (acquired, type IvW like syndrome, more commonly in O blood group patients), **impairing platelet function** (coating), and **causing platelet damage.**
- HES (especially high concentration eg 10% HES or repeated use of high MS, and MW slowly degradable HES) administration causes hyperviscous urine, tubular stasis & obstruction, osmotic nephrosis like lesions (tubular cell swelling & vacuolization) and **acute renal failure**. So it is avoided in preexisting renal dysfunction; need for monitoring of renal function and renal replacement therapy is recommended for at least 90 days. HES is also avoided in critically ill adult patients (in ICU) including those with **sepsis** (FDA).
- **Pruritis**, d/t extravascular HES deposition after large volume administration, may occur after a latency period and may persist for weeks to months.
- **Allergic (hypersensitivity) reactions** may occur with HES; however the incidence is **lowest** compared with other colloids. **Gelatins, d/t bovine origin (produced by degradation of bovine collagen)** have hypothetical potential of transmitting **prion diseases** (eg bovine spongiform encephalopathy) and have **most frequent incidence of allergic reactions among all colloids (0.35% ie 6 times highe than HES)**Q.

QUESTIONS

VENOUS AIR EMBOLISM

1. A 40 yr old male with controlled thyrotoxicosis and Carcinoma rectum was undergoing laparcopic abdominoperineal resection, during which he was found to have decreased Blood Pressure and Heart Rate. On examination, a mill-wheal murmur was heard. The end tidal pCO_2 was observed found reducing from 40 to 10. What is the most likely diagnosis?

A. Air embolism *(DNB 02; AI 01)* ☐
B. Thyroid storm ☐
C. Blood loss ☐
D. Acute hypoxia ☐

2. 5 yr old child going to sitting craniotomy while positioning in O.T. developed End Tidal CO_2 0mm Hg PO_2 80 mm Hg implies

A. Endotracheal tube in oesophagus ☐
B. E.T. blocked with secretion ☐
C. Venous air Embolism *(AIIMS 2000)* ☐
D. Left lung collapse ☐

FAT EMBOLISM

3. Factors favouring fat embolism in a patient with major trauma : *(PGI 2001)*

A. Mobility of # ☐
B. Hypovolemic shock ☐
C. Resp. failure ☐
D. Diabetes ☐

RESPIRATORY COMPLICATIONS

4. The gas which produces systemic toxicity without causing local irritation is:

A. Ammonium *(AI 2002)* ☐
B. Carbon monoxide ☐
C. Hydrocyanic acid ☐
D. Sulfur dioxide ☐

5. True about aspiration pneumonia

A. Affected by volume of aspiration ☐
B. Affected by pH of aspiration fluid ☐
C. ↑Incidence during induction ☐
D. Inflammation *(PGI June 04)* ☐
E. Infection ☐

6. Upper respiratory tract infection is a common problem in children. All of the following anesthetic complications can occur in children with respiratory infections except-

A. Bacteremia *(AI 2002)* ☐
B. Halothane granuloma ☐
C. Increased mucosal bleeding ☐
D. Laryngospasm ☐

7. Mendelson syndrome is due to: *(PGI 1998)*

A. Aspiration pneumonitis ☐
B. Chemical pneumonitis ☐
C. Oesophagitis ☐
D. Oesophageal spasm ☐

8. Surgery done to prevent aspiration: *(PGI May 13)*

A. Tracheostomy ☐
B. Tracheoesophageal division ☐
C. Total laryngectomy ☐
D. Feeding gastrostomy ☐
E. Feeding jejunostomy ☐

AIP

9. Drugs contraindicated in AIP:

A. Thiopentone *(PGI Dec 07)* ☐
B. Etomidate ☐
C. Ketamine ☐
D. Propofol ☐
E. Midazolam ☐

10. The drug which is not suitable for patients with acute porphyria for intravenous induction is: *(AIIMS May 05)*

A. Thiopentone sodium ☐
B. Propofol ☐
C. Midazolam ☐
D. Etomidate ☐

11. A patient selected for surgery was induced with Thiopentone iv through one of anti cubital vein complains of severe pain of whole hand. The next line of management *(AIIMS 2001)*

A. Give IV propofol through same needle ☐
B. IV ketamine through same needle ☐
C. IV lignocaine through same needle ☐
D. Leave it done ☐

MALIGNANT HYPERTHERMIA

12. Feature of malignant hyperthermia includes: *(PGI May 12)*

A. Tachycardia ☐
B. Hypotension ☐
C. Excessive sweating ☐
D. ↓ed E_{TCO2} ☐
E. ↓ed O_2 saturation ☐

13. Malignant hyperthermia is most common with

A. Succinyl Choline *(AIIMS 1993, AI 95)* ☐
B. Gallamine ☐
C. Dantrolene ☐
D. Ketamine ☐

14. Which of the increases chances of malignant hyperthermia: *(PGI May 13)*

A. Diazepam ☐
B. Halothane ☐
C. Suxamethoium ☐
D. Nitrous oxide ☐
E. Ketamine ☐

15. Which of the following anesthetic agents does not trigger malignant hyperthermia?

A. Halothane *(AI 06)* ☐
B. Isoflurane ☐
C. Suxamethonium ☐
D. Thiopentone ☐

16. All the following cause malignant hyperpyrexia except -

A. N_2O *(Karnataka 05)* ☐
B. Halothane ☐
C. Methoxyflurane ☐
D. Isoflurane ☐

17. All are seen in malignant hyperthermia except:

A. Bradycardia *(AIIMS May 2007)* ☐
B. Hyperkalemia ☐
C. Metabolic acidosis ☐
D. Hypertension ☐

18. Which of the following is true about malignant hyperthermia *(AIIMS May 10)*

A. Hypernatremia ☐

B. Hypercalcemia ☐
C. Hyperkalemia ☐
D. Hypothermia ☐

19. **About malignant hyperthermia true:** *(PGI June 08)*
A. Succinylcholine & Halothane predisposes ☐
B. Dantrolene usefull in all cases ☐
C. Ketanserine can be used as an alternative to Dantrolene ☐
D. Propofol is safe ☐
E. Muscle biopsy is diagnostic ☐

20. **Treatment of malignant Hyperthermia includes:**
A. Dantrolene *(PGI Dec 08)* ☐
B. Cooling ☐
C. Deepening plane of inhalational anaesthesia ☐
D. Discontinue inhalational anesthesia ☐
E. Give O_2 therapy with 100% O_2 ☐

21. **Hyperthermia is caused by:** *(PGI 2002)*
A. Anticholinnergics ☐
B. MAO inhibitors ☐
C. Lithium ☐
D. Chlorpromazine ☐
E. Carbimazole ☐

22. **Hypothermia is used in :** *(PGI 2000)*
A. Hyperpyrexia ☐
B. Prolonged surgeries ☐
C. Massive blood transfusion ☐
D. Hypertension ☐

23. **During surgery after inhalational anesthesia a patient suddenly developed, fever, increased heart rate and BP, acidosis and arrhythmia. What is your first step of intervention** *(AIIMS May 12)*
A. Dantrolene ☐
B. Sodium bicarbonate ☐
C. Procainamide ☐
D. Antipyretics ☐

24. **Which of the following agents is used for the treatment of postoperative shivering?** *(AI 06, DNB 02)*
A. Thiopentone ☐
B. Suxamethonium ☐
C. Atropine ☐
D. Pethidine ☐

25. **In a young patient who had extensive soft tissue and muscle injury, which of these muscle relaxants used for endotracheal intubation might lead to cardiac arrest :**
A. Atracurium. *(AIIMS 2003)* ☐
B. Suxamethonium. ☐
C. Vecuronium. ☐
D. Pancuronium. ☐

26. **The use of succinylcholine is not contraindicated in:**
A. Tetanus *(AIIMS 2002)* ☐
B. Closed head injury ☐
C. Cerebral stroke ☐
D. Hepatic failure ☐

27. **Adiministration of Scoline (Sch) produces dangerous hyperkalamia in** *(AIIMS 1999)*
A. Acute Renal Failure (A.R.F.) ☐
B. Raised ICT ☐
C. Fracture femur ☐
D. Paraplegia ☐

28. **The administration of succinylocholine to a paraplegic patient led to the appearance of dysarrhythmias, conduction abnormalities and finally cardiac arrest. The most likely cause is** *(AIIMS 2003)*
A. Hypercalcemia ☐
B. Hyperkalemia ☐
C. Anaphylaxis ☐
D. Hypermagnesemia ☐

29. **Hyper K^+ due to scoline is seen in all except** *(AIIMS 2000)*
A. Crush injury ☐
B. Burn ☐
C. Abdominal sepsis ☐
D. Muscular dystrophy ☐

MYSTHENIA GRAVIS

30. **In myasthenia gravis, which druges should not be used :**
A. Gallamine *(PGI 2002)* ☐
B. Neostigmine ☐
C. Aminoglycosides ☐
D. Metronidazole ☐
E. Ampiciliin ☐

TENSIONS

31. **Which of the following anaesthetic agents causes a rise in the Intracranial pressure:**
A. Sevoflurane. *(DNB 07, AI 05)* ☐
B. Thiopentone sodium. ☐
C. Lignocaine. ☐
D. Propofol. ☐

32. **↑ ICT is treated by A/E** *(AIIMS 1992)*
A. IV mannitol ☐
B. IV Frusemide ☐
C. Controlled Hyperventilation ☐
D. Addition of positive end respiratory pressure ☐

33. **Cause of post operative hypertension** *(PGI 04)*
A. Pre-operative hypertension ☐
B. Inadequate analgesia ☐
C. Phaeochromocytoma ☐
D. Hypoxemia ☐
E. Hypercarbia ☐

34. **Which of the following agents is not used to provide induced hypotension during surgery?** *(AI 06, DNB 07)*
A. Sodium nitroprusside ☐
B. Hydralazine ☐
C. Mephenteramine ☐
D. Esmolol ☐

CARDIAC COMPLICATIONS & CPR

35. **The outcome following resuscitation of cardiac arrest is worsened if during resuscitation patient is given:**
A. Ringer's lactate *(AIIMS Nov 2005)* ☐
B. Colloids ☐
C. 5% Dextrose ☐
D. Whole blood transfusion ☐

36. **The most common rhythm disturbance during early post-operative period is:** *(AIIMS 05, DNB 06)*
A. Bradycardia ☐
B. Ventricular fibrillation ☐
C. Tachycardia ☐
D. Complete heart block ☐

37. **Use of Intraarterial cannula in major surgery :** *(PGI 2005)*
A. Measurement of direct intra arterial BP ☐
B. Sample for ABG ☐
C. Drug injection ☐
D. BT ☐

38. **In an injured patient with hypovolemia intr-avenous fluid administerved is guided by:**
A. Central venous pressure *(PGI 2003)* ☐
B. Blood pressure ☐
C. Urine output ☐
D. Pulse rate ☐

39. **Importance of CVP measurements is :**
   A. Need for blood transfusion *(PGI 2001)* □
   B. Assess amount of fluid to be given □
   C. Need for inotropic support □
   D. Rate of intravenous fluid replacement □
   E. Assess need for plasma transfusion □

40. **In a patient.with cardiorespiratory arrest, basic life support is given to support which of the following systems:** *(PGI 2001)*
   A. Respiratory system □
   B. Cardiovascular system □
   C. Renal system □
   D. Gastrointestinal system □
   E. CNS □

41. **In a patient with multiple injuries, first thing to be done is:** *(PGI 1999)*
   A. Patency of airway □
   B. Maintenance of B.P □
   C. Immobilize cervical spine □
   D. Lateral position with mouth gag □

42. **First step in CPR (cardio pulmonary resuciatation) should be :** *(PGI 2000)*
   A. IV adrenaline □
   B. Intracardic atropine □
   C. Airway maintainance □
   D. Hystrectomy □

43. **True about adrenaline in CPR :** *(PGI 2001)*
   A. Can be given intratracheally □
   B. I.V. route better than intracardiac □
   C. Intracardiac route better than IV □
   D. Converts coarse fibrillation into fine ones □
   E. The dose used is 2ml. containing 1 in 1000 concentration □

44. **According to 2005 AHA guidelines true about no of chest compression in CPR:** *(PGI Dec 2007)*
   A. 80/min including neonate □
   B. 90/min including neonate □
   C. 100/min excluding neonate □
   D. 120/min including neonate □
   E. 120/min excluding neonate □

45. **During cardiac resuscitation, the follwing can occur except :** *(PGI 2001)*
   A. Rupture of Lungs □
   B. Rupture of liver □
   C. Rupture of Stomach □
   D. Rupture of Spleen □
   E. Disseminated intravascular coagulation occurs □

46. **A man posted for elective laparoscopic cholecystectomy. All pre-anesthetic check up was normal. After connecting the monitors and administering IV antibiotics, patient suddenly becomes pulseless and unresponsive. Next appropriate step:** *(AIIMS May 13)*
   A. Check for breathing □
   B. Call abulane □
   C. Start chest compression □
   D. Give two breaths □

47. **An infant with respiratory distress was intubated. The fastest and accurate method to confirm intubation:**
   A. Capnography *(AIIMS Nov 12)* □
   B. Clinically by auscultation □
   C. Chest radiography □
   D. Airway pressure measurement □

48. **Heparin interferes with which of the following results of ABG** *(DNB 03, UP 06)*
   A. PO_2 □
   B. PCO_2 □
   C. pH □
   D. HCO_3 □
   E. Anion gap □

49. **During intraoperative anaesthesia mismatch BT develops:**
   A. Increased bleeding *(PGI Dec 2007)* □
   B. Hypotension □
   C. Bronchospasm □
   D. Rash □
   E. Movements of limbs □

50. **Mismatched blood transfusion manifests intraoperatively as:** *(PGI 1999)*
   A. Rise in B.P. □
   B. Excessive bleeding □
   C. Dyspnoea □
   D. Hematuria □

51. **Drugs which interfere with anesthesia are :**
   A. Calcium channel blocker nifedipine □
   B. Beta blockers *(PGI 2001)* □
   C. Aminoglycosides □
   D. Steroid administration □
   E. D-tubocurar □

52. **Calcium channel blockers in anesthesia, True is :**
   A. Needs to be decreased as they augment hypotension & muscle relaxation *(PGI 2000)* □
   B. Withheld because they lower LES pressure □
   C. Should be given in normal doses as they prevent MI & angina □
   D. All of the above □

53. **Lithium should be stopped how many days before anesthesia?** *(AIIMS May 13)*
   A. 1 □
   B. 2 □
   C. 3 □
   D. 4 □

OTHER

54. **True statement related to use of hyroxyetheyl starch:**
   A. Cause coagulation abnormality due to factor X decidiency *(AIIMS May 13)* □
   B. It is amylopectin etherified with hyroxyethyl group □
   C. Hypersensitivity similar to gelatin □
   D. Obtained from fermentation of gelatin/collagen □

55. **In a 10 year old child presented with anaphylactic shock, drug of choice is:**
   A. I/V adrenaline *(PGI 1997)* □
   B. S.C. adrenaline □
   C. Anti histamine □
   D. Corticosteroids □

56. **In status epilepticus, drug of choice is:**
   A. I/V diazepam *(PGI 1997)* □
   B. I/M diazepam □
   C. Oral clonazepam □
   D. I/M phenytoin □

57. **In belladona poisoning, antidote is:**
   A. Physostigmine *(PGI 1997)* □
   B. Neostigmine □
   C. Anti histamine □
   D. Atropine □

58. **Atropine is used in following except:**
   A. Glaucoma *(PGI 1997)* □
   B. Mushroom poisoning □
   C. Malathion poisoning □
   D. Organophosphorous poisoning □

Answers and Explanations:

VENOUS AIR EMBOLISM

1. **A i.e. Air embolism** *[Ref: Aitkenhead 5/e p-389; Morgan 4/e p-638-39; Wylie 7/e p-665-66, 1143, 711-12]*
2. **C i.e. Venous Air embolism**

A patient undergoing *lapro/thoraco-scopy*[Q] or procedure *(eg craniotomy) in sitting, head up*[Q], park-bench, knee-chest positions that place the operative site above the right atrium carry an increased risk of VAE. ***Sudden decrease in end-tidal CO_2 concentration (E_TCO_2), sudden hypotension/circulatory arrest and Mill wheel murmur indicate the diagnosis***[Q].

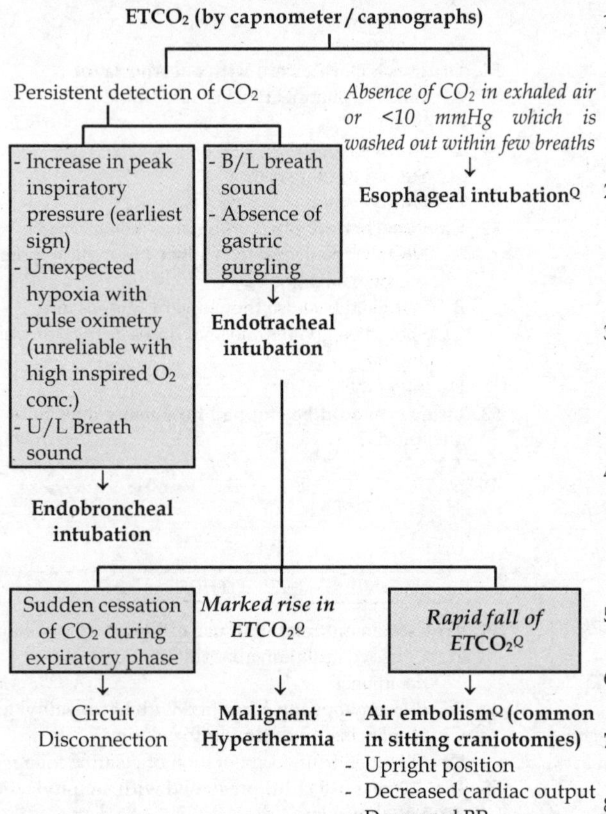

1. *Preventing esophageal intubation* depends on direct visualization of the ETT passing through vocal cord, auscultation for presence of bilateral breath sounds, absence of gastric gurgling, *analysis of exhaled gas for the presence of CO_2 (most reliable method)*, chest radiography or use of fiber optic bronchoscopy.
2. ***Capnographs (detection of $ETCO_2$) rapidly & reliably indicate esophageal intubation,*** but do not reliably detect endobronchial intubation while *there may be some CO_2 in the stomach from swallowing* ***expired air (<10 mmHg)****, this should* ***be washed out within a few breaths.***[Q]
3. *Although persistent detection of CO_2 by a capnograph is the best confirmation of tracheal placement of an endotracheal tube*[Q] (ETT); it connot exclude endobronchial intubation. ***The earliest manifestation of endobronchial intubation is an increase in peak inspiratory pressure***[Q]
4. Over insertion usually results in intubation of right main stem bronchus because of its less acute angle. Clues to the *diagnosis of endobronchial intubation include unilateral breath sounds,* ***unexpected hypoxia with pulse oximetry (unreliable with high inspired O_2 concentration)***[Q]
5. ***A rapid fall of ET CO_2 is a sensitive indicator of air embolism a major complication of sitting craniotomies.***[Q]
6. Sudden cessation of CO_2 during expiratory phase may indicate a circuit disconnection.
7. The increased metabolic rate caused by malignant hyperthermia causes marked rise in $ETCO_2$
8. *Any significant reduction in lung perfusion (eg. air embolism,* upright position, decreased cardiac output or decreased blood pressure) increases alveolar dead space, dilutes expiratory CO_2 & lessens $ETCO_2$[Q].

FAT EMBOLISM

3. **A i.e. Mobility of #; D i.e. Diabetes** *[Ref: Harsh Mohan – 123]*

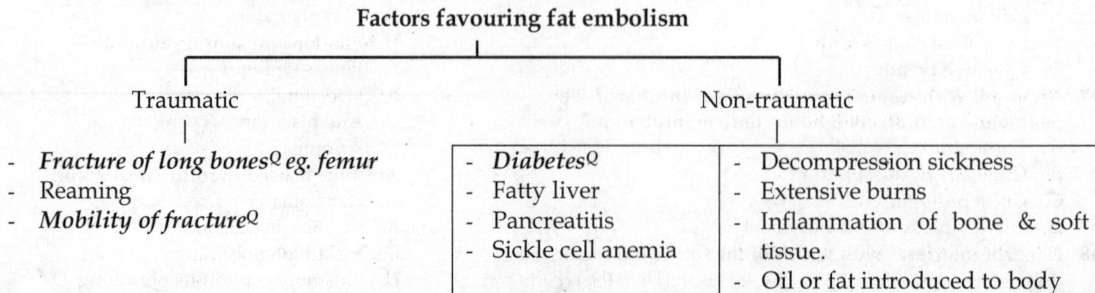

RESPIRATORY COMPLICATIONS

4. **B i.e. Carbon Monoxide** *[Ref: Harrison 15th/e P-2606; Reddy 16/e P-506; Morgan's 3/e, P-974,802, 144]*

Carbon Monoxide Poisoning

- CO is a colourless, tasteless, ***non irritant gas***Q which is produced due to incomplete combustion of carbon.
- CO poisoning is defined as > ***15 % carboxyhemoglobin***Q in blood (normal < 1.5 % in nonsmokers, < 10 % in smokers).
- Diagnosis is made by ***cooximetric*** measurements of blood not by pulse oxymeter.
- CO has *200 – 300 times* the affinity of O_2 for hemoglobin.
- It decreases the affinity of O_2 and *shifts hemoglobin dissociation curve to right.*
- Toxicity may be due to smoke inhalation or *by degradation of desflurane* by CO_2 absorbent [particularly Ba $(OH)_2$ lime but also NaOH & KOH]
- *Lower levels* produce systemic toxicity because of binding with *cytochrome-c & myoglobin* and *higher levels* produce toxicity due to binding with *Hemoglobin* leading to tissue hypoxia.

5. **All i.e. A, B, C, D, E**

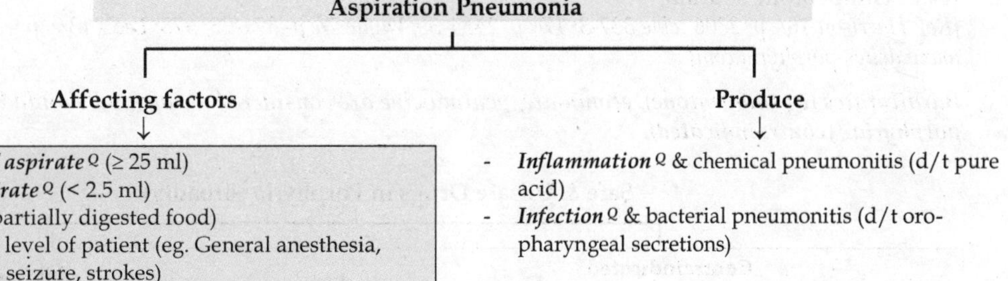

Aspiration Pneumonia
Affecting factors
Produce
- Volume of aspirate Q (≥ 25 ml)
- pH of aspirate Q (< 2.5 ml)
- Content (partially digested food)
- Conscious level of patient (eg. General anesthesia, alcoholics, seizure, strokes)
- Mechanical impediments (e.g. nasogastric or enotracheal tube)
- Inflammation Q & chemical pneumonitis (d/t pure acid)
- Infection Q & bacterial pneumonitis (d/t oro-pharyngeal secretions)

Note: ***Incidence is increased during induction of G.A.*** Q d/t introduction of tubes, and increased intraabdominal pressure.

6. **B i.e. Halothane granuloma** *[Ref: Lee's Anesthesia P-168; Morgan's clinical Anesthesiology 3/e P-140]*

- Due to local infection there is hyperemia of the local area & trauma can result in mucosal bleeding
- Due to local edema & inflammation, laryngospasm can be a complication
- Systemic infection can lead to Bacteremia
- ***Halothane toxicity more common in obese & elderly women; rare in children***Q
- Halothane
  - *attenuates airway reflexes & relaxes bronchial smooth muscles* by inhibiting intracellular Ca^{++} mobilization.
  - ***best bronchodilator***Q, this action is ***not inhibited by propranolol (B- Blocker)***
  - *depresses clearance of mucus* from respiratory tract promoting post op hypoxia & atlectasis.

7. **A i.e. Aspiration pneumonitis** *[Ref: Morgan 5/e p. 887]*

- **Sellick's manuvere** is application of *backward pressure on cricoid cartilage to prevent gastric aspiration* ***(Mandelson's syndrome).***Q
- **Mendelson's syndrome** is ***acid aspiration***Q syndrome.

8. **A i.e. Tracheotomy; B i.e. Tracheoesophageal division; D i.e. Feeding gastrostomy; E i.e. Feeding jejunostomy** *[Ref: http//emedicine.medscape.com/article; http:/www.ncbi.nim.gov/pmc/articles/PMC2494386]*

Surgery done to prevent aspiration include **partial (not total) laryngectomy, cuffed tracheotomy** (blocking respiratory tract), **trachea-oesophageal division** and **laryngo-tracheal seqeration** (separating respiratory & alimentary tract), and **feeding gastrostomy/jejunostion** (ie feeding from below the possible level of aspiration).

Surgical Management to Prevent Intractable Aspiration

Laryngeal Procedures

- Reversible laryngeal closure by epiglottic flap
- Vocal cord medialization
- Total/partial cricoidectomy
- **Laryngeal suspension**
- **Laryngectomy** (partial preferred, total avoided)

Alimentary Procedures

- ***Feeding gastrostomy***[Q]
- ***Feeding jejunostomy***[Q]
- Gastric fundoplication
- Cricopharyngeal myotomy

Tracheo-oesophageal diversion (division) and Laryngotracheal Separation Proceding

- ***Cuffed Tracheotomy***[Q]
- Endolaryngeal stent
- Supraglottic closure
- Complete separation of alimentary & respiratory tracts eg partial & subperichondrial cricoidectomy, narrow field laryngectomy[Q], **tracheo-oesophageal diversion and laryngo-tracheal separation.**

AIP

9. **A i.e. Thiopentone > B i.e. Etomidate**
10. **A i.e. Thiopentone sodium**

[Ref: Harrison 16/e p. 2306 table 337-3; 17th p. 2434-39; Wylie 7/e p- 371-73, 573; Lee's 13/e ,p – 50-51, 156, 357 www.drugs-porphyria.com]

Barbiturates (eg thiopentone), etomidate, pentazocine are considered unsafe and should be avoided in porphyria[Q] (contraindicated).

Safe & Unsafe Drugs in Porphyria (Broadly)

Contraindicated		Safe
- Alcohol	- Griseofulvin	- Narcotic analgesics
- ***Barbiturates (Thiopentone)***[Q]	- Meprobamate	- Aspirin
- Carbamazapine	- Mephenytoin	- Acetaminophen
- Danazol	- Methyprylon	- Atropine
- Ergots	- Pyrazolones	- Bromides
- Estrogens & Progesterogens	- Succinimides	- Glucocorticoids
- Glutethimide	- Sulfonamides	- Insulin
	- Valproic acid	- Streptomycin
		- Phenothiazines
		- Penicillin & derivatives

11. **C i.e. IV lignocaine through same needle** *[Ref: Lee 12/e P-180; Morgan's 3/e, P-157]*

Anticubital vein is not right place to give thiopentone injection as the artery lies adjacent to vein. ***Pain** is first symptom of intraarterial injection & **cynosis of nail with white hand** is 1st sign*[Q]. Management includes-

- ***Never remove needle***[Q]
- Through same needle give
  - Saline for dilution
  - Heparin for anticoagulation
  - Papavarin
  - ***Procaine / Xylocaine for pain***[Q]
  - Hydrocortisone
- ***Stellate ganglion / Brachial Plexus block***[Q]

MALIGNANT HYPERTHERMIA

12. **A i.e. Tachycardia; C i.e. Excessive sweating; E i.e. ↓O_2 saturation**
13. **A i.e. Succinyl choline**
14. **B, C i.e. Halothane, Suxamethoium**
15. **D i.e. Thiopentone**
16. **A i.e. N_2O**
17. **A i.e. Bradycardia**
18. **C i.e. Hyperkalemia**
19. **A. i.e. Succinyl choline & halothane predispose B. i.e. Dantrolene useful in all cases D. i.e. propofol is safe E. i.e. Muscle biopsy is diagnostic**

20. **A.i.e. Dantrolene; B. i.e. Cooling; D. i.e. Discontinue inhalational anesthesia; E. i.e. Give O_2 therapy with 100% O_2**

21. **B i.e. MAO inhibitor**

22. **A & B i.e. Hyperpyrexia & prolonged surgeries**

[Ref: Miller's 7/e p. 1180-89; Katzung 8th/e p. 428; Lee's 13/e p. 352-54; Morgan's 5/e p. 1185-90; Wylie 7/e p. 365-67]

- **Features of malignant hyperthermia** include **increased E_{TCO2} (often the first & most sensitive early sign), decreased O_2 saturation (falling SpO_2** despite increase in FiO_2), **cynosis, tachycardia, tachypnea and hypertension (or unstable BP)Q.**
- ***Thiopentone & pancuronium are protective drugs for malignant hyperthermia*Q** as these raise the triggering threshold. In malignant hyperthermia susceptible patients, safe anesthetics are **N₂O, No**ndepolarizing muscle relaxants, opiates, tranquilizers, *etomidate, barbiturates (thiopentone), benzodiazepines, propofol*Q, *ketamine*Q (Mn **"NOTE BP KIT"**) and regional anesthesia.
- Drugs causing malignant hyperthermia are – ***succinyl choline (most common cause)*Q, *halothane (mc inhalational agent)*Q**, iso/des/sevo/methoxy –flurane, lignocaine, TCA ***MAO inhibitors*Q** & phenothiazines. Pediatric age & muscle dystrophy predispose to MH.
- *Hyperthermia, hyperkalemia* (most imp), hypernatremia, hyperphosphatemia and myoglobinuria indicate muscle damage.
- ***Discontinuation of all anesthetic agents, hyperventilation with 100% O_2, dantrolene, $NaHCO_3$ and cooling measure*Q** are used in treatment.

23. **A i.e. Dantrolene**

Sudden development of fever, tachycardia, hypertension arrhythmia and acidosis after inhalational anesthesia (most probably halogenated drug) or muscle relaxant succinylcholine suggest an episode of **malignant hyperthermia**. ***The triggering agent must be stopped and dantrolene must be given immediately*Q.**

24. **D i.e. Pethidine** *[Ref: Ajay Yadav 1/e p. 101]*

- In anaesthesia, shivering occurs as a protective mechanism as inhalational agents, spinal/epidural block causes vasodilatation leading to heat loss. Shivering can be abolished by inhibition of hypothalamus.
- *Halothane most commonly leads to shivering.*
- Treatment of shivering
  1. ***Pethidine or pentazocine*Q**
  2. Oxygen inhalation. Oxygen consumption may increase upto 4 times (400%) during shivering. So oxygen inhalation during shivering is mandatory.

25. **B i.e. Suxamethonium** 26. **D i.e. Hepatic failure** 27. **D i.e. Paraplegia**

28. **B i.e. Hyperkalemia** 29. **C i.e. Abdominal sepsis**

[Ref: Ganong 21/e P-102; Millar anesthesia 5/e P-419, 420 & 423; Morgan's anesthesiology 4/e p 207-223]

- Succinyl choline may cause **life threatning hyperkalemia** in ***Burn injury*Q, *Massive trauma* Q, *Neurological disorder (ex. paraplegia)* Q, *Tetanus* Q *and Extensive soft tissue & muscle injury*Q.** Maximum chances of hyperkalemia is usually in 7-10 days following injury and between 3 days & 6 months after onset of paraplegia. Hyperkalemia may lead to cardiac arrest refractory to routine CPR. Duration of action is prolonged in Pregnancy, Hypothermia, liver failure, Renal failure, Low level of Pseudocholinestrase.
- ***The Sch is mainly metabolized by plasma pseudocholinesterase enzyme; so it is not contraindicated in hepatic failure.*Q Conditions causing susceptibility to succinylcholine induced hyperkalemia** and l/t cardiac dysarrythmias & cardiac arrest

1. Acidosis	10. Prolonged total body immobilization
2. Burns	11. Severe Parkinson's disease
3. Barre Gullian Syndrome	12. ***Severe intra abdominal infection*Q**
4. ***Closed Head injury*Q**	**13. *Spinal cord injury (paraplegia*Q)**
5. ***Cerebral Aneurysm Rupture (Cerebral stroke)* Q**	14. ***Stroke*Q**
6. Drowning (Near Drowning)	15. ***Massive Trauma*Q** *causing extensive soft tissue & muscle injury*
7. Encephalitis	16. ***Myopathy (like Duchenne's dystrophy)*Q**
8. Haemorrhagic shock with metabolic acidosis	17. Near drowning, Neurological disorders
9. Polyneuropathy	18. ***Tetanus*Q**

MYSTHENIA GRAVIS

30. A i.e. Gallamine; C i.e. Aminoglycoside *[Ref: Lee 12/e P-344-346; Harrison 15/e P-2515]*

- **Drugs C/I in myasthenia gravis are:**
  1. ***Aminoglycosides***[Q]
  2. Tetracyclines
  3. Polypeptide antibodies.
  4. Procainamide
  5. Penicillamine
  6. B-Blocker
- M.G. patients are ***hypersensitive to non depolarizing M.R.***[Q] (*ex gallamine*). So these are avoided (but small dose of short acting like mivacurium may be used). Myasthenics are **resistant** to ***depolarizing M.R. like Sch & decamethonium***[Q]. ***Neostigmine***[Q] & Pyridostigmine are used in treatment.

TENSIONS

31. A i.e. Sevoflurane **32. D i.e. Addition of positive end respiratory pressure**
[Ref: Rowbotham & Smith 4/e p159; Aitkinhead 4/e p159; Morgan 3/e p. 138, 558, 568, 569]

Intracranial pressure is increased at high inspired concentrations of sevoflurane but this effect is minimal over the 0.5-1.0 MAC range.

Management of raised intracranial tension (ICT) is:

1. ***IV Mannitol***[Q],
2. ***Loop diuretic***[Q] (*furosemide*[Q]) and other diuretics.
3. ***Hyperventilation***[Q] ($PaCO_2$ 25-30 mmHg)
4. Fluid restriction
5. Osmotic agents
6. ***Corticosteroid (Dexamethasone)***[Q] for vasogenic edema of tumors.

33. All i.e. A, B, C, D, E *[Ref: Wylie 7/e p. 214-15]*

Causes of post operative hypertension

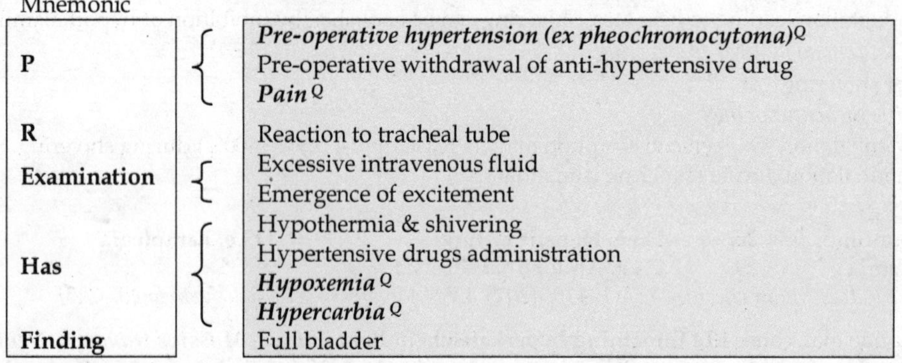

Mnemonic	
P	***Pre-operative hypertension (ex pheochromocytoma)***[Q] Pre-operative withdrawal of anti-hypertensive drug ***Pain***[Q]
R	Reaction to tracheal tube
Examination	Excessive intravenous fluid Emergence of excitement
Has	Hypothermia & shivering Hypertensive drugs administration ***Hypoxemia***[Q] ***Hypercarbia***[Q]
Finding	Full bladder

34. C i.e. Mephenteramine *[Ref: KDT 4/e p. 112]*

Sodium nitroprusside, hydralazine and esmolol are used to produce hypotension. While ***mephentermine is used to protect against hypotension during spinal anesthesia***[Q].

CARDIAC COMPLICATIONS & CPR

35. C i.e. 5% Dextrose *[Ref. Oxford surgery p-8-11]*

- ***Glucose containing solutions should not be used in I.V. lines during treatment of shock or cardiac arrest***[Q] because the amount needed to maintain B.P. would cause pulmonary edema and congestive heart failure d/t volume overload.
- ***In high risk patients, I.V. glucose solutions should be avoided***[Q] or used judiciously and blood glucose concentration should be maintained within the normoglycemic range until the patients have passed the period of high risk for hemodynamic compromise.

36. **C i.e. Tachycardia** *[Ref: Miller's anaesthesia 6/e p. 2717, 1398]*

Sinus tachycardia is most commonly occurring arrhythmia in the perioperative period.Q

It occurs with such frequency that it is not included in most incidence studies.

Postoperative dysrrthmias

Common Types	Predisposing factors
- *Sinus tachycardia (m.c.)* Q - Sinus bradycardia - Ventricular premature beats - Ventricular tachycardia - Supraventricular tachyarrhythmias	- Electrolyte imbalance(especially hypokalemia) - Hypoxia - Hypercarbia - Hyperthermia (fever) - Heart disease (preexisting) - Metabolic alkalosis and acidosis - Inadequate anesthesia - Pain

37. **A, B, C, D** *[Ref: Lee 12/e P-137, 622]*

Use of intra-arterial cannula in major surgery

1. ***Arterial blood sampling***Q (ex ABG measurement)
2. ***Intra-arterial BP measurement***Q
3. ***Drug injection***Q eg. local analgesics.
4. Expected large blood or fluid loss
5. To treat severe prolonged hypotension
6. Non pulsatile arterial flow (eg. cardiopulmonary bypass)

38. **A i.e. CVP; B i.e. BP; C i.e. U.O.; D i.e. P.R.** *[Ref: BL 23/e P-58-59]*

In hypovolemic patient, the adequacy of IV fluid replacement can be assessed by–

- ***Blood pressure***Q
- ***Pulse rate***Q
- ***Urine out put***Q
- ***Central venous pressure***Q (CVP)
- ***Pulmonary capillary wedge pressure***Q (PCWP)

39. **A i.e. Need for blood transfusion; D i.e. Rate of intravenous fluid replacement; E i.e. Assess need for plasma transfusion** *[Ref: Lee 3/e P-141]*

- CVP is useful means of assessing the circulating blood volume and therefore appropriate for
  1. ***Measuring rate of I.V. fluid replacement***Q
  2. ***Assessing need for blood & plasma transfusion***Q
- CVP is not a good guide for daily fluid requirement eg. A patient can easily be waterloaded or dehydrated in presence of normal CVP.

40. **A i.e. Respiratory system; B i.e. Cardiovascular system; E i.e. CNS**
41. **A i.e. Patency of airway**
42. **C i.e. Airway maintenance**
43. **A & B i.e. Can be given intra tracheally & I.V. route is better than intracardiac**
44. **C i.e. 100/min excluding neonate**
45. **E i.e. Disseminated intravenous coagulation**
46. **C i.e. Start chest compression** *[Ref: Harrison 18/e p. 2240-44; Pardo 6/e p. 718-726; Miller 7/e p. 2971-3001;*
47. **A i.e. Capnography** *Morgan 3/e p. 1231-37, 872-73; Wylie 7/e p. 1199-1211; Ajay Yadav 5/e p. 252-5]*

- Goal of CPR or Basic life support is **to maintain functioning of vital organ systems** – ***CNS, CVS, Respiratory***Q
- **Sequence of management in CPR / multitrauma patient / severely ill patient** is (According to ILCOR-2000). **ABCD=** ***<u>A</u>irway patency***Q**,** ***<u>B</u>reathing***Q**,** ***<u>C</u>irculation***Q**, <u>D</u>efibrillation**
- However, the **sequence of steps in CPR or CPCR or CPRECC has been changed in 2010 guidelines** (by AHA & ILCOR) **from ABC (airway and breathing first, before compression) to CAB (compression first with airway and breathing treated later)**. Both CAB and ABC sequences are in use in various parts of world. However, **circulation always takes precedence over airway and breathing in a cardiac arrest (pulseless) situation. So in this scenario, chest compression should begin prior to initial breaths.**Q

- According to **2005 AHA guidelines, number of chest compression** in CPR is **120/min in neonates; > 100/min in infants and 100/min in children and adult (ie 100 /min in all excluding neonates).**
- **Epinephrine (adrenaline)** in CPR is given in dose of **1mg (10 ml of a 1:10000 solution) repeated every 3-5 minutes through central or peripheral venous line, intra tracheal route** (dosage 2-2.5 times higher) or **intraosseous route** (in children). Contrary to general belief that **epinephrine increases the amplitude of ventricular fibrillation (β adrenergic effect) and makes defibrillation easier**, clinical studies have shown no effect on defibrillation success (Wylie). **Adrenaline converts fine fibrillations to coarse ones**Q.
- **During CPR (d/t chest compression & Heimlich maneuver), fracture of sternum and ribs** (very rarely vertebrae)**, trauma to internal viscera eg rupture of lung, liver, spleen & stomach** and **regurgitation** may occur (but not DIC). DIC is usually seen in massive trauma, burn & surgery.
- **The 2010 CPR-ECC guidelines** recommend a **TT (tracheal tube) as the airway adjunct of choice** (if persons skilled in placing it are available). And rescuers must **confirm TT placement with a PETco$_2$ detector**-an **indicator** a **capnograph** or a **capnometric device.** The **best choice for confirmation of TT placement is continuous capnographic waveform analysis**Q. All confirmation devices are considered adjuncts to clinical confirmation techniques eg auscultation.

48. **C i.e. pH** *[Ref: KDT 5/e P-561]*

Heparin is *strongest organic acid* present in body, so it can decrease **pH.**

49. **A i.e. Increased bleeding; B i.e. Hypotension; C i.e. Bronchospasm; D i.e. Rash**
50. **B i.e. Excessive bleeding** *[Ref: Lee's Synopsis of Anaesthesia 12/e p. 30]*

Mismatched blood transfusion is anesthetized patient present as:

1. *General oozing from wound (excessive bleeding)*Q
2. *Severe & progressive hypotension*Q
3. Tachycardia
4. *Urticarial rash*Q
5. *Bronchospasm*Q, raising airway pressure on intermittent positive pressure ventilation
6. Later jaundice & oliguria (5-10%)

51. **A i.e. Calcium channel blockers; B i.e. Beta Blockers; C i.e. Aminoglycoside**

- *Aminoglycoside, Tetracycline & Polypeptide antibiotics*Q (Mnemonic ATP) potentiate **neuromuscular block**
- *B Blockers & Calcium channel blocker*Q may cause **Bradycardia & AV block** with anesthesia

52. **C i.e. Should be given in normal dose as they prevent MI & Angina** *[Ref: Miller 7/e p. 525-26, 1135-36, 1140]*

Calcium channel blockers potentiate neuromuscular-block, cause lowering of muscle tone of lower esophageal sphincter but there is no such indication of stoppage of this drug during anesthesia. ***CCB's prevent MI & angina during anesthesia & should be given in normal doses (preoperatively)*Q.**

53. **B i.e. 2** *[Ref: Lee's 13/e p 26; Miller's 7/e p 886; Morgan 5/e p 625]*

- **Antihypertensive drugs** (except **ACE** & **angiotensin II receptor blockers?), antianginal drugs (calcium channel blockers or nitrates)** and **levodopa are continued upto the time of surgery** to prevent precipitation of hypotonsion, angina and Parkinsonism respectively.
- Drugs stopped before surgery include **lithium (2 days before), nonspecific MAO inhibitors (2 weeks before) and oestrogen containing combined OCP (4 weeks before surgery).**

OTHER

54. **B i.e. It is amylopection etherified with hyroxyethyl group** *[Ref: Washington Manual of Medicine 31st /40; Ajay Yadav 5/e p. 13-14; Lee 13/e p. 233; Miller 7/e p 1762-63, 2799-2800, 1727]*

HES is **amylopectin etherified with hydroxyethyl starch.** It causes coagulation abnormalities by **decreasing vWF level and factor 8 (not 10) activity**Q, impairing platelet function and causing platelet damage. Its **hypersensitivity is least among colloid; 6 times lesser than gelatins**Q**. Gelatins are obtained from degradation of bovine collagen.**

55. **A i.e. IV adrenaline** *[Ref: Lee 12/e P–294, 295; Roxburgh's 17/e p. 93]*

Intravenous adrenaline is the drug of choice in anaphylactic shock.

Treatment of Anaphylactic shock

Main stay / TOC	Other modes of t/t
- *IV-adrenaline*[Q] 1 μg/kg upto 1 mg - If IV access is not available, the *IM/ intrathecal route is used*	- *IV-Corticosteroids*[Q] - Antihistamines - Bronchodialators (aminophylline or salbutamol) - Bicarbonates (for acidosis) - IPPV

56. **A i.e. IV diazepam**
[Ref: Harrison 15/e P–2368; OPG 5/e P-413]

Status epilepticus is said to occur when seizures lasts beyond 30 minutes or seizures are repetitive, prolonged & the patient remains unconscious in between the seizures. The drug of choice is ***IV Lorazepam (Benzodiazipine)***[Q] 0.1 mg/kg at rate of 2 mg/min. Pharmacologic treatment of generalized tonic-clonic status epilepticus in adults. IV, intravenous, PE, phenytoin equivalents. The horizontal bars indicate the approximate duration of drug infusion.

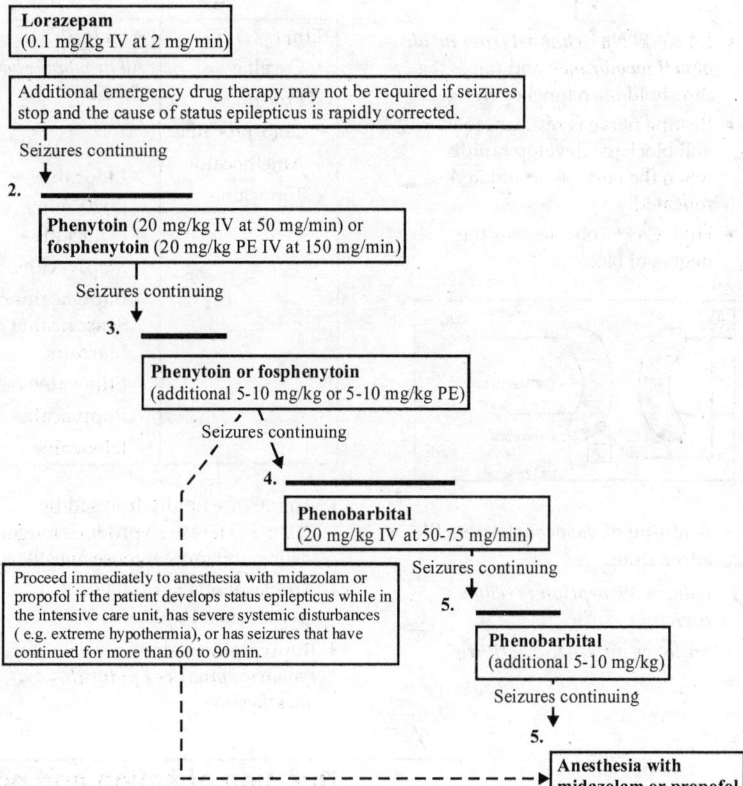

57. **A i.e. Physostigmine** *[Ref: KDT 4/e P–112]*

Belladona Poisoning

- May occur due to consumption of seeds & berries of **belladona / dhatura** plant
- Clinical presentation are due to *anticholinergic effects* i.e. Dry mouth, difficulty in swallowing & talking, dry skin, difficulty in micturation, dilated pupil, photophobia etc.
- Treatment of Belladona poisoning:

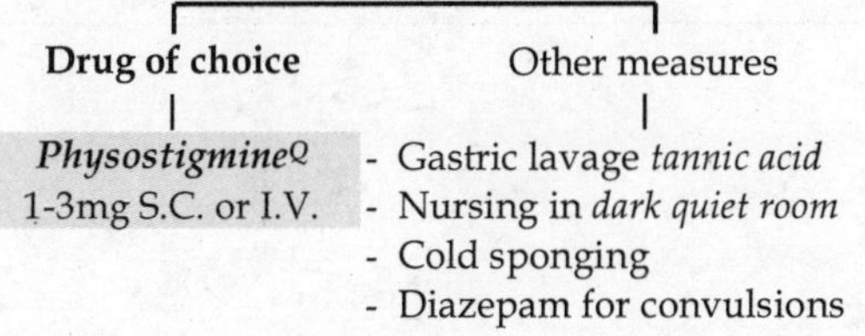

Drug of choice	Other measures
Physostigmine[Q] 1-3mg S.C. or I.V.	- Gastric lavage *tannic acid* - Nursing in *dark quiet room* - Cold sponging - Diazepam for convulsions

58. **A i.e. Glaucoma** *[Ref: KDT 4/e P–110-112]*

Atropine

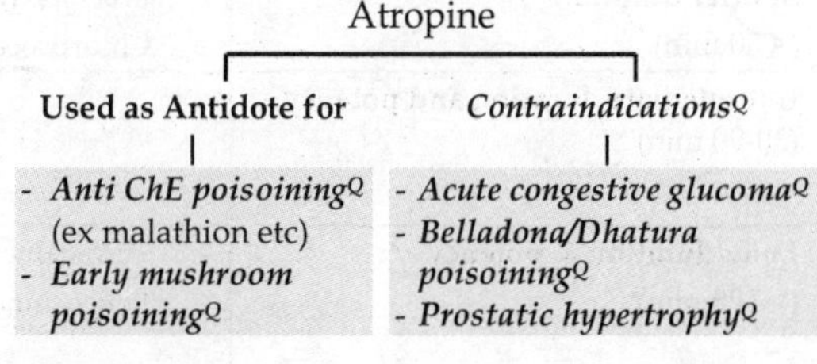

Used as Antidote for	*Contraindications*[Q]
- *Anti ChE poisoning*[Q] (ex malathion etc) - *Early mushroom poisoning*[Q]	- *Acute congestive glucoma*[Q] - *Belladona/Dhatura poisoning*[Q] - *Prostatic hypertrophy*[Q]

7 LOCAL ANAESTHETICS & BLOCKS

LOCAL ANESTHETICS

Mechanism of Action

- *LA blocks* **Na$^+$** ***channel from inside of cell membrane***[Q] and raises the threshold of channel opening
- Resting nerve is resistant to block and blockage develop rapidly when the nerve is stimulated repeatedly.
- High Ca++ conc. lessens the degree of block.

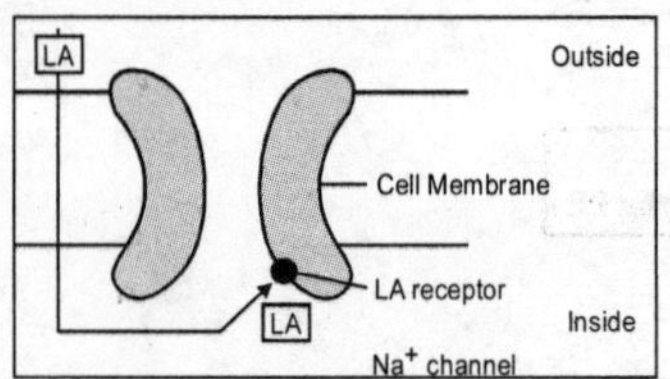

- **Addition of vasoconstrictors like adrenaline**
- ***reduces absorption & reduces toxicity***[Q]
- ***prolongs anesthetic activity***[Q]

Classification

Ethers[Q] **(1 'i')**	**Amides**[Q]
- Cocaine - Procaine - Chlorprocaine - Amethocaine - Tetracaine	*All membrane has '2i' except xylocaine* - Lignocaine/ Lidocaine (xylocaine) - Prilocaine - Mepivacaine - Bupivacaine/ Sensoricaine / Marcaine - Etidocaine - Ropivacaine - Dibucaine

- Amides are not hydrolysed by Plasma Esterase so produce longer lasting and more intense anestheisa
- Amides Binds to $\alpha 1$ acid glycoprotein in plasma.
- **Bupivacaine** is drug of choice for ***Isobaric spinal & Epidural anesthesia***[Q]

Sequence of block

1. ***Autonomic (1st) - Preganglionic sympathetic***[Q]
2. *Sensory* inorder of
   - P - Pain
   - T - Temperature
   - T - Touch
   - P - Pressure
   - In tounge Bitter taste lost Ist
     ↓
     f/b sweet & sour
     ↓
     salty (last)
3. **Motor**
   - Reversal in reverse order

- In local anesthesia nerve fibres ***Ist blocked is Type C***[Q]*, Last blocked Type A*
- *Smaller diameter* fibres and *non mylinated* fibres are *blocked more easily* and at low conc. then thicker, mylinated fibres.
- Minimum Concentration of LA, required to block a nerve fibre, is called Cm (i.e. Thicker, Mylinated fibres have greater cm)

Duration of action and potency

	Amide linked	*Ester linked*
Shorter duration (< 30 min)	- Procaine (low potency) - Chlorprocaine (intermediate potency)	
Intermediate duration and potency (30-90 min)		- Lidocaine - Mepivacaine - Prilocaine
Long duration & potency (> 120 min)	- Tetracaine - Bencocaine	- Bupivacaine - Ropivacaine - Dibucaine - Etidocaine

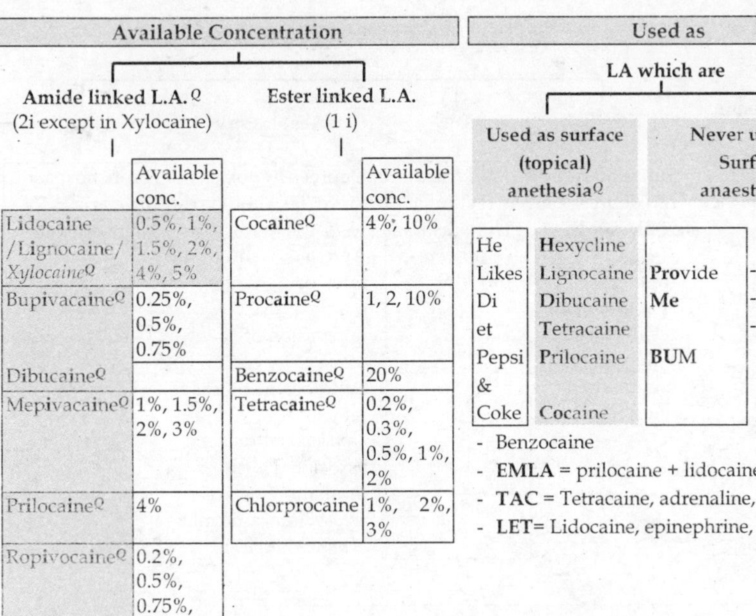

Available Concentration

Amide linked L.A.[Q] (2i except in Xylocaine)

Amide linked L.A.	Available conc.
Lidocaine /Lignocaine/ Xylocaine[Q]	0.5%, 1%, 1.5%, 2%, 4%, 5%
Bupivacaine[Q]	0.25%, 0.5%, 0.75%
Dibucaine[Q]	
Mepivacaine[Q]	1%, 1.5%, 2%, 3%
Prilocaine[Q]	4%
Ropivacaine[Q]	0.2%, 0.5%, 0.75%, 1%

Ester linked L.A. (1 i)

Ester linked L.A.	Available conc.
Cocaine[Q]	4%, 10%
Procaine[Q]	1, 2, 10%
Benzocaine[Q]	20%
Tetracaine[Q]	0.2%, 0.3%, 0.5%, 1%, 2%
Chlorprocaine	1%, 2%, 3%

Maximum Dose

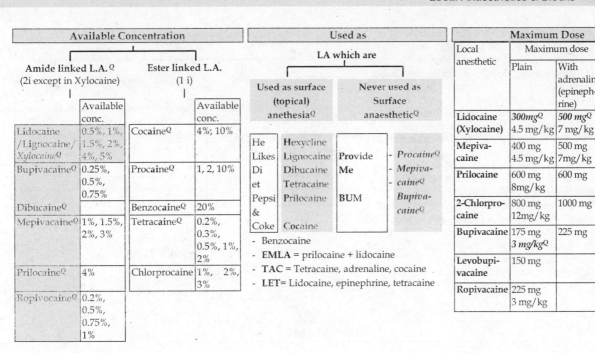

Local anesthetic	Maximum dose: Plain	Maximum dose: With adrenaline (epinephrine)	Over 24 hours
Lidocaine (Xylocaine)	*300mg*[Q] 4.5 mg/kg	***500 mg***[Q] 7 mg/kg	
Mepivacaine	400 mg 4.5 mg/kg	500 mg 7mg/kg	
Prilocaine	600 mg 8mg/kg	600 mg	
2-Chlorprocaine	800 mg 12mg/kg	1000 mg	
Bupivacaine	175 mg *3 mg/kg*[Q]	225 mg	400 mg
Levobupivacaine	150 mg		400 mg
Ropivacaine	225 mg 3 mg/kg		800 mg

EMLA

- It is ***eutectic mixture of local anesthetics (2.5% lidocaine & 2.5% prilocaine)***[Q]
- It allows anesthesia of intact skin (topical anesthetic cream). The cream must held in contact with skin for at least 1 hour and is held in place with an occlusive dressing.
- Its uses are:
  - ***to make venepuncture painless especially in children.***[Q]
  - skin grafting procedures
  - circumcision, needle phobics
- It ***should not be used in the very small child or on mucocutaneous membrane***[Q], because of the danger of syetmic absorption of prilocaine that results in methaemoglobinemia. It should not be left on the ksin for more than 5 hours. A major disadvantage is that it causes some vasoconstriction and this obscures the vein.
- **Tetracaine gel** is other agent that has *quicker onset of action and long duration of action.*

Use of Additives with Local Anesthetic Solutions

- **Sodium bicarbonate** *raises the pH* of local anesthetics (making it less acidic or closer to pKa) and *increases the unionized form of local anaesthetic.*This increases the rate of diffusion across the nerve sheath and the nerve membrane and ***increases the speed of onset of anaesthesia. It also prolongs the duration and intensity of block***[Q] *and reduces pain of injection* (which is associated with low pH & cold solution). The recommended dose is 1 ml of 8.4% $NaHCO_3$ per 10 ml of LA.
- **Epinephrine (adrenaline)** *increases speed of onset* of epidural block, *enhances both spread & quality* of block. It also *prolongs effect* of lignocaine & *reduces* peak local anesthetic *blood level & toxicity* by *reducing* the local blood supply and delaying its uptake.
- **Dextrose** 3 - 5% , is added to subarachnoid LA solutions to adjust the *baracity of solution* in relation to CSF.
- **Narcotics (opioids)** are used in intraspinal solutions as *analgesic agents.*

Lignocaine / Lidocaine / Xylocaine

- Most commonly used LA. It is ***amide linked local anaesthetic that can be used as surface anesthetic agent (i.e. through mucous membrane or skin)***[Q].
- *Vasoineffective* - Neither Vasocontrictor Nor Vasodilator
- *No mydriaris & Cycloplegia*
- Propanolol increases risk of toxicity by decreasing clearance.
- C/I in malignant hyperprexia and pt. with history of convulsions.

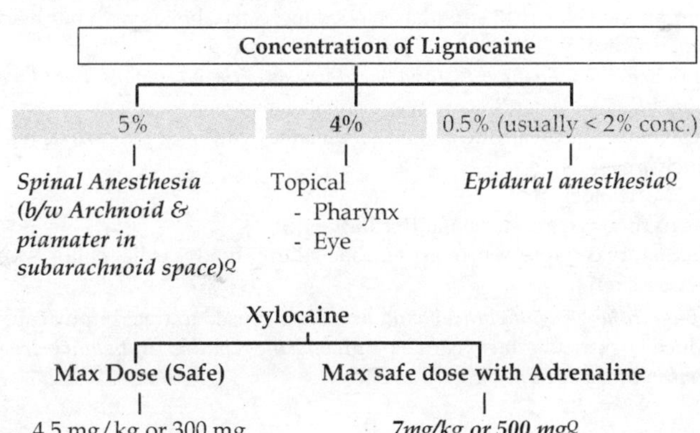

Cardiac: Antiarrhythmic Action

- ***Lidocaine (Xylocaine, lignocaine) blocks both open (active) and closed (inactivated) cardiac Na⁺ channels***[Q]**. It is well absorbed but *undergoes extensive though variable first pass hepatic metabolism***[Q] (only ~3% orally administered

ANAESTHESIA

2

drug appearing in plasma); **thus oral use of the drug is inappropriate**. Theoritically, therapeutic plasma concentrations of lidocaine may be maintained by intermittent intra muscular injections, but the **intravenous route is preferred**.

- Lidocaine is a local anesthetic that also is **useful in acute intravenous therapy of ventricular arrhythmias.** *It is not useful in atrial arrhythmias*. Lidocaine decreases the automaticity by reducing the slope of phase 4 and altering the threshold for excitability.
- Lidocaine is **least cardiotoxic antiarrhythmic**, only excessive doses cause cardiac depression & hypotension. Dose related neurological effects is main toxicity.
- It is used to **suppress ventricular tachycardia (VT) and prevent ventricular fibrillation (VF)**. Its efficiacy in chronic ventricular arrhythmia is poor but it *suppress VT d/t digitalis toxicity* (because it does not worsen AV block). However, it is not routinely prophylactically used to prevent VF in all acute MI patients because it may increase mortality.

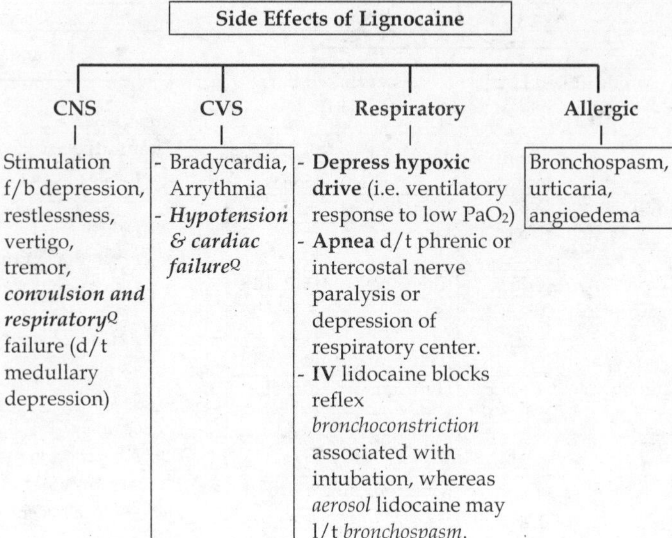

Side Effects of Lignocaine
CNS
CVS
Respiratory
Allergic
Stimulation f/b depression, restlessness, vertigo, tremor, convulsion and respiratory[Q] failure (d/t medullary depression)
- Bradycardia, Arrythmia
- Hypotension & cardiac failure[Q]
- Depress hypoxic drive (i.e. ventilatory response to low PaO2)
- Apnea d/t phrenic or intercostal nerve paralysis or depression of respiratory center.
- IV lidocaine blocks reflex bronchoconstriction associated with intubation, whereas aerosol lidocaine may l/t bronchospasm.
Bronchospasm, urticaria, angioedema

Bupivacaine

- **Bupivacaine** is a ***potent cardiotoxic and long acting (duration of action 120-240 min) amide linked local anesthetic***[Q]. It is used for infiltration, nerve block, epidural and spinal anaesthesia of long duration. Epidural anaesthesia using bupivaine is very popular. Bupivacaine is drug of choice for labour analgesia. Bupivacaine is prone to prolong QTc interval and induce ventricular tachycardia or cardiac depression. So bupivacaine is contraindicated in IV regional anaesthesia. Maximum tolerable dose is 175 mg without epinephrine and 225mg with epinephrine.
- Commercial bupivacaine is a racemic mixture of 'R' & 'S' isomer. **Levo bupivacine** being 'S' isomer has less potential for toxicity and is as effective as racemic one. **Bupivacaine** is ***most potent & best agent for isobaric spinal anesthesia but cannot be used as surface (topical) anesthetic agent.***[Q] **Bupivacaine** is ***contraindicated in regional IV anesthesia d/t fear of cardiac arrhythmia***[Q]. It can be used by following routes-
  - ***Intrathecal***[Q]
  - ***Epidural***[Q]
  - **Peripheral nerve block**
- All local anesthetics (LAs) bind & inhibit cardiac Na channels, but bupivacaine binds more avidly & longer than lignocaine. The bupivacaine R (+) isomer binds cardiac Na channels more avidly than S (-) isomer. This finding lead to development of levobupivacaine & ropivacaine. Inhibition of epinephrine – Stimulated C-AMP formation by LAs could explain the refractoriness of bupivacaine cardiovascular toxicity to standard resuscitation measures. Programmed electrical stimulation elicit more arrythmias with bupivacaine & levobupivacaine then with lidocaine or ropivacaine.
- ***Bupivacaine is most cardiotoxic local anaesthetic, so it should not be used for Beir's block.***[Q] It's cardiotoxicity is enhanced in pregnancy.
- **Intravenous bupivacaine and etidocaine** may cause severe cardiac reactions which are
  - A.V. heart block
  - Dysarythmias e.g. ventricular fibrillation.
  - Circulatory collapse & primary cardiac failure (bradycardia, pallor, sweating & hypotension)
- ***Amiodarone (drug of choice)***[Q] and *Bretylium* is used to treat bupivacaine induced ventricular tachycardias. ***Epinephrine remains first choice drug in event of circulatory collapse***[Q].
- **Bupivacaine (R,+) isomer** avidly *blocks cardiac sodium channels & dissociates very slowly*; its prolonged & high degree of protein binding makes resuscitation difficult & prolonged. At higher doses *calcium & potassium channels are also blocked*. Bupivacaine is more cardiotoxic than levobupivacaine, ropivacaine and lidocaine, particularly in presence of *acute respiratory acidosis, hypoxemia, hypercapnia in pregnancy (>>) and young children*.
- **Amiodarone** and possibly **bretylium** should be considered as preferred alternative to lidocaine in the treatment of LA induced ventricular tachyarrhythmias. **Vasopressors** may include ***epinephrine, norepinephrine and vasopressin***[Q]. ***Isoproterenol***[Q] may effectively reverse some of electrophysiological abnormalities characteristic of bupivacaine toxicity.
- If LA intoxication produces cardiac arrest, the **ACLS (advanced cardiac life support) guidelines** are reasonable; however, I suggest that ***amiodarone & vasopressin be preferred***[Q]/substituted for lidocaine & epinephrine (ACLS prefers epinephrine) – Morgan/273. With unresponsive bupivacaine toxicity, **intravenous lipid infusion** (remarkable ability to effect resuscitation from overdose even after 10 min of unsuccessful conventional resuscitation) or *cardiopulmonary bypass* may be considered.
- ***Calcium channel blockers are not recommended as these exaggerate the cardiodepressant effects***[Q].

Local Anaesthesia Systemic Toxicity (LAST)

- **Local anesthesia systemic toxicity (LAST) is increased by hypercapnia, hypoxia, acidosis (metabolic & respiratory)**Q, decreased plasma protein binding of LA (d/t increased Pa_{CO2} or decreased pH), abnormally low protein concentration (eg in neonates increasing the proportion of free drug), **extreme (advanced) age, hepatic failure** (l/t decreased clearance of amide LAs), **renal failure and cardiac failure**Q (prolonged absorption & drug accumulation), underlying cardiac pathology of ischemic heart disease, conduction block & CCF (esp in elderly) and metabolic (esp mitochondrial) disease. Severity and likelihood of LAST is also influenced by *individual patient risk factors, concurrent medication,* location/technique of block, specific LA compound and total dose (ie con. × volume), timeliness of detection and adequacy of treatment.
- **Rate of systemic absorption of LA** is related to the **vascularity of site of injection, intravenous or intra arterial** (is greatest) **> tracheal > intercostals > paracervical > caudal > epidural > brachial plexus > sciatic > subcutaneous** (Morgan). Systemic absorption of LA (ie chances of LAST) is greatest after intercostal nerve blocks and caudal anesthesia, intermediate after epidural anesthesia and least after brachial plexus blocks (Pardo). **Most rapid onset but shortest duration** of action occurs after **intrathecal or subcutaneous LA.** Whereas, the **longest latencies & durations** are observed after **brachial plexus blocks** (Miller).
- In general CNS is more susceptible and CNS toxicity occurs at lower blood levels and LA doses than CVS toxicity. Systemic toxicity of LA include - CNS toxicity, cardiovascular system, methemoglobinemia & Allergies.

Central Nervous System Toxicity

- **CNS** is particularly vulnerable to toxicity & is the site of premonitory signs of overdose in awake patients. *Cortical inhibitory pathways are most susceptible* resulting in excitatory motor phenomenon in initial stages of LA toxicity.

Early symptoms	Sensory symptoms	Excitatory signs	Ultimately CNS depression
Circumoral numbness, tongue paresthesia, dizziness & light headedness	Tinnitus, blurred vision, metallic taste, difficulty in focusing	- Restlessness, agitation, nervousness, paronia - Shivering, muscle twitching, & tremors involving face & distal extremities ultimately l/t generalized tonic clonic convulsions	- Slurred speech, drowsiness, unconsciousness - Respiratory depression & respiratory arrest

- ***Hypercapnia, respiratory & metabolic acidosis exacerbates CNS toxicity***Q. Increased $PaCO_2$ *increases cerebral blood flow* delivering greater dose of LA more rapidly to brain. And decreased intracellular pH favours formation of *non diffusable cationic (protonated)* form of LA, which is *trapped within neuron.* Finally plasma protein binding of LA is decreased in acidic environment resulting in increased availability of free drug for diffusion into brain.
- The highly perfused organs (as Brain, Lung, Liver, Kidney, heart) are responsible for initial rapid uptake **(Alpha phase)** which is followed by a slower redistribution **(Beta phase)** to moderately perfused tissues (muscle and gut).
- **Amide LA are metabolized (N-dealkylation & hydroxylation) by microsomal P450 in liver** at rate that depends on agent; prilocaine > lidocaine > mepivacaine > ropivacaine > bupivacaine (but at rate slower than ester hydrolysis of ester LA). ***Decrease in hepatic function (cirrhosis) or liver blood flow*** *(eg.* ***congestive heart failure,*** *β blockers, or H_2 receptor blockers)* ***will reduce metabolic rate*** and potentially **predispose patients to greater blood concentrations of LA and greater risk of systemic toxicity**Q.

Methemoglobinemia

- **Pilocaine** is only LA that is metabolized to o-toludine. **O-toludine metabolites of prilocaine**Q, which accumulate after large dose of drug, **covert hemoglobin to methemoglobin** and produce **methemoglobulinemia is a dose** dependent fashion (in the range of 10mg/kg).
- Younger, healthier patient develop it after lower doses of prilocaine (and at lower doses than needed in older, sicker, patients).
- *Benzocaine*Q, a common ingredient in local anesthetic sprays during endoscopic procedures also can cause methemoglobinemia.
- Treatment of Methemoglobinemia is ***IV Methylene blue***Q (1-2mg/kg of 1% solution) which reduces methemoglobin (Fe^{3+}) to hemoglobin (Fe^{2+}).

Allergy/Anaphylaxis

- True anaphylaxis d/t anesthetic agent is rare. Anaphylactoid reactions are much more common. Hypnotic agents (thiopental & propofol) and muscle relaxants (Succinyl choline, curare & atracurium) are mostly responsible for it.
- ***Esters (local anesthetics) are more likely to induce IgE/IgG mediated immune response*** *especially* ***procaine or benzocaine,*** as they are derivatives of ***p-amino benzoic acid (PABA), a known allergen.***
- ***Immunological response to amide L.A. is very rare. Methyl paraben*** a preservative agent is responsible for its most of rare allergic response.

2

ANAESTHESIA

Cardiovascular Toxicity of Local Anesthetics

CVS Toxicity

- *Inadvertent intravascular injection* of LA, or frank overdosage & systemic absorption from the site of injection can block *Na^+, K^+ and Ca^{++} channels* within conducting tissues such as in CNS and CVS.
- *Higher dose* (3 times for bupivacaine & 7 times for lidocaine) is required to cause cardio vascular complications than to cause CNS toxicity (Seizure)
- LA may cause arrhythmias & *negative inotropic* effect directly as well as can affect circulation by blockade of sympathetic or para sympathetic activity.
- Primary cardiac electrophysiological effect of LA is *decrease in the rate of spontaneous phase IV depolarization in fast conducting tissues of purkinje fibers and ventricular muscle*, due to decreased availability of fast sodium channels (i.e. Na channel blockade). *Action potential duration and effective refractory period* are also *decreased*. However ratio of effective refractory period to the duration of action potential (both in Purkinje fibers & ventricular muscle) is increased.
- *Bupivacaine binds more strongly to Na channel and depress depolarization to greater extent* than lidocaine, leading to prolonged inhibition of normal conduction.
- ***The rate of recovery is slower in bupivacaine particularly at high heart rates (tachycardia)***Q whereas, recovery from lidocaine is complete, event at rapid heart rates. These differences explain antiarrhythmic property of lidocaine and arrythmogenic potential of bupivacaine.
- High concentrations decrease myocardial contractility & conduction velocity l/t *increase PR interval & duration of QRS complex*. **Extremely high conc**.of LA depress spontaneous pacemaker activity resulting in *bradycardia & sinus arrest.*
- *Dose dependent negative* intropic effects on cardiac muscle occur in direct proportion to conduction blocking potency i.e.,

  Bupivacaine = Tetracaine > Etidocaine >> Lidocaine = Prilocaine = Mepivacaine = Cocaine > Chlorprocaine = Procaine
- *Myocardial contractility* is depressed by affecting *Ca^{++} signaling mechanism.*
- Along with Na channels, LA can also bind to *Ca & K channels, β-adrenergic receptor, NMDA* (N-methyl D-aspartate enzyme) *receptor and nicotinic acetylcholine receptor*; hence causing spinal/epidural analgesia & toxic effects.
- Refractoriness of bupivacaine to CV toxicity to standard resuscilation may be attributed to *inhibition of epinephrine –stimulated C- AMP.*
- ***Cocaine is the only LA consistently causing vaso constriction***Q others produce smooth muscle relaxation & arteriolar dilation.
- So combination of hypotesion, heart block & bradycardia may cause cardiac arrest. The usual presentation of LA overdose during GA is arrhythmia or circulatory collapse

Local Anesthetics

- **CV toxicity of bupivacaine** differs from lidocaine in that bupivacaine has
  - Lower ratio of CC/CNS i.e., dose required to cause irreversible cardiac collapse (CC) & dose producing CNS toxicity eg convulsion
  - More chances of fatal ventricualr arrhythmia after large rapid intravenous dose
  - *Pregnancy* (>> young children) predispose to bupivacaine toxicity so it is **not recommended for obstetrics anesthesia** (US).
  - *Hypoxia, respiratory acidosis & hypercapnia* predispose & potentiate toxicity
  - Cardiac resuscitation is more difficult.
- Because of evidence that myocardial toxicity is caused by *R-enantiomer of bupivacaine* (enantiomers are one pair of molecules which are *mirror images* of each other & *non-superimposable;* and racemate is an equimolar mixture of a pair of enantiomers) *levobupivacaine (S-enantiomer of bupivacaine)* and *ropivacaine* (butyl group attached to amine of bupivacaine is replaced by propyl group and presented as single S-enantiomer) are developed.
- **Ropivacaine** *shares similar onset time & duration of action with bupivacaine, but is half as lipid soluble, has lower potency provides less motor block, 70% less likely to cause severe arrhythmia i.e. has larger theraputic index and greater central nervous tolerance. The improved profile is d/t its lower lipid solubility & pure (S) isomeric form.*
- Unlike other LAs, *Cocaine inhibit re uptake of nor epinephrine at adrenergic nerve terminals;* thus potentiating adrenergic stimulation & l/t hypertension & ventricular ectopy. So it is *contraindicated in patient anesthetized with halothane*. Cocaine induced arrhythmias are successfully treated with *adrenergic & calcium channel antagonists.*
- *Cardiac resuscitation is still easiest in lidocaine.* After that resuscitation after cardiovascular collapse was better with **ropivacaine (90% success) > levobupivacaine (70%) > bupivacaine (50%)**

Prevention

- Because CPR after LA induced circulatory collapse is so difficult, ***prevention of massive intravascular injections or excessive dosing is crucial.***
- *Negative aspiration of syringe* does not always exclude intravascular placement. So *incremental, fractionated dosing* should be the rule. ECG changes are often (although not always) present and *continuous ECG monitoring* (including PR interval, QRS duration, time corrected QT interval = QTc, QT dispersion = QTd, rate, rhythm and ectopy) may be life saving by terminating injection before a lethal dose is administered.

Treatment

- **No t/t is uniformly effective for bupivacaine induced CV toxicity**. The basic principles of **CPR** i.e, securing airway, providing oxygenation, ventilation and performing chest compression if needed are followed. ***Epinephrine remains drug of first choice in case of circulatory collapse***Q
- If a patient experience profound cardiovascular depression or circulatory arrest after administration of bupivacaine, ropivacaine, or by extrapolation, other local anesthetics, then along with **initiation of basic life support** and **ACLS protocol, Weinberg recommendation** of administration of **rapid bolus of Intralipid 20%,** 1.5ml/kg (~100 mL in adults) **without delay** followed if necessary by an infusion (0.25 mL/kg/min) for next 10 minutes. It theoretically removes bupivacaine from sites of action and treats cardiac toxicity. It raise the question of whether *standard propofol in 10% lipid solution* would be used for cardiac toxicity. However, the dose of lipid in a standard induction dose of propofol would be too small & the dose of propofol would lead to unacceptable cardiac depression.
- Emergency treatment includes
  - ***Sodium bicarbonate*** to prevent metabolic acidosis
  - ***Benzodiazepine*** to prevent or treat seizure
  - Inotropic support in hemodynamic unstability

1. **IV atropine**
2. IV vasoactive agent eg. ***epinephrine, dopamine or dobutamine, vasopressin & occasionally isoprenaline***
3. Calcium chloride

- T/t of ventricualr tachycardia or fibrillation

1. Defibrillation
2. Antiarrhythmic : ***Amiodarone >> bretylium***Q is preferred to lidocaine
3. Anticonvulsant: IV diazepam, midazolam, phenytoin, thiopental & propofol

- Inotropic : IV atropine, dobutamine
- **Lipid infusion** & /or propofol infusion

Use of Additives with local anesthetic (LA) solutions

Vasoconstrictors

- **Addition of vasoconstrictor** (eg felypressin, adrenaline/epinephrine in 1:2 lacks concentration etc) to a solution of local anesthetic drug *slows the rate of its vascular absorption*, thereby allowing more LA molecules to reach the nerve membranes and thus improving **the depth and duration of anesthesia** resulting in a *profound block of prolonged duration*. It *reduces toxicity*, as well as *provides a marker for inadvertent intravascular injection*. The most common cause of life threatening systemic toxicity is an inadvertent intravascular injection of LA f/b its absolute overdose. So the single most important factor in prevention of toxicity is avoidance of accidental IV injection of LA by careful negative aspiration test repeated each time the needle is moved. However, a negative test is not an absolute guarantee, especially when a catheter technique is used. So initial injection of 2-3 ml of LA solution that contains adrenaline (1:2 lack) has been advocated, an increase in heart rate during the succeeding 1-2 min should indicate intravascular injection. False negatives and false positives can occur *in adults and children under GA, parturient in labor, and patients receiving β blockers*. An alternative to prevent toxicity is to repeat aspiration test after each 5-10 ml of solution and to inject slowly (~5ml/minute). The patient should be watched for early signs of toxicity and injection stopped before major sequale.
- **Addition of vasoconstrictor to LA** slows *its vascular absorption* thereby **reducing toxicity** (esp. in highly vascular sites intercostal> epidural> brachial) and **improving the depth and duration of anesthesia** (ie resulting in profound block of prolonged duration). However vasoconstrictors are **absolutely contraindicated** for injection close to end arteries ***(ring blocks of finger and toe digits, penis and pinna)***[Q] and in ***intravenous regional anesthesia (Bier's block)***[Q] because of the risk of ischemia. It should also be avoided (used cautiously) in *MI patients, hyperthyroidism, severe hypertension and with inhalational agents eg. halothane* which sensitizes heart to arrythmogenic action of adrenaline.
- **Epinephrine (adrenaline)** *increases speed of onset* of epidural block, *enhances both spread & quality* of block. It also *prolongs effect* of lignocaine *& reduces* peak local anesthetic *blood level & toxicity* by *reducing* the local blood supply and delaying its uptake.
- Epinephrine *significantly extends the duration* of both infiltration anesthesia and peripheral nerve block with shorter duration agents (eg lignocaine), whereas, epinephrine produces *mild intensification* of blockade but only most *modest prolongation* of epidural or peripheral blocks with bupivacaine.

Carbon dioxide (Carbonation), $NaHCO_3$ and pH Adjustment

- *To accelerate the onset and decrease the onset time and minimum concentration (Cm) required for conduction blockade*, sodium bicarbonate ($NaHCO_3$) is added to solution of LA.
- **Sodium bicarbonate** *raises the pH* of local anesthetics (making it less acidic or closer to pKa) and *increases the unionized (uncharged base) form of local anaesthetic*.This increases the rate of diffusion across the nerve sheath and the nerve membrane and ***increases the speed of onset of anaesthesia. It also prolongs the duration and intensity of block***[Q] *and reduces pain of injection* (which is associated with low pH & cold solution). The recommended dose is 1 ml of 8.4% $NaHCO_3$ per 10 ml of LA.
- In order *to speed the onset of* blockade, LA can be produced as **carbonated salt, with CO_2** dissolved under pressure. The rationale is that after injection, CO_2 lowers intracellular pH and *favours formation of more of ionized active form* of LA.

Others

- **High molecular weight very large dextran's** (esp with adrenaline) may *prolong duration of action* by forming macromolecules with LA, which are held in tissues for longer period.
- **Hyaluronidase** enzyme may aid spread by breaking drown tissue barrier (used only rarely in ophthalmic practice)
- **Narcotics (opioids)** are used as *analgesic agents in epidural and intrathecal* solutions.
- **Sodium hydroxide and hydrochloric acid** are used to **adjust the pH, sodium chloride** the *tonicity*, and **glucose and water** the *baricity of solution*.
- **Dextrose** 3 - 5% , is added to subarachnoid LA solutions to adjust the *baracity of solution* in relation to CSF.
- *Preservatives, eg. methylhydroxy benzoate* are added to multidose bottles and these *should not be used for subarachnoid or epidural block*.

Summary

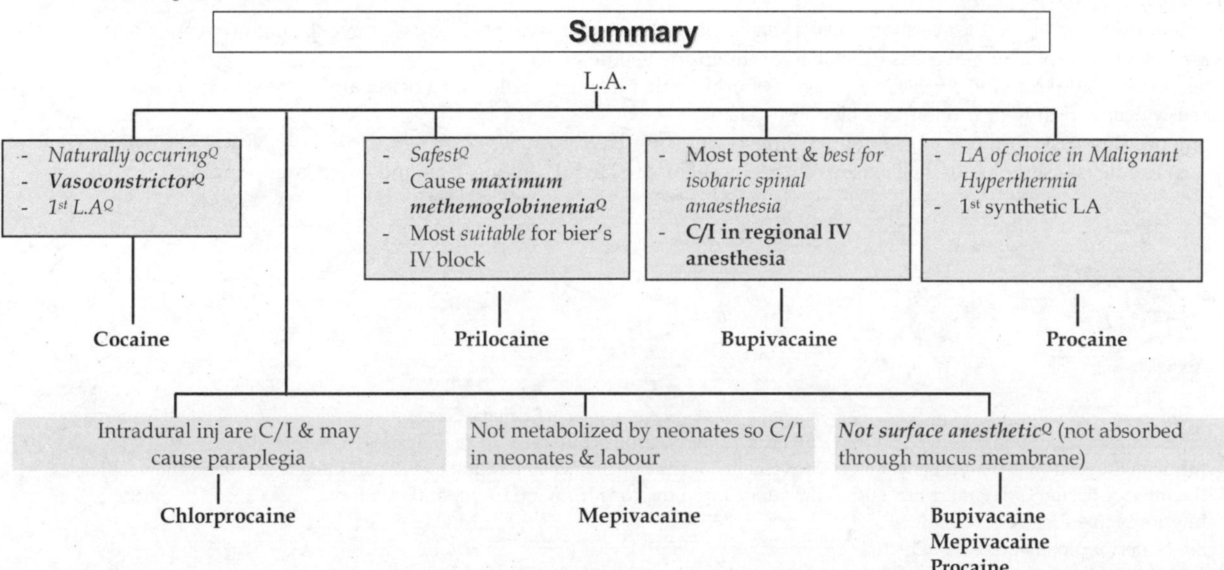

Intravenous Regional Anesthesia (IVRA) or Bier's Block

- It consists of *intravenous injection of local anesthetics in a tourniquent occluded limb*.It is mainly used for *minor upper limb orthopaedic procedures* like forearm fracture manipulations, minor surgery of forearm & hand.
- Although theorectically possible, *lower limb IVRA is not often performed* owing to the lare volumes (60-80 ml) of anesthetic required. ***IVRA is contraindicated in situations in which tourniquets are contraindicated eg sickle cell disease or Raynaud's disease and scleroderma***[Q]. Children with sickle cell anemia are prone to develop massive hemolysis in cases of low oxygen tension, or in cases where blood flow slows down. During tourniquet application in IVRA, blood flow slows down, & can precipitate **acute hemolytic crisis** in patients with sickle cell disease.
- *2 intravenous cannulas* are inserted – one *as distal* as possible in the forearm to be operated upon and second in the opposite arm to access circulation if required. A *double pneumatic tourniquet cuff* is applied to the arm after exsanguinations. The tourniquet should be inflated *100 mmHg (13.3 KPa) above the pulse occlusion pressure (better) / or systolic blood pressure.*
- Upto *40 ml of LA* is then injected distally & *slowly (at least 90 sec)* to decrease leak. A characteristic skin mottling will be seen. In Europe & UK, **prilocaine**, 0.5%, 3mg/kg (preservative free) and in USA, preservative free **lidocaine**, 0.5%, 3mg/kg are most commonly used agents. Following IVRA with prilocaine, methemoglobin levels are never >3% (Methemoglobinemia l/t cyanotic color it must be >10%)
- ***Bupivacaine is contraindicated for intravenous regional analgesia***[Q] *as it is more prone to induce prolong QTc interval, ventricular tachycardia & cardiac depression.*
- ***Bupivacaine is LA of choice for isobaric spinal anesthesia***[Q].
- In any case distal *cuff should not be deflated for atleast 20 min*. By this time, most of the anesthetics will have fixed to the tissues and there should be no overt toxicity.
- *Addition of NSAIDs eg ketorolac* improves postoperative analgesia. Addition of *sodium bicarbonate* to prilocaine is useful and produces a block of faster onset and more intense anesthesia.
- LA accumulates around antecubital fossa and so blocks the vascular nerve trunks of *median and ulnar nerves prior to blocking less vascular radial nerve*. Because the LA is carried into the vascular core of nerve trunks the *block starts distally* (innervated by more central fibers of nerve at vascular core) and progress proximally to elbow. This is opposite to nerve (brachial plexus) blockade, in which LA diffuses inwards through the nerve trunk. Thus the inner fibers supplying the distal part are affected last and block progresses distally.
- *IV regional sympathetic blockade* is obtained by using **guanethidine** (20-40 mg) which selectively interrupt sympathetic innervation to an extremity. **Reserpine** (1-1.5 mg) & **bretylium** (5mg/kg) can be used similarly. 10 ml lidocaine 0.5% can also be added to prevent burning.

Intraconal Retrobulbar Block

- Local anesthetic is injected *behind the eye into the cone* formed by extraocular muscles.
- The **optic , occulomotor** (which supplies the *superior, inferior and medial recti and the inferior oblique* muscles), **abducens** (which supplies the *lateral rectus muscle*) and the **nasociliary nerves** (innervating the corneal and perilimbal conjunctiva) as well as ciliary ganglion are all within the cone (formed by four recti muscles). The **lacrimal, frontal and infraorbital nerves** (which supply the peripheral conjuctiva) and **trochlear nerve** (***which supplies the superior oblique muscle) are outside the cone***[Q] and are thus least & last to be affected by block.
- **Retrobulbar block** anesthetizes ***ciliary nerves, ciliary ganglia and 2nd, 3rd & 6th cranial nerves***[Q], hence producing global akinesia, anesthesia and analgesia. ***Superior oblique muscle is usually not or (late & least) paralyzed as the 4th cranial nerve is outside the muscle cone***[Q].
- For a retrobulbar block, the eye should *look straight ahead in the primary gaze position*, to prevent rotation of optic nerve, vasculature, and pole of globe towards the inferotemporal needle
- Injection is made from the *inferotemporal region* of orbit, either through conjunctiva (less painful) or skin (in deep set eye, narrow orbital fissure or pronounced blepharospasm)
- Long needles (~ 38 mm previously popular) must not be used as they reach optic nerve in ~ 11%. Now 25- gauge , 2.5 cm sharp needle is inserted with the bevel towards globe, close to lateral canthus (5 cm medial to lateral canthus).

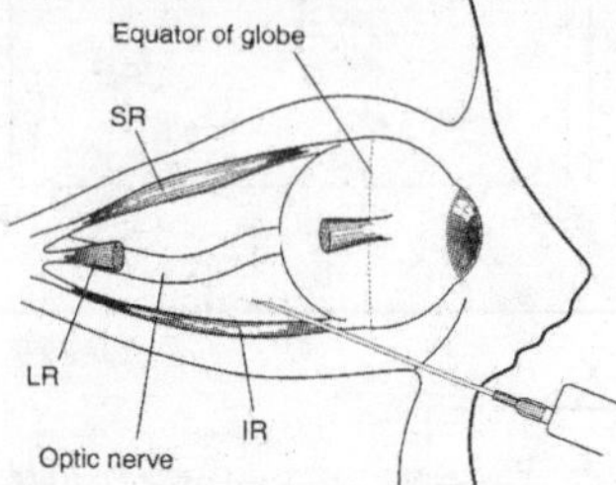

Intraconal injection is placed between the inferior border of lateral rectus and inferior rectus
SR: Superior rectus; LR: Lateral rectus; IR: Inferior rectus

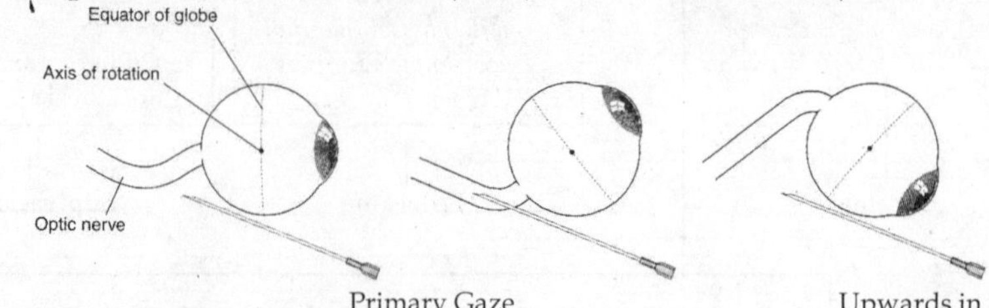

Primary Gaze Upwards in inwards Downwards & outwards

Movements of the optic nerve in relation to eye ball movement when the needle is introduced into the cone from inferitemporal quadrant.

- The tip of needle should *not cross the line of the lateral edge of iris* so that it cannot reach the optic nerve. The injection is placed between *the inferior border of lateral rectus and inferior rectus.*
- Commonly used drugs are – *lidocaine (2%) or bupivacaine (0.5 – 0.75%)* = drug of choice, prilocaine (2-4%) and *hyaluronidase* (to *enhance spread of drug*). Sodium bi carbonate (neutralises acidity, reduces sting on injection), adrenaline & vecuronium may be also added.
- Successful block is accompanied by *anesthesia, akinesia and abolishment of oculocephalic reflex* (i.e. blockade eye does not move during head turning)
- Complications may be – retrobulbar haemorrhage, globe perforation, optic nerve atrophy, frank convulsions, oculocardiac reflex, acute neurogenic pulmonary edema, trigeminal nerve block and respiratory arrest.

Stellate Ganglion (Cervico Thoracic Sympathetic) Block

It is used to treat **chronic pain syndromes** (eg phantom limb pain, refractory angina, Raynaud's syndrome, obliterative vascular insufficiency, frost bite etc)

It is also used in quinine poisoning, long QT syndrome, chest pain associated with primary pulmonary hypertention & climacteric psychosis.

Signs of successful stellate ganglion block

- ***Horner's syndrome***Q **i.e.** *miosis, enopthalmos, ptosis, anhydrosis* (over ipsilateral face & neck upto T3), and absence of cliospinal reflex and papillary dilation on sheding the eye.
- *Flushing of face, conjunctival congestion*
- *Lacrimation/Increased tear production (if superior cervical ganglion involved)*
- Injection of tympanic membrane **(Mueller's syndrome)**
- ***Stuffy nose (Guttman's sign)*** Q *(Obstruction of ipsilateral half of nose)*
- *Increased temperature of face & upper extremity on ipsilateral side of block*
- *Venodilation in the ipsilateral extremity(hand and forearm)*

Brachial Plexus Block

Interscalene Approch	Axillary Approch	Supra clavicular & Infraclavicular approches
- ***Most intense at*** C_5 ***–*** C_7 **dermatomes and *least intense at*** C_8***-*** T_1 **(ulnar nerve area)**Q - Most optimal for procedures on shoulder, arm and forearm	- *Most intense block in* C_7*-*T_1 *(ulnar nerve)* Q **distribution** *least intense in* C_5*-*C_6 *dermatome* Q - Most optimal for procedures from elbow to hand	***More even distribution*** of local anaesthesia & can be used for procedures on arm, forearm and hand

Celiac Plexus Block

The celiac plexus contains visceral afferent and efferent fibers derived from T_5 *to* T_{12} by means of *greater, lesser and least splanchnic nerves.* The plexus has no somatic fibers. It innervates most of the abdominal viscera.

It is usually given for *pain relief in gastric and pancreatic malignancy.* A celiac plexus block can be *combined with intercostals* block to provide anesthesia for intra *abdominal surgery.*

Because it results in blockade of the autonomic system, this block may help reduce stress and endocrine response to surgery.

Most common complication of **celiac plexus block** is ***postural hypotension***Q due to *lumbar sympathetic chain blockade* leading to upper abdominal vessel dilation and venous pooling. So intravenous fluids are required preblock to reduce the risk.

Other complications indude spinal, epidural or intravascular injection, bleeding d/t aorta or inferior venacava injury, pneumothorax, puncture of viscera such as kidney, ureter or gut with abscess or cyst formation, retroperitoneal hematoma, paraplegia (d/t intra arterial injection supplying spinal cord), diarrhea and sexual dysfunction (b/l sympathetic chain , block)

Orthostatic hypotension occurred more often when the *retrocrural* (50%) *or splanchnic* (52%) technique was used than when the anterocrural approach (10%) was used. Whereas **transient diarrhea** was more frequent with *anterocrural approach* (65%) > *retrocrural approach (25%)* > *splanchnic nerve block* (5%).

QUESTIONS

GENERAL

1. **Local anaesthesia acts by** *(PGI 97; DNB 03)*
   A. Na^+ channel inhibition ☐
   B. Ca^{++} channel inhibition ☐
   C. Mg^{++} channel inhibition ☐
   D. K^+ channel inhibition ☐
2. **True about local anaesthetic** *(PGI 2001)*
   A. Cocaine acts by decreasing norepinephrine ☐
   B. Act by decreasing sodium entry into cell ☐
   C. Lignocaine is a amide ☐
   D. Dibucaine is drug of choice for epidural anaesthesia ☐
3. **True statements about local anaesthesia** *(PGI 2003)*
   B. It inhibits the generation of action potential ☐
   C. Unmyelinated thin fiber are most susceptible than myelinated large fibers ☐
   D. Toxicity is reduced by addition of vasoconstrictor ☐
   E. Blocks all modalities of sensation at the same time ☐
4. **True about local anaesthetic agents** *(PGI 04; DNB 09)*
   A. Duration depends on protein binding ☐
   B. Potency depends upon lipid solubility ☐
   C. LA with low PK is more active ☐
   D. Higher dose produces more block ☐
   E. Signal transduction blockade ☐
5. **Afferent nerve fibre affected by local anesthesia first**
   A. Type A *(AIIMS 04, AI 95)* ☐
   B. Type II – B ☐
   C. Type C ☐
   D. Type II ☐
6. **Which of the following is/are not local anesthesia:**
   A. Bupivacine *(PGI Nov 09; DNB 10)* ☐
   B. Mepivacine ☐
   C. Mivacurium ☐
   D. Butorphenol ☐
   E. Bupernorphine ☐
7. **Which one of the following is not a amide**
   A. Lignocaine/Lidocaine *(AI 07, 03; AIIMS 02)* ☐
   B. Procaine ☐
   C. Bupivacaine/Mepivacaine ☐
   D. Dibucaine/Prilocaine/Etidocaine ☐
8. **Cholinesterase metabolizes following except:** *(PGI 1997)*
   A. Propanolol ☐
   B. Procaine ☐
   C. Acetyl choline ☐
   D. Bupivacaine ☐
9. **Earliest (first) L.A. used clinically** *(AIIMS 09, 96; DNB 07)*
   A. Xylocaine/Lidocaine ☐
   B. Morphine ☐
   C. Cocaine ☐
   D. Cannabis & Procaine ☐
10. **Vasoconstricator L.A. is** *(AI 1999)*
    A. Cocaine ☐
    B. Procaine ☐
    C. Lidocaine ☐
    D. Chlorprocaine ☐
11. **Which local anaesthetic causes vasoconstriction:**
    A. Cocaine *(PGI 1997)* ☐
    B. Lidocaine ☐
    C. Bupivacaine ☐
    D. Procaine ☐
12. **All are vasodilators except** *(AI 1998)*
    A. Procaine ☐
    B. Lidocaine ☐
    C. Cocaine ☐
    D. Chlorprocaine ☐
13. **The topical use of following local anesthetic is not recommended?** *(AIIMS 02; DNB 03)*
    A. Ligocaine ☐
    B. Bupivacaine ☐
    C. Cocaine ☐
    D. Dibucaine ☐
14. **Which of the following local anesthetic is /are not used for surface analgesia:** *(AIIMS May 13)*
    A. Benzocaine ☐
    B. Prilocaine ☐
    C. Mepivacaine ☐
    D. Lignocaine ☐
    E. Bupivacaine ☐
15. **True about EMLA:** *(PGI Dec 06)*
    A. Can be used for intubation ☐
    B. Mixture of local anesthesia ☐
    C. Faster acting ☐
    D. Used in children ☐
16. **Anesthetic agent with vasoconstrictor is contraindicated in?** *(AI 2011)*
    A. Finger block ☐
    B. Spinal block ☐
    C. Epidural block ☐
    D. Regional anesthesia ☐
17. **Sodium bicarbonate when given with local anaesthetics has which of the following effect?** *(AI 09)*
    A. Increases speed and quality of anaestheisa ☐
    B. Decreases diffusion of the anaesthetic drug ☐
    C. Causes rapid elimination of the local anaesthetic ☐
    D. Decreases speed and quality of anaesthesia. ☐
18. **Shortest acting local anesthetic agent is**
    A. Procaine *(AI 97, PGI 2K)* ☐
    B. Lidocaine ☐
    C. Tetracaine ☐
    D. Bupivacaine ☐
19. **Longest acting L.A** *(AI 1994)*
    A. Bupivacaine ☐
    B. Tetracaine ☐
    C. Xylocaine ☐
    D. Procaine ☐
20. **Local anasthetic acting for more than 2 hrs.**
    A. Bupivaciane *(PGI 2K; DNB 02)* ☐
    B. Etodocaine ☐
    C. Lignocaine ☐
    D. Cholorprocaine ☐
21. **Which of the following is long acting local anesthetic > 2hrs** *(PGI 05; DNB 07)*
    A. Bupivacaine ☐
    B. Prilocaine ☐
    C. Etidocaine ☐
    D. Dibucaine ☐
    E. Tetracaine ☐
22. **Which of the following statement is/are not true about Dibucaine:** *(PGI May 12)*
    A. Shorter acting than tetracaine ☐
    B. Longer acting than tetracaine ☐
    C. More potent than tetracaine ☐
    D. More potent than bupivacaine ☐
    E. Dibucaine no. < 30 indicates more quantity of atypical pseudocholinesterase ☐

LIDOCAINE

23. **Concentration of lignocaine used** *(PGI Dec 2007)*
 A. 2% ☐
 B. 4% ☐
 C. 5% ☐
 D. 10% ☐
 E. 1% ☐
24. **Xylocaine heavy in subarachnoid space has concentration of** *(AIIMS 92)*
 A. 1% ☐
 B. 2% ☐
 C. 3% ☐
 D. 5% ☐
25. **Conc. of Lidocaine used in spinal anesthesia** *(AI 1994)*
 A. 5% ☐
 B. 3% ☐
 C. 2% ☐
 D. 1% ☐
26. **Maximum does of lidocaine as local anesthesia is** *(AIIMS 1992)*
 A. 100 mg ☐
 B. 200 mg ☐
 C. 300 mg ☐
 D. 500 mg ☐
27. **Max dose of lignocaine with adrenaline is** *(AIIMS May 12; AI 92)*
 A. 3 mg/kg ☐
 B. 4 mg/kg ☐
 C. 5 mg/kg ☐
 D. 7 mg/kg ☐
28. **About lidocaine, all are true except :** *(PGI 1998)*
 A. LA effect ☐
 B. Cardiac arrhythmia ☐
 C. Ester ☐
 D. Acts on mucous membranes ☐
29. **Lignocaine in high dose produces** *(PGI June 2004)*
 A. Convulsion ☐
 B. Respiratory depression ☐
 C. Hypotension ☐
 D. Cardiac arrest ☐
 E. Hypothermia ☐
30. **All are true about lidocaine except:** *(AIIMS Nov 12)*
 A. It acts on sodium channels in both active and inactive state ☐
 B. It is most cardiotoxic local anesthetic ☐
 C. It is given IV in cardiac arrhythmias ☐
 D. Extensive first pass metabolism ☐

TOXICITY

31. **L.A. causing Meth Haemoglobinemia** *(AIIMS May 10, AI 1994)*
 A. Procaine ☐
 B. Prilocaine ☐
 C. Bupivacaine ☐
 D. Cocaine ☐
32. **Which of the following local anaesthetics is most likely to produce an allergic reaction:** *(Jipmer 05)*
 A. Prilocaine ☐
 B. Ropivacaine ☐
 C. Etidocaine ☐
 D. Benzocaine ☐
33. **A 25 year old male with roadside accident underwent debridement and reduction of fractured both bones right forearm under axillary block.**
 On the second postoperative day the patient complained of persistent numbness and paresthesia in the right forearm and the hand. The commonest cause of this neurological dysfunction could be all of the following except : *(AI 2004)*
 A. Crush injury to the hand and lacerated nerves ☐
 B. A tight cast or dressing ☐
 C. Systemic toxicity of local anaesthetics ☐
 D. Tourniquet pressure ☐
34. **Cardiac or central nervous system toxicity may result when standard lidocaine doses are administered to patients with circulatory failure. This may be due to the following reason:** *(AI 2003)*
 A. Lidocaine concentration are initially higher in relatively well perfused tissues such as brain and heart ☐
 B. Histamine receptors in brain and heart gets suddenly activated in circulatory failure ☐
 C. There is a sudden out-burst of release of adreneline, noradreneline and dopamine in brain and heart ☐
 D. Lidocaine is converted into a toxic meta-bolite due to its longer stay in liver. ☐
35. **Which one of the following local anaesthetic is highly cardiotoxic:** *(AIIMS May 2005)*
 A. Lignocaine ☐
 B. Procaine ☐
 C. Mepivacaine ☐
 D. Bupivacaine ☐
36. **Correct statement regarding bupivacaine includes:** *(PGI Dec 2005)*
 A. Less carditoxic than prilocaine ☐
 B. It is an amide ☐
 C. The maximum tolerable dose is 8mg/kg body wt ☐
 D. Duration more than 2 hrs ☐
37. **Levo-bupivacaine is administered by which of the following route:** *(PGI June 2004)*
 A. Nasogastric ☐
 B. Epidural ☐
 C. Intravenous ☐
 D. Intra-theccal ☐
 E. Oral ☐
38. **Buoivacaine toxicity treated with:** *(PGI Dec 07)*
 A. Esmolol ☐
 B. Epinephrine ☐
 C. Lignociaine ☐
 D. 5 percent dextrose ☐
 E. Benzodiazepines ☐
39. **Treatment of bupivacaine toxicity includes:** *(PGI May 11, Nov 10)*
 A. Isoproterenol ☐
 B. Epinephrine ☐
 C. Bretylium ☐
 D. Metoprolol ☐
 E. Lignocaine/Calcium channel blockers ☐
40. **Local anesthetic system toxicity (LAST) is/are increased by:** *(PGI May 12)*
 A. Hypoxia ☐
 B. Metabolic acidosis ☐
 C. Extreme age ☐
 D. Renal failure ☐

IV REGIONAL BLOCK

41. **Bier's block is** *(AIIMS May 12)*
 A. Subarachnoid block ☐
 B. Infiltration and surface block ☐
 C. Intravenous block ☐
 D. Peripheral nerve and nerve root block ☐
42. **Which anaesthetic modality is to be avoided in sickle cell disease** *(AI 2011)*
 A. General anaesthesia ☐
 B. Brachial plexus block ☐
 C. I.V. Regional Anaesthesia ☐
 D. Spinal ☐

43. A 30 year old lady is to undergo surgery under intravenous regional anesthesia for her left 'trigger finger'. Which one of the following should not be used for patient?
A. Lignocaine (*AIIMS May 2004*) ☐
B. Bupivacaine ☐
C. Prilocaine ☐
D. Lignocaine + ketorolac. ☐

44. A young boy has sickle cell trait. Which of the following anaesthesia is contraindicated: (*AIIMS May 2010*)
A. IV regional anaesthesia (IVRA) ☐
B. Brachal plexus block by infraclavicular approach ☐
C. Brachial plexus block by infraclavicular approach ☐
D. Brachial plexus block by axillary approach ☐

RETROBULBAR BLOCK

45. In general, the last muscle to be rendered akinetic with a retrobulbar anesthetic block is:
A. Superior rectus (*AIIMS May 2006*) ☐
B. Superior oblique ☐
C. Inferior oblique ☐
D. Levator palpebral superioris ☐

46. Least affected cranial nerve in retro-orbital block:
A. 1 CN (*AIIMS May 13*) ☐
B. 2 CN ☐
C. 3 CN ☐
D. 4 CN ☐
E. 6 CN ☐

47. Complication of peribulbar block- (*PGI Dec 2004*)
A. Retrobulbar hemorrhage ☐
B. Globe rupture ☐
C. Optic neuritis ☐
D. Local anaesthetic solution can migrate to brain ☐
E. Vasovagal syncope ☐

STELLATE GANGLION BLOCK

48. Which of the following is not a sign of successful stellate ganglion block? (*AI 2009*)
A. Nasal stuffiness ☐
B. Guttman sign ☐
C. Horner's syndrome ☐
D. Bradycardia ☐

49. A patient in ICU was on invasive monitoring with intra arterial canulation through right radial artery for last 3 days. Later he developed swelling and discolouration of right hand. The next line of management is
A. Stellate ganglion block (*AIIMS 2001*) ☐
B. Brachial Block ☐
C. Radial Nerve block ☐
D. Celiac plexus block ☐

50. From which of the following routes absorption of local anaesthetic is maximum? (*AIIMS Nov 08*)
A. Intercostal ☐
B. Epidural ☐
C. Branchial ☐
D. Caudal ☐

BRACHIAL PLEXUS BLOCK

51. Interscalene approach to brachial plexus block does not provide optimal surgical anaesthesia in the area of distribution of which of the following nerve
A. Musculocutaneous (*AI 2003*) ☐
B. Ulnar ☐
C. Radial ☐
D. Median ☐

52. Pneumothorax is a complication of (*AI 1992*)
A. Axillary block ☐
B. Brachial plexus block ☐
C. Epidural block ☐
D. High Spinal block ☐

53. Pudendal Nerve Block Involve (*AI 1993*)
A. $L_1L_2L_3$ ☐
B. $L_2L_3L_4$ ☐
C. $S_1S_2S_3$ ☐
D. $S_2S_3S_4$ ☐

54. Most common complication of celiac plexus block:
A. Pneumothorax (*AIIMS May 09*) ☐
B. Postural hypotension ☐
C. Retroperitoneal hemorrhage ☐
D. Intra-arterial injection ☐

Answers and Explanations:

GENERAL

1. **A i.e. Na^+ channel inhibition** 2. **B i.e. Act by decreasing sodium entry into cell; C i.e. Lignocaine is amide**
3. **A i.e. It inhibits generation of action potential; C i.e. Toxicity is reduced by addition of vasoconstrictor**
4. **All i.e. A, B, C, D, E** *[Ref: Lee's 13/e p. 370-75; Miller's 6/e p. 579-95]*

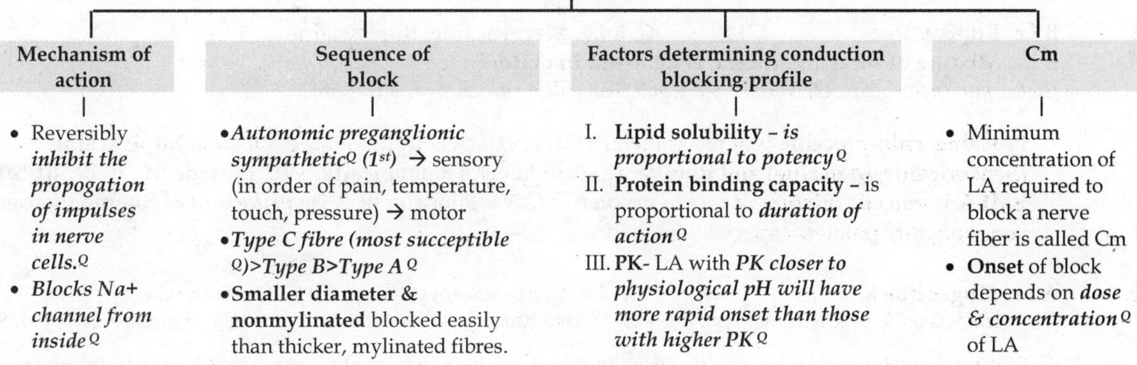

Local Anesthesia
Mechanism of action
• Reversibly inhibit the propogation of impulses in nerve cells.[Q]
• Blocks Na+ channel from inside[Q]
Sequence of block
• Autonomic preganglionic sympathetic[Q] (1st) → sensory (in order of pain, temperature, touch, pressure) → motor
• Type C fibre (most succeptible [Q])>Type B>Type A [Q]
• Smaller diameter & nonmylinated blocked easily than thicker, mylinated fibres.
Factors determining conduction blocking profile
I. Lipid solubility – is proportional to potency[Q]
II. Protein binding capacity – is proportional to duration of action[Q]
III. PK- LA with PK closer to physiological pH will have more rapid onset than those with higher PK[Q]
Cm
• Minimum concentration of LA required to block a nerve fiber is called Cm
• Onset of block depends on dose & concentration[Q] of LA

5. **C i.e. Type C** *[Ref: Ganong 20/e P-59]*

- Local Anesthetics (C>B>A) — max. affects – C; min affects – A
- O2 difficiency (Hypoxia) — max. affects – B; min affects – C
- Presure (A>B>C) — max. affects – A; min affects – C

Mnemonic	
LOCAL	Local anesthesia maximally affects C; minimally affects A
OBC	O_2 deficiency (i.e. hypoxia max. aff. B; min. aff. C)
PAC	Pressure max. affect A; minimally aff. C

Susceptibility	Most susceptible	Intermediate	Least susceptible
Local Anesthetic (LA) = CBA	*C*[Q]	B	*A*[Q]
O_2 deficiency (Hypoxia) = BAC	*B*[Q]	A	*C*[Q]
Pressure = ABC	*A*[Q]	B	*C*[Q]

6. **C, D, E i.e. Mivacurium, Butorphenol, Bupernorphine** 7. **B i.e. Procaine** 8. **D i.e. Bupivacaine**
[Ref: Morgan 4/e p. 270; Stoelting & Miller 4/e p 195; Lee 12/e P–593-95; Wylie 7/e pg-557]

- Mivacurium is short acting muscle relaxant. Whereas buprenorphine and nalorphine like drugs (including nalorphine, pentazocine, nalbuphine, and butorphanol) are partial agonists at both μ and k opioid receptors. However, slow dissociation from μ receptors and an unusual bell shaped dose response curve give buprenorphine a unique pharmacological profile. Nalorphine like drugs were originally (previously) believed to be μ antagonist & k agonists.
- All amide L.A. has '2i' in their name but lignocaine is also k/a Xylocaine which has only one 'i' in spelling.
- **Features of amide local anaesthetic** (compared to ester LA)
  - ***Produce more intense & longer lasting anesthesia***[Q]
  - Bind to α_1 acid glycoprotein in plasma
  - ***Not hydrolysed by plasma esterases***[Q]
  - ***Rarely cause hypersensitivity reactions***[Q], no cross sensitivity with ester LAs

9. **C i.e. Cocaine** 10. **A i.e. Cocaine** 11. **A i.e. Cocaine** 12. **C i.e. Cocaine**
[Ref: Lee 12/e, P-592]

- Cocaine, ***a natural alkaloid***[Q] from Erythroxylon coca leaves, was the ***earliest used***[Q] local anaesthesia (1st time used in 1884 for ocular surgery.)
- Cocaine is ***earliest*** used, ***naturally*** *occurring* ***easter linked***[Q] local anesthetic.
- It *blocks uptake of NA and Adrenaline* causing ***sympathomimetic effect***[Q] – Vasoconstriction[Q] etc.
- It ***should not be used with adrenaline***[Q] as it increases chances of *cardiac arrythmias & ventricular fibrillation*[Q].
- Cocaine has '2C' i.e. - **constrictor** of vessels and **contraindicated** with **adrenaline** as may *l/t* cardiac arythmias and V.T.

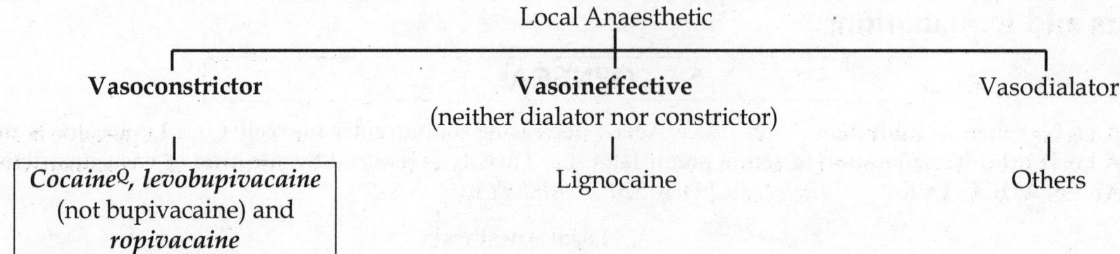

13. **B i.e. Bupivacaine** **14.** **C, E i.e. Mepivacaine, Bupivacaine**

15. **B i.e. Mixture of local anesthesia; D i.e. Used in children**

[Ref: Ajay Yadav 5/e p. 42; Miller's 6/e p.589; Aitkenhead 4/e, p. 575, 657, 666]

- Procaine, chlorprocaine (not recommended d/t poor penetration), **Mepivacaine, Bupivacaine (Sensoricaine, Marcaine) and Ropivacaine are never used topically**. Mn "**Provide Me BUR/BUS/BUM**".
- **EMLA** is eutectic ***mixture of local anesthetics (2.5% lidocaine & 2.5% prilocaine)***[Q] commonly used to make venepuncture painless especially in children.

16. **A i.e. Finger block** **17.** **A i.e. Increases speed & quality of anesthesia**

[Ref. Aitkenhead 5/e, p.61-62, Morgan 4/e, p 341, Ajay yadav 2/e, p 106; Millar 7/e, p 925; Katzung 10/e, p 419]

- ***Sodium bicarbonate increases the speed of onset of anaesthesia and improves its quality by increasing the intensity and duration of block.***
- **Addition of *vasoconstrictor* to LA** slows *its vascular absorption* thereby **reducing toxicity** (esp. in highly vascular sites intercostal> epidural> brachial) and **improving the depth and duration of anesthesia** (ie resulting in profound block of prolonged duration). However vasoconstrictors are **absolutely contraindicated** for injection close to end arteries ***(ring blocks of finger and toe digits, penis and pinna)***[Q] and in ***intravenous regional anesthesia (Bier's block)***[Q] because of the risk of ischemia. It should also be avoided (used cautiously) in *MI patients, hyperthyroidism, severe hypertension and with inhalational agents eg. halothane* which sensitizes heart to arrythmogenic action of adrenaline.

18. **A i.e. Procaine** **19.** **B i.e. Tetracaine**

20. **A & B i.e. Bupivacaine & Etodocaine** **21.** **A, C, D & E**

[Ref: Lee 12/e p. 592; KDT 5/e P-166; Morgan's 3/e P-238]

- Duration of action of various L.A. in descending order are:
  Dibucaine (Cinchocaine) >Tetracaine (Amethocaiene) >Bupivacaine >Lidocaine >Procaine
  Mnemonic: Delhi To Bombay
- Shortest acting LA – ***chlorprocaine***[Q]
- Intradural injection is contraindicated & may cause paraplegia – ***chlorprocaine***[Q]
- Longest acting LA – ***Dibucaine (Cinchocaine)***[Q]
- Only naturally occurring LA- ***Cocaine***[Q]
- Only vasoconstrictor LA - ***Cocaine***
- Safest LA / causes maximum methaemoglobinemia – ***Prilocaine***[Q]
- Best LA for regional block & isobaric spinal analgesia –***Bupivacaine***[Q]

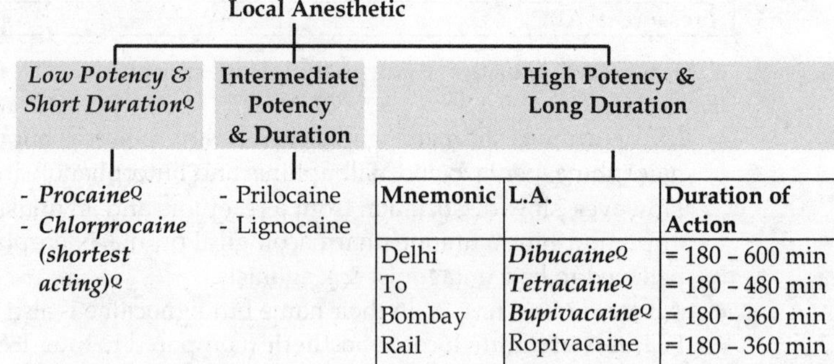

Mnemonic	L.A.	Duration of Action
Delhi	***Dibucaine***[Q]	= 180 – 600 min
To	***Tetracaine***[Q]	= 180 – 480 min
Bombay	***Bupivacaine***[Q]	= 180 – 360 min
Rail	Ropivacaine	= 180 – 360 min

Also remember:

- C fibre are most susceptible to local anaesthetic
- A fibre are least susceptible to local anaesthetic
- Potency of local anaesthetic (in increasing order) – Procaine < Mepivacaine < Prilocaine < Lidocaine < Chlorprocaine < Teracaine = Bupicaine = Etidocaine < Dibucaine

22. **A i.e. Shorter acting than tetracaine** *[Ref: KDT 7/e p 366-67; Miller 7/e p 1044, 863-64, 915]*

Dibucaine (Cinchocaine) is most potent, most toxic and longest acting local anesthetic[Q]***.***
Dibucaine number <30 indicates more quantity of atypical pseudocholinesterase[Q]***.***

Lidocaine

23. **A i.e., 2% B i.e., 4% C i.e., 5% E i.e., 1%**
24. **D i.e. 5%** **25.** **A i.e. 5%** **26.** **D i.e. 500 mg**
27. **D i.e. 7mg/kg** **28.** **C i.e. Ester** *[Ref: Lee's 13/e p. 386; Morgan's 4/e p. 270]*
29. **A i.e. Convulsion; B i.e. Respiratory depression; C i.e. Hypotension; D i.e. Cardiac arrest**

- Xylocaine is available in concentration of **5%** (for **subarachnoid-spinal anesthesia**), **4%** (**topical**) and **≤2%** (2, 1.5, 1 and **0.5%**) of which 0.5% is usually used for **epidural**.
- If it is asked that what is the max dose of Xylocaine with adrenaline the answer will be same i.e. **500 mg**Q and ans. will be **300 mg**Q when max dose of lignocaine without adrenaline is asked.
- Lidocaine is an amide and can l/t ***convulsions, bronchospasm, respiratory failure, depress hypoxia drive, and can cause apnea, bradycardia, hypotension & cardiac failure***Q.

30. **B i.e. It is most cardiotoxic local anesthetic** *[Ref: Goodman 12/e p 841-42, 565-73; KDT 7/e p 531]*

Lidocaine (xylocaine) ***acts on Na^+ channel in both active (open) and inactive (closed) state***Q. ***Because of extensive & variable 1st pass heptic metabolism*** oral use of drug is inappropriate. It is ***least cardiotoxic antiarrhythmic*** used intravenously to treat VT & prevent VF.

Toxicity

31. **B i.e. Prilocaine** **32.** **D i.e. Benzocaine**
33. **C i.e. Systemic toxicity of Local Anaesthetics**
34. **A i.e. Lidocaine concentration are initially higher in relatively well perfused tissues such as brain and heart**

- *Amide Local anaesthetics* (lidocaine) are metabolzied by *Microsomal enzymes in liver*

35. **D i.e. Bupivacaine** **36.** **B & D i.e. It is an amide, Duration more than 2 hrs**
37. **B & D i.e. (Epidural) & (Intratheccal)** **38.** **B i.e. Epinephrine; E i.eBenzodiazepines**
39. **B i.e. Epinephrine, C i.e. Bretylium, A i.e. Isoproterenol** **40.** **All**
[Ref: Miller 7/e p. 913, 932-35; Wylie 7/e p. 272-73; Morgan 5.e p. 270-74; Pardo 6/e p. 136-38; Barash 6/e p. 545; Goodman & Gillman 10/e p. 17, 962; Sataskar 17/e p. 384]

- **Procaine** and **benzocaine** are metabolized to **PABA**, which have been a/w rare **anaphylactic (allergic) reactions**Q.
- **Prilocaine (metabolized to O-toluidine) and benzocaine** can cause **methemoglobinemia**Q.
- **Local anesthesia systemic toxicity (LAST)** is increased by **hypoxia, hypercapnia, metabolic & respiratory acidosis, decreased hepatic function**Q (cirrhosis, liver failure) or **decreased liver blood flow** (CHF, β-blocker, H_2 receptor blockers). **Renal failure, advanged age** & genetically abnormal pseudocholinesterase (theoreticaly) would also increase LAST.
- **Bupivacaine** is **most cardiotoxic LA**Q. It is **long acting (2-4 h) amide, contraindicated in intravenous regional anesthesia or Bier's block**Q. It can be used in **peripheral nerve blocks, epidural and intrathecal routes**Q. Toxicity is treated by **amiodarone (doc), bretylium** (for VT), vaspressors eg **epinephrine, vasopressin** (for circulatory collapse), **isoproterenol and benzodiazepines (sedative)**.
- **LAST causes central nervous system not PNS symptoms/signs.** But the involvement of the peripheral nerve is characterized by parathesies, numbness, hypaesthesia, pain and neurological dysfunction. So, this patient is having peripheral nerve injury. It could have happened d/t: Open (crush) injury l/t laceration of nerves. As the patient underwent debriment, so he is a case of open injury, Nerve injury during debriment, Nerve injury during reduction & manipulation, Tourniquet pressure palsy, Nerve injury d/t tight bandage or cast.
- ***CNS or CVS systemic toxicity may result when standard lidocaine dose is administered to patient with circulatory failure because its concentration is initially higher in relatilvely well perfused tissue such as brain & heart***Q. And reduced cardiac output (in CHF) slows delivery of lildocaine (amide LA) to liver **reducing their metabolism (to MEGX**=mono ethyl glycine xylidide) prolonging Lidocaine's plasma half life. Toxicity of Lidocaine is due to it's own concentration in blood not due to it's toxic metabolite that is why option 4 is wrong. MEGX can cause seizures in neonates.

IV Regional Block

41. **C i.e. Intravenous block** 42. **C i.e. I.V. Regional Anaesthesia**
43. **B i.e. Bupivacaine** 44. **A i.e. IV regional anaesthesia (IVRA)**

[Ref: Aitkenhead 5/e p-320-21; Morgan 4/e p-387, 269-274; Wylie 7/e p-622-23; Paul 4/e p-198-99]

Intravenous Regional Anesthesia (IVRA or Bier's block) is ***contraindicated in situations in which tourniquets are contraindicated (eg sickle cell or Raynaud's disease)***Q. ***Bupivacaine is contraindicated in IVRA***Q owing to deaths from cardiotoxicity.

Retrobulbar Block

45. **B i.e. Superior Oblique** *[Ref: Morgan's 4/e p. 831; Lee's 13/e p-684-86; Wiley 7/e p-849-51; Aitkenhead 4/e, P- 600–602; Khurana 5/e p. 604-605]*
46. **A i.e. 1 CN >> D i.e. 4 CN**

Retrobulbar block anesthetizes ***ciliary nerves, ciliary ganglia and 2nd, 3rd & 6th cranial nerves***Q, hence producing global akinesia, anesthesia and analgesia. ***Superior oblique muscle is usually not or (late & least) paralyzed as the 4th cranial nerve is outside the muscle cone***Q.

In retrobulbar block, a good sign of correct needle placement is the *onset of ptosis* during the injection. This may be used as the end *point to limit the injection volume*. This volume should ***block all the relevant sensory nerves and the motor nerves to all structures, except perhaps the orbicularis oculi and the superior oblique***Q, which are out side the muscle cone. Orbicularis oculi can be blocked by nasal peribulbar injection.

47. **All** *[Ref: Parson 19th/602]*

Complications of peribulbar block are:

- Conjunctival damage
- Globe perforation
- Retrobulbar hemorrhage
- Extraocular muscle paralysis
- LA toxicity
- Syncope

Stellate Ganglion Block

48. **D i.e. Bradycardia:** *[Ref: Ajay Yadav : Anesthesia 4th/126; Anesthesiology by Zopol(2007)/2084]*

Bradycardia is not an established sign of successful stellate ganglion block.

49. **A i.e. Stellate ganglion block** *[Ref: Morgan's 3/e, P-332 & 93]*

- The patient has developed vasospasm (reflex sympathetic dystrophy) as indicated by development of swelling & discolouration of hand
- **Stellate (Cervicothoracic) Block** in reality blocks upper thoracic and cervical ganglion. It is indicated in :
  - ***Reflex sympathetic dystrophy***Q
  - ***Vasospastic disorder of upper extremity***Q
  - Head, Neck, Arm & Upper chest pain

50. **A. i.e. Intercostal** *Ref: Miller's aneshthesia 7/e p- 1639- 67;926-27 ; Ajay yadav 3/e p-118*

- Systemic absorption is directly proportional to blood supply. ***Local Anesthetic is absorbed very rapidly in intercostals block d/t close location of blood vessels around the nerve***Q. Highest blood level of LA is achieved per volume of drug injected in intercostals block.
- Sites of greatest absorption include: intrapleural > intercostals > pudendal > caudal > epidural > brachial > infiltration.

Brachial Plexus Block

51. **B i.e. Ulnar Nerve** *[Ref. Morgan 3/e p. 288; Miller 3/e vol.1 p.1408]* 52. **B i.e. Brachial Plexus block**

Brachial plexus block with **interscalene approach** provides **most** intense anesthesia in C_5-C_7 **dermatomes** and **least** intense in C_8-T_1 **(ulnar nerve)** area. Whereas the viceversa is true for **axillary approach.**

Brachial Plexus Block	**Phrenic Nerve Block**
Needle is passed **lateral to Subclavian Artery**Q with a risk of **Pneumothorax**Q	By infiltrating **scalenus anterior**Q

53. **D i.e. S_2 S_3 S_4** *[Ref: Morgan's 3/e P-331]*

- **Nucleus ambigaus** = 9, 10, 11 – cranial nerves nuclei
- **Nu. Solitarious** = 9, 10 & 7 Cranial nerve nuclei
- Phrenic Nerve = C_{345}
- Phrenic nerve block is done by infiltrating **scalenus anterior**
- **Erb's point/Axillary Nerve** has root value of C_{56}
- **Musculocutaneous Never** C567
- **Radial N** = C_{5678} T_1
- **Ulanar N** = $C_{(7)8}$ T_1
- Pudendal N = S_2 S_3 S_4

54. **B i.e. Postural Hypotenson** *[Ref: Millers Anesthesia 7/e p. 1669; Ajay Yadav 4/e p. 129]*

Most common complication of celiac plexus block is postural hypotension[Q]

2

ANAESTHESIA

8 SPINAL, EPIDURAL AND CAUDAL ANAESTHESIA

Central Neural (Neuraxial) Blockade

- **Epidural anaesthesia** is given in ***epidural space***Q (extending from foramen magnum to sacral hiatus) not in ***subarachnoid space***Q (which is used for **intrathecal – spinal anesthesia**).
- In comparison to spinal anesthesia, the volume of drug given is larger, ***onset on effect is delayed (5-20 min) and duration of action is prolonged***Q in epidural anesthesia. Both epidural & spinal anesthesia *block sympathetic outflow* (T_{12} – L_2). This produces ***dilation of resistance and capacitance vessels decreasing venous return & causing hypo-tension***Q. However, this fall is sudden & profound in spinal anesthesia, whereas slower & profound in epidural anesthesia.
- Epidural anesthesia is provided by **the effect of LA on the spinal nerve roots** as they pass from spinal cord to the periphery through the extradural space to unite in intervertebral foramen to form segmental nerves. Epidural analgesia produces effect by same mechanism, although opioids also acts on *spinal cord receptors*. Whereas, in spinal anesthesia, injection of LA into CSF produces anesthesia/analgesia of lower limbs & torso. And opioids modify the modulation of noxious stimuli as they are transmitted to brain via the spinal cord.

Feature	Epidural/Extradural (Caudal, Lumbar, Thoracic)	Intrathecal (Spinal)
Given in	Epidural space	***Subarachnoid space***Q
Technique	Single injection; or catheter	Single injection
Onset	***Late (5-20min)*** Q	***Early***Q (5 min)
Duration	2-4 hours (single shot); many days (via catheter)	2-3 hours (single shot)
Volume	10-20 ml	1-4 ml
Dose of drug	More	Less
CVS effects	Fall in BP is slower but can be profound with larger doses of LA. Bradycardia with high/thoracic blocks	BP fall is sudden & profound. Bradycardia with high block
Headache	Unlikely unless accidental dural tap	Low incidence (<2%) with modern needles (but higher than epidural)

Contraindications of Centrineuraxial (Spinal /Epidural) Anesthesia

Absolute Contraindications

- ***Patient's refusal***Q
- Patient's inability to maintain stillness during the needle puncture (eg. dementia, psychosis)
- ***Raised intra cranial pressure***Q (papilledema, cerebral edema, tumors in posterior fossa, suspected subarachnoid hemorrhage)/acute neurological disease.
- ***Severe hypovolemia***Q
- Severe stenotic valvular heart disease, the patient may be unable to compensate for vasodilation because of a fixed cardiac output.
- Marked skin sepsis & marked spinal deformity
- ***Marked coagulopathy, blood dyscariasis or full anticoagulant therapy***Q

Relative contraindications

- Un coperative patient (may be performed in conjuction with GA)
- Pre existing neurological deficit (eg demyelinating lesions) d/t medicolegal problems
- All severe & marked diseases in lesser degree i.e. spinal deformity, sepsis etc.
- Pre eclamptic toxaemia – epidural block has been used with great benefit in this condition, but a platelet count of less than 100 $\times 10^9$ L^{-1} usually preclude epidural or subarachnoid block.
- ***Mildly impaired coagulation***Q
- ***Patients with platelet <8000 /ml***Q

Centri – Neuraxial – Blockade

(NB) In setting of Anticoagulant & Antiplatelet Agents

- ***Oral anti coagulants (warfarin)***Q must be stopped & normal PT & INR should be documented prior to block in
  - Long term therapy
  - Initial dose was given more than 24 hours prior to block
  - More than one dose was given
- NB is best avoided if a patient has recieved **fibrinolytic or thrombolytic therapy**
- NB should be avoided in patients on ***theraputic dose of standard heparin***Q & with increased PTT. If the patient is started on heparin after placement of epidural catheter, the catheter should be removed only after discontinuation of heparin & evaluation of coagulation status.
- **Low molecular weight heparin (LMWH)** : catheter should be removed at least 10 hr after a dose and subsequent dosing should not occur for another 2 hours.

Neuraxial anesthesia best avoided

- ***Most antiplatelets (aspirin & NSAIDS) do not appear to increase the risk of spinal hematoma from neuraxial anesthesia or epidural catheter removal***Q. In contrast, more potent agents should be stopped & NB should be administered only after their effects have worn off. The waiting periods are
  - Ticlopidine = 14 days
  - Clopidgrel = 7 days
  - Abciximab = 48 hours
  - Eptifibatide = 8 hours
- **Minidose subcutaneous prophylaxis with standard (unfractioned) heparin** is not a contrain dication. For patients who are to receive heparin intraoperatively, block may be performed 1 h or more before and catheter removal should occur 1 hr prior to, or 4 hr following subsequent heparin dosing.

Neuraxial anesthesia can be given

High or Total Spinal Anaesthesia

- It occurs *following attempted epidural/caudal anaesthesia,* if there is *inadvertent intrathecal injection (i.e. subarachnoid injection).* Onset is usually rapid because the amount of anaesthetic required for epidural and caudal anaesthesia is 5-10 times that required for spinal anaesthesia. Due to ***inadvertent intrathecal injection of large amount of drug***Q; spinal anesthesia asecent into cervical levels k/a ***high or total spinal anesthesia***Q.
- Block extending above T_4 level may result in severe cardiovascular problems, with **bradycardia & marked hypotension**, which should be managed by aggressive IV fluids, chronotropic & vasoconstrictor drugs.
- Higher extending block **affecting phrenic nerve (C_3, C_4 & C_5)** may cause **respiratory difficulty & tingling/numbness in hands**. It is managed by intubation, ventilation & some form of general anesthesia to maintain unconsciousness (which facilitates intubation) until the block wanes & spontaneous ventilation returns.
- If the block is high enough then **unconsciousness, apnoea and dilated pupils** will occur, but consciousness may return before the patient can breathe spontaneously.

Clinical manifestation
- ***Marked hypotension***Q
- ***Bradycardia***Q
- ***Respiratory difficulty***
- ***Tingling/numbness in hands***
- ***Apnoea***Q
- Unconsciousness
- Dilated pupils

Prevention
- Careful aspiration
- Use of test dose
- Incrimental injection technique

Treatment
- Subarachnoid lavage by repeated withdraw of 5ml of CSF & replacement with preservative free NaCl
- IV fluids & vasopressor
- Immediate intubation & 100% O_2, assisted/ mechanical ventilation
- ***Hypotension by rapid IV fluid***Q ***head down position***Q, ***aggressive use of vasopressors***Q (eg – ephedrine, phenylephrine, metaraminol, *Dopamine* & epinephrine)
- Bradycardia by *atropine*

Epidural Analgesic

- **Spinal analgesia** includes *intrathecal & epidural administration of morphine.*
- **Morphine** has *poor lipid solubility* and converts to active metabolite *morphine 6 glucuronide.* The *slow onset & prolonged duration of action* which is disadvantageous, when attempting to titrate analgesic effects of interavenous morphine, confer a unique role in spinal analgesia. The systemic absorption of morphine after spinal analgesia is very slow resulting in long duration of analgesia and low plasma levels of drug. So the effect of spinal morphine are mediated by direct penetration into the CNS, not absorption into the circulation & subsequent redistribution to CNS. The therapeutic effect occur *mainly within spinal cord,* although large doe reach brain via CSF and *depress respiratory centre.*

- Effects of lipophilic (highly lipid soluble) opioids such as fentanyl analogues in general are subsequently the same whether given intravenously or spinally i.e. both produce similar plasma concentrations and comparable analgesia (in other words has no advantages).
- Extended release **liposomal formulation of morphine (Depo Dur)** can provide analgesia for upto 48 hrs but approved only for epidural administration following hip arthroplasty (15mg), lower abdomen surgery (10-15 mg) & cesarian section (10mg).
- Whether given epidurally or intrathecally, opiate penetration into spinal cord is both time & concentration dependent. Epidurally administered **hydrophilic agents** (such as **morphine**) produce analgesia at much lower blood levels than **lipophilic agents** (such as **fentanyl**). The fentanyl may produce segmental effects & thus should generally *be used only when catheter tip is close to incisional dermatome.* Systemic blood levels of fentanyl during epidural infusions are nearly equivalent to those during IV administrations. So the efficacy of epidural alfentanyl (& sufentanil) appears to be almost entirely due to systemic absorption.
- *Hydrophilic agents (morphine) spread rostrally (cranially) with time* thus low lumbar morphine injections can provide good (but delayed) analgesia for upper abdominal & thoracic procedures.
- Location of catheter tip to incisional dermatome and age influence the opiate dose requirement – closer location & older age require less drug.
- For **epidural continuous infusions**, local anesthetics **bupivacaine, levobupivacaine, or ropivacaine** are the drugs of choice (b/o low toxicity). Ropivacaine and levobupivacaine are considered to be safer alternatives to racemic bupivacaine, particularly with regard to cardiotoxicity following inadvertent intravenous administration.
- Either LA or opioids or frequently a combination of both may be used epidurally. ***Opioids are most suited for post operative analgesia***Q but are inadequate for surgery in most cases. Almost all opioids have been tried by epidural route with success but ***diamorphone or fentanyl are the most common additives***Q in UK (Aitkenhead). ***Fentanyl is the most commonly used lipophilic agent***Q (Morgan). Morphine, hydromorphone, fentanyl, clonidine & nalbuphine all can be used.

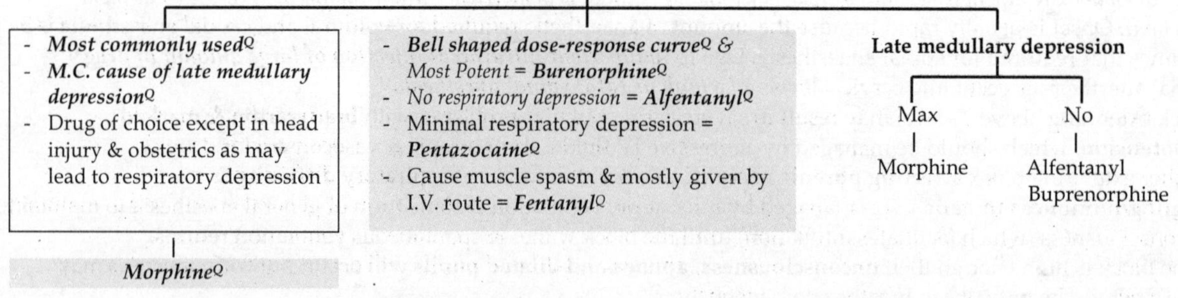

- *Most commonly used*Q
- *M.C. cause of late medullary depression*Q
- Drug of choice except in head injury & obstetrics as may lead to respiratory depression
*Morphine*Q
- *Bell shaped dose-response curve*Q &
*Most Potent = Burenorphine*Q
- *No respiratory depression = Alfentanyl*Q
- Minimal respiratory depression = *Pentazocaine*Q
- Cause muscle spasm & mostly given by I.V. route = *Fentanyl*Q
Late medullary depression
Max
Morphine
No
Alfentanyl
Buprenorphine

Post Dural Puncture Headache (PDPH)

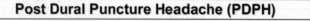

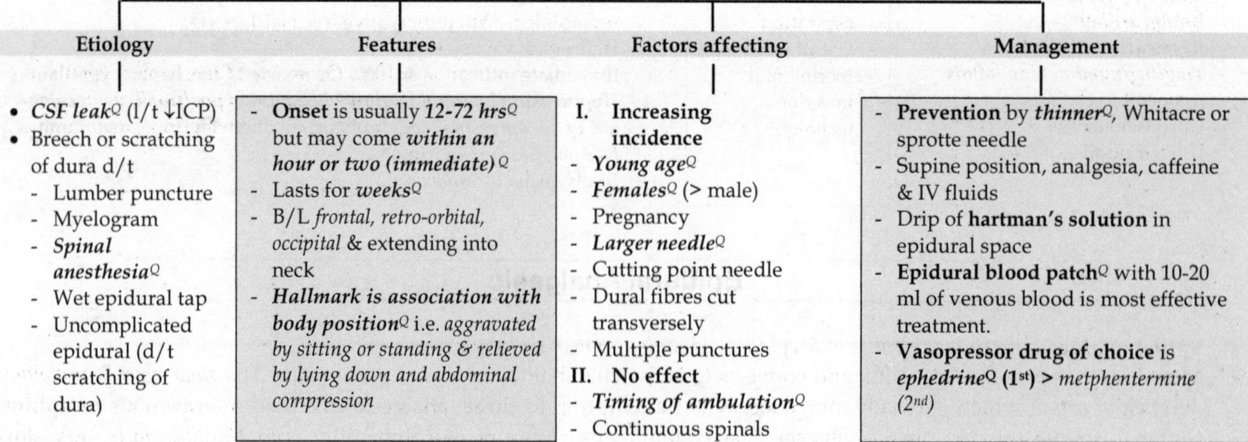

Etiology
- *CSF leak*Q (l/t ↓ICP)
- Breech or scratching of dura d/t
- Lumber puncture
- Myelogram
- *Spinal anesthesia*Q
- Wet epidural tap
- Uncomplicated epidural (d/t scratching of dura)
Features
- **Onset** is usually *12-72 hrs*Q but may come *within an hour or two (immediate)*Q
- Lasts for *weeks*Q
- B/L *frontal, retro-orbital, occipital* & extending into neck
- ***Hallmark is association with body position***Q i.e. *aggravated by sitting or standing & relieved by lying down and abdominal compression*
Factors affecting
I. **Increasing incidence**
- *Young age*Q
- *Females*Q (> male)
- Pregnancy
- *Larger needle*Q
- Cutting point needle
- Dural fibres cut transversely
- Multiple punctures
II. **No effect**
- *Timing of ambulation*Q
- Continuous spinals
Management
- **Prevention** by *thinner*Q, Whitacre or sprotte needle
- Supine position, analgesia, caffeine & IV fluids
- Drip of **hartman's solution** in epidural space
- **Epidural blood patch**Q with 10-20 ml of venous blood is most effective treatment.
- **Vasopressor drug of choice** is *ephedrine*Q (1st) > *metphentermine (2nd)*

PAIN MEASUREMENT & MANAGEMENT/ANALGESICS

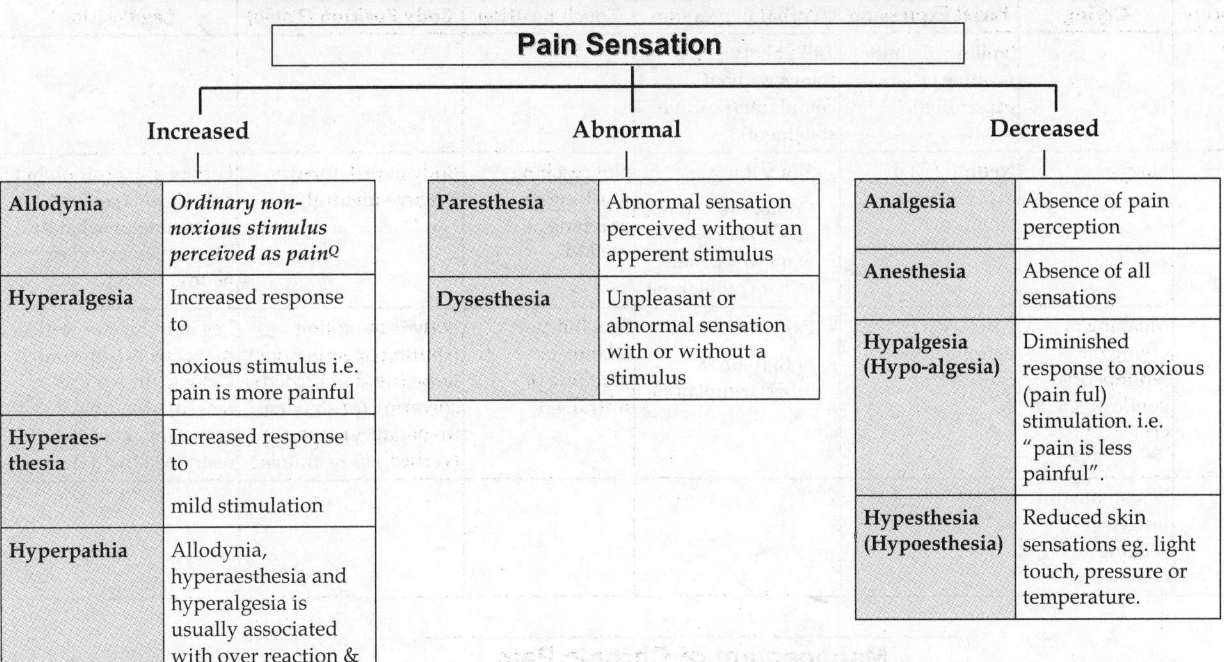

Pain Sensation

Increased

Allodynia	*Ordinary non-noxious stimulus perceived as pain*[Q]
Hyperalgesia	Increased response to noxious stimulus i.e. pain is more painful
Hyperaes-thesia	Increased response to mild stimulation
Hyperpathia	Allodynia, hyperaesthesia and hyperalgesia is usually associated with over reaction & *persistence of sensation after the stimulus*[Q].

Abnormal

Paresthesia	Abnormal sensation perceived without an apperent stimulus
Dysesthesia	Unpleasant or abnormal sensation with or without a stimulus

Decreased

Analgesia	Absence of pain perception
Anesthesia	Absence of all sensations
Hypalgesia (Hypo-algesia)	Diminished response to noxious (pain ful) stimulation. i.e. "pain is less painful".
Hypesthesia (Hypoesthesia)	Reduced skin sensations eg. light touch, pressure or temperature.

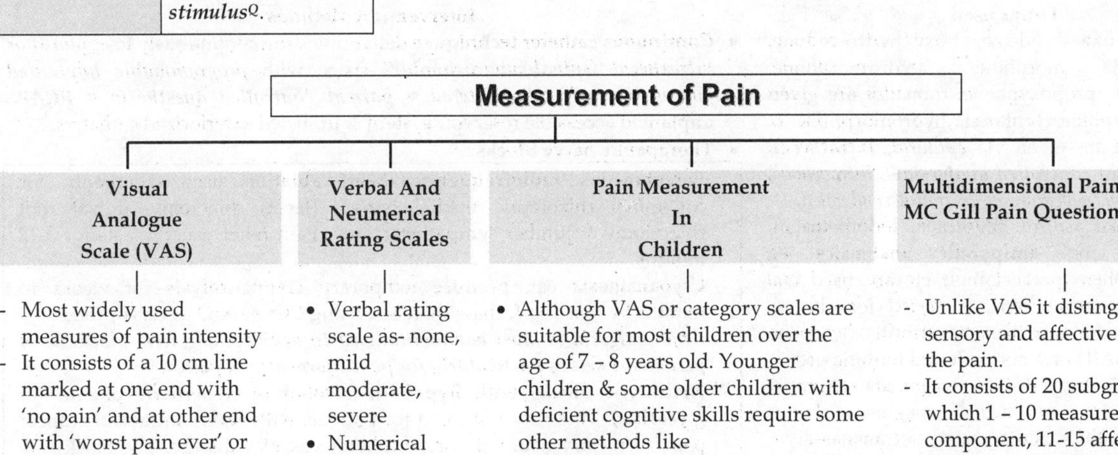

Measurement of Pain

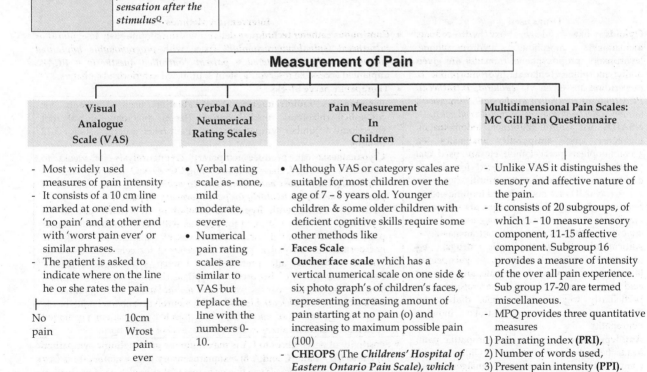

Visual Analogue Scale (VAS)

- Most widely used measures of pain intensity
- It consists of a 10 cm line marked at one end with 'no pain' and at other end with 'worst pain ever' or similar phrases.
- The patient is asked to indicate where on the line he or she rates the pain

No pain — 10cm — Wrost pain ever

1 2 3 4 5

Verbal And Neumerical Rating Scales

- Verbal rating scale as- none, mild moderate, severe
- Numerical pain rating scales are similar to VAS but replace the line with the numbers 0-10.

Pain Measurement In Children

- Although VAS or category scales are suitable for most children over the age of 7 – 8 years old. Younger children & some older children with deficient cognitive skills require some other methods like
- **Faces Scale**
- **Oucher face scale** which has a vertical numerical scale on one side & six photo graph's of children's faces, representing increasing amount of pain starting at no pain (o) and increasing to maximum possible pain (100)
- **CHEOPS** (The *Childrens' Hospital of Eastern Ontario Pain Scale), which measures crying, facial expression, body position (torso), verbal expression, touch position & leg position*[Q]. It is suitable for wide range of ages, including children too young to be able to use face.

Multidimensional Pain Scales: MC Gill Pain Questionnaire

- Unlike VAS it distinguishes the sensory and affective nature of the pain.
- It consists of 20 subgroups, of which 1 – 10 measure sensory component, 11-15 affective component. Subgroup 16 provides a measure of intensity of the over all pain experience. Sub group 17-20 are termed miscellaneous.
- MPQ provides three quantitative measures
  1) Pain rating index **(PRI),**
  2) Number of words used,
  3) Present pain intensity **(PPI).**
- ***Best tool for clinical and research work***[Q]

CHEOPS is recommended for *children 1 – 7 years old.* And a *score* > 4 indicates pain. It has *6 components.*

Score	Crying	Facial Expression	Verbal Expression	Touch position	Body Position (Torso)	Leg Position
O		Smiling (definite positive facial expression)	Talks about other things without complaint (positive statement)			
1	No cry	Neutral facial expression (composed)	- Not talking - Complains but not about pain eg. I want to see mom. (other complaints)	Not reaching, touching or grabbing at wound	Body at rest, torso is inactive (neutral)	Legs in any position but are relaxed (gentle swimming or separate like movements) i.e. neutral
2.	Moaning or crying (i.e. whimpering, gentle or silent cry)	Grimace (i.e. definite negative expression)	- Pain complaints, - Both (pain & other) complaints	Reaching, or toching or grabbing or restrained	Body is in motion (shifting or serpentine), tense (rigid or arched), shivering (or shaking involuantry), upright (vertical) or restrained	Leg in uneasy or restless movements (squirming, kicking, drawn up, tensed), standing, crouching, kneeling, restrained (held down).
3	Screaming (full lunged cry), sobbing (± complaints)		-			

Management of Chronic Pain

Drugs used

- **Opioids** like codeine, oxy/hydro-codone, methadone, morphine, hydromorphone, levorphanol, propoxyphene, tramadol are given orally; morphine, **fentanyl**, hydromorphone & meperidine are given via ***epidural, intrathecal, PCA (patient controlled analgesia)***Q, *intravenous, intramuscular, subcutaneous or transdermal patch.*
- **NSAIDs** like aspirin, ibuprofen, indomethacin, diclofenac and **antipyretic analgesics** eg acetaminophen (paracetamol) etc are used *oral (mostly), parenteral, rectal or topical* for chronic degenerative disease like osteoarthritis, headache & fever. NSAIDs are not preferred for long use.
- **Serotonergic drugs (5-HT$_{1B/1D}$ agonists - triptans)** are used in *neurovascular (migrane, cluster) headaches* orally, subcutaneously or transnassaly.
- **Anticonvulsants (antiepileptic drugs)** eg carbamazepine, clonazepam, gabapentin, lamotrigine, phenytoin, topiramate, and valproic acid are extremely useful in *neuropathic pain* particularly trigeminal neuralgia, diabetic or herpetic neuropathy and stroke induced neuropathy.
- **Antidepressants** are used for neuropathic pain, headache and cancer related pain. Older tricyclic compounds are more effective analgesics and SSRIs are better antidepressants.
- **Systemic local anesthetics** eg *lidocaine, procaine & chloroprocaine* are occasionally used in neuropathic pain to produce sedation, central analgesia & break pain cycle. Patients who respond to this (but not to anticonvulsants) may benefit from **chronic oral antiarrhythmic** *therapy (mostly mexiletine).*
- **Epidural or intrathecal local anesthetics** eg ***bupivacaine, levobupivacaine & ropivacaine***Q.

Intervention Methods

- **Continuous catheter techniques** delivering drug continuously to ***epidural or intrathecal (spinal/subarachnoid)***Q space with ***programmable implanted pumps (i.e. self administered = patient controlled anesthesia = PCA)***Q, implanted accessible reservoir system & tunneled exteriorized catheters.
- **Therapeutic nerve blocks**
  - **Percutaneous radiofrequency (heat) ablation** used commonly for trigeminal rhizotomy, medial branch (facet) rhizotomy, dorsal root rhizodomy & lumber sympathetectomy. Pain relief usually lasts for 3-12 months.
  - **Cryoanalgesia** can produce temporary **cryoneurolysis** for weeks to months by freezing & thawing tissue using CO_2 or N_2O gas cryoprobe.
  - ***Cryoanalgesia is most commonly used to achieve long term blockade of peripheral nerves particularly for post thoracotomy pain***Q.
  - **Neurolytic blocks with hypobaric alcohol or hyperbaric phenol (in glycerine).** These are indicated for patients with severe intractable cancer pain, refractory neuralgia or peripheral vascular disease. The blocks are not permanent. Alcohol is painful & preferred for celiac plexus block. Phenol is painless and preferred for lumbar sympathetic blockade. Neurolytic blocks are also used for hypogastric plexus, ganglion impar, somatic or cranial nerves or ***even neural axial (i.e. epidural & subarachnoid/intrathecal) blocks***Q. With neurolytic subarachnoid block, very small amounts of agent (0.1ml) is injected and patient positioned such that solution localizes to appropriate level of dorsal horn.

★ Sensitivity of nerve fibres to LA is maximum for **preganglionic sympathetic (β) fibres f/b > pain (C and A δ) > somatosensory (Aβ) > motor fibres (Aα).** *Differential epidural blockade* use this principle to distinguish pain mechanisms (sympathetic, somatic or psychogenic). If pain disappears *after saline* injection it is either *psychogenic (profound long lasting effect) or placebo effect (short lasting usually).* If pain relief (after epidural 0.5 lignocaine) coincides with signs of sympathetic blockade (i.e. *decreased BP*) it is mediated by *sympathetic fibres.* If pain relief (1% xylocaine) follows somatosensory blockade (pinprick & light touch) it is likely mediated by somatic fibres. Lastly, if pain persists even after motor blockade (by 2% epidural xylocaine), the pain is either *central (supraspinal) or psychogenic.*

- **Anterolateral cordotomy**

- α_2 **adrenergic agonists** eg *clonidine via epidural or intrathecal route* are effective in neuropathic pain and opioid tolerance.
- **Botulin toxin** in painful involuntary contractions of skeleton muscles eg *focal dystonia & spasticity.*
- **Neuroleptics** like fluphenazine, haloperidol, chlorpromazine & perphenazine
- ***Ketamine***[Q]

- **Therapeutic adjunct** include –
  - *Psychological interventions* like cognitive therapy, behavioural therapy, biofeedback, relaxation technique & hypnosis;
  - Physical therapy: *superficial heating modalities* include *conductive (hot packs; paraffin baths, fluidotherapy), convective (hydrotherapy), and radiant (infrared) techniques. Deep heating* modalities include *ultrasound, as well as short wave & microwave diathermy.*
  - Electric stimulation of nervous system like *transcutaneous electrical nerve stimulation (TENS), spinal cord stimulation (SCS) or dorsal column stimulation & intracerebral stimulation.*
  - Acupuncture.

2

Postoperative Analgesia for Thoracic Surgery

- After thoracotomy adequate postoperative analgesia is important not only for patient *comfort, but also to minimize pulmonary complications (atelectasis, pneumonia, respiratory failure), allowing the patient to breathe deeply, cough effectively and ambulate.* Major respiratory complications occur mostly within the first 3 days after thoracic surgery and their incidence have overall declined from 20% (prior to 1990) to 10% specifically b/o pain management.
- The multiple sensory afferents include the *intercostal nerves* T_4*-*T_6 (incision), T_7-T_8 (chest drains), *vagus nerve and CNX* (meditational pleura), *phrenic nerve and* C_3-C_5 (central diaphragmatic pleura) and brachial plexus (ipsilateral shoulder), There *is no one analgesic technique that can block* all these various pain afferents, so *analgesia should be multimodal.* The optimal choice depends on patient factors (preferences, contraindication), type of incision and available support. Main classes of drugs used are ***local anesthetics (regional), opioids (neuroxial/systemic) NSAIDS, ketamine and dexmedetomide (systemic)***[Q]**.**

ANAESTHESIA

Neuraxial (Epidural and Intrathecal) Analgesia (Opioids ± LA)

- *Neuraxial (both epidural and intrathecal) opioid analgesia* when compared with parenteral opioids, improves pulmonary function and oxygenation and *reduces post operative complication.*
- Unlike LA, neuraxial opioids are selective and have no hemodynamic or motor effects. However, *combination of opioids and LA provide better epidural analgesia at lower doses than either drug alone.* This suggest that the LA facilitate entery of opioids from epidural space to CSF and increase he affinity of narcotic for opioid receptor. A low concentration of LA (0.1% or 0.05% bupivacaine) used (b/o synergistic effect of opioid) can reduce sympathetic blockade that can occur, with a more concentrated LA alone. Addition of **epinephrine** (1:3 lack) decrease the amount of opioid needed for analgesia.
- **Epidural route is preferred** since the incidence of respiratory depression is less than with intrathecal (spinal/subarachnoid) opioids and the **presence of a catheter** allows for continuous, prolonged drug administration and avoids use of large bolus injections. The risks of *respiratory depression (dlt opioid), hemodynamic instability (hypotension) and motor blockade (d/t LA)* are largely d/t the use of bolus dose. So these are avoided with epidural infusions. **Patient controlled epidural opioid analgesia** is also possible if a catheter is present.
- The advantage of neuraxial opioid compared to systemic opiates include *selective blockade of spinal pain* receptors with minimal sympathetic blockade, no loss of motor function and greater predictability of pain relief.
- Depending on the opioid selected, a catheter can be placed at *lumbar or thoracic levels.* However, in order to reduce the volume required to produce an effect and lessen the chance of hypotension and motor weakness, *the catheter can be placed as close as possible to the*

Systemic Analgesia (Opioids and NSAIDs)

- Systemic opioids alone are effective in controlling *back ground pain,* but the acute component a/w cough or movement requires high plasma levels that *produce sedation and hypoventilation* in most patients.
- When used as a single modality, systemic opioids require plasma concentrations that are usually a/w *sedation, respiratory depression hypoventilation cough inhibition and reduced sighing.* They have very narrow therapeutic window. Even when used as patient controlled analgesia, **pain control is often suboptimal** b/o fluctuations in durg plasma concentration and patients have *interrupted sleep pattern* and are *unwilling to cough and clear secretion)with inadequate pain relief* (d/t sub-therapeutic opioid levels).
- **NSAIDs** such as *diclofenac, ketoprofen, ketorolac, indomethacin and acetaminophen* can reduce opioid consumption more than 30% and can be used as adjuvant to systemic opioids, particularly for treatment of *shoulder pain a/w chest tube placement* (that is often present post-operatively and is poorly controlled with epidural analgesia).
- **Low dose intramusaslar** (1mg/kg) **or intravenous infusion** (0.2 μg/kg/hr) **ketamine** can be used as an adjuvant in chronic/refractory pains.
- Intravenous (0.2-0.5 μg/kg/hr) **dexmedetomidine,** a selective adrenergic α_2 receptor agonist, is a useful adjuvant. It *potentiates analgesia* and significantly *decrease the requirement for opioids.* It is a/w hypotension and bradycardia but preserves renal function.

Paravertebral Block (PB)

- Paravertebral is a potential space deep to endothoracic facia that the intercostal nerve traverses as it passes from *intervertebral foramen to intercostal space.* It is bounded anteriorly by endothoracic facia & parietal pleura, posteriorly by costotransverse ligaments and heads of ribs and medially by vertebral body.
- A thoracic paravertebral block can be administered as a single injection (high failure rate & more S/E) or as a continuous infusion through a catheter (which can be placed either percutaneously or by approaching the space directly when the chest is open). Possible sites of analgesia include ***direct somatic nerve, sympathetic nerve & epidural blockade***[Q]**.**
- Thoracic paravertebral block is most promising technique and may ***provide analgesia equal or superior to that with thoracic epidural***[Q] and is a valuable alternative to it (Miller 2272). Paravertebral local

dermatome to be covered.

- Potential complications of thoracic epidural technique can be related to the placement (inadvertent dural puncture, trauma to spinal cord, hematoma) or drug administration (iv LA with resultant CVS and CNS toxicity). Epidural narcotics may, cause *respiratory depression (most serious), urinary retention, pruritus, nausea and vomiting*. The antagonist naloxone can reverse all side effects but will reverse analgesia also.

	Lipophilic Opioids	Hydorphilic Opioids
Drugs	*Fentanyl, sufentanil*Q	*Morphine, hydromorphone*Q
CSF diffusion onset and duration of action	**Rapidly diffuse** across the dura into CSF, bind to spinal opiate receptor and produce a **rapid onset (5-10 min)** and **short duration (2-4 hr)** analgesia	Diffuse more **slowly** into CSF, so their **onset** of action is **delayed (30-60 min)** but duration of action is **longer (6-24 hr)**
CSF spread	**Minimal** CSF spread is responsible for **narrow band analgesia**	**Extensive** CSF spread l/t **wide band analgesia**
Administration	By **continuous infusion** (b/o short duration of action) and *as close as possible to the dermatome* (b/o narrow band). The more lipid soluble the agent, the *more potent* it is.	By**constant infusion**, their low lipid solubility allows these drugs to be given *at either thoracic or lumber levels* (b/o wide band). However these agents are **preferred when a continuous infusion is not possible**
Site of action	Spinal ± systemic	**Primarily spinal**
Potency	Relatively low *potency versus systemic*	Neuraxial hydrophilic opioid has relatively *high potency vs. Systemic*
Nause, vomiting and pruritis	Lower incidence	Higher incidence
Respiratory depression (RD)	Rapid absorption into systemic and cerebral circulation may l/t **primarily acute (early severe) RD; minimal delayed.**	Both early (<6 hr) and delayed (>6 hr) RD possible, intrathecal> thoracic epidural > lumbar epidural
Tachyphylaxis	More	-

anesthetics ***provide a multilevel intercostal blockage that tends to be unilateral with a low tendency to spread to the epidural space***Q.

- Advantages of PVB in comparison to epidural analgesia include *comparable analgesia, unilateral effect, fewer failed blocks* (d/t under direct vision placement of catheter), *decreased risk of neuraxial hematoma, and less hypotension, vomiting, nausea and urinary retention*. Potential risks of PVB include pneumothorax (if repeated b/l blocks attempted), LA toxicity (b/o high vascularity), hypotension and inadvertent total spinal (both less than the epidural). At therapeutic doses, serum bupivacaine level can approach toxic levels by 4 days.
- **Paravertebral infusion in combination with NSAIDS and systemic opioids** are a reasonable alternative to epidural analgesia in **children or patients with contraindications to neuraxial blockade (eg patients on anticoagulants and tumor involvement of epidural space)**. However, the decrease in respiratory morbidity in high risk cases is shown by thoracic epidural analgesia but not by PVB.

Intercostal Nerve Block

- Like other techniques continuous catheter infusion is preferred over repeated injections, similarly blocks (catheter placement) under direct vision before chest closure is preffered over percutaneous method.
- The intercostal nerves to be blocked are at the level of *and 2 or 3 inter spaces above and below*. The quality of analgesia with this technique alone is *inferior to that of epidural and paravertebral analgesia* but may reduce opioid requirements. So it is used as a part of multimodality treatment when neuraxial blocks are contraindicated or for minimally invasive procedures (i.e. pain a/w *multiple small port incisions and chest drains following VATS*). It is important to place the block **near posterior axillary line** to be certain to block the lateral *cutaneous branch of intercostal nerve* and avoid injection into intercostal vessels, which are adjacent to nerve in intercostal groove. There is increased risk of systemic toxicity because the rate of systemic absorption of LA from intercostal space is quite high.

Intrapleural Analgesia

- It is performed by injecting LA *b/w parietal and visceral pleura* either by percutaneous catherter or *chest drainage tube*. The analgesia is extremely variable, unfavourable and ***inferior to epidural and paravertebral analgesia for control of pain and so for preservation of lung function and reduction for post operative pulmonary complication***Q.
- The analgesia is extremely dependent on patient position (in sitting LA pools in CP angles), chest drains (LA can be lost), infusion volumes (diluted by extravascated blood and tissue fluid in pleural space) and type surgery (sequestered and channelled b/o decreased movement operated lung), limiting the quality of analgesia. It can be used in video assisted thoracoscopic surgery (VATS) but is rarely used on routine basis.

Cryoanalgesia

- Long lasting (3 weeks to 6 months) intercostal nerve block can be obtained by cryoablation (applying - 60°C probe to intercostal nerves intraoperatively).
- It is moderately efficicent in decreasing postoperative pain but is a/w an incidence of ***chronic neuralgia that has led many centers to abandon it***Q (Miller 1879). Cryoanalgesia can be used for postoperative analgesia after thoracotomy but like intrapleural analgesia and intercostal blocks, does not appear to provide any analgesic advantage over epidural analgesia, is not effective for other types of postoperative pain, and is short lived (Miller 2772). Although cryoanalgesia was shown to effectively relieve pain and improve postoperative pulmonary function, more detailed studies have revealed a *significant* incidence of *paraesthesia and posthoracotomy pain syndrome* (Yaa-50).

TENS

- May be useful in mild to moderate pain (of VATS) but is ineffective in severe pain. It does not reduce opioid requirements or improve pulmonary functions.

QUESTIONS

CENTRINEURAXIAL ANESTHESIA

1. **In all of the following conditions neuraxial blockade is absolutely contraindicated, except:** *(DNB 05, AI 03)*
   A. Patient refusal ☐
   B. Coagulopathy ☐
   C. Severe hypovolemia ☐
   D. Pre-existing neurological deficits ☐
2. **Centrineuraxial (spinal and epidural) anaesthesia is not contraindicated in –** *(AI 07; DNB 09)*
   A. Platelets < 80,000 ☐
   B. Patient on aspirin ☐
   C. Patient on oral anticoagulants ☐
   D. Patient on LMH (heparin) ☐

EPIDURAL ANESTHESIA

3. **True about Epidural anesthesia:** *(PGI 10; DNB 11)*
   A. Effects start immediately ☐
   B. C/I in coagulopathies ☐
   C. Given in subarachnoid space ☐
   D. Venous return decreases ☐
4. **True about epidural narcotics (opioids) are all except**
   A. Nausea, vomiting (gi side effects) *(AI 11)* ☐
   B. Pruritis (itching) ☐
   C. Respiratory depression ☐
   D. Act on dorsal horn cells ☐
5. **Site of action of epidural analgesia**
   A. Sensory nerve endings *(AIIMS 98; DNB 02)* ☐
   B. Ventral horn ☐
   C. Substantia gelatinosa ☐
   D. Cortex ☐
6. **Epidural narcotic is preferred over epidural LA because it causes** *(DNB 04; AIIMS 96)*
   A. Less respiratory depression ☐
   B. Less dose is required ☐
   C. No motor paralysis ☐
   D. No retention of urine ☐
7. **Drug used for Epidural Analgesic**
   A. Morphine *(AI 93)* ☐
   B. Fentanyl ☐
   C. Piroxicam ☐
   D. NSAID'S ☐
8. **True about epidural anaesthesia in pregnancy**
   A. Given through subarachnoid space ☐
   B. Increases cardiac output *(PGI 03; DNB 04)* ☐
   C. Decreases venous return ☐
   D. Venous pooling ☐
   E. Decreased placental circulation ☐
9. **A patient was admitted epidural anaesthesia with 15 ml of 1.5%. Lignocaine with adrenaline for hernia surgery. He devoled hypotension and respiratory depression within 3 minutes after administration of block. The most common cause would be:** *(AIIMS May 05,03)*
   A. Allergy to drug administered ☐
   B. Systemic toxicity to drug administered ☐
   C. Patient got vasovagal shock ☐
   D. Drug has entered the subarachnoid space ☐
10. **An anesthesia resident was givnig spinal anesthesia when the patient had sudden aphonia and loss of consciousness. What could have happened?** *(AI 11)*
    A. Total spinal ☐
    B. Partial spinal ☐
    C. Vaso vagal attack ☐
    D. Intra vascular injection ☐
11. **In high spinal anaesthesia what is seen** *(AIIMS 2001)*
    A. Hypotension & Bradycardia ☐
    B. Hypotension & Tachycardia ☐
    C. Hypertension & Bradycardia ☐
    D. Hypertension & Tachycardia ☐

CAUDAL ANESTHESIA

12. **A Lower Segment Caesarean section (LSCS) can be carried out under all the following techniques of anaesthesia except:** *(AI 05; CMC 08)*
    A. General anaesthesia. ☐
    B. Spinal anaesthesia. ☐
    C. Caudal anaesthesia. ☐
    D. Combined Spinal Epidural anaesthesia. ☐
13. The **anesthetic drug injected for paravertebral block is least likely to diffuse to:** *(AI 09)*
    A. Epidural space ☐
    B. Subarachnoid space ☐
    C. Intercostal space ☐
    D. Superior and inferior paravertebral spaces ☐

SPINAL ANESTHESIA

14. **Structure (s) pierce in Lumbar spinal puncture is/are:**
    A. Ligamentum flavum *(PGI June 09)* ☐
    B. Duramater ☐
    C. Supraspinous ligament ☐
    D. Anterior longitudinal ligament ☐
    E. Posterior longitudinal ligament ☐
15. **In spinal anesthesia which fiber is lost first** *(AIIMS 92)*
    A. Sympathetic ☐
    B. Sensory ☐
    C. Motor ☐
    D. Propiorecption ☐
16. **Spinal anesthesia should be injected into the space between** *(AI 97)*
    A. T_{12} - L_1 ☐
    B. L_1 – L_2 ☐
    C. L_3 – L_4 ☐
    D. L_5 – S_1 ☐
17. **Spinal anesthesia is given at which of the following levels :** *(AI 11)*
    A. L1-2 ☐
    B. L2-4 ☐
    C. Midline of thorax ☐
    D. Below L5 (caudal) ☐
18. **Most common complication of spinal anesthesia is**
    A. Hypotension *(DNB 96, AIIMS 94)* ☐
    B. Headache ☐
    C. Meningitis ☐
    D. Arrythmia ☐
19. **Best way to prevent hypotension during spinal anesthesia**
    A. Preloading with crystalloids ☐
    B. Mephentermine *(DNB 2K, AI 95)* ☐
    C. Dopamine ☐
    D. Tredelenbug's position ☐
20. **Following spinal subarachnoid block a patient develops hypotension. This can be managed by the following means except:** *(AIIMS 2003)*
    A. Lowering the head end ☐
    B. Administration of 1000 ml of Ringers lacate before the block ☐
    C. Vasopressor drug like methoxamine ☐
    D. Use of ionotrope like dopamine. ☐

2

ANAESTHESIA

21. Vasopressor of choice in hypotension produced during sub-arachnoidblock *(PGI 04; DNB 05)*
A. Ephedrine ☐
B. Mephenteramine ☐
C. Adrenaline ☐
D. Dopamine ☐
E. Steroids ☐

22. Post spinal headache is due to *(AI 1995)*
A. Meningitis ☐
B. Encephaletics ☐
C. CSF leak ☐
D. Increased ICT ☐

23. Post Spinal Headache can last for *(AI 1994)*
A. Upto 10 min ☐
B. Upto 10 hours ☐
C. 7 - 10 days ☐
D. Upto 10 months ☐

24. True about post spinal headache *(AI 1992)*
A. Frontal ☐
B. More in lying down ☐
C. Low incidence with thin (25 G) needle ☐
D. Increased by abdominal compression ☐

25. Post dural puncture headache, true about -
A. Common in elderly *(PGI 04; DNB 05)* ☐
B. Small bore needle prevents it ☐
C. Early ambulation increases incidence ☐
D. Occurs immediately after spinal anaesthesia ☐
E. Blood patch is the first line of treatment ☐

26. Which is the true statement regarding post-dural anesthetic headache: *(PGI 2001)*
A. Blood patch is the first line of treatment ☐
B. Occurs due to low CSF pressure ☐
C. Increased incidence with early mobilization of patient ☐
D. Use of small guage needle prevents headache ☐
E. Common in old age ☐

PAIN MEASUREMENT AND MANAGEMENT

27. Which one of the following is the description used for the term allodynia during pain management? *(AIIMS May 06)*
A. Absence of pain perception ☐
B. Complete lack of pain sensation ☐
C. Unpleasant sensation with or without a stimulus ☐
D. Perception of an ordinarily non-noxious sitmulus as severe pain ☐

28. Perception of ordinarily non noxious stimuli as pain, is better known as : *(PGI 2K, SGPGI 03; DNB 05)*
A. Allodynia ☐
B. Huperalgesia ☐
C. Hyperesthesia ☐
D. Radiculopathy ☐

29. Pain rating index is provided by
A. Faces scale *(PGI 02; JIPMER 02; DNB 04)* ☐
B. Visual analogue scale ☐
C. Mc Gill questionniare ☐
D. CHEOP scale ☐

30. Best Scale to measure pain in children of 5 years age would be *(SGPGI 02; DNB 06)*
A. VAS ☐
B. Mc Gill Scale ☐
C. Faces Scale ☐
D. CHEOPS ☐

31. Visual analogue scale (VAS) most widely used to measure
A. Sleep *(AI 10; DNB 11)* ☐
B. Sedation ☐
C. Pain intensity ☐
D. Depth of Anaesthesia ☐

32. A children hospital Eastern Ontaria Pain Scale (CHEOPS) for rating potoperative pain in children includes all except
A. Cry *(AIIMS Nov 08)* ☐
B. Touch ☐
C. Torso ☐
D. Oxygen saturation ☐

33. Which one of the following is the shortest acting intravenous analgesic: *(AIIMS 2003)*
A. Remifantanil ☐
B. Fentanyl ☐
C. Alfentanil ☐
D. Sufentanil ☐

34. Narcotic of choice for out patient anesthesia: *(AIIMS 1994)*
A. Morphine ☐
B. Alfentanyl ☐
C. Fentanyl ☐
D. Pethidine ☐

35. Least analgesic *(AIIMS 1994)*
A. N_2O ☐
B. Ether ☐
C. Halothane ☐
D. Cyclopropane ☐

36. Which of the following have analgesic property?
A. N_2O *(PGI June 08)* ☐
B. Ketamine ☐
C. Thiopentone ☐
D. Etomidate ☐

37. Which of the following anesthetic agents have analgesic property: *(PGI 2001)*
A. Ketamine ☐
B. Nitrous oxide ☐
C. Thiopentone ☐
D. Propofol ☐
E. Midazolam ☐

38. All are opioid agonist – antagonist compounds except
A. Buprenorphine *(JIPMER 01, PGI 02, DNB 01)* ☐
B. Nalbuphine ☐
C. Pentazocine ☐
D. Nalmefene ☐
E. Papaverine ☐

39. True regarding morphine *(PGI June 06)*
A. Tolerance develps for all except miosis and constipation ☐
B. Tolerance to all effects develops with chronic usage ☐
C. Tolerance develops for all except euphoria and sedation ☐
D. Tolerance can develop to all effects in high doses ☐

40. Best antagonist of morphine is *(AIIMS 97)*
A. Nalorphine ☐
B. Naloxone ☐
C. Buprenorphine ☐
D. Pentazocine ☐

41. Drug with Ceiling effect: *(AI 1994)*
A. Morphine ☐
B. Buprenorphine ☐
C. Fentanyl ☐
D. Alfentanyl ☐

42. Management of chronic pain includes: *(PGI Nov 2010)*
A. Intra-thecal hyperbaric phenol ☐
B. Antrolateral cordotomy ☐
C. Epidural fentanyl ☐
D. Patient controlled analgesia(PCA) ☐
E. Anticonvulsant drugs ☐

43. A patient after undergoing thoracotomy complains of severe pain. He can be managed by *(AIIMS Nov 2010)*
A. Intercostal cryoanalgesia ☐
B. I.V fentanyl ☐
C. Oral morphine ☐
D. Oral brufen ☐

Answers and Exlanations:

CENTRINEURAXIAL ANESTHESIA

1. **D ie Pre existing Neurological defect**
2. **B i.e. Patient on aspirin** *[Ref: Lee's 13/e p-477–84, 658, 661-62, 369, 17; Morgan's 4/e p. 299; Aitkenhead 5/e, p. 323; Miller's 6/e p-1654]*

- *Centrineuraxial anesthesia is not associated with increased risk with most antiplatelet agents (eg. aspirin*[Q] & NSAIDs).
- **Neuroxial block** is combined name given to *Spinal, Epidural and Caudal Blocks*. Principal site of action for neuroaxial blok is **Nerve root** [Q].
- **Absolute contraindications are**[Q]-
  - ***Patient Refusal***[Q]
  - ***Bleeding Diathesis***[Q]
  - ***Severe Hypovolemia***[Q]
  - Raised ICT
  - Infection at site of injection
  - Severe stenotic valvular Heart disease & fixed cardiac output states

EPIDURAL ANESTHESIA

3. **B i.e. C/I in coagulopathies, D i.e. Venous return decreases**
[Ref: Aitkenhead 5/e p. 321, 328-31, 768-9, 10, 632; Wylie 7/e p. 613-17, 926-28; Morgan 4/e p. 396-98]

- **Epidural anaesthesia** is given in ***epidural space***[Q] (extending from foramen magnum to sacral hiatus) not in ***subarachnoid space***[Q] (which is used for **intrathecal – spinal anesthesia**).
- In comparison to spinal anesthesia, the volume of drug given is larger, ***onset on effect is delayed (5-20 min) and duration of action is prolonged***[Q] in epidural anesthesia. Both epidural & spinal anesthesia *block sympathetic outflow (T_{12} – L_2)*. This produces ***dilation of resistance and capacitance vessels decreasing venous return & causing hypo-tension***[Q]. However, this fall is sudden & profound in spinal anesthesia, whereas slower & profound in epidural anesthesia.
- Centrineuraxial (spinal & epidural) anesthesia is **contraindicated** in *coagulopathy, blood dyscariasis, full anticoagulant (oral warfarin, LMW heparin & fibrinolytic) therapy* but can be given to patients on antiplatelet agents like aspirin & NSAIDs.

4. **D i.e. Act on dorsal horn cells** *[Ref. Morgan 4/e p 398-96]*
5. **C i.e. Substantia gelatinosa**

- **Opoid receptors are maximum in Lamina 2 (substantia gelatinosa) Lamina 5** of spinal cord. So Epidural Narcotics acts mainly on substantia gelatinosa
- **Common side effects** of intraspinal/ epidural opioids are ***pruritis (itching), nausea – vomiting, urinary retention, sedation, ileus and dose dependent respiratory depression (most serious)***[Q]

6. **C i.e. No motor paralysis**
7. **A i.e. Morphine; B i.e. Fentanyl** *[Ref: Aitkenhead 5/e, p. 333; Wylie 7/e p. 555, Morgan's 4/e p. 192-196]*

- *Spinal Anesthesia is preferred in lower abdominal surgeries as* ***it shrinks the intestines*** *so other viscera can be seen very well.*[Q]
- *Narcotic* ***(morphine)***[Q] *are preferred over LA* ***as motor function is maintained*** *and patient may co-operate in surgery.*[Q]

8. **C i.e. Decrease venous return; D i.e. Venous pooling** *[Ref: Wylie 5/e P-862,1037; Shridev 3/e P-37]*

- In **epidural anesthesia,** the anesthetic drug is injected in ***epidural space***[Q]& in **spinal anesthesia** the drug is injected in ***subarachnoid space***[Q].
- CVS changes that occur after epidural anesthesia are summarized in box-
- **Hypotension** (20-30% ↓ in B.P. or systolic B.P. <100 mmHg) is the ***most common S/E***[Q]. It is treated by ***IV ephedrine, IV fluids, IV phenylepherine, O_2 supplement & left uterine displacement***[Q] ***Use of head down (Trendelenburg) position is controversial because of its potentially detrimental effects on pulmonary gas exchange.***[Q]
- In the absence of hypotension neither epidural nor spinal have any effect on the uterine blood flow. (placental circulation)

Epidural anesthesia
↓
Loss of sympathetic vasomotor tone
↓
Vasodilation
↓
Peripheral pooling of blood[Q]
↓
Reduced venous return[Q]
↓
Reduced cardiac output[Q]
↓
Hypotension

9. D i.e. Drug has entered the sub arachnoid space.
[Ref: Morgan's 4/e p. 277, 317-319; Lee's 12/e p684; Paul's 4/e p217]

Marked hypotension & apnoea after epidural anaesthesia

Earlyonset (< 5 minutes)	Delayed onset (15-30 minutes)
*Total spinal anaesthesia i.e. inadvertent intrathecal/sub arachnoid injection.*Q	*Sub dural injection*Q

10. C i.e. Vaso vagal attack
[Ref. Wylie 7/e p 662; Miller 7/e p 932-30; Aitkenhead 5/e p 316-17, 54; Stoelting 5/e 129-31; Yao 7/e p 1027]

Total spinal anesthesia
- Ocurs if the large volume of LA used for epidural anesthesia is injected into subarachnoid space i.e. **it occurs following epidural/caudal anesthesia**, if there is inadvertent intrathecal injection of large volume of drugs.
- It occurs after (not during injection)

Vasovagal attack or emotional fainting (Syncope)
- Likely to occur particularly in **an anxious patient** with a rapidly ascending **spinal block.** It may occur ***instantaneously even during the procedure (e.g. spinal)***Q.
- Pallor, nausea and (neurocardiogenic) bradycardia or asystole are a/w hypotension and fainting. Rapid resolution results from placing the patient in head down position and administration of iv ephedrine or atropine.

Systemic toxicity
- If large amount of LA reach the tissues of heart and brain they exert the same membrane stabilizing effect as on nerve resulting in **progressive depression** of function. The **earliest feature is numbness or tingling of tongue and circumoral area**; b/o rich blood supply to these tissue depositing enough drug to have an effect on nerve endings. The patient may beome *light headed, anxious, drowsy and or complain of tinnitus. Convulsions, loss of consciousness, coma and apnoea* may develop subsequently. Cardiovascular collapse may result from direct myocardial depression and vasodilation or hypoxemia d/t apnoea.
- The most ommon cause is ***accidental intravascular injection***Q but it may also result from absolute overdose during blocks. System absorption of LA is greatest after **intercostal nerve block and caudal anesthesia;** intermediate after **epidural anesthesia >** brachial plexus > sciatic & femoral nerve block; and least after infiltration anesthesia.

11. A i.e. Hypotension & Bradycardia *[Ref: Morgan's 3/e, P-277]*

- Spinal anesthesia ascending into cervical levels causing *severe **hypotension**Q, **bradycardia**Q, **respiratory insufficiency**Q & **unconsciousness**Q is known as* **high or total spinal anesthesia.**
- It can also occur following attempted epidural/caudal anethesia, if there is inadvertent intrathecal injection of large amount of anesthetic intended for epidural space.

Local Anesthesia in high dose

In Heart cause	**In Blood Vessels** cause
- ↓ Automacity - ↓ Excitability - ↓ Contractility - ↓ Conductivity - ↑ Eff. Refractory Period ↓ 1/t *Bradycardia*Q	**Fall in BP d/t** - Sympathetic blockage - In high doses d/t direct relaxation of arterior smooth muscle ↓ *Hypotension*Q

CAUDAL ANESTHESIA

12. C i.e. Caudal anesthesia *[Ref: Aitkin Head 4/e p 568, 641, 643, 52]*

Caudal anaesthesia is used for *perineal operations.* It is ***unpopular for LSCS (lower segment caesarian section) because of the risk of introducing needle passing through mother's sacrum and rectum into fetal presenting parts.***Q

Anaesthesia for cesarian section

Regional Anaesthesia	General Anaesthesia
• It is the *technique of choice*Q for elective cesarian section. • Methods available are: - ***Spinal anaesthesia***Q - Epidural anaesthesia - ***Combined spinal-epidural anesthesia***Q	• The primary advantage is reliability and rapidity of onset of a state in which the operation is performed. • It is required in following situations: - Extreme emergency eg severe fetal distress or maternal haemorrhage - Contraindications or refusal to regional anaesthesia.

13. **B i.e. Subarachnoid Space:** *[Ref: Complications of Regional Anesthesia by Finucane 2nd/108; Irwin and Rippe's intensive care medicine 6th/217; Miller 7/e p. 1881]*

The subarachnoid space is not in direct continuity with the paravertebral space and hence the anesthetic drug injected for a paravertebral block is least likely to diffuse into this space amongst the options provided. The subarachnoid space is not in direct communication with the paravertebral, intercostal or epidural space and diffusion to this space is least likely.

Paravertebral Space and Block

- The paravertebral space is the area spinal nerves enter as they leave the intervertebral foramen.
- The paravertebral space is continuous laterally with the intercostal space and medially with the epidural space via the intervertebral neural foramina.
- Anesthetic injected for a Paravertebral block may flow laterally into the intercostals space as well as up and down into the ipsilateral *paravertebral space*. Epidural spread is also always possible through the intervertebral neural foramen if enough volume is injected.

'Injection into a paravertebral catheter causes flow laterally into the intercostals space as well as up and down into the ipsilateral paravertebral space'- Irwin and Rippe's intensive care medicine 6th/217

'Because the paravertebral space is contiguous with the epidural space via the intervertebral neural foramina, epidural spread is also always possible if enough volume is injected.'- Complications of Regional Anesthesia by Finucane 2nd/108

SPINAL ANESTHESIA

14. **A, B, C i.e. Ligamentum flavum; Duramater; Supraspinous ligament**
15. **A i.e. Sympathetic**
16. **C i.e. $L_3 - L_4$** *[Ref: Morgan 4/e pg-291-93]*

- Anterior and posterior longitudinal ligaments are not pierced in lumbar puncture as these lie anterior (ventral) to spinal cord. Whereas the **supraspinous ligament, interspinous ligament** (both thickened in cervical region to form **ligamentum nuche**), and **ligamentum flavum** lie posterior (dorsal) to spinal cord so the needle passes through these dorsal structures in **epidural & spinal anesthesia**. ***Duramater & arachnoid are additional structures pierced in spinal anesthesia***Q.

Order of Block in Spinal Anesthesia

A	*Autonomic Preganglionic Sympathetic*Q
Temple	Temperature
Prayer	Prick
Pays	Pain
Tough	Touch
Precious	Pressure
Moral	Motor
Values	Vibration

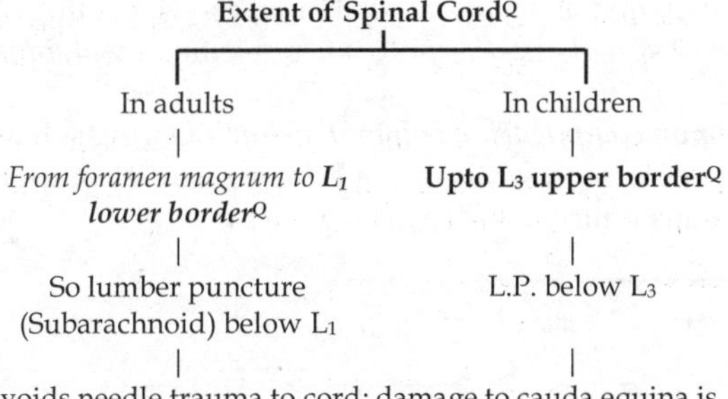

Avoids needle trauma to cord; damage to cauda equina is unlikely as these nerve do not float in dural sac and tend to be pushed away by advancing needle.

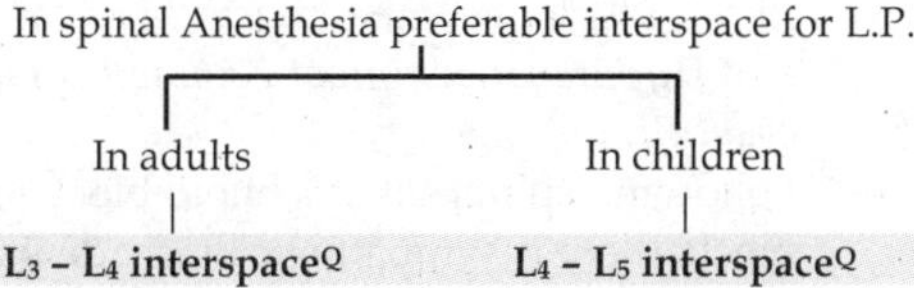

17. **B i.e. L_{2-4}**
[Ref: Wylie 7/e p. 609; Morgan 4/e p. 293; Miller 7/e p. 1620]

Spinal anesthesia is usually injected at L_{2-3}, L_{3-4} ***or sometimes L_{4-5} space in adults***Q.

Normal Extent of Spinal Cord
(from foramen magnum to)

- **Lower border of L_1 vertebrae in adults**
  - Therefore, performing a **lumbar (subarachnoid) puncture, dural puncture, spinal (intrathecal) anesthesia** below L_1 ***usually at L_2-L_3, L_3-L_4 or sometimes L_{4-5} space***Q in adults avoids potential needle trauma to spinal cord.
- **Upper border of L_3 vertebrae in infants**
  - Spinal needle puncture **below L_3, usually in L_{4-5} space** avoids trauma to spinal cord. Damage to cauda equine is unlikely as these nerve roots float in the dural sac and tend to be pushed away (rather than pierced) by advancing needle.

Extent of Dural sac, subdural and sub-arachnoid space

- **S_2 in adults**
- **S_3 in children**

★ Because of lower extent & smaller body size caudal anesthesia carries a greater risk of subarachnoid injection in children than in adults.

★ Nerve blocks close to intervertebral foramen carry a risk of subdural or subarachnoid injection because *dural sheath/duramater/theca* invests nerve roots for a small distance even after they exit the spinal cord.

★ **Filum terminale**, an extension of piamater, penetrates the duramater and attaches the terminal end of spinal cord (conus medullaris) to periostium of coccyx. Because spinal cord ends at L_1/L_3, lower nerve roots course some distance (forming **cauda equina/ horse's tail**) before exiting intervertebral foramina.

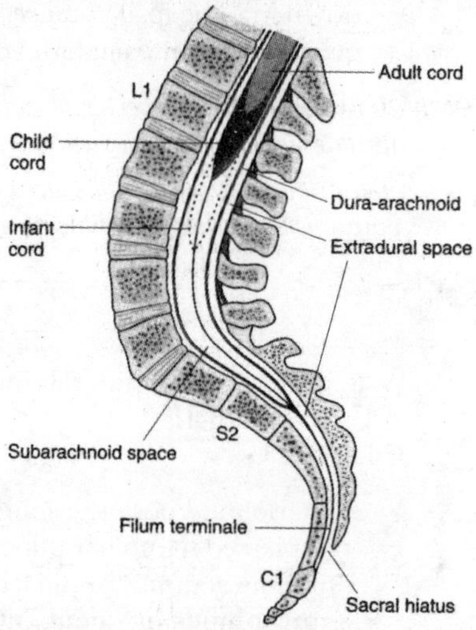

★ **Piamater** is innermost highly vascular membrane. **Arachnoidmater** is a delicate, nonvascular membrane attached to outermost layer dura which functions as the principal barrier to drugs crossing in & out of CSF. **Subdural space** (b/w dura & arachnoidmater) contains only small amount of serous fluid and an injection into it during spinal anesthesia may l/t failed spinal anesthesia; and rarely total spinal after epidural anesthesia when there is no indication of errant injection of LA into CSF.

★ Spinal, caudal, epidural anesthesia is also known as ***neuraxial anesthesia.*** The principal site of action for neuraxial block is ***nerve root in cauda equina***Q. ***Differential block*** typically results in Sympathetic block (judged by temperature sensitivity) that may be two segments higher than sensory block (pain, light touch) which in turn two segments higher than motor blockade. ***Autonomic Preganglionic Sympathetic B fibers***Q are most sensitive.

18. **A i.e. Hypotension**
19. **A i.e. Preloading with crystalloids**
20. **A. i.e. Lowering the head end**
21. **A i.e. Ephedrine**

[Ref. Morgan's 3/e p-260, 61, 267; Lee anesthesia 12/e p-680; Bailey & Love 23/e p83]

- Most common complication of spinal anesthesia is ***hypotension***Q, which can be prevented by ***preloading with crystalloid.*** In spinal anesthesia ***autonomic preganglionic sympathetic fibres***Q are the earliest blocked fibres. Block of sympathetic nerves causes vasodialation of venous capacitance vessels, pooling of blood and ***Hypotension***Q ***(most common complication of spinal anesthesia***Q***).*** It is prevented by ***preloading with crystalloid.***
- Following spinal subarachnoid block ***most common complication is hypotension***Q. During sub-arachnoid block, there is sympathetic blockade producing decreased venous return & hence, cardiac output and BP falls. The main aim of treatment is to restore venous return, which can be done by-

Prevented by

- ***Preloading with 10-20 ml/kg of intravenous fluid***Q ***(method of choice)***
- Left uterine displacement in third trimester of pregnancy

Managed by

- Increased intravenous fluid administration
- ***Autotransfusion accomplished by placing the patient in head down position***Q.
- Bradycardia treated with ***atropine***
- Hypotension with ***vasopressors***Q. ***Ephedrine is vasopressor choice***Q. It acts on ∝ and β both receptors. *Mephentermine ($\alpha_1\beta$ action) is 2nd choice.* Phenyephrine & Methoxamine (α action) preferred when tachycardia is present, IV adrenaline is last measure given to avoid cardiac arrest.
- If profound hypotension or bradycardia persist despite these interventions ***epinephrine*** should be used.

- So the patient can be managed by all the four means but the least effective & most controversial mean is lowering head end. The specific gravity (baricity) of CSF is ***l.003 - 1.008***[Q] at 37°C. A **hyper baric** solution of LA is ***denser* than CSF** & **hypobaric** solution of LA is ***Lighter* than CSF.** A LA solution can be made hyperbaric by adding *glucose* & hypobaric by addition of *sterile water.* Most important factors affecting **level of spinal anesthesia** are: ***Baricity***[Q], ***Position of patient - during & immediately after injection,***[Q] *drug dose & site of injection.* Thus *with a head down position a hyperbaric solution spreads cephald & hypobaric solution moves caudad and vice versa.* And in this Q baricity of LA & time passed after injecting spinal anesthesia is not mentioned, so lowering the head end is weakest option.

22. **C i.e. CSF leak** **23.** **C i.e. 7-10 days**
24. **C i.e. Low incidence with thin needle**
25. **B & D i.e. (Small bore needle prevents it) & (Occurs immediately after spinal anesthesia)**
26. **B i.e. Occurs due to low CSF pressure; D i.e. Use of small gauge needle prevents headache**
[Ref. Morgan's 3/e p. 275; Lee 12/e p. 685 to 687; Wylie 7/e p. 612]

Post Dural Puncture Headache (PDPH)

- Any breach of dura may result in PDPH. This may follow a *lumber puncture, myelogram,* ***spinal anesthesia***[Q], ***wet epidural tap***[Q] (in which epidural needle pierced dura) *or uncomplicated epidural* (dlt scratching of dura).
- **It result from decreased intracranial pressure as CSF leaks from dural defect at a greater rate than it is being produced.**[Q]
- The headache is *BIL, frontal or retro-orbital, occipital & extending into neck.* It may be throbbing & associated with photophobia & nausea. The onset is usually ***12-72 hours***[Q] following procedure **(in first 3 days)** may ***last for 1-2 weeks***[Q]. **The hallmark is its association with body position**[Q] (i.e. *aggravated by sitting or standing & relieved by lying down)*[Q]
- The incidence increases with -
  1. ***Larger needle***[Q]
  2. *Cutting point* (in comparision to pencil point) needle.
  3. ***Young age, Female sex, Pregnancy***[Q]
- So, max incidence is expected in a wet epidural tap with a large epidural needle in an obstetric patient. Lowest incidence would be expected with an elderly male using 27 gauge pencil point needle.

Management of PDPH

1. ***Prevention by thinner needle***[Q] (whitacre needle)
2. Supine position, intravenous fluids & caffeine and analgesia.
3. ***Epidural blood Patch*** is most effective treatment.

Pain Measurement & Management

27. **D i.e. Perception of an ordinarily non-noxious sitmulus as severe pain**
28. **A i.e. Allodynia** *[Ref: Morgan's Anesthesia 4/e p. 361; Aitkenhead 4/e, P--214]*

Term	Description
Allodynia	*Perception of ordinarily non- noxious stimulus as pain*[Q]
Analgesia	Absence of pain perception
Anesthesia	Absence of all sensation
Anesthesia dolorosa	Pain in area that lacks sensation
Dysesthesia	Unpleasant or abnormal sensation with or without a stimulus
Hypalgesia (Hypoalgesia)	Diminished response to noxious stimulation (eg. pinprick)
Hyperalgesia	*Increased response to noxious stimulation*[Q]
Hyperesthesia	*Increased response to mild stimulation*[Q]
Hyperpathia	Presence of hyperesthesia, allodynia, and hyperalgesia usually associated with over reaction, and persistence of the sensation after the stimulus.
Hypesthesia (Hypoesthesia)	Reduced cutaneous sensation (eg. light touch, pressure, or temperature)
Neuralgia	Pain in the distribution of a nerve or a group of nerve
Paresthesia	Abnormal sensation perceived without an apparent stimulus
Rediculopathy	Functional abnormality of one or more nerve root.

29. **C i.e. Mc Gill questionnaire** **30.** **D i.e. CHEOPS**
31. **C i.e. Pain intensity** **32.** **D. i.e. Oxygen satyration**
[Ref: Miller's 6/e p-407-22; Morgan's 4/e p. 192-198; Aitkenhead 4/e, p. 213-218; KDT 5/e p. 58; Harrison 15th/e p-495; www.anes.ucla.edu/pain/assessment_tool-cheops.htm]

ANAESTHESIA

2

- *10 division visual analogue scale* is used to indicate the ***severity of pain***Q. **Mc Gill questionnaire** provide pain rating index.
- **CHEOPS**, which measures ***crying, facial expression, verbal expression, touch position, body position (torso) and leg position***Q, is suitable for wide range of ages including ***children***Q.

33. **A i.e. Remifentanil** *[Ref. Lee's 12/e p-188, 189, 190, 417; Morgan's 3/e, P-173, 884; Aitknenhead 4/e P-617]*
34. **B i.e. Alfentanyl**

All of these are short acting narcotic analgesics the shortest acting among them is Remifentanil.

Drug	Onset	Duration of action
Remifentanil	30 - 60 second	3 - 5 minute
Alfentanil	0.5 minute	5 - 10 minute
Fentanyl & Sufentanil	1 - 4 minute	30 minute .

- ***Remifentanyl, Alfentanyl & Sufentanil*** have short duration of action so can be used as outpatient anesthetic agents.
- ***Desflurane & Sevoflurane*** provide the **fastest wake up time** among volatile anesthetic outpatient agents.

35. **C i.e. Halothane**
36. **A. i.e. N_2O, B. i.e. Ketamine**
37. **A i.e. Ketamine; B i.e. Nitrous oxide** *[Ref: Lee 12/e P-167; Morgan's 3/e P-139-140; KDT 6/e p-370-77]*

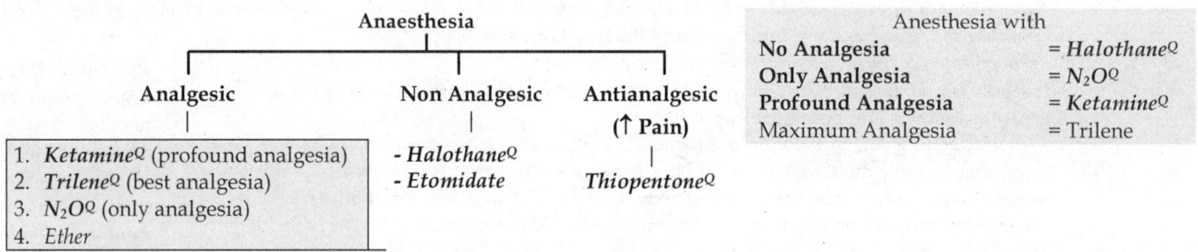

38. **D i.e. Nalmefene; E i.e. Papaverine**
39. **A i.e. Toerance develops for all except miosis & constipation**
40. **B i.e. Naloxone** *[Ref: Miller's 6/e p-407–22; Morgan's 4/e p. 192- 198; Aitkenhead 4/e, p. 213- 18; KDT 5/e P- 58]*

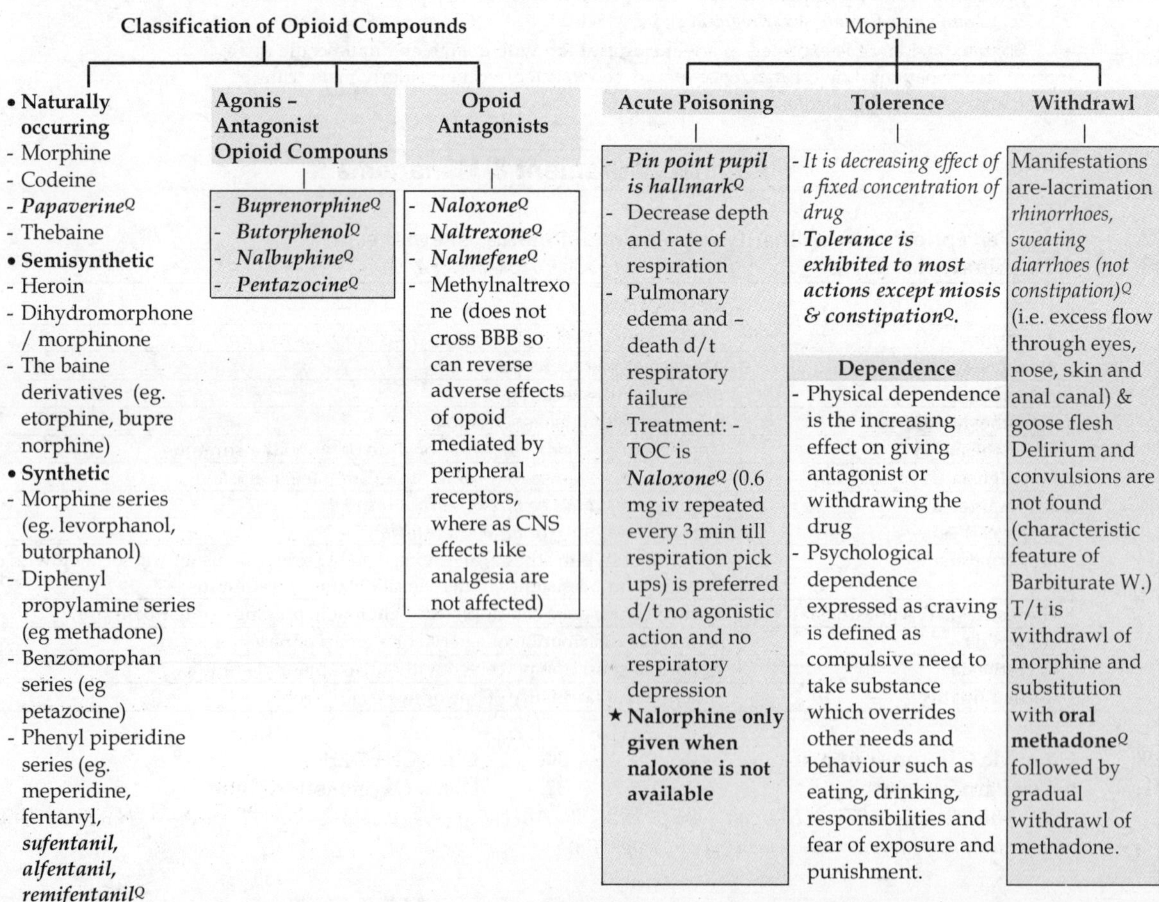

41. **B i.e. Buprenorphine** *[Ref: Miller's Anesthesia 6/e p-418-22]*

- **Ceiling effect** means particular effect of drug increases with dose of drug, and when the ceiling (roof) is reached further incriment in dose not result in increase in effect.
- ***Opioid agonist – antagonist compounds produce respiratory depression (& anelgesia) with a ceiling effect***[Q]. which means higher doses do not produce further respiratory depression and may actually result in increased ventilation (d/t predominance of antagonist actions)

Drug	Correlation of Respiratory Depression (RD) with Dose	
Morphine	Increase proportionally with dose	R.D. / Morphine / Dose
Buprenorphine **Butorphanol** **Nalbuphine**	} *Produce ceiling effect*[Q]	RD / *Buprenorphine*[Q] / Ceiling Effect
Pentazocine	*Ceiling effect suggested* but difficult to study, because of Psychotomimetic effects	

MANAGEMENT OF CHRONIC PAIN

42. **A i.e. Intra-thecal hyperbaric phenol, B i.e. Antrolateral cordotomy, C i.e. Epidural fentanyl, D i.e. Patient controlled analgesia(PCA), E i.e. Anticonvulsant drugs**
[Ref: Miller 7/e p. 1802-8; Barash 6/e p. 1515-30; Morgan 4/e p. 389-410]

Management of chronic pain includes *patient controlled analgesia (PCA), epidural or intrathecal opioid (fentanyl) & local anesthetic, neurolytic blocks by hypobaric alcohol or hyperbaric phenol, anterolateral cordotomy and various drugs like anticonvulsants, antidepressants, neuroleptics, opioids, serotonergic drugs and α_2 adrenergic agonist*[Q].

43. **B i.e. IV fentanyl** *[Ref. Miller 7/e, p. 1829, 1877-81, 2772, Wylie's 7/e, p. 798-99, Yao and Artusio's 7/e, p 48-50]*

Post thoracostomy pain can best managed by **continuous epidural analgesia** *with opioids* **± local anesthetics by catherter tip placed as close as possible to the incisional dermatome** (may be patient controlled analgesia) > **Paravertebral block** (with continuous infusion of LA by catheter) in combination with NSAIDS and systemic opioids > **Systemic analgesia by opioids and NSAIDS > Intercostal nerve block (by catheter) > TENS, cryoanalgesia and intrapleural block.**

NOTES

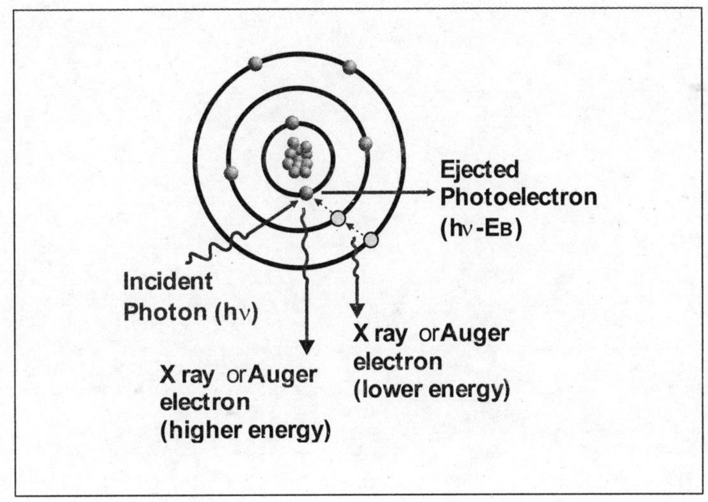

Radiotherapy

Electromagnetic Radiation/Photon

- **Electromagnetic radiation or photon waves** are **non particulate (0-mass), non charged (0-charge)** waves, that **do not require a medium to travel** (i.e. can travel in vaccum) and transfer energy from one location to another at the **speed of light** (c= 3×10^8 m/s).
- The **major difference** between various forms of photons/electromagnetic radiation **lies in their wave length (λ) and frequency (n)**, which accounts for their differences in energy carried. $E \propto n/\lambda$

  So Xrays with shorter wave length in comparison to visible light carries 5000 times higher energies. Because for EM waves energy is proportional to frequency (n) and inversly proportional to wave length (λ).
- EM radiation spectrum consists of *photons with wave length, frequency and energy ranges over 10 orders of magnitude* (the range is really infinite). **From low energy to high energy** these are <u>R</u>adar waves, <u>M</u>icrowaves, <u>I</u>nfra-red, <u>L</u>ight (visible photons), <u>U</u>ltraviolet, <u>**X**</u> rays and <u>G</u>amma rays. (Mn- "Reliance **MILL X**tra **G**rand").
- Photons are named by their wave lengths (eg radio & microwaves) and origins (eg **Xrays originate from** ***within the atom***[Q] as a result of atomic transformation or **gamma rays** from within the **nucleus** as a r/o nuclear transformations).

Photon Interactions: X rays & Gamma rays

- When ionizing photon radiation (i.e. radiation of sufficient energy to cause ionization or removal of electron from atom) fall on matter, it can *undergo interactions with atomic electrons or nuclei* and are removed from the primary beam (an effect called **attenuation**) or do not interact and instead exit the material (k/a **transmitted photons**).
- **Beam quality** describes the amount of penetration by a photon radiation beam and is indicated by **beam energy** (defined by *acclerating potential, effective energy or gamma ray energy)* and **half value life (HVL).** HVL is the thickness of a material that reduces the transmitted intensity to one half of the original intensity. Similarly, the **tenth value layer (TVL)** is the thickness required to reduce the number, intensity, or exposure by a factor 10.
- Megavoltage photon interaction probabilities are <1 and vary with energy of incident photon and atomic number of interaction material. A/t physical law, the fractional number of unattenuated photons interacting per unit thickness of material is constant, such that ΔN is change in no of photons d/t attenuation, N is no of incident photon, ΔX is thickness traversed by photons for attenuation, and μ is constant fractional attenuation per thickness also k/a **linear attenuation co-efficient**. Minus indicates result is negative & results in fewer photons. And $\mu = 0.693/HVL$

$$\frac{\Delta N / N}{\Delta X} = -\mu$$

- For *monoenergetic photons HVL & μ are constant* but for *polyenergetic photons* μ is not constant instead *decreases with increasing depth.* This happens because the low enegy photons are attenuated preferentially, compared with high energy photons (i.e. b/o *increased attenuation at low energies*). As the depth increases, the ratio of high energy to low energy photons increases resulting in increased beam penetration or **beam hardening**. After large number of low energy photons are attenuated at depth, beam hardening is minimal and μ becomes constant. *Because μ changes with depth, HVL also changes and the greatest HVL is found at maximum depth* (i.e. $HVL_1 < HVL_2 < HVL_3$ and so on)
- Mass attenuation coefficient, is the linear attenuation coefficient (μ) divided by material's density (ρ). It is independent of material density.
- So when a photon beam falls it can either **exit (transmitted photons)** or interact (attenuate) with increasing amount of energy in 5 possible ways: **Cohert scattering (COH), photo electric effect (PE), Compton effect (CE), pair production (PP) and photodisintegration (PD)**. So total linear and mass attenuation coefficients are sum of their components.

$$\mu_{ToT} = \mu_{COH} + \mu_{PE} + \mu_{CE} + \mu_{PP} + \mu_{PD}$$

Coherent Scattering (COH)

- It occurs at **very low energy levels (<10 KeV)** of photons.
- In COH, a photon is *scattered (deflected) off* an outer orbital electron *with a change in direction and no change in energy*

Photo electric Effect (PE)

- It occurs at **low energy** (upto **60 KeV**) levels in water and *strongly depends on photon energy ($1/E_\gamma^3$) and atomic number of material (Z^3)*. It is used in diagnostic radiology.
- In this process, the *most tightly bound inner orbital electron* (with binding energy E_B) *completely absorbs all energy of falling (incident) photon,* so much so that the photon ceases to exist, and the orbital electron now called **photoelectron** is **ejected** (with kinetic energy = $E\gamma - E_B$)
- Ejection of orbital electron leaves a ***vacancy in the inner***

Pair Production

- PP occurs at **very high energy levels** (photon energies **> 1.022 MeV**), dominates above 10 MeV in water and *linearly depends on atomic number (z) and photon energies.* 1.022 MeV is threshold energy or the energy needed to create 2 electrons (rest energy of an electron is 0.511 MeV).

- The amount of COH is negligible in the diagnostic and therapeutic energy ranges.

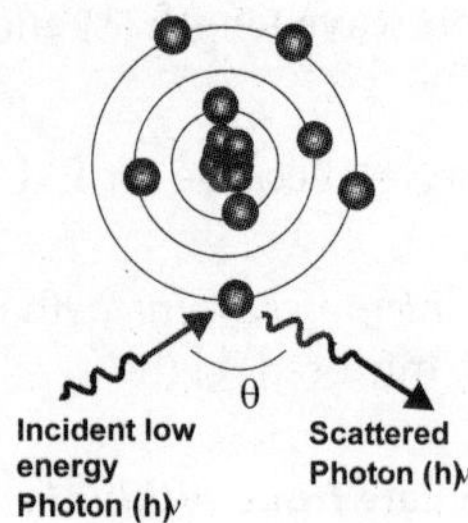

Coherent Scattering

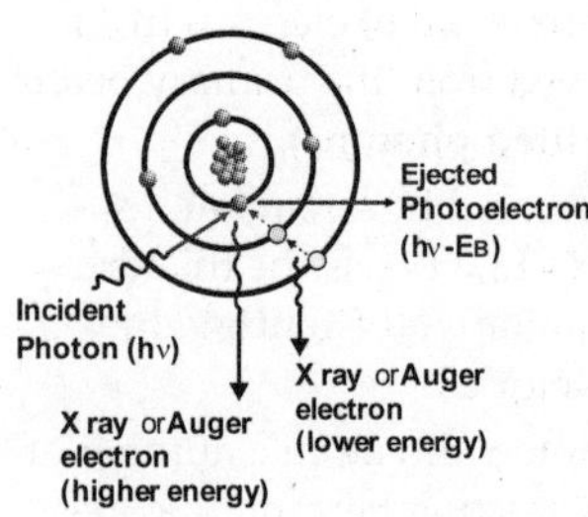

Photo electric effect

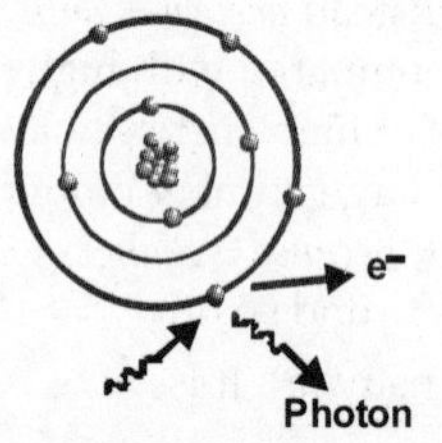

Compton Scattering

electron shell. This is filled by an electron form outer orbit, with **simultaneous emission** of characteristic **X ray** with an energy equal to the differences of two electron binding energies (E_{B1} – E_{B2}). And sometimes this X-ray energy is transferred to one of the nearby orbital electrons l/t **ejection of this Auger electron with no x-ray emission.**

- This process leaves a new vacancy in outer orbital shell, which is filled by electron from an orbital beyond, with emission of second X-ray or Auger electron of lower energy than first. This **cascade of vacancy creation, filling and x-ray /Auger electron emission** continues until the most outer orbital vacancy is filled by a free or unbound electron.
- PE occurs only when the photon energy exceeds the electron binding energy l/t sharp increase in (μ/ρ_{PE}), called an absorption edge.

Compton / Recoil Effect (CE)

- CE dominates from **60 keV to 10 MeV** (in water) i.e. occur at *higher than COH & PE energy levels* and is used in *therapeutic radiology (RT)*. CE only depends on the **number of electrons per gram (electron density)**, which is almost constant for all materials (=3×10^{23}) except **hydrogen** (for which it is 6×10^{23}). CE is *independent of atomic number and has only a slight dependency on incident photon enrgy* (decreasing as energy increases through the megavoltage range). So except for small energy dependency and ***increased scattering probabilities for hydrogen laden materials***Q, compton mass attenuation coefficient is constant across energy & atomic numbers (Z) esp for low Z biological materials tissue.
- In **Compton scattering**, incident photon ***transfers only a part of its energy to a loosely bound, outer orbital electron and is deflect or scattered off in a new direction with lower energy***Q. The orbi electron (now called **recoil** or **Compton electron**) is ejected (with kinetic energy equal to the difference b/w the incident and scattered photon) and the photon will subsequently undergo either another Compton or PE process.
- Because of interaction with negligible binding energy outer shell electron **no x-rays or Auger** (pronounced oh – jhay) **electrons are produced.**
- Minimum energy transfer occurs for a **O-degree photon scatter;** there is no interaction and scattered photon has the same energy as the incident photon. The electron is scattered at 90° with zero energy. *Maximum energy transfer* occurs for a **direct hit** with a **180° back scattered photon** and yields *minimal scattered photon energy* but the *electron has maximum energy* and travels in the *forward direction.*
- At *diagnostic photon energies*, image contrast is determined primarily by differences in *atomic numbers (Z) of materials* being imaged, because PE depends strongly on Z. Material thickness and density are secondary determinants. Whereas at therapeutic *photon energies*, image contrast is determined by *densities of material* being imaged because the *compton effect depends on electron densities* not the atomic number of materials.

- In PP, *incident photon* with > 1.022 MeV energy spontaneously *disappears when passes near a heavy nucleus*. The energy is absorbed ***creating an electron (e⁻) – positron (e⁺) pair*** in its place. The total kinetic energy of pair = energy of photon - 1.022 MeV.
- The electron and position (anti-particle of an electron) do not have equal energies and travel off in no particular direction. The electron gradually slowing down and stopping in material, whereas positron slows down very quickly and annihilates with a free electron, giving of **annihilation radiation** (i.e. *two 0.511 MeV photons that travel in opposite direction at 180°*).

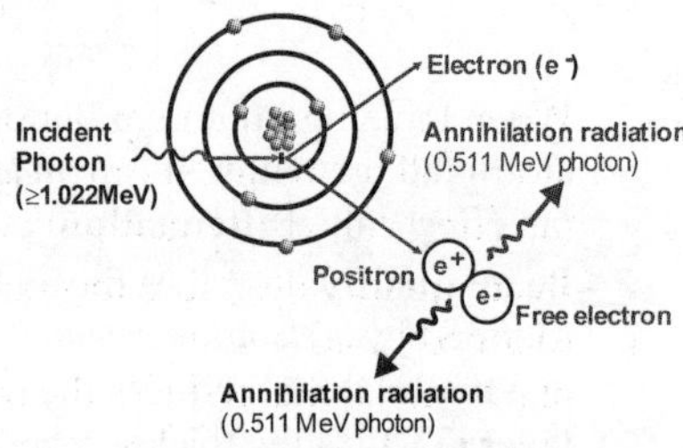

Photodisintegration (PD)

- PD occurs at **very high photon energies (above 10 MeV)** and is responsible for *creation of neutrons in a linear accelerator* facility.
- In PD, very energetic photon (> 8-10 MeV) penetrates the atomic nucleus and is absorbed resulting in emission of a neutron, thereby leaving a *fragmented (possibly unstable i.e. radioactive) nucleus*, giving the name PD.

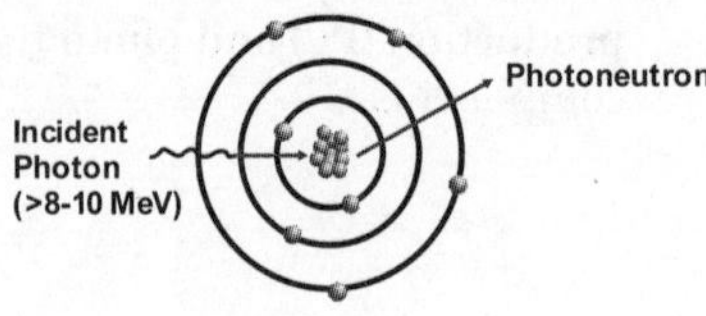

Particle Interactions and Clinical Applications

Particle with kinetic energy undergo inelastic and elastic interactions with an absorbing material. **Inelastic interactions** (i.e. *collisional & radiative processes*) result in *loss of energy*, whereas **elastic** *do not* as the particle is scattered by electron or nucleus (for charged particles)/ by nucleus (uncharged particles), resulting in a change of direction but no loss of energy.

Charged - Light Particle (eg electron) Interactions

- Electron interactions result in a large amount of scattering, caused by the light mass of electron relative to the nuclear mass of any absorber.
- The interaction probability for charged particfle is 1 (i.e. particle interacts at every opportunity) The **stopping power** (dE/dx) is the *rate of energy loss (dE) that occur over distance travelled (dx) for inelastic collisions.* **Mass stopping power is** independent of absorber density (dE / ρdx). Because energy loss is almost continuous, particles travel finite distance (**k/a particle range**) to obtain zero kinetic energy (or stop).
- *Collisional energy losses* increase by square of incident *particles atomic number* and as the *particle velocity decreases*. Increased atomic number results in a greater Coulomb force and decreased velocity increases the amount of interaction time. Collisional energy loss increases as the *absorber atomic number decreases* (because with decreasing Z there is increase in number of electrons pergram). **So electrons are stopped sooner in low Z than in high Z material.**

Collisional energy loss	$\propto \dfrac{\text{particles } Z^2}{V^2} \times$ **No of electrons/cc³ in absorber**

- The electron mass is small and it undergoes 4 types of particle interactions (*i.e. excitation, ionization of outer & inner shell and interaction with nuclear field)* with large amount of scattering. Collisional interactions **with atomic electrons result** in loss of energy causing **excitation** (to higher energy orbits) or **ionization. Ionization of outer shell electron** l/t its ejection only, whereas ionization of inner shell electron is also associated with *production of characteristic X-ray*. Ionization of inner shell (K) electron creates a vacancy, which is filled by fall of outer orbital (eg L or M) electron to inner orbit. In doing so, the difference in binding energies of two shells is radiated as photons, which is called **characteristic radiation**. So a **characteristic (or line) x-ray spectrum** consists of x-ray photons of **only few (discrete) energies.**

Bremsstrahlung (or Braking) Radiation (BR)

- Radiatiative interaction result in x-ray emission. When *a high energy electron (β-particle or Auger electron) passes close tothe nucleus's positive electrical field (of another /target atom), it is abruptly deflected & decelerated by electrostatic attraction and loses energy in the form of x-ray photons* (called **bremsstrahlung** or **braking radiation**)
- The electron may have 1 or more such interactions resulting in partial or complete loss of energy. The energy of bremsstrahlung radiation is determined by *the distance b/w the electron and the nucleus. At very large distances,* the Coulombic force is *weak*, only *low energy x-ray* is created, but this interaction has *high probability* to

Charged - Heavy Particle (eg proton and α particle) Interactions

- Heavy charged particles (eg **proton and alpha particles**) mainly experience *inelastic collisions with a high rate of energy loss resulting in short ranges.*
- There is only *little scattering with most trajectories in forward direction* (in water/tissue); because the particle mass is similar to that of interacting material, and *very few large angle direction changes* occur, in contrast to the large amount of scattering experienced by (light mass) electrons.
- Because of dependency on Z^2 and $1/V^2$, heavy charged particles *exhibit rapidly increasing and large energy losses near the end of their ranges.* This increase in energy loss result in a *dramatic increase in ionization at the end (tail) of particle track* length after a relatively constant loss, a phenomenon called **Bragg-peak.**
- Although observed mainly for protons and alpha particles, Bragg peak is exhibited by all charged particles including electrons. However, electrons are light enough such that multiple scatters occur and ionization paths are randomly oriented, blurring any observable effect.
- The proton finite range can be modulated through a physical attenuator to decrease the range from the maximum. If the range modulation is done continuously, while the beam is on, the Bragg peak will be swept over a range and produce a high dose platue. The width of high dose platue can be designed to match a tumor size at a certain depth and demonstrates the attractiveness of proton for radiotherapy.

Charged Particle Radiotherapy

- **Charged particle (eg proton) radiotherapy** has *superior dose distribution*; i.e. energy loss per unit path length is relatively small and constant until near the end of range where the residual energy is lost over a short distance, resulting in a steep rise in the absorbed dose (energy absorbed per unit mass). This portion of particle track, where energy is lost rapidly over a short distance is k/a **Bragg peak**. The initial low dose region (i.e. ~ 30% of Bragg peak maximum dose) in the depth dose curve, before Bragg peak is k/a platue of dose distribution.
- Because Bragg peak is too narrow for clinical application, the beam energy is modulated to achieve a uniform dose over a significant volume by super imposing several Bragg peaks of descending energies (ranges) and weights *to create a region of uniform dose for irradiation of most tumors.* These extended regions of uniform peak doses are called **spread out Bragg peaks (SOBP)**.
- Although the beam modulation used to spread out the Bragg peaks, increase the entrance dose, but the proton dose distribution is still characterized by a ***lower dose region in normal tissue proximal to tumor; a uniform high dose region in the tumor depth (d/t accumulation of many Bragg peaks or SOBP) and zero dose beyond the tumor***Q.
- With the development of hospital based-**cyclotrons** (a **high energy spiral accelerator which can accelerate protons, deutrons & alpha particles**) *producing higher energy proton beams* (of 230-250 MeV) ***capable of reching deep seated tumors (upto 30 to 40cm)***Q, field sizes comparable to those of linear accelerator and rotational gantries, with *precise dose delivery reducing integral dose, second cancers, late effects and morbidity* – the use of **proton therapy is becoming the the treatment of choice for deep seated tumors**.
- Proton beam RT provides greatest benefit for larger target in younger patient where reduction in second cancer and late effects make this therapy cost effective. With minimization of normal tissue dose, protons may allow for better tolerance of combined chemotherapy & radiotherapy reigemens. For smaller targets in older patients, such as prostate cancer, even when protons will permit a 10-Gy escalation of prostate dose compared with IMRT photons, proton beam therapy is not cost effective (50,000 $ per quality adjusted life year).
- **Heavier charged particles like carbon ions** have high linear energy transfer (LET) radiation. There is an initial increase in relative biological effectiveness (RBE) with an increase in LET; carbon ions have RBE of 3 whereas protons have 1.1. Higher-LET radiation is less influenced by tissue oxygenation & less sensitive to the variations in the cell cycle & DNA repair. So carbon ions have a slight physical advantage over protons in that they will have a sharper (narrow) penumbra particularly for deep seated tumors and may also confer a biological

occur. When electron passes *close to nucleus,* more kinetic energy is lost l/t a *high energy x-ray production,* but this process has *lower probability* to occur. Therefore, breamsstrahlung radiation is a continuous spectrum *consisting of x-ray photons of all energies upto the maximum* in a *continuous fashion.*

- The *maximum energy and directin of emission of BR photons* is determined by the (maximum) kinetic energy of incident electron. BR production increases with increase in incident electron energy and atomic number (Z) of absorber. Radiative interactions are the mechanism by which x-rays are *produced in diagnostic x-ray tubes and linear accelerators.*
- The probability of collisional & /or radiative interactions depends on electron energy and atomic number of incident material. For electrons **collisional energy losses dominate at lower energies** (at 100KeV, 99% collision & 1% radiative resulting in mainly heat production), whereas **radiative losses dominate at higher energies** (at 10 MeV, both are 50% r/i more efficient x-ray production). Above 10 MeV, BR production exceeds colisional losses.
- ***Loss of energy of electron increases as the electron slows down (i.e. its kinetic energy decreases below 1 MeV)***Q. In water or tissue, megavoltage (>1MeV) electrons lose about **2 MeV/cm** traveled (so range can be found by dividing energy in MeV by 2). So a 10 MeV electron has a range 5 cm in water. This can be used to scale density, as the higher than water density materials (eg bone) cause electron to stop earlier.

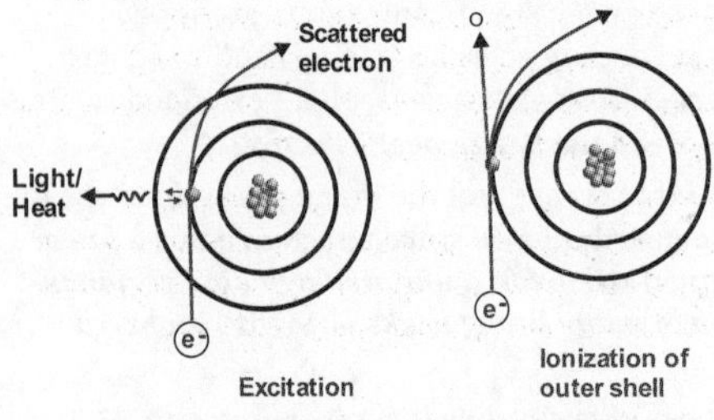

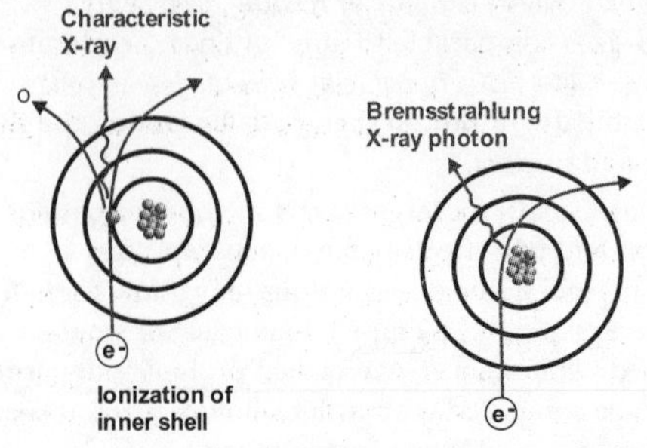

advantage against tumor b/o the higher RBE and differential effects on hypoxic cells. On the other hand carbon ions also produce some spallation products deep to Bragg peak.

Uncharged - Heavy Particle (eg neutron) Interactions

- Neutrons have no charge and donot undergo coulomb interactions like charged particles, instead they interact by inelastic and elastic collisions with nuclei.
- For lower Z materials, a neutron penetrates nucleus and is absorbed f/b ejection of proton (n-p reaction). They new neucleus may be radioactive (process called *neutron activation*) or show *nuclear disintegration.* For very heavy neuclei, neutrons may cause *fission* (used for power production in nuclear reactors)
- Neutrons do not have a finite range. Elastic scattering of neutron is also common. Type of collision (elastic or inelastic) that a neutron experiences depends on the neutron energy and absorber atomic number. Example includes

Fast Neutron Radiotherapy (FNRT)

- FNRT uses *neutrons of tens of megaelectron volts (MeV) energy.* These are generated by accelerating either protons or deutrons with **cyclotrons** or particle accelerators and then delivering them to appropriate target (mostly beryllium). Fission neutrons (1-2 MeV) from neuclear reactors can also be used to treat patients.
- For neutrons of energies used in RT, about 85% of deposited energy is via a *knock on reaction (billard ball type collision)* involving the hydrogen nucleus (^{1}H) meaning that kinetic energy release in matter (KERMA) is **larger in high hydrogen content tissue such as fat or myelin.**
- The resulting energy transfer is in the range of *20 to 100 KeV/μm* compared with 0.2 - 2 KeV/μm for megavoltage photons and electrons used in conventional RT. It is the higher energy transfer that gives rise to the different radiobiological properties of FNRT. The higher RBE accounts for the different clinical response observed with neutrons as opposed to conventional photon irradiation. Fast neutrons have RBEs 3 to 3.5 in terms of most normal tissue late effects, RBEs 4 to 4.5 in terms of damage to CNS and **RBEs 8 for salivary gland malignant tumors.**
- Neutron therapy is best used in the treatment of certain tumor that exhibit a resistance to standart low LET radiotherapy - a small niche, but it remains a very important treatment option for small number of patients for whom it appears to be better than tradition forms of treatment. Example includes.

1. ***Patients with inoperable or recurrent salivary gland malignant tumors***Q or in high risk situations where there has been an *incomplete surgical extirpation* or
2. Where *inoperable or incompletely resected sarcomas of bone, cartilage and soft tissue or locally advanced prostate cancers* particularly those that are not hormonally responsive have been found.
3. May also be beneficial in *metastases from melanoma & renal cell carcinoma.*

Boron Neutron Capture Therapy (BNCT)

- It is under research, *magic bullet* approch to treating tumors. Pure beams of very low energy neutrons do not directly deposit much energy in tissue. The basic idea is to *selectively attach a nuclide with a large cross section for capturing thermal neutrons [eg boron-10 (^{10}B) or gadolinium - 157 (^{157}Gd)]* to the cancer cells.
- The nucleide then undergoes a nuclear reaction with the localized release of substantial amount of energy and *kills the tagged cancer cells but does not damage the surrounding untagged normal cells.*
- At present moderated neutron beams from nuclear reactors are used but there is ongoing work in developing *high current particle accelerator to produce low energy thermal or epithermal beams* for BNCT.

Californium-252 (^{252}CF) Neutron Brachytherapy

- Beneficial for tumors in which **hypoxia** is thought to be a factor in limiting tumor control with standard treatment.

External Beam Radiation / Teletherapy

External beam radiation therapy (with a radiation source outside the patient) from distance (tele = at a distance) produce **ionizing radiation** (i.e. radiation of sufficient energy to cause ionization upon interaction) by two methods.

Radiation production by radioactive decay of nucleide	Radiation production by linear accelerators (LA)
- *Gamma (γ) rays / photons*[Q] are emitted from a daughter nucleus formed after *radiactive decay of an unstable parent nucleus.* Each γ ray has a *unique energy* that relates to the immediately preceding nuclear transformation and this unique energy can be used to identify the daughter (& therefore the parent nucleide). - **^{226}Ra, ^{137}Cs, and most commonly ^{60}Co** have been used for teletherapy units. ^{137}Cs & ^{60}Co are manufactured by neutron activation & as a by product of fission in nuclear reactor. - ^{60}Co decays to ^{60}Ni with emission of gamma ray photon spectra of 1.17 & 1.33 MeV each. Typical activity is 9000 Ci (3.33x10^{14} Bq) for a dose rate of 3 Gy/min at 80 cm (& 2Gy/min at 100 cm) from source. The source decays with t½ of 5.263 years & is *replaced every 5-7 years* when the dose rate becomes too low.	- **Linear accelerator** (Linac) is *a particle accelerator which greatly increase the velocity of charged ions or subatomic particles (eg electrons)* by subjecting them to a series of oscillating electrical potential along a linear beamline. Linac can be used **to achieve highest kinetic energy for election/protons in particle** physics or as particle injectors for high energy accelerator, or **to generate X-rays and high energy electrons for RT.** - In linear accelerator, *electrons are accelerated electronically to high energy* and are allowed to exit the machine as an ***electron beam***[Q] or are directed into a high Z target to produce ***X-rays***[Q] by bremsstrahlung interaction. - Electrons are accelerated in LA down a wave guide by use of *alternating microwave fields.* **Klystrons** (> 10 MeV) and **magnetrons** (< 10 MeV) provide accelerating potential & amplitude (power) and act as a *source of microwaves* whereas wave guide conveys the microwave power to accelerator structure and so wave guide length is a function of maximum acceleration energy (longer is higher) & frequency of microwave field. The most common frequency is *2.998 GHz (S band microwave).* The shorter waveguides are possible at *9.3 GHz (X-band microwave)* that produce megavoltage energies above 6 MeV.
- ^{60}Co source is *always on* & *decay always occurs,* the source must be moved to an unshielded condition to start irradiation.	- In LA, **no source is present** until the unit is energiezed and the irradiation is on or off with a flip of electronic button.
- In ^{60}Co, two **monoenergetic gamma rays** at **1.17** and **1.33 MeV** each (average 1.25 MeV) are emitted	- LA provides a **continuous X-ray spectrum** through bremsstrahlung interaction with energy ranging from maximum to zero (average is 1/3rd of Emax). LA is a high energy mechine and provide *megavoltage therapy.*
- *Gamma (γ) rays (photons)*[Q] are produced by beta decay but beta particles (electrons) are stopped by capsule & cannot be used for treatment.	- *LA provides both electron beam & X-rays (photons) for treatment*[Q]
- Lower cost, simple design, with lower requirements for operating environment. So ^{60}Co tele therapy devices are used world wide in regions with limited resources.	- Computer controlled, enabling better optimized close distribution, in room verification of target location through remote sensing & image guided approches (IGRT=image guided radiation therapy; tomotherapy using CT). Developed nations use mostly L.A. - Other higher energy particles such as electrons, protons, neutrons & higher Z ions are produced using other accelerator techiques like **betatron, Vande Graaff accelerators, cyclotrons,** & race track **microtron** etc.

- **^{226}Ra, ^{137}Cs and most commonly ^{60}Co** have been used for teletherapy (i.e. external beam radiotherapy from distance). Until 1951, all isotope machines were **teleradium (radium bomb) units** using radium as radiation source. But these units have many drawbacks. Apart from the *high cost of radium,* it has *large self absorption, low gamma ray constant (0.8 MeV) and high risk due to the radon gas leak,* produced as by product. The outputs were also very low. Because of these reasons teleradium units could never become standard teletherapy unit in real sense. And now its use is **obsolete *due to its very long half life (~1600 years) and associated hazards***[Q].
- **Telecesium units (gamma chambers)** use ^{137}Cs as radiation source which has 30.2 years t½, 0.662 MeV gamma ray energy, 0.34 Rhr^{-1} m^{-2} gamma ray constant and 79 Ci/gm specific activity Because of *low gamma ray constant and low specific activity,* telecesium unit are not proved to be useful and are now used mainly for radiobiological studies involving irradiation of small animals. However, very few units are still in clinical use in India. **Ir^{192}** can also be used for animals.
- **Tele cobalt units** using **^{60}Co** are the ***teletherapy units of choice in developing countries***[Q]. The half life is 5.28 years, average photon energy is 1.25 MeV, gamma ray constant is 1.3 Rhr^{-1} m^{-2} at 1 meter distance from 1Ci of source. The specific activity & gamma ray constant of ^{60}Co are very high. Thus it provides fairly high radiation outputs at treatment distance as large as 80-100cm. However in developed countries cobalt units are preferrably replaced by **4-8 MV linear accelerator (linac).**
- Basic components of all external beam treatment machines include a radiation source, stored in a shielded head of machine mounted on gantry; a **collimating system** (consisting of interleaved bars of high Z material) to form and direct a radiation beam, and define the field size, inherent or added **shielding** for radiation protecting, a control system to turn the beam on & off, **cross -hair & field-light** to delineate visibly the radiation field to be treated (i.e. field dimensions) & central ray, a *means to rotate the beam* or otherwise change its direction and a support for patient (couch), all assembled in a *isocentric geometry.*

- ^{60}Co is produced by irradiating ordinary stable ^{59}Co with neutrons in a reactor or nuclear pile.
- **Contact Therapy** is treatment with x-rays produced at 40 to 50 kv, **superficial** therapy is 50-150 kv, **orthovoltage or deep therapy** is treatment with 150–500 KV Xrays, **supervoltage** or **high voltage therapy** is treatment with 500-1000 KV.
- **Megavoltage therapy** is treatment with x ray beams of energy **> 1 mev** such as produced by Van de graff generator, betatron, linear accelerator, microton. Sometimes gamma rays of >1 Mev produced by radionuclide (^{60}Co) are also included although term strictly applies to x ray beams.
- **Van de graff accelerators** accelerate electrons to produce x-rays (2-10 mev). But b/o large size and required high voltage insulation (provided by N_2 and CO_2 mixture) these are no longer in clinical use.
- **Linear accelerator (linac)** and **betatron** can accelerate electrons to produce **electron beam** for therapy or may be directed against a target to produce **megavoltage X-ray beam** for therapy. Because of low x-ray output, large size, field size restrictions (max 20×20 cm at 100 cm source to skin distance =SSD), betatrons could never become a popular teletherapy machine in radiotherapy.
- **Microtron** is an electron accelerator which *combines the principles of both linear accelerator* (ie e^- are accelerated by oscillating electric field of a single microwave cavity) and *cyclotron* (electrons are moved in circular orbit of increasing radius = circular microtron; or e^- are moved in *D shaped hollow conducting semicircular multicavity accelerating structure =racetrack microtrons*). The advantage of microtrons over linac of same energy is its simplicity, easy energy selection, small beam energy spred and smaller size of machine.
- **Cyclotron** is a charged particle accelerator, which can accelerate protons, deuterons, alpha particles, high energy Z ions etc and ***produce photons, protons or neutrons for clinical use***[Q]. It is also used as a particle accelerator for production of certain *(artificial) radio nucleotides such as ^{125}I, ^{198}Au* etc. It is the major source of radiation for nuclear physic research.

Brachy-Therapy

- Brachytherapy is *short distance radiotherapy* in which radioactive source of small size is placed *very close to tumor (as surface mold)* or *in the tumor (as interstitial or intracavitary implants)* for treatment. Implants can also be divided into- *permanent and temporary types*, on the basis of duration they stay in body.
- Brachytherapy source may be constructed as *sealed source in the form of needles, tubes or seeds.* The solid radioactive material in a stable inorganic or organic chemical form, adsorbed onto a material, or possibly as a liquid or gas *is sealed into a metal source capsule by welds* or other means *that prevent leakage of material.* Most radioactive sources are β emitters, and useful radiation for treatment of cancer are **gamma rays** or **characteristic X-rays** emitted after beta decay. Besides containment and prevention of leakage of source material, the metal encapsulation *also stops all beta (and alpha) emissions* and allow only the gamma or x-ray to be transmitted. Sources can also be used in unsealed (liquid) form or for their beta emissions (i.e. Sr-90).

Properties of ideal brachy therapy source

1. Source should emit γ-rays of energy high enough to avoid increased energy deposition in bone by photoelectric effect and at the same time γ ray energy should be low enough to minimize radiation protection requirements. Optimum range is **0.2 to 0.4 MeV** (monoenergetic γ rays)
2. *Absence of charged particle (β, α) emission* or it should be easily screened
3. Half life should be such that correction for decay during treatment is minimal (ie low for permanent implants and *higher for temporary implants to avoid decay during treatment and frequent replacements*)
4. *No gaseous disintegration* product to prevent physical damage to the source and to avoid source contamination
5. Specific activity should be high and proto yield adequate
6. Material should be available in *insoluble and nontoxic* form, should *withstand sterilization* process, and *can be made in different shapes and sizes* (such as tubes, needles, spheres, and flexible wires) to suit various clinical needs. It should *not be in powder form* and costly.

Advantages in comparison to teletherapy

- *Steep dose gradient* b/o inverse square relation b/w dose decrease and distance increase. So a *confined high dose* (thousands of centigrays) *is delivered near a source* to small tumor volume, whereas *a few centimetres away the dose is low* (tens of centigrays)
- Photons emitted by brachytherapy source have relatively low energies and greater attenuation in tissue compared with photons used for external beam treatment. This *increased attenuation concentrates dose near the source and minimizes dose at distance.*
- *Prescribed dose rates are low (~0.40 Gy/h to 0.80 Gy/h)* and it takes many days to deliver the prescribed dose. It allows *treatment of all cells in each phase of cell cycle* for radiobiological advantage.
- *High dose rate remote after loading brachytherapy* with dose rates of *2 Gy/min* at the prescription point, comparable to external beam dose rate are also used.

After loading systems and High dose are (HDR) afterloading

- Earlier the applicators were preloaded with radioactive nuclide sources resulting in *unnecessary radiation exposure* to medical persons involved in procedure. Now a days, the applicators are first inserted into patient with more care and deliberation and its position is checked radiographically. And later the radiation source is inserted (loaded) into these applicators – a process k/a **after loading**. As the source does not come in direct contact with the body tissue, sterilization of source is not essential and the *probability of loss of source is also minimal*. The after loading is carried out either manually or **remote controlled** from outside the treatment room (*preferable method* provides complete radiation safety).
- Remote after loading systems (RAL) are available in low dose rate (LDR) ie 0.4–2 Gy/h at the point of dose prescription, medium dose rate (MDR) ie >2 Gy/h to <12 Gy/h and high dose rate (HDR) ie >12 Gy/h. For **LDR**, **Cs-137**[Q] source and for **HDR**, **Ir-192**[Q] source are most commonly used.

Permanent Implant	Temporary Implants
- Implant stays in place forever - The implant (seed) releases small doses of radiation slowly, until the radioactivity gradually fades away - The radiation affects only a very small area around the implant - Permanent implants are performed with relatively short t ½ like ***I-125, Palladium – 103***, Au-198, Cs-131Q.	- Does not stay in place forever - Sources are either inserted directly into tissue or afterloaded in hollow needles or plastic catheter placed in the body. - They can either low-dose rate or high-dose rate eg. Cs-137, Ir-192, Str-90

Element	Isotope	Half-life	Source	Implant	
Gold	AU – 198	2.7 days	Seeds	Permanent	**Not used now**
Cesium-131	Cs-131	9.7 days	Seeds	Permanent	1st choice
Palladium	Pd – 103	17 days	Seeds	Permanent	2nd choice
Iodine	I – 125	60 days	Seeds	Permanent	3rd choice
Iridium	Ir – 192	74 days	Seeds, wire	Temporary	
Cesium	Cs – 137	30 years	Tubes	Temporary	
Strontium	Sr – 90	29 years	Plaque	Temporary	

★ Biological effective dose (BED) & associated cell kill is the lowest for Au – 198; whereas *Pd – 103, I – 125* implants are more effective for *fast growth and slow growth tumors respectively.*

Radiotherapy

Teletherapy

When Radiation source is far from patient ex.
- **Cobalt (Co)^{60} = best & most**Q commonly used radionucleide source, mainly in developing nations.
- **Cesium (Cs)^{137}** = ***rarely used***Q mainly for human teletherapy.
- **Iridium (Ir)^{192}** = used for animal research/treatment
- **Radium (Ra)^{226}** = ***obsolete & abandoned***Q d/t high associated hazards.
- Deep X-ray therapy
- **Linear accelerator provide *electron beam and/or bremsstrahlung X rays* for therapy (*best & most commonly used method in developed nations*Q).**

Brachy Therapy

Intracavitary: Source is inserted into body cavities by means of applicator devices. Sites include oral, rectal, vaginal & uterine cavities and tracheal & bronchial lumina. Ex. Cs^{137} in Ca Cervix

Interstitial: Source is implanted in malignant tissue directly or within catheter ex.

Mold: Source in mold that conforms to patients surface is used. It is not commonly performed except in *ocular melanoma (I ^{125})* and is replaced by total electron therapy.

Permanent Implant
- Pallidium (Pd)^{103}
- Iodine (I)^{125}
- Gold (Au)^{198} = not used now b/o high cost
- Cesium (Cs)^{131}

Mn- **"PIG – Ce i.e. see Pig"**

Temporary Implant
- **Ytterbium (Yb)^{169}** is HDR source
- **Yttrium (Y)^{90}**
- **Cesium (Cs)^{137}** Q
- **Cobalt (Co)^{60}** = ***not preferred for interstitial therapy***Q b/o risk of needle breakage & loss of source with long t½ (is **HDR source**)
- Strontium (Sr)^{90}
- Samarium (Sm)^{145}
- **Iridium (Ir)^{192}** = ***most common HDR source***Q
- Tantalum (Ta)^{182}
- Americium (Am) – 241
- **Radon (Rn)^{222}** } *abandoned & obsolete*Q
- **Radium (Rs)^{226}**

Mn- **"Y² – C² – S²ITAR² i.e. why se SITAR"**

Systemic Radionucleide

I-131	Thyroid ca
Strontium (Sr)-89Q **Smarium (Sm)-153**Q **Phosphorous (P)-32**Q **Rhenium (Re)-186**Q Tin (Sn) - 117	**Bone metastasis** (pain)
I^{131} labeled anti CD20 & Yttrium labeled anti CD20	B cell lymphoma

Other brachytherapy techniques

- Include molds using **I^{125}** seeds for **ocular melanosis, biliary stent** implants using **^{192}Ir**; ultrasound guided **prostate brachytherapy** using **^{103}Pd** or **^{125}I**; endovascular brachytherapy using **^{90}Sr, ^{192}Ir** and other nucleides, and treatment of pterygium using *^{89}Sr.*
- β emitting nuclides are used for therapy as they deliver most of radiation dose locally eg. P^{32} for polycythemia vera, ***I^{131} for thyrotoxicosis and thyroid cancer***Q, Yttrium – 90 for arthritic conditions.
- Measurement of GFR with chromium -51 (^{51}Cr) EDTA, diagnosis of vitamin B$_{12}$ malabsorption (Schilling's test) by urinary excretion of *cyanocobalamin labelled with cobalt -57.* RBC labelled with ^{51}Cr is used to document splenic sequestruction and decreased red cell survival in patient with suspected hemolysis, or increased RBC in polycthemia vera.

Radioisotopes: Types & t½

Rays	Radioactive Elements		t½	Energy (MeV)
α, β, γ	**Ra-226**	**Radium**	*1602-1622 years (longest)*Q	**0.8**
	U-235	Uranium	7.1 x 10^8 year	
β	P-32	Phosphorous	14.3 days	0.698
	Sr-90	Strontium	28 years	
	Y-90	Yttrium	2.54 days	
	H3	Tritium	12.5 years	
β, γ	Au-198	Gold	2.7 days	0.411
	I - 131	**Iodine (mainly β)**	**8 days**Q	
	Co-60	Cobalt	**5.2 years**Q	**1.173**
	Tc-99	Technitium	**6 hours**Q	
	Cs-137	Cesium	**30 years**Q	**0.662**
	Ir-192	Iridium	**74.5 days**Q	***0.47***Q
	Mn-56	Manganese	2.6 hrs	
	Mo-99	Molybdenum	66.7 hrs	
	Gd-153	Gadolinium	242 days	
	Sm - 153	Samarium	446.3 hrs	
	Sn - 117	Tin	13.6 hrs	
	Re - 186	Rhenium	3.8 days	
γ	Xe-133	Xenon	5.2 days	
	I-123	Iodine	**13 hours**	
	I-132	Iodine	**2.3 hours**	
	Tc-99	Technitium	6 hours	
	Ga-70	Gallium citrate	3.2 days	
	Tl-201	Thallous chloride	3.1 days	
	Rn-222	**Radon**	3-6 days	
	Cr-51	Chromium		
	K-81	Krypton		
	Se	Selenium		
N, γ	Cf - 252	Californium	2.6 years	
	Ta-182	Tantulum	4 months	

★ I^{125} has 60 days t½ & 0.027 MeV energy.

Physical Quantity	S.I. Unit		Non S.I. Unit	Conversion
Radioactivity Mn: "**RBC**"	**Disintegration/ second**	*Becquerel (Bq)*	*Curie*Q *(Ci)*	1Ci = 3.7 × 10^{10} Bq 1Bq = 2.703 × 10^{-11}Ci
Absorbed dose Mn: "**A**rterial **B**lood Gas Reading"	*Joule / Kg*	Gray (Gy)	**Rad**	1Gy = 100 rads 1rad = 0.01 Gy.
Dose equivalent	*Joule / Kg*	Sievert (Sv)	Rem	1Sr = 100 rem 1 Rem = 0.01 sv
Exposure	-	Coulombs/Kg	Roentgen	

Radiation Dosimetry

Absorbed Dose (D)

- It is ***total amount (quantity) of radiation energy delivered or deposited to per unit volume of organ (tissue)***Q.
- Define the quantity of radiation delivered to a specific point (organ / tissue) in radiation field.
- **Does not** include the *type of radiation & sensitivity* of organ in its description
- And so does not consider the *biological damage* (effect) caused by radiation.

Equivalent Dose (Hsv)

- It is a *measure of biological damage caused to an organ (tissue) by radiation* equal to absorbed **dose depending on the relative effectiveness** of incident radiation to produce biological damage.
- Because biological damage depends both on amount of radiation *absorbed (i.e. absorbed dose=D) and type of radiation (or weighting factor=wt)*
- So equivalent dose (Hsv) is calculated by

Hsv=D (GY) X Wt

Radiation Type	Wt
X rays, γ-rays, Electron	1
Proton	2
Neutron	10
Alpha (α) particle	20

- So biological damage caused by proton/neutron/ α-particle is 2/10/20 times more than. X-rays for the same absorbed dose (D).

Effective Dose (E)

- It is an *imaginary total body dose used* to translate a partial body exposure (eg cardiac CT or head irradiation) to an equivalent uniform total body dose *as if the radiation given to partial body (exposure to specific organ)' was spread uniformly across the whole body.*
- *It measures the risk of carcinogenesis & genetic defects*
- It is calculated by estimating the doses to all other organs in the body from radiation to specific organ/field and then multiplying by a risk factor (Wi) based on the sensitivity of each organ.

$$E = \sum H_i \times W_i$$

Radiotherapy & Cell survival

- **X rays** generated by linear accelerators, **& gamma (γ) rays** generated from decay of atomic nuclei of radioisotope eg. Ra, Co; are *most commonly used radiation to treat cancer.* X-rays & γ-rays are *electromagnetic , non particulate waves,* which behaves biologically as packets of energy (photons) to cause ejection of orbital (outer shell) electron, when absorbed. This orbital electron ejection is k/a ionization.
- Particulate form of radiation such as *electron beam & neutron beam* are used to treat *mycosis fungoides & salivary gland tumors respectively.*
- The dose response curve for cells undergoing radiation exposure has

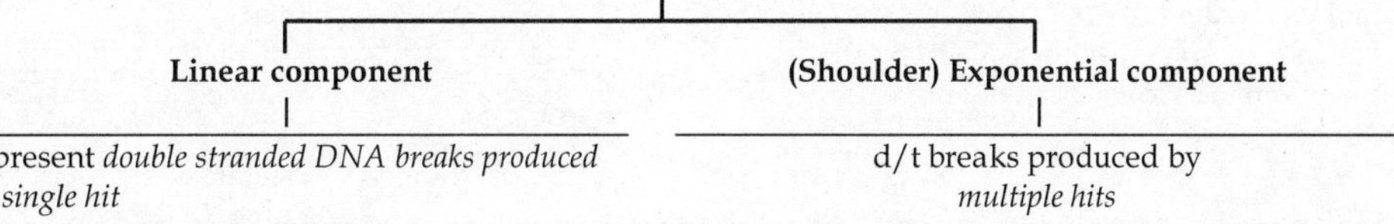

- For *X-ray & γ -rays* the curve has *shoulder, followed by linear portion.* Whereas for *alpha (α) particles or lower energy neutrons,* the curve is *straight line from origin.* According to latest view, the cell must undergo double stranded DNA break to be killed.
- Four important processes that occur after radiotherapy are Mn **"4R"** repair (temperature dependent process), reoxygenation, repopulation& redistribution.
- The factors that influence tumor killing are:

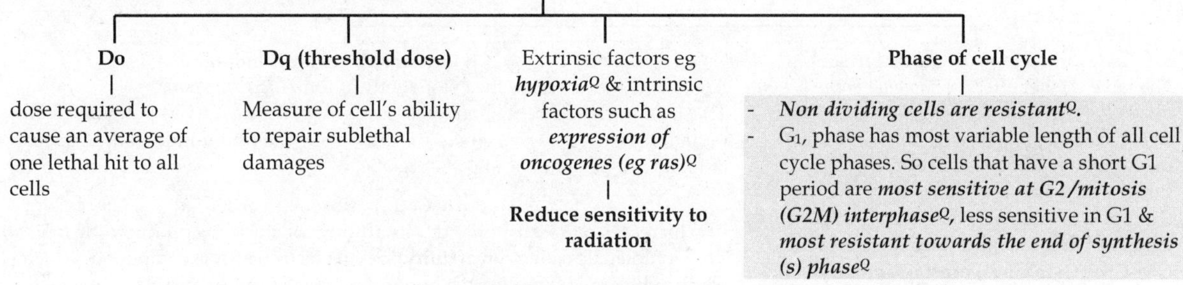

Do
dose required to cause an average of one lethal hit to all cells
Dq (threshold dose)
Measure of cell's ability to repair sublethal damages
Extrinsic factors eg hypoxia[Q] & intrinsic factors such as expression of oncogenes (eg ras)[Q]
Reduce sensitivity to radiation
Phase of cell cycle
- Non dividing cells are resistant[Q].
- G1, phase has most variable length of all cell cycle phases. So cells that have a short G1 period are most sensitive at G2 /mitosis (G2M) interphase[Q], less sensitive in G1 & most resistant towards the end of synthesis (s) phase[Q]

Radiosensitivity

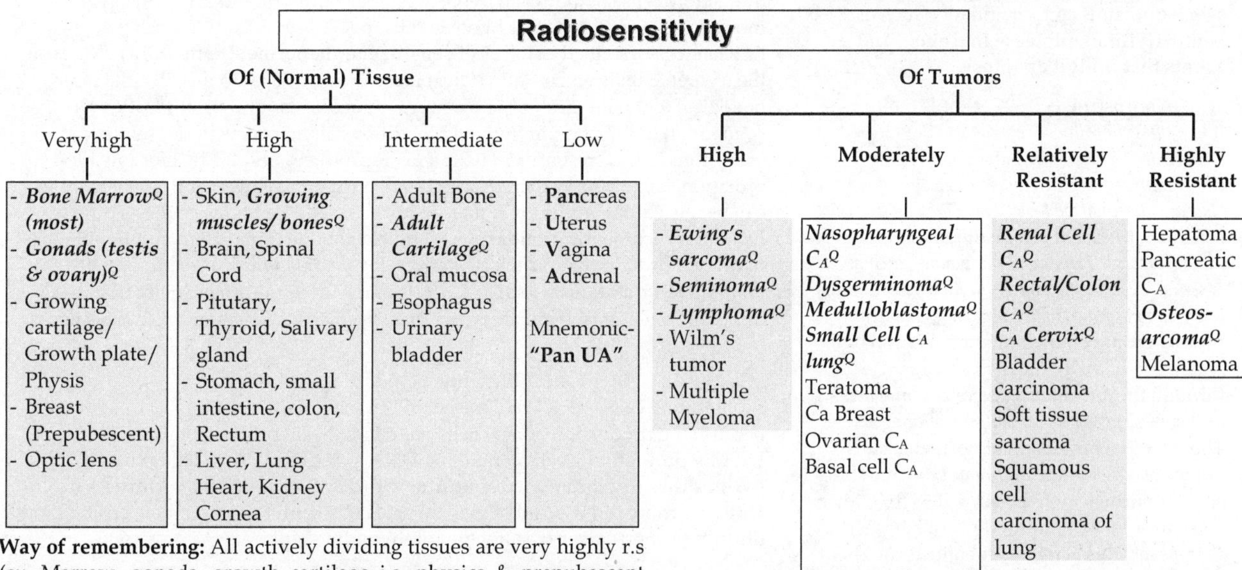

Way of remembering: All actively dividing tissues are very highly r.s (ex. Marrow, gonads, growth cartilage i.e. physics & prepubescent breast) except for growing muscle & bones (which are highly r.s.)

- Least r.s. is seen in: **Pan Ultra Voilet A** (i.e. Pancreas, uterus, vagina, adrenals)
- In highly r.s. group all vital organs (long, liver, heart, kidney), most of GI tract (stomach, s. intestine & rectum), CNS (Brain, s.cord) & growing musculo-skeletal system (skin, muscle, bone) & cornea comes.
- Grown (Adult) Bone & Cartilage with upper GI (oral mucosa & (esophagus) & bladder are intermediate R.S.

★ Neuroblastoma is very sensitive to ionizng radiation.

Chemotherapy

Highly sensitive cancers	Highly resistant cancers
- Acute Leukemias (AML, ALL) - Lymphoma - ***Small Cell lung CA***Q - Ovarian CA - Germ cell neoplasm (Seminoma, dysgerminoma, chorio CA, embryonal CA, Terato CA) - Pediatric neoplasm (***Ewings***Q, Wilm's, Neuroblastoma, embryonal rhabdomyosarcoma, peripheral neuroepithelioma)	- ***Melanoma***Q - Thyroid - Non small cell lung (some) - Thyroid - Hepatocellular - Biliary tract - **Pancreatic** - Colorectal - Renal - Prostate - Vulva

Radioprotection and Sensitization

Radiation damage is dependeat on O_2. Hypoxia (deficiency of O_2) in tumor cells cause them to become more radioresistant and protect them from radiotherapyQ. To overcome this radiotherapy resistance 2 classes of drugs are used.

Radioprotectors (of normal tissue)

- The have the net effect of *allowing normal tissues to better tolerate higher doses of radiation and chemotherapy*, which negates (balances) the relative readioresistance of hypoxic tumor cells.
- Examples include ***amifostine (WR-2721)***Q. Other apparent readioprotectors are – **IL-1, GM-CSF, Cytokines, prostaglandins** (such as **misoprostol**), anti coagulants (such as **pentoxifylline), protease inhibitors and agents that inhibit apoptosis.**

Amifostine (Wr- 2721) or Ethyol

- It is a *phosphorothioate compound* developed by US army. It is a *prodrug* that is dephosphorylated by *plasma membrane alkaline phosphatese to active metabolite free thiol WR 1065*. Modeled after *naturally occurring radioprotective sulfhydryl compounds such as cysteine, cysteamine and glutathione*; amifostine has *free SH group, which scavenges the free radicals* produced by ionizing radiation (RT).
- It can also detoxify other reactive species through the *formation of thioester conjugates* and so also used as a *chemprotective agent.*
- The selective protection of normal tissues apparently results from *tumor being both less able to convert amiostine to WR 1065* (b/o lower concentrations of required phosphatases) *and to transport* this active metabolite throughout the cell. Because the tumor vascularization is not as complete as normal tissue, the amifostine will mainly diffuse to normal tissue.
- **Dose reduction factor (DFR)** (i.e. the ratio of radiation doses to produce an isoeffect in the presence versus the absence of radioprotector), is in the range of *1.5 to 3.5 for normal tissue*, whereas it seldom exceeds *1.5 for tumors*. Normal tissue exhibiting the

Radiosensitizers (of tumors)

Are agents that increase the cytotoxicity of ionizing radiation.
True radiosensitizers being non toxic themselves, acting only as potentiators of radiation toxicity. *Apparent radiosensitizer* make the tumor more radioresponsive but may not be nontoxic and synergistic.

Hypoxic Cell Radiosensitizer (HCR)

- O_2 increases radiosensitivity d/t its affinity for electrons produced by ionization of biomolecules **(electron affinity)**. So an electron affinic compound, which is not utilized by cells should reach hypoxic regions of tumor and act in on **oxygen-mimetic** fashion to sensitize hypoxic cells to RT.
- Efficiency is described in terms of **sensitizer enhancement ratio (SER)**. Where as the oxygen enhancement ratio (OER) is the ratio of doses to produce the same biological end point under hypoxic versus aerobic conditions, the SER is the dose ratio for an isoeffect under hypoxic conditions alone versus under hypoxic conditions in the presence of HCR. If HCR produces SER **2.5 to 3** for low LET radiation, it can be considered *"as effective as oxygen"*. However in some cases it can be misleading as the HCR dose required would be higher then the dose of O_2.
- Examples include **nitroimidazoles** (with electophile nitro group and lipophilic hydrocarbon side chain) such as ***metronidazole, misonidazole, etanidazole, pimonidazole and nimorazole***Q. Unfortunately dose limiting toxicity of fairly lipophilic agent misonidazole is *peripheral neuropathy*. So etaindozole is designed to be less lipophilic.

Proliferating cell Radiosensitizer

- Proliferating cells are not radioresistant but may seem refractory to treatment because the production of new cells out paces the cytotoxic action of RT.
- Rapidly proliferating cells containing DNA substituded with **halogenated pyrimidines (e.g. bromodeoxy uridine – BrdUdR or iododeoxyuridine = Id UdR)** are more radiosensitive than normal cells, with the amount of sensitization directly proportional to the fraction of thymidine replaced.

Bioreductive (Hypoxia specific cytotoxic) Drugs

- These *kill rather than sensitize hypoxic cells*; the net effect of combining them with RT is apparent sensitization of tumor d/t elimination of otherwise radioresistant cell population. They are *selectively toxic to hypoxic cells* and also sensitize (apparently) tumors to anticancer drugs.
- All require bioreductive activation by *nitoreductase enzyme* such as *cytochrome P-450, DT-diaphorase, and NO synthase* to reduce the parent compound to its cytotoxic intermediate, usually an oxidizing free radicle capable of damaging DNA. Whereas, the active species is either not formed or else is immediately back oxidized to non-toxic parent compound in presence of O_2, which accounts for its

highest DRFs (=max radioprotection) include *bone marrow, gastrointestinal tract, liver testicular and salivary gland tissues.* Oral mucosa is only marginally protected. ***Because amifostine does not cross blood brain barrier, it offers no protection to central nervous system (i.e. brain and spinal cord)***Q.

- It provides comparable protection against *cisplatin and cyclophosphamide.* While peripheral nervous tissue, haematological and non haematological (renal, cardiac) tissues are protected, it provides no protection to CNS.
- FDA approved indications are protection against **nephrotoxicity and ototoxicity of platinum drugs (cisplatin)**, and reduction of incidence and severity of **Xerostomia** in head and neck cancer (secondary to exposure of parotid glands). It was developed as *antiradiation agent for astronauts.*
- Subcutaneous dose is better tolerated than IV; dose limiting tioxicities include hypotension, emesis, generalized weakness and fatigue.

preferential toxicity under hypoxic conditions.

- Examples include 3 classes of drugs.

1. **Nitroheterocyclic drugs** include **misonidazole, etanidazole and dual functioning agent RSU 1069** (also activates alkylating moiety capable of cross linking DNA).
2. **Quinone antibiotics e.g. mitomycin C and its analogues porfiromycin and EO 9.**
3. **Organic nitroxides** e.g. **tirapazamine** (SR 4233). Its hypoxic cytotoxicity ratio is highest and it retains its hypoxia selective toxicity over a wide range of low O_2 conc. Trials are ongoing for its combination with RT and cisplatin.

Other Radiosensitizers

- ***Oxygen (most potent)***Q, hypebaric O_2 breathig, artificial blood substitutes with increased O_2 carrying capacity, hyperthermia, vasoactive agents as *nicotinamide* and agents that modify the O_2-Hb dissociation curve e.g. *pentoxifylline.*
- **Anticancer agent: Mn-A,B,C,D, - 5F GH, Pac, M,T,V"**

- *Actinomycin-D*Q ***(Dactinomycin)***Q	- Gemcitabine
- Bleomycin, Buthione-sulfoxamine	- *Hydroxy* ***urea***Q
- ***Cisplatin***Q, ***Cytarabine***	- Paclitaxel
- Doxorubicin	- Mitomycin – C
- *5-**Fu***Q	- Topotecan
- Fludarabine	- Vinorelbine

- *Busulphan, cisplatin and nitrosourea are radiomimetic agents.*

Conformal Therapy & IMRT

- A radiotherapy (RT) treatment that creates *a high dose volume that is shaped to closely conform to the desired target volume* while minimizing the dose to critical normal tissue is called conformal therapy. It includes a treatment plan in which
  1. *target volumes are defined in 3 dimensional planes using* CT/MRI etc
  2. *multiple beam directions are used to cross fire* on the targets
  3. individual *beams are shaped or intensity modulated* to create a dose distribution that *conforms in shape and dose to the target volume shape and desired dose levels.*
  4. deviations from planned treatment are minimized by appropriate use of image guidance, accurate patient setup and immobilization and management of motions (eg respiratory) and other changes.
- **Three dimensional conformal radiotherapy (3DCRT)** was first conformal therapy technique based on use of 3D planning. A new technique **inverse planning**, involves creation of RT plan using mathematical optimization techniques, **intensity modulated beams** (ie beams with complex intensity distribution) are used. The combination of inverse planning and intensity modulated beams is called **intensity modulated radiation therapy (IMRT)**. The uses of integrated megavoltage and/or kilovoltage diagnostic imaging with modern treatment accelerators has led to **image guided radiation therapy (IGRT)**, which typically implies the *integration of image based patient positioning or monitoring with modern IMRT or 3DCRT.* Active consideration of patient and respiratory motion in the planning or treatment is k/a **four dimensional (4D) imaging and 4D planning.**
- The advantage of IMRT in comparison to 3DCRT is its ***ability to form concave, horse-shoe like dose distributions***Q, desirable in cases in which the target partly encircles a critical involved structure whose tolerance is less than the desired target dose such as
  1. **Head and neck cancers** in which targets are *arranged anterior and lateral to spinal cord* and are bound laterally by the *major salivary glands.*
  2. **Prostate cancers**Q, in which the rectum invaginates into the target.
  3. **Lung cancers**, in which target usually the mediastinal lungh nodes may lay close to the oesophagus.
  4. **Oesophageal cancers**, in which sparing the lungs from high doses is an objective.
  5. **Gynecological cancer**, in which the lymph node targets are arranged lateral to and posterior to the small bowel.
  6. **Left sided breast cancer**, in which target is concave anterior to part of lung and heart.
  7. **Brain tumors** near the optic pathways, **medulloblastoma** in which posterior fossa partly surrounds the inner ear.
  8. **Retreatment of recurrent cancer** in which minimizing the extent of the tissues receiving a high dose (at the *expense of higher volumes receiving low doses*) is likely to be beneficial.
- **Although IMRT reduces the tissue volumes receiving high doses, larger tissue volume receives low doses, larger tissue volume receives low doses** compared with the standard RT or 3DCRT. This is due to *use of many beams* (primarily), many MUs, and leakage through MLC leaves, and **increase the risk of radiation therapy related mutations and carcinogenesis** (because this risk is higher at intermediate rather than high doses). This risk is especially relevant for young patients. Another theoretical negative aspect of IMRT is the *loss of biological effect* of RT when treatment delivery time is prolonged (a characteristic of some IMRT). There is also *increased uncertainities regarding the accurate positioning* of targets and adjacent normal tissue *in chest and abdomen and to lesser degree in pelvis* d/t poor immobilization and breathing related motion.

Stereotactic Radiosurgery (SRS), Stereotactic Radiotherapy (SRT) and Sterotactic Body Radiotherapy (SBRT)

- These are *radiotherapy performed under conditions of high accuracy & precision using stereotactic imaging & rigid immobilization* or remote *monitoring & positioning systems.* Stereotactic imaging refers to immobilization or fixation of patient with a rigid-stable system coupled with same day imaging, to establish *a patient specific image based coordinate system* for the entire treatment process.
- **SRS** refers to the use of *one (single) fraction, small field, high dose* (12-20 Gy margin dose) focal radiation for treatment of relatively small intra or extra cranial tumors. By two irradiation approaches, a relatively large number of radiation fields are aimed accurately to focus (intersect) a common point at which target (tumor) is positioned. Whereas **SRT** refers to use of **>1 (usually 2 to 5) fractions,** small fields & high dose (5-20 Gy margin dose per fraction) using similar techniques. SRS & SRT can use high doses because the *total irradiation volume is small (< 20cc for CNS tumors)* & peripheral dose is spread over a large volume.
- Radiosurgery uses **Gamma Stereotactic Radiosurgery (GSR) unit or Gamma Knife**. In GSR devices, **gamma rays** from very large number of ***C^{60} sources***Q (30-200 sources) arranged in hemisphere or torus within a heavily shielded dose unit are focused at a *a common point (focus or isocenter) with high accuracy* (< 0.3mm error). With all gamma ray beams on (all collimators open) one irradiation is called a "shot" delivers a spherical dose distribution with slight variations in 3 orthogonal (coronal, axial, saggital) planes.
- **SRS is used in *(brain metastases, gliomas, meningioma, acoustic neuroma, pituitary adenoma and AVM).***

Vascular Lesions (15%)	Benign CNS Tumors (30%)	Malignant CNS Tumors (45%)	Functional Disorders (10%)
- **Arteriovenous (AV) malformation** Q. (mc) - Cavernous angiomas - Others	- **Meningiomas** (mc) - Vestibular schwannomas - Pituitary adenoma - Craniopharyngioma - Chemodectoma	- **Metastasis**Q (mc) - Glioblastoma multiforme - Low grade astrocytoma & recurrent gliomas - Choroidal melanomas etc.	- **Trigeminal neuralgia** (mc) - Cluster headache - OCD - Parkinssris disease - Epilepsy

- SRS performed using a linear accelerator is called **linac radiosurgery (LSR)**. Its shot diameter is 4-40mm in comparison to 4-18 mm of gamma knife.
- ***Stereotactic body radiotherapy (SBRT)*** applies principles of radio surgery to **outside brain** and involves precise delivery of high doses of radiation over 1 to 5 fractions using 4 dimensional CT scans, fluoroscopic motion studies, PET, FDG-PET imaging etc. to provide accurate planning target volume. It usually involves 3-D conformal radiotherapy with multiple beam arrangement, often noncoplanar or *intensity modulated radiotherapy (IMRT)* to produce distribution of RT with a very rapid fall off.
- SBRT is used as ***aggressive local therapy for oligometastatic disease and ablation of clinically localized, early stage malignant tumors***Q. It is currently being investigated for ***non operable early stage non-small cell lung cancer and lung metastases***Q, *prostate cancer, bone and spinal metastases, liver metastases, hepatocellular carcinoma, pancreatic cancer, renal cell carcinoma, and other abdominal tumors.*

Method

- SRS use a *stereotaxic frame (3 – Dimensional coordinates +* Mechanical platform to mount instruments) fixed to patient head and brain images (CT / MRI); to locate site to be operated.
- In it ***focused high dose of radiation (usually gamma knife) is administered to a precisely defined volume of tissue in a single treatment***Q.
- Correct identification of target is confirmed by *intra – operative physiological studies* such as neuronal recording with microelectrodes.
- The *neurological status of patient* (such as strength vision and improvement of motor function) must be monitored frequently during the procedure.
- It contains ***Co-60***Q sources of approximately 30 Curis placed in a circular array in a heavily shielded unit. The unit directs the gamma rays to the target.
- SRS uses **numerous beamlets** of radiation aimed precisely at an immobilized target to deliver a single session of high dose radiation. *Although no single beamlet carries significant dose of radiation, a large dose is deposited* at the intersection of these beamlets with a steep dose fall off outside the target **Radiosurgery becomes prohibitive** at sizes in excess of 4-5cm; as dose fall of becomes shallower **resulting in unacceptable increase in dose to adjacent normal brain tissue.**
- Radiosurgery differs from conventional fractionated RT in that it implies a single treatment and normal brain tissue adjacent to target not receiving nearly full dose of radiation.
- Radiosurgery differs from neurosurgery in that it does not require craniotomy or general anesthesia and is an OPD procedure.
- Radiosurgery can be performed using many devices including **multi cobalt unit (gamma knife /GK),** ***particle beam devices or modified linear accelerator.***

Gamma Knife	Linac RS
>3 decade experience, submillimeter accuracy, about equal treatment time.	>2 decade experience, submillimete accuracy, about equal treatment time
Dedicated machine, fewer quality assurance (QA) checks, **high price as Co source must be replaced every 5-7 years**	Usually not a dedicated machine, requiring more QA checks but providing less expansive treatment
Cannot be used for extracranial RS. **Difficult** to radiate peripheral lesions. Frationated treatments **not** practicle.	Can be used for **extracranial RS,** Can treat **peripheral lesions** Can treat with **fractionated regimens**
Longer experience in functional disorders	Shorter experience in functional disorders.

Advantages

- Achieve tumor ablation *without surgery.*
- *Damage to near by structure is minimized* as it delivers radiation to focused area.
- Used primarily in *neurosurgery.*

Limitations

- Can be used for relatively small tumors, generally < 3cm in diameter.

★ **Interstitial brachytherapy** (implantation of radioactive beads into the tumor mass), is generally reserved for ***tumor reccurence***Q of brain tumors because of its toxicity – necrosis of adjacent brain tissue.

Craniospinal Irradiation

Craniospinal radiation therapy is used as a *treatment* for cases of *neuraxial dissemination*. And **prophylactic cranio- spinal irradiation** is used in any malignancy with high risk of CNS spread or ***CNS tumors which show high propensity for dissemination via CSF (i.e. neuroxial dissemination)*** like

- **Most embryonal tumors** eg infratentorial primitive neuroectodermal tumor (PNET) including ***medulloblastoma***Q; supratentorial PNET including ***pineoblastoma***Q and atypical teratoid rhabdoid tumor.
- **Some germ cell tumors** eg ***malignant germinoma & malignant non-graminomatous germ cell tumors***Q like embryonal carcinoma, choriocarcinoma, yolk sac tumor, teratoma, mixed germ cell tumors.
- **Glioma WHO grade III (*anaplastic astrocytoma and anaplastic oligodendroglioma)*Q grade IV (*glioblastoma multiforme*)Q**
- ***Ependymoma***Q
- ***Acute lymphoblastic leukemia (ALL)***Q
- ***Non Hodgkin's lymphoma***Q (★ Given generally when older than 3 years of age)
- ***Small cell carcinoma of lung***Q
- ***Leptomeningeal rhabdomyosarcoma***Q

Biological Effect of RT

Acute Toxicity (less serious)

- Occuring **within days** of RT
- Radiation sickness
- Acute radiation syndrome ***(nausea, vomiting, headache, lethargy*Q*)***
- Acute cerebral toxicity occurs during RT to brain causing transient disruption of BBB; and can be prevented or treated with glucocorticoid administration. ***Spinal cord is not affected in adult RT***Q

Delayed Toxicity

Early delayed toxicity occurs in **weeks to months** and **more serious often irreversible late delayed toxicities** develop in *years*. These include

CNS

- **Focal demyelination** (causing pseudoprogression) and **somnolence syndrome** (marked sleepiness seen mainly in children) d/t brain toxicity and **Lhermitte symptoms** (i.e. paresthesias of limbs or along the spine on flexion of neck) d/t spinal cord toxicity are *early-delayed toxicity of RT.*
- Focal demyelination may be asymptomatic or take form of worsening or reappearance of a preexisting neurological deficit and cause contrast enhanced MRI/CT lesions mimicking tumor **(pseudoprogression)**; seen mostly in *malignant glioma and when chemotherapy particularly temozolomide* is given concurrently with RT.
- **Radiation necrosis and leukoencephalopathy** are late delayed toxicities. Radiation necrosis (appear identical to pseudoprogression but unlike it) is *always symptomatic and appears mother to years after RT*. It is a focal mass of necrotic tissue (caused d/t fibrinoid necrosis and occlusion of cerebral vasculature) that is *contrast inhancing of MRI/CT* (i.e mimic tumor radiographically) but unlike tumor is typically *hypometabolic on PET scan and has reduced perfusion on perfusion MR scan.* Clinical features include seizures & lateralizing findings based on location of mass.
- Leukoencephalopathy is seen *most commonly after whole brain RT* (as opposed to focal RT) and more oftenly in patients with *increased age*. Patients present with *cognitive impairment, gait disorder, and later urinary incontinence* (all of which can progress over time). – i.e. symptoms mimicking normal pressure hydrocephalus. On MR (T_2 or FLAIR sequences) there is *diffuse increased signal seen throughout hemisphere white matter, often bilaterally and symmetrically*, with periventricular predominance, atrophy and *ventricular enlargement*. Ventriculoperitoneal shunts can improve function in some patients but does not reverse the deficit completely.

Other Somatic and Genetic effects

- **Endocrine dysfunction;**
  - GH >> ACTH and gonadotropin > TSH
  - Thyroid, Ovarian failure
- **Second Cancer**
  - *Leukemia (MC), thyroid cancer*Q, brest cancer
- **Vascular**
  - Accelerated atherosrerosis l/t stroke
- **Peripheral nervous system**
  - Peripheral nerves are relatively resistant (rarely affected) but **plexopathy** develop more commonly in *brachial distribution* than in lumbosacral distribution
- **Skin**
  - Radiation dermatitis
  - Basal cell/ squamous cell C_A
- **Heart**
  - ***Pericarditis (constrictive)***Q
  - MI & fibrosis
- **Kidney & U.B**
  - Peritubular fibrosis
  - Hyalinization of glomeruli
  - Vascular damage
- **Lungs**
  - ***Radiation pneumonitis***Q
- **Gonads**
  - ***Infertility & mutations***Q
- **G.I.T.**
  - Eosophagitis, gastritis, ***enteritis***Q, colitis, Proctitis
  - Vascular damage l/t ischemia, ***ulceration & atrophy of mucosa & fibrosis***Q causing strictures & obstruction.
- **Eyes & CNS**
  - Cataract, Retinal damage
- **Genetic**
  - Point mutation
  - ***Chromosomal mutation***Q

In Radiotherapy

- Most commonly affected – ***Skin*** (more commonly moist *areas*)Q
- Most common skin menifestation – ***Erythema***Q
- Most sensitive Blood Cell - ***Lymphocyte***Q
- Most resistant Blood Cell - ***Platelets***Q
- **Most sensitive body tissue** – *Bone marrow, Male testis, Female ovary*
- Most resistant body organ – Bone
- Organs with less need for cell renewal such as heart, *skeletal muscle & nerves are more resistant* to radiation. In radio-resistant organs, *vascular endothelium* is most sensitive component.
- Organs with more self renewal d/t normal homeostasis such as *hematopoietic system & mucosal lining of intestine* are more sensitive.
- Most sensitive cell in CNS – Neuron
- Most sensitive CNS part – Mid brain, Medulla, Spinal Cord
- Most sensitive abdominal organ – Kidney
- Most Sensitive mucosa – Intestinal mucosa

Whole-Body Irradiation Syndromes

- These are *early effects of high radiation exposure, occur only when most or all of the body is irradiated* (such as seen in victims of Chernobyl, Hiroschima and Nagasaki etc)
- The *radiosensities of target cells* determine the effective *threshold dose* below which the syndrome does not occur, whereas the *onset time of individual symptoms* is dependent on the *proliferative organization of tissue.* It is important to understand that a particular organ/tissue contains >1 type target cells, each with its own radiosensitivity, so *severity of one complication does not necessarily predict the severity of another complication,* even within the same tissue and therefore radiosensitivity of tissue's cells and radioresponsiveness of tissue as a whole are not necessarily same always. For example *depletion of basal cells of epidermis* result in *desquamation* (dry/moist) of skin, depletion of *dermal fibroblast* in *fibrosis* and *damage to small dermal blood vessels* in *telangectasia.*
- **LD_{50}** or **mean lethal dose** is whole body dose that results in mortality for 50% of an irradiated population and is often expressed in terms of time scale (eg 30 or 60 days following irradiation). $LD_{50/60}$ is **~3.5Gy** in absence of medical intervention and ~7Gy with careful medical management. LD_{50} is inversely related to LET (ie LD_{50} increases with decreasing LET).
- **Prodromal syndrome** consists of ≥1 transient gastrointestinal and neuromuscular symptoms beginning soon after irradiation and persisting for upto several hours. Symptoms include *anorexia, nausea, vomiting, diarrhoea, fatigue, disorientation and hypotension,* and their sensitivity duration increase with increasing doses.

Hematopoietic Syndrome	Gastrointestinal Syndrome	Cerebrovasuler Syndrome	Teratogenesis
- Acute doses **> 1 to 2.5 Gy** (1 in Walter; 1.5-2 in ACEP; 2.5 in Ganderson; **kill bone marrow stemcells and lymphocytes** and produce hematopoietic syndrome. - It is characterized by a *precipitous (within 1-2 days) fall in peripheral blood lymphocyte count* f/b *gradual* reduction (over period of 2 to 3 weeks) in the number of circulating *leukocytes, platelets, and erythrocytes.* The *granulocytopenia and thrombocytopenia* reach a maximum within 30 days after irradiations, and death (if occurs) is usually d/t *infection or haemorrhage* - Treatments include antibiotics, blood transfusion and bone marrow transplantation.	- Acute dose **>5 to 8 Gy** (5 in Walter; 6-7 in ACEP; 8 in Gunderson) principally kill the **crypt stem cells of gut epithelium** and l/t gastrointestinal syndrome. As mature cells of vill, are lost over period of several days, no new cells are available to replace them, so villi begin to shorten and eventually become completely denuded. - It is characterized by *lethargy, vomiting, and diarrhoea, dehydration, electrolyte imbalance,* malabsorption, weight loss, and ultimately bleeding and sepsis - Symptoms begin to appear within a few days of irradiation and are progressive in nature, culminating in death in 5 to 10 days. To date no one has survived ≥10 Gy whole body dose of low LET radiation.	- Acute dose **>20 to 50 Gy** (20 in Walter; 20-30 in ACEP; and 50 in Gunderson; l/t cerebro vascular syndrome. - The *onset of features is almost immediate* following exposure, consisting of severe gastrointestinal and neuromuscular disturbances including *nausea, vomiting, disorientation, ataxia, and convulsions. It in invariably fatal* and survival is seldom >48hrs. - Target cells remain unclear. The immediate cause of death, however, is *vascular damage* l/t progressive brain edema, hemorrage and/ or cardiovascular shock, meningitis, myelitis and encephalitis. Such acute high doses, even kills radioresistant cells such as neurons and parenchymal cells of other tissues and glial cells etc.	- Radiation induced excess relative risk of teratogenesis during the most sensitive phase of gestation is **40% per Gy**. - Most common anomalies include microcephaly, mental retardation, other neurological defects and growth retardation. Although still births, miscarriage, cataract, ocular defects, gross malformation and sterility all are reported. Each effect has a temporal relation to the stage of gestation as, well as dependency on dose and dose rate. - **Within 10 days** of conception during (preimplantation stage) *lethality* is most common consequence; between **10 to 14 days (implantation stage)** growth retardation; and during **organogenesis period (15 to 50 days** after conception) the embryo is most sensitive to lethal, teratogenic and growth retardation effects. Gross abnormality of major organ system do not occur *during fetal period (> 40 days),* although >1 Gy doses can cause generalized growth retardation and neurological defects.

Complications of RT in Children

Long term complications are central to decision about the use of radiotherapy in children CNS tumor. RT for pediatric CNS tumor may affect ***neurological, endocrine, and congnitive functions and l/t somatic effects, parenchymal or vascular damage and secondary neoplasms***Q. The risk of S/E is governed by ***age of patient, prescribed dose and volume of RT***Q, time after treatment and the location of primary tumor. The *effects of tumor* (e.g. hydrocephalus and irreversible neurological impairment) *and prior treatment* (including surgery and chemotherapy) i.e. combinations of clinical and treatment factors increase S/E.

Cognitive Effects

- Predictions regarding side effects are driven by factors of *treatment site, total dose, and the targeted volume*. The weight of age is greater than the effect of dose on *cognitive effects (i.e. global intelligence, learning, memory, attention and bhaviour)*. The adverse cognitive effects of RT in children with brain tumor occur only in patients who received *whole brain irradiation to dose levels of 18, 24 and 36 Gy (commonly used in treatment of medulloblastoma)*. Age has the greatest impact on cognitive outcome after irradiation. **Young age** at the time of irradiation is the most important prognostic factor regardless of dose. **Volume of irradiation** is an important prognostic factor for the functional outcome. *Children treated with partial brain irradiation* were more likely to have in IQ>90 at 5 years (with no decline in memory, IQ and academic achievement even in children younger than 3 years) compared to who received craniospinal irradiation (CSI). Fear of cognitive deficits has been the driving force in medulloblastoma patients receiving CSI. And there is a move to increase the age at which CSI is considered acceptable **from age 3 years to 5 year at the time of treatment**.
- Summary: **Effect of RT on cognitive functions (i.e. global intelligence, IQ, learning, memory, attention and behavior)** depends on ***age (< 3-5 years) of patient, volume of irradiation (CSI) > and dose (36>24>18)***Q.

- **Endocrinal deficiencies (GH>> ACTH and gonadotropin > TSH l/t hypothyroidism)** can occur d/t irradiation of hypothalamic – pituitary axis. Total dose and differential sensitivity of hypothalamic nuclei are important determinant. *Hypothalmic obesity, diabetes insipidus and hyperprolactinemia* are more often d/t local tumor effects and surgery. *Thyroid and ovarian failure* often occurs d/t CSI d/t incidental irradiation of these organs.
- **Hearing loss** (d/t conducting system damage >> sensorineural damage of choclea) and *dental complications (d/t CSI affecting salivary glands* or medicines of seizure disorder) can occur.
- Other long term **somatic complications** include permanent hair loss, wound healing problems, ***softening of bone and ligaments of spine and spinal growth impairment and small head size (musculo-skeletal problems)***Q.
- **Second tumors, increased incidence of vasculopathy** (after RT in craniopharyngioma and optic pathway glioma), *microangiopathy with calcifications, lacunar infarcts and transient or permanent enhancement or T2 signal abnormalities* (mostly but not always in regions that received the highest dose).

Radiatilon Detection & Dose Measurement

Gas Filled Detector (GFD)

These measure exposure by collecting ionization in air or gas chamber. Photon entering GFD, ionizes the gas atom into an electron (negative ion) and a positive (atom minus an electron) pair. The positive ion moves toward cathode and e- towards anode (producing **small current or output signal in anode). Voltage regions of GFD include.**

I	**Recombination region** has voltage not high enough to separate the ion pairs.
II	**Ionization (Saturation) region** has voltage high enough to collect almost 100% of **ionization.** A GFD operating in this region is called **ionization chamber** (thimble or farmer chamber & parallel palte chamber a/t design; **Xenon gas ionization chamber** used in some rotate-rotate 3rd generation CT scans). In these low voltage GFD, the *current is directly proportional to intensity of incoming radiation.*
III	**Proportional (Gas Amplification) region** has voltage high enough to accelerate the ionized electrons to an energy that causes **additional secondary ionization** of gas atoms, amplifying the actual amount of initial ionization by a factor M. GFD operating in this made is called **proportional counter**. *Secondary ionization & so the output signal is proportional to energy of photon.*

Solid State Detectors (SSD)

Thermoluminescent Dosimeters (TLD)

- Small crystalline solid absorbs energy from ionizing radiation and raises **an electron-hole pair to an excited but trapped (unfilled) state** (ie valence band bound electron jumps to conduction band leaving a positive hole in valence band). Heating the crystal enables the *electron-hole pair to leave the trap and return to de-excited state with emission of light* that is proportional to the amount of radiation dose.

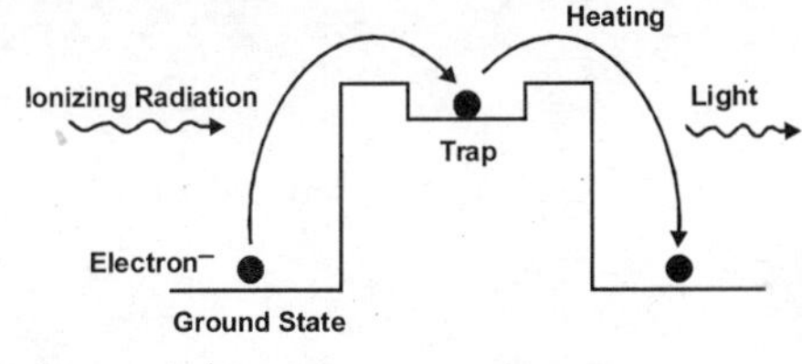

- Most common types of TLD are **lithium fluoride** (LiF, almost tissue equivalent) and **calcium fluoride** (CaF, not tissue equivalent).

Films: Silver halide Films and Radiochromic Films

MOSFET DETECTORS

- A semiconductor device called **metal oxide silicon semiconductor field effect transistor** (MOSFET) is very small size point dosimeter for in vivo patients (both as implantable and surface placed dosimeter).

Scintillation Detectors

- SD detects radiation by measuring amount of light produced in a special crystalline material by ionizining radiation.
- **Sodium iodine (NaI)** is the most common material followed by **cesium iodide (CsI), bismuth germinate (BGO)** and **cadmium tungstate ($CdWO_4$)**
- All rotate fixed (4th generation) and some rotate-rotate (3rd G) CT scanners use scintillation crystal detectors.

RADIOTHERAPY 3

IV	**Geiger-Miller (GM) region:** With higher voltage, the secondary ionization is so large that *the energy proportionality is lost and all coming photons register the same size pulse.* Whether low or high energy the amount of **ionization that occurs is the** same, as the entire gas is ionized each time a photon hits the detector. **GM counter** emits a large click/signal for each photon seen and is a **photon counting device** (hand carried survey meters).
V	**Continous discharge region:** The voltage is very high to spontaneously ionize the detector gas. GFD is not useful as ionization continues & continues.

Semiconductor: Germanium (GeLi) and Silicon (SiLi) Detectors

Absolute Dosimeters

- Do not require caliberation and measure the amount of dose directly

Calorimeter

Chemical or Frickle Dosimeter

Personal Dosimetry

- Previously **TLD badge/ring and film badge**[Q] have been used for monitoring of dose for radiation safety purpose by occupational workers.
- **OSL (Optically stimulated luminescence)** by thin matrix material of **aluminum oxide (Al_2O_3:C) wafer** is primary dosimeter.
- Badge is worn at waist or neck during work. Filters that overlay the dosimeter enable discrimination between electrons or low energy photons and high energy photons.

QUESTIONS

Principles of Radiotherapy

1. **Which of the following statements best describes 'Background Radiation'** *(AI 10)*
   A. Radiation in the background of nuclear reactors ☐
   B. Radiation in the background during radiological investigations ☐
   C. Radiation present constantly from natural sources ☐
   D. Radiation from nuclear fall out ☐
2. **At t=0 there are 6×10^{23} radioactive atoms of a substance, which decay with a disintegration constant (λ) equal to 0.01/sec. What would be the initial decay rate?**
   A. 6×10^{23} *(AI 05; DNB 07)* ☐
   B. 6×10^{22} ☐
   C. 6×10^{21} ☐
   D. 6×10^{20} ☐
3. **The major difference between X-Rays and Light is:**
   A. Energy *(AI 10)* ☐
   B. Mass ☐
   C. Speed ☐
   D. Type of wave ☐
4. **Photon transferring some of its energy to electron is**
   A. Photoelectric effect *(Jipmer 06, DNB 09)* ☐
   B. Bremsstrahlung effect ☐
   C. Compton effect ☐
   D. Ionization ☐
5. **Photoelectric effect is** *(AI 08)*
   A. Interaction between high energy incident photon and the inner shell electron ☐
   B. Interaction between incident photon and the outer shell electron ☐
   C. Interaction of the incident photon with the nucleus ☐
   D. Interaction between a photon and electric current ☐
6. **True about Electromagnetic radiation:**
   A. Pair production occur for low energy ☐
   B. Infrared is a EM radiation *(PGI 11, DNB 11)* ☐
   C. Compton scattering occur for intemediate energy ☐
   D. X-ray is EM radiation ☐
7. **Maximum scattering in X Ray plate occurs in**
   A. Carbon *(AI 96, DNB 02)* ☐
   B. Mercury ☐
   C. H^+ ☐
   D. Ca^{++} ☐
8. **Which of the following best estimates the amount of radiation delivered to an organ in the radiation field:**
   A. Absorbed dose *(AI 2010)* ☐
   B. Equivalent dose ☐
   C. Effective dose ☐
   D. Exposure dose ☐
9. **All are feature of radiaiton except** *(AI 91; DNB 09)*
   A. Biological ☐
   B. Photographic ☐
   C. Fluorescent ☐
   D. Non penetrating ☐
10. **Which of the following is the most ionizing radiation:**
    A. Alpha *(AI 2010)* ☐
    B. Beta ☐
    C. X-Ray ☐
    D. Gamma ☐
11. **Which one of the following has the maximum ionization potential?** *(AI 2006)*
    A. Electron ☐
    B. Proton ☐
    C. Helium ion ☐
    D. Gamma (γ) – photon ☐
12. **Which of the following has most penetrating power?**
    A. α-particle *(AI 2002)* ☐
    B. β-particle ☐
    C. γ-radiation ☐
    D. Electron beam ☐
13. **Which of the following is the most penetration beam?**
    A. Electron beam *(AI 04; DNB 05)* ☐
    B. 8 MV photons ☐
    C. 18 MV photons ☐
    D. Proton beam ☐
14. **Ionization radiation acts on tissue leading to**
    A. Linear acceleration injury *(AI 98; DNB 01)* ☐
    B. Excitation of electron from orbit ☐
    C. Formation of pyramidine dimer ☐
    D. Thermal injury ☐
15. **Principle used in radiotherapy is** *(AI 1997)*
    A. Cytoplasmic coagulation ☐
    B. Ionization of molecule ☐
    C. DNA damage ☐
    D. Necrosis of tissue ☐
16. **Functional basis of ionising radiation depends on:**
    A. Pyramidine base pairing *(AIIMS 96; DNB 97)* ☐
    B. Removal of orbital electron ☐
    C. Linear energy transfer ☐
    D. Adding orbital electron ☐
17. **Principles used in Radio Therapy is:**
    A. Infrared rays *(AIIMS 1994)* ☐
    B. Ionizing molecules ☐
    C. Charring of nucleoprotein ☐
    D. Ultrasonic effect ☐
18. **Radiation produces its effect on tissue by**
    A. Coagulation of cytoplasm *(AIIMS 93)* ☐
    B. Increasing the temperature ☐
    C. Charring of nucleoprotein ☐
    D. Hydrolysis ☐
19. **Which is not a deep heat therapy.** *(AI 2007)*
    A. Short wave diathermy ☐
    B. Infra Red ☐
    C. USG ☐
    D. Microwave ☐
20. **What is atomic number :** *(PGI 2001)*
    A. Proton ☐
    B. Electrons + protons ☐
    C. Protons + neutrons ☐
    D. Protons + protons ☐
21. **Gray equals** *(PGI June 07; DNB 03)*
    A. 100 rad ☐
    B. 1000 rad ☐
    C. 10000 rad ☐
22. **Which of the following is true about Gray (G):**
    A. G=SI unit for absorbed dose *(AIIMS May 13)* ☐
    B. 1G=Joule/Kilogram ☐
    C. 1G=10Joule/kilogram ☐
    D. 1G=100Joule/Kilogram ☐

E. 1G=100Rad

23. **Curie is unit of:** *(PGI 97; DNB 98)*
A. Radiation exposure ☐
B. Radiation absorption ☐
C. Radioactivity ☐
D. All of the above ☐

24. **1 becquerel is equal (Disinegration/sec) to:**
A. 3.7×10^{10} *(PGI May 2010)* ☐
B. 2.7×10^{10} ☐
C. 1.7×10^{10} ☐
D. 3.7×10^{-2} ☐

25. **Regarding particle interaction true is** *(PGI Nov 11)*
A. Bragg peak observed with light mass electrons ☐
B. Bremsstrahlung photons produced by α particles ☐
C. Electron scatter less than protons ☐
D. Electrons stop sooner in low atomic number (than higher Z) materials ☐
E. X-ray production increases with high energy electrons ☐

X-Rays

26. **X-rays are produced when:** *(AIIMS 2002)*
A. Electron beam strike the nucleus of the atom ☐
B. Electron beam strikes the anode ☐
C. Electron beam reacts with the electromagnetic field. ☐
D. Electron beam strikes the cathode ☐

27. **Which is provided by linear accelerator**
A. Electron *(AIIMS 1995)* ☐
B. Neurtron ☐
C. Proton ☐
D. Infrared rays ☐

28. **↑ energy linear acceleration used in**
A. X-ray *(PGI June 2004)* ☐
B. Cathode rays ☐
C. Photon rays ☐
D. α- rays ☐
E. γ - rays ☐

29. **High energy accelerator produces:** *(PGI May 2011)*
A. X-ray ☐
B. Electron beam ☐
C. Gamma rays ☐
D. Neutron ☐
E. Proton ☐

30. **Principles of Linear accelerators is used in**
A. X-rays *(PGI 06; DNB 07)* ☐
B. Gamma-rays ☐
C. Alpha rays ☐
D. Infrared rays ☐
E. Alpha particles ☐

31. **Radioactive emissions used in radiotherapy are**
A. α-Particles *(DNB 02; PGI 03, 01)* ☐
B. β-Particles ☐
C. γ-rays ☐
D. X-ray ☐
E. Infrared rays ☐

32. **Most common used rays for radiotherapy:**
A. X rays *(DNB 05; PGI 06, 02; AIIMS 99)* ☐
B. γ rays ☐
C. α rays ☐
D. β rays (electrons) ☐

33. **Most commonly used radiation(s) in modern radiation therapy:** *(PGI May 13)*
A. X-ray ☐
B. Gamma ray ☐
C. Alpha beam ☐
D. Electron Beam ☐
E. Proton beam ☐

34. **Beams can be used for cancer treatment are**
A. γ-rays *(PGI 02)* ☐
B. α-rays ☐
C. Neutrons ☐
D. Protons ☐
E. X-rays ☐

35. **In radiation therapy rays used are:**
A. α, β *(PGI 1999)* ☐
B. α, γ ☐
C. β, γ ☐
D. γ, α, β ☐

36. **Most harmful to individual cell :** *(PGI 98)*
A. X-rays ☐
B. α - particles ☐
C. β - particles ☐
D. X- rays (gamma rays) ☐

37. **Whole body electron therapy is useful in Mx of** *(AI 12)*
A. NHL ☐
B. Sezary syndrome ☐
C. Mycosis fungoides ☐
D. Hodgkin's disease ☐

38. **What contrast is needed for proper radiographic image in a heavy bony built person?** *(AI 2002)*
A. ↑ed ma ☐
B. ↑ kvp ☐
C. ↑ed exposure time ☐
D. ↑ed developing time ☐

Radio Isotopes : Teletherapy

39. **For teletherapy, isotopes commonly used are**
A. I-123 *(PGI 02; DNB 01)* ☐
B. Cs-137 ☐
C. Co-60 ☐
D. Tc-99 ☐
E. Ir-191

40. **Which of the following is obsolete in modern day clinical use?** *(AIIMS Nov 09)*
A. Ra^{226} ☐
B. Co^{60} ☐
C. $Ir1^{92}$ ☐
D. Cs^{137} ☐

41. **Which of the following radioisotopes is commonly used as a source for external beam radiotherapy in the treatment of cancer patients**
A. Strontium – 89 *(AI 2003)* ☐
B. Radium – 226 ☐
C. Cobalt – 59 ☐
D. Cobalt – 60 ☐

42. **In Teletherapy setup all are used except**
A. Irridium-191 *(AIIMS 1998)* ☐
B. Co – 60 ☐
C. Simulator ☐
D. Computer ☐

43. **Radionucleotide (s) used in external beam therapy:**
A. Iodine-131 *(PGI Nov 2010)* ☐
B. Co-60 ☐
C. Cs137 ☐
D. Ra226 ☐
E. Ir192 ☐

3 RADIOTHERAPY

Brachytherapy

44. Advantage of brachytherapy *(PGI 04; DNB 05)*
A. Non-invasive ☐
B. Less radiation hazard to normal tissue ☐
C. Max.radiation to diseased tissue ☐
D. Can be given in all malignancies ☐
E. Doesn't require trained personnel ☐

45. Features of intestitial therapy are all except:
A. Only used in head & neck *(PGI June 2006)* ☐
B. ↓ Damage to normal tissue ☐
C. Temporary or permanent ☐
D. Only iridium used ☐
E. Used for easily accessible organ ☐

46. Which of the following radioactive isotopes is not used for brachytherapy:
A. Iodine-125 *(AIIMS 2005)* ☐
B. Iodine – 131 ☐
C. Cobalt – 60 ☐
D. Iridium – 192 ☐

47. Which one of the following radioisotope is not used as permanent implant:
A. Iodine-125. *(AI 2005)* ☐
B. Palladium-103. ☐
C. Gold-198. ☐
D. Caesium-137. ☐

48. All may be used in interstitial brachytherapy except
A. Cs ^{137} *(AI 1999)* ☐
B. Au ^{198} ☐
C. Ir ^{192} ☐
D. Co ^{60} ☐

49. Isotope (s) used in high brachytherapy: *(PGI June 09)*
A. Ir192 ☐
B. C0-60 ☐
C. Cs133 ☐
D. Ra226 ☐
E. Pd103 ☐

50. Radioactive isotopes that are used in treatment of cancer are *(PGI 2003)*
A. Cesium ☐
B. Cobalt ☐
C. Carbon ☐
D. Technetium ☐
E. Nitrogen ☐

51. Which is used in teletherapy & Brachytherapy both
A. Iridium 127 *(AIIMS 1998)* ☐
B. Cobalt 60 ☐
C. Pallidium ☐
D. Iodine 131 ☐

52. Which is/are false about T½ of radioisotopes: *(PGI 10)*
A. Ra-226: 1626 years ☐
B. I-131: 60 years ☐
C. Co-60: 5.26 tears ☐
D. Cs-137: 30 years ☐

53. Longest half life is seen in *(AIIMS 1997)*
A. Radon ☐
B. Radium ☐
C. Uranium ☐
D. Cobalt ☐

54. The half life of Cobalt -60 is *(AIIMS 1997)*
A. 3.4 years ☐
B. 5.2 years ☐
C. 1.2 years ☐
D. 2.3 years ☐

55. Half life of I^{131} is *(AI 1994)*
A. 4 hours ☐
B. 8 days ☐
C. 4 days ☐
D. 10 days ☐

56. Half life of Technetium is *(AI 1993)*
A. 6 hours ☐
B. 12 hours ☐
C. 24 hours ☐
D. 26 hours ☐

57. Artificial radioisotops: *(PGI 2002)*
A. Radium ☐
B. Uranium ☐
C. Plutonium ☐
D. Iridium ☐
E. Cobalt ☐

58. Radium emits which of the following radiations:
A. Alpha rays *(DNB 09; PGI 10, 01, 2K)* ☐
B. Beta rays ☐
C. Gamma rays ☐
D. X-rays ☐
E. Neutrons ☐

59. Phosphorous-32 emits: *(AI 2006)*
A. Beta particles ☐
B. Alfa particles ☐
C. Neutrons ☐
D. X-rays ☐

60. Radiation emitts by Ir- 192: *(PGI Dec 07)*
A. 0.5 Mev ☐
B. 0.6 Mev ☐
C. 0.66 Mev ☐
D. 0.666Mev ☐
E. 0.47 Mev ☐

61. True about Cobalt 60 is A/E *(PGI Dec 2004)*
A. Natural radioactive agent ☐
B. At.wt.59 ☐
C. Emits β and γ-rays ☐
D. Half life is 5.3 yrs. ☐
E. Used in both brachy & teletherapy ☐

62. All are pure beta emitters except: *(AIIMS May 2011)*
A. Yttrium-90 ☐
B. Phosphorus-32 ☐
C. Strontium-90 ☐
D. Samarium-153 ☐

63. Isotope used in RAIU *(AI 2007)*
A. I^{131} ☐
B. I^{123} ☐
C. I^{125} ☐
D. I^{127} ☐

64. Most suitable radioisotope of Iodine for treating hyperthyroidism is: *(AI 2003)*
A. I^{123} ☐
B. I^{125} ☐
C. I131 ☐
D. I^{132} ☐

65. Radio isotopes are used in the following techniques except: *(AI 2004)*
A. Mass spectroscopy ☐
B. RIA ☐
C. ELISA ☐
D. Sequencing of nucleic acid ☐

Radiosensitivity of Tissues

66. Maximum dose of radiation per year in a human which is safe *(AI 1992)*
A. 1 rads ☐
B. 5 rads ☐
C. 10 rads ☐
D. 20 rads ☐

67. Maximum permissible radiation dose in pregnancy is:
A. 0.5 rad. *(AIIMS 2003)* ☐
B. 1.0 rad. ☐
C. 1.5 rad. ☐
D. rad. ☐

68. Most sensitive tissue to Radiaton is
A. Liver *(AIIMS 1995)* ☐
B. Gonads ☐
C. Spleen ☐
D. Skin ☐

69. Organs sensitive to radiation are *(PGI 03)*
A. Gonad ☐
B. Bone marrow ☐
C. Liver ☐
D. Fat ☐
E. Nervous tissue ☐

70. The cell most sensitive to RT:
A. Neutrophill *(AIIMS 1993)* ☐
B. Lymphocyte ☐
C. Basophill ☐
D. Platelett ☐

71. The radiation tolerance of whole liver as :
A. 15 Gy *(AI 2004)* ☐
B. 30 Gy ☐
C. 40 Gy ☐
D. 45 Gy ☐

72. Most sensitive structure in cell for radiotherapy is :
A. Cellmembrane *(PGI 2002)* ☐
B. Mitochondrial membrane ☐
C. DNA ☐
D. Enzymes ☐
E. ER ☐

73. Ionoising radiation most sensitive in-
A. Hypoxia *(PGI June 2005)* ☐
B. S phage ☐
C. G_2M phage ☐
D. Activating cell ☐

74. Most Radio sensitive stage *(DNB 06; AI 98, 96, 07; AIIMS 2002, PGI 97)*
A. S phase ☐
B. G_1 phase ☐
C. G_2 phase ☐
D. G_2M phase ☐

75. The phase of Cell cycle, most sensitive to radiation is /are: *(DNB 02, PGI 09)*
A. M phase ☐
B. G_2 phase ☐
C. S phase ☐
D. Early G_1 phase ☐
E. G_0 phase ☐

76. Most radiosensitive stage of cell cycle
A. G_0G_1 *(AIIMS Nov 12, DNB 04; PGI 05)* ☐
B. G_2M interphase ☐
C. Late S phase, G_2S ☐
D. Late S_1 phase ☐
E. M phase ☐

77. What is radioresistant *(AIIMS 1997)*
A. Cartilage ☐
B. Seminoma ☐
C. Ewings sarcoma ☐
D. GI epithelium ☐

Radiosensitivity of Tumors

78. Which of the following is the most radiosensitive tumour? *(AIIMS May 2005)*
A. Ewing Tumour ☐
B. Hodgkin's disease ☐
C. Carcinoma cervix ☐
D. Malignant fibrous histocytoma ☐

79. Radiosensitive tumors are *(PGI June 2006)*
A. Seminoma ☐
B. Lymphoma ☐
C. Sarcoma ☐
D. Ewing's sarcoma ☐
E. Leukemia ☐

80. Most Radiosenstitive ovarian tumor is
A. Serus cystadenoma *(AIIMS 1997)* ☐
B. Dysgerminoma ☐
C. Dermoid cyst ☐
D. Teratoma ☐

81. Highly radiosensitive tumor(s) is/are: *(PGI May 12)*
A. Dysgerminoma ☐
B. Seminoma ☐
C. Wilm's tumor ☐
D. Lymphoma ☐
E. Osteosarcoma ☐

82. Most Radiosensitive tumor *(AIIMS 1995)*
A. Brenner's tumor ☐
B. Dysgerminoma ☐
C. Mucinous cystadenoma ☐
D. Teratoma ☐

83. Most Radiosensitive testicular tumor is
A. Yolk Sack Tumor *(AIIMS 1993)* ☐
B. Embryonal cell tumor ☐
C. Teratoma ☐
D. Seminoma ☐

84. The most radiosensitive tumour among the following is:
A. Bronchogenic carcinoma *(AI 2006)* ☐
B. Carcinoma parotid ☐
C. Dysgerminoma ☐
D. Osteogenic sarcoma ☐

85. Tumor(s) most responding to radiotherapy
A. Sarcoma *(PGI 2003)* ☐
B. Seminoma ☐
C. Lymphoma ☐
D. Leukaemia ☐

86. Tumor responding best to radiation include following:
A. Melanoma *(PGI 1997)* ☐
B. Dysgerminoma ☐
C. Teratoma ☐
D. Choriocarcinoma ☐

87. Most radiosensitive brain tumor is
A. Astrocytoma *(AIIMS 1997)* ☐
B. Ependymoma ☐
C. Medulloblastoma ☐
D. Craniopharyngeoma ☐

88. Most Radiosensitive lung CA is
A. Sqamous cell *(AIIMS 1993)* ☐
B. Small cell ☐
C. Adeno ☐
D. Large cell ☐

89. Most radiorestistant tumor among following is:
A. Ewing carcinoms *(PGI May 13)* ☐
B. Osteosarcoma ☐
C. Cervical ca ☐
D. Lymphoma ☐
E. Rhabdomyosarcoma ☐

90. Which of these tumors is least radiosensitive
A. Ewing's sarcoma *(AIIMS May 07)* ☐
B. Osteosarcoma ☐
C. Wilm's tumor ☐
D. Neuroblastoma ☐

91. **All are highly radiosensitive except:**
A. Osteogenic sarcoma (AIIMS 1993)
B. Lymphoma
C. Ewing's sarcoma
D. Seminoma

92. **Which of the following malignant tumors is radio resistant?** (AI 2006)
A. Ewing's sarcoma
B. Retinoblastoma
C. Osteosarcoma
D. Neuroblastoma

93. **Most Radiosensitive tumor of the following is:** (AI 2001)
A. Ca Kidney
B. Ca Colon
C. Ca Pancreas
D. Ca Cervix

Chemotherapy

94. **Tumors that are sensitive to chemotherapy**
A. Lymphoma (PGI 2003)
B. Germ cell tumor
C. Leukaemia
D. Choriocarcinoma

95. **Poor wound Healing is seen in** (AIIMS 1993)
A. Adriamycin
B. 5-FU
C. Methotrexate
D. Nitrogen mustard

96. **Chemotherapeutic agent of choice in CA pancreas**
A. Mitomycin (AIIMS 1993)
B. 5-FU
C. Streptozocin
D. Adriamycin

97. **All are Chemosensitive except** (AIIMS 97)
A. Small Cell CA
B. Ca Cervix
C. Ewing's tumor
D. Malignant melanoma

Therapeutic

98. **Hypoxia cause cell to become:** (AIIMS May 13)
A. More radiosensitive
B. More radioresistance
C. No effect on radiosensitivity
D. May increase or decrease radiosensitivity

99. **Radiation therapy to hypoxic tissues may be potentiated by the treatment with:** (AIIMS 2003)
A. Mycostatin
B. Metronidazole
C. Methotrexate
D. Melphalan

100. **All are radiosensitizer except** (AIIMS 1997)
A. 5-Fu
B. BUDR
C. Cyclophosphamide
D. Hydroxyurea

101. **A patient with cancer received extreme degree of radiation toxicity. Further history revealed that the dose adjustment of a particular drug was missed during the course of radiotherapy. Which of the following drugs required a dose adjustment in that patient during radiotherapy in order to prevent radiation toxicity**
A. Vincristine (AIIMS May 2004)
B. Dactinomycin
C. Cyclophosphamide
D. 6-Mercaptopurine

102. **Radioprotective drug is** (AI 12, 01)
A. Paclitaxem
B. Vincristine
C. Amifostine
D. Etoposide

103. **Amifostine, protects all of the following except:** (AI 2009)
A. CNS
B. Salivary glands
C. Kidneys
D. GIT

104. **The technique employed in radiotherapy to counteract the effect of tumour motion due to breathing is known as:** (AI 2005)
A. Arc technique
B. Modulation
C. Gating
D. Shunting

105. **Radiation exposure during infancy has been linked to which one of the follwing carcinoma** (AI 2003)
A. Breast
B. Melanoma
C. Thyroid
D. Lung

106. **Least amneable to screening is**
A. Breast CA (AIIMS 1993)
B. Cervix CA
C. Lung CA
D. Oral cavity CA

107. **Craniospinal irradiation is used in the Treatment of-**
A. Oligodendroglioma (AI 2002)
B. Pilocytic astrocytoma
C. Mixed oigoastrocytoma
D. Meduloblastoma

108. **Prophylactic cranial irradiation not indicated in treatment of-** (AI 2002)
A. Small cell Ca of lung
B. ALL
C. Hodgkin's lymphoma
D. NHL

109. **Prophylactic intracranial irradiations are given in :**
A. Small cell Ca of lung (PGI 1998)
B. Testicular Ca
C. Ca breast
D. Ca stomach

110. **Prophylactic cranial irradiation is/are given in:**
A. AMI (PGI Nov 12)
B. ALL
C. Small cell Ca of lung
D. Glioblastoma multiforme
E. Non-Hodgkin's lymphoma

111. **Stereotactic surgery is used for treatment of:**
A. Brain tumor (AIIMS Nov12)
B. Lungs carcinoma
C. Cervix cancer
D. Renal carcinoma

112. **Stereotactic radiosurgery is/are indicated in:** (PGI Nov 12)
A. Multiple cerebral metastasis
B. Arteriovenous malformation
C. Carcinoma lung
D. Primary CNS tumor

113. **Stereotactic Radio-surgery is a form of:** (AIIMS 2003)
A. Radiotherapy

B. Radioiodine therapy
C. Robotic surgery
D. Cryo Surgery

114. **Gamma knife** *(PGI June 06)*
A. Steel knife
B. Used for cutting tumours in difficult location
C. Cobalt is used
D. Recovery delayed

115. **Stereotactic radiotherapy is most useful for**
A. Inoperable lung tumor stage-1 *(AIIMS May 12)*
B. Base of tonge carcinoma with enlarged lymph nodes
C. Lymphangiocarcinomatosis
D. Miliary lung metastasis

116. **Which of the following is not an indication of RT in Pleomorphic adenoma of parotid:** *(AI 2004)*
A. Involvement of deep lobe
B. 2nd histologically benign recurrence
C. Microscopically positive margins
D. Malignant transformation

117. **For mobile tumor of vocal cord treatment of choice is:**
A. Surgery *(AIIMS 1992)*
B. Chemotherapy
C. Radiotherapy
D. None

118. **What dose of radiation therapy is recomme-nded for pain relief in bone metastases** *(AIIMS May 04)*
A. 8 Gy in one fraction
B. 20 Gy in 5 fractions
C. 30 Gy in 10 fractions
D. Above 70 Gy

119. **All of the following radioisotopes are used an systemic radionucleide, except:**
A. Phosphorus-32 *(DNB 04, AI 06)*
B. Strontium-89
C. Iridium-192
D. Samarium-153

120. **Isotopes used in relief of metastatic bone pain includes:** *(PGI May 2010)*
A. Strontium-89
B. I-131
C. Gold-198
D. P-32
E. Rhenium-186

121. **Radiotherapy is used for which stage-I cancer** *(PGI 2001)*
A. Colon
B. Larynx
C. Anterior 2/3 of tongue
D. Lung
E. Stomach

122. **Radiotherapy is Rx of choice for:** *(AIIMS Nov 09)*
A. Nasopharyngeal Carcinoma T3N1
B. Supraglottic Carcinoma T3NO
C. Glottic Carcinoma T3N1
D. Subglottic Carcinoma T3NO

123. **Which of the following is used in the treatment of differentiated thyroid cancer?** *(AI 2006)*
A. ^{131}I
B. ^{99}Tc
C. ^{32}P
D. ^{131}I-MIBG

124. **Which one of the following therapeutic mode is commonly employed in intra-operative radiotherapy?** *(AIIMS 2003)*
A. Electron
B. Photon
C. X-ray
D. Gamma rays

125. **Intraoperative RT is given in** *(AIIMS 1998)*
A. Ca Cervix
B. Ca Breast
C. Ca Pancreas
D. Ca Thyroid

126. **For the treatment of deep seated tumors, the following rays are used.** *(AIIMS 2003)*
A. X- rays and Gamma- rays
B. Proton beam therapy
C. Electrons and positrons
D. High power laser beams

127. **In which malignancy postoperative radiotherapy is minimally used?** *(AI 2004)*
A. Head and neck
B. Stomach
C. Colon
D. Soft tissue sarcomas

128. **The ideal timing of radiotherapy for Wilms Tumour after surgery is:** *(AI 2006)*
A. Within 10 days
B. Within 2 weeks
C. Within 3 weeks
D. Any time after surgery

129. **Intercavitatory radiotherapy is treatment modality for**
A. Ca Cervix *(AIIMS 1999)*
B. Ca Oesophagus
C. Ca Stomach
D. Renal cell CA

130. **Point B in treatment of Ca cervix corresponds to**
A. Mackenrodts ligament *(AIIMS 1993)*
B. Obturator Lymph node
C. Isheal tuberosity
D. Round ligament

131. **Emergency radiotherapy is given in-** *(PGI June 2005)*
A. Superior vena cava syndrome
B. Pericardial temponade
C. Increased ICP
D. Spinal cord compression

Side Effects

132. **Long term effect of RT for CNS tumor in children are all except** *(AI 12)*
A. Reduced IQ and learning
B. Endocrine dysfunction
C. Musculoskeletal problems
D. Neuropsychological effects are independent of radiation dose.

133. **True about effects of RT on a child's brain** *(AI 12)*
A. IQ not significantly affected
B. Behaviour changes are common
C. Recurrent seizure common
D. No memory loss

134. **Most common hormone deficiency seen after intracranial radiation therapy –**
A. Prolactin *(AIIMS May 07)*
B. Gonadotropins
C. ACTH
D. Growth hormone

135. **MC cancer due to Radiation :**
A. Leukaemia *(PGI Dec 07)*
B. Bronchogenic Ca
C. Thyroid Ca
D. Breast cancer
E. Bone tumour

136. **Most common presentation of radiation carditis is :**
A. Pyogenic Pericarditis *(AI 1997)*

B. Pericardial Effusion ☐
C. Myocardial Fibrosis ☐
D. Atheromatous Plaque ☐

137. Late effects of radiation thearpy: *(PGI 2002)*
A. Mucositis ☐
B. Enteritis ☐
C. Nausea and vomiting ☐
D. Pnueumonia ☐
E. Somatic mutations ☐

138. Most common skin manifestation seen after 2 days of radiation therapy is-
A. Erythema *(AI 1998)* ☐
B. Atopy ☐
C. Hyperpigmentation ☐
D. Dermatitis ☐

139. Which of the following statements about 'Stochastic effects' of radiation is true
A. Severity of effect is a function of dose ☐
B. Probability of effect is a function of dose ☐
C. It has a threshold ☐
D. Erythema and cataract are common examples ☐

IMRT

140. For which malignancy, Intensity Modulated Radiotherapy (IMRT) is the most suitable:
A. Lung *(AIIMS Nov 2005)* ☐
B. Prostate ☐
C. Leukemias ☐
D. Stomach ☐

141. Low dose radiation cause: *(PGI Nov 2010)*
A. Lung cancer ☐
B. AML ☐
C. Cervical cancer ☐
D. Glioma ☐
E. Meningioma ☐

142. Dose of radiation during whole body exposure that leads to haematological syndrome is: *(AI 2011)*
A. 2 Gy ☐
B. 10 Gy ☐
C. 100 Gy ☐
D. 200 Gy ☐

143. Radiation exposure can be measured by: *(PGI May 13)*
A. TLD badge ☐
B. Gamma Camera ☐
C. Auger emission ☐
D. Linear accelerator ☐
E. Film badge ☐

Answers and Explanations:

PRINCIPLES OF RADIOTHERAPY

1. **C i.e. Radiation present constantly from natural sources** *[Ref: Thayalan 1/e p-206-7]*

Back ground radiation is ***a low level, wide spread (ubiquitous), constantly present radiation from natural sources that is usually not detrimental to life***[Q].

Radiation according to sources

Natural Background Radiation	Artificial man made Radiation
- Extra terrestrial (cosmic rays) - Terrestrial (i.e. radioactive substances like uranium, thorium, radon etc present in earth crest/rock/sand and radioactive gases) - Radionucleotides present in diet & human body	- Radioactive materials used in industry, research & medicine - Diagnostic x-rays/CT - Nuclear fall outs (accidents & explosions) - Consumer products (Smoke detectors)

2. **C i.e., 6×10^{21}** *[Ref. Radioactive decay equation – Lee ESCI – 480 2003; Chapter 3A]*

Radioactive Decay Law

The **Rate of Decay of a radioactive substance**, 'N', is given by $\boxed{\frac{dN}{dt} = \lambda N}$

where N = no. of undecayed radioactive atoms
t = time in seconds
λ = decay constant, which represents the probability per unit time for one atom to decay. It is assumed that the probability of decay is constant and does not depend on time or number of radioactive atoms present.

Now so

$\lambda = 0.01/\text{sec}$ Decay rate $= \frac{dN}{dt}$

$N = 6 \times 10^{23}$ $= 6 \times 10^{23} \times 0.01$
$= 6 \times 10^{23} \times 10^{-2}$
$= 6 \times 10^{21}$

The initial rate of decay therefore will be 6×10^{21}.

3. **A i.e. Energy** 4. **C i.e., Compton effect**
5. **A i.e., Interaction between incident photon & the outer shell electron**
6. **B i.e. Infrared is a EM radiation; C i.e. Compton scattering occur for intemediate energy; D i.e. X-ray is EM radiation**
7. **C i.e. H^+** *[Ref: Gunderson 3/e p 97; Campeau 3/e p 161-62; Thayalon p 53-54; Christe4nsen's 4/e p 64; Grainger 5/e p 133-34]*

Major difference between x-rays & light are wave length (λ) & energy[Q]

- **Electromagnetic radiation or photon waves** are **non particulate (0-mass), non charged (0-charge)** waves, that **do not require a medium to travel** (i.e. can travel in vaccum) and transfer energy from one location to another at the **speed of light** (c= 3×10^8 m/s).
- The **major difference** between various forms of photons/electromagnetic radiation **lies in their wave length (λ) and frequency (n)**, which accounts for their differences in energy carried. $\boxed{E \propto n/\lambda}$

  So Xrays with shorter wave length in comparison to visible light carries 5000 times higher energies. Because for EM waves energy is proportional to frequency (n) and inversly proportional to wave length (λ).
- EM radiation spectrum consists of *photons with wave length, frequency and energy ranges over 10 orders of magnitude* (the range is really infinite). **From low energy to high energy** these are Radar waves, Microwaves, Infra-red, Light (visible photons), Ultraviolet, **X** rays and Gamma rays. (Mn- "Reliance **MILL Xtra** Grand").
- When a photon beam falls, it can exit (**transmitted electrons**) or interact with matter (**attenuation**). **With increasing amount of photon energy** 5 possible interactions are possible, which are **coherent scattering (very low energy** electrons; <10KeV), **photoelectric effect (low energy** electrons; < 60 KeV), **Compton/ Recoil scattering (higher energy**; 60 KeV – 10MeV), **pair production (very high energy**; > 1.022 to > 10 MeV), and **photodisintegration (very high energy**; > 8-10 MeV)
- ***Maximum compton scattering occurs with hydrogen***[Q] b/o highest electron density.
- In **photoelectric effect**, the ***most tightly bound-inner most electron completely absorbs all energy of falling low energy photon***[Q], so much so that the photon is completely absorbed and no longer exists and inner orbital electron (now called photoelectron) is ejected. The interaction can occur with other orbital electrons but the most probable interaction is with inner most shell electron. The vacency created in inner shell is filled by an electron from outer orbit with simultraneous emission of **X-ray** or **Auger electron**.

- In **Compton Scattering** incident *higher energy photon transfers only a part of its energy to a loosely bound outer shell electron*Q. and is deflected or scattered off in a new direction with lower energy. The outer shell electron (now called **compton /recoil** electron) is ejected **with no production of X-ray or Auger electron.**
- **Charged heavy particles** (such as **protons and α-particles**) have a finite range and *experience a rapid increase in energy loss near the end of their track (range/path), dumping most of their remaining energies quickly and producing an ionization* curve with a peak near end (K/a **Bragg peak**).
- When a **light mass-charged particle (such as electron or β-particle**) with high energy passes close to the nucleus's positive electrical field, it is deflected & decelerated by electro static attractions and loses energy in form of X-ray photons called ***bremsstrahlung or braking radiation. So Bragg peak is produced by charged heavy particles mainly, whereas Bremsstrahlung radiation is produced by charged light particles***Q.
- ***Collisional energy losses (& heat production) dominate at lower energyies, whereas radiative losses dominate at higher energies (l/t more efficient X-ray production)***Q.
- ***Because of dependency on atomic number (Z^2) and 1/velocity^2; collisional energy losses increases as atomic number increases and particle velocity decreases. So electrons are stopped sooner in low Z than high Z materials***Q.

8. **A i.e. Absorbed dose** *[Ref: Farr 2/e p-17; Christian 3/e p-25]*

Amount of radiation delivered to an organ is defined as absorbed doseQ. Whereas **equivalent dose** is a *measure of biological damage* caused by the absorbed dose *depending on the relative effectiveness of type of radiation*; and **effective dose** is a *measure to assess the risk of carcinogenesis & genetic defect* by calculating an imaginary total body dose depending on equivalent dose for each organ and *relative sensitivity of each organ to radation.*

9. **D i.e. Non penetrating** *[Ref: K. Parks-SPM 17/e P-52]*

There is nothing to explain as radiation may be *penetrating* also. (Example gamma rays)

10. **A i.e. Alpha** 11. **C i.e., Helium ion** 12. **C i.e. γ Radiation** 13. **C i.e. 18 MeV photons**
[Ref: Grainger & Allison's diagnostic Radiology 4/e P-139; Park 17/e P-521; K.N.Sharma Chemistry]

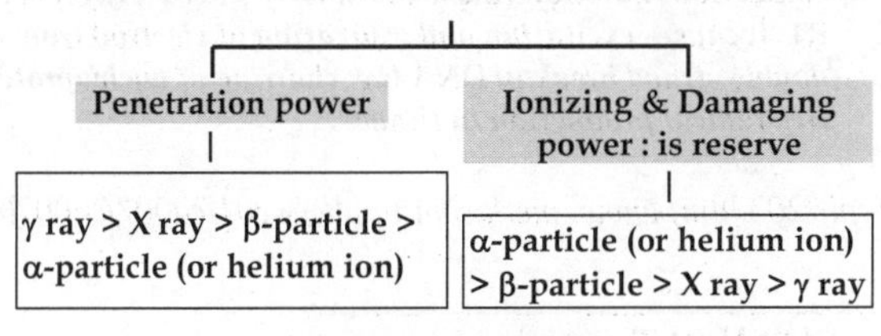

Penetrating Power

Neutrons > γ rays (very high energy photons) > X Rays (low energy photons) β-rays (high energy electrons) > α-particle (helium nuclei ie 2 protons & 2 neutrons).

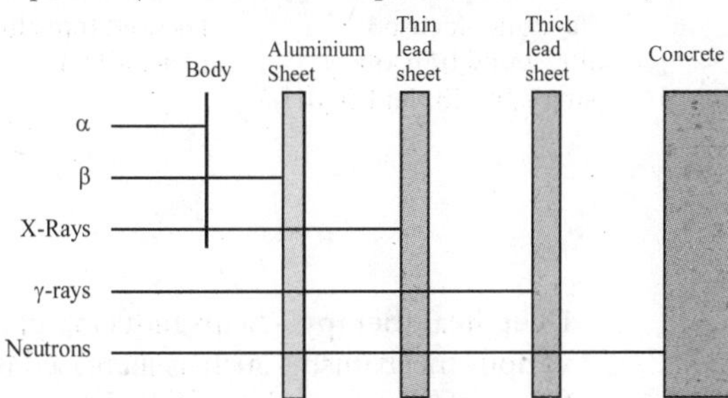

Radiation	Content	Penetrating Power	Ionizing Power	Damaging Power
α-particle	Helium nuclei (i.e. 2 protons & 2 neutrons)	***Poorest***Q **(1)**	***Maximum***Q	***Most damaging***Q
β-particle	Either high energy electron or antimatter counter part positron	Greater than α-particle (100)	Lesser than α-particle	< α-particle
X-Ray	*Low energy photons*Q	More than β-particles	Lesser than β-particle	< β-particle
γ-radiation	*Very high energy photons*Q	**More than X Rays (10000)** i.e. ***Most Penetrating***Q	***Minimum Ionizing***Q	***Least damaging***Q

14. **B i.e. Excitation of electron from orbit**
15. **B i.e. ionization of molecule**
16. **B i.e. Removing orbital electrons**
17. **B i.e. Ionizing molecules**
18. **C i.e. Charring of nucleoprotein**

Radiotherapy is treatment of malignant tumors with ***ionizing radiation (m.c. γ rays)***Q ; which causes ***excitation or ionization (ejection of electron from orbit) of electron***Q and kills tumor cells by producing ***double strand breaks in DNA*** (direct) or *free radicles* **(indirect). So *ionizing* Radio Therapy** acts (on tissue) by- **Excitation** of electron (to higher energy levels without actual ejection) **- and Ionization of electron (Removal of orbital e-).**

Ionizing radiation is of two types – *electromagnetic (photon)* and *particulate radiation.*

Type	Mass	Charge	Comment
Electromagnetic			X Ray & γ ray do not differ except in the source. γ rays are produced intranuclearly and X rays are produced extranuclearly (i.e. mechanical)
X Ray	0	0	
Gamma Ray	0	0	
Particulate			
Electron (e)	e	-1	-
Proton (p)	2000xe	+1	Exhibit *Bragg peak* (most of energy is given abruptly causing ionization)
Neutron (n)	2000xe	0	Can't be accelerated by an electrical field
Alpha particle	2p+2n (8000xe)	+2	*Helium Particle* (2p+2n)

- The biological effects produced by a radiation is quantified as **relative biological effectiveness (RBE),** which compairs them to effects produced by **250KV photon radiation** as a standard.
- RBE value depends on **Linear energy transfer (LET**; is amount of ionization occurring per unit length of radiation tract), dose, dose rate & nature of biological system.
- ***Absorption of energy from radiation in tissue leads to ionization &/or excitation leading to various biological effects*** Q.

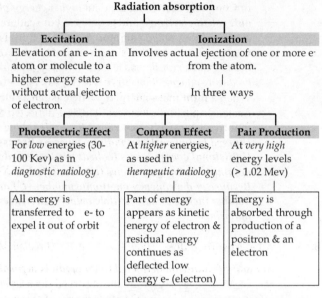

Radiation absorption

- **Excitation**: Elevation of an e- in an atom or molecule to a higher energy state without actual ejection of electron.
- **Ionization**: Involves actual ejection of one or more e⁻ from the atom. In three ways
  - **Photoelectric Effect**: For *low* energies (30-100 Kev) as in *diagnostic radiology* → All energy is transferred to e- to expel it out of orbit
  - **Compton Effect**: At *higher* energies, as used in *therapeutic radiology* → Part of energy appears as kinetic energy of electron & residual energy continues as deflected low energy e- (electron)
  - **Pair Production**: At *very high* energy levels (> 1.02 Mev) → Energy is absorbed through production of a positron & an electron

- Radiation must produce *double-strand breaks (not single-strand) in DNA* to kill a cell. It can indirectly kill by producing *free radicles.*
- **Chromosomal abnormalities** occur in cells irradiated in G_1 *Phase* of cell cycle before doubling of genetic material.
- **Chromatid aberration** occurs in cells irradiated in G_2 *Phase.* **Most sensitive** ***phase to radiation is M > G₂M interphase***Q. ***Most resistant phase to radiation is end of S phase***Q. ***Lymphocyte analysis provides evidence of recent total body exposure.***
- **Ionization radiation (most commonly γ rays/X rays)** is used for RT. It ***causes excitation and ionization of electron from orbit l/t double strand break in DNA (i.e. charring of nucleoprotein) and free radical production in tissue***Q.

19. B i.e. Infra red *[Ref: http://www.emedicine.com/ pmr/topic 203.htm, www. merk.com/mmhe/sec01/ch007/ch007b-htm; Gunderson 3/e p. 391]*

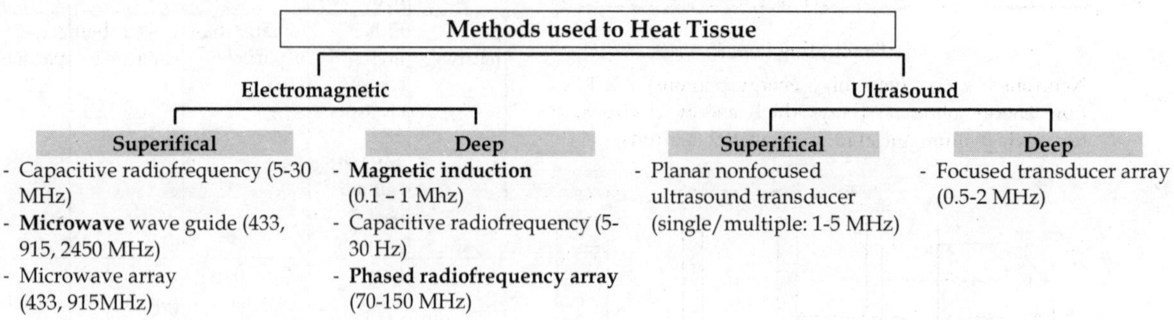

Heat therapy

Superficial heat therapy
- Heat packs
- ***Infra red***Q
- Paraffin bath
  Hydrotherapy

Deep heat therapy
- ***Short wave diathermy***Q
  - High radiofrequency electrical currents
- ***Micrwave diathermy***Q
  - Electromagnetic radiation
- ***Ultrasound***Q
  - 0.8-1 mHz frequency

Deep heat therapy – helps reducing pain by various mechanisms such as increased blood flow, enhanced cellular metabolism, reversible nerve conduction block & relief of muscle spasm.

It is indicated in conditions associated with pain such as inflammation of joints or tissue, muscle spasm, sprain, neurogenic pain.

20. **A i.e. Proton** *[Radiological science for technologists 7/e P-41; D P Tondon – Chemistery P-80]*

Atomic number	*Number of protons*Q *Number of electron*Q
Mass number	*No. of protons + No. of neutrons*Q

21. **A i.e., 100 rads** *[Ref: Harrison 18/e p 1788, 691, 17/e p 135-61]*
22. **A i.e. G=SI unit for absorbed dose; B i.e. 1G=Joule/Kilogram; E i.e. 1G=100 Rad**

Rad (radiation absorbed dose) is energy deposited within living matter & is equal to *100 ergs/gm of tissue.* Whereas, **1 gray is absorption of** ***1 joule energy by 1 kg*** **living matter**Q. **Gray (Gy) is the Systeme International (SI) unit for absorbed dose**Q.

1 Gray (Gy=G; SI unit) = 1 Joule/Kilogram = 100 Rad= 100 cGy (centigray)

23. **C i.e. Radioactivity** 24. **E i.e. 1** *[Ref: Thayalon p 93; Grainger 5/e p 131, 101]*

Becquerel (Bq) or disintegration per second is the **SI unit** of radioactivity whereas, **Curie (Ci)** is **non-SI unit** of radioactivity. The rate of radioactive decay of a sample is called radioactivity. SI unit of activity is the Bequerel *(Bq), defined as one nuclear disintegration per second*Q. The **Curie (Ci)** is defined as **3.7×10^{10} disintegrations** per second, thought to be the number of disintegrations found in *1 gm of radium.*

1 mili Ci = 37 MBq; 1 mCi = 3.7×10^7 dps;	1 Micro Ci = 0.037 MBq 1 μ Ci = 3.7×10^4 dps

25. **D i.e. Electrons stop sooner in low atomic number (than higher Z) materials; E i.e. X-ray production increases with high energy electrons**

X-Rays

26. **B i.e. Electron beam strikes the anode** 27. **A i.e. Electron**
28. **A i.e. X-ray** 29. **[A,B > D, E] i.e. (X-ray, Electron beam > Neutron, Proton)**
30. **A i.e. X –ray** 31. **C i.e. γ-rays; D i.e. X Rays > A i.e. α- Particle; B i.e. β particle**
32. **B i.e. Gamma Rays > A i.e. X- Rays** 33. **A i.e. X-ray; B i.e. Gamma ray**
34. **A i.e. Gamma rays; B i.e. α-rays; C i.e. Neutron; D i.e. Protons; E i.e. X Rays**
35. **D i.e. γ, α, β** 36. **B i.e. α-particles** 37. **C i.e. Mycosis fungoides**

[Ref: Gunderson 3/e p 345-90; Oxford onchology 2/e p 398; Thayalan p 184-86; 97, 53-54; Harrison 18/e p 691]

- **High energy linear accelerators** produce ***electron beam (β-particle) and high energy (megavoltage) X-rays by bremsstrahlung interaction***Q. **High energy cyclotron** accelerates proton, deutron & α particles producing ***high energy proton beams or fast neutrons***Q.
- In **linear accelerator, electrons** are accelerated in straight line to high energy & are allowed to exit the machine as **electron beam** (for treatment of ***superficial cancers eg mycosis funguides***Q as particle therapy) or are directed to a target to produce **high energy (megavoltage) bremsstrahlung X-rays** (to treat deep seated tumors). Betatron & Van de Graff accelerator also accelerate electrons.
- **Cyclotron** can accelerate **proton, dentron and alpha particles** spirally to 35 MeV energy and can generate ***proton & neutrons beams***Q and other high energy charged particles
- **Gamma rays (γ) photons** are generated from decay of atomic nuclei of radioisotopes such as Cobalt & radium.
- X-Rays was first produced by Rontgen in 1895. Now a days X-Rays are produced by cooling tube. **X Rays** are produced when fast moving *stream of* ***electron produced by cathode***Q (negative charged tungsten filament) ***strikes the anode***Q (positive charged tungsten or molybdenum containing copper block).
- Scattering depends on *Electron/Nucleus ratio.* X-Ray is most scattered by ***H^+ ion***Q. The period when **fetus is most sensitive to radiation** is ***8-15 weeks of gestations***Q.
- ***X Rays***Q ***& Gamma rays***Q are the forms of radiation ***most commonly used to treat cancer.***
- **Xrays** (generated by *linear accelerator*) and **gamma rays** (generated by decay of *atomic nuclei of radio isotopes*) are both electromagnetic, non-particulate, non charged, zero mass, packets of energy (photons) waves that

cause ejection of an orbital electron when absorbed (i.e. ionization) and kill-tumor cells by producing double strand breaks in DNA (direct) or free radicle production (indirect).

- **Particulate forms of radiation** are also use in certain circumstances. **Total skin electron treatment (TSET)** which is similar to total body irradiation (TBI) except that electrons are used instead of photons. TSET have a very low tissue penetration and are used to treat skin cancer such as ***mycosis fungoides***Q. The main advantage of liner accelerator is the ability to produce X-rays and electrons of varying energy within the same machine.

Rays used in radiotherapy

Low LET (linear energy transfer)

LET, is the rate of energy loss by the practice in tissue

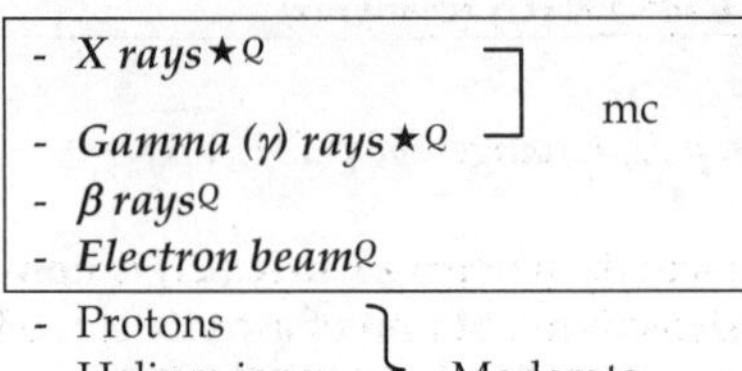

- *X rays*★Q
mc
- *Gamma (γ) rays*★Q
- *β rays*Q
- *Electron beam*Q

- Protons
- Helium ions
- *α particles*Q

Moderate LET

High LET

More tissue damage, less influenced by tissue oxygenation & less sensitive to variations in cell cycle & DNA repair.

High LET radiation is les sensitive to reduce cell killing effect of hypoxia, with there being ~ equal cell killing under normoxic & hypoxic condition. It causes a dense change of ionization in both strands of DNA & therefore makes DNA repair more difficult.

Example includes

- Neon ions
- Carbon ions
- Negative π mesons (pions)
- **Neutron**★ (neutral particles produced from beryllium & cause knock-on or billiard ball collision)

38. A i.e. Increase ma *[Ref: Christensens 3/e p. 164]*

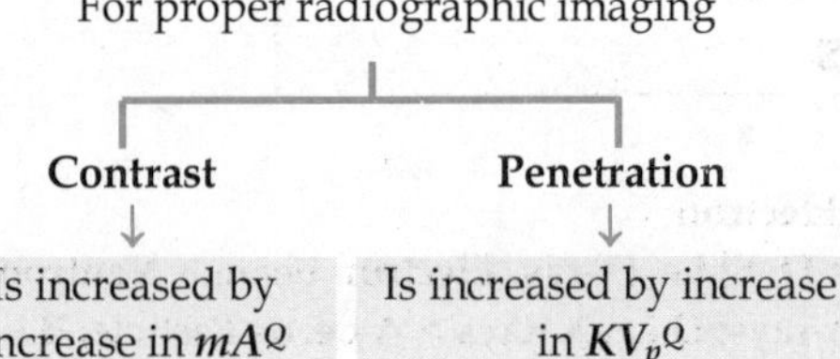

- ***Low KV_p gives high subject contrast while mA controls film blackening (density)***Q.
- **Contrast** is increased by increasing intensity of X Ray, which depends on number of electrons striking the target (i.e. rate of emission of electrons); which is controlled by varying filament current.
  So increase in current leads to increase in contrastQ.
- **Penetration** of X Ray is enhanced by enhancing ***voltage***Q, On the basis of penetration, X Rays are of two type
  Hard X Rays = High penetrating X Rays
  Soft X Rays = Low penetrating X Ray

Radio Isotopes

39. C i.e. Co^{60} >>> B i.e. Cs^{137}

40. A i.e. Ra226

41. D i.e. Cobalt 60

42. A i.e. Irridium

43. B >>C >>>E i.e. Co-60 >> Cs^{137} >>> Ir^{192}

[Ref: Gunderson 3/p 98; Ruth 1/e 124-27; Thayalan 1/e p 178-80; Armstrong RT p 698]

In **external beam radiotherapy (or teletherapy)**, ***Cobalt (^{60}Co)***Q is the most commonly used radioisotope. Cs^{137} and rarely Ir^{192} can be used for animals. But ***Ra^{226} is obsolete and avoided***Q b/o associated hazards. So order of preference is

^{60}**Co (best)** >>>> ^{137}**Cs** (rare clinical use) >>> ^{192}**Ir** >>> ^{226}**Ra (avoided)** no clinical use

Computer is used for planning of RT & for record keeping of RT. Simulator is used for localization of RT to maximize therapeutic gain and minimize the radiation hazard to adjacent normal tissue.

Brachytherapy

44. **B i.e. Less radiation hazard to normal tissue; C i.e. Max.radiation to diseased tissue**
45. **A i.e. Only used in head & neck; D i.e. Only iridium is used; E i.e. Used for easily accessible organs**
46. **B i.e. Iodine – 131** **47.** **D i.e. Cesium – 137** **48.** **D i.e. CO^{60}**
49. **A, B i.e. Ir^{192}, Co^{60}** **50.** **A i.e. Cesium; B i.e. Cobalt** **51.** **B i.e. Cobalt-60**

[Ref: Ruth's 1/e p. 98-100; Gunderson 3/e, p 96-98; Radiation in Medicine: A need for Regulatory reform (1996) pg 71 published by the Institute of medicine http//www.iom.edu; Radiation oncology Biophysis 1992; 23(1):81; D.C Dutta 3e/P 466; Walter Miller 5/e p-80]

- In brachytherapy the source of radiation is placed very close to the site of action. It can be invasive technique as it needs the implantation of needle into the tumor (interstitial) or in the cavity (intracavitary). It is often used in brain tumors & cervical cancers. It requires trained perssonels. Maximum radiation effect can be obtained in diseased tissue. Minimum risk of radiation exposure to the normal tissue.
- **Interstitial brachy therapy** uses *variety of rodionucleide implants (not only Ir) inserted into the tumors like sauamous cell carcinoma of head and neck region, skin, breast tumor, soft tissue sarcomas and many others.* These implants are allowed to remain their for a definite period (**temporary implants**) or indefinitely (**permanent implants**). It decreases damage to normal tissue.
- **Radium-226** is a radioactive *decay product of **uranium- 238** series and is the precursor of **radon – 222**. It decays very slowly by emitting α-particles.* Earlier it was used for brachytherapy etc but ***now its use is obsolete due to its very long half life (1600 years)***Q and associated hazards. ***Now radium (Ra-226) and radon (Rn-222) have been completely abondened for clinical use***Q.
- ***I^{125} (not I^{131}) is used for brachytherapy.***
- ***Cesium-131 (t½ 10 days) is used as permanent implant for brachytherapy not Cs-137 (half life 30 years)***Q.
- ***Because of the hazard of breaking the needle within tissue substance, the utility of ^{60}Co as interstitial implant remained questionable***Q. Presently use of Co-60 in brachytherapy is restricted to ophthalmic applicators or for certain after loading systems where small sources are loaded into spherical form.
- **High dose rate (HDR) brachytherapy** uses a dose of *≥ 20c Gy/minute*. Isotopes used for HDR remote after loaders are ***Ir 192 (now most commonly used), Yb 169 and Co60***Q (used in early version of HDR).
- ***Co-60***Q ***& Cesium 137***Q are used in Brachy & Teletherapy both. Carbon is used in carbon dating. Tc is used for bone scanning.

52. **B i.e. I^{131}, D i.e. Ir^{192}** **53.** **B i.e. Radium** **54.** **B i.e. 5.2 years**
55. **B i.e. 8 days** **56.** **A i.e. 6 hours**

[Ref: Wolfgang 7/e p 1092-93; Thayalan p 92-96, 156; Harrison 17/e p 1360; Merdith radiation physics & nuclear medicine p 28; Dutta Gynaecology 5/e p 484]

Half life ($t_{1/2}$) of radium (Ra^{226}) is ***1602-1626 years (longest)***Q; ***Cesium (^{137}Cs) is 30 years***Q; **Cobalt (^{60}Co)** is **5.2 *years***Q; iridium (^{192}Ir) is ***74.5 days***Q; Iodine (I^{131}) is ***8 days***Q; **I^{123}** is ***13 hours***Q; ***technitium (Tc^{99}) is 6 hours***Q; and **I^{132}** is ***2.3 hours***Q.

Half life
- Minimum: I^{132} *(2.3 hours)*Q
- Maximum: **Radium** *(1622 yr)*Q

Isotope	t½
Co-60	*5.2 years*Q
Tritium	12 years
Cs (Cesium)	30 years
Ra (Radium)	1622 years

Isotope	Half life
I^{132}	**2.3 *hours*Q**
I^{123}	***13 hours*Q**
I^{131}	***8 days*Q**

Isotope	Half life
I^{132}	**2.3 *hrs(minimum)*Q**
Tc^{99}	***6 hours*Q**
I^{123}	***13 hours*Q**
Rn (Radon)	3.8 days
I^{131}	***8 days*Q**
Tritium	12 years
Cs (Cesium)	30 years
Ra (Radium)	***1622 years (longest)*Q**

57. **D i.e. Iridium; E i.e. Cobalt** **58.** **A i.e. α rays; B i.e. β-rays; C i.e. ϒ -rays**
59. **A i.e. Beta particles** **60.** **E i.e. 0.47 Mev**
61. **A i.e. Natural radioactive agent** *[Ref: Dorland's pocket dictionary 25/e P-687]*

- **Radium** has ***longest half life***Q (1622 years). It emits ***α, β & ϒ rays***Q and it decays to radon. ***P-32, Sr-90 & Y-90 emits β particles.***Q

- Energy of radiation emitted by **Co-60 is 1.173 Mev**[Q]; Ra-226 is 0.8 Mev; P-32 is 0.698 Mev; **Cs-137** is **O.662 Mev** and **Ir-192** is **0.47 Mev**[Q]
- **Co^{60}** is ***artificially made radeonucliode***[Q] produced by irradiating ordinary naturally occurring Co-59 with neutrons. Co-60 has atomic number-27, ***atomic weight 58.93***[Q], ***half life 5.3 years***[Q] and ***emits both β and γ rays***[Q]***. It is used in both teletherapy (source of choice) and brachytherapy (but avoided in interstitial implantation)***[Q].
- Naturally occurring radioactive nucleide elements belong to one of the 3 series ie
  1. Uronium series; 2. Thorium series; 3. Actinum series
- $Cobalt^{60}$ and Ir^{192} are artificial isotopes

62. **D i.e. Samarium-153** *[Ref: Gunderson 3/e p 429-30]*

- **Pure beta (β) emitters** (radionuclides) are ***phosphorus-32, strontium-90, Yttrium-90 and tritium-30***[Q]. Whereas *Samarium-153 & Rhenium-186 are mixed β and γ emitters*[Q].
- **Systemic radionuclide therapy for bone metastases and pain** include ***^{89}Sr, ^{32}P, ^{186}Rh and ^{153}Sa***[Q]. Phosphorus-32 the first agent to be used is now rarely used b/o risk of myelo suppression, pancytopenia & acute leukemia. Strontium-89 decays by β emission to yttrium-89 with a half life of 50.6 days (β energy 1.46MeV). It is quickly taken up by mineral material of bone b/o chemical similarity to calcium and b/o extremely little γ radiation patient is not a radiation hazard to family members & hospital staff.
- **Samarium-153** is a artificial radionuclide that emits **β particles** of 0.81 MeV (20%), 0.71 Mev (30%), 0.64 MeV (50%) and **gamma photons** of 103 KeV (28%). It has a short half life of 46.3 hours and is chelated with EDTMP to produce bone seaking complex.
- **Rhenium-186** emits **β particles** of 1.07 MeV and a 137 KeV **gamma rays.** It has a short half life of *3.8 days* and is chelated with *HEDP* to produce bone seeking complex.

63. **B i.e. I^{123}**

- **Iodine $(I)^{123}$** is ***agent of choice for thyroid imaging and radioactive iodine uptake (RAIU)***[Q]/thyroid counts/capsule counts because of low radiation exposure.
- **Iodine $(I)^{131}$** is ***agent of choice for treatment of hyperthyroidism***[Q] (esp after 35 years of age and when patient is not fit for surgery d/t medical problems) ***treatment of functioning thyroid cancer***[Q] *and imaging and functioning of metastases.*

64. **C i.e. (I^{131})** *[Ref: Wolfgang 7/e, p 1112-14]*

The various modalities of thyroid scintigraphy are:

a) Tc 99 m pertechnitate scan
b) I^{123} scan [Agent of choice][Q]
c) I^{121}

RAIU i.e. **Radio active iodine uptake/ Thyroid count /capsule count** is a thyroid imaging method that measures the fraction of orally administered iodine isotope taken up by the thyroid. It is measured at intervals of 4 & 24 hours after administration of the isotope

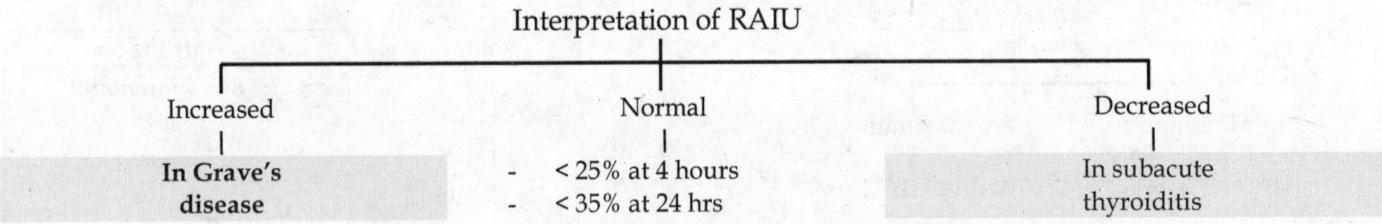

∗ However this test is not diagnostic of hyper thyroidism without measurement of hormones

65. **C i.e. ELISA** *[Ref: Harper 25/e P-13; Anant Narayan 5/e P-78]*

Concept: **ELISA (Enzyme Linked Immunoabsorbent Assay)** is an enzyme based immnoassy; the similar test which uses radioactive isotope in place of enzyme is known as **Radioimmunoassay (RIA)**
So I don't think any need of learning that- *Nucleic acid sequencing, mass spectroscopy & RIA* are tests using radio isotopes.

Radiosensitivity Of Tissues

66. **B i.e. 5 rads** *[Ref: K Park SPM 17/e P-522]*

- Amount of radiation received from out space = **0.1 rad/*year***[Q]
- Additional permissible dose = **<5 rads/*year***[Q]

67. **A i.e. 0.5 rad** *[Ref: Christensens physics of diagnostic radiology; Williams 2/e P-1150]*

- **Maximal permissible radiation dose:** is the dose of radiation which if received each year for a 50 years working life time would not be expected to produce any harmful effect.
- The recommended occupational limit of maternal exposure to radiation from all sources is ***500 milli rads (0.5 rads)***[Q] for entire 40 weeks of gestation.
- **10 days rule** advices that any **X Ray** examination involving the **abdomen** of a women of child bearing age should be carriedout ***with the 10 days of menstruation.***[Q]
- Fetus is most sensitive to the effects of radiation during ***8-15 weeks of gestation***[Q].

68. **B i.e. Gonads** *[Ref: Anderson Pathology 10/e P-489 Harrison 15/e P-533]*
69. **A i.e. Gonad; B i.e. Bone marrow**
70. **B i.e. Lymphocyte** *[Ref: Anderson pathology 10/e P-489]*

- ***Lymphocyte*** is most sensitive to RT so ***Lymphocytic Predominant Hodgkins*** has best prognosis
- ***Platelett*** is mot resistant to RT.

71. **C i.e. 40 Gy** *[Ref: Harrison 15/e P-2588; Gunderson & Tepper radiation onchology P-715)]*

Whole Organ	TD 50/5
Fetus	400
Bone marrow	450
Kidney	2000 (whole strip) 2500 (whole)
Lung	2500
Liver	2000 (whole strip) *4000*[Q] (whole)
Brain	6000

T_D 50/5 = **maximal tolerance dose** = i.e. the dose that results in a rate of severe complications of 50% or less within 5 years of treatment.

T_D 5/5 = **minimal tolerance dose** = i.e. the dose that results in a rate of severe complications of 5% or less with in 5 years of treatment.

72. **C i.e. DNA**

Dividing part of cell is most sensitive to radiotherapy, so **nucleoprotein – DNA & RNA** are highly radiosensitive.

73. **C i.e, G_2M phage D i.e., Activating cell** *[Ref: Harrison 16/e P 484-85; 17/e p – 516 – 17].*
74. **D i.e. G_2M phase**
75. **A i.e. M phase; B i.e. G_2 phase**
76. **B i.e. G_2M** *[Ref: Harrison 17/e p. 516; Principles of radiation therapy Washington Lever 2/e p. 85; Abeloff's Clinical Onchology 4/e p. 428]*

- ***Most sensitive period is junction of G_2M phase in actively dividing cells.***[Q]
- **Susceptibility of various phase of cell cycle to radiation is G_2M** (late G_2 and M) **> Late G_1** and **Early S > Mid G_1 > Mid – Late S** and **Early G_2 phase**

Most sensitive	Moderate sensitive	Moderate Resistant	Most Resistant
Late G_2 and M (mitosis)	Late G_1 Early S	Mid G_1	Mid-Late S Early G_2

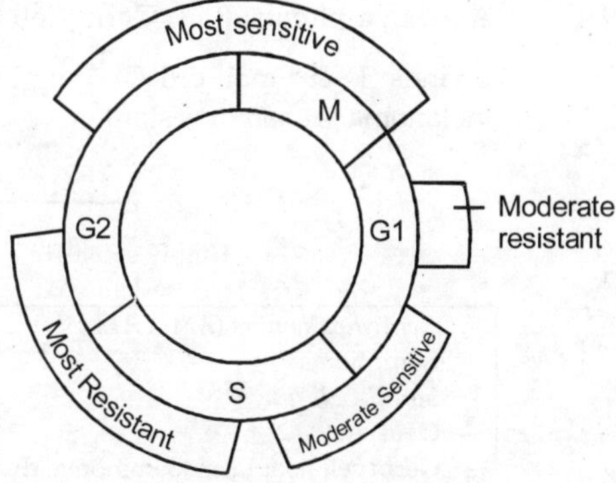

- Radiation energy is absorbed by tissue causing ***ionization or excitation***[Q], which are responsible for various biological effects.

Phase of Cell Cycle	Comment
G_2M > M	*Most* ***sensitive***[Q] to radiation
End of S phase and early G_2	*Most* ***resistance***[Q] to radiation
G_1	Radiation exposure l/t *chromosomal* aberration
G_2	Radiation exposure l/t *chromatid* aberration

77. **A i.e. Cartilage**

- We already know Seminoma & Ewing's sarcoma are highly radiosensitive tumors
- Intestinal Epithelium is most sensitive mucous membrane to Radiography.
- Actively dividing cells are highly radiosensitive (Ex. GI epithelium, Bone marrow, hair follicles, germ cells)
- Non dividing stable cells are radio resistant (Ex. Cartilage, Nerves, muscles)

3 RADIOTHERAPY

Radiosensitivity Of Tumors

78. **A i.e. Ewing's tumour**

79. **A i.e. Seminoma; B i.e. Lymphoma; D i.e. Ewing's sarcoma** **80.** **B i.e. Dysgerminoma**

81. **B i.e. Seminoma; C i.e. Willm's tumor; D i.e. Lymphoma >> A i.e. Dysgerminoma**

82. **B i.e. Dysgerminoma**

83. **D i.e. Seminoma** **84.** **C i.e. Dysgerminoma**

[Ref: Rozer's Radiotherapy 3/e Table 11.3; Essentials of radiology: Bhadury 1/e p. 502; Devita's Oncology 7/e p. 1907]

Highly radiosensitive tumors are:

Multi millionare	**Multiple Myeloma**
Wills	**Wilm's tumor**
Love	**Lymphoma**
Seminal	*Seminoma*Q
Evenings	**Ewing's** *sarcoma*Q

Most radiosensitive
- Ovarian tumor → ***Dysgerminoma***Q (otherwise moderately radiosensitive)
- Testicular tumor → ***Seminoma***Q (highly radiosensitive)

85. **B i.e. Seminoma; C i.e. Lymphoma** **86.** **B i.e. Dysgerminoma**

87. **C i.e. Medulloblastoma** **88.** **B i.e. Small Cell**

- Most radiosensitive kidney tumor - Willm's tumor
- Most radiosensitive Bone tumor - ***Ewings*** S_A ***& Multiple myeloma***Q.
- Most radio sensitive Testicular tumor - ***Seminoma***Q

— **Highly radio sensitive**

- Most radio sensitive Ovarian tumor – ***Dysgerminoma***Q ***> teratoma***
- Most radio sensitive Brain tumor - ***Meduloblastoma***Q
- Most radio sensitive Lung tumor – ***Small Cell*** C_AQ

— moderatively radio sensitive otherwise

89. **B i.e. Osteosarcoma** **90.** **B i.e Osteosarcoma** **91.** **A i.e. Osteosarcoma** **92.** **C i.e. Osteosarcoma**

*Osteosarcoma*Q, Melanoma, Pancreatic carcinoma and Hepatoma are **highly radio-resistant tumors.**

93. **D i.e. CA Cervix** *[Ref: Rozers Radiotherapy 3/e Table 11.3]*

- So the problem is as it was because except C_A pancreas other three are in same group
- This is a good question based on the fact that *TOC in Ca Cervix beyond stage II B is Radiotherapy and in others (Ca Colon, Ca Kidney, Ca Pancreas) Surgery is the best palliative treatment (in late stage).*

Chemotherapy

94. **A i.e. Lymphoma; B i.e. Germ Cell tumor; C i.e. Leukemia** *[Ref: Harrison 15/e P-534]*

Ewings S_A & Small cell C_A lung are highly chemosensitive, in C_A cervix cisplatin is used for palliation but melanoma is chemoresistant

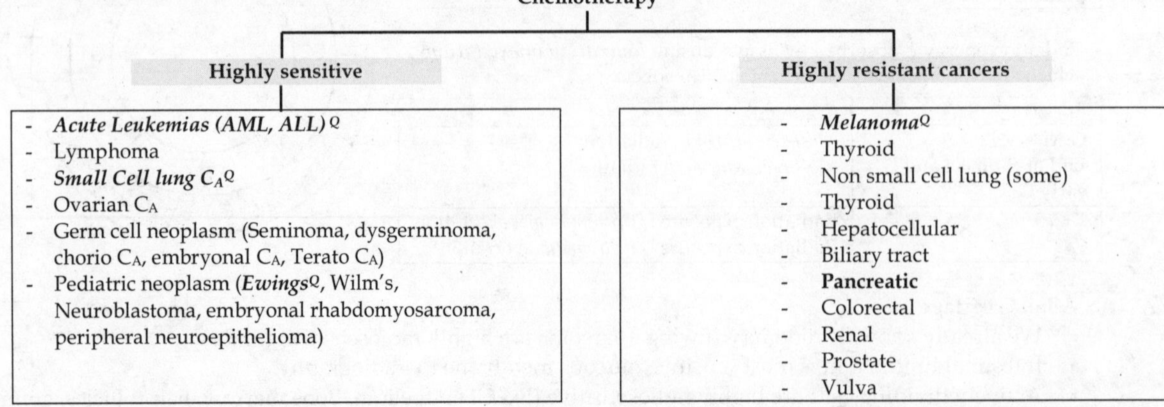

95. **D i.e. Nitrogen musturd** *[Ref: Harrison 15/e P-536]*

Drug	Comment
Nitrosourea	Cross Blood Brain Barrier
5 - FU	***Hand-Foot Syndrome***Q (other causes coxakie A 16, Entero 71 virus & sickell cell anemia
Nitrogen Mustard	Vesicant ***(Poor wound healing***Q***)***
Busulfan	Lymphocyte sparing myelosuppression

96. **B i.e. 5-FU** *[Ref: Harrison 15/e P-593; Love & Bailey 24/e P-1130]*

Disease	Chemo Therapeutic agent of Choice
- Retinoblastoma	Vincristine
- Willim's tumor	ActinomycinD
- Chorio C_A	***Methotrexate***Q
- Chorio CA with liver ds	***ActinomycinD***Q
- C_A Pancreas	***5 Fluro Uracil***Q **/ Gemcitabine**

97. **D i.e. Malignant melanoma** *[Ref: Harrison 15/e P-534]*

Ewings S_A & Small cell C_A lung are highly chemosensitive, in C_A cervix cisplatin is used for palliation but melanoma is chemoresistant.

Therapeutic

RADIOSENSITIZERS

98. **B i.e. More radioresistance**

Radiation damage is dependeat on O_2. Hypoxia (deficiency of O_2) in tumor cells cause them to become more radioresistant and protect them from radiotherapy.Q

99. **B i.e. Metronidazole** **100.** **C i.e. Cyclophosphamide** **101.** **B i.e. Dactinomycin**
102. **C i.e. Amifostine** **103.** **A i.e. CNS**

[Ref: Radiation Oncology' 8th/41; Outcomes in Radiation Therapy (2001)/207; Comprehensive Geriatric Oncology 2nd/494; Gunderson 3/e p. 25-28; Oxford oncology 2/e p 462; Rozer's 3/e p 161; Harrison 18/e p 691]

Metronidazole & other nitroimidazolesQ can sensitize hypoxic tumor cells to the effect of ionization radiation. ***Actinomycin – D***Q ***(Dactinomycin)***Q***, 5FU, BUDR & hydroxy urea are*** *well* known radiosensitizer. So its dose should be reduced during radiotherapy to prevent radiation toxicity.
Amifostine is a ***radioprotector drug but it does not corss BBB and therefore offers no protection to CNS.***

GATING

104. **C i.e. Gating** *[Ref: How Respiratory Gating Works: Respiratory Gating: The Latest Technique in Radiation Therapy. Article by Carol L. Kornmehl, MD, FACRO Radiation Oncologist Valley Hospital, Ridgewood, NJ]*

- **Respiratory gating** is one of the latest techniques in radiation therapy and ***involves matching radiation treatment to a patient's own respiratory pattern.*** In it radiation beam is gated i.e. turned on only when the target is in correct location based either on external markers or internal markers.
- *When one breathes, the chest wall moves in and out, and any structures inside the chest and upper abdomen also move. Organ motion during the respiratory cycle is known to be a source of inaccuracy in treatment delivery because it leads to tumor displacement and sub optimal dose delivery.* ***Respiratory gating is one of the latest techniques in radiation therapy and involves matching radiation treatment to a patient's own respiratory pattern.*** *With respiratory gating, radiation treatment is timed to an individual's breathing pattern, targeting the tumor only when it is the best range. This approach decreases possible complications and side effects, while using higher doses and getting better outcomes.* Respiratory gating, involves tracking the patient's natural breathing cycle via computer and determining an algorithm to control radiation administration at the optimum moments – the ***"gate"*** – to deliver dose. The computer synchronizes the beam to switch on only when the target area is within the calculated parameters. The patient's respiration is continuously monitored and the beam switches off as the tumor moves out of the target range.

- Methods to handle motion & set up effects are – active breathing controls (ABC), **gating radiation beam**, real time tracking with radiographic & radio frequency transponders, creating internal target volume (i.e. defining volume extent at both ends of respiration cycle) and imaging with 4DCT, fast helical CT, fast MRI, 4D CBCT (respiratory correlated) using daily set up correction (IGRT).

105. C i.e. Thyroid *[Ref: Harrison's 15/e P-2590]*

- ***Papillary carcinoma thyroid may develop due to radiation exposure in infancy***Q.
- Papillary carcinoma is ***most common variety with best prognosis;***Q ***lymph node metastasis is most common in this variety.***Q
- ***Thyrogglassol cyst & Hashimoto ds***Q predispose to papillary C_A thyroid

Types of Exposure	Associated Cancers
Neck Radiation during infancyQ	*Thyroid (Papillary)* C_AQ
Brush licking by **radial** dial painters	*Bone Sarcomas*Q
Uranium	Lung C_A
Inutero Exposure	Leukemia
Asbestos (amphibole i.e. crocidolite, amosite, anthophyllite)Q	*Mesothalioma*Q, G.I. tract (Oropharynx, oesophagus, large bowel), *Lung* C_AQ, laryngeal C_A, Renal tract & peritoneal

106. C i.e. Lung C_A

- Carcinoma Cx screened by PAP smear
- Ca Breast by Mamography & xeroradiography
- Oral lesions are screened by direct visualization of leukoplakia & erythroplakia
- Lungs are deep structure and evidence suggestive of lung Ca in sputum are seen only in late stages.

CRANIOSPINAL IRRADIATION

107. A i.e. Medulloblastoma *[Ref: Gunderson 3/e p. 1482-84, 1411-12, 1419, 518-20; Harrison 18/e p. 3383-90]*
108. C i.e. Hodgkin's Lymphoma **109. A i.e. Small cell C_A of lung**
110. B i.e. ALL; C i.e. Small Cell Ca lung; D i.e. Glioblastoma multiforme; E i.e. NHL

Craniospinal irradiation is used in treatment of most ***embryonal tumors such as medullablastoma (infratentorial PNET) and pineoblastoma (supratentorial PNET)***Q; some (malignant) grem cell tumors (germinoma & nongerminoma), ependymoma and WHO grade III/IV gliomas (ie anaplastic astrocytoma &oligodendroglimo/glioblastoma multiforma), ***non Hodgkins lymphoma (NHL), ALL and small cell carcinoma of lung***Q.

STEREOTACTIC RADIOSURGERY

111. A i.e. Brain tumor
112. A i.e. Multiple Cerebral Metastasis; B i.e. AV mal formation; C i.e. Ca lung; D i.e. Primary CNS tumor
113. A i.e. Radiotherapy **114. B i.e. Used for cutting tumours in difficult location; C i.e. Cobalt is used**
115. A i.e. Inoperable lung tumor stage-1 *[Ref: Gunderson 3/e p. 138-40; 330-43; Schwartz 7/e p. 1627; CSDT (2003) 944]*

- **SRS** can be used in **vascular malformation** such as **AVM** & cavernous hemangiomas; **primary benign CNS tumors** such as meningioma, vestibular schwannomas, pituitary adenomas, craniopharyngeomas, chemodectomas; **primary malignant CNS tumors** like glioblastoma multiforme, low grade astrocytomas, recurrent gliomas, choroidal melanomas; **malignant CNS metastasis,** and **functional disorders** like trigeminal neuralgia, cluster headache, OCD, Parkinson's disease and epilepsy.
- **SBRT** is used in **Ca lung**, lung metastasis, prostate cancer, hepatocellular Ca, pancreatic cancer, renal cell ca other abdominal tumors, and bone, spinal, lung & liver metastases.
- **Sterotactic Radio surgery (SRS) and Stercotactic Radio Therapy (SRT) are used for treatment of intracranial brain tumors**Q**, by focusing single or multiple fractions (respectively) of high dose radiation (gamma knife).**
- **Steriotactic body radiosurgery** is image directed *precisely focused radiotherapy*Q, which uses **gamma knife** ***(or gamma rays from very large number of*** ^{60}***Co source)***Q to treat ***relatively small (<3 cm), clinically localized, in operable early stage malignant tumors eg. early stage non small cell lung cancers***Q.
- SRS is ***image directed focal radiotherapy***Q, used for relatively *small tumors* (<3 *cm* diameter) and achieve tumor ablation *without surgery* by administration of focused ***high dose of radiation (usually gamma knife)***Q to a precisely *defined volume of tissue in single treatment.*

116. D i.e. Malignant transformation *[Ref: Cancer Principles & Practise of Onchology by Devitta 6/e P-894-3]*

- ***Radiotherapy may lead to malignant transformation & RT is not indicated in treatment of it.*** Q
- The management of pleomorphic adenoma that recur despite surgical removal, includes **radiotherapy after appropriate surgical excision,** in ***high risk conditions (for both benign and malignant histological types)*** Q
  - Multifocality
  - ***Positive surgical margins*** Q
  - ***Deep lobe tumors*** Q

Indications of postoperative radiotherapy for salivary gland tumors are:

Advanced primary tumor stage	Inappropriate surgery indicated by	**Recurrence (benign or malignant) despite surgical removal** with high risk condition
- Unresectable / inoperable / gross residual tumor - Regional metastasis i.e. involvement of skin, bone nerve, extra glandular extension & periglandular soft tissue invasion - ***Facial nerve involvement*** Q - Lymph node metastases (i.e. positive neck nodes) - ***High grade histology*** Q - ***Deep lobe involvement*** Q	- Tumor spillage during operation - Positive surgical margins	- Multifocality - ***Positive surgical margins*** Q - ***Deep lobe tumors*** Q

117. C i.e. Radiotherapy *[Ref: Schwartz 7/e P-651]*

- In Ca larynx (vocal cord), there are 2 modes of treatment - surgery and radiotherapy.
- Vocal cord tumor is mobile i.e. tumor is localized.
- In this case surgery will lead to cure but voice will be affected (patient left with no voice)
- And after RT there is 90% cure rate with advantage of preservation of voice.
- **RT is TOC for** - Mobile cord lesions
  - No invasion of cartilage
  - No cervical lymph node involvement

118. A i.e. 8 Gy in one fraction *[Ref: Cancer Pain by Arnold – 284]*

- Radiation therapy is an important means of treating malignant bone pains; which can be used in 3 ways:
  30 Gy in 10 fraction
  20 Gy in 5 fraction
  *8 Gy in one fraction*Q ***(most preferred*** according to latest trial by UK collaborative group)
- All trials have demonstrated that low dose radiation with single dose or at most two doses (i.e. 8 Gy in one fraction) of treatment, are as effective as more prolonged treatments (30 Gy x 10, 20 Gy x 5) in all parameters of pain relief including rate of onset & over all incidence of pain relief.

119. C i.e. Iridium –192 **120. A i.e. Strontium-89; D i.e. P-32; E i.e. Rhenium-186**
[Ref. Walter-Miller 6/e, p 245-47, www. buzzle.com; Harrison 18/e, p 72-73, Wolfgang 7/3, p 1112]

- **Strontium (Sr)- 89, phosphorus (P)-32, samarium (Sm) 153, tin (Sn)-117, and rhenium (Re) – 186** are used for pain relief in metastatic bone disease. **I**^{131} is used for thyroid uptake study, thyroid imaging, treatment of hyperthyroidism, treatment of functioning thyroid cancer, imaging and treatment of functioning metastases (and pain)
- Ir -192 is not used as systemic radionuclide
- **Radiation therapy** can treat bone pain from single metastatic lesion. Bone pain from multiple metastasis is amenable to **Sr 89** and **Sm 153. Biphosphonate** (eg pamidronate) and **calcitonin** also provide relief from bone pain but have onset of action of days

121. B i.e. Larynx; C i.e. Ant 2/3 of tongue *[Ref: B&L 24/e P-712]*

- **Radiotherapy** is reserved for ***early larynx C_A which has not involved cartilage or cervical lymphnodes & don't impair cord mobility***Q.

RADIOTHERAPY 3

- Surgery is the treatment of choice for early lesions suitable for simple intra oral excision, for tumors on the tip of tongue but brachy therapy with iridium wires has the advantage of preserving the tongue.
- Stomach, colon, lung C_A in early stage are treated by surgery.

122. **A i.e. Nasopharyngeal Carcinoma T3N1** *[Ref: Diagnostic Radiology; Neuroradiology 3rd/ed pg-454, pg-461]*

Radiotherapy is the ***standard treatment of nasopharyngeal carcinoma***Q***, as surgery is not fesible***Q. Patient with advanced disease also receive concurrent chemotherapy.

Radical Radiotherapy is preferred treatment for *early supraglottic carcinomas* (i.e. small (< 6ml) tumor mass and absence of cartilage invasion). In unfavourable conditions *voice preserving supraglottic laryngectomy* (surgery) is preferred. Tumors involving the true vocal cords or cartilage are treated with supracricoid laryngectomy & for advanced tumors total laryngectomy is required. *Cord fixation is an indirect evidence of cricoarytenoid joint involvement. It upstages the tumor to T3 and precludes voice preserving surgery in all laryngeal cancers.*

Radiotherapy is *preferred modality for definitive treatment of early glottic carcinoma (T2 NO)* as it allows voice preservation. Hemilaryngectomy is the usual surgical procedure in early glottic cancers and supracricoid laryngectomy is performed if there is imaging evidence of invasion of anterior or posterior commissure, contra lateral true vocal cord, false vocal cord or parglottic fat invasion.

123. **A i.e. ^{131}I** *[Ref: Textbook of radiation oncology: principles and practice: Rath & Mohanti p. 5936; KDT 5/e p. 234; Harrison 16/e p 2125]*

The differentiated thyroid cancer and even the metastatic burden can be effectively controlled by I^{131} therapy.Q

Radio Iodine Treatment in Thyroid Cancer

- Well-differentiated thyroid cancer still incorporates radio iodine, but less efficiently than normal tissue. The retention time for Radioactivity is influenced by the extent to which the tumour retains **differentiated functions** such as *Iodine trapping and organification.* It is indicated for tumours that take up iodine, ^{131}I treatment can reduce or eliminate residual **disease.**
- **Thyroid ablation + ^{131}*I treatment in:***
  - *Large papillary* tumour
  - Lymph node involvement
  - FTC
  - Evidence of metastasis

124. **C i.e. X Ray** *[Ref:Oxford Onchology 2/eP-408; Gunderson 3/e p. 315-28; Clifford 2/e P-35]*

Intraoperative – Radiotherapy

- It is a specialized radiation technique for treating deeply situated cancer with large single dose, while avoiding irradiation of norml tissue. It has been, and still is, applied ***with orthovoltage X Ray***Q (external beam RT) > intraoperative electron radiation therapy (IOERT).
- Intraoperative **electron *beam used as a boost* followed by photon beam (X Rays & γ rays)** treatment is an innervative regimen for ***pancreatic***Q**, gastric & rectal cancers; retroperitoneal sarcomas; head & neck cancers; and genitourinary and some gynecological cancer.**

125. **C i.e. Carcinoma Pancreas**

Intraoperative radiotherapy is used in carcinoma pancreasQ. Because of poor local control achieved with postoperative EBRT & chemotherapy, the use of *intraoperative RT in pancreatic cancers in rational.* The cpmbination of *EBRT plus IOERT* in locally advanced/ unresectable *pancreatic adenocarcinoma* result in improvement in local control and survival.

126. **B i.e. Proton beam therapy > A i.e. X Rays & Gamma rays**

- **Penetrating Power**
  Gamma raysQ ***(high energy photons***Q***)*** > *X-Rays* (low energy photons) > *β-particles* (electron) > *α-rays* (helium nucleus)
- **For deep seated tumors,** *X Rays & gamma rays*Q are used, since high energy penetrating beam deliver a less intense superficial dose & *spares the skin* (least damage to skin).
- ***Electron beams***Q have very low penetrance and are used to treat **skin conditions like mycosis fungoides.**
- X-Rays are generated by ***linear accelerator***Q, when ***electron beam strikes the anode***Q.
- Gamma rays are produced by decay of atomic nuclei in radioisotopes as Cobalt & radium.

127. **B i.e. Stomach** *[Ref: Schwartz 7/e P-336; Gunderson & Tepper radiation onchology]*

- There is no role of radiotherapy in carcinoma stomach except for palliation of pain.
- In Head & neck, colon & soft tissue sarcomas, RT is given as adjuvant therapy to surgery.

128. **A i.e. With in 10 days** *[Ref. Rath & Mohanti p. 679*

The **postoperative radiotherapy in** Willm's tumor is started ***within 10 days of surgery***. Delay in starting RT beyond 10 days leads to tumor cell repopulation and increase in relapse rate.

Indication of RT in Willim's tumor are:

1. Stage II, III, IV with unfavourable histology (UH)
2. Stage III & IV with favourable histology (FH)
3. Metastatic disease
4. Clear cell sarcoma of kidney in all stages.

129. **A i.e. Ca Cervix** *[Ref: Shaws 12/e P-337]*

Intracavitatory RT is most commonly used in Ca cervix in form of Cs-137 rods[Q]

130. **B i.e. Obturator Lymph node** *[Ref: Shaws 13/e P-410]*

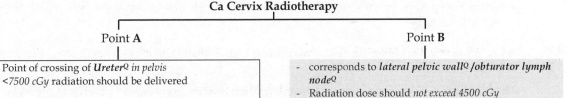

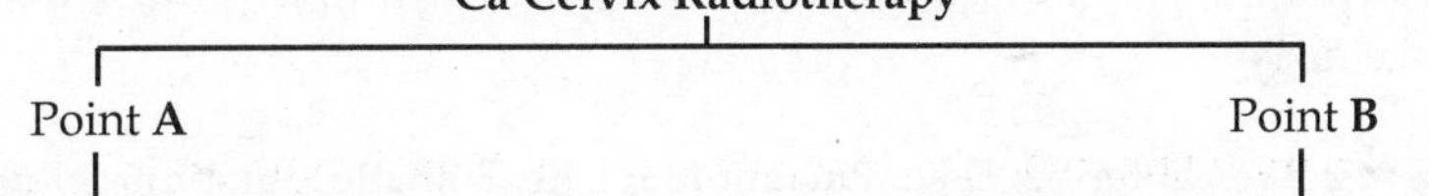

Point A
- Point of crossing of ***Ureter***[Q] *in pelvis*
- *<7500 cGy* radiation should be delivered

Point B
- corresponds to ***lateral pelvic wall***[Q] ***/obturator lymph node***[Q]
- Radiation dose should *not exceed 4500 cGy*

131. **All**

Emergency radiotherapy is given in following conditions-

1. Neoplastic ***cardiac temponade***[Q]
2. Acute epidural ***spinal cord compression***[Q]
3. Severe hypercalcemia
4. ***Superior vena cava syndrome***[Q]
5. ***Tumor lysis syndrome***[Q]

SIDE EFFECTS

132. **D i.e. Neuropsychological effects are independent of radiation dose**

133. **B i.e. Behaviour changes are common** *[Ref: Gunderson 3/e p 1420-22, 1412-11 Harriso 18/e p-3393]*

- **Effect of RT on cognitive functions (i.e. global intelligence, IQ, learning, memory, attention and behavior)** depends on *age (< 3-5 years) of patient, volume of irradiation (CSI) > and dose (36>24>18)*[Q].
- **Endocrinal deficiencies (GH>> ACTH and gonadotropin > TSH l/t hypothyroidism)** can occur d/t irradiation of hypothalamic – pituitary axis. Total dose and differential sensitivity of hypothalamic nuclei are important determinant. *Hypothalmic obesity, diabetes insipidus and hyperprolactinemia* are more often d/t local tumor effects and surgery. *Thyroid and ovarian failure* often occurs d/t CSI d/t incidental irradiation of these organs.
- Other long term **somatic complications** include permanent hair loss, wound healing problems, ***softening of bone and ligaments of spine and spinal growth impairment and small head size (musculo-skeletal problems)***[Q].

134. **D i.e. Growth hormone** *[Ref: Harrison 17/e p. 2610]*

Growth hormone deficiency is most common endocrinal complication of intracranial radiotherapy[Q].

<u>Endocranial dysfunction in intracranial radiotherapy</u>

Hypopituitarism frequently occurs after exposure of *hyothalmus or pituitary gland* to therapeutic radiation; especially in *children & adolescent*. It develops usually after *5- 15 years* and reflects *hypothalmic damage rather* than absolute destruction of pituitary cells. *Irradiation dose & time interval* after completion of radiotherapy strongly correlates with the development of hormonal abnormalities.

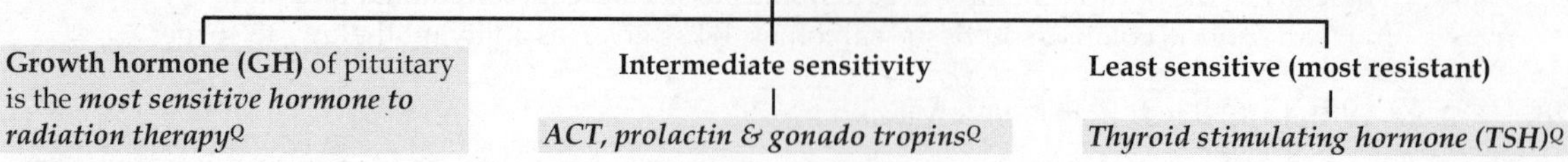

135. **A i.e., Leukemia** *[Ref: Harrison 17/e p. 517, 2610]*

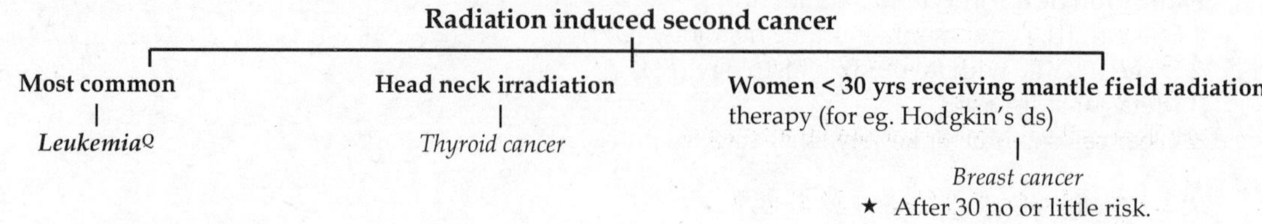

136. **B i.e. Pericardial Effusion** *[Ref: Harrison 15/e P-2588-9]*

- ***Asymptomatic Pericardial effusion***[Q] is the most common presentation of radiation carditis which is *best diagnosed by **Echocardiography***[Q]
- Radiation exposure may also cause *acute pericarditis* which presents as chest pain, fever, with or without pericardial effusion.

137. **A i.e. Mucositis; B i.e. Enteritis; D i.e. Pneumonia; E i.e. Somatic mutation** *[Ref: Harrison 18/e p. 3393, 691]*

138. **A i.e. Erythema**

Most common early (acute) manifestation of local skin reaction is erythema[Q] which is followed by desquamation.

139. **B i.e. Probability of effect is a function of dose** *[Ref: Christian 3/e p-181; Farr's 2/e p-25-26; Thayalan 1/e p-207-8]*

The ***probability of occurrence of late stochastic effects (like cancer & hereditary genetic defects) increases with increasing absorbed cumulative dose***[Q]. However there is **no threshold dose** below which it is certain that the stochastic effect can not occur.

Effects of Radiation

Feature	Acute (non stochastic) deterministic Effects	Late Stochastic Effect
Threshold dose below which it does not occur	Present	***Absent/No***[Q]
Dose (exposure) & effect relationship	*Clear* *The severity (magnitude) of effect is directly proportional to the size of dose*	Not clear, occur by chance. The ***probability that effect will occur increases with dose***[Q]. However, at no time even with higher doses it is certain that the effect with occur
Associate with	Definitely a/w *radiation exposure*	*Not definitely a/w radiation exposure* and can also occur in individuals that have not exposed to radiation above background levels.
Occur in	*Irradiated people*	*Irradiated & normal population both*
Examples	***Erythema, cataract***[Q], Alopecia, impaired fertility, Myelosuppression etc.	Cancers Hereditary genetic diseases/effects

140. **B i.e. Prostate**

141. **A i.e. Lung cancer; B i.e. AML; C i.e. Cervical cancer; D i.e. Glioma; E i.e. Meningioma**
[Ref: Wolfgang 7/e p. 154, 313, 408, 574; Gundersun 3/e, p 35-36, 353, 373, 417, 1485, Hollenfrei 6/e, 98 P. 98, Harrison 18/e p. 839-42, 934-35, 3383]

- **Intensity modulated RT(IMRT)** ***is most suitable for prostate cancers***[Q] **(b/o reduced rectal toxicity) ≥ gynaecological cancer eg endometrial cancer (d/t reduced gastrointestinal > genitourinary and bone marrow toxicity) ≥ *large lung tumors close to esophagus* (but issues regarding lung motion, dose calculation accuracy need to be addressed and clinical data is sparse).**
- Reducing rectal toxicity is major dose limiting factor in therapy of prostate cancer, may allow dose escalation and a potential for improved cure rates. Partial sparing of rectal wall seems to be a the major

advantage of IMRT, which allow higher than standard doses to be delivered to the prostate. So **IMRT with daily image guidance** has **become routine to treat definitive prostate cancer**.

- Radiation induced cancers include ***thyroid carcinoma, breast carcinoma and sarcomas***Q (osteogenic sarcoma> fibrosarcoma> chondrosarcoma> malignant fibrous histiocytoma)- *Wolfgang*
- Secondary malignant tumors after total body irradiation (TBI) include ***acute myelogenous leukemia (AML)***Q, *myelodysplastic disease (MDS), post* hematopoietic stem cell *transplant lymphoproliferative disorder (PTLD),* and solid tumors such as oral cavity, pharyngeal, liver, central nervous system, thyroid, bone and soft tissue cancers and melanomas.
- Risk of radiation induced second malignancy is higher in certain patients including *children and young adults,* those *with known genetic predisposition to cancer* (eg Li-Fraumeni, Lynch, Cowden and Gardner's syndrome), immuno compromized individuals and those with known exposure to other carcinogen (eg chemotherapy tobacco, alcohol etc). Use of **highly conformal, intensity modulated radiation therapy** designed specifically to deliver lower doses to normal tissues immediately surrounding the tumor, but at the expense of direct, leaked or scattered dose to larger volumes of body (ie **large volumes and low doses**) tend to be those most associated with radiation carcinogenesis.
- Hodgkin's lymphoma surviors have risk of ***breast and lung cancer***Q, cervical carcinoma surviors have risk of ***leukemia and sarcoma***Q, and long term surviors of childhood retinoblastoma have risk of *sarcomas* as second malignancy.
- Exposure to ionizing radiation (RT) may cause ***meningiomas, gliomas***Qand ***schwannomas***Q and immunosuppression is a risk factor for primary CNS lymphoma (*Harrison 3383*). There is ***increased risk of secondary neoplasia in any organ***Q (eg bone, soft tissues, brain **thyroid**, salivary glands, eyes, heart, **lung,** kidney, liver, intestine, **gonads** etc), depending on the irradiation field after radiation therapy (*Harrison 839 table*).

142. **A i.e. 2 Gy** *[Ref. Gunderson 3/e, p 32, 349, 355-59; Walter-Miller 6/e, p 304; Emergency medicine (ACEP) 6/e, p 53-55]*

Total (whole) body irradiation dose ≥ 1 to 2.5 Gy predominatly leads to *hematopoietic syndrome*Q; dose ≥ 5 to 8 Gy predominantly leads to *gastrointestinal syndrome*Q and doses ≥ 20 to 50Gy predominantly leads *to cardiovascular syndrome*Q.

143. **A i.e. TLD badge; E i.e. Film badge**
[Ref: Tepper 3/e p. 113-16; Christensen's 4/e p 298-300]

- **Thermo luminescent dosimeters (TLD) badge, film badge, pocket chamber (pencil) dosimeterQ can measure accumulated radiation exposure to gamma radiations. Geiger counter can detect gamma and beta radiation.** Alpha radiation is harder to detect because of its poor penetration.
- **Linear accelerator, (Linac),** ***a subatomic charged particle accelerator is used to generate X rays and high energy electrons for radiotherapy***Q.
- **Gamma camera,** imaging the radiation emitted from radioisotope traces introduced in patient's body, is used *for functional nuclear scans of brain, thyroid, lung, liver, gall bladder, kidney & bones.*
- **Auger electron emission** is photoelectric effect of photon interaction. **Auger emission spectroscopy (AES) or Auger failure analysis** is used for identification of elements present on surface of sample.

NOTES

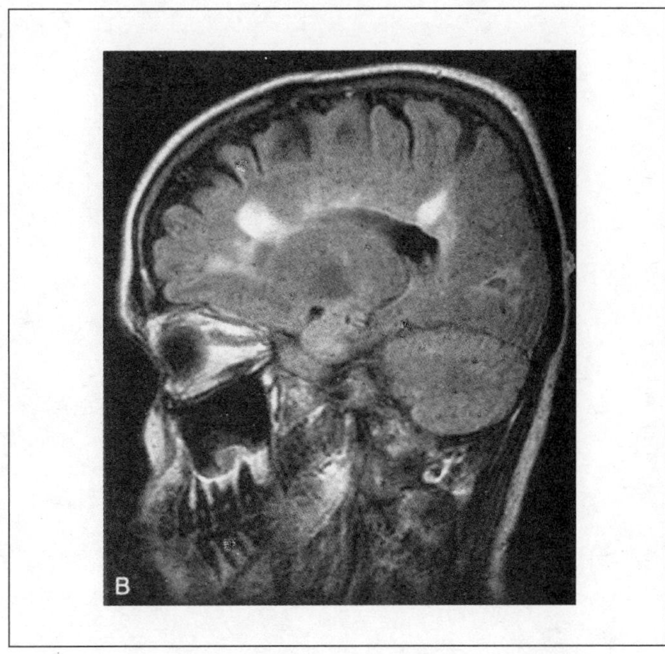

Nuclear Medicine

BONE SCAN (Scintigraphy)

- **Technetium – 99m (99m Tc)** is most commonly used radioisotope for bone scanning and it has replaced long half life and high energy gamma photon isotopes such as *Strontium 85 (^{85}Sr), Fluorine-18 (^{18}F), and Calcium-47 (^{47}Ca)* etc. Ethylenehydroxy diphosphonate (EHDP), Mehylene diphosphaonate (MDP) and hydroxymthylene diphosphonate (HDP) radiopharmaceuticals can be labelled with Tc^{99m}. **99m Tc-MDP** is ***most commonly used radiopharmaceuitcal in bone scintigraphy***^Q^.
- Tc-labelled phosphate/phosphonate compounds are mainly ***taken up in mineral phase of skeleton at the site of reactive bone formation***^Q^**.** 3-4 hours after IV injection 25-30% of radiotracer is retained in normal bones and rest is excreted in urine via kidneys.
- It can be perfomed in 3 ways: 1) **Multiphase** (*flow phase* is multiple images upto 1-2 minutes after iv injection; *blood pool phase* = static image at 5min.; *delayed phase* = static image after 2-4hours) is procedure of choice for most lesions including osteomyelitis and primary bone tumor; 2) **Static image** for evaluation of presence of bone metastasis in patient with known maligency; 3) **SPECT bone imaging** gives 3D picture and is beneficial in patients with equivocal findings esp in thoracolumbar spine, skull and pelvis.
- **Normal bone scan** shows symmetrical uptake in all bones with minimal soft tissue activity. Enhanced (markedly increased) uptake is seen in growing regions (epiphyseal and apophyseal growth centers) and the axial joints as compared to surrounding bone. Mild activity in both kidneys and urinary bladder is almost always visualized.

Super Scan

- *In diffuse involvement of bone d/t metabolic disease* or widespread bone lesions. (e.g. metastases) bone scan shows *intense uptake of radiotracer through out skeleton with diminished renal activity and minimal or no background radiotracer activity*. It is k/a super scan.
- More common involvement of *calvarium and long bones* differentiate metabolic bone causes from metastasis. Causes of superscan include.

Metabolic bone Disease	Widespread bone lesions
- Renal osteodystrophy - ***Osteomalacia***^Q^ - Hyperparthyroidims - Hyperthyroidism - Widespread Paget's disease	- ***Diffuse skeletal metastases***^Q^ (mc from prostate, breast) - Myelofibrosis/myelosclerosis - Aplastic anemia, leukemia - Waldenstrom macroglobilinemia - Systemic mastocytosis

Long Segmental Diaphyseal Uptake (Seen in)

Bilateral Symmetric
- Hypertrophic pulmonary osteoarthropathy (HPOA)
- Mechanical enthesopathy (thigh/shin splints)
- Ribbing disease
- Engelmann disease. (progressive diaphyseal dysplasia)

Unilateral
- Vitamin A toxicity
- Melorheostosis
- Osteogenesis imperfect
- Osteomyelitis
- Pagets disease
- Fibrous dysplasia
- Chronic venous stasis
- Inadvertent arterial injection

Hot Bone Scan

All conditions with tendency of bone formation leads to hot bone scan (↑ tracer uptake) example – Mnemonic – "**NATI-MAN**" = **N**eoplasm (primary bone tumor), **A**rthropathy, **T**rauma, **I**nfection (osteomyelitis), **M**etastasis (sclerotic), **A**vascular **N**ecrosis.

Photon Deficient Bone lesions

Indicate *decreased radio tracer uptake* by lesion (**=Cold spot**). It is seen in bone lesions d/t (Mn **"His New TRAMS"**)

- **His**tiocytosis X
- **Neu**roblastoma
- **T**hyroid carcinoma
- **R**enal cell carcinoma
- **R**adiation therapy
- **R**eticulum cell sarcoma/**A**naplastic tumor
- ***Multiple myeloma***^Q^
- Sickle cell crisis

Benign lesions can be differianted on the basis of osteoblastic activity (tracer uptake)

NO Tracer uptake	**Increased** tracer uptake (osteoblastic activity)
1. ***Fibrous cortical defect***^Q^ 2. ***Non ossifying fibroma*** 3. Osteopoikilosis 4. Osteopathia straita 5. Bone island	1. ***Fibrous dysplasia***^Q^ 2. ***Paget's disease***^Q^ 3. Eosinophillic granuloma 4. Melorheostosis 5. Exostosis 6. Enchondroma 7. ***Osteoid osteoma***^Q^

★ In osteomyelitis and painful prosthesis bone scan is combined with white cell or **gallium scintigraphy** (^{67}Ga citrate/^{99m}Tc or ^{111}In-leucocytes).

RENAL SCAN / Renal Scintigrapy

Morphological/Anatomical Scanning

99m Tc DMSA (Dimercaptosuccinic acid) is **agent of choice** for imaging
- ***Renal anatomy, functional renal parenchymal (cortical) mass and scarring (non-functional tissue)***Q.
- Indentifying renal ectopic & anomalies.
- Differentiating renal masses from pseudomasses (abscess, cyst, tumor).

GFR Measurement and Assessment	**Inulin** (Most accurate but costly) **Creatinine clearance** (Used most widely clinically) **Urea clearance**
	^{99}Tc MAG3 (Preferred) ^{99}Tc DTPA (Cost effective and accurate) ^{123}I-OIH ***EDTA labelled with chromium 51***Q

Functional/Dynamic Scanning

- ^{99m}Tc DTPA (100% glomerular filtration) and ^{123}I-hippuran (80% tubular secretion and 20% GF) have been superseded by **^{99m}Tc MAG3** (99% tubular secretion) to assess the ***function of nephron or renal excretory function. i.e. renal perfusion, renal plasma flow, glomerular filtration and tubular secretion***Q except in emergency situations (when **^{99m}Tc DTPA is preferred**).
- Functional scanning is done in:
  - Urinary tract obstruction (Obstructive uropathy)
  - Vesico-ureteral reflux
  - Renovascular hypertension
  - Acute renal failure (anuria/obliguria)
  - Renal transplant

Radionuclide Imaging of Kidney

Radioactive traces that are *retained* in kidney are used to *demonstrate renal anatomy*, while *tracer* that are *excreted* by kidney are used to access renal *excretory function & perfusion.*

Renal tracers

- **DMSA** (dimercaptosuccinic acid) ***labelled with Tc 99m is best for imaging renal anatomy and scarring***Q.
- ***Tc 99m – MAG3***Q (mercapto acetyl glycyl glycine) is ***best for investigating renal perfusion & excretion***Q. It is preferred to earlier tracer excreted solely by *glomerular filtration (eg* ***DTPA****)* or by *tubular secretion* **(orthoiodohippurate labeled with iodine – 131 or iodine – 123)**

Stressing agents
- *Diuretics* reveal minor obstructions by increasing urinary flow rates
- *ACE inhibitors* are used to magnify disturbances associated with renal arterial disease.

DMSA Scintigraphy

- Tc99m – DMSA is excreted by & bound in the *parenchymal cells of PCT*.
- Patient's level of hydration has little influence, so *no patient preparation is needed.*
- **Optimum imaging time**, (with maximum kidney: back ground ratio) is 2 – *3 hour in children & 3- 4 hours* (after iv injection) *in adults.*
- *Posterior & posterior oblique (right & left)* views are obtained for normal anatomy, while *anterior view* is also obtained in patients with *marked renal asymmetry esp ectopic & transplanted kidney.*
- It is most accurate (noinvasive) method for ***estimating distribution of function b/w two kidneys***Q. For symmetrical kidneys only posterior view is used for estimation, whereas posterior & anterior both views are used for asymmetrical kidneys.
- It is used ***to locate functional renal tissue***Q, *differentiate renal cortex from soft tissue masses in or near kidney ,* ***to find scar, or non functioning areas of renal parenchyma and to estimate the functional contribution of each/ abnormal kidney***Q.
- It identifies renal ectopia & anomalies, & differentiate b/w renal mass & pseudomasses
- *Tumor, cysts or abscess show no uptake of DMSA (photon deficient areas). Infection* eg acute pyelonephritis *produces diminished function & segmental wedge* of renal cortex, whereas, *scarring produce total non functional (no uptake) area* seen as *discontinuity or indentation* in cortical image.
- It must be remembered that acute infection & permanent scarring can not be distinguished

Dynamic Renal Imaging (Study)

- Because nephron under most circumstances act as individual functional units, so that when any part of nephron is diseased, the function of whole nephron is affected. It is not necessary to investigate perfusion, filtration, reabsorption and transit functions independently. Whatever the primary site of pathology, whether at arterial, arteriolar, glomerular, tubular or ureteric levels, the functional deficit can be assessed by the same technique (except in acute tubular necrosis and some enzyme deficiencies when filtration and excretory functions may be dissociated). So in most circumstances, radiotracers which are handled differently by kidney will produce similar results in the estimation of renal uptake and clearance.
- **Tc99m MAG3** has superseded Tc99m DTPA (excreted almost entirely by GF) & I^{123} hippuran (excreted mostly by tubular secretion)
- ***MAG3 is better than DTPA***Q because the later has slower excretion, inferior count statistics (poor image) & higher amount of activity needs to be administered.
- With MAG 3, the images obtained during the first pass of the tracer illustrate *vascular anomalies in the abdomen* as well as *perfusion of kidneys*. Images obtained 3-5min after injection illustrates the *size, shape and location of kidneys*. Serial images obtained during the excretion phase give a visual impression of relative renal function, rate of transit of activity through the renal pelvis, drainage from the pelvis in the sitting position and the residual bladder volume after micturition. The distinction between *obstruction and the reservoir effect of an un-obstructed but dilated renal pelvis* can usually be made from the **response to dieresis.** With the normal (unobstructed) kidney, administration of furosemide 20min after MAG3 produces, a rapid increase in urine flow with decreased activity and count rate in baggy renal pelvis. If the *activity falls by >50%* within 20min of diuretic then *obstruction is very unlikely*. If the activity *remains constant or increases, then obstruction is extremely likely*. Activity falling <50% in 20 min

Measurement of GFR

- DPTA & EDTA are excreted almost entirely by glomerular filtration
- **GFR** is measured by either ***Tc99m – DTPA or Cr-51 EDTA***[Q]

by this method as both may produce total non function. DMSA imaging ***at the time of infection or shortly afterwards*** indicate the ***extent of infection.*** Whereas, if the aim of DMSA imaging is ***to detect and monitor renal scarring,*** it is important ***to delay the examination*** for long enough (at last 3 ***months & probably 6 months***) **after infection** to allow functional recovery to reach a maximum.

- Most true renal masses ae satisfactorily investigated by **anatomical imaging** but occasionaly esp in bilateral diseases **functional imaging with DMSA** is needed to *establish distribution of functional renal tissue.* It may tell which of the two kidneys with b/l tumor should be operated on first or whether the residual function of one side justifies a conservative surgical procedure eg. partial nephrectomy.

may suggest low grade *obstruction or a failing kidney unable to concentrate urine* and so unresponsive to diuretic. Low grade obstruction also shows an *incomplete fall off* in response to a diuretic stimulus, and then starts raising again – the **delyed double peak (Homsy) sign** on renogram.

- **99m Tc- DTPA** is less costly and also quicker and easier to prepare than ^{99m}Tc-MAG3, and so it ***may be used in emergent situations where a rapid result is needed, particulary in respect of perfusion, e.g. with acute oliguria in renal transplant recipient***[Q]. In comparison to MAG3, excretion is slower, count statistics are inferior and larger amount of activity needs to be administered.
- **Diphosphonate** (eg Tc99 medronate) can satisfactorily obtain renal study (in first 30 –40 min) & bone imaging (2- 3hr. later) in single visit.
- Dynamic (perfusion & excretion) studies are used in ***urinary tract obstruction, renal vascular hypertension, acute renal failure, renal transplantation & reflux disease***[Q].
- For **excretion studies** 100 MBq MAG 3 & 300 MBq DTPA and for **perfusion imaging** 200 MBq of MAG3 & 800 MBq of DTPA is requirement

Clinical problem	Imaging	Radionuclide	Behaviour
Renal scarring	Static renal scintigraphy	Tc99m- **DMSA**	Glomerular filtration & proximal tubular uptake
Renovascular hypertension	**Captopril Scintigraphy** (renography)	Tc99 m- **MAG3**	
Renal tract obstruction	**Diuresis renography**	Tc99m – **DTPA** Tc99m – **MAG3**	*GFR*[Q] Proximal tubular secretion
Vesicoureteric reflux	**Indirect micturating cystogram**	Tc99m – **MAG3**	Compartment localization
Adrenal medullary tumor Adrenal cortical tumor	Adrenal study	I_{123} – **MIBG** I_{123} – **Iodocholesterol**	NA transporter uptake Hormone metabolism incorporation

MAG3/DTPA (Renogram)	DMSA Isotope Scanning
- DTPA is freely filtered at glomerulus with no tubular reabsorption or excretion (i.e. GFR = Excretory function) and so used for dynamic scanning - The patient is given intravenous injection & a series of images of kidney are taken immediately thereafter with the help of a gamma camera which shows: 1) Angiographic phase 2) Parenchymal phase 3) Drainage phase - DTPA is useful for ***evaluating perfusion (blood flow to kidney) and function of each kidney*** *(for production of urine) and to find out if there* ***are any obstructions in urine output***[Q] - Indications: 1. Measurement of ***relative renal function***[Q] ***in each kidney.*** **2. *Urinary tract obstruction***[Q] 3. Diagnosis of ***Renovascular cause of hypertension***[Q] 4. Investigation of ***Renal transplant***[Q]	- Tc.99 DMSA is used for ***Renal morphological imaging***[Q] - This compound gets fixed in renal tubules & images may be obtained after 1-2 hours of injection – Lesions such as ***tumors & benign lesions as cysts show filling defect***[Q] - Used to assess ***cortical function of Kidney***[Q]

PARATHYROID SCAN

- The **most preferred radiopharmaceutical** for **parathyroid imaging** is **^{99m}Tc-methoxyisobutyl-isonitrile (MIBI)**, an agent which is specifically extracted by *myocardial tissue and parathyroid glands.* It is also taken up by *thyroid* but the tracer washes out of thyroid quickly and retained more avidly in parathyroid tissue/abnormal parathyroid (need for dual phase study at 10 min and 3 to 4 hours).
- **Thallium-201 (^{201}Tl)** as **thallous chloride** or **^{99m}Tc-thallium substraction imaging** is less preferred (than MIBI or ^{99m}Tc sestamibi scan) bacause of higher radiation dose.
- **^{99m}Tc-tetrafosmin** (cardiac agent) and ^{11}C-methionine PET/CT are other methods of parathyroid imaging and may be used in patients with negative conventional parathyroid scan.
- In **substraction technique** the image of thyroid gland as shown by previous ^{99m}Tc or ^{123}I is removed with the *after use of ^{99m}Tc-MIBI or ^{201}Tl scan.*
- Preferred agent for parathyroid scan is **MIBI (^{99m}Tc sestamibi) > ^{99m}Tc-thalium substraction imaging >** ^{99m}Tc tetra fosmin and ^{11}C-methionine PET/CT.

THYROID SCAN

- Thyroid imaging can be done by ^{99m}Tc **pertechnetate** and ^{123}I. Pertechnetate is *most widely used first line imaging agent* in the evaluation of thyroid because it is *readily available, inexpensive,* the radiation dose delivered is relatively low and the photon flux is greater (ie detectability of small thyroid lesions >8 mm is improved). However it has *less favourable high neck background* (target to background ratio) than with iodine. And unlike iodide it is *not incorporated into thyroglobulin.* It is *less suitable for assessment of thyroid function* than it is for imaging as uptake measurements *cannot reliably seperate normal from hypo functioning glands,* although hyper functioning can be recognized. Tc-pertechnetate is given IV and image taken after 20 min.

- **Radioisotopes of iodine** permit **studies of entire metabolic pathway** of iodine (ie trapping, organification, coupling, hormone storage and secretion) with in the thyroid. *Oral iodides, iodine containing drugs and radiographic contrast media compete* with these isotopes *and should be avoided* before studies with iodine radioisotopes. **^{123}I** is the ***agent of choice for thyroid imaging***[Q] whereas **^{131}I** is a preferred ***therapeutic agent for hyperthyroidism and functioning thyroid cancer***[Q]**.**

- ^{123}I is ***excellent radiotracer for functional evaluation of thyroid***[Q]. Imaging is performed 2-6 hrs and 18-24 hrs after IV administration, at which time the most of iodine within the thyroid is present as radio-iodo tyrosine residues on thyroglobulin, reflecting hormonogenesis. ^{123}I is ***prefered for imaging retrosternal or ectopic thyroid tissue***[Q], *in neonatal or childhood hypothyroidism, and in the follow up of patients who have had surgery for thyroid malignancy.* The disadvantages of ^{123}I are its *limited availability and high production cost,* as it requires a cyclotron.

- Both iodine and pertechnetate cross the placenta and they are both secreted in milk, so thyroid imaging is *relatively contraindicated in pregnancy and lactation.*

- Thyrotoxicosis d/t diffuse toxic goiter (Grave's disease), which accounts for 80% cases show *diffusely increased uptake of either $^{99}TcO_4$ (pertechnetate) or ^{123}I and pyramidal lobe* is more often apperent than in euthyroid patient. While *autonomous toxic nodule (Plummer's disease)* appears as *intensely active foci within a thyroid which is partly or totally suppressed.*

- Suppression of hot nodule following T_3/T_4 administration (**suppression scan**) is proof that autonomy of nodule does not exist. Administration of TSH (**stimulation scan**) demonstrate thyroid tissue suppressed by hyper functioning nodule.

- Demonstration of **a cold nodule within a toxic gland** is an indication of **ultrasound guided FNA biopsy** as such nodules have a higher incidence of malignancy than similar nodules in nontoxic glands. Malignancy is more likely in *males in <20 or >60 years, family h/o thyroid cancer, with previous irradiation of head and neek and in solitary nodule.* Other pointers to malignancy include hardness to palpation, rapid growth, laryngeal nerve involvement and lymph node enlargement of neck

- **Thyroid cancers** concentrate less iodine (only 1%) than normal thyroid tissue and hence appear **cold** in the presence of normal thyroid tissue. Rarely well differentiated thyroid cancers have preserved trapping function, but virtually no capacity for iodine organification, therefor giving the appearance of function on early imaging (trapping phase) but *becoming cold on delayed images. Most cold nodules are adenomas, colloid nodules, foci of thyroiditis, intrathyroid lymph nodes, lymphoma or metastasis.* **US guided FNAC** is most reliable non operative method for obtaiing definitive diagnosis.

- **Perchlorate washout (discharge) test**, detect disorders characterized by a failure to organify the trapped iodide (eg *Pendred's syndrome*). In this repeat measurement of radioiodine uptake(ie thyroid scan) following oral potassium perchlorate (which rapidly discharges unbound iodine from gland) shows lower values/thyroid activity if organification defect present.

- **[F-18]-2 fluoro-2-deoxy glucose ([F-18] FDG)** is transported into caner cell like glucose and has become *most commonly used radiopharmaceutical for clinical PET in thyroid cancer patients.* The main indication is in patient with *residual or recurrent thyroid cancer* with raised thyroglobulin and a negative radioiodine whole body survey (^{201}Tl scan has same indication). It may also be helpful in anaplastic and some medullary carcinoma thyroid.

- **^{201}Tl (preferred)**, **^{99m}Tc-MIBI** (better images but considerable hepatic and abdominal activity) an **^{99m}Tc-tetrofosmin** can also be used to detect residual thyroid tissue, and these donot require the withdrawl of thyroid suppressive treatment unlike radioiodine.

- In medullary thyroid cancer, ^{123}I –Metaiodobenzyl guanidine (**^{123}I-MIBG**), **pentavalent ^{99m}Tc DMSA** and Indium-111-diethylenetri aminepentaacetic acid-octreotide (**^{III} In-DTPA-octreotide**) or **[F-18] FDG-PET** (with rising calcitonin and other tests negative) may be used.

Brain Scan

Clinical Condition	Imaging technique	Radionuclide	Biological behaviour
Hydrocephalus CSF rihinorrhoea	CSF study	^{111} **In DTPA** (intrathecal)	*Marker of CSF flow*[Q]
Encephalitis	BBB study	^{99m}**Tc HMPAO**	*Passage across disrupted BBB*[Q]
Cerebrovascular accident (CVA)	**Cerebral perfusion SPECT**	^{99m}**Tc HMPAO**	*Uptake proportional to cerebral blood flow*[Q]
Dementia	Cerebral perfusion SPECT **Cerebral Metabolism PET**	^{99m}Tc HMPAO **18 F-fluorodeoxy glucose (FDG)**	*Uptake proportional to cerebral blood flow*[Q] *Marker of glucose metabolism*[Q]
Epilepsy (presurgical localization)	**Ictal SPECT** **Inter-ictal PET**	^{99m}Tc HMPAO **18F – FDG**	Uptake proportional to blood flow Marker of glucose metabolism

Endocrine Scan

Clinical Condition	Imaging technique	Radionuclide	Biological behaviour
Thyrotoxicosis, Thyroid nodule, Ectopic thyroid	**Thyroid Scan**	^{123}**I** (Sodium iodide) ^{99m}**Tc –pertechnetate**	Active uptake (^{123}I and ^{99m}Tc) f/b organification (of ^{123}I)
Hyper parathyroidism (presugical localization of parathyroid)	**Parathyroid Scan**	^{99m}**Tc MIBI**	Differential expression (of p-glycoprotein) b/w parathyroid adenoma and thyroid
Dry mouth (Connective tissue disease)	**Salivary gland study**	^{99m}**Tc pertechnetate**	Secretion in saliva

Heart Scan

Clinical Condition	Imaging technique	Radionuclide	Biological behaviour
Chest pain	**Mycardial perfusion scan**	^{201}**Tl** (thalous chloride) = **agent of choice**	K^{43} is not suitable; so K^+ analogue **indicating perfusion (ischemic heart disease)** is used (delayed uptake reflects *myocardial viability*)
		^{99m}**Tc isonitriles**	Cationic complexes *taken up by myocytes* in proportion to blood flow
		^{99m}**Tc teboroxime**	Lipophilic boronic acid oxine complex which accumulates by diffusion
		^{99m}**Tc phosphines e.g. tetrofosmin, furifosmin** (Q12), Q3	Uptake proportional to blood flow
Cardic Failure	**Mycordiac Viability Study**	^{18}**F-FDG**	Demonstrates shift from metabolism of fatty acids to glucose
	Cardiac ventriculography (gated study)	^{99m}**Tc RBCs**	Blood pool label
Congenital heart disease	**Quantitiative shunt study**	^{99m}Tc RBCs	Blood pool label

Lung Scan

Clinical Condition	Imaging technique	Radionuclide	Biological behaviour
Pulmonary embolism	**Ventilation perfusion (V/Q) Scan**	^{123}I fatty acids **Perfusion:** ^{99m}Tc albumin, Macroaggregates **Ventilation:** ^{99m}Tc aerosols, ^{133}**Xe gas;** ^{81m}Kr gas	- Pulmonary artery blockade - Distributes in lung in proportion to gas regional ventilation
Solitary pulmonary nodule	**Tumor imaging**	^{18}**F – FDG**	Marker of glucose metabolism
Occult lung disease (alveolitis)	Alveolar permeability study	^{99m}**Tc DPTA aerosol**	Passage accoss alveolar membrane into blood

4

NUCLEAR MEDICINE

GI Scan

Clinical Condition	Imaging technique	Radionuclide	Biological behaviour
Difficulty in swallowing	Oesophagal transit time and reflux	**^{99m}Tc Sulphur colloid**	Transit of labelled material
Vomiting (gastro-paresis); Dumping	Gastric emptying study	**^{99m}Tc sulphur colloid in egg** (solid phase) or **^{111}In DTPA in orange** juice (liquid)	Comparment localization of labblled material
GI bleed	GI bleed study	^{99m}Tc sulpur colloid ^{99m}Tc labelled red cells	Blood pool label extravasting into bowel
Ectopic gastric mucosa	**Meckel's diverticulum scan**	**^{99m}Tc pertechnetate**	Active uptake by ectopic gastric mucosa
Diarrhoea (IBD)	White cell scan	**^{99m}Tc leucocytes**	Leucocyte migaration

Liver Scan

Clinical Condition	Imaging technique	Radionuclide	Biological behaviour
Focal liver lesion (Heamangioma)	RBC Study	^{99}Tc labelled RBC	RBC pooling
Cholecystitis, biliary atresia/dyskinesia, Bile leak (Post-op)	**Hepato biliary** study	**^{99m}Tc iminodiacetic acid derivatives**	Uptake by hepatocytes and excretion into bile.

Spleen Scan

Clinical Condition	Imaging technique	Radionuclide	Biological behaviour
Sleenic tissue (ectopic)	**Spleen Scan**	***Heat damaged ^{99m}Tc labelled RBC***[Q]	Spleenic trapping of damaged cells
Abdominal sepsis; pyrexia of unknown origin	**White cell or gallium scan**	**^{99m}Tc/^{111}In leucocytes** **^{67}Gallium citrate**	Leucocyte migration Binds to transferrin and leaks into extravascular space

Cancer Scan

Clinical Condition	Imaging technique	Radionuclide	Biological behaviour
Tumor staging; Tumor recurrence; Tumor response assessment (of t/t)	**Tumor imaging**	*^{18}F- FDG*[Q]	***Tumor glucose metabolism***[Q]
Tumor Hypoxia	**Hypoxia imaging**	**^{18}F-fluromisonidazole**	Trapped in hypox cells
Space occupying lesion (SOL) in brain; and soft tissue mass (sarcoma)	**Tumor Imaging**	**^{201}Tl** (thalous chloride) **^{18}F – FDG**	K+ analogue indicating perfusion Marker of glucose metabolism
Insulinoma; Carcinoid tumor	**Somatostatin receptor study**	**^{111}In pentetreotide** (octreotide)	Binds to somatostatin receptor
Neuroblastoma	**MIBG Scan**	**^{123}I –MIBG**	Uptake by noradrenaline transporter
Thyroid Cancer	**Whole body iodine scan**	**^{131}I sodium iodide**	Uptake by Na/I transporter
Skeletal metastasis	Bone scan	^{99m}Tc Polyphosphate	Osteoblastic response
Sentinel node Detection	**Lymphoscintigraphy**	**^{99m}Tc nanocolloid**	Lymphatic uptake and trapping

Uses of ^{99m}Tc Radiopharmaceutical

^{99}Tc is the most commonly used radiopharmaceutical, for imaging in nuclear medicine, it is used with different ligands for imaging of different sites.

Radiopharmaceutical	Primary used for
^{99}Tc bound diphosphonate ligands eg ***Tc – 99m Medronate (MDP ie Methylene diphosphonate) is most common**, Tc - 99m Oxidronate (HMDP ie* Hydroxy methele diphosphonate) , *Tc – 99m HEDP* (ie Hydroxy ethylene dphosphonate)	**Bone (Skeletal) imaging**
Tc 99 – m Bicisate (ECD), Tc 99 – m Exametazine (HMPAO)	**Cerebral perfusion imaging**
Tc 99 – m Disofenin (DISIDA), Tc 99 – m Lidofenin (HIDA or IODIDA), Tc 99 – m Mibrofenin	**Hypato-biliary imaging**
Tc - 99 m Albumin colloid Tc - 99 m Sulfur colloid (SC)	RES (liver, spleen) imaging RES (liver, spleen) imaging, gastric emptying, GI bleed
Tc - 99 m Labelled Red Blood Cells (RBLs)	Imaging of GI bleed, ***spleenic disease***Q**, *cardiac*** *chambers*
Tc - 99 m - **Human Serum Albumin**	- Imaging of cardiac chambers - *Cardiac ventriculography (myocardiad function)* Q
Tc - 99 m **Pyrophosphate (PYP)**	***Avid infarct imaging ie in acute myocardial infarction hot spots are seen (hot spots in acute MI).***
Tc - 99 m Teboroxime, Tc - 99 m Tetrfosmin, ***Thallium scan***	**Myocardial perfusion imaging**
Tc - 99 m Sestamibi	Myocardial perfusion imaging Breast tumor imaging
Tc - 99 m Gluceptate Tc - 99 m Metriatide *Tc - 99 m Succimer (DMSA)*	**Renal imaging** ***DTPA is used for GFR (excretory function) & DMSA for cortical functions.***
Tc - 99 m Pentate (DTPA)	**Renal imaging & functional studies** Radioaerosol ventilation imaging
Tc - 99 m Macroaggregated Albumin (MAA) Tc - 99 m Depreotide Tc - 99 m Nofetumomab Merpentan (NR – LU – 10)	Pulmonary perfusion Somatostatin receptor – bearing pulmonary masses Monoclonal antibody Fab fragment for imaging Small cell cancer
Tc - 99 m Acritumomab	Monoclonal antibody for colorectal cancer
Tc - 99 m Apcitide	Peptide imaging for DVT (deep vein thrombosis)
Tc – Thallium substraction scan (MIBI Scan)	***Parathyroid gland***

Positron Emission Tomography (PET)

Concept & Instrument

- PET measures distribution of position emitting radionuclide labelled biocompound as a function of time, after injecting it into patient. PET permits **noninvasive invivo functional examination of glucose metabolism, blood flow (perfusion), electricl activity, neurochemistry & receptor density.**
- Each postiron gives rise to **two photons of 511 Kev (each) travelling in exactly opposite directions,** detected by coincidence circuitry through simultaneous arrival at detectors on apposite side of patients, allowing the position of source of radiation to be determined. PET detectors use crystals such as **bismuth germinate (BGO), lutetium orthosilicate (LSO) and**

PET Tracers & their Use

- **Positron emitters ^{11}C, ^{13}N and ^{15}O** isotopes of caron, nitrogen & oxygen are **short lived** so they can only be used near the cyclotron in which they are produced. They are only used for **physiological** (by labelling naturally occurring small organic molecules) and *pharmacological* research.
- Only PET tracer used for clinical purpose is **fluorine-18 of ^{18}FDG (18 fluoro deoxyglucose=glucose analogue tracer 2**Q **= [fluorine 18] fluoro 2 deoxy D glucose).**
  - **Malignant cells have increased rate of glucose metabolism** because of abnormally large numbers of **cell surface glucose transporters** together with **increased hexokinase mediated glycolysis** and a **reduced level of dephosphorylation by glucose 6 phosphate**. So FDG competes with serum glucose for entery, undergoes high rate of glycolysis in tumor cells but trapped intracellularly as FDG 6 phosphate because dephosphorylation of FDG-6-P is relatively slow. Fasting and blood glucose level < 200 mg/dl (in diabetics) are required as FDG tumor uptake is diminished by an elevated serum glucose.
  - Imaging is carried out after **45-60min**, when rate of dephosphorylation equals rate of uptake and FDG (intracellular) concentration reaches a platue.
  - **Liver (hepatocytes)** have low levels of hexokinase and higher concentration of

gadolinium orthosilicate (GSO) in electronic collimation through coincidence circuit. Due to electronic collimation not requiring collimators (as opposed to lead collimation of gamma camera in SPECT), *PET is 30-100 times more sensitive and has higher resolution than SPECT (single photon emission computed tomography).*

- *PET lacks anatomical landmarks*, particularly in thorax, abdomen and pelvis, so in oncology, PET images need to be interpreted in cojuction with CT or MRI, anatomy.
- Although using **gamma camera** (coincidence detector) for PET allows performance of SPECT & PET by same machine but the performance of this machine is inferior (esp for detection of small < 2 cm lesions).
- Because of difference in sizes, body composition & glucose metabolism, absolute measurement of glucose uptake into lesion or specific organ is difficult. Approximate quantitation is achieved by using the **standardized uptake value (SUV)** which is estimate of uptake of FDG into the lesion or organ of interest compared with mean uptake in rest of body.

glucose 6 phosphatase resulting in **faster (rapid) dephosphorylation (clearance or washout) of FDG.**

- **Kidney does not recognize FDG as glucose**, so it is largely excreted by glomerular filtration, although there is some reabsorption in proximal tubule. In normal person, 50% of injected activity excreted unmetabolized in urine in 2-2.5 h.
- **Brain and heart** contain little G-6 phosphatase resulting in high concentrations of FDG
- There is **intense accumulation of FDG** in brain, myocardium, intrarenal collecting system, ureter and bladder; **moderate accumulation** of FDG in liver, spleen, bone marrow, renal cortex, mediastinal blood pool. However, more specifically in brain areas of high metabolic activity ie cerebral > cerebellar cortex, basal ganglia, thalamus show intense uptake; cervical & upper thoracic spine show moderate uptake than areas of low metabolic activity such as white metter and CSF.

- **^{18}FDG-PET** can be used for **detecting occult primary tumors, staging, response** to **treatment** and **identification of recurrence after surgery or RT** and **detecting distant metastase** of many tumors especially **lung tumors (non small cell lung Ca** > small cell Ca), **malignant melanoma, colorectal cancer, lymphoma, head and neck cancers, breast cancer, eosophageal tumors.** It can also be used in **locating temporal lobe (brain) lesions** in patients with **refractory epilepsy**, where surgical excision is planned.

Radioisotope PET Tracer	Use
Fluorine (F)-18 in form glucose analogue ^{18}FDG	***Glucose uptake & metabolism***[Q] *eg in* ***tumor staging, recurrence & response to treatment***[Q]
Oxygen (O)-15	**Oxygen metabolism** using $^{15}O_2$, ; **perfusion (blood flow)** using $H_2{}^{15}O$
Nitrogen (N)-13	Perfusion of $^{13}NH_3$ (ammonia)
Carbon (C)-11	Carbon metabolism using ^{11}CO, $^{11}CO_2$
Rubidium (Rb)82	-

QUESTIONS

1. **True about FDG-PET scan:** *(PGI May 13)*
   A. FDG is anolouge of glucose ☐
   B. Malignant cells shows high uptake due to increased metabolism ☐
   C. It cannot be used to detect brain metastasis ☐
   D. Used to detect tumor recurrence in patients who have undergone surgery for brain tumors ☐
   E. Helpful in investigating lesion. ☐
2. **Gamma camera in Nuclear Medicine is used for:**
   A. Organ imaging. *(AI 05)* ☐
   B. Measuring the radioactivity. ☐
   C. Monitoring the surface contamination. ☐
   D. RIA. ☐

Bone Scan

3. **On 3 phase 99mTc-MDP bone scan, which of the following bone lesions will show least osteoblastic activity.** *(DNB 04; AIIMS 03)*
   A. Paget's disease ☐
   B. Osteoid Osteoma ☐
   C. Fibrous Dysplasia ☐
   D. Fibrous cortical defect ☐
4. **Bone scan in multiple myeloma shows-:**
   A. Hot spot *(AIIMS Nov 06)* ☐
   B. Cold spot ☐
   C. Diffusely increased uptake ☐
   D. Diffusely decreased uptake ☐
5. **Increased Radioisotope uptake is seen in A/E**
   A. Primary bone tumor *(AI 1993)* ☐
   B. Osteomylitis ☐
   C. Paget's disease ☐
   D. Pseudoarthrosis ☐
6. **In Radionuclide imaging the most useful radio pharamaceutical for skeletal imaging is:**
   (DNB 09, 08; AI 05, 95, 94; AIIMS 95; PGI 03, 02, 00)
   A. Gallium 67 (^{67}Ga). ☐
   B. Technetium-sulphur-colloid (^{99m}Tc-Sc) ☐
   C. Technetium-99m (^{99m}Tc). ☐
   D. Technetium-99m linked to Methylene disphosphonate (^{99m}Tc-MDP). ☐
7. **Best investigation for bone metastasia is:** *(AI 2011)*
   A. MRI ☐
   B. CT ☐
   C. Bone scan ☐
   D. X-ray ☐

Renal Scan

8. **Distribution of functional renal tissue is seen by**
   A. DMSA *(JIPMER 05, PGI 05, DNB 03)* ☐
   B. DTPA ☐
   C. MAG3 - Tc 99 ☐
   D. I123 iodocholesterol ☐
9. **The gold standard method for detection of renal scarring in patient with recurrent urinary tract infection is:** *(AI 2012)*
   A. 99 Tc- DMSA scan ☐
   B. 99 Tc-DTPA scan ☐
   C. 99Tc-MIBG Scan ☐
   D. 99Tc-MDP scan ☐
10. **Vesicoureteric reflux is demonstrated by using**
    A. DMSA *(DNB 09, JIPMER 06, TN 04)* ☐
    B. DTPA ☐
    C. MAG3 - Tc 99 ☐
    D. I^{123} iodocholesterol ☐
11. **Impared Renal Function is assessed by**
    A. MAG3 *(DNB 99, AI 99)* ☐
    B. IodoHippurate ☐
    C. DMSA Scan ☐
    D. DTPA ☐
12. **GFR is measured with which of the following?**
    A. Iodohippurate *(AI 08)* ☐
    B. Tc99m-DTPA ☐
    C. Tc99m-MAG3 ☐
    D. Tc99m-DMSA ☐
13. **Renal GFR is best measured by**
    A. Tc^{99} DMSA *(DNB 02, PGI 05)* ☐
    B. Tc^{99} Pyrophosphate scan ☐
    C. Tc^{99} DTPA ☐
    D. Creatinine clearance ☐
    E. Tc^{99} albumin scan ☐
14. **A patient presents with acute renal failure (ARF) and complete anuria. The USG is normal. Which of the following investigation will give best information regarding renal function.** *(AI 10, 99)*
    A. Intravenous Pyelogram ☐
    B. Retrograde Pyelography ☐
    C. Antegrade Pyelography ☐
    D. DTPA scan (Radiorenogram) ☐
15. **Renal GFR is estimated by** *(AI 1995)*
    A. TC^{99} DMCA ☐
    B. TC^{99} DMSA ☐
    C. Tc^{99} DTPA ☐
    D. Tc^{99} – Gallium ☐

Endocrine : Parathyroid Scan Scan

16. **Best imaging modality for neuroendocrinal tumors-**
    A. PET *(AIIMS 2001)* ☐
    B. CECT ☐
    C. Radio nucleotide Scan ☐
    D. MRI with gadolinium scan ☐
17. **Sestamibi Scan is used in** *(DNB 01, PGI 03)*
    A. Ectopic thyroid ☐
    B. Ectopic parathyroid ☐
    C. Parathyroid adenoma ☐
    D. Extra adrenal pheochromocytoma ☐
    E. Adrenal pheochromocytoma ☐
18. **Investigation of choice for locating Parathyroid gland:**
    A. Tc Thallium substraction scan *(AIIMS 91, DNB 95)* ☐
    B. CAT Scan ☐
    C. USG ☐
    D. Angiography ☐

Thyroid Scan Scan

19. **All isotopes are used for thyroid except:**
    A. I-131 *(PGI 2002)* ☐
    B. I-123 ☐
    C. I-122 ☐
    D. I-125 ☐
    E. I-129
20. **Isotope for thyroid scaning:** *(PGI 2K, DNB 01)*
    A. I^{129} ☐

B. I^{131} ☐
C. Technetium^{99} ☐
D. Selenium ☐

21. **Amount of I131 used for thyroid scan is**
A. 5 Microcuries *(AIIMS 94, DNB 96)* ☐
B. 50 Microcuries ☐
C. 50 Milicuries ☐
D. 500 Milicuries ☐

Heart Scan

22. **Hot spot in acute MI is seen in:** *(DNB 99, AI 98)*
A. Thallium ☐
B. Stroncium ☐
C. Tc99 Strontium Pyrophosphate ☐
D. Gallium citrate ☐

23. **Hot spot in MI is seen in** *(AIIMS 1996)*
A. Th-201 ☐
B. Gallium ☐
C. Pyrophosphate Tc99 ☐
D. Albumin ☐

24. **Which test is performed to detect reversible myocardial ischemia?** *(AIIMS 03)*
A. Coronary angiography. ☐
B. MUGA scan. ☐
C. Thallium scan. ☐
D. Resting echocardiography ☐

25. **Isotope used in ventriculography is**
A. Gallium *(AIIMS 1994)* ☐
B. Lipoidate ☐
C. Technetium (Tc) ☐
D. Diatrizoate ☐

GI Imaging

26. **Tc labelled RBC's are used for** *(AI 95, DNB 97)*
A. Biliary tree ☐
B. Renal disease ☐
C. Pulmonary embolism ☐
D. Spleenic disease ☐

27. **In Pancreatic scanning radio isotope used is**
A. Cr51 *(DNB 96, AIIMS 94)* ☐
B. Se 75 ☐
C. Tc 99 ☐
D. I 131 ☐

28. **All are used to diagnose protein losing enteropathy except:** *(AIIMS May 2011)*
A. Tc albumin ☐
B. Tc dentran ☐
C. In-transferrin ☐
D. Tc-seclosumab & Tc Fab ☐

Brain Scan

29. **Which of the following technique is the best for differentiating recurrence of brain tumour from radiation therapy induced necrosis?** *(AIIMSNov 09, 05)*
A. MRI ☐
B. Contrast enhanced MRI ☐
C. PET scan ☐
D. CT scan ☐

30. **A patient presented with a 4 cm tumour in the left pariental lobe for which he underwent surgery and radiotherapy. After 2 months, he presented with headache and vomiting. Which of the following would best characterize the lesion in this patient?:** *(AI 2012)*
A. Gd-enhanced MRI ☐
B. ^{99}T-HMPAO SPECT brain ☐
C. Digital subtraction angiography with dual source CT scan ☐
D. ^{18}FDG PET Scan ☐

31. **Which one of the following is the most preferred route to perform cerebral angiography?** *(AI 2005)*
A. Transfemoral route. ☐
B. Transaxillary route. ☐
C. Direct carotid puncture. ☐
D. Transbrachial route. ☐

Answers and Explanations:

1. **A i.e. FDG is anolouge of glucose; B i.e. Malignant cells shows high uptake due to increased metabolism; D i.e. Used to detect tumor recurrence in patients who have undergone surgery for brain tumors; E i.e. Helpful in investigating lesion** *[Ref: Wolfgang 7/e p 1096-98; Lange 3/e p 205; Sutton 7/e p 1829-31; Grainger 5/e p 137-38, 1255]*

^{18}FDG is analogue of glucose. So ^{18}FDG PET scan shows increased uptake & metabolism by malignant cellsQ. It can be used to **detect distant (eg brain) metastasis, tumor recurrence** (after surgery or RT), **treatment response & staging of various tumors** esp lung (non small cell) Ca, colorectal ca, lymphoma, head & neck ca, breast cancer, malignant melanoma, and oesophageal ca. It is also helpful in preoperative localization **of temporal lobe (brain) lesion in refractory epilepsy**Q.

2. **B i.e. Measuring the radioactivity** *[Ref: Oxford surgery 6/e p 6.7, 33.2; Sutton 7/e p-1504; Wolfgang 5/e p-1068–70]*

A gamma camera, ***measures radioactivity***Q of the substance that is taken up by specific organ or tissue of interest, *by detecting gamma rays*

Working of gamma camera

- Nuclear medicine studies require the *oral or intravenous* introduction of very low level radioactive material (called *radio pharmaceuticals, radionuclide or radiotracess*) into the body; which is *taken up by a particular organ* or tissue.
- The decay of radiotracer then leads to *emission of γ (gamma) rays,* which are measured by gamma camera with the help of its *crystal detector* (or *scintillation crystal*).

BONE SCAN

3. **D i.e. Fibrous cortical defect** 4. **B i.e. Cold spot**
5. **D i.e. Pseudoarthrosis** 6. **D i.e. Technetium–99m linked to Methylene diphosphonate (^{99}Tc– MDP)**

[Ref: Wofgang 7/e p. 1105-8; Harrison 18/e p. 3137, 803; Berry 2/e p. 38-48]

- **Increased ratiosotope uptake (i.e. hot spot)** is seen in ***primary bone tumors e.g. ostieoid osteoma, infection (osteomyelitis), fibrosis dysplasia and paget's disease (all a/w increased osteoblastic activity)***Q. Where as **multiple myeloma** and **fibrous cortical defects** present with *decreased/no tracer* uptake l/t **cold spot** (at the affected site not diffuse)
- **Technetium - 99m linked to Methylene di phosphonate (^{99}Tc-MDP)** has the highest affinity for osteogenic bone sites. So it is the *most widely used* diphosphonate bound *radiopharmaceutical for skeletal imaging*).

7. **C i.e. Bone Scan** *[Ref: Grainger 5/e p. 1035, 1801, 907, 927, 1070-73; Sutton 7/e p. 1251-55; Daldrup et al: Whole body MRI for detection of bone metastases in children and young adults: comparison with skeletal scintigraphy]*

- **Radio nucleotide bone scintigraphy (bone scan)** *is* ***highly sensitive, and most common investigation for evaluation of cancer patients for bone metastasis***Q. *It is preferred because it examines the entire skeleton* and is more sensitive than CT in detecting small and early metastatic lesions
- Areas corresponding to **sites of persistent hemotopoiesis** ie **spine, pelvis and ribs >> proximal humerus and femur** are most commonly involved in metastasis. The tumors most likely to metastasize to the bone include those of ***breast, prostate, lungs, thyroid, kidney and neuroblastoma***Q. Most common bone scan pattern of metastasis is **multiple (wide spread), diffuse, hot lesions** distributed randomly throughout the skeleton. A lytic lesion on x-ray d/t metastasis usually presents as **photopenic area** with increased activity at the edge of lesion. This is seen in patients of **multiple myeloma** and few patients of *renal cell carcinoma, thyroid carcinoma and anaplastic tumors (reticulum cell sarcoma)* where lesions show *poor metabolic activity.*
- Major role of ***MRI*** *is* ***in local staging***Q, particularly for high grade malignant tumors (such as osteosarcoma) where it identifies intraosseous extent, skip lesions, involvement of neurovascular bundle, adjacent joint and soft tissue with great accuracy - ie information vital for planning surgical management. **Dynamic contrast enhanced MRI** has been advocated for determining chemotherapeutic response. In presence of purely lytic lesions, MRI may help in lesion diagnosis and characterization. For example vascular nature of **renal metastasis** demonstrate **flow-void sign; aneurysmal bone cyst** show completely filled with fluid levels; *hemangioma and intraosseous lipoma* demonstrate *fatty matrix* on MRI; chronic haemorrhage seen with giant cell tumor demonstrate low signal intensity (SI) on T_2W MRI; and *osteoid osteoma, osteoblastoma, chondrablastoma, and Brodie's abscess* demonstrate reactive medullary and soft tissue edema.

- Bone scan has only very little role in the diagnostic workup of a suspected primary bone tumor, with the possible exception of **osteoid osteoma** or **osteoblastoma**, *particularly in the spine.* However, bone scintigraphy is still useful for identification of skeletal metastases, although its role has recently been challenged by **whole body MRI** (not MRI).

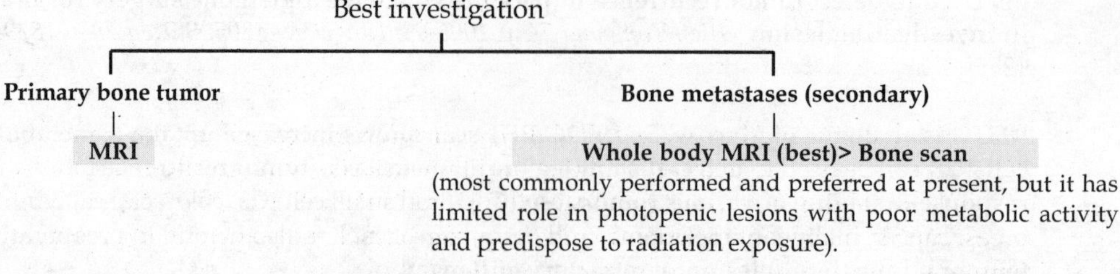

(most commonly performed and preferred at present, but it has limited role in photopenic lesions with poor metabolic activity and predispose to radiation exposure).

RENAL SCAN

8. **A. i.e. DMSA**
9. **A i.e. 99 Tc- DMSA scan**
10. **C i.e. MAG3 – Tc99**
11. **A i.e. MAG3**
12. **C i.e. Tc99m-MAG3 > B i.e., Tc 99m – DTPA**
13. **C i.e. Tc^{99} DTPA**

[Ref: Grainger 5/ep 141-46, 150,846,850,873-72 Sutton 7/e p: 912-21, AMP: Genitourinary series 3/e p 344-41; RRm 6/e P 1121; Wolfgang 7/e p 1138-42]

- **^{99m}Tc DMSA** (gold standard) and ^{99m}Tc- GHA are **morphologic agents. Dimercaptosuccinic acid (DMSA) labelled with technetium-99m** is most satisfactory tracer for ***imaging renal anatomy***[Q] (e.g. in renal ectopia and anomalies like horseshoe kidney), ***differentiating functional renal masses (with radiotracer uptake) from pseudomasses***[Q] (abscess, cysts or tumors which show no uptake of DMSA and appear photon deficient on renal images) and ***detecting infection and scarring***[Q].
- **^{99}Tc-DMSA scan** is **most accurate** (non invasive) method for estimating ***distribution of function between two kidneys***[Q]. It is used ***to locate functional renal tissue, to find out scar or non-functioning areas of renal parenchyma***[Q] (or to differentiate renal cortex form soft tissue masses in or near kidney) and to estimate the functional contribution of each abnormal kidney.
- **Dimercaptosuccinic acid (DMSA) labelled with technetium-99m** is most satisfactory tracer for ***imaging renal anatomy***[Q] (e.g. in renal ectopia and anomalies like horseshoe kidney), ***differentiating renal masses (with radiotracer uptake) from pseudomasses***[Q] abscess, cysts or tumors which show no uptake of DMSA and appear photon deficient on renal images) and ***detecting infection and scarring***[Q].
- **^{99m}Tc – MAG3 (preferred), ^{99m}Tc-DTPA (preferred in emergency)** and **^{131}I OIH**, (orthoiodohippurate) are **functional agents**. Functional agents are used for assessment of *renal perfusion, renal plasma flow, glomerular filtration and tubular secretion* and are applied in dynamic radionuclide studies of **urinary tract obstruction. (obstructive uropathy), vesico-ureteral reflux, renovascular hypertension, and acute renal failure. (anuria/oliguria).**
- **Radionucleide that are excreted almost entirely by glomerular filtration can be used to estimate GFR and these are** - ***Tc99 m- labelled DTPA (diethylenetriaminepenta acetic acid)***[Q] and ***Chromium 51- labelled – EDTA***[Q]

14. **D i.e. DTPA scan**

- **Antegrade pyelography (AP) & retrograde pyelography (RP)** are invasive techniques. Percutaneous AP done by puncturing the collecting system & injecting contrast is rarely performed for diagnostic imaging purpose as ultrasound or CT may be used to visualize the ureter even in presence of abnormal renal function. However the indications of AP may be percutaneous nephrostomy (Whitaker test), to obtain renal urine for cyto/bactero-logical examination, to pinpoint obstruction level in dialated urinary system not adequately opacified by IVU/or after failed RP.

  Retrograde ureteropyelography (RP) is valuable when (IVU/IVP) is suboptimal owing to poor renal function & in cases where IV contrast administration is contraindicated. **Intravenous urography/pyelography (IVU/IVP)** is intravenous administration of iodinated contrast and taking renal x-rays. It is initial technique in evaluation of possible urinary obstruction. For taking additional radiographs rule of 8 (i.e. if no contrast appears in collecting system by 15 min after injection, there is a little reason to obtain next film until 2 hours (=15x8) later) prevent multiple exposure. There has been a significant decline in use of IVU as dominant imaging technique in obstruction d/t fear of contrast induced nephrotoxicity and d/t growth of renal sonography & low dose CT. The main draw back of IVU is that it is time consuming.

- **Conventional gray scale sonography** is good screening method for detecting subacute and chronic obstruction as demonstrated by *pyelocaliectasis* however, in acute obstruction pyelocaliectasis is minimal or absent. Another drawback is its *inability to realibly distinguish mild hydronephrosis from normal or prominent extrarenal pelvis.* **Duplex & color Doppler ultrasound** have yielded advances in:
  - distinguishing mild pyelectasis from prominent central renal blood vessels.
  - detecting high grade acute ureteric obstruction through analysis of ureteral jets (normal *ureteral jets* i.e. ejection of urine from ureter into urinary bladder are bilaterally symmetrical).
  - estabilishing renal resistive index (RI) as an independent hemodynamic measure of urinary obstruction.
- **CT scan** has emerged as an effective imaging tool in evaluation of *acute renal obstruction* esp in screening patients with *acute flank pain / azotemia* who are strongly suspected as having obstruction and in establishing the etiology of ureteral obstruction when other investigations have failed. Non contrast low dose CT is very quick & useful in determining the presence or absence of obstruction and have higher sensitivity for detection of ureteric stones as compared to IVU.
  The radionale for **CT urography** is that *high risk patients or patients with hematuria* can be fully investigated by a single imaging technique with a high degree of sensitivity & specificity. The major disadvantage is the radiation dose of CTU which is upto 5 times higher than IVU.
- **Radionuclide renography** has limited role in evaluation of acute obstruction as it lacks precise anatomical delineation of obstruction as well as ability to define the cause of obstruction. Its major use is in differentiation of a dilated non obstructed system from a partially obstructed system. When IVU demonstrates a dilated collecting system and there is doubt about the presence or absence of obstruction **diuresis (frusemide) renography with Tc99 DTPA or MAG-3** will usually help to distinguish obstructive from non-obstructive dilatation & will localize the site of obstruction. The collecting system activity washes out with in 10minutes in non obstructive after diuresis challenge but no or partial response is seen in obstructive cases. ***Measurement of differential renal function can be made during diuresis renography or as a separate procedure using Tc99 DMSA examination***Q.
- **MR urography** is *an ideal technique in pregnancy, where there is contrast allergy, renal failure patients & if radiation dose is an issue.* The level of obstruction is always identified however ureteric abnormalities (if < 4mm) are poorly defined & that includes stones.

15. **C i.e. Tc^{99} DTPA**

- **DTPA** is *freely filtered at globerulus with no tubular reabsorption or excretion.* Thus its ***excretion rate measures GFR***Q. **DTPA Scan** is useful for evaluation of ***perfusion and function of each kidney***Q. It is also indicated in ***Urinary tract obstruction***Q, ***Renovascular cause of hypertension***Q ***and Renal transplant.***Q
- **DMSA scan** is used to assess ***cortical functions of kidney***Q and ***morphology***Q ***(Structure) Mn = "S".***

PARATHYROID SCAN

16. **C i.e. Radionucleotide Scan** *[Ref: Harrison 15/e P-602 to 594]*

Neuroendocrinal tumors (NET) are derived from diffuse neuroendocrine system of gastrointestinal (GI) tract, which is composed of amine & acid producing cells with different hormonal profiles, depending on the site of origin.

NET refers to two type of tumors

Name	Biologically active peptide secreted
I. Carcinoid Tumor	***Serotonin***Q, possibly tachykinin, motilin, Prostaglandin
II. Pancreatic Endocrinal Tumor (PET)	
- Zollinger-Ellison Syndrome	***Gastrin***Q
- Insulinoma	Insulin
- Glucagonoma	Glucagon
- Somatostatinoma	Somatostatin
- GRF-oma	***Growth Harmone Releasing Harmone***Q
- ACTH-oma	ACTH
- VIP oma (Verner Morrison Syndrome/WDHA, Pancreatic cholera)	Vasoactive intestinal peptide (VIP)
- PET causing Carcinoid syndrome	Serotonin, ? tachykinin
- PET causing hypercalcemia	PTHrP

- Because of its greater sensitivity than conventional imaging (CT, MRI, USG) and its ability to localize tumor throughout the body at one time. ***SRS (Somatostatin receptor Scintigraphy)*** is now ***the imaging modality of choice for localizing both primary and metastatic NET tumors***Q. ***(except for Insulinoma)***Q.
- ***Best modality of localizing Insulinoma is endoscopic U/S.***
- Somatostatin receptors are of 5 types, radiolabeled octreotide binds with highest affinity to *SS_2 receptor*.
- SRS is not a diagnostic investigation. Diagnosis is confirmed by detecting peptides or amines (or their metabolites) secreted by the tumors in urine or serum.

17. **C i.e. Parathyroid gland**

18. **A i.e. Tc-Thallium Substraction Scan**

[Ref: Sutton 7/e, p. 1507-10; Wolfgang 7/e p 1113-14; Bailey and Love 24/e, p 809; Grainger 5/e, p 142, 1717-18]

Investigation of choice for locating parathyroid gland (normal/abnormal):

1st. = *Fusion Scan (MIBI Scans & CT combined)*Q.
2st = *MIBI Scan & SPECT*Q
3rd = *Tc – Thalium substration scan* Q

- Preferred agent for parathyroid scan is **MIBI (^{99m}Tc sestamibi) > ^{99m}Tc-thalium substraction imaging >** ^{99m}Tc tetra fosmin and ^{11}C-methionine PET/CT.

THYROID SCAN

19. **C i.e. I-122; D i.e. I-125; E i.e. I-129**

20. **B i.e. I^{131}; C i.e. Technetium**

21. **B i.e. 50 Microcurie** *[Ref: Sutton 7/e P-1504; Wofgang 7/e p. 1112, 1091]*

Thyroid scanning can use radionuclides such as ***^{99m}Tc pertechnetate***Q **(most commonly used for imaging but not for function),** ***123 Iodine***Q ***(radiotracer of choice for functional evaluation)***Q**, 131 Iodine** ***(most favoured for therapeutic purpose like thyrotoxicosis and malignancy)***Q**, [F18] FDG-PET (for thyroid cancers), ^{201}Tl, ^{99m}Tc MIBI, ^{99m}Tc-tetrofosmin, ^{123}I-MIBG, pentavalent ^{99m}Tc DMSA and 111 In-DTPA-octreotide.**

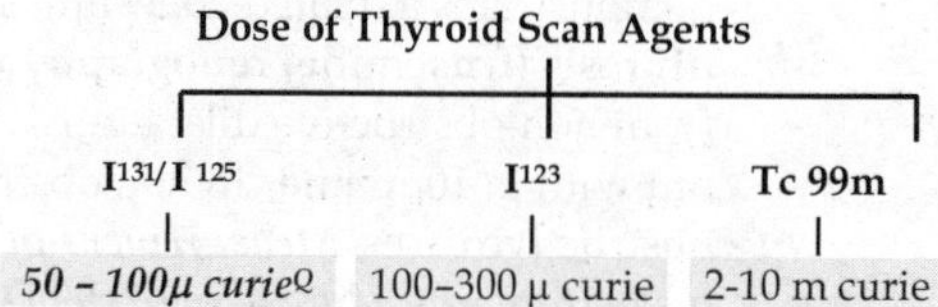

HEART SCAN

22. **C i.e. Tc^{99} – Strontium Pyrophosphate**

23. **C i.e. Pyrophosphate Tc^{99}**

24. **C i.e. Thallium scan** *[Ref: Sutton 7/e P-34. Grainger 5/e P-145; Braunwald heart disease 6/e p 279; Wofgang 7/e p. 1128-32]*

- **Infarct – Avid – Imaging /Hot spot Imaging** is done in ***myocardial infarction***Q. The ***standard agent is Tc-99-pyrophosphate***Q. It shows doughnut pattern i.e. central cold defect (d/t necrosis in large infarct).
- Only tumor producing hot nodules is ***wartheims tumor/adenolymphoma***Q.
- For **myocardial perfusion imaging** agent of choice is ***Thallium – 201 – chloride***Q.
- Interpretation of stress thalium image

Immediate Image	Delayed Image	Diagnosis
Normal	Normal	Normal
Defect	Fill-in	*Reversible/Exerctional Ischemia*Q
Defect	Defect persist	*Myocardial – scar*
Defect	Partial fill-in	*Scar + Persististent Ischemia*

Cardiac – Imaging for

- **Myocardial Perfusion**
  - ***Thallium Scan***Q
- **Myocardial Infarct**
  - **Cold – Spot/Nonavid infarct imaging**: *TI – 201 (< 12-48 hrs) post infarct*
  - **Hot Spot / Avid infarct imaging**: ***Tc – 99m Pyrophosphate***Q (> 10-12 hours post infarct)
- **Ventriculography (cardiac-function)**
  - ***Tc-99m albumin***Q (almost any Tc-99 m labelled compound as albumin, pyrophosphate, pertechnetate etc can be used except lung scanning particles.)

25. **C i.e. Technetium** *[Ref: Grainger 4/e P-722, 729]*

Radionuclide	Used In
Technetium (Tc) 99	*Ventriculography*Q, *Bone scan*Q, *Liver scan*Q, Kidney
Thallium - 201	**Myocardiol** *perfusion*Q
Tc **99-pyrophosphate**	**Myocardial Infarction** *(MI) = hot spot in acute MI*Q
Tc - albumin	*Myocardial function (ventriculography)*Q
Tc- Thallium – substraction scan MIBI –Scan (preferred)	**Parathyroid** *Gland*Q

T_C - labelled - RBC	**Splenic *disease*^Q**
MIBG Scan (using I^{123}/I^{131})	**Extra-adrenal /Ectopic /Metastatic / Locally recurrent *pheochromocytoma*^Q**
Selenium 75 methionine	***Pancreas*^Q**
I^{131} & I^{132}	**Placental *function*^Q**
I^{131} & Selenium	Thyroid
I^{131} orthohippurate	Kidney
Gallium scan	Abscess

GI Imaging

26. **D i.e. Splenic disease** *[Ref: Grainger 4/e P-145; Wofgang 5/e P-1088]*

Tc^{99} - labelled RBCs provides information about red cell pooling, so it is used in :

1. *Haemingioma* detection
2. ***Gastrointestinal bleeding*^Q**
3. ***Spleenic disease*^Q**
4. *Cardiac ventriculography*

27. **B i.e. Se 75** *[Ref: Grainger 4/e P-722 to 729]*

- ***Selenium^75 methionine*^Q** is used for pancreatic scanning
- In pancreatic carcinoma – **5 – *Fluro-uracil & intra-operative radiotherapy*^Q** is used.

28. **D i.e. Tc seclosumab & Tc Fab** *[Ref: GI Imaging (AMPIS) 3/e p 8-9; Wolfgang 7/e p 1101, 1132; Harrison 18/e p. 2474-76; Radionuclides by Francis 6/e p 218]*

- **^{99M}Tc antimyosin Fab fragments** are ***specific markers of myocyte damage*^Q** with a sensitivity of 95%. It is taken up only in acute infarct with decreasing intensity as the infarct heals.
- **Infarct avid imaging (hot spot imaging)** of *myocardial infarction*, uses radionuclide agents such as **^{99M}Tc-pyrophosphate (standard)**, *^{99M}Tc tetracycline, ^{99M}Tc –glucoheptonate*, ^{99M}Tc *antimyosin Fab fragment*, 203Hg-chlormerodrin, 18F- sodium fluoride, ^{111}Indium antimyosin (murine monoclonal antibodies to myosin).
- **^{201}Thallium chloride** used for **nonavid infarct imaging (cold spot imaging)** is the radionuclide *agent of choice to assess myocardial viability and to study myocardial perfusion* for acute MI. ^{201}Tl uptake depends on *quality of regional perfusion and viability of myocardial cells with cellular integrity of Na/K pump*. So it is used in coronary artery disease & acute MI. Cold defects at rest may represent transient ischemia in unstable angina. However, it cannot distinguish between recent & remote infarction.
- Protein losing enteropathy is a group of gastrointestinal & non gastrointestinal disorders with excessive protein loss into the gi tract resulting in hypoproteinemia & edema in absence of either proteinuria or defect in protein synthesis (eg liver cirrhosis). The protein loss into git may be due to-
  1- Exudation through ulcerative lesion eg UC, gi carcinoma & peptic ulcers;
  2- Altered permeabitily through nonulcerated mucosa eg menetrier's disease and ;
  3- Lymphatic dysfunction eg d/t enlarged lymph node or primary lymphatic disease. The diagnosis is suggested by *peripheral edema*, **low serum albumin & globulin leves (both)**, in absence of kidney & liver disease (selective loss almost excludes the diagnosis). *Relative lymphopenia (d/t loss of lymphocytes via lymphatics)* may also occur.
- **Protein loss in GIT is documented and established** by **administration of radionuclide labeled proteins** and its quantification in stools during a 24-or 48-hr period. Radionuclides that are tried include ^{111}Indium (In) chloride, **^{111}In –transferrin ^{99M}Tc-albumin** (HSA = human serum albumin), ^{99M}Tc *human immunoglobulin*, **^{99M}Tc dextran**, ^{131}I polyvinyl pyrrolidone, ^{125}I polyvinyl pyrrolidone, ^{125}I **albumin**, ^{51}Cr chromic chloride, ^{51}Cr-**albumin** and **α-1 antitrypsin clearance**. Broadly you can remember that ***albumin, dextran, transferrin and α_1- antitrypsin*** **(all proteins) lobelled with ^{99M}Tc / ^{111}In / ^{125}I / ^{131}I / ^{51}Cr** are used to detect protein losing enteropathy.

BRAIN SCAN

29. **C i.e., PET scan** *[Ref. Harrison 18/e pg 3393]*

MRI or CT scan are often unable to distinguish radiation necrosis from recurrent tumour
***PET or SPECT scans may demonstrate that glucose metabolism is increased in tumour tissue but decreased in radiation necrosis, used to distinguish recurrence from radiation necrosis*^Q.**

4

NUCLEAR MEDICINE

30. **D i.e. [18]FDG PET Scan** *[Ref: Grainger 5/e p. 144; Wolfgang 7/e p 1097, 1110]*

- **18 FDG-PET scan** detects cerebral metabolism and is used for *tumor grading, estimation of prognosis, localization of optimal biopsy site* (most malignant areas show maximum F18 fluoro-deoxy-glucose uptake), ***assessment of response to therapy and detection of recurrence (versus radionecrosis)***Q in brain tumor.
- **99mTc HMPAO-SPECT** Scan detects **uptake** / *distribution of lipophilic radio pharmaceutical (99mTc HMPAO) across functioning BBB proportional to cerebral blood flow (with no redistribution)*. It is indicated in *acute cerebral infarct imaging* before evidence of CT/MRI pathology (and gives positive finding with in 1 hr of event), *stroke* (shows *flip flop phenomenon* ie decreased arterial, equal capillary, and increased perfusion/activity in venous phase secondary to slow washout and late arrival of blood via collaterals), dementia, seizure and blood brain barrier study.

31. **A i.e. Transfemoral route** *[Ref: Grainger and Allison's 4/e p 2311]*

- ***The most preferred route to perform cerebral angiography is the transfemoral route***Q.
- Puncture of the axillary artery or direct puncture of the carotid artery are rarely performed.

4

NUCLEAR MEDICINE

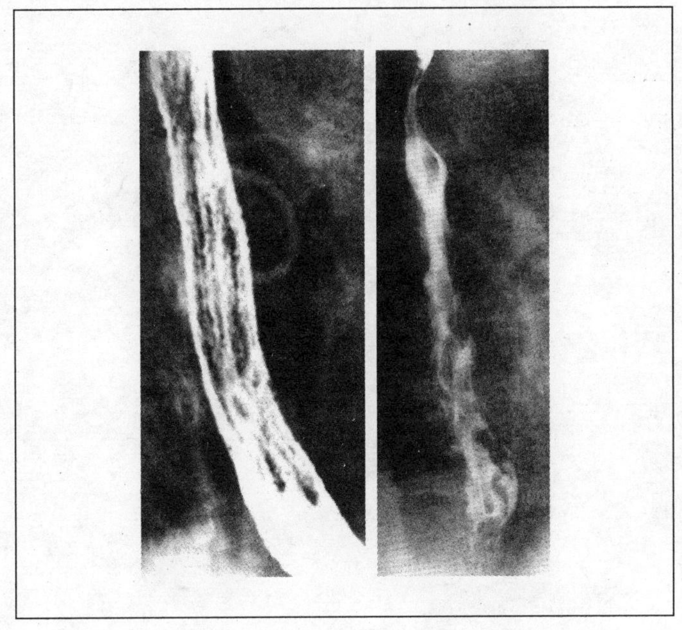

Radiodiagnosis

1 PHYSICS AND TECHNIQUES

Contrast Agents

Intravascular Radiological Iodinated Contrast Media

- All are tri-iodo benzene ring derivatives with *3 atoms of iodine* at 2, 4, 6 position (*in monomers) & 6 atoms of I_2 per molecule of ring anion (in dimers). They have low lipid solubility, low toxicity, low binding affinitie for protein, receptors or membranes, low molecular wt (<2000) and are very hydrophilic.* On iv injection, b/o high capillary permeability, all are distributed rapidly into **extravascular**, ***extracellular space (except in CNS)***[Q]. They *do not enter the interior of blood cells or tissue cells* and are rapidly excreted (>90% by GFR within 12 hrs). They are *used purely as imaging and not therapeutic agents (no pharmacological actions)*
- All *ionic agents* are salts of *sodium or meglumine (N-methyl glucomine)* and dissociate in water in 2 *ions (osmotic particles)* per molecule whereas, *non-ionic agents* do not ionize or dissociate. All *monomers* contain *1* and *dimers contain 2* tri-iodinated radio opaque anion benzene ring (*i.e. 3 & 6 I_2 atoms* per molecule) respectively. *Ionic monomers are high osmolar contrast media (HOCM)* with a 3:2 iodine per particle ration; whereas nonionic monomer, ionic dimer (both 3:1 ratio) and nonionic dimer (6:1 I_2 per particle ratio; physiologically isotonic) are **low osmolar contrast media (LOCM)**.
- **High osmolar contrast agents (HOCM)** are all ***ionic monomers***[Q]; whereas **low osmolar contrast agents (LOCM)** ***may be ionic dimers, and nonionic monomers or dimers (i.e. both ionic & nonionic)***[Q]. HOCM have osmolality in range of **1500** mosmols/kg water at concentrations of 300 mg I_2/ml. Whereas LOCM have osmolality which is *less than half of the osmolality of HOCM* (i.e. 600-700 for nonionic monomer, 560 for ionic dimer and 300 for nonionic dimer). So compred *to physiological osmolality of 300 mosmols/kg water,* ***nonionic dimers are physiologically isotonic*** in solution at 300 mg iodine/ml. Normal plasma osmollity is 300 mosmols/kg water at iodine concentration of 300mg/ml.
- So LOCM means that osmolality is lower than the HOCM (not physiological). *Lowest osmolality/osmolarity is seen in* ***non ionic dimer*** *agents* which becomes almost ***physiologically isotonic or iso-osmolar***[Q] (visipaque 320 is 290 mosmol/kg and isovist 300 is 320 mosmol/kgH_2O;320 & 300 are iodine concentrations).
- **Contrast agent ratio (CAR)** which indicates the osmolality of an agent, is derived by dividing the number of particles in solution.

$$\text{CAR} = \frac{\text{Number of iodine atoms}}{\text{Number of particles in solution}}$$

Osmolality is proportional to **the ratio of iodine atoms to the number of particles in solution**. The contrast agent with **lower ratio (3:2)** are **HOCM** and they have more particles in solution per iodine atom (or in other words less iodine atoms per particle). And agents with ***higher ratio (3:1 or 6:2 and 6:1)*** are **LOCM**.

Extracellular MRI Contrast Agent

Iodinated contrast agents have low lipid solubility, low toxicity, low binding affinities for protein, receptor or membranes, low moleculer wt & are very hydrophilic. On iv injection b/o high capillary permeability they all are ***distributed rapidly into extravascular, extracellular interstitial space (except in CNS)***[Q] but do not enter blood or tissue cells. **Pharmacokinetics of all extracellular MRI contrast agents (all gadolinium except Gd-BOPTA) are similar to iodinated water soluble contrast media**. They ***donot cross the blood brain barrier unless the barrier is disrupted***[Q]. These agents accumulate in tissues with abnormal vascularity (inflammation & malignancy) and in regions where BBB is disrupted.

Owing to their rapid equilibration in interstial space of both normal & inflammatory/tumor tissues, the use of dynamic MR imaging after bolus injection makes the best use of narrow imaging window with a transiently increased tumor /inflammatory to normal tissue contrast.

These agents are well tolerated with no differences in the safety of various agents except when it comes to extravasation in soft tissues; then the osmolality is important and ***high osmolar agents are likely to induce more local dmage***. In blood, the osmotic load of all Gd-based contrast media is very low, compared to iodinated contrast media, because only a small amount of contrast agent is required to produce a diagnostic MRI.

The pharmacokinetics of all agents except **Gd-BOPTA** (gadobenate dimeglumine) are similar to iodinated water soluble contrast media. Unlike all other Gd- chelates, Gd-BOPTA has a capacity for weak & transient protein binding & is eleminated through both the renal & hepatobiliary pathways. So it behaves *as a conventional extrcellular contrast agent in first few minutes* following iv administration and as a *liver specific agent in a later delayed phase* (40-120 min after administration) when it i taken up specifically by normal functioning hepatocytes.

These are *more nephrotoxic than iodinated contrast medium in equimolar dose*. However, nephrotoxicity after contrast enhanced (CE) MRI is not common even in patients with renal disease as the *dose required is small in comparison to the doses of iodinated contrast media* that are used for CT or other radiographic examinations.

Nephrogenic systemic fibrosis (NSF) is characterized by indurated scleroderma like skin changes mainly affecting limbs & trunks. It can progress to cause flexion contractures of joints & fibrotic changes affecting other organs such as muscles, heart, liver and lungs. NSF is most commonly a/w *administration of less stable, nonionic-linear chelates (gadodimide >> gadovesetamide;* l/t release of highly toxic Gd^{+++} ion) in patients with *advanced renal failure (GFR < 30ml/min) including those on dialysis.* A more stable Gd-CA such as macrocyclic Gd chelates might prove less hazardous if CEMRI is thought to be necessary in such a group of patients, including *pregnant & lactating women with end stage renal failure.*

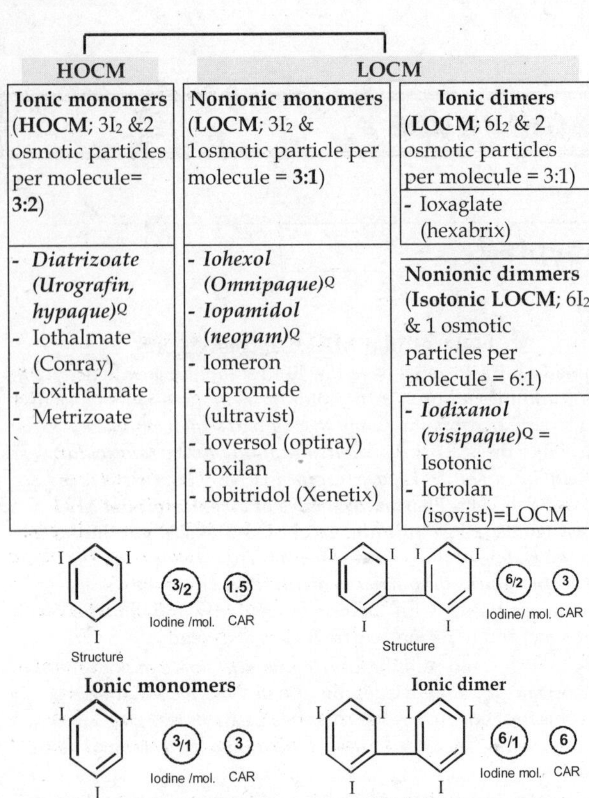

HOCM	LOCM	
Ionic monomers (**HOCM**; $3I_2$ &2 osmotic particles per molecule= **3:2**)	**Nonionic monomers** (**LOCM**; $3I_2$ & 1osmotic particle per molecule = **3:1**)	**Ionic dimers** (**LOCM**; $6I_2$ & 2 osmotic particles per molecule = 3:1) - Ioxaglate (hexabrix)
- ***Diatrizoate (Urografin, hypaque)***Q - Iothalmate (Conray) - Ioxithalmate - Metrizoate	- ***Iohexol (Omnipaque)***Q - ***Iopamidol (neopam)***Q - Iomeron - Iopromide (ultravist) - Ioversol (optiray) - Ioxilan - Iobitridol (Xenetix)	**Nonionic dimmers (Isotonic LOCM**; $6I_2$ & 1 osmotic particles per molecule = 6:1) - ***Iodixanol (visipaque)***Q = Isotonic - Iotrolan (isovist)=LOCM

Extracellular MRI-CA (with osmolality in mosmol kg H_2O)	MR Contrasts for liver imaging
• **Linear ionic** - Gadopentate dimeglumine (Gd-DPTA)=1960 - Gadobenate dimeglumine (Gd-BOPTA)=1970 • **Linear –nonionic** - Gadodiamide (Gd – DPTA - BMA)= 650 - Gadovesetamide (Gd-DTPA-BMEA)=1110 • **Cyclic–ionic** - Gadoterate meglumine (Gd-DOTA)= 1350 • **Cyclic–nonionic** - Gadoteridol (Gd-HP-DO3A)= 630 - Gadobutrol (Gd-BT-DO3A)= 1600	• Non specific Gd-chelates eg omniscan, gadovist distribute in extracellular space • **Hepatocyte selective Gd-chelates** eg **Gd-BOPTA** & **Gd – EOB-DTPA** (multihance, primovist) initially distribute in EC space but undergo hepatic excretion • **Non Gd – based contrasts** - **Magafodipir trisodium (Mn DPDP) eg manganese based** teslascan is selectively taken by **hepatocytes** & excreted into bile ducts - **Superparamagnetic iron oxide particles (ferrumoxide** 80-150nm)eg endorem is selectively taken up by **Kuffer cells** - **Ferucarbotran** (60 nm iron oxide particles) eg resovist (by Kuffer cells)

Adverse Reactions to Radiological Contrast Media (RCM)

Factors Significantly Predisposing to adverse drug (contrast) reactions

All adverse reactions are significantly more frequent with **HOCM** and in patients with

- *Previous adverse reaction* (excluding mild reactions like flushing, nausea) to contrast and h/o *asthma or bronchospasm* are two most dangerous predisposing factors.
- H/o allergy or atopy
- Cardiac patients in failure, with decompensation (CCF), unstable arrhythmia, recent MI
- ***Renal patients in failure (creatinine > 2mg%), diabetic nephropathy, on metformin***Q
- Feeble infants, aged patients, patient with severe general debility, ***dehydration***Q
- Anxiety, apprehension, very nervous.
- ***Hematological eg sickle cell anemia***Q & metabolic conditions.
- Menifest hyperthyroidism, thyrotoxic-goitrous patients (**absolute contraindication** to RCM administration).
- Delayed adverse reactions (more common in LOCM & dimmers than HOCM &/or monomers)

Guidelines to Prevent generalized RCM reactions

- ***Use nonionic agents***Q
- Premedication (with *corticosteroid / prednisolone* orally 12 hr & 2hr before RCM *along with anti histamines) in high risk patients* especially when ionic agents are used.

Types of Adverse Reaction

- **Idiosyncratic (anaphylactoid) reactions** are most serious & fatal complications that occur without warning are *not dose*

Renal Adverse Reactions (Contrast Nephropathy)

- It is reduction in renal function induced by contrast agent. It classically presents with rise in BUN & creatinine (>25% or 44 µmol/L within 3 days of IV constrast).
- Patients at **highest risk** for developing contrast induced ARF are those with

1. ***Pre-existing renal impairment/failure (>132µmol/L) and oliguria***Q.
2. ***Diabetic nephropathy***Q (DM without renal impairment is not a risk factor)
3. ***Dehydrated (hypovolemic)patient***Q.
4. Large doses and multiple injections within 72 hours (usually upto 25 g and maximally upto 70 gm of iodine i.e. 1 gm iodine per Kg body weight is advisible even in well hydrated patients with good renal function).
5. Intra arterial injection (in renal arteries or aorta) is more nephrotoxic than intravenous injection.
6. Nephrotoxic drugs (diuretics, antibiotics, NSAIDs, cytotoxic therapy) may enhance nephrotoxicity.
7. ***Myelomatosis, multiple myeloma***Q (b/o tubular obstruction d/t proteinaceous casts).
8. **Metformin (phen formin)**, an *oval biguanide hyperglycemic therapy* for diabetes mellitus type 2, in patients with severe renal impaiment.
9. **HOCM** are more nephrotoxic and large doses may damage renal medulla & reduce intramedullary blood flow in patients with acute calculus renal colic.

dependent.

- **Non-idiosyncratic reactions** are *dose dependent* & therefore relate to the chemical composition, osmolality & concentration of contrast agent and the volume, speed & multiplicity of the injection. Examples include
- **Hyperosmolar reactions** such as *erythrocyte damage* (d/t loss of intra RBC water), ***endothelial damage and blood brain barrier damage*** occur in HOCM, that have very high osmolality (5-8 times the physiological osmollity). Other hyperosmolar reactions are **vasodilatation** (l/t local heat, warmth, discomfort or severe pain during peripheral arteriography; and severe systemic hypotension, peripheral venous pooling, decreased venous return & cardiac failure), **hypervolemia** (l/t decreased hemoglobin concentration and increasing stress on left ventricle) and **cardiac depression** (esp after coronary angiography). All these are reduced by use of LOCM.
- **Chemotoxic reactions** are d/t anion rather than to its iodine content as it is very firmly bound to benzene ring. Chemotoxicity increases as the number of carboxyl group increases & number of hydroxyl group decreases. Chemotoxicity may l/t allergic like symptoms, cardiac, neurological & renal toxicity as well as vascular manifestations.
- **Cationic toxicity** may result from changes (either greater or lesser) in *sodium or calcium ion concentration*
- **Vasomotor reactions** like severe hypotension, tachy or bradycardia, marked apprehension, anxiety, sweating, and depression of myocardiac contraction, and reduced cardiac output l/t unconsciousness, collapse & death are *combined idosyncratic & non-idosyncratic reactions.*

- *Metformin is primarily excreted by kidney as an active compound.* In patients with severe renal impairment, intravascular accumulation of biguanide may occur ofter RCM precipitating a **potentially fatal – biguanide lactic acidosis** (*vomiting, diarrhoea, somnolence*). RCM related lactic acidosis is extremely rare in diabetics receiving metformin, if the patient has normal renal function before RCM. It is therefore recommended that metformin is *only discontinued if there is pre-existing renal impaiment* and it may be *recommenced 48 hr later* (after reassurance of good renal function after RCM).
- It is an established concept, that HOCMs are more nephrotoxic and ***LOCMs are preferred for all patients considered to be at increased risk of contrast nephropathy***[Q], (especially with diabetic nephropathy). However, it is not yet established whether nonionic **monomer** LOCM or nonionic **dimer** LOCM (i.e. iso-osmolar agents) have the *lower renal toxicity.*
- **Delayed reactions like** arm pain, delayed rash, flu like symptoms, *salivary gland swelling (iodide mumps), delayed vasculitisw, disseminated LE and Steven Johnson syndrome* are more common in women and with **LOCM** and **dimers**. Presumbly the reaction is *idiosyncratic and non dose dependent.* Because of this nonionic dimer – iotrolan has been with drawn from clinical use.
- Patients with **thrombotic tendency (like severe polycethmia)** may have an increased risk *esp after arterial injection of nonionic LOCM.* HOCM inhibits thrombosis more than LOCM.
- Patients with **pheochromocytoma** may develop hypertensive crisis, therefore, *preliminary alpha - & beta – adrenergic blockade* is advisible.
- It is clear that all RCM can cause nephropathy in patients with risk factor. Although **hemodialysis** can safely remove iodinated contrast media from the body, it does not prevent nephrotoxicity & nephropathy of poorly functioning kidneys. In contrast **hemofiltration** is effective in reducing this complication.

CAT Scan: Concept, Evolution and Hounsfield Unit/CT number (CTn)

CAT Scan: Concept and Evolution

- In conventional projection radiography (e.g. X-ray), structures further from film are superimposed on those closer to the film. This causes an overall reduction in contrast b/w objectects of smilar composition and l/t an inability to determine the depth and shap of an object.
- **Tomography** literally means a **sectional imaging** or **slice (transverse section) view**[Q] of a patient. In tomography only structures in a selected slice, parallel to the film are imaged sharply. Those above and below are deliberately blurred (so as to be unrecognizable) by simultaneous movement, of two of the three following: tube, film, patient during the exposure. In **conventional linear tomography** the contrast is poor because of influence of overlying tissue.
- **Computed tomography** (**CT scan** or originally k/a **computed axial tomography = CAT Scan)** generates image in ***transaxial section***[Q], i.e. perpendicular to the axis of rotation of x-ray tube about the body and generally **perpendicular to crano-caudal axis of patients body**. Unlike linear tomography, CAT images are not influenced by the properties of neighbouring regions of body and therefore, display true contracts within the imaged section. The only limitation being imposed is by width/thickness of section.
- Most CT had are performed in supine position with the plane of section at **10-25° to Reid's baseline (canthomeatal line)** to avoid radiation through eyes (esp. senstive lens).
- Three factors significantly improve the spatial resolution of CT such that it can be described as high resolution CT **(HRCT).**

Hounsfield unit / CT number

- **CT** is ***a special type of X-ray procedure***[Q], that involves the measurement of the weakening, or attenuation of X-ray beams by body structure at numerous positions located within the patient. These attenuation values are named **Hounsfield unit (CTn)** in honour of **Godfrey Hounsfied**, the inventor of CT Scanning.
- CT mages are mostly calculated on 512×512 (rarely 256 × 256 or 1024 × 1024) pixel matter. Each **pixel** or more correctly described as **voxel** is a volume element having 3 dimensions with *a depth that is equal to thickness of the section.* The value stored in each pixel/voxel, the CT number represents the average liner attenuation coefficient of tissue (μ_t) in the voxel.
- CTn is an *arbitrary unit of X-ray attenuation* used for CT scan, and it *depends on average linear attenuation coeficient of the matter* and is given by

$$HU = \frac{\mu_t - \mu_{H_2O}}{\mu_{H_2O}} \times 1000$$

μ_t = Attenuation coefficient of tissue of interest

μ_{H2O} = Attenuation coefficient of water

- By definition, **water has CTn equal to 0**, and **air** (b/o its *very low density* giving it and *attenuation coefficient of zero*) has a ***CTn equal to -1000***[Q]. Air and water are used as fixed points for calibration of CTn scale, which approximately ranges from *–1000 to +3000 (i.e. 400 levels of grey)* or more accurately from -1024 to +3071 (4096 levels of grey).

A CT number **-1000** is represented as **black** and **+3000** as **white**, with **all shades of grey displayed between**. However, the human eye cannot differentiate >50 grey shades. So **windowing** is done to bring out hidden details in image. For example -900 to -400 window range (which coincides with CTn of lung – 300 to - 800) display

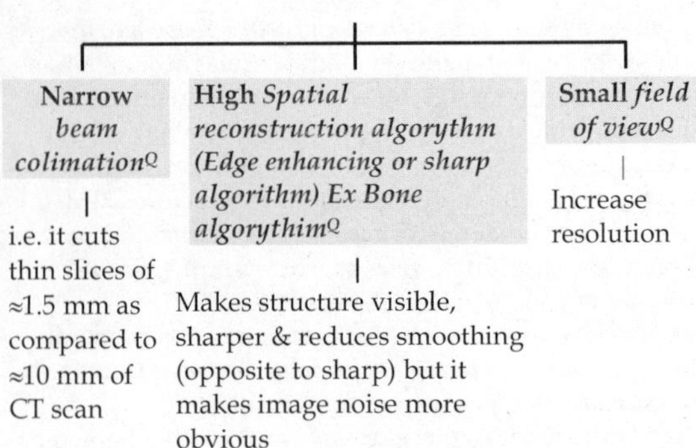

Narrow beam colimationQ
High Spatial reconstruction algorythm (Edge enhancing or sharp algorithm) Ex Bone algorythimQ
Small field of viewQ
i.e. it cuts thin slices of ≈1.5 mm as compared to ≈10 mm of CT scan
Makes structure visible, sharper & reduces smoothing (opposite to sharp) but it makes image noise more obvious
Increase resolution

detailed lung structure but same section with -240 to + 300 window range provides no information of lung but show good structural detail outside.

- **CTn (or HU)** for various tissues is.

CTn above 0 i.e. positive

Bone	500-1000
Contrast	130
Calcification	100
Muscle	40-60
Blood (congealed)	55-75
Grey matter (brain)	35-45
White matter (brain)	20-30

CTn ≤ 0 (i.e. Negative)

Water	0
Fat	-50 to -150
Lung	-300 to 800

Colonography & Virtual Colonoscopy

- **CT colonography (virtual colonoscopy)** is an innovative technique which combines MD-CT examination of entire colon and computerized processing of raw data to obtain 3 ***dimensional volume rendered images of colonic lumen*** *typically resembling colonoscopy like endoluminal fly through view.* **MR clonography** (virtual colonoscopy) acquire 2D and/or 3D fast imaging with steady state precession **(FISP)** MR sequence, 3D T1 W images after iv gadolinium and T1W 2D **FLASH** (fast low angle shot) sequence in axial plane during single breath hold scans. Advantages of MR colonography is lack of inoizing radiation and superior soft tissue contrast and disadvantages include *lower spatial resolution, high susceptibility to motion artifacts, longer examination time* and limited availability.
- **Barium studies** and **sigmoidscopy/colonoscopy** provides excellent visualization of mucosa. However, *they cannot determine the depth of mural (wall) invasion,extra luminal tumor spread, and extent of lymph node and distant metastasis.* By virtue of cross sectional imaging format, **CT and MRI** can determine these features and have ***become the primary means for radiological preoperative staging of colorectal carcinoma***Q. *Tumor recurrence and complications* (of surgery or primary colonic malignancy) such as obstruction, perforation and fistula formation can also be readily visualized with CT. In general, ***CT is most widely used for staging colorectal cancers***Q.

The **accuracy of CT for colonic evaluation is improved by**

- Administration of IV *smooth muscle relaxants (antispasmodic agents) like hyoscine/buscopan* (more effective but should be used with caution because *glaucoma, cardiac ischemia and urinary retention* may be precipitated and *dry mouth and blurred vision* may occur) or *glucagon* (less effective).
- **Colonic distension** by automated **CO_2** insufflation is safer and causes less post procedural discomfort (than **room air** insufflation) b/o rapid absorption of CO_2 through colonic mucosa. It (CT-pneumocolon)

Interpretation of Results

- The wall thickness in a well distended (with oral contrast) normal colon is **≤3mm**. Wall thickness b/w **>3 to 6mm** is considered indeterminate (i.e suggest phathology) and **>6mm** is definitely abnormal. However, with air contrast technique, measurements of *3mm for rectum and 2mm for colon* are the upper limit of normal. Both *luminal (mucosal) and outer margins of colon should be smooth and sharply delineated* by contrast/air and surrounding homogenous pericolic fat respectively. On CT or MRI, a colorectal cancer appears as a *discrete mass or irregular surface of focal or short segmental asymmetrical wall thickening.*
- *Most colorectal cancers are considered to arise in adenomatous polyps;* therefore, colorectal cancers can be prevented by early detection & removal of polyp. Because **polyp size** is clinically the single most important feature, indicating risk of cancer development, the size should be measured accurately and reliably. **CT colonographyis more reliable and accurate than colonoscopy for polyp measurement.** Guideline using CT colonography reporting and data system (C-RADS) suggest

Co: Inadequate study/awaiting prior comparisons	**C1: Normal colon or benign lesion**	**C2: Indeterminate polyp or finding**	**C3: Polyp possibly advanced adenoma**	**C4: Colonic mass; likely malignant**
- Inadequate insufflation (≥1 collapsed colonic segments on both views) - Inadequate preparation owing to presence of fluid and feces cannot exclude lesions ≥ 10mm - Awaiting prior colon studies for comparision	- No visible abnormality or **polyp ≥ 6mm** - Lipoma or inverted diverticulum or colonic diverticula (non-neoplastic finding)	- **6-9mm, polyp <3 in number** - Cannot exclude ≥6mm polyp in adequate exam	- **Polyp≥ 10mm** - **≥3polyps; each 6-9mm**	- Compromise bowel lumen - Demonstrate extracolonic invasion
	↓ Continue **routine screening every 5-10years**; reporting of **≤5mm** polyp is not recommended because they are mostly nonneoplastic and false positive.	↓ **Surveillance** or **follow up colonoslopy** that can be delayed at least **3years**	↓ **Immediate follow up (therapeutic colonoscopy re-commended)**	↓ Surgical consultation recommended

Indications and Contraindication

- **Indications** of CT colonography are

1. Incomplete colonoscopy d/t colonic tortuosity, adhesion, severe diverticular disease, patient intolerance or occlusive ness or stricture preventing examination of proximal colon.

improves CT colongraphic visualization because a suboptimally distended colon can obscure and miss a fairly large lesion as well as mimic a lesion.

- **Complete bowel cleansing** using **colonic purgation** and rectal enema. **Dry preparation** with **sodium phosphate** (phospho-soda) and **magnesium citrate** (smaller dose and leaves little fluid in colon) is preferred and advantageous in comparison to **wet preparation** with **polyethylene glycol** as large (4L) volume of PEG has to be taken which leaves a large amount of luminal fluid that can impair visualization of colonic lesions. **Bisacodyl** is often used in dry preparation as it stimulates parasymathetic reflexes to induce evacuation of stools. *Sodium phosphate* is a *high sodium preparation* and rarely can l/t significant *electrolyte disbalance*. So it is *contraindicated in renal failure, congestive heart failure, pre-existing electrolyte abnormalities, ascites and paralytic ileus.*
- **Laxative free CT colonography** can be successfully performed with no/reduced bowel preparation (purgation). In it *radiopaque, oral contrast agent like barium sulphate, sodium amidotrizoate and meglumine amidortrizoate (gastrograffin)* is administered at each meal, typically the day before CT colonography *to label residual feces and colonic fluid*, a procedure called ***fecal or fluid tagging***. On CT, labelled fecal material appears hyperdense or white making it *easily distinguishable from the homogynous soft tissue density of colonic polyps and masses*. It improves diagnostic performance (accuracy 100% for ≥ 10mm polyps), substantially decreases patient discomfort and increases acceptance by eliminating the inconvienience of rigorous dietary restriction and colonic purgation. Gastrograffin very rarely may cause anaphyloctoid reaction in *blunt trauma patient without bowel disease and in patients with pseudomembranous colitis*; and 3% amount is absorbed and eliminated via kidneys. Hence, it should not be used in patients with *hypersensitivity to iodine, decreased renal function or manifest hyperthyroidism.*

2. Patient adamantly refusing diagnostic colonoscopy (but have strong indication) or there is inability to perform colonoscopy d/t requirement for anticoagulant therapy or risk of sedation.

- **Contraindication** for CT colonogrphy are *allergy to contrast, suspected colonic perforation, acute colonic infection,* (acute diverticulitis, severe infective colitis), *acute lower GI bleeding, complete colonic obstruction, very recent colonic surgery (<1 week),* medically unstable patient and refusal to undergo colonic preparation.

Procedure

- Images are taken in **supine** and **prone position** on *a helical CT scanner using low dose technique*. One should use the *thinnest slice possible* to cover the entire abdomen in single breath-hold. *A slice collimation of ≤3mm with a reconstruction interval of ≤1.5mm* is required and achieved easily with modern *16 or 64 detector MDCT scanners*. Because of intrinsic high contrast b/w colonic mucosa and luminal air detailed images of endoluminal surface can be obtained even with the use of very low dose radiation (1.8m Sv in men and 2.4 m Sv in women) which is ***less than half the radiation dose of barium enema***[Q].
- **Intravenous contrast enhancement** is usually not required for screening purpose. However, it improves detection of medium sized polyps (6-9mm) esp in soboptimally prepared colon. IV contrast enhancement is necessary in *patients with known or suspicious colorectal cancer, those who are undergoing followup-after curative surgery* for colorectal cancer and those with symptoms that suggest and *increased prevalence of extra colonic abnormalities* (standard radiation dose for body CT is used for extrcolonic evaluation).
- *Role of colonic distension in staging rectal cancer is controversial.* Although colonic distension improves lesion visualization but may alter the distance between the outer tumor margin and mesorectal fascia, confounding (confusing) the assessment of extramural depth of tumor invasion.
- Lesions can be searched by using **2D (cross section)** and **3D (virtual colonoscopic) views**. Polyp detection is greatly enhances on 3D endoluminal view compared to 2D view which requires a higher level of reader concentration, experience and effort. However, 3D review is less time efficient and maynot work well with fecal tagging and reduced purgation protocol that leaves large amount of fecal residue in colon. Internal air density, a higher density than soft tissue attenuation and ***movability (i.e. positional change b/w supine and prone position)*** are specific signs of residual feces. **Flat** adenomatous lesions (~40%) appear as *nodular mucosal surfaces, plaque shaped mucosal elevations and thickened haustral folds* at CT colonography and are more difficult to detect (in comparison to sessile or pedunculated lesions).

Colour Doppler USG

- **Colour doppler** permits accurate **detection of vessels (arteries and veins), confirming their patency and direction of flow** (where relevant eg in portal vein) and **obtain useful velocity information**, such as *peak systolic velocity, mean velocity & turbulence*. It permits the detection of very small vessels (that even could not be studied in 2D images) and the **assessment of number and distribution of vessels with in a tissue volume.**
- Color doppler can **identify segments of**

Neck Vessel Examination

- Color doppler can be used for **evaluation of neck vessels (carotid & vertebral arteries)** *in patients with transient ischemic attacks (TIA) or reversible ischemic neurological deficits (RINDs),* who may benefit from carotid endaterectomy surgery. It is usually not indicated in patients with established and completed strokes, unless there are milder-resolving strokes in younger patients.
- Stenosis or absent segment in one **vertebral vessel** in neck is not usually of clinical significance as the basilar circulation can be maintained from the other artery. However, a **reversed flow** (sometimes exercise of

stenosis or occlusion (by directly measuring *diameter reduction or cross sectional area reduction* in large vessels or indirectly quantifying stenosis by the *increase in velocity* that occurs as blood passes through stenosis), **detect false aneurysm** (by to and fro patterns as blood flows in and out of flase aneurysm during the cardiac cycle) **and define plaques/thrombus** (smooth, echogenic plaques are likely to be fibrotic and stable, whereas irregular, hypoechoic plaques are more likely to be unstable and act as a source of **emboli**).

- Color doppler can be used for **evaluation of neck vessels (carotid & vertebral arteries)**, pulsatile neck masses, **peripheral arteries/veins of extremities (lower & upper limb), large abdominal vessels** (such as **portal vein, hepatic artery, hepatic vein, renal artery, renal vein, aorta & IVC**), **blood flow to ovaries, uterus, testis and prostate** (in pelvis; through trans abdominal, trans vaginal or transrectal approaches). Color doppler can also be used to evaluate **vascular complications** of **renal transplant** and to identify **ureteric jets** as urine enters the bladder at vesico-ureteric junctions. In patients with obstructed ureter the jets on affected side will be less frequent or absent.
- **In Colour doppler colours** are used to represent ***direction of flow***Q towards & away from the transducer; usually **red is towards & blue is away from transducer.** Mn "BART or jV AB= Blue – Away; Red - Towards". **Shades (intensity of colour)** represent *velocity of flow*Q; the paler shades representing higher velocity.
- **Power doppler** is good for *showing areas of flowing blood*, particularly when it is *moving slowly or in small vessels*; but *at the expense of losing directional & velocity information.*

ipsilateral arm muscles may be required to produce it) **is a sign of occluded or severely stenotic subclavian artery (subclavian steal syndrome).**

Abdominal & Pelvic Vessel Examination

- Color doppler USG examination of abdominal vessels is little more challenging than peripheral & neck vessel examination because of their *deeper location, presence of respiratory motion and bowel gas interferences.*
- **Blood to uterus and ovaries** varies with ovulation with increased flow and decreased pulsality near ovulation; it is used to monitor **infertility treatment**. Increased vascularity with low RI (<0.6) is seen in **ectopic pregnancy** (d/t trophoblastic tissue) and **trophoblastic disease**; return of wave form and RI to normal correlates well with successful treatment. Increased uterine artery RI during established pregnancy (a sign of increased resistance in placenta) reflects **intra uterine growth retardation.**
- Color doppler USG is also useful in differentiating **ovarian/testicular torsion** (decreased blood flow) from **inflammation (epididymo-orchitis)** and tumors (increased blood flow), **varicoceles** (multiple serpiginous cystic areas in epididymis).

Transcranial Doppler Examination

- **Transcranial color doppler USG examination of neonatal and fetal brain** through the fontanelles and thin calvarial bones to detect fetal abnormalities. **In adults, transcranial approach** is more difficult esp. in females, back skinned and elderly and **can examine main cerebral arteries (not veins) only** through thin squamous temporal bone in front of ear. The main indication for transcranial color doppler in adults include **monitoring of spasm and flow after** stroke and subarachnoid hemorrhage, assessment of intracranial collateral pathways and detection of stenosis (>65%) and aneurysm (>5mm) of main cerebral arteries.

Peripheral Vessel Examination

- Peripheral vessels (arteries & veins) can be evaluated for stenosis or occlusion in **patients with claudication**, and **peripheral vascular disease;** for abnormal flow in **varicose veins** and to reveal thrombosis/plaque in ***deep vein thrombosis***Q.

QUESTIONS

Contrast Agents

1. **In cerebral angiography the dye is injected through:** *(AI 1999)*
   A. Femoral Artery
   B. Brachial Artery
   C. Axillary Artery
   D. Radial Artery
2. **Which artery is disected most frequently following arteriography by femoral route:** *(AIIMS May 2011)*
   A. Celiac trunk
   B. Superior mesenteric artery
   C. Inferior mesentric artery
   D. Gastroduodenal artery
3. **Which of the following contrast agent is non iodinated:** *(AIIMS May 2011)*
   A. Iohexol
   B. Diatrizoate
   C. Gadolinium
   D. Visipaque
4. **Contrast used in CT :** *(PGI 2K)*
   A. Gadolinium
   B. Technitium
   C. Iodine
   D. Chromium
5. **Contrast used for MRI :** *(PGI 2K, DNB 01)*
   A. Iodine
   B. Gadolinium
   C. Metvazamide
   D. Omnipaque
6. **Contrast dye(s) used in MRI:** *(PGI May 12)*
   A. Gadolinium
   B. Iodine
   C. Myodinium
   D. Technitium
   E. Indium
7. **Which of the following statements about contrast in radiography is true:** *(AI 2011)*
   A. Ionic monomers have three iodine atoms per two particles in solution
   B. Osmolar contrast agents may be ionic or non ionic
   C. Gadolinum may cross the blood brain barrier
   D. Iohexol is a high osmolar contrast media
8. **Contrast material used in the diagnosis of esophageal atresia is** *(PGI 1997)*
   A. Gastrograffin
   B. Conray 420
   C. Dianosil
   D. Myodii
9. **Contrast media of choice for myelogram is** *(AIIMS 93, DNB 95)*
   A. Urografin 75%
   B. Conray 470
   C. Iohexol
   D. Biligrafin
10. **Most common complication of myelography is** *(AI 99, DNB 98)*
    A. Allergic reaction
    B. Headache
    C. Focal neurological deficit
    D. Arachanoiditis
11. **Radiocontrast is contraindicated in all except –** *(AI 2007)*
    A. Renal failure
    B. Ptient on metformin
    C. Dehydration
    D. Obesity
12. **Which of the following contrast agents is preferred in a patient with decreased renal function to avoid contrast nephropathy:** *(AI 2011)*
    A. Acetylcystine
    B. Fenoldapam
    C. Mannitol
    D. Low osmolar contrast
13. **Excretory urography should be cautiously performed in** *(AI 91, DNB 94)*
    A. Bone 2°
    B. Multiple myeloma
    C. Neuroblastoma
    D. Leukemia

Oral Cholecystography

14. **True about OCG is :** *(PGI 2000)*
    A. First done by Graham Cole in 1942
    B. Dye ingested at rate of 1 ml/kg
    C. USG has replaced it
    D. Dye used is telepaque
15. **Which is Not required for visualisation of gall bladder in oral cholecystography:** *(AIIMS 1995)*
    A. Functioning liver
    B. Motor mechanisms of gall bladder
    C. Patency of cystic duct
    D. Ability to absorb water

Ultrasonography

16. **Contrasts used in USG:** *(PGI Dec 07)*
    A. Urograffin
    B. Ultragraffin
    C. Sonavist
    D. Conray
    E. Barium
17. **Which of the following techniques use piezoelectric crystals?** *(AIIMS 04, DNB 06)*
    A. Ultrasonography
    B. X-ray diffraction
    C. NMR imaging
    D. Xeroradiography
18. **Radiation hazard is absent in:** *(PGI June 2006)*
    A. MRI
    B. Doppler USG
    C. Digital substraction Angiography
    D. Tc 99 scan
19. **Acoustic shadow in USG is due to** *(AI 94, DNB 95)*
    A. Artefact
    B. Absorption
    C. Reflection
    D. Refraction
20. **Ultrasound frequency used for diagnostic purposes in obstetrics :** *(PGI 2001)*
    A. 1-20 MHz
    B. 20-40 MHz
    C. 40-60 MHz
    D. 60-80 MHz
    E. 80-100 MHz

21. USG is sensitive in *(PGI June 2004)*
A. Ureteric colic
B. Gall stone
C. Blunt abdominal trauma
D. Appendicitis
E. Pancreatic pathology

22. Piezoelectric crystals are made use of in which modality that is safe from radiation also: *(PGI 1998)*
A. MRI
B. US
C. CT
D. All

23. The intensity of colour in Doppler is determined by:
A. Direction flow *(PGI 1998)*
B. Velocity of flow
C. Strength of returning echo
D. None of the above

24. Colour Doppler is/are used in diagnosis of: *(PGI May 13)*
A. Peripheral vascular disease
B. Deep vein thrombosis
C. Pulmonary embolism
D. Bone tumors
E. Fetal abnormality

MRI

25. All of them use non-ionizing radiation except: *(AI 2006)*
A. Ultrasonography
B. Thermography
C. MRI
D. Radiography

26. Radiation exposure occurs in all except
A. CT Scan, PET scan *(AI 93, DNB 95, PGI 97)*
B. MRI
C. Fluroscopy
D. Plain X-Ray

27. NMR based in the principle of -
A. Electron beam *(AIIMS 2K, AI 99)*
B. Proton beam
C. Magnetic field
D. Neutron beam

28. In MRI, images are produced due to *(AIIMS 93, DNB 96)*
A. H^+ (proton)
B. CO_2
C. N_2O
D. K^+

29. In MRI the field used is *(AI 97, DNB 99)*
A. 0.05 tesla
B. 100 tesla
C. 1.1 tesla
D. 11 tesla

30. MRI is not better than CT for detection of :
A. Ligament Injury *(AIIMS May 2012)*
B. Soft tissue tumors
C. Meningeal pathology
D. Calcified lesions

31. All of the following about MRI are correct except: *(AI 12)*
A. MRI is contraindicated in patients with pacemakers
B. MRI is useful for evaluating bone marrow
C. MRI is better for calcified lesions
D. MRI is useful for localizing small lesione in the brain

32. An absolute contraindication of MRI is:
A. Pacemaker wires *(AIIMS May 08)*
B. Intravascular stents
C. Prosthetic cardiac valves
D. Severe hypertension

33. Absolute C/I of MRI is- *(PGI June 2005)*
A. Pacemaker
B. Preganancy at 1st trimester
C. Aneurysmal clip
D. Phobia

34. Patient with a metallic foreign body in eye, which investigation is not done.
A. MRI *(PGI Dec 2006)*
B. USG
C. X-ray
D. CT

35. Metallic foreign body in eye can be detected by:
A. X-ray *(PGI May 13)*
B. CT
C. MRI
D. Color Doppler
E. USG

36. The EEG cabins should be completely shielded by a continuous sheet of wire mesh of copper to avoid the picking of noise from external electromagnetic disturbances. Such a shielding is called as:
A. Maxwell cage *(AIIMS Nov 2004)*
B. Edison's cage
C. Faraday cage
D. Ohm's cage

37. MRI rooms are shielded completely by a continuous sheet or wire mesh of copper or aluminum to shield the imager from external electromagnetic radiations, etc. It is called.
A. Maxwell cage *(AIIMS 2003)*
B. Faraday cage
C. Edison's cage
D. Ohms cage

CT Scan

38. MRI is better than CT scan to detect lesions located in:
A. Head and neck tumour *(PGI May 13)*
B. Extremity
C. Thorax
D. Retroperitoneum
E. It is equally effective for all above

39. Hounsfield Units depends on: *(AIIMS May 09)*
A. Electron density
B. Mass density
C. Effective atomic number
D. Attenuation coefficient

40. In computed tomography (CT), the attenuation value are measured in Hounsefield units (HU). An attenuation value of '0' (zero) HV corresponds to:
A. Water *(AIIMS Nov 2004)*
B. Very dense bone structure
C. AIR
D. Fat

41. Attenuation Value (Hounsfield Unit) of < Zero (i.e. negative) on CT is seen in: *(PGI May 2011)*
A. Muscle
B. Bone
C. Fat
D. Air
E. Blood

42. Walls of the CT scanner room are coated with: *(AI 2010)*
A. Lead
B. Glass
C. Tungsten
D. Iron

43. High – resolution CT of the lung is a specialized CT technique for greater detail of lung parenchyma and it utilizes:
A. Special lung filters *(AIIMS 2002)* ☐
B. Thick collimation ☐
C. Bone algorithm for image reconstruction ☐
D. Large filed of view ☐

44. Slice of tissue X-rays is: *(PGI 1999)*
A. Tomography ☐
B. Mammography ☐
C. Contrast studies ☐
D. All of the above ☐

45. CT dose index, True is: *(AIIMS Nov 08)*
A. By reducing KVP by 50% radiation dose is reduced to half ☐
B. In pediatric patients dose should be reduced ☐
C. CT dose index is not useful for control exposure in multi-slice CT ☐
D. KV has no control over CT dose index ☐

46. Which one of the following imaging techniques gives maximum radiation exposure to the patient?
A. Chest X-ray *(AIIMS May 12, AI 06, DNB 07)* ☐
B. MRI ☐
C. CT scan ☐
D. Bone scan ☐

47. High resolution computed tomography of the chest is the ideal modality for evaluating: *(AI 2003)*
A. Pleural effusion ☐
B. Interstitial lung disease ☐
C. Lung mass ☐
D. Mediastinal adenopathy ☐

Colonography & Virtual colonoscopy

48. True about virtual colonoscopy *(PGI Nov 10, 09)*
A. Provide endoluminal view ☐
B. Biopsy can be taken ☐
C. CT and MRI use ☐
D. Used even when conventional colonoscopy fails ☐
E. Used for screening of ca colon ☐

Computers in Radiology

49. PACS in medical imaging stands for: *(AIIMS May 08)*
A. Portal Archiving Common System ☐
B. Photo Archiving Computerized System ☐
C. Picture archieving communication system ☐
D. Planning archiving communication scheme ☐

Answers and Explanations:

Contrast Agents

1. **A i.e. Femoral Artery** *[Ref: Sutton 7/e p. 418; Harrison 18/e p. 303, 3291-93, 3249-50]*

- In **cerebral angiography, dye** is injected through – ***Femoral Artery***Q (M.C. route).
- In **Fluorscein angiography, dye** is injected through ***Cubital Vein***Q

2. **C i.e. Inferior mesentric artery** *[Ref: GI-Imaging (AMPIS) 3/e p 215,; Sutton 7/e p 447-60; 418-31; Grainger 5/e p 118-24; Haga 5/e p 1263-65; Armstrong 5/e p 429-30; AJR (78 march)130:455-60]*

- **Direct catheter arteriography (angiography)** is *percutaneous arterial* catheterization based on original work of *Seldinger* (in Stockholm, 1953). The most useful and commonly used sites for insertion of catheter into the arterial tree are 1) **femoral artery (most preferred & most common route)** and 2) **axillary artery** (although *most proximal portion of brachial artery* is punctured rather than axillary artery, so **high brachial** is preferred term).
- The **most common vessel** punctured for diagnostic and therapeutic angiography is **common femoral artery. Retrograde** femoral artery puncture is the most common technique used to approch arteries above inguinal ligament (such as coronary, carotid etc). **Antegrade** femoral artery puncture is used when performing ipsilateral superficial femoral, popliteal or infragenicular artery angioplasty.
- In practice, femoral & axillary arteries permit investigation of most areas so other sites like popliteal, lower brachial, radial artery, common carotid, etc are used in special circumstances (eg if femoral approach is not possible d/t iliac-occlusive disease). In recent years, there has been a *trend toward a greater use of upper extremity access* even in those individuals with patent femoral vessels because of lower morbidity caused by small caliber catheters (and DSA technique enables adequate studies to be obtained by injection through small caliber catheters).
- **Digital substraction angiography (DSA)**, digitally substract (manipuletes via computer) the shadow that are present on plain films from the films taken after contrast injection resulting in an image containing detalis of opacified structures only.
- **Selective catheterization** of renal artery, coeliac axis etc is done by fluoroscopic manipulation of special shape catheters like straight flush/pigtail/cobra/sidewinder. **Superselective (or subselective) catheterization** is *catheterization of small subsidiary arteries that themselves arise from named branch arteries* mostly during *embolization procedure*. A **co-axial catheter** (one that passes through the lumen of a diagnostic or guiding catheter) is often used for catheterization of these small vessels.
- *Damage to arterial wall (like subintimal stripping) leading to dissection* occurs during puncture, manipulation and injection of saline/large volumes of contrast. The decreasing order of artery damaged during femoral route celiac angiography is **external iliac artery > internal iliac artery > inferior mesenteric > gastroduodenal > celiac trunk > superior mesenteric artery**.

3. **C i.e. Gadolinium** 4. **C i.e. Iodine** 5. **B i.e. Gadolinium**
6. **A i.e. Gadolinum** 7. **A i.e. Ionic monomers have three iodine atoms per two particles in solution**
[Ref: Grainger 5/e p 32-51, 1249-53; Berry 3/e p 70, 104-110; Sutton 7/e p 419-21; Contrast Media 2/e p 4; Wolfgang 7/e p 1147]

- ***Ionic contrast agents** dissociate (ionize) in water in 2 ioins (or osmotic particles) per molecule whereas **nonionic agents** do not ionize or dissociate.* All **monomers** contain **1** ***benzene ring with 3 iodine atoms*** and **dimers** contains **2 benzene rings with 6 iodine atoms** per molecule. Therefore ***ionic monomers have 3 iodine atoms per 2 ionic/osmotic particles in solution***Q and a contrast agent ratio of **3:2 (i.e. 1.5)**. And **ionic dimers** have **6 iodine atoms per 2 ionic/osmotic particles** in solution with a contrast agent ratio of **6:2** or **3:1.**
- **Nonionic agents** donot ionize so they have only **1 osmotic particle** per molecule. And similarly **monomers** contain **3 iodine atom** and **dimers** contain **6 iodine atoms** per molecule of contrast agent. Therefore contrast agent ratio of **nonionic monomers is 3:1** and **nonionic dimers** is **6:1.**
- **High osmolar contrast agents (HOCM)** are all *ionic monomers*Q; whereas **low osmolar contrast agents (LOCM)** ***may be ionic dimers, and nonionic monomers or dimers (i.e. both ionic & nonionic)***Q. HOCM have osmolality in range of **1500** mosmols/kg water at concentrations of 300 mg I_2/ml. Whereas LOCM have osmolality which is *less than half of the osmolality of HOCM* (i.e. 600-700 for nonionic monomer, 560 for ionic dimer and 300 for nonionic dimer). So compred *to physiological osmolality of 300 mosmols/kg water*, ***nonionic***

dimers are physiologically isotonic in solution at 300 mg iodine/ml. Normal plasma osmollity is 300 mosmols/kg water at iodine concentration of 300mg/ml.

- So LOCM means that osmolality is lower than the HOCM (not physiological). *Lowest osmolality/osmolarity is seen in* ***non ionic dimer*** *agents* which becomes almost ***physiologically isotonic or iso-osmolar***[Q] (visipaque 320 is 290 mosmol/kg and isovist 300 is 320 mosmol/kgH_2O; 320 & 300 are iodine concentrations).
- **Osmolality** is proportional to **the ratio of iodine atoms to the number of particles in solution**. The contrast agent with **lower ratio (3:2)** are **HOCM** and they have more particles in solution per iodine atom (or in other words less iodine atoms per particle). And agents with ***higher ratio (3:1 or 6:2 and 6:1)*** are **LOCM**.
- **Iohexol (omnipaque)** is a ***nonionic monomer (LOCM with 3:1 ratio)***[Q]
- **Iodinated contrast agents** have low lipid solubility, low toxicity, low binding affinities for protein, receptor or membranes, low moleculer wt & are very hydrophilic. On iv injection b/o high capillary permeability they all are ***distributed rapidly into extravascular, extracellular interstitial space (except in CNS)***[Q] but do not enter blood or tissue cells.
- **Pharmacokinetics of all extracellular MRI contrast agents (all gadolinium except Gd-BOPTA) are similar to iodinated water soluble contrast media.** They ***donot cross the blood brain barrier unless the barrier is disrupted***[Q]. These agents accumulate in tissues with abnormal vascularity (inflammation & malignancy) and in regions where BBB is disrupted.
- **Contrast enhanced CT scans** use intravenous injection of ***iodinated contrast medium***[Q]; whereas **contrast enhanced MRI** use ***non iodinated contrast medium containing paramagnetic metal ions gadolinium (Gd^{3+}), Copper (Cu^{2+}) or manganese (Mn^{2+})***[Q]. Gd is the most powerful (with 7 unpaired electrons) but unfortunately most toxic of these ions and therefore it is necessary to encapsulate it by a chelate such as DTPA (diethylene triamine pentaacetic acid salt) forming Gd-DTPA.
- Paramagnetic agents are mainly positive enhancers that reduce the T_1 & T_2 relaxation times, *increase tissue signal intensity on T_1 weighted images & almost have no effect on T_2 weighted MR images.*

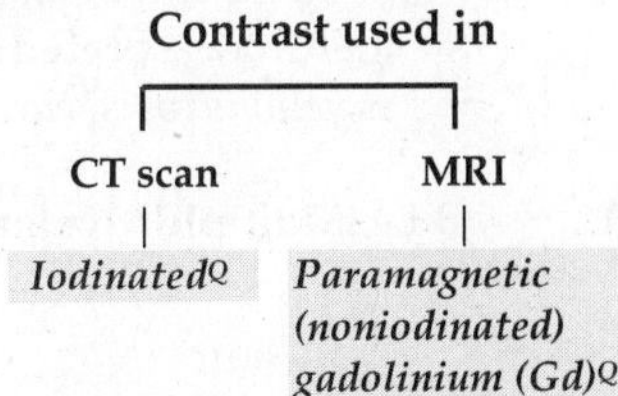

8. C i.e. Dianosil
9. C i.e. Iohexol *[Ref: Grainger 5/e p 39; Sutton 7/e p 1645-47; Adams & Victor 7/e p- 26]*

- **Dianosil** is used in ***oesophageal atresia***[Q], as in most cases it is frequently associated with tracheo-oesophageal fistula; so on instillation of contrast media, there is risk of flooding in the lungs.
- **Water soluble-nonionic LOCM** are licenced for **intrathecal** use ***eg Iohexol (omnipaque) and Iopamidol (neopam)***[Q] and are contrast agents of ***choice for myelography***[Q]. These are non neurotoxic, donot cause epileptic fits, can be used without withdrawing other drugs & are devoid of arachioid toxicity and anticonvulsant cover is unnecessary. Whereas ionic contrast media (both HOCM & LOCM) are very very toxic & often fatal when injected into subarachnoid space.

Condition	Dye
Myelography, Ventriculography & DSA Mnemonic: **I^2 M^2**	- ***Iopamidol***[Q] } I^2 - ***Iohexol (Omnipaque)***[Q] } I^2 - **Myodil**[Q] (abandoned d/t risk of arachnoiditis) } M^2 - Metrizamide (cause flapping tremor) } M^2
Patency & integrity of recent surgical anastamosis, Idiopathic mega colon/Hirschprung's ds.	- ***Gastrograffin enema***[Q]
Oesophageal atresia	- ***Dianosil***[Q]

10. **B i.e. Headache** *[Ref: Grainger 5/e p. 34-36]*

Complication from myelography are due to needle puncture & reaction to contrast agent; complications include-

1. ***Headache***[Q]***, nausea & vomitting, arm pain, flushing, pruritis;*** are the ***most common complications of dural puncture & myelography***[Q] ***(38%). These occur more commonly with HOCM & less commony with LOCM.***
2. Allergic reactions are most serious complications.
3. Others are – arachnoiditis, vasovagal syncope, postural hypotension, hearing loss, puncture of spinal cord, infection, hyperthermia, hallucination, depression, anxiety.

Pathology	Appearance on Myelography
Extradural block	Feathered appearance
Intradural-extramedullary block	Meniscus sign
Intramedullary block	Widening of cord (Trouser leg appearance)

11. D i.e. Obesity **12. D i.e. Low osmolar contrast**

[Ref. Harrison 18/e p. 1854, 2298, 2300; Sutton 7/e P- 927, Grainger 5/e p. 37-38; Canon Review of radiology p. 627; Emergency Medicine 6/e p. 642]

- **Radiocontrast agent is contraindicated** in ***patients with previous adverse reactions to contrast***[Q], (excluding mild reactions like nausea and flushing), in ***patients with renal failure, diabetic nephropathy on metformin***[Q] and in feeble elderly / infant ***patients with dehydration***[Q]. However, contrast agents are not ***contraindicated in obese***[Q].
- Measures recommended to reduce the incidence of **contrast medium induced nephropathy** include adequate **hydration** (*most important safe gaurd*), volume expansion with IV normal saline / or half strength sline solution, infusion of sodium bicarbonate instead of normal saline, ***infusion of mannitol***[Q], pharmacological manipulation (***prostaglandin, infusion, acetyl-cystine, fenoldapam mesylate infusion***[Q], theophylline and replete magnesium), ***use of LOCM instead of HOCM***[Q], hemodialysis rapidly after contrast administration and avoiding short intervals (< 48 hrs) between procedures requiring IV administration of contrast agent.
- **HOCM are avoided in cardiac disease** (b/o high sodium content), **pre-existing renal impairment (failure), myelomatosis** (because HOCM are more toxic & more protein binding possibly promoting renal tubular obstruction & renal failure d/t proteinaceous casts and precipitation of Bence Jones and Tamm Horsfall protein) and **hematological & metabolic conditions** (HOCM may l/t **fatal sickling in sickle cell anemia).**
- **LOCM are preferred contrast agents** especially if the patient has **preexisting renal impairment,** ***myelomatosis, cardiac disease and hematological & metabolic conditions like sickle cell anemia***[Q].

13. B i.e. Multiple Myeloma *[Ref: Sutton 7/e P-894]*

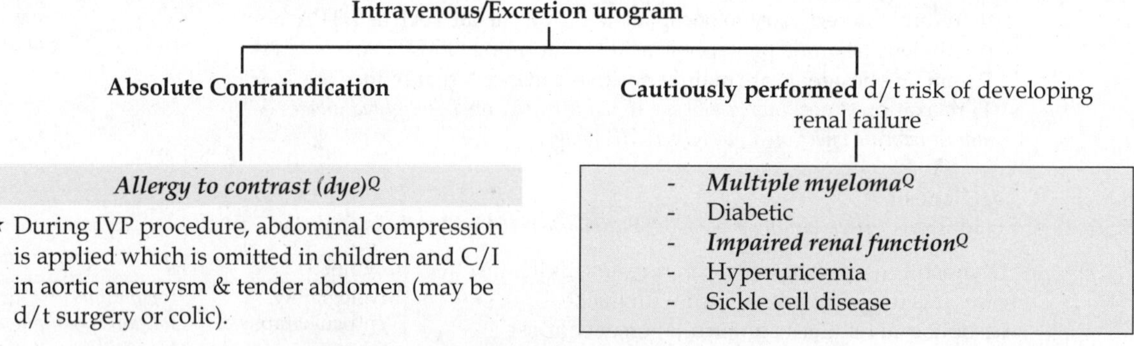

Intravenous/Excretion urogram
Absolute Contraindication
Cautiously performed d/t risk of developing renal failure
Allergy to contrast (dye)[Q]
★ During IVP procedure, abdominal compression is applied which is omitted in children and C/I in aortic aneurysm & tender abdomen (may be d/t surgery or colic).
- Multiple myeloma[Q]
- Diabetic
- Impaired renal function[Q]
- Hyperuricemia
- Sickle cell disease

Oral Chlecystography

14. C i.e. USG has replaced it; D i.e. Dye used is telepaque **15. B i.e. Motor mechanism of Gall bladdar**

[Ref: S. Das, text book 4/e P-892. Sutton 7/e P-718; Schwartz 7/e P-1443; Grainger 4/e P-1282; Bailey & Love 24/e P-1096]

Oral Cholecystography (Graham – Cole – Test)

- OCG was introduced in *1924* by *Graham & Cole.*
- ***Na/Ca-Iopanoic acid (Telepaque***[Q] / Biloptin/ Solubiloptine) dye is used as contrast media.
- ***3 gm***[Q] of dye is given & X Rays are taken at an interval of 12-15 hours.
- ***USG has replaced it***[Q].

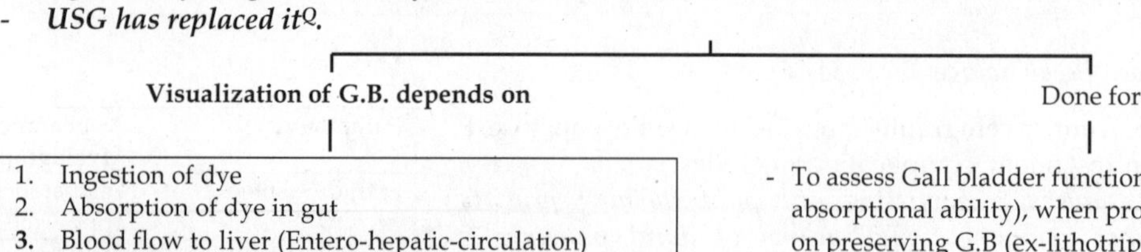

Visualization of G.B. depends on
1. Ingestion of dye
2. Absorption of dye in gut
3. Blood flow to liver (Entero-hepatic-circulation)
4. Take up in liver[Q] (functional liver)
Ability of liver to excrete dye into the bile[Q] (functional liver)
5. Ability of gall bladder to concentrate the excreted dye (by absorbing water[Q])
6. Patency of hepatic & cystic duct system[Q]
Done for

- To assess Gall bladder function (contractility, patency, absorptional ability), when proposed therapy is based on preserving G.B (ex-lithotripsy, gall stone dissolution)
- Gold standard for demonstrating gall stones in G.B.

Ultrasonography (USG)

16. **C i.e. Sonavist** *[Ref: Goldberg & Forsberg : US contrast agents basic principles & clinical approch 2/e p – 15 – 12]*

Ultrasound contrast agents (UCAs)

- It consists of microbubbles filled with air or gases, which acts as *echo – enhancer* by *increasing acoustic impedence at the interface b/w gas & blood.*
- The ideal USCA, should have:
  no biological effect with repeat doses.
  low : attenuation, blood gas solubility & diffusivity.
  high : echogenicity & ability to pass through pulmonary circulation.

A typical USCA has thin flexible /rigid shell of albumin /lipid/ polymer containing a gas such as N2/perfluro carbon. Some examples are:

Sona / Levo / Ima – vistQ (all IV)
Sona / Echo – gen (both IV)
Quanti / Opti – son (both IV)
Filmix, Omalex, Sonovue, Bisphere, Definity (all IV)
Sono Rx (oral), Myomap (IC)

17. **A i.e. Ultrosonograpphy** *[Ref. Christensen's 4/e p 328; Sutton 6/e P-12; Grainger 4/e P-102]*
18. **A i.e. MRI; B i.e. Doppler USG**

USG is based on ***piezoelectric effect***Q of lead-zirconate titanate and **MRI** is based on ***gyromagnetic property of proton (hydrogen nucleus)***Q. ***Both are associated with no risk of radiation exposure***Q.
Nuclear scans (Tc 99 scan) and digital substraction angiography encompass the risk of radiationQ.

Piezoelectric Effect

The ability of certain materials to change their physical dimensions when an electric voltage is applied to them. They are thus able to convert electric voltage to sound energy and vice-versa. This effect is ***used in ultrasonography to produce the ultrasound beam***Q. Piezoelectric crystals used now a days in USG is ***lead zirconate titanate***Q.

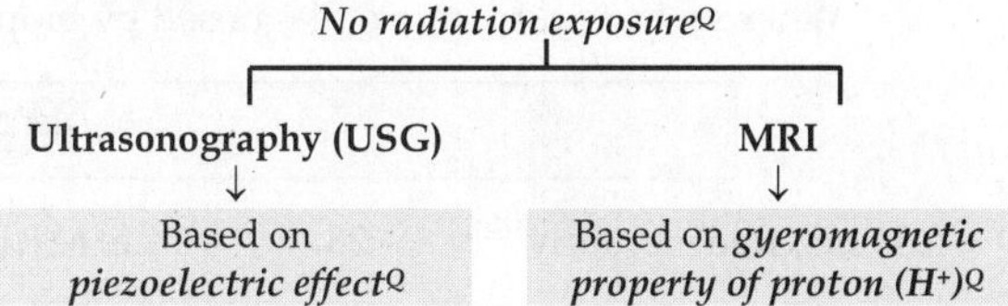

19. **C i.e. Reflection** *[Ref: Grainger 4/e P-53]*

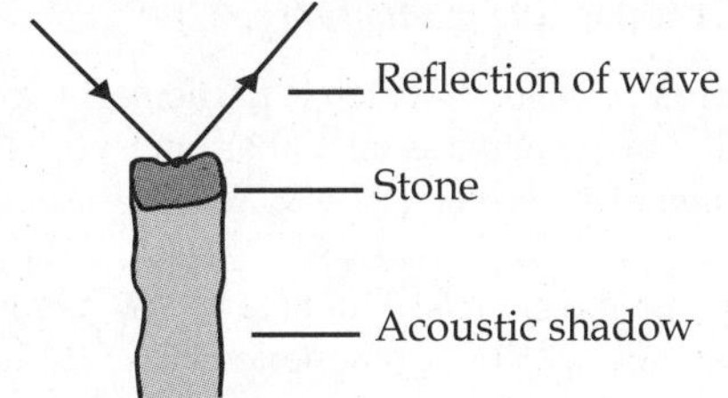

Shadowing occurs when little or no ultrasound can penetrate a structure and results in dark band over the deeper tissue. It may be d/t *reflection (by hard structure as stone)* or *absorption (fibrous tissue & fat* has higher than average absorption or attenuation as compared to surrounding tissue) of ultrasound.

USG Finding	Cause	Interpretation
Acoustic shadow	*Reflection*Q	• *Stone* (60% reflection) • *Tissue gas interface* (100% reflection so more dense shadow)
	Absorption or attenuation	• Fibrous tissue (ex behind scars, scirrhous breast C_A) • Fat (fatty liver)
Edge Shadows	*Refraction (deep to strongly curved surface)*	• Cysts • Fetal skull • Neck of gall bladder • Cooper's ligament of breast
Increased through transmission	Opposite to attenuation shadow (lesser absorption by the tissue as compared to surrounding)	The tissue has lower than average attenuation, so echoes from deeper tissues are over amplified (Brighter zone inspite of dark shadow of stone) *Hallmark of Cystic space.*

So don't get confused guys. The answer for this, Q is same but when more specific Q is asked, like cause of acoustic shadow in fatty liver or C_A breast or scar then the answer will be absorption or attenuation.

20. **A i.e. 1-20 MHz** 21. **B, C & D i.e. (Gall Stone), (Blunt abdominal trauma) & (Appendicitis)**
22. **B i.e. US** *[Ref: Sutton 7/e p. 650, 691, 684, 715, 967, 1791, 1039; Dutta-686]*

Type of USG	USG frequency
- Trans abdominal USG for obstetric purpose - Trans vaginal USG for obstetric purpose	*3-5 MHz*[Q] *5- 7.5 MHz*[Q]
- USG for breast - Endoscopic USG for gutwall - To image vessel wall via cathater	15 MHz 7.5 – 20 MHz 20 MHz

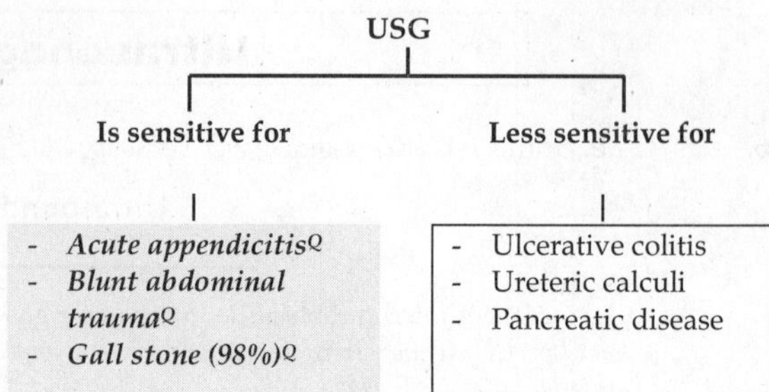

USG
Is sensitive for
Less sensitive for
- Acute appendicitis[Q]
- Blunt abdominal trauma[Q]
- Gall stone (98%)[Q]
- Ulcerative colitis
- Ureteric calculi
- Pancreatic disease

23. B i.e. Velocity of flow *[Ref: Sutton 7/e p. 460-72; Grainger 5/e p. 69-70]*

24. A i.e. Peripheral vascular disease; B i.e. Deep vein thrombosis; E i.e. Fetal abnormality

- **In color doppler, intensity (shades) of color represent velocity of flow** (paler color = highr velocity) and **color** itself **represent direction of flow (blue = away and red = towards transducer).**
- Color doppler can **identify stenosis,** ***occlusion, plaque, thrombus, aneurysm, varicosity, abnormal flow and measure diameter/cross sectional area reduction*** **and flow velocity** in **peripheral (extrimity), neck (carotid, vertebral), and major abdominal & pelvic vessels** as well as in **main cerebral arteries** (through trans cranial USG **in fetus, neonates ± adults).** In this way, it can ***diagnose peripheral vascular disease, deep vein thrombosis, intrauterine growth retardation and fetal abnormality***[Q].
- ***Pulmonary embolism and bone tumors can nnot be diagnosed by color doppler.*** PE is diagnosed by chest CT, lung scanning, pulmonary angiography, CR-MR & chest Xray; venous USG only helps in diagnosing DVT. Whereas bone tumors are diagnosed by biopsy, Xray & MRI.

MRI

25. D i.e., Radiography **26. B i.e. MRI** *[Ref: Grainger 4/e P-606; Mendith radiation physics]*

- ***Radiography use X-rays, which are ionizing radiation.***[Q]
- **Thermography** or **thermal imaging** is a type of ***infrared imaging***[Q]. Thermographic cameras detect radiation in the infrared range of the electromagnetic spectrum (roughly 900-14,000 nanometer or 0.9-14 μm)
- **MRI & USG** ***has no radiation risk***[Q].

27. B i.e. Proton Beam **28. A i.e. H^+ (proton)** **29. C i.e. 1.1 tesla** *[Ref: Sutton 7/e p. 17]*

- MRI is based on ***gyromagnetic property of proton (or hydrogen nucleus)***[Q], which is particularly favourable nucleus from MRI stand point and is present in virtually all biological material. Other nuclei of interest include- *carbon* (^{13}C), *phosphorus* (^{31}P), *Sodium* (^{23}Na), *Potassium* (^{39}K), *helium* (^{3}He) & *Xenon* (^{129}Xe) **(all have** ***odd number of protons or neutrons*** **& possess a** ***net charge*****).**
- **Magnetic field strength** used for clinical imaging currently range from ***0.02 Tesla (T) to 8T***[Q] as compared with **earth's magnetic field** of *0.5 Gauss*[Q]. According to old books, MRI use magnetic field of ***0.15 to 1.5 T (1,500 to 15,000 gauss).***
- M.C. contrast agent in MRI is ***Gadolinium DTPA***[Q].

30. D i.e. Calcified lesions **31. C i.e. MRI is better for calcified lesions**
[Ref: Hagg 5/e p 2195, 1189, 1194, 1420-22, 1939, 1916-17; Breast Imeging (AMPIS) 3/e p 530]

- **MRI is very poor in detection of calcification.** It is *inferior to CT scan, mammography and x-ray* in detecting calcification. That is why it ***lags behind mammography in early detection of noninvasive ductal carcinoma in situ (DCIS)***[Q], which most commonly has *microcalcification* as its only presenting feature. And similarly it has ***a very limited role in detection of renal stones and gall stones***[Q]. However, it is important to note that only upto 60% of gall stones have enough calcium density (more than that of bile) to get visualized on CT.
- Becaus of its **superior calcification detection abilities, MDCT** is used in **Agatston scoring (Coronary calcium scoring)** of *calcified plaques of coronary artery* using coronary calcium as a surrogate marker to detect the presence and measure the amount of coronary atherosclerosis. Because with *exception of patients with renal failure calcification of arteries occurs exclusively in context of atherosclerosis.*
- Similarly **nonenhanced helical CT** is ***superior to all other imaging modalities in diagnosis of urinary tract calculi***[Q] but at the cost of higher radiation exposure.
- Now there is no need to say that MRI is better that CT for evaluation of bone marrow, small brain lesions, meniscus/ ligament injuries, soft tissue tumors and meningeal pathology. But MRI is very poor in detection of calcification.

32. **A i.e. Pacemaker Wires** 33. **A i.e. Pacemaker; C i.e. Aneurysmal clip**

34. **A i.e. MRI** *[Ref: Grainger & Allison's 5/e p- 105; Harrison 16th/ 2353,2356]*

Common C/I of MRI are following-

- *Cardiac pacemakers*Q & internal defibrillatory device
- *Intracranial aneurysm clips*Q (some but not all)
- Cochlear prosthesis
- Bone growth & spinal cord stimulators
- Mc Gee stapedectomy piston prosthesis
- Omniphase penile implant
- Electronic infusion devices
- ***Ocular metallic foreign bodies*Q*/implants***
- Magnetic sphincters/stoma plug/dental implants
- Swan Ganz catheter
- Ferromagnetic IVC filters/Coils/Stents (safe after 6 weeks of implantation)
- Tatooed eyeliner

- **Ferromagnetic objects** mainly containing *iron, nickel or cobalt,* experience a force of attraction in magnetic field. So ***cardiac pace makers absolutely contraindicate the entery*Q *as*** do intracranial aneurysm clips of ferromagnetic / unknown composition.
- In very high fields (>1.5 T), mild *sensory stimulation* such as *visual magnetophospheres , balance alteration , unpleasant peripheral nerve stimulation , & acoustic noise (upto 108dBA)* may happen. *Energy deposition* d/t radio frequency field is expressed in *specific absorption rate (SAR) in watts /kg.* SAR have been set to limit tissue heating to <1°C *over 15 – min period;* to avoid burn.
- MR is not advised during 1st trimester (pregnancy) as a precautionary measure.

35. **A i.e. X-ray; B i.e. CT; E i.e. USG** *[Ref: A. K. Khurana 5/e p. 438-39]*

X-ray (eg limbal ring method), CT scan and ultrasonography (but not color doppler) can be used to detect and locate intraocular foreign body. **MRI is contraindicated** in this scenario.

36. **C i.e. Faraday Cage** 37. **B i.e. Faraday cage** *[Ref: - http://www.ezresult.com/article/faraday-cage]*

Faraday cage is an electrical apparatus designed ***to prevent the passage of electromagnetic waves*Q**, either containing them in or excluding them from its interior space.

Mu – Copper foils, which can be applied as wall paper for **electromagnetic shielding of rooms** (MRI Rooms, faraday chamber, computer rooms, EMC – test rooms, anechoic chambers etc), an existing room can be transformed easily into a ***Faraday cage*Q** with an attenuation level of **40 to 80 dB**
For magnetic shielding, monitor protection & shielding of transformers & cable trunks **MU- Ferro plates** are available.

38. **A i.e. Head and neck tumour; B i.e. Extremity** *[Ref: Sutton 7/ep 38, 830]*

- **CT is better for thorax and retroperitoneum because CT is less sensitive to patient's, respiratory motions**Q **(as it is performed much more rapidly than MRI)** and the soft tissues in thorax & retroperitoneum are larger and easily discriminable.
- **MRI is better than CT for head & neck, spine and extremity soft tissue lesions (such as tumors, arthritis, AVN, ligament-tendon injuries, spinal cord injury, bone marrow involvement)** because MRI depicts anatomy in greater detail, has much greater range of availabe soft tissue contrast and is more sensitive & specific. The soft tissues in these parts are not moved during respiratory movements so MRI can be easily performed and provides greater anatomical, details (than CT), which is mostly required in head, neck, spine, extremities and joints.

CT- Scan

39. **D i.e. Attenuation coefficient** 40. **A i.e. Water**

41. **C i.e. Fat; D i.e. Blood** 42. **A i.e. Lead**

43. **C i.e. Bone – algorithm for image reconstruction** 44. **A i.e. Tomography**

[Ref: Farr's 2/ep 103-118; Thaylan 1/e p 214; Christensen's 4/ep 289-322; Haga 5/e p7; Sutton 7/e p 30-32, 1723-24; Grainger 5/e p 187-93]

- **Hounsfield units (CT number)** represent ***average linear attenuation coefficient*Q**. The Hounsfield scale is an arbitray one with ***air at-1000 and water at 0 units as fixed points*Q**. **Fat** which is less dense than water also has a **negative value (- 20 to – 100 range).**
- **CT** has been designated *a high dose procedure* as it exposes 50-500 times higher radiation doses than a conventional radiograph. ***Lead shielding or coating (1/16 inch) is most common way of protection*Q**. Other protective agents include *concrete* (4-6 inch standard density i.e. 147 pounds/cubic foot), *brick blocks and barium plaster.*
- ***Narrow beam collimation, high spatial reconstruction algorhythm like bone algorhythm and small field of view improve spatial resolution of HRCT*Q.**

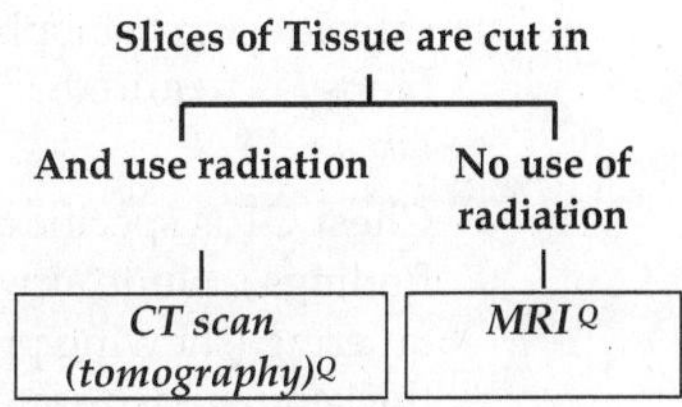

RADIODIAGNOSIS 5

45. **B. i.e. In pediatrics patient dose should be reduced**
[Ref: Essential physics of medical imaging 2/e p. 23-24; Christensen's 4/e p. 317-318]

Because ionizing radiation causes more biological effect in children, it is important to adapt CT technical parameters to minimize radiation doseQ.

CT Dose index (CTDI)

- ***Is most common parmeter to estimate and minimize patient dose in CT***Q.
- Integrates the dose delivered both within & beyond the scan volume.

Factors that influence radiation dose from CT:

KVp (Kilovoltage)	- has ***nonlinear relationship with radiation dose***Q - An ↑ ***in 120-130 KVp can double radiation dose***Q.
Tube current (mAs)	- has *linear relationship* with radiation dose - ↑ *mAs by 50% : ↑es radiation twice*
Pitch (Slice thickness/Table speed)	- is *inversely proportional* to radiation dose.

46. **C i.e. CT Scan** *[Ref: Grainger 5/e p. 164]*

- Patient's radiation exposure for fluoroscopy & radiography are measured by *DAP (dose area product) meter and thermo-luminesent dosimeters (TLDs).* The DAP meter measures the product of dose exiting the x-ray tube (D) and the area (A) of x-ray tube, which d/t inverse square law is the same as the product of the dose at the entrance surface of patient and the area of tissue irradiated. Which means as the patient goes away from tube the dose decreases (D/2) in same proportion as the area increases (2A); so DAP remains DXA.
- TLD_5 measures *entrance surface dose (ESD)*, suitable for single view radiography. ESD can also be calculated based on knowledge of x-ray out put from quality assurance measurement & individual exposure factors.
- The radiation exposure in decreasing order is ***CT abdomen or pelvis > CT chest > Barium enema***Q > Dynamic cardiac ^{99m}Tc scan > PET head 18FDG > ***Bone ^{99m}Tc scan***Q >Barium follow through > Barium meal > **IVU (intravenous urogram) > CT head > Barium swallow** > Thyroid ^{99M}Tc = Kidney ^{99M}Tc = Lung perfusion ^{99M}Tc scan > X-ray lumbar spine > X-ray thoracic spine = Abdomen = pelvis > X-ray hip > Lung ventilation ^{133}Xe scan > X-ray skull > **Xray chest PA > Xray limbs & joints (except hip)**. The **MRI and USG** have no radiation exposure.
- But if we dont specifig & speak broadly the decreasing order can be said as : **CT scan > Barium enema > Dynamic cardiac scan > PET > Bone scan > IVU > Xray**. However, it is important to note that CT scan head has lesser radiation exposure than IVU.
- CT abdomen or pelvis exposes to a dose of 10 mSv which is equivalent to 500 chest Xrays or 4.5 years of background exposure; bone scan exposes to 4 mSv (200 Xray chest or 1.5 yr background exposure); CT head (2 mSv, 100 Xray chest or 10 month be) ; chest Xray (0.02 mSv equivalent to 3 days of be) and Xray limbs (<0.01 mSv, < 0.5 Xray chest or < 1.5 day be).

47. **B i.e. Interstitial Lung disease**
[Ref: Harrison 18/e p. 2118, 2095, 2143-67; Armstrong -5381 Grainger 5/e p. 192]

- **Routine chest CT** examinations consist of adjacent *8-10 mm sections* through the area of interest. Intravenous contrast medium may be injected when the primary purpose of examination is to show the mediastinum or hilar structures. **High resolution CT (HRCT)** uses very thin *1-2 mm **thick.***Q
- **High resolution chest CT (HRCT chest)** is the ***procedure of choice for hyper sensitivity pneumonitis (HP) or extrinsic allergic alveolitis***Q such as farmer's / mushroom worker's / bird fancier's / chemical worker's / hot tub / coffee worker's etc – lung.
- HRCT – chest is superior to plain Xray chest for early detection and confirmation of suspected ***interstial lung disease (ILD)***Q such as fibrosing alveolitis, lymphangitic carcinoma, idiopathic pulmonary fibrosis, sarcoidosis, eosinophilic granuloma, asbestosis, berylliosis and other industrial lung diseases etc. When lung biopsy is required, HRCT is useful for determining *most appropriate area from which biopsy sample should be taken.*
- **Chest CT** is specific and ***imaging modality of choice for confirming diagnosis of bronchiectasis***Q. CT findings include airway dilation (detected as **"parallel tram tracks"** or **"signet ring sign"**), lack of bronchial tapering (showing presence of tubular structure within 1 cm from pleural surface), bronchial wall thickening, inspissated secretions (**tree-in-bud pattern**), or cysts originating from bronchial wall.
- **Helical CT scanning** allows collection of continuous data over a larger volume of lung during a single breath holding maneuver (faster scan with improved contrast enhancement & thinner collimation) that

allows less motion artifact. Data from single imaging procedure can be reconstructed as images in planes other than the traditional axial (cross-sectional) view, including coronal, or saggital planes or even **3D representation (virtual bronchoscopy)** mimicking visualization through a bronchoscope.

- **Multidetector CT (MDCT)** uses higher number of detectors (upto 64) along scanning (Z) axis to obtain multiple slices in a single rotation that are *thinner and can be acquired in a shorter period of time, resulting in enhanced resolution and increased image reconstruction ability*. Shorter breath holds are especially beneficial for *children, elderly and critically ill patients*, however, at the risk of increased radiation dose. MDCT has led to improved imaging of *pulmonary vasculature* and the *ability to detect segmental & subsegmental emboli*. In contrast to pulmonary angiography, **CT pulmonary angiography (CTPA)** by MDCT usually allows simultaneous detection of parenchymal abnormalities; and has rapidly become the ***test of choice in evaluation of pulmonary embolism***Q (b/o equal accuracy and less risk in comparison to pulmonary angiography).

Colonography & Virtual colonoscopy

48. **A i.e. Provide endoluminal view, C i.e. CT and MRI use; D i.e. Used even when conventional colonoscopy fails; E i.e. Used for screening of ca colon**
[Ref: Peter Armstrong 5/e p 170, 186; AMPIS 3/e p 167-69, Haga 5/e p 1320-31; Grainger 5/ep 680-81]

Virtual colonoscopy is computer reconstructed three dimensional ***(3D) display of (endoluminal view) of CT or MRI-colonography***Q. It can be used even when ***conventional colonoscopy or barium enema has failed or can not be done, as a screening tool for colorectal cancer***Q.
But the main ***disadvantage is that the biopsy (samples) cannot be taken***Q, as there is no real colonoscope in the lumen.

Computer Radiology

49. **C i.e. Picture archiving communication system** *[Ref: Sutton 7/e p. 1841-43]*

- **Picture archiving & communication system (PACS)** makes *hospitals filmless*; as it uses *digital imaging modalities like ultrasound, CT, MRI and digital x-ray (rather than traditional x ray films).*
- **Electronic patient record (EPR)** or **Electronic medical record (EMR)** accommodate electronic patient case notes, discharge summaries, clinical letters & prescription data.
- **Hospital or clinical information system (HIS/CIS) or patient administration system (PAS)** is a computer system holding data such as patient demographics (name, address, family doctor name, hospital number, other personal information), neumerical results from laboratory tests (biochemistry, bacteriology), virology, immunology, haematology), and reports of clinical investigations (endoscopy, bronchoscopy, biopsy) as well as scheduling information eg out patent clinic appointments, hospital admissions, bed state & occupancy and patient discharge information. It is the *most important system of hospital & major part of EPR.*
- **Remote requesting system (RRS) / Remote order entery and order communications (order comms)** is an electronic means of requesting & booking investigations from a remote location eg. wards, OPD etc.
- **Radiological information system (RIS)** is responsible for scheduling & booking examinations in various rooms within the imaging department. It serves as repository of radiological reports once they have been typed.
- **Digital imaging and communication in medicine (DICOM) & Health level 7 (HL7).**

2 SYSTEMIC RADIODIAGNOSIS I: NEUROLOGY & NEPHROLOGY

These chapters also include complete description of pathology, medicinal & surgical aspects of relevant topics

CENTRAL NERVOUS SYSTEM

Amyotrophic Lateral Sclerosis (Motor Neuron Disease: MND)

Pathology

- **Pathological hallmark** of MND is **death of lower motor neurons** (LMN consisting of **anterior horn cell** in spinal cord & their brainstem homologues innervating bulbar muscles) and **upper (corticospinal) motor neurons** (UMN, originating in *layer 5 of motor cortex & descending via the pyriamidal tract* to synapse with LMN, either directly or indirectly via interneurons).
- In ALS, the motor neuron *cytoskeleton* is affected early l/t frequent *focal enlargements (spheroid* composed of accumulation of neurofilaments & other proteins). The affected *motor neuron undrgoes shrinkage with accumulation of lipofuscin* (=pigmented lipid that normally develop with advancing age) and *proliferation of astroglia & microglia* (inevitable accompaniment of all CNS degenerative process).
- Due to loss of cortical motor neurons, there is **thinning of corticospinal tracts** (that travel via *internal capsule, brainstem, and lateral & anterior white matter columns of spinal cord*). The loss of fibers in lateral column & resulting fibrillary gliosis imparts a particular **firmness (lateral sclerosis)**.
- As *denervation progresses* (d/t death of motor neurons and less reinnervation, in comparison to polio & peripheral neuropathy, by nearby nerve), *muscle atrophy* (i.e. **amyotrophy**) is recognized on clinical examination & muscle biopsy.
- **Selectivity of neuronal cell death** is a remarkable feature. On light microscopy, the **entire sensory apparatus, regulatory mechanisms for control & coordination of movement**, and components of brain needed for **cognitive processes** remain intact. Within the motor system there is some selectivity of involvement – therefore, **motor neurons required for ocular motality** and **parasympathetic neurons is sacral spinal cord (the nucleus of onufrowicz or Onuf) that innervate the spincter of bowel and bladder** remain unaffected. However, immunostaining & glucose metabolism studies indicate neuronal dysfunction of nonmotor neurons also.

Classification of MNDs (on the basis of involvement)

Both UMN & LMN	More UMN	Predominant LMN
- *Amyotrophic lateral sclerosis*[Q]	- *Primary lateral sclerosis (PLS)* - Familial spastic paraplegia (FSP) - Pseudobulbar palsy	- **Progressive mucular atrophy (spinal muscular atrophy = SMA)** - Bulbar palsy - Multifocal motor neuropathy with condiction block - Motor neuropathy with paraproteinemia or cancer - Motor predominant peripheral neuropathies

Clinical Features

- Manifestations of ALS are *variable depending on whether UMN (corticospinal tract) or LMN (anterior horn cell) are more predominently involved.*
- **Predominant /early LMN** involvement causes insidious development of **asymmetric weakness** (initially usually first evident distally in one of the limbs, a/w *cramping* (caused by volitional movements), **progressive wasting and atrophy of muscles** and spontaneous **twitching of motor units** or **fasciculations.**
- LMN involvement of bulbar (rather than limb) muscles causes *difficulty with chewing, swallowing and movements of face and tongue. Early involvement of respiratory muscles l/t death* before the disease is far advanced elsewhere.
- With **prominent corticospinal UMN involvement**, there is *hyperactivity of muscle stretch reflexes (**exaggerated tendon jerks**) and often spastic resistance to passive movements* of affected limb (**spastacity**). Patients complain of **muscle *stiffness*** *often out of proportion to weakness.* Degeneration of **cortico-bulbar UMN** projections innervating the brainstem result in **dysarthria** and **exaggeration of motor expressions of emotions** (l/t *involuntary excess in weeping or laughing* =**pseudobulbar affect**).
- Virtually any muscle group may be first involved but *ultimately* the disorder takes on a *symmetrical distribution in all regions.* Although at its onset ALS may predominantly /selectively involve UMN or LMN but it is *characteristic of ALS that both will eventually be involved.*
- ***Sensory, bladder-bowel and cognitive functions are preserved***[Q], even in the late stages of ALS. **Ocular motility is spared**, even when there is severe brainstem disease. **Dementia** does not occur in sporadic ALS. However, *in familial ALS, fronto-temporal dementia may be co-inherited.*
- A/t CWFN guidelines, essential criteria for diagnosis of ALS is **simultaneous upper & lower motor neuron involvement with progressive weakness** & exclusion of all, alternative diagnoses. The ALS is ranked *definite (when* 3 or 4)/probable (when 2)/ possible (when 1) of the following site are involved: **bulbar, cervical, thoracic and lumbo-sacral motor neurons**. An exception is made for those who have progressive upper & lower motor neuron signs at only one site and a *mutation in gene encoding superoxide dismutase (SOD1).*
- **Familial ALS (FALS)** is AD trait that is clinically indistinguishable fromsporadic ALS. It occur d/t *mutation in gene encoding cytoplasmic enzyme SOD1 (most common) > RNA binding protein TDP-43* (encoded by TAR-DNA binding protein gene) and FUS/TLS (fused in sarcoma/translocated in liposarcoma) >> *vesicle binding protein, senataxin (helicase) > dynactin,* a cellular accessory motor protein (predominantly LMN disease with early hoarseness) > *alsin,* a guanine exchange factor (predominantly UMN disease that starts in first decade). *Kennedy's disease (androgen receptor defect), hexominase deficiency and Pompe's disease (infantile α-glucosidase deficiency)* are other causes of hereditary MND that may mimic ALS.
- **T2WI (MRI)** reveal ***abnormal high signal intensity within corticospinal /cortico-bulbar tracts***[Q] representing an increase in water content in myelin tracts udergoing Wallerian degeneration secondary to cortical motor neuron loss. It is commonly present in *ALS* but can also be seen in *AIDS related encephalopathy, infarction* or other disese processes that produce corticospinal neuronal loss in symmetric fashion.

Multiple Sclerosis (MS)

Demyelinating disorder characterized by inflammation & ***selective destruction of CNS myelin predominantly of white matter long tracts***[Q]. Characteristic pathological triad include – inflammation, demyelination & gliosis (scarring).

Pathogenesis

- Perivenular cuffing with inflammatory T cells and macrophages, which also infiltrate the surrounding **white matter**
- At site of Inflammation, **BBB** is **disrupted**
- Myelin specific auto antibodies promote **demyelination** & stimulate macrophages & microglial cells.
- As lesion evolves, Astrocytes proliferates (**gliosis**)

Clinical Presentation

- Age of onset is between **20 & 40 years** (slightly later in men) with a **F:M ratio of 3:1**. Course is *relapsing/remitting/progressive*.
- **Sensory symptoms** include *paresthesia* (eg tingling, prickling, formications, pins & needles, or painful burning), *unplesant sensations* (feelings that body parts are swollen, raw, wet or tightly wrapped), *pain and hypesthesia* (reduced sensation, numbness or dead feelings).
- **Weakness of muscles** may mainfest as *loss of strength, speed, or dexterity, as fatigue or gait disturbance*, Exercise induced weakness is characteristic symptoms of MS. Weakness is of UMN type and is usually a/w the signs of pyramidal signs. **Spasticity** is commonly seen with *painful muscle spasms*.
- **Optic neuritis** presents as *decreased visual acuity and color perception* (desaturation) in central field of vision and rearely complete loss of light perception. The symptoms are generally monocular, preeded/accompanied by *periorbital pain (aggerevated by eye movements)* and accompanying afferent pupillary defect, papilliti and ultimately optic atrophy.
- **Diplopia** (double vision) may result from *internuclear opthalmoplegia (INO)* of cranial nerve (6 >3, 4) palsy. INO consists of *impaired adduction* of one eye (d/t *ipsilateral medial longitudinal fasciculus lesion*) often a/w prominent nystagmus & small skew deviation of abducting eye. Gaze disturbances common in MS include *bilateral INO horizontal gaze palsy, one & a half syndrome* (horizontal gaze palsy and INO), and acquired pendular nystagmus.
- *Visual blurring*, ataxia, *bladder dysfunction* (eg detrusor hyper reflexia, detrusor sphincter dyssynergia occurs in >90%), *constipation, cognitive dysfunction*, depression, fatigue, facial weakness, vertigo, *sexual dysfunction* (like decreased libido/sensation, impotence in men and decreased lubrication or adductor spasm in women).
- Heat sensitivity (eg visual blurring d/t hot shower/ exercise = **Unthoff's symptom**), Lhermitte's symptom, **paroxysmal symptoms** (high frequency i.e. 5-40/day, brief duration i.e. 10 s-2 min), trigeminal neuralgia, hemifacial spasm, glossopharyngeal neuralgia & facial myokymia (rapid flickering).

Diagnosis of MS

- It requires **≥2 episodes** of **symptoms** and **≥2signs** that reflect pathlogy in **anatomically non contiguous white matter tracts** of the CNS.
- Symptoms must **last for >24hr** and occurs as distinct episode that are **seperated by ≥1month**.
- **At least 1 sign** must be present on **neurological** examination and the **other may be** documented by

MRI Findings

- MRI has revolutionized the diagnosis & management of MS. Characteristic abnormalities are found in **>95%** of patients, although **>90%** of lesions visualized by MRI are asymptomatic.
- Early MS lesions show **gadolinium (Gd) enhancement** d/t increased vascular permeability caused by inflammatory breakdown of BBB. Such *leakage of IV-Gd into parenchyma* occurs early, severs as a marker of inflammation and persists for 1 month; and residual MS plaque remains visible indefinitely as a focal area of **hyper intensity** (a lesion) **on spin echo (T_2WI) and proton density images.**
- Lesions are frequently oriented ***perpendicular to the ventricular surface,*** corresponding to the pathological pattern of previous **demyelination (Dawson's fingers).** Lesions are **multifocal** within the brain, brainstem & spinal cord. **Lesions >6mm** located in **corpus callosum, periventricular white matter, brain stem, cerebellum, or spinal cord (i.e. juxtacortical, periventricular, infratentorial or spinal cord) are MS- typical lesion- locations** (regions) and perticularly helpful diagnostically.
- Total volume of T2W signal abnormality **(burden of disease)** shows a significant correlation with clinical disability, as do brain atrophy.

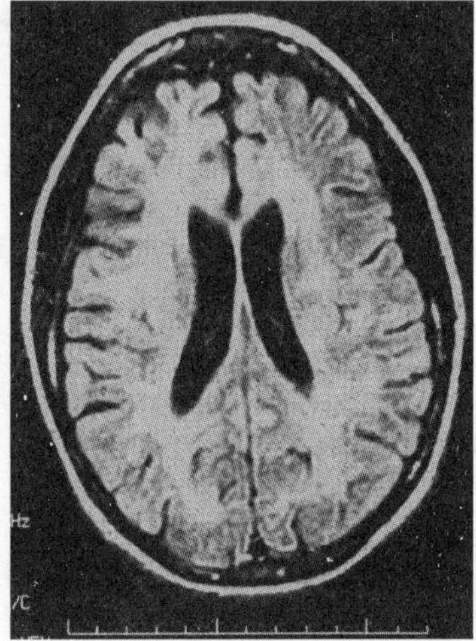

Multiple Sclerosis as shown of a FLAIR MR image

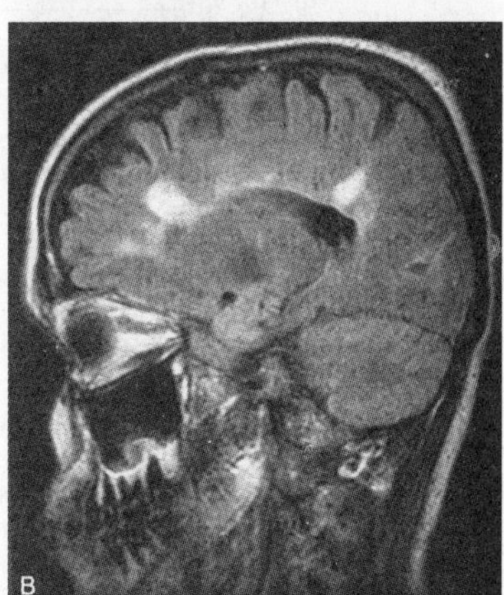

Parasagittal FLAIR MR image

- Few (1/3rd) T2W lesios appear as **black holes** (*hypointense lesions*) on T1WI, which may be a marker of irreversible demyelination & axonal loss.
- Magnetization transfer ratio (**MTR**) imaging & proton magnetic response spectroscipic imaging (**MRSI**) may ultimately serve as *surrogate marker of clinical disability*. MRSI *may differentiate demyelination from edema* and can quantitate molecules such as *N-acetyl aspartate, which is a marker of axonal integrity*.

Evoked Potentials (EP)

- EP testing of *visual, auditory, somatosensory or efferent/motor-CNS pathways* provide most information. When the pathways studied are clinically uninvolved
- It *is not specific* to MS, although *a marked delay in latency* of a specific EP component (as opposed to reduced amplitude or distorted wave shape) is suggestive of demyelination.

abnormal paraclinical tests such as **MRI or EPs**

- A/t most recent diagnostic scheme, **the 2nd clinical episode** (event in time) may be supported by *paraclinical test usually* development of new *focal white matter lesions on MRI.*
- *In insidious / gradual neurological progression of disabiity for ≥6 months* without superimposed relapse, documentation of ***intrathecal IgG synthesis may be used to support the diagnosis*** Q ***(assessed by presence of oligoclonal banding or CSF-IgG index)*** Q.

CSF

- Mononuclear cell pleocytosis and **an increased level of intrathecally synthesized IgG** (assessed by **oligoclonal banding/OCB** &/or **CSF-IgG index**). CSF IgG index expresses the ratio of IgG to albumin in CSF divided by the same ratio in serum. 2 or more OCB on agarose gel electrophoresis are found in >75-90% MS patients.
- Pleocytosis of >75 cells / μL, presence of polymorphonuclear leukocytes or protein concentration >1gm/L should raise concern that diagnosis is not MS.

Leukodystrophies & Disorders of White Matter

- **White matter** abnormalities are described in terms of *location* (lobar involvement, centrifugal or centripetal distribution & A-P gradient), *juxtacortical U fiber involvement, deep white matter* involvement *such as internal capsule, corpus callosum & pyramidal tract* as it decends from motor strip (precentral gyrus) through posterior limb of internal capsule and cerebral peduncles to the decussation within medulla & then into spinal cord.
- **Grey matter** assessment include analysis of *cerebral & cerebellar cortex , basal ganglia,* thalmi, and *deep grey structures such as red neuclei , subthalmic and dentate nuclei.*
- **Macrocephaly** is seen in – **G**M-2 gangliosidosis (Tay sachs disease), **g**lutaric acid uria type 1, L-2 hydroxy – **g**lutaric aciduria, **A**lexanders leuko encephalopathies, **M**egalencephalic Leukodystrophy with subcortical cyst (**M**LC), **C**anavan's (spongiform) Leuko dystrophy. Mn – "**GAMC**"
- Myelination is energy dependent. So hypomyelination is also seen in *developmental delay, cardiorespiratory illness & metabolic disorder.*

Dysmyelinating

Where there is *abnormal formation or maintenance* of myelin.

X- Linked leukodystrophies

- **Adrenoleuko dystrophy (ALD)**
  - It affects *boys aged 4- 10 years* & presents with learning difficulties, behaviour problems, impaired visuospatial perception , deteriorating gait, progressing to ataxia, dementia, cortical blindness, spasticity & adrenal insufficiency.
  - Involvement of *parieto – occipital regions and thin serrated or curvilinear rim of contrast enhancement* at leading edge of demyelination, representing perivascular inflammation.
  - ***Posterior central white matter, (specifically splenium & peritrigonal*** w.m. progressing to cortico spinal tracts visual & auditory pathways) showing low attenuation (density) on CT low signal on T_1 image and high signal (hype intensity) in T_2 weighted MRI.
  - Dystrophic calcification in affected white matter
- **Aelrenomyeloneuropathy**

• Alexander's disease

- *Sporadic leukodystrophy* characterized histopathologically by abundant ***presence of Rosenthal fibers*** *in affected brain.* So definitive diagnosis depends on *biopsy*
- *Extensive , bilateral (± symmetrical) deep & subcortical* white matter abnormality ***begining in & predominantly involving frontal & periventricular white matter*** Q
- Large cystic cavities in frontal & temporal regions
- *Basal ganglion* involvement (some)
- *Contrast enhancement along ventricular ependyma, periventricular area & caudate nuclei.*

• Krabbe's disease (globoid leukodystrophy)

- ***Increased density in basal ganglia & thalmus*** Q
- Hypodensity of white matter. White matter

• Metachromatic Leukodystrophy

- *Confluent & symmetrical hypodensity in deep & peripheral supratentorial white matter in CT*
- *Widespread* low density in white matter in T_2 (w) MR.

• MLC

- ***Bilaterl symmetrical involvement of globus pallidus with sparing of thalmi & rest of basal ganglia*** Q
- Cerebral cortex is normal
- *B/L T_2 hyperintensity* showing palladial involvement is also seen in *Kernicterus, Co poisoning,LHGA, GAMT (guanidino acetate methyl transferase deficiency) &* ***Kearns – Sayer syndrome.***
- However, in Kearns – Sayer syndrome hyper intensity is also present in *caudate nucleus, thami, cerebellar dentate nuclei,* frontal white matter & dorsal midbrain.

• L-2 hydroxyglutarica-ciduria *(LHGA)*

- Peripheral white matter involvement *particularly subcortical U fibers,*

Demyelinating (Myelinoclastic)

Where there is *destruction of normally* formed myelin.

Multiple Sclerosis

- Sites of involvement are ***periventricular white matter (commonest)***, optic pathway, juxta cortical, subcortical U fibers, infratentorial (brain stem, cerebellar white matter & peduncle, spinal cord).
- Typical lesions are *periventricular nodular hyperintense ovoid lesions* on T_2 images with *long axis oriented perpendicular to ventricle wall.*
- Lesions of *corpus callosum (at calloseptal interface & subcallosal striation)* are characteristic & best shown on FLAIR images
- Infratentorial lesions are best seen in T_2 imaging
- Lesions show solid or ring enhancement with IV gadolinium (upto 3 months) and reduced magnetic transfer ratio (MTR) reflecting decreased levels of myelin.
- Disbility correlates better with number of low signal lesion on T_1 weighted MRI (black holes) and poorly with T_2W lesions.
- MRI has 100% accuracy & ***demonstrates lesion disseminated in time*** (i.e.,

Schilder's disease (diffuse sclerosis)

- Histologically, lesions are similar to MS, but are more extensive, continuously progressive & fulminant rather than intermittent & relapsing.
- ***Main lesions extend through corpus callosum into both parieto – occipital regions,*** and enlarge progressively but not symmetrically.

Marchiafava – Bignami disease

- ***Corpus callosum*** is mainly affected and other central pathways may be involved.
- Associated with *chronic alcoholism,* & chronic cyanide intoxication produce similar lesions.

Central pontine myelinosis

- ***Pontine white matter*** is primarily

- Variant of ALD, more commonly involving *cerebellum* & less frequently cerebral hemisphere.
- **Pelizaeus – Merzbacher disease**
- T2 images show more severe hypomyelination as compared to T_1 images
- Considerable atrophy

changes are more severe ***posteriorly & centrally***
- ***Involve cerebellar white matter (sparing dentate nuclei) and pyramidal tact within brain stem***[Q].

internal, external & extreme capsules with a slight frontal predominance, and sparing periventricular white matter & corpus callosum.
- Grey matter involvement ***affecting basal ganglia and sparing thalami***[Q]

detection of new lesion 30 days & /or gadolinium enhancement 3 months apart) and ***disseminated in space*** (i.e., at least 1 periventricular / Juxtacortical / or infratentorial lesion & 1 gadolinium enhancing or 9 T2 hyperintense lesion).

involved. CT shows low density in advanced lesion and there is increase in T1 & T2 on MRI.
- *Midbrain, thalmi and subcortical white matter* may be involved.

- **Leigh's Disease (mitochondrial disorder)**
- *Bilateral typically symmetrical signal change within brainstem, deep cerebellar grey matter, subthalmic nuclei & basal ganglia* (hyper intensity in T2 & coronal FLAIR)
- **Panda face** is *midbrain* changes with involvement of *substentia nigra & tegmentum*
- Medulla is frequently involved.

Mesial Temporal Sclerosis (MTS)

- MTS refers to marked neuronal loss and gliosis of hippocampus/mesial temporal lobe, caused by long standing temporal lobe epilepsy.
- This is considered to be the most common cause of temporal lobe epilepsy which results from generation of an epileptogenic focus from reorganization of neuronal pathways.

Mechanism of Excitotoxicity induced neuronal death

Seizure → excessive neuronal depolarization → over production of excitatory aminoacid NT → excessive activation of NMDA receptors → unregulated entery of Ca^{++} → neuronal swelling with cytotoxic edema.

MRI features include

- Mesial temporal sclerosis can now be accurately predicted by MRI.
- *Decreased volume of hippocampus* **(*Hippocampus atrophy*)** *and increased signal intensity on T2WI*[Q] compared to contralateral side.

Associated limbic system finding

- ***Atrophy of fornix***[Q] (ipsilateral) – 55%
- ***Atrophy of mamillary body***[Q] (ipsilateral) – 26%
- *Atrophy of amygdala and ipsilateral parahippocampal white matter tract*

Associated extrahippocampal abnormality

- *Small temporal lobe*
- *Enlarged temporal horn*
- Increased signal intensity of anterior temporal lobe cortex (38%)
- Cerebral hemiatrophy (1%)

Intracranial Vascular Malformations

Arterio-Venous Malformations

- **AVM** represents a *direct communication between dilated feeding arteries and tortuous veins without intervening capillaries.* The communicating vascular channels k/a **nidus** is larger then capillaries yet smller than fistula, represents the *central compact closely packed recemose tangle of pathological low resistance vessels constituting the junction of feeding arteries & draining veins.* The nidus does not contain normal brain parenchyma and has no mass effect, although the enlarged feeding arteries & draining veins can traverse normal tissue.
- The AVM nidus volume, presence of fistulas, the chronicity of lesons (age of patient) and flow rate determine the size & tortuosity of feeding arteries & draining veins.
- **Spetzler & Martin AVM grading system** is based on the size of nidus (<3 cm=1; 3-6 = 2; >6 cm = 3), the location of nidus in relation to eloquent functional brain (=1; noneloquent=0) and the venous drainage (superficial=0; deep =1)
- It is focal collection of *mixed density (iso/hyper) irregular lesion* which shows occasional calcification (25-30%), surrounding edema, mass effect or adjacent brain atrophy on NE-CT. Typical **bag of worms appearance** or **dense serpentine/serpiginous enhancement** is seen in contrast enhanced (CE)-CT.
- *Non contrast-MRI is the investigation of choice,* which can demonstrate nidus, evaluate its size and identify

Cavernous Angioma

- Cavernous angioma (hamangioma) or cavernoma is a benign vascular malformation that is composed of *well circumscribed, nonencapsulated compact or racemose (honey-comb like) network* of multiple endothelium lined, sinusoidal, nonuniform vascular channels containing *thrombosed blood of varying age.* The endothelium demonstrates large intercellular gaps, fenestrations & internal vesicles. Compartment walls contain no basement membrane or muscularis or elastic lamina layers or intervening (interposed) brain tissue and are irregularly thickened with collagen, hyalin & calcium deposition.
- MRI typically demonstrates a mass characterized as **"popcorn" in appearance** owing to the *varying ages of internal hemorrhages* (also k/a) **variegated or inhomogenous reticulated appearance or mulberry shaped lesion**). The low signal peripheral rim that completely surrounds the lesion is typical with cavernous angiomas and is produced by hemosiderin & ferritin residua of previous (chronic) hemorrhage. It is seen in T2 weighted spin echo or fast/turbo spin echo and *blooms (or becomes more prominent)* on **T2 weighted gradient echo studies**. So this should always be performed as in few cases it may be the only imaging study that identifies cavernous angioma. The hemosiderin & ferritin may cause a **dark flaring appearance** extending into adjacent brain parenchyma because macrophage & astrocytes remove these & other blood breakdown products along white matter fibers.
- On MRI typical **mulberry shaped mixed density lesion** is caused by *extracellular methemoglobin /slow blood flow /thrombosis* producing **increased signal intensity** and *intracelular methemoglobin /deoxyhemoglobin /hemosiderin /ferittin /fibrin /collagen /calcification*

5

RADIODIAGNOSIS

supplying arteries & draining veins, and is crucial for localized the AVM in relation to eloquent cortex. The nidus vessels demonstrate flow / signal void on spin echo or fast/turbo-spin echo pulse sequences and bright signal intensity (hyperintense) on gradient echo sequences. **Diffusion tensor tractography** (an MRI technique) is used to confirm AVM involvement of nearby white matter tracts.

- MR perfusion imaging, PET & SPECT scintigraphy can illustrate AVM steal phenomena.

*producing **decreased signal intensity***.

- Cavernomas are k/a **cryptic** or **occult vascular malformations** because of *negative angiography*; which lacks a **Medusa head pattern** of *dilated medullary veins coverging in an enlarged transcortical collector draining vein with* normal arterial phase & late capillary blush seen in *venous angiomas* (Medusa is Greek god whose hair was turned into a mass of hissing snake); or *a tightly packed mass of enlarged feeding arteries and dilated tortuous draining veins with little or no intervening brain parenchyma (no mass effect) with in the AVM nidus*. (i.e. dilated arteries feeding and tortuous vein draining the definite nidus) seen in parenchymal or pial true arteriovenous malformations (AVMs).

Vein of Galen Malformation (VOGM)

Etio-Pathology

- Vein of Galen (great cerebral vein) is large deep vein at the base of brain that curves posteriorly under the splenium of corpus callosum. It is located under cerebral hemisphere & drains anterior & central regions of brain into sinuses of posterior cerebral fossa. ***It unites with inferior sagital sinus to form the straight sinus***Q.
- VOGM is hetrogenous group of anomalies a/w *enlarged deep venous* structures of *galenic system* that are *fed by abnormal midline arterio-venous communications.*
- *Aneurysmal dilatation of VOG is most common pathological finding*. The hugely dilated central venous structure is a persistent embryonic vein k/a *median vein of prosencephalon.*
- VOGM are located in *subarachoid space* and may be:
  Type 1= AV malformation fed by enlarged arterial branches l/t dilatation of VOG + straight sinus + trocular herophili
  Type 2= angiomatous malformation involving basal ganglia + thalmi ± mid brain draining into VOG
  Type 3= transitional AVM with both features
- Feeding vessels of VOGM are
  - *Posterior cerebral artery, posterior choroidal artery (90%)*
  - Anterior cerebral artery & anterior choroidal artery
  - Middle cerebral artery + lenticulostriatal + thalamic perforating arteries (least common; nidus type).

Clinical Presentation

- *Can be detected in utero >30 weeks* gestation age
- Male: Female = 2: 1 and *loud intracranial bruit*Q may be heard b/o blood turbulence
- **Neonatal pattern of presentation** (0-1 month) is ***high output cardiac failure***Q d/t massive shunting.
- **Infantile** (1-12 months) pattern includes ***macrocrania from obstructive hydrocephalus and seizures***Q.
- Adult (>1year) pattern of presentation is *headache, focal neurological defecits* (5%) d/t steal of blood from surrounding structures (steal phenomenon) ± *hydrocephalus* ± *intracranial haemorrhage*
- It may be a/w –
  - ***Smoothy marginated midline mass, posterior to indented 3rd ventricle***Q
  - ***Dilatation of lateral & third ventricle***Q (37%), straight + transverse sinus & trocular herophili.
  - Prominent serpiginous network in basal ganglia, thalami and mid brain.
  - Porencephaly & nonimmune hydrops.
- **Obs/ Trans fontanellar USG** shows ***median tubular hypoechoic cystic space with high velocity turbulent bidirectional flow***Q (on pulsed / color doppler). B mode USG shows sonolucent posterior *3rd ventricular mass & obstructive hydrocephalus.*
- **Angiography** shows *enlarged choroidal / thalamoperforating arteries*, VOG
- On **NECT,** round well circumscribed homogenous hyperdense/isodense mass in region of 3rd ventricle outlet, hyperdense intracerebral hematoma (ruptured AVM), hyperdense focal zones (ischemic) & rim calcification. *Strong enhancement on contrast enhanced CT.*
- **MRI** shows *areas of high velocity signal loss (signal void).*

Signs of Raised Intracranial Tension (ICT)

In children

- *Suture diastasis (1st & Most prominent)* Q
- ***Increased convolutional markings or copper beating of skull vault***Q. However, **it is not necessarily pathological** & n*ormal children particularly b/w 4-10 years* as well as children with craniostenosis may show this sign.
- *Sellar erosion* is a late sign of long standing raised ICT usually in children above 10 years of age.

★ Manifestations of **localizing evidence** of presence of cerebral tumor are *localized skull (vault) erosion, intracranial calcification, hyperostosis, abnormal vascular markings and pineal displacement.*

In adults

- *Thinning or erosion of dorsal sellae*Q **(cardinal sign)**.
- Erosion starts as *slight porosis* of anterior cortex of dorsum & sellar floor (best seen in lateral view). It progresses to ***loss of lamina dura (definition of cortex***Q**)** & eventually frank erosion.
- **Pineal displacement** (>3mm from midline in PA and Towne's view) is a strong evidence of mass lesion displacing pineal away from affected hemisphere.
- Suture diastasis is not seen in adults.

Types of Injuries

	Diffuse Axonal Injuries (DAI)	Cortical/Cerebral/ Brain Contusion	Epidural Hematoma (EDH)	Subdural Hematoma (SDH)	Multiple Infarcts
Etiology	*High velocity severe closed head injury* with *sudden acceleration deceleration or rotational force* produce *axonal shear strain deformation* often at grey-white junction (d/t differing tissue density or fixation) Characteristic microscopic findings are *axonal bulbs or retraction balls (hallmark)* & perivascular hemorrhage Gross pathological markers are *disruptions of penetrating blood vessels at corticomedullary junctions, corpus callosum, internal capsule, deep grey matter & upper brain stem producing numerous small haemorrhagic foci*	Focal brain lesions primarily involving *superficial grey matter*, with relative sparing of white matter d/t *linear acceleration deceleration forces or penetrating trauma* Punctate or linear hemorrhages occur along gyral crests *d/t brain striking on stationary osseous ridge or less often a dural fold.* **Coup** (*same side as impact*) is *small* area of *direct* impact on stationary brain a/w skull fracture **Countre coup** (*180⁰ opposite to side of impact*) is *broad* area of impact as a result of moving brain against stationary calvarium a/w fall.	Blood collects *b/w inner table of skull and dura* (calvarial periosteal layer) which is bound to cranium at sutural margins Source of bleeding are ***middle meningeal artery tear (most common)***[Q] or less commonly venous d/t *rupture of dural venous sinuses or diploic veins* Mostly a/w *skull fractures* (in squamous part of temporal bone) but in children EDH can occur without fracture or invisible (ping pong). #	Blood Collects b/w inner dural layer & leptomeninges (arachnoid-pia mater) i.e. *epiarachnoid space* Generally venous in origin, ***from laceration of bridging cortical veins***[Q]. Less common causes are injury to pial vessels & pacchionian granulations and rapid decompression of obstructive hydrocephalus *History of trauma* may be *lacking* particularly in *elderly*	A gradual & global reduction in cortical blood flow of *normal aging subjects* (vascular dementia)
Location/Presentation	It is characterized by ***loss/severe impairment of consciousness beginning, at the moment of direct impact***[Q]. Tend to be *diffuse, bilateral & in very predictable locations* depending on severity of trauma - **Grade I**- at peripheral *grey-white junctions of lobar white matter* (parasaggital frontal & periventricular temporal lobes) - **Grade II**- also involves *corpus callosum* (particularly posterior body & splenium) - **Grade III**- DAI also involves *dorsolateral upper brain stem (mid brain)*	Compared to DAI, CC are *less frequently a/w initial loss of consciousness & poor prognosis* unless they are extensive or occur with shearing or brainstem injury Multiple, bilateral lesions characteristically on **temporal lobes** (just above petrous bone or posterior to greater sphenoid wing) and **frontal lobes** (in orbito frontal, inferior frontal & rectal gyri above cribriform plate, planum spenoidale and lesser sphenoid wing) and less so the **parasaggital convexity (gliding contusion** as sub cortical tissue glides more than cortex).	95% are *unilateral & occur above tentorium in temporoparietal* area As it force fully strips the dura away from inner table, an EDH assumes a characteristic focal ***biconvex or lentiform shape***[Q]. EDH may cross dural *attachments but not sutures* More common in *younger (20-40 yrs)* as dura is easily stripped away and presents with *transient loss of consciousness* (from brain stem concussion)**, *lucid interval***[Q], delayed somnolence 24-96 hrs after accident (d/t accumulation of EDH) and *progressive deterioration of consciousness to coma.*	Usually more extensive than EDH & *may cross suture line but not dural attachments* *95% are supratentorial* (frontoparietal, convexity, middle fossa most common) Bilateral, inter hemispheric parafalcial SDH is common in child abuse *More common in elderly* d/t prominent extra axial space (b/o cerebral atrophy) which allows increase motion.	Often asymmetrical - Frontal - Temporal - Parietal lobe with multiple areas of diminished flow
CT	Initial CT are often *normal* in 50-80% DAI Unfortunately only 20% DAI lesions contain sufficient hemorrhage to be detectiable on CT as *multiple small*	CT 24-48 hrs after injury often show more lesions than initial normal/subtle scan Hemorrhagic contusions are more easily identified & appear as small *foci of high attenuation (hyerdense)*	***Well defined, homogenous, hyperdense, biconvex (lenticular or elliptical) extra axial fluid collection***[Q]. It is *usually a/w overlying*	**Acute** SDH is seen as ***homogenously hyperdense, crescent shaped exteraaxial collection***[Q] that spreads diffusely over the affected hemisphere	- Cortical & subcortical infarct - Large ventricles and cortical sulci - White matter leucencies

	petechial hemorrhage at grey-white junction & corpus callosum[Q]	within superficial gray matter of frontal or temporal lobes. They may be surrounded by larger irregular areas of low attenuation from associated edema. Characteristic **salt & pepper lesion** or **mottled /speckled densities** d/t mixed areas of hyperdensity (petechial hemorrhage) & hypodensity (edema) *Edema & mass effect increase* in first few days & delayed hemorrhage may develop *Show contrast enhancement*	*skull fracture, does not cross suture lines.* However at vertex, where the periosteum that forms the outer wall of sagittal sinus is not tightly attached to the *saggital suture*, the EDH can cross midline *Only EDH displace falx & venous sinuses away from inner table.* *Mass effect with sulcal effacement & midline shift* is frequent **Swirl sign** predicting poor outcome/rapid expansion of EDH is *presence of low attenuation areas of active bleeding with in hyperdense hematoma*	**Sub acute SDH** is nearly *isodense* with cortex. In such cases *displaced gray white matter interface, midline shift, effacement of adjacent sulci, sulci not traceable to brain surface, ipsilateral ventricle compression or distortion, thickening of ipsilateral portion of skull, contrast enhancement and window setting* usually permit detection of SDH	
MRI	***Most sensitive modality***[Q] is MRI Spin echo T_2 weighted MR esp FLAIR imaging can detect many non hemorrhagic foci of DAI *but still under estimates the true extent of injury* Nonhemorrhagic DAI lesions appear as *multiple small foci of increased signal on T_2WI & DWI* images and as decreased signal intensity on T_1 WI with in white matter Patechial hemorrhage causes *a central hypointensity on T2 & hyperintensity on T1 weighted images.*	*MR is investigation of choice* Non hemorrhagic lesions are hypo intense on T_1 and hyper intense on T_2WI Hemorrhagic lesions are - *hypointense* (deoxy Hb) *surrounded by hyper intense* (edema) on T_2 WI in *acute phase* - hyperintense (met Hb) on T_1 and T_2 in sub acute phase - *hyperintense* (gliosis) + *hypointense* (hemosiderin) on T_2 in *chronic phase.*	-	-	-

CNS Infection: Meningitis

Tubercular Meningitis

- In contrast to bacterial (acute-septic) meningitis, tuberculous infections is a/w a ***more insidious onset***[Q], fewer changes in CSF profile, and ***higher rate of mortality & complications such as infarction***[Q]. Although the TB tends to involve the **basal meninges, tuberculoma** may occur with in the *brain parenchyma or subarachnoid, subdural or epidural spaces.* MRI of tuberculous **meningitis denonstrates meningeal *enhancemen most often in the basal cisterns***[Q], reflecting the known predilection of ***TB for the base of brain***[Q]. **Calcification of basal meninges** may be seen (CT better than MRI for calcification)
- **Tubercular meningitis** pridominantly involves the ***basal cisterns, inter hemispheric fissure, sylvian fissure, sulci of cerebral convexities***[Q] and characteristically l/t complications like

Viral Meningitis

- **Viral meningoencephalitis**, and especially **herpes simplex virus (HSV) encephalitis** can mimic the clinical presentation of acute bacterial meningitis. HSV encephalitis typically presents with *headache, fever, altered consciousness, focal neurological defecit (eg dysphasia & hemiparesis) and focal or generalized seizures.* CSF studies, neuroimaging & EEG distinguish HSV encephalitis from acute bacterial meningitis. The typical CSF picture of viral CNS infection is a *lymphocytic pleocytosis with a normal glucose concentration*, in contrast to *polymorphonuclear (PMN) pleocytosis and hypoglycorrhachia* characteristic of bacterial *meningitis.* ***MRI abnormalities other than meningeal enhancement are not seen in uncomplicated bacterial meningites***[Q]. By contrast, in HSV encephalitis, on T2 weighted and FLAIR (fluid-attenuated

hydrocephalus (mostly communicating & rarely obstructive) and ***ischemic infarcts of basal ganglia and internal capsule***Q (d/t vascular compression or occlusive panarteritis in basal cisterns; mostly in MCA distribution). Spinal TB meningitis may l/t *syringomyelia & syringobulbia.*

- Sequelae of chronic meningitis, particularly tuberculosis include **pachymeningitis, ischemia, infarction, atrophy and calcification**. 75% infarctions occur in regions supplied by *medial lenticulostriate and thalamoperforating arteries;* 25% involve the cerebral cortex. Bilateral infarction occurs in 70% cases.
- Non contrast CT in chronic meningitis shows ***en plaque dural thickening and popcorn like dural calcification particularly around basal cistern***Q. Contrast enhanced CT may show **abnormal meningeal enhancement** (even years after treatment of initial infection). Sequelae of chronic meningitis may be striking and include ***cerebral atrophy & infarction***Q
- *TB and other chronic meningitides (like Coccidiodomycosis and Cryptococcus) have a predilection* for basal cisterns.

Fungal Meningitis

- **Fungal meningitis** is often seen in immuno compromised hosts. **Aspergillosis** (usually in *organ transplant recepient*) may be a/w *focal, thick dural arachnoid enhancement that resolves with treatment.* **Cryptococcus** (usually in AIDS) only *occasionally causes meningeal-enhancement*; probably b/o blunted host response. Cryptococcal infection tends to spread from the *basal cisterns via perivscular spaces to the basal ganglia, brain stem, internal capsule and thalamus.* This produces a characteristic appearance on MRI scans of ***nonenhancing dilated perivascular spaces*** caused by infestation with the gelatinous pseudocysts of cryptococcal material. In contrast to cryptococcus, **Coccidioidal meningitis** causes MRI enhancement of meninges most prominent in *basilar cisterns, the sylvian and interhemispheric fissures, and upper cervical SAS.*

Spirochetal Infection

- Spirochetal infections may exhibit *both localized & diffuse meningeal enhancement. Similarly, smooth, diffuse, pia – SAS enhancement of brain stem & entire spinal cord* is seen in **Lyme disease**, even in absence of MRI evidence of parenchymal disease.

Toxoplasmosis

- **Toxoplasma** is *most common oppurtunistic CNS infection in AIDS* patient. The *basal ganglia and cerebral hemispheres* near the *corticomedullary junction* are most common sites, resulting in focal or diffuse necrotizing encephalitis.
- Toxoplasma gondii lesions are characterized by *no capsule with three distinct zones (innermost zone of coagulative necrosis* with few organism, *intermediate hypervascular zone* of neumerous inflammatory cells mixed with tachyzoites and encysted organisms, and *peripheral zone* mostly composed of encysted organisms). *Vasogenic edema typically surrounds the mass.*
- CECT shows solitary or *multiple ring-enhancing masses with peripheral edema and target or bull's appearance.* Focal nodular or rim enhancement patterns are seen on CE-MRI

Neurocysticercosis

- Neurocysticercosis (Taenia solium larva) is most common CNS parasitic infection. Brain parenchyma (corticomedullary junction) > intraventricular (4th ventricle mostly) >> subarachnoid space are usually involved.
- Parenchymal cysticercosis have 4 stages with imaging manifestations varrying a/t stage : **vesicular stage** (i.e. viable larva in clear fluid containing bladder without inflammation l/t **nonenhancing CSF like cyst with a mural nodule** that represents head/scolex of larva, edema & contrast enhancement is very rare); ***colloidal vesicular stage*** (larva dies & degenerate, fluid becomes turbid / colloidal, cyst shrinks & capsule thickens evoking

inversion recovery) images, high signal intensity lesions are seen in **orbitofrontal, anterior and medial temporal lobes** in majority of patients (>90%) within 48 hrs of symptom onset. ***The absence of temporal lobe lesions on MR reduces the likelihood of HSV encephalitis and should prompt consideration of other diagnostic possibilities***Q. *Bilateral lesions* are more common but may be quite *asymmetric* in their intensity with *predominant involvement of gray matter.* Some patients with HSVencephalitis have a *distinctive periodic pattern on EEG. The* ***diagnostic procedure of choice*** in these patients is **CSF-PCR analysis** for HSV.

- HSV encephaliti should be considered when clinical features suggesting involvement of **inferomedial fronto-temporal regions of brain** are present icluding *prominent olfactory or gustatory hallucinations, anosmia, unusual or bizzhare behavior or personality alterations or memory disturbance.* **Focal findings** in patient with encephalitis that should always raise the possiblity of HSV encephalitis include (1) areas of *increased signal intensity in fronto-temporal, cingulate or insular* regions of the brain on *T2 WI, FLAIR or diffusion weighted MRI*; (2) focal areas of *low absorption, mass effect, and contrast enhancement on CT*; or (3) *periodic focal temporal lobe spikes* on a background of slow or low amplitude (flattened) activity on EEG. 10% of patients have normal MRI, 10% have extra temporal & frontal lesions (more often in children) and 80% show *hyperintense temporal lobe lesion on T_2WI* (addition of FLAIR & diffusion WI) increase sensitivity. Typical EEG pattern consist of *periodic, stereo-typed, sharp and slow complexes* originating in one or both temporal lobes & *repeating at regular intervals of 2-3 sec.* The periodic complexes are typically noted *between days 2 and 15* of the illness (in $2/3^{rd}$ patients).
- HSE characteristically involves **inferomedial temporal lobe > frontal** > parietal lobes; with propensity for **limbic system** (olfactory tract, temporal lobes, cingulate gyrus and insular cortex) and initially is predominantly unilateral.
- Patients with **rapidly progressive encephalitis** & **prominent brain stem** signs, symptoms or neuro imaging abnormalities may be infected by **flavi-viruses** (*WNV, St.Louis encephalitis virus, Japenese encephalitis virus), HSV, rabies or L.monocytogenes.* Significant involvement of **deep gray matter structures**, including the **basal ganglia and thalamus**, should also suggest possible flavivirus infection. These patient may prsent clinically with **prominent movement disorders** (*tremors, myoclonus*) or *parkinsonian features.* Patients with *WNV infection, enterovirus 71 and less commonly other enteroviruses* can also present with **poliomyelitis like acute flaccid paralysis** (i.e. *acute onset of a LMN type weakness with flaccid tone, reduced or absent reflexes and relatively preserved sensation*).
- MRI abnormalities in **WNV encephalitis** involve **deep brain structures**, including **thalamus, basal ganglia, and brain stem** rather than cortex and may only be apparent on **FLAIR images**. (seen in $2/3^{rd}$ patients). EEG in WNV encephalitis typically shows generalized slowing that may be more anteriorly predominent rather then temporally predominant pattern of sharp or periodic discharges more characteristic of HSV encephalitis.
- Involvement of *subcortical white matter of both hemisphere* (assumetrical) and *($\pm$) brainstem / posterior fossa* is seen in **acute disseminated encephalomyelitis (ADEM) / postviral leukoencephalopathy and flavi-virus encephalitis. Rabies encephalitis** shows *hyperintensity in brainstem, hippocampus and hypothalamus.* **Japanese encephalitis** may show *bilateral thalamic hemorrhage.*
- *Diffuse enhancement of cauda equina with polyradiculomyelitis* may indicate *CMV or varicella- zoster virus infection* in patients with AIDS

inflammation, **edema** & disruption of BBB l/t **ring like enhancement); granular nodular stage** (scolex calcifies l/t isodense cyst with **hyperdense calcified scolex on NECT; edema** & enhancement still persists with **nodular or micro ring enhancement** pattern suggesting granuloma, occasionally **target or bull's eye** appearance is seen); **nodular calcified stage** (completely mineralized & shrunken l/t ***small calcified*** nodules without mass effect or enhancement, **starry sky appearance** on NECT).

- Immunocompromised adult patiens with **CMV** often show **enlarged ventricles** with areas of **increased T2 signals outlining the ventricles and sub ependymal enhancement** on T1 weighted post contrast MR images.
- Patients with **VZV encephalits** shows **multifocal areas of hemorrhagic & ischemic infarction**, reflecting the tendency of VZV to produce a CNS vasculopathy rather than a true encephalitis.

Epidermoid (Inclusion) Cyst or Tumor

- It is actually a **benign-nonneoplastic epidermal (ectodermal epithelial elements) inclusion cyst**, which may be congenital or acquired, and proliferates with extremely slow linear growth rate comparable to normal epidermis.
- **Congenital epidermoid cysts** arise d/t inclusion of ectodermal tissue from *pharyngeal pouch of Rathke / pleuripotent cells during closure of neural tube (5th week)* or during *formation of secondary cerebral vesicles.* Early inclusions r/i midline lesion & later inclusions r/i more lateral location.
- **Acquired EC** occur d/t implantation of epidermis as a result of trauma *mostly in lumbo sacral spine following nonstylet needle puncture.*
- It is *well delineated cystic lesion* with **irregular – lobulated** or **cauliflower-like** outer surface that often has a **shiny mother of pearl appearance. It insinuates along CSF-cisterns, encase (intimately surrounds) vessels and engulf cranial nerves** (rather than displacing them, l/t limited resectability)
- EC wall is composed of *simple stratified cuboid squamous epithelium that desquamates regularly* l/t production of *lamellar appearance* and soft flanky center filled with desquamated *keratinaceous debris rich in solid crystalline cholesterol & triglyceride* (**primary / congenital cholesteatoma**). In contrast to EC, dermoids (cyst) contain dermal elements including skin appendages such as hair follicles & sebacedous glands also. Teratoid cysts (teratoma) contain all 3 germ layers with tissues of other organ system suchas teeth also.
- 90% are *intradural primarily in basal subarachnoid space* (offmidline or lateral >> midline); 40-50% EC occurs in **CP angle cisterns** (making it 3rd most common CPA mass after acoustic schwannoma & meningioma) >> **supra & para-sellar** (cavernous sinus or middle cranial fossa) region >> cerebral hemisphere, ventricle, brain stem (rare). Extradural (10%) are mostly *intradiploic* in frontal, parietal or occipital & rarely sphenoid bone.
- EC typically occur between 10-60 year (peak 4th & 5th decade) with no gender predelection (M:F = 1:1). They expand slowly to become symptomatic in adulthood. It may l/t visual & endocrine abnormalities (DI) and hydrocephalus in supraseller EC; cranial nerve palsies in CP angle EC and chemical meningitis.
- EC is *avascular lesion with little / no mass effect, edema & hydrocephalus.* It is characteristically a lobulated round ***homogenous mass with density (on CT) / intensity (on MRI) similar to CSF which shows no contrast enhancement.*** On MRI it shows *lamellated layer on layer onion skin appearance with hypointense T_1 and hyperintense T_2 images. Calcification* is present in 10-25% cases. Occasionally EC appears *hyperdense on CT* d/t hemorrhage, high protein content, sopanification of cyst debris to calcium soap or deposition of iron containing pigment; or hyperintense on T_1 & T_2 both d/t presence of triglycrides & polyunsaturated FA; or rarely hypointense on T_2 d/t calcification, low hydration and iron containing pigment. Similarly *peripheral rim enhancement* is somtimes observed.
- **Steady state free precession (SSFP & diffusion weighted (DW) MR sequences** can differentiate epidermoids from arachnoid cysts. ***Because epidermoids consists of closely packed keratin cells, the diffusion is restricted, producing high signal intensity*** **on DW images**Q. The **apparent diffusion coefficient (ADC)** of epidermoid is similar to brain parenchyma, whereas the ADC of arachnoid cyst is similar to stationary water. **Proton density weighted image** (is a first echo of T_2 image with

Feature	Epidermoid tumor	Arachnoid Cyst
Etiology	Ectodermal inclusion cyst	Meningeal maldevelopment
Gross pathology	Irregular lobulated ***(cauliflower like), shiny mother of pearl appearance containing desquamated keratin debris & cholesterol***	Thin, transparent wall containing clear CSF
Location	*Intradural CP angle > supra & paracellar*	Middle cranial fossa (50%) >> suprasellar, quadrigeminal cistern, cerebral convexities & posterior fossa (CP Angle)
Age & Gender	10-60 yrs (peak 4th or 5th decade); M:F=1:1	Any; but 75% in children M:F = 3:1
Vessels & nerves	Intimatelly surrounds (engulfs) limiting resectability	Displaced
Symptoms	In adulthood	Often asymptomatic (Wolfgang)
Calcification **Enhancement**	Upto 25% No, peripheral-rim enhancement rarely	No No
Margins	Scalloped	Smoth
CT density	± hyperdense to CSF	CSF like
Proton density, FLAIR image	**Hyperintense (slightly)** to CSF	CSF like
ADC	Similar to brain parenchyma	Similar to stationary water
Diffusion	***Restricted***Q	**CSF like**
Diffusion weighted images (DWI)	***Hyperintense***Q **(characteristic)**	CSF like

Epidermoid	Dermoid
Contain **solid** Crystalline cholesterol but no dermal appendage; rupture rarely	Contain **dermal appendages, liquid** cholesterol & **commonly ruptures**
Common; involve 20-60 yrs M=F	Uncommon; involve 30-50yrs M>F
Off midline; mostly in CP angle	Midline; parasellar, frontobasal (mc) > vermis, 4th ventricle

shorter echo time or TE; or is a mixture of T_1 & T_2). FLAIR (fluid attenuated inversion recovery) images are T_2 images with attenuated (no) signals arising from CSF, therefore CSF which normally is white on T_2 images appears black on FLAIR resulting in better contrast / visualization of periventricular pathologies and cysts with CSF. ***So epidermoid tumors which usually follow CSF signal intensity on all pulse (T_1 & T_2) sequence may appear slightly hyperintense on proton density images and FLAIR sequences***Q. Whereas arachnoid cyst follows CSF density / intensity on all sequences. EC may show signal intensity suppression on fat - suppression sequence, however, lipome which is characteristically hyperintense on T_1 and less hyper intense on T_2 exhibits more fat suppression.

On NECT, **low density (like CSF)**, calcification uncommon (<25%)	On CT, **very low density (like fat), calcification common**
T_1 and T_2 are often like (iso-intense to) CSF i.e. EC is hypo intense on T_1 and hyperintense on T_2 weighted images like CSF	**T1 is typically hyperintense (d/t lipid)** or isointense to muscle. T2WI are variable ranging from hypointense (d/t calcification) to heterogenously hyperintense **Sac of marbles appearance** representing multiple fat nodules in cyst is **pthognomic;** rarely *fluid-fluid levels* are seen

Meningioma

Incidence & Location

- It is *most common nonglial primary brain tumor,* ***most common intracranial extra axial tumor,*** *most common primary extracerebral (extra-axial) tumors of CNS & most common radiation induced CNS tumor* with 20-35 years latency. It is 2nd most common tumor in *intradural extramedullary* region (spine).
- Most meningiomas are **intracranial extra axial dural based** lesions.
- 90% of which are **supratentorial** and most frequent sites are *parasagital* (medial hemisphere) > *Frontal & parietal convexity* (lateral hemisphere) > *sphenoid ridge* > *frontobasal at olfactory groove,* sylvian fissure & parasellar.
- **Infratentorial** (at cerebellar convexity, CP angle and clivus) tumors occur in 10%.
- **Spine (thoracic** > cervical > lumbar) with **intradural** (90%)> dumbbell (5%)=extradural (5%) lesions are seen in 10%

Age & Gender predilictions

- Meningioma is **most common primary tumor arising from the leptomeninges**. A **hormonal** influence is implicated in pathogenesis because they are *more common in women* than in men, occur *more often in patients with breast cancer and may become symptomatic during pregnancy.* **Radiation** is also a causative factor esp in patients treated for *vascular nevi or tinea capitis* in childhood.
- Predominantly occurs in middle & old age with a peak incidence in the **fifth through seventh decades of life** (Haga)/ **40-60 years** (osborn)/ **45 years (range 35-70 yr)** (Danhart) with definite **female predominance (M:F=1:2 to 1:4)**
- Multiple meningiomas in children is a/w ***neurofibromatosis (NF)2.*** Chromosome 22 monosomy / long arm deletion are common associations. Meningiomas a/w hereditary syndromes occur in younger patients and do not demonstrate a gender predilection.

Pathology

- Meningiomas are *solid, well circumscribed, well encapsulated, slow growing, highly cellular tumors* that are *usually benign (WHO grade I).* They are derived from **meningothelial cells** called **arachnoid cap cells** concentrated in arachnoid (granulations) villi. Vill are numerous in large dural sinuses, in smaller veins, along root sleeves of existing cranial /spinal nerves, choroids plexus.
- Meningiomas assume two basic gross morphological types:
  a) **Globular (spherical or lobulated) mass = globose meningioma** (most common)
  b) **Flatter, carpet like en plaque lesion** mostly arising in *sphenoid wing & base of skull* (**=meningioma en plaque**) that infiltrate dura and also sometimes invades underlying bone and causes **pronounced hyperostosis, thickening & sclerosis (meningioma bone)**.- There is considerable controversy, clinicians are divided and some regard this

Imaging Features

- **Plain X-Ray**
  - **Hyperostosis** at sites close to/within bone (**exostosis, enostosis, sclerosis**) such as skull vault or sphenoid ridge. It does not indicate tumor infiltration
  - **Enlarged meningeal grooves/vascular channels** leading upto the site of attachment (if location in vault), *enlarged foramen spinosum*
  - **Tumor calcification *(psammoma/sand bodies)*** characteristically **amorphous parasaggital** or less typical *speckled or nodular calcification.*
  - **Pneumosinus dilatans** (blistering at ethmoid, sphenoid paranasal sinuses ± sclerosis) is expanded paranasal sinuses
  - **Erosion of overlying bone (least common)**
- **Myelography** (of spine)
  - ***Intradural, extramedullary mass***Q
  - Subarchanoid space on the side of lesion is widened
  - Sharp meniscus is seen where contrast caps the lesion
- **Angiography**
  - ***Dual vascular supply*** (dural to central and pial to periphery of tumor)
  - ***Sunburst or spokewheel or radial pattern of tumor vascularity*** *with hypervascular cloud like stain*
  - **Mother in law (prolonged vascular stain) phenomenon** i.e. contrast material shows up early and stays late into venous phase or **prominent, homogenous, prolonged vascular blush.**
  - Occasionally AV *shunting with early opacification of draining veins and dural sinus occlusion occurs* (in angioblastic meningioma). En plaque meningioma is poorly vascularized.
- **CT scan (Non contrast enhanced & Contrast enhanced)**
  - **On noncontrast CT**, meningiomas appear as **sharply circumscribed**, rounded & sometimes lobulated ***homogenous masses of slightly increased density (hyperdense 40-50HU) compared with adjacent brain (75%)***Q/isodenese (10-25%)/ or very rarely hypodense (1-5%) that *abuts a dural surface, usually at an* ***obtuse angle. The characteristic homogenous hyperdensity*** is related to *dense cellularity of meningiomas* and does not reflect psammomatous changes. Meningiomas typically have a ***broad base on a dural surface***Q. So mostly **homogenous hyperdense mass with broad dural base** displaces and compresses the underlying brain and

bony sclerosis & thickening as highly indicative of tumor *infiltration into the haversian canals of calvaria*, whereas others state that hyperostosis is *reactive phenomenon* & does not indicate tumor infiltration.

- **Dural attachment** that underlies most meningiomas can be **broad**, giving rise to a *sessile appearing tumor* or **narrow or stalk like** with a pedunculated tumor mass. Meningiomas have lobulated or bosselated surface and are sharply circumscribed lesions with **well delineated tumor brain interface**. A distinct **cleft of arachnoid with trapped CSF and prominent vessels** that surround the extra-axial (i.e. extra-parenchymal) mass is often observed.
- ***Most meningiomas are characteristically homognously solid tumors***Q, but *foci of necrosis and scarring* (probably secondary to ischemia), *microcystic changes, hemorrhagic foci*, or *areas of heavy lipid storage* (lipomatous /lipoblastic meningiomas) *and xanthomatous changes* are sometimes observed (5-15% of excised tumors). A collar of reactive thickened dura often surrounds the meningioma base.
- **Vasogenic edema** of adjacent cerebral white matter (i.e. **peritumoral intra cerebral edema**), which may be secondary to compressive ischemia, venous stasis, or aggressive growth or parasitization of pial vessels, occurs in 50-75% of meningiomas. It is *more common* in patients with *lateral convexity tumors and indicates poor resectability & poor prognosis*; although there is no correlation between tumor size & extent of edema. The **most important factor in clinical outcome** of meningiomas are ***location and resectability***Q.

Clinical Picture

Mostly meningiomas project inwards from dura, indenting & compressing the underlying brain, causing neurological symptoms and signs through compression of adjacent cortex. *Less than 10%* ever cause symptoms and present with *seizure, hemiparesis* (parasagittal, convexity tumors), visual field defects (bisphenoidal), multiple cranial nerve palsies (cavernous sinus tumor), anosmia (frontal cribriform plate meningioma) and *sensory-motor deficit & bladder bowel dysfunction* (in spinal meningiomas)

Differential Diagnosis

- Arachnoid contributes embryologically to formation of choroid plexus, so **intraventricular meningiomas** may arise within *choroid plexus of lateral ventricles (80%) or 3rd ventricle (15%) rarely* and locally expand the ventricles to conform to the size & shape of tumor. The normally compact *choroid glomus calcifications may be fragmented & spread apart* by expanding tumor mass. These tumors *show characteristic imaging features* of extracerebral meningiomas and are *differentiated from choroid plexus papilloma* on the basis of

Feature	Intraventricular Meningioma	Choroid Plexus Papilloma
Age	Middle aged & old adults	Infants & very young children
Tumor surface	Smoothly rounded	Nodular, irregular margin
Cerebral ventricles-size & shape	Focal enlargement	Diffuse enlargement of all ventricles

- Like meningiomas, **hemangiopericytomas** are *well circumscribed, highly cellular, dural based extra axial rounded masses* (that were *formerly considered angioblastic meningioma* b/o high vascularity). Now despite many gross histopathological & imaging similarities to meningioma, they are considered a seperate entity and are differentiated on the basis of

Features	Hemangiopericytoma	Meningioma
Cell of origin	**Pericyte**, a perivascular cell of mesenchymal origin	**Meningothelial (arachnoid cap) cells**

causes *flattening (buckling) of underlying brain cortex* (in 40% cases). A **hypodense cleft** representing *trapped CSF & occasionally blood vessels or arachnoid cysts seperates it from parenchyma* and indicates its **extra axial (i.e. extraparenchymal) location**. About 10-25% meningiomas may be isodense with adjacent brain and 1-5% contain areas of hypodensity that correlates pathologically with foci of ischemic scar, microcysts or lipoblastic and xanthomatous changes.

- On NE (non contrast/non enhanced) CT, ***a thick band of hypodensity representing peritumoral vasogenic edema***Q of adjacent cerebral cortex & white matter is seen in 50-75% of meningioma. **Hyperostosis & thickening** of adjacent ***bone in sphenoid wing (temporal bone)***, base of skull etc can be ***clearly delineated by CT scan***Q (in a bone window setting calcification is seen in 20-25% and can be psammomatous (sand like), sunburst, globular, or even rimlike.
- On **contrast enhanced (CE) CT**, ***meningiomas characteristically display strikingly intense and homogenous (uniform) contrast enhancement***Q (in most ~ 90% cases). Even occasional meningiomas that are isodnse on CT also exhibit this **intense opacification**. However, meningiomas that are predominantly *microcystic may not enhance strongly or uniformly*. In 5-15% cases, *focal areas of nonenhancement* canbe identified within the tumor mass (which correlates with regions of *necrosis, old hemorrhage, scarring, cystic degeneation and lipoblastic changes*): but they usually do not interfere with accuracy of diagnosis (i.e. do not l/t sufficient heterogeneity). Occasionally, however, heterogeneity of contrast enhancement may be sufficient to raise the differential of glioblastoma.
- Large parasaggital meningiomas may ***compress or invade the adjacent superior saggital sinus***Q; interruption of the sinus can be identified on coronal post contrast CT or non contrast MRI. **Indistinct irregular tumor margins** (& tumor brain interface), **inhomogenous contrast enhancement, mushrooming** (i.e. a mushroom like extension of opacified tumor well away from main ovoid tumor mass), & **prominent venous drainage** centrally from the tumor are CT & MRI signs that may suggest *an aggressive anaplastic or malignant meningioma* invading the brain. Malignant & benign meningiomas cannot be distinguished solely on the basis of CT.
- *Hyperdense* (75%), *calcified (25%),* ***enhance intensily & uniformly (90%)***, *minimal peritumoral edema (60%), cystic areas (10%). Sharply demarcated well circumscribed* slowly growing mass *with wide attachment to dura* & causing **cortical buckling** of underlying brain.
- It may be extramedullary-intradural spinal mass that is iso- or moderately hyperdense compared to muscle.

- **MRI** (100% detection rate with *gadolinium DTPA)*

- On **noncontrast MRI**, most meningiomas present a **homogenous appearance** (similar to that seen on CT). On **T1** weighted images **(T1WI)** meningioma tends to be *isointense (50%) and slightly hypointene (50%)* to adjacent cortex. Whereas, on **T2** weighted images it is *isointense (50%) and mildly hyperintense* (50%). Others say it is **isointense (60%)** with **grey matter on T1 and T2 images** and remaining 40% are mildly hypointense on T1 and hyperintense on T2 images. *On T2 weighted images, signal intensity may have histological correlation –*

Histology	Highly cellular with moderate nuclear atypia & prominent mitotic activity comparable to malignant anaplastic meningioma. Highly vascular (more than meningioma) branching vascular channels (***Staghorn sinusoids***) *with perivascular fibrosis* is prominent microscopic finding	**Benign WHO grade I** slowly growing tumor may show *psammomatous calcification*, whorls & lobules of meningothelial cells, ***storiform appearance*** of spindle shaped cells.
Invasion & destruction (erosion) of overlying bone, infiltration of underlying brain parenchyma, Recurrence	More common *Tend to metastasize* beyond cranial cavity to lung, bone & liver	Less/Extremely rare
Hyperostotic (meningioma bone)	Do not form	***Common***Q
Lobulation & location	*More lobulated; Occipital region* near confluence of dural venous sinus	Less lobulated; *Fronto-parietal parasaggital convexity* (in close a/w *falx cerebri*)
Incidence, Age, Sex	50 times less common, occurs in *younger patients* (in their 40s) and **M:F=1.4:1**	**More common**, occurs in 5th through 7th decade and **M:F=1:2 to 1:4**
Imaging (NE-CT & NE MRI); contrast enhancement is intense & homogenous in both.	Greater frequency of **internal heterogeneity & external lobulation. Narrow base of dural attachment. Absence of tumor calcificaition & hyperostosis**	More homogenous internally & less lobulated externally Broad dural base Calcification & hyperotosis present

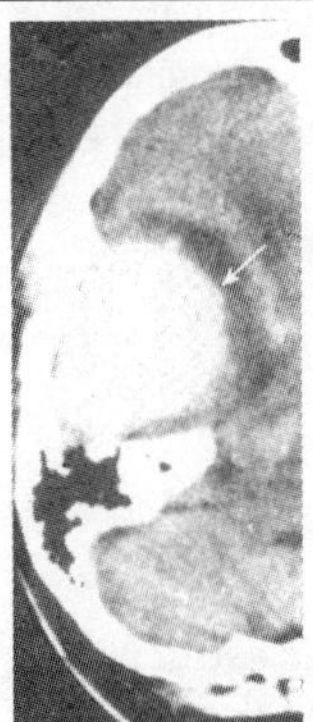

Axial postcontrast CT image demonstrates intense homogenous contrast enhancement of a large round extracerebral tumor with its base on the right greater sphenoid wing

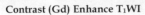

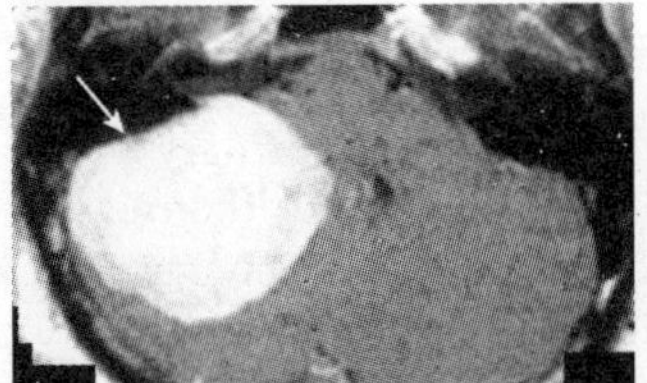

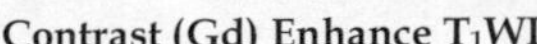

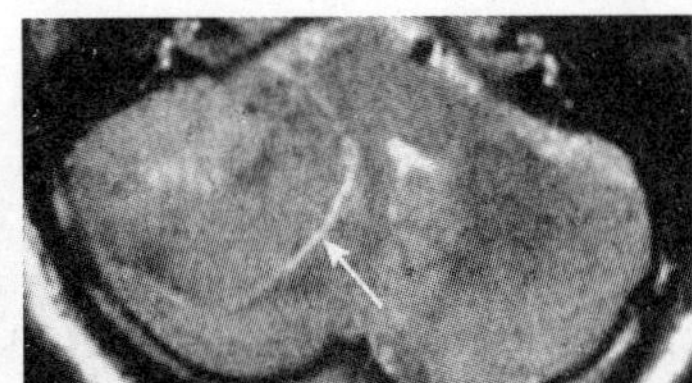

Contrast (Gd) Enhance T_1WI **T_2WI**

i.e. *syncytial or angioblastic meningiomas show hyperintensity* (in 75% cases), whereas fibroblastic and transitional meningiomas failed to demonstrate hyperintensity (or were hypointense) in 90% cases. Very few meningiomas appear heterogenous on both T1 & T2 b/o presence of intratumoral lipoblastic/cystic changes, or calcification or prominent vessels.

- *MRI is more accurate for localization & evaluation of meningiomas.* It shows grey whit matter *buckling/displacement (arcuate bowing of* white matter & *cortical effacement).* A **cleft or pseudocapsule of CSF or interposing vessels** surround the mass seperating it from brain (i.e. **demarcate the brain tumor interface) and confirm its extraaxial location**. Enlarged displaced arterier & pial veins show **flow voids**. Invasion of adjacent brain by meningiomas can be recognized as a *breech in hypointense dural rim at tumor margin.* Finally **arterial encasement** and partial **dural venous sinus invasion** are more easily & accurately depicted by the *contrast between the flow void and tumor tissue* (on MRI). Peritumoral edema is seen in 2/3rd cases. ***Meningioma show broad (wide) based dural attachment.***Q.
- As on CT, meningiomas ***characteristically demonstrate rapid and intensely/strikingly pronounced and homogenous contrast enhancement***Q on CE-MRI.
- **Dural tail sign** (i.e. presence of *homogenously enhancing collar of dural thickening* surrounding the dural attachment) seen in 60% is highly suggestive but not pathognomic (specific for meningioma)
- ***>95% enhance strongly***Q ***& homogenously;*** heterogenous enhancement is common.
- Dural tail may be d/t proliferative dural reaction or indicate tumor infiltration. Because a *major prognostic factor in the recurrence* of meningiomas after surgery is the *extent of tumor resection;* therefore *careful assessment must be done in preoperative post contrast MRI for presence of a dural tail. However, acoustic schwannomas, glioblastoma multiforme, metastases, chloroma, primary CNS lymphoma, sarcoidosis and syphilitic gumma* occasionally are a/w dural tail.

Features	Intra axial	Extra axial
Dural relationship	No attachment (until advanced)	Contiguous
Local bony change	Uncommon	Common
Feeding arterier	Pial	Dural
Subarachnoid cistern	Effaced	Widened, CSF cleft
Cortex displacement	Towards bone	Away from bone with buckling of gray & white matter and displacement of vessels
Examples	Brain parenchymal neoplasms like *astrocytoma (glioma), oligodendroglioma, ependymoma etc.*	Extraparenchymal neoplasms like ***meningioma***Q, and low attenuation lesions such as *acoustic schwannoma, epidermoid cyst and arachnoid cyst*

5

RADIODIAGNOSIS

Schwannoma

- **Schwannoma** is a *benign (WHO grade I) extraaxial encapsulated tumor* that arise from *Schwann cells* of cranial/spinal nerve sheath. Most common site of intracranial involvement is *vestibular division of 8th cranial nerve (at transition zone b/w central=oligodendroglial and peripheral=Schwann cell portion,* which lies within internal auditory canal) and is k/a **acoustic neuroma or nurinoma**. It is the *most common cause of cerebello-pontine angle mass* (80-85%). It presents with symptoms of CP angle mass, including tinnitus, sensorineural hearing loss & facial paresthesia. Despite the tumor's origin from vestibular nerve vestibular dysfunction do not become manifest until relatively late.
- **Trigeminal nerve Schwannomas** are much less common with facial, abducent & trochlear nerve tumors very rare. ***1st and 2nd CN lack schwann cell sheaths and are therefore spared***Q. Involvement of *sensory nerve root is common but motor uncommon.*
- Intracranial Schwannomas occur in all age but the peak incidence is in ***4th through 7th decade***Q with ***female predilection*** *(F:M=2:1)*Q; although no such prediliction occurs in spinal schwannoma.
- **NF-2** (ch-*22 mutation*) presents with *multiple inherited schwannomas, meningiomas & ependymomas (MISME)* in 2nd & 3rd decades of life.
- On gross schwannomas are focal, well circumscribed globular/ovoid mass that donot infiltrate nerve but rather grow eccentrically displacing it to side. As tumor grows it becomes heterogenous d/t cystic degeneration, lipid accumulation, Xanthomatous change or intermixed areas of hyper & hypocellularity. **So tumors upto about 1mm** typically demonstrate **homogenous density and homogenous strong contrast enhancement but larger tumor** *often demonstrate* ***heterogeneity of both density and contrast enhancement.***
- **On T1WI**, tumors **<5mm** appear *homogenously mildly hypointense or isointense* (to adjacent brain) intracanalicular mass with *intense homogenous contrast enhancement.* On T2 weighted pulsing sequences small tumors appear **mildly to markedly hyperintense**. With tumor enlargment heterogeneity increases.

Features		Meningioma	Schwannoma (esp acoustic neuroma
Angle with dura/petrous ridge		Obtuse (because are eccentric to IAC)	Acute
Dural tail		Frequent (specific but not pathognomic)	Rare
Calcification		Common (20%)	Very rare
Cystic degeneration/Necrosis		Rare	10%
Heterogeniety		Rare	Common in large tumors
Contrast enhancement		***Homogenous (uniform)***Q	***Hetrogenous (non uniform)*** 32%Q; homogenou in 2/3rd
Cerebellopontine angel mass		Only 10%	***Most common cause***Q (80-85%)
Internal auditory canal (IAC) involvement		Rare; extension into IAC is uncommon but not unknown; *hyperstosis*Q	Common (80%): cause ***fusiform widening & erosion***Q. On axial MRI tumor is **comma shaped (ice-cream cup appearance)** with globular cisternal mass medially & short tapered fusiform extension laterally into IAC
NE-CT		***Homogenous hyperdense mass with broad dural base***Q	***Homogenous (<1mm) or heterogenous (>1mm), hypodense to isodense mass***Q
CECT/CE MRI (T1WI)		**Uniform intense enhancement (90%)**	**Heterogenous** enhancement in large tumors (30-40%); enhancement may be very intense in small tumors
MRI	**T2WI**	Iso/Mildly hyper	**Hyper**tense
	T1WI	Hypo / Iso	Hypo / Iso

Astrocytomas: Types & Features

- **Astrocytomas** are *infiltrative tumors of glial cell origin. Cell type has great prognostic significance* eg pilocytic astrocytoma rarely become malignant, whereas others eg fibrillary atrocytoma are eventually fatal even though they may have low grade initially.
- **Focal (circumscribed) astrocytoma** are found in specific locations and include **grade I astrocytomas** (such as **pilocytic astrocytoma**, *subependymal giant cell tumor*) and pleomorphic xanthoastrocytoma. **Diffuse (fibrillary) astrocytomas** include low *grade (II) astrocytoma*, and high grade III (anaplastic) and IV (glioblastoma multiforme, gliomatosis cerebri & gliosarcoma). Anaplastic can be further divided into *gemistocytic astrocytoma* (that contain plump cells with abundant eosinophilic cytoplasm) and protoplasmic astrocytoma (satellite cells with delicate process).

RADIODIAGNOSIS 5

Tumor	Low grade Astrocytoma	Anaplastic (Malignant) Astrocytoma	Gliblastoma Multiforme	Pilocytic Astrocytoma	Pleomorphic Xanthoastrocytoma	Subependymal Giant cell Astrocytoma
Age	Children & adults (20 to 40 yrs)	Usually **older (40-60yrs)**	Usually **older (>50yrs)**; rare <30yrs	**Mostly <20yrs**	*Children & young adults* (mostly in **2nd or 3rd decade)** rarely upto 5th decade	Mostly **<20yrs**
Incidence	10-15% of astrocytomas (uncommon)	One third (33%) of all astrocytoma	***Commonest of all primary brain tumor***Q; 50% of all astrocytomas	5-10% of adult & 33% of pediatric gliomas; overall 2nd most common pediatric brain tumor	Rare (<1%)	10-15% in patients with ***tuberous sclerosis***Q
Location	**Cerebral hemisphere in proportion to white matter ±** often involve adjacent cortex	**Cerebral hemisphere white matter** (mostly in frontal & temporal lobe *peripherally)*	*Cerebral hemispheric white matter*Q (mostly in frontal & temporal lobe, *deeply)*; multilobed & bihemispheric tumors crossing corpus callosum are common	**Cerebellar (hemisphere > vermis) > optic pathway & hypothalamus** i.e. around 3rd & 4th ventricles	**Superficial cortical** location is typical; usually **abuts leptomeninges. Temporal lobe** (most common) >> parietal, occipital, frontal lobes	*Foramen of Monro*Q; vistually never found anywhere else.
Imaging	- Because of slow growth ***calcification is common*** *(15-20%) but edema, hemorrhage & cystic degeneration are rare and necrosis not seen* - **Hypodense/ hypo intense** on NECT/T1WI an hyper intense on T2WI - ***Contrast enhancement is absent/mild and inhomogenous***Q	- On NECT & MR (T1/T2-WI), AA is poorly delineated **inhomogenous (heterogenous) mixed density/intensity** mass; calcification uncommon, hemorrhagic foci occasional and *peripheral edema common.* - On T2WI, a *central hyperintense core* surrounded by *isointense rim* with peripheral *finger like hyperintense projections* secondary to vasogenic edema is common appearance. - **Strong but non-uniform** contrast enhancement; *irregular rim/peripheral ring like enhancement is common.*	- **Highly vascular, very heterogenous** tumor with *central necrosis, cyst formation & hemorrhage of different age and peripheral edema.* Calcification is rare - NECT, T1 & T2-WI all show ***very inhomogenous mixed. density/intensity signals.*** - **Strong (marked) but inhomogenous contrast enhancement**; *thick irregular rim enhancement* is common & *prominent flow voids* are often present	Almost like PXA but **calcification** is more common (10%) and so is **heterogeniety** i.e. mural nodules & solid tumors **enhance strongly** but some what **more inhomogenously** (variable enhancement.	- **Well delineated partially cystic mass** with a **peripheral mural nodule**; calcification is unusual - PXA are **hypodense** cystic masses on CT, **hypo-or isointense** (compared to normal brain) on T_1WI and are **hyper intense** (both nodule & cyst) on **proton density & T_2WI** - **Strong/marked contrast enhancement** of mural nodule is typical	- **Partially calcified & partially cystic-heterogenous, focal mass at formamen of monro** (FOM) - Calcified subependymal nodule along striothalamic groove (FOM) with enlarged lateral ventricles & cyst formation - Heterogeniety l/t *mixed hypo & isodense (CT);* mixed *hypo & isointense* on T_1 WI and iso to hyper intense on T_2WI. - ***Strong but heterogenous (in homogenous) contrast enhancement***Q

Pilocytic Astrocytoma / Hemangioblastoma

Pilocytic Astrocytoma (Juvenile PA or Polar Spongioblastoma)	Hemangioblastoma (HB)
- PA are the *most common tumor of childhood* (Harrison). It is *most common pediatric glioma* (Danhert). *Optico-chiasmatic-hypothalmic PAs* are one of the most common *supratentorial neoplasm* in children, and *cerebellar astrocytomas* are most common *posterior fossa* tumor in this age group (in some series *medulloblastoma is most common pediatric infra tentorial tumor*). PAs are 2nd most common pediatric brain	- Although relatively uncommon overall (1-2.5% of all primary CNS neoplasm), HB is the **most common primary intra-axial (i.e. parenchymal) infratentorial/posterior fossa tumor in adults.** - Most (85%) of HB are **sporadic & solitary** with a predominantly male (M>F) involvement. They typically present clinically **in**

5

RADIODIAGNOSIS

tumor (Osborn). - PAs are typically tumors of **children & young adults**; most becoming *symptomatic during first two decades of life* and have a peak incidense at *age 10 for cerebellar & optic pathway* lesions and 20 for cerebral hemisphere PAs. It may be a/w **neurofibromatosis type 1** and present earlier in childhood.	**young adults** with a peak incidence **in 3rd to 5th decade of life (i.e. 20-50 years age)**, and are rare in children. - 10-20% HB are multiple & occur ***as a part of von Hippel Lindau (VHL) syndrome***[Q]. And 10-40% of all VHL patients eventually *develop multiple CNS hemangioblastoma.* VHL is characterized by ***multiple CNS hemangioblastomas in a/w retinal HB, clear cell renal carcinoma, pheochrommocytoma, and pancreatic, renal & hepatic cysts***[Q]. Multiple HB are seen only with VHL. VHL associated HB **become symptomatic at an earlier age** (Mean age 29yr = Haga/39yrs = Osborn) than those with solitory - sporadic HB with a F >M predominence; and relatively more childhood lesions.
- It mostly (60%) occurs in **cerebellum (hemisphere >vermis)** with a peak age b/w 5 to 15 years. PA also frequently occurs in **optic pathway and adjucent hypothalami** often in a/w **NF1** usually in slightly younger children (2-3 years)-Haga - PAs are characteristically located **around the 3rd & 4th ventricles.** Nearly ½ are found in **optic chiasma & hypothalmus** and 1/3rd are in **cerebellar vermis or hemisphere**. Less common locations include brain stem, basal ganglia >> cerebral hemisphere (esp frontal lobe), intraventricular, subependymal (Osborn). PAs occur typically in cerebellum but may also be found in neuraxis including **optic nerves** & brainstem (Harrison).	- *Most (85%) of CNS-HB occur in* ***cerebellum (paravermian hemisphere)***[Q] >> *spinal cord* (10-15%). ***Medulla (2-3%), supra tentorial (1%) like cerebral hemisphere HB are uncommon***[Q]. - Symptoms are usually related to obstruction of CSF flow (in 4th ventricle) and associated *raised ICT such as headache, nausea, vomiting, dizziness, vertigo and ataxia (disequilibrium).* Some tumors *secrete* erythropoietin and stimulate erythropoiesis l/t erythrocythemia.
- Grossly cerebellar PAs are *well circumscribed but unencapsulated masses that typically have large cyst with a small, reddish tan mural nodule Opticochiasmatic hypothalmic PAs are wellcircumscribed, lobulated but microscopically infiltating tumors.* - PA is a well circumscribed brain neoplasm but *lacks a true tumor capsule and grows mainly by expansion rather than by infiltration.* It is a benign (biologically stable) grade I neoplasm which may be densely cellular &/or with intervening microcysts. *Mitoses are rare and necrosis are not seen. Intratumoral* calcification is occasionally seen (5-25%) but hemorrhage into or adjacent to tumor is rare. *Cysts are common but necrosis is absent* - Most often tumor represents a mural nodule in the wall of well circumscribed cyst. *Wall of cyst consists of compacted normal brain or non neoplastic gliotic tissue.* Fluid is proteinaceous & is secreted from capillaries in nodular tumor. - Histology shows *hair like pilocytic process*, spongiform foci with *stellate astrocytes, microcysts,* ***Rosenthal fibers***, small amorphous *eosinophilic bead like or* ***Corkscrew shaped hyaline bodies*** and low/absent mitotic activity.	- HB are *well demarcated (well circumscribed), highly vascularized, potentially curable, slowly growing, small* (5-10mm) rounded lesion located mostly in cerebellum, usually abutting a pial surface. 60% of tumors are cystic with a mural (tumor) nodule and 40% are solid. *Despite prominent vascularity, hemorrhage, necrosis and calcification are rare in HB.* - Just like cyst a/w juvenile pilocytic astrocytoma, the cyst a/w HB is extratumoral, lacking any tumor tissue inits margin except for eccentrically located solid mural nodule and the *cysts wall is composed of compressed brain parechyma or reactive gliosis.* - HB are *benign (WHO grade I) vascular neoplasm* of uncertain origin that consists of *abundant endothelial pericytes* forming rich capillary network *intermixed with vacuolated (lipid containing) stromal cells.*
- They mostly appear as **cystic lesions with intensely homogenous enhancing mural nodule**. Enhancement may be variable or inhomogenous in some cases d/t calcification. *Nonneoplastic cyst wall typically does not enhance* although may be enhancing also in few cases. - On CT typical cystic cerebellar PA appears as **round/oval sharply demorcated (well defined), smoothly marginated hypodense cyst like mass with less hypodense (rarely isodense) tumor nodule** on one wall. The cyst fluid is less hypodense than CSF because of high protein concentration. This means cyst appears more black (hypodense) in comparison to brain but less black (less hypodense) in comparision to dark black CSF. Whereas tumor nodule is isodense (similar to brain) or less hypodense (not as black as cyst). Typically after IV contrast administration ***dense homogenous contrast enhancement of mural nodule but not of cyst wall is seen.*** CSF Cyst Mural (tumor nodule) Brain tissue **CT: Cerebellar PA**	- Characteristic **angiographic** finding is *a large avascular posterior fossa mass with a smal highly vascular mural nodule showing intense & prolonged stain.* A-V shunting with early draining veins some times occurs. Because of intense vascularity of even the smallest solid tumor nodules, angiography may be more sensitive than. CT/MRI in detection of HB. **Mother in law phenomenon** = tumor blush comes early, stays late, very dense. - **Noncontrast CT** demonstrate large, sharply marginated cystic cerebellar hemispheric mass with *hypodense (dark) cyst and less hypodense* (i.e. more dense = more like gray matter) rounded mural nodule. There is little or no peritumoral edema and the solid tumor or mural nodule may not be distinguishable from surrounding normal cerebellar parenchyma (i.e. tumor is almost *isodense)* - *B/O almost lack of calcification, necrosis & hemorrhage,* after IV administration of iodinated contrast (CE CT), ***the solid tumor or mural nodule enhances homogenously and intensely***[Q] adjacent to a pial surface.

- On MRI, mural nodule appears **homogenously hyperintense** to grey matter on **T2WI** and **hypointense** to isointense on **T1WI**. Cystic portion is even more hyperintense on T_2 and more hypointense on T1 images. *Calcification may l/t heterogenous appearance.* **Homogenous contrast enhancement** of tumor (mural) nodule is **characteristic**, although a *calcific focus*, if present, *does not demonstrate enhancement (& may l/t hetrogenous (variable enhancement).*

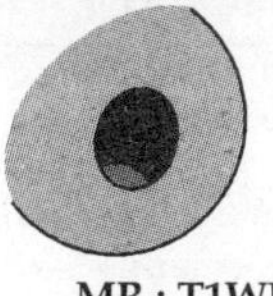
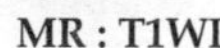

MR : T1WI

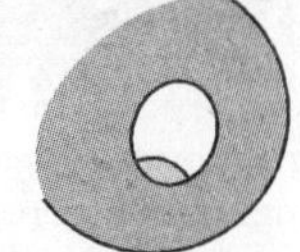

MR: T2WI

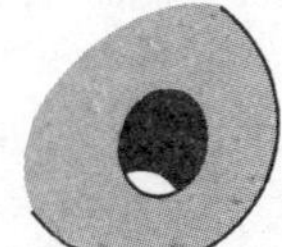

Contrast Enhanced MRI

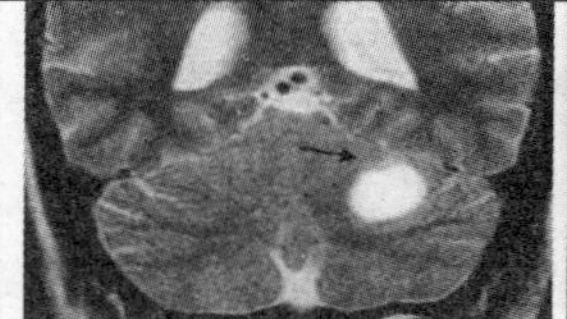

T2-MRI

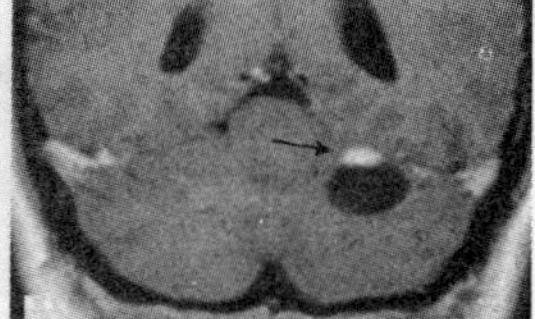

Contrast Enhanced T1W1

- On MRI, cyst typically are sharply & smoothly marginated and **homogenously hypointense** *relative to adjacent brain parenchyma and slightly hyperintense to CSF* on **T1WI** (i.e. on T1 images cyst looks black but relatively lesser than CSF). Cyst appears **hyperintense** (to brain) on T2WI (i.e. on T2 images cyst appears white). The *mural nodule is more variabdle;* most are **inhomogenously isointense** to normal grey matter on **T1** and **slightly hyperintense on T2** weighted MR images. Hyperintense areas (= increased signal) within nodule or cyst on T1WI are occasionly noted secondary to hemorrhage. **Prominenet serpentine flow (signal) voids** d/t enlarged vessels supplying & draining tumor may be seen at periphery of mass or nodule and ***strongly support the diagnosis HB***[Q]. As with CT, ***contrast enhancement of mural nodule or solid tumor on T1WI is characteristically homogenous and intense***[Q].

Intraventricular CNS Tumors

Central Neurocytoma (CN)

- A relatively *rare, benign, slow growing (WHO grad II), well defined, sharply circumscribed lobulated* intraventricular tumor mass that typically lies adjacent **to foramen of Monro** or **septum pellucidum. Intratumoral necrosis, calcification** and **multiple cyst** (formation) are common, but hemorrhage (intratumoral or intraventricular) & extensive vascularization are unusual.
- Histologically (on light microscopy) CN is **indistinguishable from oligodendroglioma** and shows nests of small well differentiated cells seperated by thin fibrovascular septa. Its ***neuronal origin is determined only with electron microscopy (by demonstrating neurosecretory granules, synapses, microtubules & nuritic processes) and immunohistochemistry (uniform & consistent expression of neuronal marker proteins, neuron specific enolase and synaptophysin)***[Q].
- CN are tumor of **young adults (average age 31yr; range 17-53** yrs) and are rare in children and older adults.
- It occurs almost exclusively in **lateral ventricle** (arising from the anterior portion of superolateral ventricular wall and extending medially) **adjacent to septum pellucidum** & **foramen of Monro**. All (almost) cases remain confined to ventricles and entension through FM into 3rd ventricle is very unusual. No tumor have been reported arising in 3rd or 4th ventricles, occipital or temporal horns or atria of lateral ventricles and only few hemispheric lesions) have been found.
- Imaging demonstrates a **sharply marginated, heterogenous (inhomogenous) intraventricular mass with a broad based attachment** to the wall of *frontal horn or anterior body of lateral ventricle* adjacent to (abutting) **septum pellucidum & foramen of Monro**. Most tumors demonstrate **calcification** (clumped, coarse or globular), *multiple small cysts* and obstructive hydrocephalus. **Contrast enhancement is mild to moderate and inhomogenous**.
- *Heterogenous pattern (heterogeniety) of CN* is demonstrated as *isodense to slightly hyperdense mass* with hypodense areas of cysts on NE-CT; and as *intermixed foci of isointensity*

Ependymoma

- **Ependyma** is a thin layer of ciliated cuboidal or columnar epithelium that lines ventricular walls and central canal of spinal cord. Ependymal cells are embryologically *related to both epithelial and glial cells*.
- Ependymomas are usually *slow growing tumors of moderate malignancy (WHO grade II)* but the prognosis is gaurded b/o their notable *tendency to recur locally & exhibit features of anaplasia* (high mitotic rate, pleomorphism & intratumoral **necrosis** in 25% cases & are considered grade III) and to *disseminate via the subarachnoid space CSF* (10%; more in infratentorial tumors).
- Ependymomas are **heterogenous tumors** commonly a/w **intratumoral calcification & cyst formation** (20-80%), **necrosis** and **peritumoral edema**. Intra tumoral hemorrhage is less common (<20%).
- Ependymomas are highly cellular with small fusiform uniform cells that tend to form characteristic ***perivascular pseudo-rosttes***[Q]. Although they do not invade through ventricular walls, they are firmly attached to floor, and complete resection of tumor base is frequently not possible. On the basis of location they can be

Infratentorial ependymoma (IE)	Supratentorial ependymoma (SE)
- Most (60-70%) ependymomas are **infratentorial (in posterior fossa)**; > 90% of which occur in the ependyma lining the floor of **4th ventricle**. Remaining (<10%) occur in *medulla & cerebellopontine angle cisterns*. - IE are well *circumscribed, lobulated, soft exophytic masses that expand within the cavity of 4th ventricle* (rather than infiltrate in to surrounding parenchyma). They often *extend in a tongue like fashion and protrude / extrude/ooze through the outlet foramina into the adjacent CSF cisterns (k/a* ***plastic ependymoma****)*. They extend antero- inferiorly into cisterna magna, anterolaterally through the lateral recesses into lateral medullary & CP angle cisterns or into **foramen**	- 30-40% ependymomas occur above the tentorium (supratentorial) arising mainly from the ***extraventricular/ paraventricular ependymal cell rests in the cerebral white matter (parenchyma) near the atrium of left ventricle or foramen of Monro***[Q]. Intraventricular location is less common than extraventricular site. - Cyst and calcification are more common (80%), whereas CSF seeding is less common. - Occur mainly in the **2nd through 4th decades of life** (peak in mid-30s).

RADIODIAGNOSIS

5

(compared to gray matter) and *hypointensity* (b/o calcification & cysts) on T1 WI and isointensity to hyperintensity on T2 weighted images. More solid portions of CN (i.e. iso to hyperdense CT regions / isointense T1 zones) demonstrate *inhomogenous faint contrast enhancement.*
- The **absence of deep extension** into adjacent brain parenchyma, **nodular tubers and intratumoral hemorrhage** and relatively young age of patient favors the diagnosis of CN (and excludes other lesions around FM like SGCA & subependymoma).

Subependymal Giant Cell Astrocytoma (SGCA)

- SGCA is a low grade (WHO grade I) tumor that ***occurs almost exclusively in patients with tuberous sclerosis***Q; 10-15% patients of TS develop SGCA.
- Subependymal hamartomatous proliferation along the *caudothalamic groove* are common in TS. By convention, *sybependymal nodules > 1cm diameter or that become symptomatic* are considered SGCA. Characteristic tumor location (FM), it larger size & presence of contrast enhancement suggest SGCA (contrast enhamcement is not seen in nontumorous nodules).
- SGCA arise from *subependymal nodules located on the lateral walls of lateral ventricles overlying the head of caudate nucleus.* The tumor does not invade the underlying caudate head but rather grows exophytically into the ventricular lumen ***near the foramen of monro***Q; however, overlying ependyma remains intact and dissemination via CSF is very rare.
- Histologically, SGCA contain *large multinucleated giant cells* of uncertain origin some of which may *display GFAP (glial fibrillary acidic protein) reactivity*, a feature of astrocytic origin, whereas others contain *neuron specific enolase* a finding consistent with neuronal origin. *Swollen astrocytes with abundant glassy eosinophilic cytoplasm*, prominent thick processes & benign appearing nuclei are present.
- SGCA is sharply delineated lobulated **heterogenous tumor**. ***Intratumor heavy calcification is common***Q and tumors are often vascular.
- ***SGCA almost always occur at foramen of Monro***Q, and most patients become symptomatic **before age 20** due to obstruction of FM l/t raised ICT/obstructive hydrocephalus.
- Imaging features of SGCA include: **heterogenous (partially cystic, partially heavily calcified) mass at foramen of Monro** which shows **strong but heterogenous contrast enhancement**.
- So SGCA appears as large heterogenous hypodense, polypoidal, sharply delineated intraventricular mass at foramen of Monro, with *areas of heavy calcification* and other menifestations of tuberous sclerosis like *cortical tubers & subependymal hemartomatous nodules.* on non contrast CT. On MRI, SGCA appears as *heterogenous, sharply demarcated intaventricular mass* that is mildly hyperintense on T2 and hypo-or isointense on T1 weighted images. It is located within the *frontal horn of lateral ventricle without evidence for deep invasion or spread within basal ganglia.* It may obstruct FM unilaterally or bilaterally, causing gross enlargement of one or both ventricles. On both CT & MRI, It shows **intense but heterogenous contrast enhancement**. Heterogenous signal on MRI both wih or without contrast is d/t presence of dense calcification in tumor (i.e. noncalcified portion is homogenous).

of Magendie into vellecula, and down through *foramen magnum* into upper cervical spine behind cerricomedullary junction. Tumor growth l/t occlusion & obstructive hydrocephalus - Predominantly occurs in **children between 1 to 6 years age**Q.	★ **Infratentorial (posterior fossa) ependymona** are 3rd or 4th most common posterior fossa tumor of childhood, exceeded only by *pilocytic astrocytoma, medulloblastoma, & probably brain stem glioma.*

- Imaging fetures of ependymoma are: a **heterogenous (mixed density/intensity) mass** demonstrating **calcification, cysts (>50%) and peritumoral edema.** Solid portions & cyst wall of tumor exhibit **mild to moderate but variable heterogenous contrast enhancement**.
- So on NE-CT, 4th ventricle ependymomas appear as heterogenous (hypo-to isodense) well circumscribed rounded mass partially or completely obliterating the cavity which is surrounded by *prominent hypodense halo of peritumar edema.* Calcifications & focal lucencies (d/t cyst) are common; although they are larger & more common in supratentorial lesions. MRI appearance is heterogenous reflecting mixed signals from calcification, cysts & hemorrhage; and tumors are usully *iso-to hypointense on T_1 and iso-to hyper intense on T_2* weighted images (relative to white matter). Supratentorial extraventricular ependymomas resemble astrocytoma.
- Ependymoma of 4th ventricle may closely resemble medulloblestoma & pilocytic astrocytoma. However, **ependymomas have greater incidence and extent of intratumoral calcification & heterogeneity** (of density on CT or intensity or MRI) and propensity for **tumor extension into the 4th ventricular recesses**, in comparison to medulloblastoma & astrocytoma. In general, **medulloblastomas** appear *more dense* on CT with a *lower frequency of intratumoral calcification*, and they exhibit *more homogenous contrast enhancement*.

Subependymoma (SE)

- It is a rare variant of ependymoma that actually consists of highly differentiated ependymal cells & astrocytes. It is classified as a *benign WHO grade I glial neoplasm*. SEs are typically **firm (solid), avascular and homogenous, well delineated intraventricular mass**. It is considered to arise from beneath the ventricular lining and projects into ventricular cavity but *does not extend deeply from its base into the adjacent brain parenchyma*.
- It is **charcteristically homogenous**, although larger tumor may contain *calcification, microcystic changes and intratumoral hemorrhage*. Microscopically it is a sparsely cellular neoplasm with a prominent fibrillary background. Microcysts are common but rosette formation, hypercellularity, mitoses, neovascularity and necrosis are absent (all *indicating homogenous –benign nature*).
- SE mostly arise from **lower medulla and project into the caudal 4th ventricle** (60%) > frontal horn of ***lateral ventricles in relation to septum pellucidum & foramen of Monro***Q >>> and rarely in region of aqueduct.
- It is a rare tumor of middle /elderly adults; most are found incidently. Average age of *symptomatic* group (*lateral ventricle* tumors mostly become symptomatic) is *40 years*, whereas of *asymptomatic* patient (mostly *4th ventricle* tumor) is *60 years*.
- Imaging features of SE are: a well **delineated homogenous, avascular/hypovascular nonenhancing mass**. So they appear *homogenously isodense or slightly hypodense on CT; homogenously hypo – to iso intense on T_1* and hyperintense on T_2 weighted MRI images. However large tumors may sometimes exhibit heterogeneity of density & intensity owing to intratumoral calcification & hemorrhage. There is *variable (no or minimal) contrast enhancement*.

Leptomeningeal–Metastases/Carcinomatous-Meningitis/Meningeal carcinomatosis

- **Solid tumors** like *breast (MC) lung (2MC), stomach (gastrointestinal carcinoma), malignant melanoma and genitourinary carcinoma*; and **hematologic neoplasm** such as *leukemia & lymphoma* are most common neoplasms inclined to CSF spread / meningeal dissemination.
- Primary CNS neoplasms such as *medulloblastoma, primitive neuroectodermal tumor (PNET), pineoblastoma / pineocytoma, anaplastic glioma, glioblastoma multiformae, germinoma (germ cell tumor), ependymoma (after local recurrence; infratentorial >> supratentorial)*. Mn – "**ME – 3PAG** i.e. 3P & 3G" = **Dropmetastases**
- **Poor differenetiation** (indicated by *poor GFAP staining* of primary CNS tumor), *close proximity to CSF spaces*, previous surgery, extended survival and *presence of other metastatic foci* (for non-CNS neoplasm) are risk factors for leptomeningeal dissemination of neoplasm. Metastases in *vertebral body* (esp in breast carcinoma), *bone marrow & liver* metastases (esp in lung carcinoma) is commonly present before their dissemination to CNS. The most common source of *brain metastases are lung >> breast* carcinoma; melanoma has the greatest propensity to metastasize to brain (80%). Most (85%) brain metastases are *supratentorial, in gray matter – white matter junction in the water shed distribution*; and 15% occur in posterior fossa (infratentorial).
- Neoplasms may involve duramater &/or leptomeninges (& CSF), both by direct extension or hematogenous spread (via arterial circulation or occasionally through retrograde flow in venous system). Hematogenous spread to dura is usually through *Batson's plexus* as a sequela of bone metastases. Whereas hematogenous spread to leptomeninges & CSF may occur via

1. hematogenous seeding of choroid plexus r/i tumor deposits that are sloughed into CSF;
2. via parenchymal blood vessels in **Virchow-Robin (perivascular) spaces** to the piamater & then to the SAS; r/i tumor spread either to or from the SAS);
3. hematological (>solid) neoplasm may *interrupt the thin walls of microscopic vessels in the arachnoid to enter SAS.*

- Once CSF has been seeded, neoplasm has the potential to disseminate widely throughout the arachnoid & pia mater, through perivascular (Virchow-Robin) spaces, along the sleves of cranial nerves and spinal nerve roots. **Carcinomatous encephaltis** refers to rare occurance of diffuse perivascular (V-R space) infiltration resulting in ischemia.
- **Before and after gadolinium administration, (i.e. contrast enhanced /Gd-) MRI** plays an important role in diagnosis of meningeal neoplasm *in asymtomatic patients when CSF examination is equivocal or when lumbar puncture is contraindicated.* However, **imaging does not replace CSF examination in diagnosis of meningeal neoplasm.** ***Demonstration of tumor cells in CSF is definitive and often considered the gold standard***Q. However, CSF cytology is positive only in 50% (12-63% range) patients on first lumbar puncture; and still misses 10% after 3 CSF samples (i.e. CSF examination has *moderate sensitivity*). CSF cytological examination is most useful in *hematological malignancies, and diffuse (leptomeningeal involvement with CSF spread).* ***Detection of chromosomal/molecular markers (in hematological malignancy) & tumor markers (in solid tumor) in CSF*** is definitive but also has suboptimal sensitivity & specificity. Accompanying CSF abnormalities include *elevated protein concentration, elevated white count & hypoglycorrhachia*
- *MRI is substantially more sensitive than CT* for visualizing both normal & abnormal meninges. Signs of meningeal or SAS neoplasm are *hydrocephalus, enhancement / signal abnormality of dura, leptomeninges (pia & SAS) and cranial nerves.* MRI can be definitive in *patients with focal spread of neoplasm to meninges or SAS. (i.e. with clear tumor nodule adherent* to spinal cord, cauda equine etc). MRI is diagnostic in ~75% patients (90% of solid & 55% of hematologic neoplasm); therefore MRI is **more sensitive in detecting** meningeal involvement resulting from **solid tumors** than hematologic neoplasm. MRI has an advantage over CSF examination inits *ability to characterize bulky neoplastic disease that may be more responsive to radiotherapy*. It can also assess outcome, in that a diffuse involvement (on MRI) confers a poor prognosis.

Genetic Syndromes associated with Primary Brain Tumors

Von Hippel Lindau Syndrome	Gorlin syndrome (Basal cell neves syndrome)	Li-Fraumeni syndrome	Turcot's syndrome	Gardner's syndrome	Familial Schwannoma-tosis	MEN1 (Werner's syndrome)
AD; **Chromosom 3**p25 (VHL gene)	AD; **Ch 9**$_q$ 22.3 (patched 1 gene)	AD; **Ch 17**p 13.1 (p 53gene)	AD; **Ch 5** (APC gene) **AR; Ch 3**p21 (hMLH1)	AD; **Ch5** q21 (APC)	Sporadic; **Ch22**q 11 (IN1/SNF5 gene)	AD; **Ch11**q 13 (menin gene)
- ***Hemangioblastomas***Q - Retinal angiomas, renal cell carcinoma, pheochromocytoma, pancreatic tumor & cysts, endolymphatic sac tumors of middle ear	- **Medulloblestomas** - Basal cell carcinoma	- **Medullo blastomas , gliomas** - Sarcomas, leukemias , breast cancer, others	- **Medullablastomas , gliomas** - Adenomatous polyposis coli (APC), adenocarcinoma	-**Medulloblastoma, glioblastoma, craniopharyngeoma** -Familial polyposis, multiple osteomas, skin & soft tissue tumor	- **Schwannomas, gliomas**	- **Malignant schwannoma, pituitary adenoma** - Parathyroid & pancreatic islet cell tumors

Neurofibromatosis type 1 (Von-Reklinghausen's disease)	NF-2 (Central neurofibromatosis)	Tuberous sclerosis (TSC) (Bourneville's disease)	Cowden's syndrome
AD; **Ch17**q 12-22 (NF1, neurofibromin)	AD; **Ch22**q12 (NF-2, merlin)	AD; **Ch9q** 34/16 (TSC 1/TSC2)	AD; **Ch10** p23 (PTEN)
- **Schwannomas, astrocytomas, meningiomas, optic nerve gliomas, neurofibromas, neurofibrosarcomas**	- Multiple inherited vestibular Schwannomas, Meningiomas (multiple), Ependymoma **(MISME)**, astrocytoma - Misnomer as there is no neurofibroma	- ***Subependymal giant cell astrocytoma (SEGA), ependymomas, glioma, ganglioneuroma, hamartoma***	- **Dysplastic cerebellar gangliocytoma (Lhermitte-Duclos disease), meningioma, astrocytoma** - Breast, endometrial, thyroid cancer, trichilemmomas

Von-Hippel – Lindau – Syndrome (Retino-Cerebellar Angiomatosis)

Inheritance

Autosomal dominant (**AD**) disorder with defective **(VHL) gene** located on **chromosome 3** (P-25-P26) with *incomplete (80-100%) penetrance and variable delayed expressivity.*

Diagmpstoc Criteria

a. ***>1 Hemangioblastoma of CNS (craniospinal axis)***[Q]
b. **1 Hemangioblastoma + Visceral manifestation**
c. **1 Centra or visceral manifestation** in a patient with **known family history** (i.e. an affected first order family member)

Sub classification

Type I = Renal & pancreatic cyst, high risk for renal all carcinoma, **No phenochromocytoma**
Type IIA = Pheochromocytoma, pancreatic islet cell tumor **(typically without cyst)**
Type IIB = Pheochromocytoma + renal + pancreatic disease

Age of Onset & Cause of Death

- Variable but *uncommon before puberty (mid teens)*. Retinal angiomas become symptomatic in 20s; hemangioblastoma of CNS in mid to late 30s and renal cell carcinoma develop by early to mid 40s.
- **Hemangioblastoma** of CNS is *most common* cause of morbidity & mortality; frequent recurrences are common after resection.
- **Renal cell carcinoma** is 2nd most **common cause of mortality**.

Clinical Presentation

It is a *heriditary phakomatosis* (although skin is not involved) presenting as *a multi systemic disease* characterized by **multiple cysts, angiomas and neoplasms of CNS & abdominal viscera**. It includes

- **Retinal angiomatosis (or hemangioblastoma of retina = von Hippel tumor)**
  - Earliest manifestation of disease
  - Occurs in >50% VHL patients. Bilateral in upto 50% and multiple in upto 66% cases
- **Hemangioblastoma of CNS = Lindau tumor**
  - Benign nonglial neoplasm is *most common manifestation* seen in 40-80% cases
  - 90% of HB occur in ***posterior fossa (infratentorial). The most common location is cerebellum***[Q] (65%) >brain stem (20%) > spinal cord (15%). Most cerebellar lesions are cystic
  - 10% of **hemangioblastomas have multiple lesions** (a feature considered **diagnostic of VHL)**. 42% patients of VHL associaed hemangioblastoma show multiple **lesions**.
  - ***Supratentorial HB are uncommon***[Q] and more often solid than cystic
- **Multiple organ cysts**
  Are seen in **kidney** (multiple cortical cysts is most common), **pancreas** (numerous cysts; 2nd mc), liver, spleen omentum, mesentery, epididymis, adrenals, lung, bone (*virtually any organ*)
- **Multiple organ neoplasm**
  - **Kidney** = ***renal cell carcinoma***[Q], renal adenoma, renal hemangioma
  - *Adrenals* = ***pheochromocytoma***[Q]
  - Liver = adenoma, hemangioma
  - **Pancreas** = cystadenoma, cystadeno carcinoma, **islet cell tumor, hemangioblastoma**
  - Epididymis = Cystadenoma
  - Heart = rhabdomyoma
  - Labyrinth = endolymphatic sac neoplasm (sensorineural hearing loss)
  - Paraganglioma

Skeletal Manifestation of Neurofibromatosis type 1

Spinal, Nerve root, Spinal cord lesions

- **Enlargement (widening) of one or more neural foramina** is characteristically seen in nearly 60% patients of **neurofibromatosis type1 (NF-1, peripheral neurofibromatosis or von Recklinghausen disease)**. Most often widening of neural foramina *is secondary to dumbbell neurofibroma along the exiting spinal nerve root* or in rare casese it is caused by ***dural ectasia or arachnoid cyst or lateral meningocele***[Q].
- Other spinal anomalies in NF1 include **scalloping of posterior vertebral bodies** (nearly always secondary to *dural dysplasia*/ectasia not neurofibroma), *spinal deformities (mostly kyphoscoliosis)*, multilevel outpouching of dura & CSF,

Skull Lesions

- **Skull lesions** in NF-1 include *macrocrania (+ macrocephaly), calvarial defects* (usually left and adjacent to *lambdoid suture*), *sutural defects, hypoplasia of greater sphenoid ala* (with temporal lobe herniation into the orbit), *dural ectasia and enlargement of internal auditory canals* (secondary to dysplastic dural enlargement, not acoustic Schwannoma which is a feture & cause of IAC enlargement in NF-2)

Orbital Lesions

- **Orbital Features** of NF1 include ***empty orbit***[Q], **Harlequin appearance of orbit** (d/t partial absence of greater & lesser wing of sphenoid bone & orbital plate of frontal bone b/o failure of development of membranous bone), *hypoplasia & elevation of lesser*

meningoceles, *lateral thoracic meningocele (**pulsion diverticula**,* l/t marked posterior scalloping or erosion; & **widening of neural foramina** d/t protrusion of spinal meninges), asymptomatic **intradural-extramedullary** masses typically *neurofibroma* on the exiting nerves (k/a **dumbbell tumor** but a/t Haga dumbbell tumors have *combined intra and extradural location); multiple arachnoid cysts* and intramedullary spinal cord lesions like low grade astrocytoma & hamartomas.

- Osseous & dural lesions of NF1 most likely represent independent derivatives of a common mesenchymal dysplasia. For example *dural ectasia secondary to weakened/dysplastic meninges allowing transmission* of normal CSF pulsations may l/t *posterior scalloping of vertebral bodies and widening or enlargement of neural foramina.* (However, widening is mostly d/t *dumbbell neurofibroma*).

wing of sphenoid, extension of middle cranial fossa structures into orbit (d/t defect in sphenoid bone).

- Concentric enlargement of optic foramen (d/t optic glioma), enlargement of orbital margins & superior orbital fissure (d/t plexiform neurofibroma of peripheral & sympathetic nerves within orbit /optic nerve glioma) and sclerosis in vicinity of optic oframen (d/t optic nerve sheath meningioma).

Appendicular & Thoracic lesions

- Appendicular skeletal abnormalities of NF-1 include anterolateral bowing of lower half of tibia (mc) $\underline{+}$ fibula, ***pseudoarthrosis***Q, atrophied / thinned/absent fibula, *bone erosions/multiple cystic lesions/multiple nonossifying fibroma, focal gigantism (overgrowth)* and **twisted ribbon like ribs**.

Lateral Meningocele

- **Meningocele** is protrusion of *meninges (lined by arachnoid ± durameter) and CSF with no neural (solid) components.* **Myelo-meningocele** is protrusion of *meninges, CSF and neural components.* **Lipo-myelo-meningocels** is protrusion of *meninges, CSF, neural components and fat.* So meningocele is herniation of meninges with subarachnoid space containing CSF.
- **Cephalocele** is *herniation or protrusion of intracranial contents* through a midline defect in skull base & duramater. An anomaly that contains neural elements is k/a **encephalocele**; neural elements & mninges is k/a **meningoencephalocele**; and **meninges & subarachnoid** space is k/a **meningocele**.
- **Lateral meningocele** is *outpouching /herniation/protrusion of leptomeninges* (arachnoid & duramater with CSF) ***through enlarged intervertebral foramen***Q into ***paraspinal, intrathoracic-extra pleural, retroperitoneal space and even into subcutaneous tissue (very rarely)***Q. It may be *unilateral (R>L)* or bilateral, *thoracic (more common)* or lumbar, solitary or multiple and *asymptomatic or symptomatic* (sensory/motor deficiencies d/t root compression).
- Lateral meningocele may be a/w *mesenchymal disorders* such as **neurofibromatosis (type 1** most common; 85%), **Marfan syndrome, Ehlers – Danlos syndrome**.
- Dysplastic meninges are focally stretched by CSF pulsations and because of pressure difference between the thorax and subarachnoid space, a pulsion diverticula called lateral meningocele can develop and protude through the adjacent neural foramina. B/o high pressure differnece thoracic location is most common.
- Mass effect of lateral meningocele l/t secondary bony changes such as ***erosion of bony elements with marked posterior scalloping (i.e. erosion of posterior surface or vertebral body), thinning of neural /vertebral arches, expansion (widening)of spinal canal and neural foramen***Q, erosion of pedicle, thinning of ribs and kyphoscoliosis.
- It manifests radiologically as ***well circumscribed paravertebral/paraspinal masses of water attenuation usually on convex side of scolisis with typical enlargement of adjacent neural formen***Q. They are differentiated from low attenuation neurofibromas by **demonstrating communication with the subarachnoid space** on CT myelography. **MRI** can also differentiated because meningoceles have low signal intensity on T1WI and high signal intensity on T2WI and donot enhance after gadolinium administration. **Cardiac gated MR images** of meningoceles reveal *pulsatile motion owing to communication with subarachnoid space.* Spinal US may show cystic mass in expanded spinal canal displacing spinal cord.

NEPHROLOGY

Approach of Urogenital Imaging

Painful Hematuria (Renal Stone)

Patients suspected to have **urolithiasis (renal stone)** present with *painful hematuria or recurrent urinary tract infection.* Their radiological evaluation includes

- **Plain X-ray abdomen KUB** is usually the **first base line investigation**. Its diagnostic accuracy depends on chemical composition, size & location of stone, however, it is still good for base line study and followup after treatment.
- **Ultrasound** is highly sensitive in detecting dilated collecting system but can easily *miss stone < 5mm and stones associated with undilated collecting system.* However, combination of Xray KUB and US provide

Painless Asymptomatic Hematuria

Painless asymptomatic hematuria needs evaluation of both renal parenchyma and urothelium to *rule out urinary tract malignancy.* Their evaluation includes.

- Traditionally IVU is the base line investigation. Americal Urological Association Best Practice Policy guidelines include either **IVU** or **CT**

Children presenting with repeated attacks of UTI

- Traditionally investigated with **IVU and cystourethrography** with aim to diagnose any *underlying congenital renal anomaly that may predispose* to recurrent UTI and *detect renal scarring and vesico-ureteric reflux.* However, radiation risks of IVU outweight it unacceptably low (8.3%) diagnostic yield and there is thus a strong case for **withdrawl of routine IVU as a screening test** in patients with recurrent UTI.
- **Renal scan** using ^{99m}**Tc DMSA** is superior to

similar information as that obtained by IVU, indicating that *IVU is unlikely to be helpful if KUB/US tests were negative.*

- **Unenhanced CT** ***can detect virtually all stons regardless of their composition in kidney & ureter***Q with high sensitiviey and specificity (95-97%). Fast spiral/helical CT are specially useful in emergency setting. It can also detect *perinephric edema, ureteral obstruction and chances of spontaneous passage* of ureteral stone with 94% accuracy. So **unenhanced spiral CT** has replaced IVU & KUB for diagnosis of stones in urinary tract (developed contries). However, **IVU/IVP** is still the best investigation if CT is not available (developing nations).
- ***US/KUB is the initial screening modality f/b spiral CT***Q if the KUB and US are negative. However, it has been postulated that CT would not add useful information after a negative KUB/US study because all the missed cases had spontaneous passage of stone.

Trauma Patient

- In renal trauma patients, US, CT and arteriography are main modalities. IVU the main diagnostic tool in the past, is no longer used now.
- ***CT is the modality of choice***Q for detection & characterization of renal injuries and for assessment of vascular status.
- **Angiography** is reserved for patient requiring interventional treatment such as *embolization of traumatic pseudoaneurysm or AV fistula.*
- **Contrast cystography, micturating cystourethrography** and **retrograde urethrography** continue to be the techniques of choice for diagnosing bladder & urethral injuries and urethral strictues.

urogrophy as the initial imaging test for asymptomatic microscopic hematuria. However, it is chear as refinement of CT urography continues, it will eventually replace IVU.

- Imaging with **US/CT/MRI** is superior to IVU for detection and characterization of *renal masses.* US is the best modality for evaluating *renal volume and morphology.*
- **Urogram** or **retrograde pyelogram** may be required to visualize the urothelium of ureter & renal collecting system in patients when there is suspicion of urothelial neoplasm.

Renal Tuberculosis

- **Intravenous urography** (IVU) is the only modality to detect early changes in renal calyces in ***tuberculosis, papillary necrosis***Q etc. US, MRI, CT may be normal in early cases, hence, in a suspected case of **urinary tract TB,** ***IVU is the first imaging modality for diagnosis and subsequent follow ups***Q. However, it is advisable to integrate it with cross sectional imaging.

IVU for renal scarring detection. However, conventional **contrast voiding cysto urethrography (VCUG)** ***continues to be the gold standard for detecting and grading of vesico-ureteric reflux (VUR)***Q. Radionuclide cystograpphy (RNC) has a lower radiation dose than VCUG, but low spatial resolution & poor grading accuracy can not identify the anatomical abnormalities of urethra, bladder & ureters.

- RNC is recommended for follow up of VUR and for screening the asymptomatic siblings of patients with VUR and for initial evaluation of VUR in girls but not in boys b/o inadequate anatomic imaging of urethra & bladder by RNC; only VCUG is used.

Obstructive Uropathy in Pregnant & Children

- **MR Urography** is preferred over **IVU** d/t absence of radiation exposure. T2WI (static fluid urography) and T1WI (excretory urography) sequences are used.
- Its accuracy in detecting level of obstruction & congenital ureteropelvic junction obstruction is 100%, strictures (98.5%), hydronephrosis (98%) and stones is 68.9%. Stones are better detected in excretory than (static) sequences.

Pretransplant Work up of Renal Donor

- To know precise information of number of ureters, site of joining in case of duplication of ureter and vascular anatomy, **IVU** and **conventional angiography** (or preferably **MDCT angiography)** are used.

Various patterns of Excretory Nephrogram

Non visualization/Absence of Nephrogram

- **Global absence of nephrogram**

Occurs in anatomical absence of kidney or completely nonfunctional kidney i.e. ***complete renal ischemia secondary to occlusion of main renal artery***Q; which may be d/t

- *Renal artery dissection* (spontaneous, traumatic or iatrogenic)
- *Injury to vascular pedicle* during blunt abdominal trauma
- Thrombo-embolism

- **Segmental absence of nephrogram**

- **Focal renal infarction** caused by *focal arterial thrombo-*

Striated Nephrogram

Streaky linear bands of alternating hyper & hypo-attenuation parallel to the axis of tubules & collecting ducts during excretory phase is seen d/t *stasis of contrast material in dilated collecting ducts on back ground of edematous renal parenchyma* with diminished contrast in obstructed ischemic tubules. It is seen in

- **Unilateral (U/L)**

- ***Acute ureteric obstruction***Q
- Renal vein

Increasingly Dense Nephrogram

Initially faint nephrogram becomes increasingly dense over hours to days b/o

1. *Diminished perfusion* l/t diminished plasma clearance of contrast material eg
   - ***Acute systemic hypotension***Q (B/L)
   - Acute renal vein thrombosis
   - Severe main renal artery stenosis
   - Acute papillary necrosis (range)
   - ***Acute tubular necrosis***Q
2. Leakage of contrast material into the renal interstial space eg
   - Acute glomerulo nephritis
   - Acute pyelonephritis
3. **Increase in tubulr transit time** d/t obstruction
   - Acute obstruction like acute urate nephropathy, myeloma nephropathy (d/t Bence-Jones protein), amyloid,
   - **Severe dehydration** in infants & children (Tamm-Horsfall protein)
   - Ureter calculus

Immediate Persistent (Dense) Nephrogram

- **Bilateral Global**

- **Tubular obstruction** (from BJ/TH proteins, myoglobin) or **tubular damage** by contrast material
- ***Systemic hypotension***Q (uncommon)
- Other causes of acute renal failure (or acute on chronic renal failure) like

embolism, vasculitis, collagen vascular disease, sickle cell anemia, septic shock and ***renal vein thrombosis***[Q]
- **Space occupying lesions** such as cyst, abscess, neoplasm.

Rim Nephrogram
- *2-4mm peripheral rim (band) of cortical opacification* is seen (from capsular, peripelvic and periureteric vessels supplying it). It is **most specific indicator of renovascular compromise** and is seen in
- ***Acute complete (total) main renal artery occlusion***[Q] (smooth nephrogram)
- Renal vein thrombosis
- Acute tubular necrosis
- Severe chronic urinary obstruction
- **Severe hydronephrosis** *(Scalloped/shell nephrogram* with negative pyelogram)

thrombosis
- Renal contusion

• **U/L or B/L**
- Acute nephritis/ pyelonephritis

• **Bilateral (B/L)**
- **Infantile AR polycystic kidney diease (PCKD)**
- **Medullary sponge kidney, medullary cystic disease** (parallel or fan shaped streaks radiating from papilla to periphery, in medulla)
- Intratubular obstruction (Bence-Jones/Tamm-Horsfall protein uria, rhabdomyolysis with myoglobinuria)
- Systemic hypotension

severe dehydration[Q]

• **Unilateral Global**
- ***Renal artery stenosis***[Q]
- ***Renal vein thrombosis***[Q]
- ***Urinnary tract obstruction***[Q]

• **Segmental**
- ***Obstruction d/t duplicated collecting system***[Q], renal calculus, & neoplasm
- Focal stricture
- Focal parenchymal disease eg tubulo interstitial infection.

Immediate Faint Persistent Neghrogram
- Proliferative/necrotizing disorders eg acute glomerulonephritis
- Renal vein thrombosis
- Chronic severe ischemia

Unilateral Delayed Nephrogram
- Obstructive uropathy
- Reduced renal blood flow d/t renal artery stenosis or renal vein thrombosis

Phase of IVU study

- Pyelogram
  - ✶ Reduced GFR from any cause or stasis of urine leads to obligatory reabsorption of Na^+ & H_2O resulting in concentration of the radiopaque contrast material in the renal tubules and an increasingly dense nephrogram.
- Nephrogram
  - **Tubular Nephrogram**
    - For Renal function
    - For Plasma contrast
    - For Concentration
  - **Vascular Nephrogram**

Renal Papillary Necrosis (Necrotizing Papillitis)

- *Ischemic necrobiosis* (coagulative necrosis) of renal papilla (i.e. loops of Henle + vasa recta), secondary to interstitial nephritis (interstitial edema) or intrinsic vascular obstruction. Diabetes (50%), sickle cell anemia and analgesics are the most important causes.
- In papillary necrosis, part or all of necrotic renal papilla sloughs and may fall into the pelvicaliceal system, which may remain there (and get calcified) or may be voided down the ureter (often causing obstruction).
- If papilla is only *partially necrotic, contrast tracks around or onto it*, whereas if papilla is *totally sloughed* the calyx appears *spherical (with loss of papillary indentation)* and as *filling defect.*

Caused by: [Mn: "ADIPOSE-CAT"]

A	- ***A**nalgesics*[Q], ***A**cute tubular necrosis*
D	- ***DM***[Q], ***D**ehydration*, ***D**iarrhoea (severe)*
I	- Infant in shock
P	- Pyelonephritis, Post partum
O	- Obstruction
S	- *Sickle cell disease*[Q]
E	- ***Ethanol (Alcohol)***[Q]
C	- Coagulopathy, Christmas disease, hemophilia
A	- Alcoholism = Cirrhosis
T	- Trauma, TB, Thrombosis of renal vein, Transplant rejection

Imaging features

• **Plain X-Ray**
- **Ring shaped calcification** in sloughed papilla

• **IVP/Excretory Urography (best investigation)**
- Thin and short **(bulbous) cavitation of papilla** and widened fornix (d/t necrotic shrinkage of papilla)
- **Ball in cup or egg in cup or signet ring sign** or **ring shadow of papilla** (caused by contrast outlining detached sloughed papilla within a contrast material filled cavity)
- **Club shaped (saccular) calyx** (d/t sloughed papilla)
- **Lobster claw sign** is subtle linear streaks of contrast material extending from fornix parallel to long axis of papilla inside calyceal void left by sloughed papilla.
- Intraluminal **nonopaque filling defects** in calyx/pelvis/ureter (d/t passing down of sloughed papilla)
- ***Diminished density of contrast material in nephrogram***[Q]; very rarely increasingly dense (not hyper dense).
- Displaced collecting system, wasted parenchymal thickness
- Extracalyceal contrast excavation, ill defined, irregular & distorted calyces with few ***ampulated calyces and formation of multiple cavities.***

RADIODIAGNOSIS

5

Renal Artery Stenosis (RAS) & Renovascular Hypertension (RVHT)

Definition

- RVHT is renin dependent elevation of BP, secondary to renal ischemia caused by RAS. It is a potentially curable form of hypertension that often improves or resolves after correction of RAS.

Pathophysiology

- **RAS → Reduced intra arterial pressure & perfusion to the glomerulus** is sensed by **baroreceptors** in juxtaglomerular apparatus (JGA) of afferent arterioles, resulting in **renin release by JGA**.→ Renin converts angiotensinogen to angiotensin I which is converted to **angiotensin II** by ACE (angiotensin converting enzyme) in lungs → **Angiotensin II** is a potent arteriolar constrictor and tries to **restore GFR by contraction of efferent arterioles** but at the same time it **also increases BP** by stimulating **aldosterone** secretion l/t salt water retention and by systemic arteriolar contraction.
- In unilateral RAS, there is decreased GFR sodium excretion and renin production by nonaffected contralateral kidney b/o high renin & angiotensin II levels. However, increased BP ultimately results in pressure natriuresis from nonaffected kidney resulting in classic *high renin-normal volume pattern of U/L RAS*. Whereas, in B/L RAS there is volume overload also.
- **ACE inhibitors (like captopril)** and *angiotensin II receptor blocker does not affect GFR in patients with normal renal arteries or those with essential hypertension*. But these agents decrease GFR (and hence urine flow) in stenotic kidney (with RAS), owing to efferent arteriolar dilation. In the presence of B/L RAS or RAS to a solitary kidney, use of these agents may result in *progressive (but generally reversible) renal insufficiency*.
- Untreated, prolonged RAS l/t nephrosclerosis and renoprival or azotemic renovascular disease with inability to excrete sodium & water, and then treatment of RAS does not relieve hypertension.

Etiology

- The most common **etiology of RAS** is **atherosclerosis** (60-90%) followed by **fibromuscular dysplasia** (10-30%) and then **nonspecific aorto arteritis (Takayasu's disease)**. However, in Indian subcontinent the order is reverse i.e. Takayasu's disease (61%) > fibromuscular dysplasia (28%) > atherosclerosis (8%). The incidence of atherosclerosis is rising in urban population.
- Atherosclerosis *mostly affects >50 year men* and *involve the origin (ostial) or the proximal third of renal artery*. Obstruction is mostly bilateral and usually results from aortic plaque engulfing the renal ostium (i.e. with in 4mm of aortic lumen). Less commonly plaques develop independently in proximal third of renal artery. **CT gives more accurate assessment of ostial stenosis than angiography** (which underestimates it). **Post**

Imaging Modalities and Assessment

IVP and Renal Scintigraphy

- **Radionuclide renal scintigraphy** (using **^{99m}Tc MAG3 ≥ ^{99m}Tc DTPA >> ^{131}I OIH**) classicaly demonstrates *small kidney with decreased uptake & delayed traser transit and excretion* and have unacceptably high rate of both false positive and negative. And it is not significantly better than IVP (which classically demonstrates *delayed appearance of contrast material* d/t decreased GFR, *increased density of contrast* d/t increased water reabsorption, *delayed washout* d/t prolonged transit time and notching of proximal ureter d/t enlarged colleteral vessels). Both IVP and RRS are no longer used for screening.

Captopril Enhanced Radionuclide Renal Scintigraphy

- **Captopril (ACEI) enhanced radionuclide renal scintigraphy (CERRS)** is highly sensitive and accurate in detection of **unilateral RAS** with normal renal function & normal base line renogram (90% sensitivity & specificity) but its accuracy/specificity falls (to 50% in patients suffering from *bilateral RAS or azotemia (with abnormal renal function with abnormal baseline renogram* and in patients with single functioning kidney.)
- A base line dynamic renogram (without ACEI) f/b captopril enhanced renogram is taken and positive ACE renogram will show a decrease in total or relative function of affected kidney (>5-10%) and/or a delayed time to peak maximum activity and prolonged intrarenal transit time (**i.e. delayed uptake & delayed washout on affected side with decreased relative uptake which is <40% of total by involved kidney**).
- CE RRS can be used as a screening test to establish the hemodynamic significances of RAS, to predict the out come of revascularization and in follow up after successful revascularization. A positive test suggest a cure or improvemnt after intervention.
- Disadvantages of CERRS include *low sensitivity in azotemia, renal dysfunction and in bilateral RAS*. ***Branch artery stenosis cannot be diagnosed and provides functional not anatomical data***[Q]. Captopril induced severe hypotension may l/t false positive results (symmetircal parenchymal retention). Advantages include low cost, *noninvasive nature* and overall high sensitivity & specificity (>90%) in detection of unilateral RAS and establishing hemodynamic (functional) significance.

Ultrasound

- **Ultrasound** is an essential part of noninvasive radiological screen but the renal size may be normal unless the stenosis is >60%. In the absence of any other renal disease, a significant difference in size of two kidneys should suggest RAS, although a normal appearance does not exclude the presence of significant unilateral or bilateral RAS.
- **Intravascular USG** is best modality for correct evaluation of stenosis & plaque morphology but b/o being invasive & expansive it is highly unlikely to become a screening modality.

Coller Doppler or Duplex

- **Coller doppler flow imaging (CDFI) or Duplex ultrasound** (more recently **contrast enhanced**) is widely performed non-invasive modality used for screening RAS by direct evaluation of renal arteries as well as indirect trans renal doppler waveform. Its **sensitvity** varies from 50-92% and is **highly observer dependent**.
- **Direct signs** require *visualization of entire main renal artery (which is not seen in 42% cases – a main draw back) include*

1. Increased **peak systolic vlocity** (>150 &180 cm/sec for angles <60° & >70° respectively)
2. **Ratio of peak renal artery to aorta velocity (RAR)** > 3.5 increases accuracy of diagnosis and RAS is considered significant
3. Post stenotic turbulent flow, spectral broadening ± flow reversal.
4. Absence of blood flow during distole (>50%RAS) and *visualization of renal artery without detectable doppler signal* (indicate arterial occlusion).

stenotic dilatation *may be present on angiography, but this is not a good indicator of the severity of disease.* It is unlikely that there will be benefit from any intervention in atherosclerotic RAS if there is *evidence of distal disease and kidney is small on ultrasound.*

- **Fibromuscular dysplasia** typically occur in (20-50yr) *young (white) women,* is frequently *bilateral* and in contrast to atherosclerotic renovascular disease, tend to affect ***more distal*** *portions of renal artery* (mainly involving distal main artery and major branches). It may involve any layer of artery but the **medial fibroplasia** is the commonest form. On angiography it presents with **strings of beads appearance** (*d/t alternating stenosis and dilatations*). It can also involve visceral, peripheral, carotid and vertebral arteries but tends to spare the intracranial vessels. Beaded artery dilates easily on percutaneous transluminal renal angioplasty (PTRA) and there are excellent long term results.
- **Takayasu's arteritis** tends to affect young females (mostly <35 years) particularly in India & southeast Asia. It ma be a/w involvement of *aortic arch & its branches (type I), descending thoracic & upper abdominal aorta (type 2,* both (type 3) and *pulmonary artery (type 4).* **CT and MR** can demonstrate **arterial wall thickening** and narrowed lumen. Initial success after dilatation can be upto 95% but surgery is often required eventually.

Hemodynamic significance

Significant renal artery stenosis *(reduction of the internal diameter by at least 60%)* is a potentially treatable cause of hypertension. Hemodynamic significane is determined by:

1. Elevated rennin levels in ipsilateral renal vein ≥ 1.5 : 1.
2. ***Presence of collateral vessels. (most important sign on angiography)***[Q]
3. Greater than 70% stenosis with poststenotic dilatation.
4. Trans stenotic pressure gradient ≥ 40 mmHg.
5. Decrease in renal size.

Screening

- Hypertension is common but RVHT is not, so **screening** should be reserved for **moderate-high risk patients**. i.e.

1. Abrupt onset or severe/malignant hypertension or *hypertension uncontrolled by 3 drug therapy* or hypertension in infants with an umblical artery catheter/children or *onset of HTN <20-30 yrs or >50-55 years.*
2. ***Worsening renal function after treatment with ACE inhibitors***[Q]
3. Recurrent pulmonary edema/unexplained azotemia in elederly with HTN or occlusive disease in other vascular bed eg peripheral vascular disease
4. ***Abdominal or flank bruit (systolic or diastolic) or grade ¾ hypertensive retinopathy***[Q]

- Intrarenal vessels are easily identified in most patients and normal waveform has a *rapid systolic upstroke with a small peak in early systole (ESP=early systolic peak).* **Indirect signs** obtained from *analysis of intrarenal segmental arterial Doppler wave forms* (from upper, mid & lower poles) indicating RAS include **pattern recognization** (1, 2, 3) & **quantitative creteria** (4, 5).

1. **Dampened appearance** or **tardus-parvus waveform** i.e. in the presence of significant RAS, there is *slowing of systolic upstroke acceleration & late arrival* k/a tardus and *low amplitude of systolic peak/attenuated peak* k/a parvus. This wave form can be produced by abdominal coarctation (false positive).
2. *Loss of ESP & early systolic acceleration* (later is best predictor)
3. Segmental arterial flow is detectable even with renal artery occlusion d/t collateral circulation.
4. **Acceleration time (AT) delay** > 0.05-0.08 sec and /or **decreased acceleration index AI**; single most sensitive screening parameter) <370-470 cm/S^2 indicate significant RAS. AT or pulse rise time is the time from start to peak of systoloe and AI is the slope of upstroke.
5. *Decreased resistive index (RI) and pulsatility index.*

For >60% RAS	Sensitivity	Specificity	Accuracy
Absent ESP	92	96	95
AI <300 cm/S^2	89	86	87
AT > 0.07 sec	81	95	91

CT Angiography (CTA)

- **After percutaneous arteriography**, the ***next most sensitive and specific screening test for diagnosis of RAS is CT angiography***[Q] (using spiral and more recently **multidetector CT**) almost equvalent to DSA. However, it requires use of large amount of iodinated contrast medium (like IVP) precluding its use in renal insufficiency and also exposes to ionizing radiation.
- **CT angiography (CTA)** is a noninvasive technique with a sensitivity of almost 100% for identifying main & accessory renal arteries. It **demonstrates the wall of aorta unlike angiography which only visualizes the lumen of vessel,** important in cases of *atherosclerosis & aorto arteritis* where the lumen may appear angiographically normal but may show vessel wall involvement in cross sectional studies. It demonstrates the *extent of plaque projecting into vessels lumen,* aiding in determining the form of intervention planned such as angioplasty and primary stent placement. **CTA is best for diagnosing ostial stenosis** the most difficult place to evaluate during arteriography and primary stent placement. CTA is best for diagnosing ostial stenosis the most difficult place to evaluate during arteriography and improves the differentiation b/w ostial & truncal stenosis. MDCT CTA can also detect collaterals and unlike MRA, can be used to determine the patency of vessels that have been dilated by intravascular stents (however, intrastent diameter was under estimated in comparison to catheter angiography).

MR Angiography (MRA)

- **Contrast (Gadolinium) enhanced magnetic resonance angiography (CEMRA)** is also very sensitive for proximal renal artery **but may miss distal lesions**. And b/o risk of gadolinium induced **nephrogenic systemic fibrosis** (NSF) in patients with deranged renal functions, CEMRA as a screening test is being avoided. **Dynamic** (3D spoiled gradient echo imaging) **CE MRI** provides functional imaging similar to scintigraphy and can evaluate the kidney after placement of stent which otherwise cannot be assessed d/t susceptibility artifacts.
- **Steady State Free Precession (SSFP) non contrast enhanced MRI angiography** (either breath hold or navigator gated) can be performed as a *1st line MRA to rule out RAS* especially in patients with high risk of NSF. If SSPF is negative for high grade RAS (>50%), RAS can be excluded without using any gadolinium based contrast agents, and if SSPF is positive then further studies (CE-MRI, DSA, CTA) can be done for better delineation of stenosis.

Conventional Renal Angiography

- **Conventional contrast renal arteriography** (or **digital substraction angiography or intraarterial catheter angiography**) is the **gold standard** for ***diagnosis of renal artery stenosis***[Q] against which all other modalities are compared.

RADIODIAGNOSIS

5

Radiological Imaging in Acute Pyelonephritis

IVU

- Limited role as 75% case have normal urogram.
- May show **global/focal renal enlargement** with *decreased, delayed and persistent nephrogram*, minimal dilation of pelvicalyceal system and attenuation of calyces.

CT-Nephrogram (CTN)

- CTN at 20-45 sec is superior & best in depicting and describing the full extent of disease
- **Secretory phase** (after 2 min) detects **sloughed papilla or fungus ball**.
- CE-CT shows **bilateral enlarged kidney with striated nephrogram** ie transverse areas of **alternate bands with increased and decreased density** representing microstriations d/t *vasoconstriction and renal edema*. It shows ***wedge shaped areas of decreased attenuation radiating from papilla** (d/t hypoperfusion or vasocontriction) in **enlarged kidnely**.*
- Delayed CT outlines true extent of renal infection and can be of 3 types.

1. Focal staining or hyperdense rim surrounding abscesses
2. Wedge shaped high denstiy area seen at the same site as the reduced density on early scans.
3. Focal areas of increased density distant from low density areas on early scan

Ultra sonagraphy

- ***Focal or diffuse enlargement of kidney with focal or segmental hypoechogencity***[Q] (low level echoes) and loss of corticomedullary (CM) differentiation.
- **Focal areas of hypoperfusion**[Q] d/t arteriolar vasocontrition and interstilial edema. Areas of poor perfusion are better demonstrated by power doppler (> color doppler) and with use of contrast.
- **Perinephric fluid collection**[Q], obstruciton, renal enlargement & inflammatory masses. However, CE CT (bi or triphasic) is superior to USG & IVP in detection of these features.
- **USG is modality of choice for pregnant patients**
- **Gas bubbles** incollecting system or renal parenchyma is seen in **emphysematous pyelonephritis** (commonly in **diabetes**).

Renal Cortical Scintigraphy (^{99m}Tc DMSA)

- Reveals wedge shaped cortical defects and is superior to USG and IVP in diagnosis

MRI

- Affected area has **low signal** on **T1** and **increased signal on T2** WI with loss of CMD.

Radiological Evaluation of Prostatic Cancer

Ultrasound

- **Screening** for prostate carcinoma consist of digital rectal examination *(DRE) and measurement of PSA levels*, and **diagnosis** is usully made by ***needle biopsy, which is best performed using TRUS (trans rectal ultra sonography) guidance***[Q]. While TRUS is an excellent adjunct to physical examination, it does not serve as a screening investigation because the *combination of DRE & PSA is more sensitive than TRUS for screening prostatic carcinoma.* ***Once suspected, prostatic carcinoma is most effectively confirmed by TRUS guided needle biopsy***[Q] and this should involve both lesion-guided and systemic sampling. Intraprostatic disease can be identified by trans rectal or transurethral approch but not by trans abdominal US. On TRUS, prostatic carcinoma most commonly demonstrates a **hypoechoic** echo texture usually in peripheral zone (however, also seen in benign conditions). Color & power doppler US improve the detection of prostate cancer.
- Accurate tumor staging is essential to determine the extent of disease & thus the choice of treatment because carcinoma confined to prostate gland are theoretically considered curable by radical prostatectomy (removal of entire prostate &

Radionucleide Scan

- **Radionucleide bone scan (not CT)** is ***preferred to screen for bony metastasis because it is more sensitive in detecting small & early lesion***[Q].

e-MRI and ^{1}H-3D-MRSI

- Major role of **MRI** in prostate cancer is in ***local staging of disease (i.e. tumor extention, capsular/seminal vesicular and bladder involvement)***[Q]. **Endorectal coil MRI (eMRI)** is better than external surface coil or body coil images. Prostatic carcinoma mostly demonstrates ***lower signal intensity*** (can be shown by other benign conditions also), *so histological diagnosis remains essential.* Tumor detection is excellent in peripheral zone but hampered by inherent heterogeneity & low signal intensity changes caused by BPH within the transitional & central zone. MRI performed significantly better in detecting cancer thn DRE *in apex mid gland, base and anterior prostate*; and significantly better than *TRUS guided biopsy in midgland & base.*
- Criteria for detecting **extracapsular extension** of tumor (on T2 weighted images) include *obliteration of rectoprostatic angle, asymmetry of neurovascular bundle (both most important), irregular capsular bulge, angulation or step off appearance of prostate contour, focal capsular retraction & thickening*, broad (>12mm) capsular tumor contact, breech of capsule with evidence of direct tumor extension.

seminal vesicle). Because **tumor volume** governs prognosis & treatment, both *TRUS & MRI have been used* for accurate assessment. But studies demonstrate that both methods can ***significantly over & under estimate tumor volumes***Q.

- US features suggestive of extracapsular extension include *contour deformity of capsule, irregularity and evidence of direct tumor extension into the periprostatic fat*. However, ***TRUS has very limited ability to detect seminal vesicle invasion & bladder neck invasion and cannot be used for detection of lymph node metastases***Q.
- Because of large discrepancies in the reported value of the accuracy of TRUS for the evaluation of prostate cancer, ***its main role in assessment of prostate cancer continues to be in biopsy guidance***Q.

CT scan

- CT is not recommended & not used for routine tumor staging because it is insensitive, nonspecific, costly & highly radiating procedure. However, it is *useful in advanced cancer particularly in evaluation of lymphadenopathy (based on size)*. It cannot detect micro invasion in normal/small nodes (<10mm) l/t **false negative** results and make **false positive** diagnosis in hyperplastic nodes (>10mm). When pelvic CT does not reveal any lymphadenopathy, abdominal CT of paraaortic nodes is unnecessary, therefore, CT examination for staging prostatic carcinoma need *only be carried to the aortic bifuracation*. However, **CT to search for nodal metastasis is reserved for high risk patients. Percutaneous CT guided needle biopsy** is recommended for confirming metastatis in patients with enlarged or suspicious lymph nodes. A negative finding does not eliminate the need for lymphadenectomy.

- **Seminal vesicle invasion criteria** include direct tumor extension into & around seminal vesicle and *tumor extension along ejaculatory ducts*, resulting in low signal intensity on T2WI & non visualization of ejaculatory ducts. The use of **Gd-DTPA** IV may facilitate demonstration of seminal vesicle invasion. **Bladder base invasion** is diagnosed on sagittal plane T2WI, in which tumor invasion results in *interruption of low signal intensity of bladder wall*.
- *MRI staging accuracy is decreased within 3weeks of biopsy*. But when e-MRI is used with **3D-^{1}H-MR spectroscopic imaging (^{1}H-3D-MRSI)** the detection of prostate cancer and accuracy of staging of local tumor post biopsy are improved. MRSI provides a *3D metabolic map of prostate gland by displaying concentrations of cellular metabolites citrate, creatine & choline. Normal prostate tissue contains high levels of citrate whereas cancer demonstrates elevated choline and decreased citrate (therefore* ***increased choline to citrate ratio) and a decreased or absent level of polyamines***.
- Addition of ^{1}H3DMRSI to eMRI can improve evaluation of extracapsular invasion, decrease interobserver variability, improves accuracy in monitoring patients who have undergone cryosurgery & hormone or radiation therapy and is useful for targeting biopsy esp for patient with previous negative biopsy results yet persistently elevated PSA levels; this occurs mostly with lesions in anterior peripheral, transition or central zones i.e. regions not palpable by DRE and often not routinely sampled during biopsy.
- 1H3D MRSI can suggest **aggressiveness (Gleason grade)** with increasing choline & decreasing citrate levels. eMRI improves staging accuracy, assist in surgical planning (eg to spare or resect neurovascular bundle), predict intra operative blood loss and urinary continence after radicle retropubic prostatectomy.

Monitoring after therapy

- **Measurements of PSA levels** is the primary method of follow up after surgery, radiation or hormonal therapy, and imaging is only done when the PSA is elevated.

QUESTIONS

CENTRAL NERVOUS SYSTEM

Embryology

1. **Insult during neuronal migration results in delayed neuroneal migration and organization, which results in certain disorders. The least likely possibility is:**
   A. Polymicrogyria *(AIIMS Nov 2011)* ☐
   B. Schizencephaly ☐
   C. Lissencephaly ☐
   D. Focal cortical dysplasia without ballon cells. ☐
2. **J-shaped sella is/are seen in:** *(PGI Nov 2011)*
   A. Mucopolysaccharidoses ☐
   B. Achondroplasia ☐
   C. Optic chiasm glioma ☐
   D. Neurofibromatosis I ☐
   E. Hydrocephalus ☐
3. **A middle aged man presents with progressive atrophy & weakness of hand & forearms. On examination he is found to have slight spasticity of the leg, genera-lized hyperreflexia and increased signal in the cortico-spinal tracts on T2 weighted MRI. The most likely diagnosis is:**
   A. Multiple Sclerosis *(AIIMS Nov 2004)* ☐
   B. Amyotrophic lateral sclerosis ☐
   C. Subacute combined degeneration ☐
   D. Progressive spinal muscular atrophy ☐
4. **Hyperintense corticospinal tract on T2WI MRI is/are:** *(PGI May 12)*
   A. Astrocytoma ☐
   B. Amyotrophic lateral sclerosis ☐
   C. Hemochondromatosis ☐
   D. Wilson disease ☐
   E. Multiple lacunar infarcts of the brain ☐
5. **All/except are true about MS:** *(DNB 10, PGI Nov 2011)*
   A. Corpus callosum lesions are characteristic ☐
   B. Periventricular white matter distribution with decreased CT attenuation ☐
   C. T1WI are most diagnostic for acute plaques ☐
   D. 4th ventricle, 5th nerve entery site & brachium pontis involved ☐
   E. Hyper intense T2WI ☐
6. **The MR imaging in multiple sclerosis will show lesions in:** *(AI 06)*
   A. White matter ☐
   B. Grey matter ☐
   C. Thalamus ☐
   D. Basal ganglia ☐
7. **A child presented with clinical features of demyelination. The chances of progression to MS is least with which of the following:** *(AIIMS Nov 2011)*
   A. Absent oligoclonal band ☐
   B. Bilateral visual loss ☐
   C. Poor recovery ☐
   D. Cord complete transaction ☐
8. **Extensive involvement of deep white matter with bilateral hyperdense thalami on non-contrast CT scan of the brain is virtually diagnostic of:** *(AIIMS Nov 07)*
   A. Alexander's disease ☐
   B. Krabbe's disease. ☐
   C. Canavan's disease ☐
   D. Metachromatic leukodystrophy ☐
9. **Which of the following is not a MRI feature of Mesial temporal sclerosis?** *(AI 2009)*
   A. Atrophy of mammilary body ☐
   B. Atrophy of fornix ☐
   C. Blurring of Grey white matter junction of ipsilateral temporal lobe ☐
   D. Atrohy of hippocampus ☐
10. **A new born presents with congestive heart failure resistant to treatment, on examination has bulging anterior fontanelle with a bruit on auscultation. Transfontanellar USG shows a hypoechoic midline mass with dilated lateral ventricles. Most likely diagnosis is**
    A. Encephalocele *(AIIMS Nov 11, May 10)* ☐
    B. Medulloblastoma ☐
    C. Arachnoid cyst ☐
    D. Vein of Galen malformation ☐
11. **All are the characteristics of raised ICT on a plain radiology except:** *(AIIMS May 08)*
    A. Erosion of dorsum sellae ☐
    B. Ballooning of sella ☐
    C. Increased convolutons ☐
    D. Sutural diastasis ☐
12. **A male was brought unconscious to the hospital with external injuries. CT shows no midline shift, but basal cisterns were full (compressed) with multiple small haemorrhage. The most probable diagnosis is:**
    A. Brain contusion *(AI 07, AIIMS Nov 06, 10)* ☐
    B. Diffuse axonal injury ☐
    C. Subdural hemorrhage ☐
    D. Multiple infarct. ☐
13. **A 15 year old boy had 10-12 partial complex seizures per day in spite of adequate 4 drug antiepileptic regime. He had history of repeated high grade fever in childhood. MRI for epilepsy protocol revealed normal brain scan. What should be the best non-invasive strategy to make a definite diagnosis so that he can be prepared to undergo epilepsy surgery.** *(AIIMS 2002)*
    A. Interictal scalp EEG. ☐
    B. Video EEG ☐
    C. Interictal ^{18}F-FDg PET. ☐
    D. Video EEG with Ictal ^{99}m Tc-HMPAO Brain SPECT. ☐
14. **Investigation which should not be done in a patient with brain tumor:** *(AI 1997)*
    A. CT Scan ☐
    B. Lumber Puncture ☐
    C. MRI ☐
    D. X – Ray ☐

INFECTION

15. **Basal exudates, infarcts and hydrocephalus on computed tomography are seen in:** *(AI 2012)*
    A. Tuberculosis meningitis ☐
    B. Viral meningitis ☐
    C. Herpes simplex encephalitis ☐
    D. Cerebral malaria / Neurocysticercosis ☐

16. **Local cerebral lesion with ring on CT scan is caused by:**
A. Toxoplasmosis *(PGI 2002)* ☐
B. Intracranial haemorrhage ☐
C. Cysts ☐
D. Hamartoma ☐

EPIDERMOID

17. **Epidermoids can be differentiated from arachnoid cyst on MRI by:** *(AIIMS Nov 2011)*
A. Contrast enhancement ☐
B. Smooth margins ☐
C. Restricted diffusion ☐
D. CSF signal on FLAIR ☐

CALCIFICATION

18. **Physiological calcification of Skull in X ray is seen in:**
A. Pineal gland *(PGI 2001)* ☐
B. Choroid plexus ☐
C. Red nucleus ☐
D. Basal ganglion ☐

19. **Which one of the following tumors shows calcification on CT Scan:** *(AI 05)*
A. Ependymoma. ☐
B. Meduloblastoma. ☐
C. Meningioma. ☐
D. CNS lymphoma. ☐

20. **Periventricular calcification is often due to:**
A. Toxoplasmosis *(DNB 03; PGI 97)* ☐
B. Cytomegalic infection ☐
C. Congenital syphilis ☐
D. All of the above ☐

21. **Intracranial calcification with cystic lesion in plain X-Ray skull is seen in** *(AIIMS 96, DNB 98)*
A. Meningioma ☐
B. Glioma ☐
C. Craniopharyngioma ☐
D. Meduloblastoma ☐

22. **Suprasellar calcification is characteristic of:** *(AI 12, 92)*
A. Toxoplasmosis, CMV, Cysticercosis ☐
B. Medulloblastoma ☐
C. Craniopharyngioma ☐
D. Meningioma ☐
E. Ependymoma ☐

23. **Bracket clacification in skull X-ray is seen in:**
A. Meningioma *(AIIMS May 2012)* ☐
B. Lipoma of carpus callosum ☐
C. Tuberous sclerosis ☐
D. Sturge weber syndrome ☐

24. **Calcification of basal ganglia is seen in A/E:**
A. Berry's aneurysm *(AIIMS 97, DNB 01)* ☐
B. Cysticercosis ☐
C. Idiopathic hyperparathroidism ☐
D. Wilson's disease ☐

25. **Basal ganglia calcification is seen in all except:** *(AI 2007)*
A. Hypoparathyroidism ☐
B. Wilson's disease ☐
C. Perinatal hypoxia ☐
D. Fahr's syndrome ☐

26. **Basal ganglia calcification is seen in**
A. Hyperparathyrodism *(PGI 2003)* ☐
B. Hyperthyroidism ☐
C. Hypoparathyroidism ☐
D. Hypothyroidism ☐
E. Acromegaly ☐

CRANIOPHARYNGIOMA

27. **Suprasellar calcification with growth retardation is seen in** *(AIIMS 95, DNB 96)*
A. Pineal body tumor ☐
B. Pituitory tumor ☐
C. Thalmic tumor ☐
D. Craniopharyngioma ☐

28. **Commonest calcifying brain tumor in a child is:**
A. Medulloblastoma *(AIIMS 93, DNB 98)* ☐
B. Craniopharyngioma ☐
C. Glioma ☐
D. Meningioma ☐

29. **Which of the following is the most common cause of a mixed cystic and solid suprasellar mass seen on cranial MR scan of a 10 years old child:** *(AIIMS May 2005)*
A. Pituitary Adenoma ☐
B. Craniopharyngioma ☐
C. Optic chiasma glioma ☐
D. Germinoma ☐

30. **A 6 year old boy has been complaining of headache, ignoring to see the objects on the side for 4 months. On Examination, he is not mentally retarded, his grades at school are good & visual acuity is diminished in both the eyes, visual charting showed significant field defect. CT scan of the head showed suprasellar mass with calcification. Which of the following is the most probable diagnosis?** *(AI 12, AIIMS 04)*
A. Astrocytoma ☐
B. Craniopharyngioma ☐
C. Pituitary adenoma ☐
D. Meningioma ☐

31. **Intracranial calcification with cystic lesion in plain X-Ray skull is seen in**
A. Meningioma *(AIIMS 97, DNB 99)* ☐
B. Glioma ☐
C. Craniopharyngioma ☐
D. Meduloblastoma ☐

INTRACRANIAL VASCULAR MALFORMATIONS

32. **Cavernous hemangioma is characterized by:** *(AIIMS Nov 2011)*
A. Reticulated popcorn like configuration ☐
B. Well defined nidus ☐
C. Well defined arterial feeder ☐
D. Phlebectasis ☐

INTRACRANIAL TUMORS

33. **A 40-years-old female patient presented with recurrent headaches. MRI showd an extra-aixal, dural based and enhancing lesion. The most likely diagnosis is:**
A. Meningioma *(AIIMS May 10, 06)* ☐
B. Glioma ☐
C. Schwannoma ☐
D. Pituitary adenoma ☐

34. A 45 year old female presented with progressive lower limb weakness, spasticity, urinary hesitancy and mid dorsal (thoracic) extra axial, dural based, intradural enhancing mass in MRI. What is the diagnosis – *(AI 12, 07, AIIMS Nov 11, 06, DNB 99, 08)*

A. Intradural lipoma ☐
B. Meningioma ☐
C. Dermoid cyst ☐
D. Neuroepithelial cyst. ☐

35. **A 48 yr old woman comes with b/l progressive weakness of both lower limbs, spasticity & mild impairment of respiratory movements. MRI shows an intradural mid-dorsal midline enhancing lesion. What is the likely diagnosis:** *(AIIMS May 2010)*

A. Intradural lipoma ☐
B. Meningioma ☐
C. Neuroenteric cyst ☐
D. Dermoid cyst ☐

36. Finding in meningioma are all except:

A. Vascular markings around falx ☐
B. Calcification *(PGI 97, DNB 02)* ☐
C. Erosion ☐
D. Osteosclerosis ☐

37. **Meningioma on plain radiography reveals:** *(PGI June 09)*

A. Calcification ☐
B. Erosion ☐
C. Sutural diastasis ☐
D. Osteosclerosis ☐
E. Vascular erosion ☐

38. A 20 yr female come with a mass in the cavernous sinus & 6th cranial nerve palsy. In T2W MRI Hyperintense shadow is present which shows homogenous contrast enhancement. Diagnosis is: *(AIIMS Nov 2010)*

A. Schwannoma ☐
B. Meningioma ☐
C. Astrocytoma ☐
D. Cavernous sinus hemangioma ☐

39. **Tumor associated with extracranial spread**

A. Ependymoma *(AIIMS May 10)* ☐
B. Medulloblastoma ☐
C. Glioblastoma multiformae ☐
D. Choroid plexus papilloma ☐

40. **In 7 year old posterior fossa mass with cyst formation, hypodense on CT, hyper intense on T2WI and showing post gadolinium nodule enhancement is**

A. Medulloblastoma *(AIIMS May 10)* ☐
B. Ependymoma ☐
C. Astrocytoma ☐
D. Cysticercous ☐

41. 35 years old patients presents with complaints of headache, vomiting (raised ICT) and ataxia. MRI findings are well - demarcated cysric lesion with a mural nodule in the right cerebellar hemisphere with homogenous contrast enhancement. The most likely diagnosis is: *(AI 012)*

A. Ependymoma ☐
B. Hemangioblastoma ☐
C. Pilocytic-Astrocytoma ☐
D. Medulloblastoma ☐

42. Which of the following tumor is typically a/w VLH:

A. Hemangioblastoma *(AI 2012)* ☐
B. Hemangioendothelioma ☐
C. Neurofibroma ☐
D. Glioma ☐

43. All is true about von Hippel Lindau syndrome except: *(AI 2012)*

A. Hemangioblastomas seen in craniospinal axis ☐
B. Multiple tumors common ☐
C. Tumors of Schwann cells are common ☐
D. Supratentorial lesions are uncommon ☐

44. A child presents with raised ICT. On CT scan a lesion is seen around foramen of monro with multiple periventricular calcific foci. What could be probable diagnosis: *(AIIMS Nov 2011)*

A. Subependymal giant cell astrocytoma (SGCA) ☐
B. Subependymoma or Ependymoma ☐
C. Pilocytic astrocytoma ☐
D. Neurocytoma ☐

45. Investigation of choice for meningeal carcinomatosis in CNS: *(AIIMS Nov 2011)*

A. NE-CT ☐
B. PET ☐
C. SPECT ☐
D. Gd-MRI ☐

46. Investigation of choice for a lesion of temporal bone:

A. CT *(AIIMS May 2010)* ☐
B. MRI ☐
C. USG ☐
D. Plain X-ray ☐

47. Wide neuralforamina is associated with: *(AI 2012)*

A. Neurofibromatosis type 1 ☐
B. Sturge-Weber syndrome ☐
C. Von Hipple Lindau disease ☐
D. Tuberous sclerosis ☐

48. True about MRI/CT appearance of lateral meningocele:

A. Solid dural masses *(AI 2012)* ☐
B. Usually outside the spinal canal ☐
C. Widened neural foramen ☐
D. Generally there is no spinal cord compression & deformity ☐

49. Mesencephalo-oculo-facial-angiomatosis is seen in:

A. KTW Syndrome *(AI 2012)* ☐
B. NF-1 & 2 ☐
C. Sturge-Weber syndrome ☐
D. Wyburn-Mason syndrome ☐

50. Tram track appearance on CT scan of head is seen in:

A. Sturge Weber Syndrome (AIIMS 2001) ☐
B. Von Hipple Lindau Syndrome ☐
C. Tuberous sclerosis ☐
D. Neurofibroma ☐

NEPHROLOGY

Kidney

51. Which of the following is not seen on utrasound in acute pyelonephritis? *(AIIMS May 13)*

A. Grosslly enlarged kidney
B. Focal area of hypoechogenecity
C. Perinephric collection pus in the perinephric space
D. Increased vascularity

52. For renal stone, diagnosis is not done by: *(PGI May 2010)*

A. IVP ☐
B. MRI ☐
C. PET-Scan ☐
D. CT scan ☐

53. The most sensitive imaging modality for diagnosis of Ureteric stones in a patient with acute colic is: *(AI 2005)*

A. X-ray KUB region. ☐
B. Ultrasonogram. ☐

C. Non contrast CT scan of the abdomen. ☐
D. Contrast enhanced CT scan of the abdomen. ☐

54. Calcification is best detected by
A. X-ray *(PGI 2003)* ☐
B. USG ☐
C. CT Scen ☐
D. MRI ☐
E. PET Scen ☐

55. Which of the following imaging modality is most sensitive (investigation of choice) to detect early renal tuberculosis. *(AIIMS 04, 03, 02, 98; AI 06, DNB 03, 05, 07)*
A. Intravenous urography ☐
B. Ultrasound ☐
C. Computed tomography ☐
D. Magnetic resonance imaging ☐

56. Most important investigation for posterior urethralvalve is *(AIIMS 97)*
A. Urethroscopy ☐
B. IVP ☐
C. Retrograde cystogram ☐
D. Micturating cystogram (MCU) ☐

57. The posterior urethra is best visualized by-
A. Static cystogram *(AIIMS Nov 2005)* ☐
B. Retrograde urethrogram ☐
C. Voiding cystogram ☐
D. CT cystogram ☐

58. Investigation of choice to demonstrate vesico ureteral reflux *(AI 1992)*
A. Isotope cystogram ☐
B. Contrast Micturating Cysto Urethrogram ☐
C. IVP ☐
D. Cystoscopy ☐

59. Radiation exposure is the least in the following procedure: *(AIIMS Nov 2010)*
A. Micturating cystourethrogram ☐
B. IVP ☐
C. Bilateral nephrostogram ☐
D. Spiral CT for stones ☐

60. All of the following form radiolucent stones except:
A. Xanthine. *(AIIMS 2003)* ☐
B. Cysteine. ☐
C. Allopurinol. ☐
D. Orotic acid. ☐

61. A dense persistent nephrogram may be seen in all of the following except:
A. Acute ureteral obstruction ☐
B. Systemic hypertension *(AIIMS 02)* ☐
C. Severe hydronephrosis ☐
D. Dehydration ☐

62. Non-visualisation of kidney in excretory urogram is seen in
A. Duplication *(PGI Dec 2004, 05)* ☐
B. Renal vein thrombosis ☐
C. Hydronephrosis ☐
D. Hypoplasia ☐
E. Amyloidosis ☐

63. A dense renogram is obtained by *(AI 2010)*
A. Dehydrating the patient ☐
B. Increasing the dose of contrast media ☐
C. Rapid (Bolus) injection of dye ☐
D. Using non ionic media ☐

64. Papillary necrosis features are all except:
A. Egg in cup *(AIIMS May 09)* ☐
B. Hyperdense nephrogram ☐
C. Calyceal horns ☐
D. "Ring shadows" ☐

65. The most important sign of significance of renal artery stenosis on an angiogram is: *(AI 2006)*
A. A percentage diameter stenosis >70% ☐
B. Presence of collaterals ☐
C. A systolic pressure gradient >20 mmHg across the lesion
D. Post stenotic dilatation of the renal artery ☐

66. Most sensitive and specific investigation for screening of Renovascular hypertension *(AIIMS 01)*
A. MRI ☐
B. Captopril enhanced radionuclide scan ☐
C. Spiral CT angiography (CTA) ☐
D. Duplex - Doppler flow study ☐

67. Abdominal Ultra-sonography in a 3 year old boy show a soild circumscribed hypoechnoic renal mass. Most likely diagnosis is- *(AI 02)*
A. Wilm's tumor ☐
B. Renal cell carcinoma ☐
C. Mesoblastic nephroma ☐
D. Onceocytoma ☐

Urethra

68. Which of the following is not an appropriate investigation for anterior urethral stricture? *(AIIMS 2003)*
A. Magnetic Resonance Imaging ☐
B. Retrograde urethrogram ☐
C. Micturating cystourethrogram ☐
D. High frequency ultrasound ☐

Bladder

69. Teardrop bladder are seen in: *(PGI May2010)*
A. Pelvic hematoma ☐
B. Pelvic lipomatoma ☐
C. T. B ☐
D. Neurogenic bladder ☐
E. Intraperitoneal bladder rupture

70. Causes of bladder calcification are:
A. Schistosmosis *(PGI Dec 2006)* ☐
B. Urethral cell ☐
C. TB ☐
D. Carcinoma ☐

Prostate

71. Transrectal ultrasonography in carcinoma prostate is most useful for *(AI 08)*
A. Guided prostatic biopsies ☐
B. Seminal vesicle involvement ☐
C. Measurement of prostatic volume ☐
D. To detect hypoechoic area ☐

72. Hypoechoic lesion within prostate in USG seen in-
A. Adeno CA *(PGI Dec 2004)* ☐
B. Normal prostate tissue ☐
C. Infertility ☐
D. Urethral obstruction ☐
E. BPH ☐

Answers and Explanations:

CENTRAL NERVOUS SYSTEM

EMBRYOLOGY

1. **D i.e. Focal cortical dysplasia without ballon cells** *[Ref: Osborn 3/e p 7; Wolfgang 7/e p 255]*

- **Formation & maturation of brain neocortex** involve *neuronal proliferation, differentiation & migration.* Cerebral hemisphere first appear as bilateral outpouching (diverticula) of telencephalon at 35 days of gestation. With their expansion, *germinal matrix* forms at 7 weeks gestational age *d/t subependymal neuronal proliferation*, lines the lateral & third ventricles and involutes at 28 to 30 weeks (although persists in form of focal cell clustures upto 36 to 39 weeks). During this period cells form in germinal matrix, differentiate (to neuronal & glial precursor and form embryonic cortex) and then migrate peripherally *along specialized radial glial fibers* that span the entire thickness of hemisphere from ventricular surface to pia (a process called neuronal migration).
- With the exception of outer layer, neurons migrate from germinal matrix to cortex in an inside out sequence: i.e. those that will **form the deepest cortical layer (6) migrate first**, followed by layers 5, 4, 3 and finally layer 2 (layer 1 will not migrate). This **neuronal migration & layering process** occurs from weeks 6 to 7 through 24 to 26, when full 6 layered cortex is achieved. So a **brain insult during neuronal migration** can result in abnormalities ranging from ***lissencephaly (smooth brain), to schizencephaly (split brain), polymicrogyria, and laminar or focal heterotopias***Q.

2. **All i.e. Mucopolysaccharidoses, Achondroplasia, Optic chiasm glioma, Neurofibromatosis I, Hydrocephalus** *[Ref: Osborn 1/ep 460-74; Chapman 5/e p 288, 325; Wolfgang 7/e p 251; Grainge 5/e p 1248-49, 1706-10]*

- **Sella turcica** is a *cup shaped depression* in the central basisphenoid bone that *contains the pituitary gland and inferior part of the infundibular stalk. Flattened tuberculum sellae with a prominent sulcus chiasmaticus* are the factors responsible for sella looking J shaped on lateral skull x-ray. The normal dorsal sellae forms the loop of J.
- **J shaped sella turcica** is seen in : Mn – **"COMAND"** or **"CONMAN Must Die"**

- *Chronic hydrocephalus*Q (d/t enlarged anterior aspect of 3rd ventricle)
- Osteogenesis imperfecta, *Optic (chiasm) glioma*Q (glioma may be bilateral l/t *W or omega shped sella;* if chiasmatic sulcus is very depressed).
- *Mucopolysaccharidoses*Q (eg Hurler syndrome >> Hunter syndrome)
- *Achondroplasia*Q
- *Neurofibromatosis*Q (type 1 is usually a/w slowly growing optic glioma which may extend upto chiasma); Normal variant (5%)
- Dysostosis multiplex (defect in carbohydrate metabolism).
- Hajdu-Cheney syndrome & congenital hypothyroidism are other rare causes

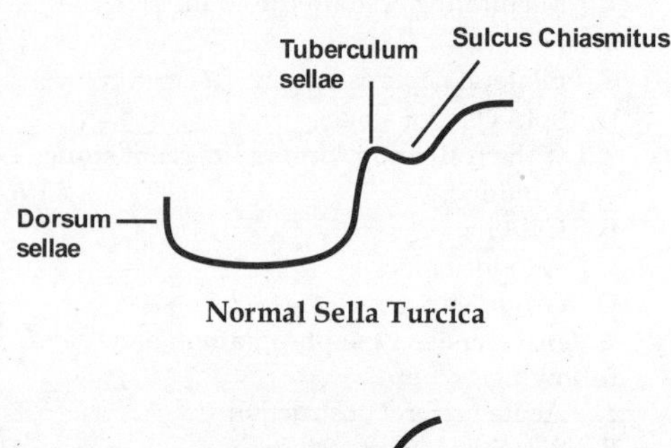

Normal Sella Turcica

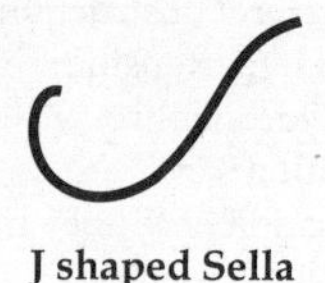
J shaped Sella

3. **B i.e., Amyotrophic Lateral Sclerosis** *[Ref. Harrison 18/e pg 3345-50]*

The presence of **both lower motor neuron signs (progressive atrophy & weakness of hands) and upper motor neuron signs (spasticity & hyperreflexia)** in the patient ***with increased signals (hyperintensity) of corticospinal tracts on T2WI of MRI***Q leads us to the diagnosis of **Amyotrophic lateral sclerosis.**

4. **B i.e. ALS >> E i.e. MLIB**
[Ref: Harrison 18/e p 3346-47; Wolfgang 7/e p 246-47, 269, 273, 305; Haga 5/e p 357, 379-81; Grainger 5/e p 1336-37]

- **Hyperintense corticospinal tracts (ie high signal intensity) on T_2 weighted images of MRI** is seen in neurodegenerative disorders of white matter involving corticospinal tracts. *It represents an increase in water content in myelin tracts undergoing wllerian degeneration secondary to cortical motor neuronal loss (ie reduced myelin, axonal loss,* astrocytic gliosis).
- **Hyperintense corticospinal tracts (corona radiata, corpus callosum, posterior limb of internal capsule, ventral aspect of brain stem, anterolateral column of spinal cord)** along with low signal intensity in motor cortex (d/t iron deposition) on T_2 WI is seen ***in amyotrophic lateral sclerosis***[Q].
- **Hyperintense corticospinal tracts on T_2 WI** is commonly seen in **ALS**. But the finding can also be seen in disease processes that produce cortiocospinal neuronal loss in a symmetric fashion eg **vascular infarctions** (as seen in **lacunar infarcts, arteriosclerosis, migrane, vasculitis, APA** etc,) **infections & inflammations** (such as **HIV encephalopathy, Lyme encephalopathy, neurocysticercosis**, cryptococcosis), **demyelinating diseases** (eg **multiple sclerosis**, ADEM, multifocal leukoencephalopathy, lymphomatoid granulomatrosis), metabolic (eg vitamin B_{12} deficiency) etc. In **Wilson's disease**, commonest MRI finding is **hyperintense putamen on T_2 WI**; lesions also occur in pons mid brain, cerebellum and subcortical wahite matter.
- **In hemochromatosis (iron overload),** on MRI there is **reduction in hepatic signal intensity on in phase** compared with out of phase images (opposite to steatosis) owing to paramagnetic effect of ferric ions (Fe^{+3}). There is **shortening of T_1, T_2 and gradient echo T_2 proportional to iron deposition**.

5. **C i.e. T1WI are most diagnostic for acute plaques**
6. **A i.e. White matter**
7. **A i.e. Absent olgoclonal band** *[Ref. Harrison 18/e p. 3395-3405; Haga 5/e p. 455-65]*

- **Multiple sclerosis** is a **demyelination** disorder characterized by selective destruction of CNS myelin ***predominantly of white matter long tract***[Q]. Diagnosis suggestive MRI findings include **≥1 hyperintense T2 lesion in at least 2 out of & MS typical regions** of CNS (i.e. **periventricular, juxta cortical, infratentorial or spinal cord**) and **Gd-enhancement**. Lesions **>6mm** located in corpus callosum (juxtacortical), **periventricular white matter**, brainstem & cerebellum (infratentorial) and spinal cord are particularly helpful diagnostically. (Harrison 18/e p 3399). However when the Q was asked Harrison 16/e p 2461 mentioned - ***confirmatory MRI must have either 4 lesions involving the white matter or 3 lesion if periventricular in location***[Q]. Acceptable lesion must be > 3 mm in diameter.
- *CT findings of MS* include focal **decreased attenuation in periventricular** ***white matter*** (most characteristic), *contrast enhancing plaques* (enhancement may be decreased or abolished by corticosteroid administration) and *cerebral atrophy*.
- MRI is imaging modality of choice and most characteristic diagnostic feature of MS plaque is not their **high signal intensity (on T2WI)** but their **anatomical distribution**. There is a **predilection for periventricular distribution & ependymal surface** (especially along *occipital horns >frontal horns)*. If not pathognomic, **corpus callosum lesions** are so characteristic of MS to be almost specific. Other MS sites are *corona radiata, internal capsule, centrum semiovale; and surface of pons* esp near 5th CN entery zone, *middle cerebral paduncle (brachium pontis), floor of 4th ventricle and colliculi* in posterior cranial fossa.
- **T1WI are less sensitive** but *chronic plaques of MS (esp in corpus callosum are often well shown* as ***black holes*** *(low signal lesions) surrounded by a very thin halo of mildly increased signal intensity.*
- Progression to MS is more likely ***with presence of oligoclonal band***[Q] (not absent), bilateral optic neuritis, poor recovery & complete cord transection.

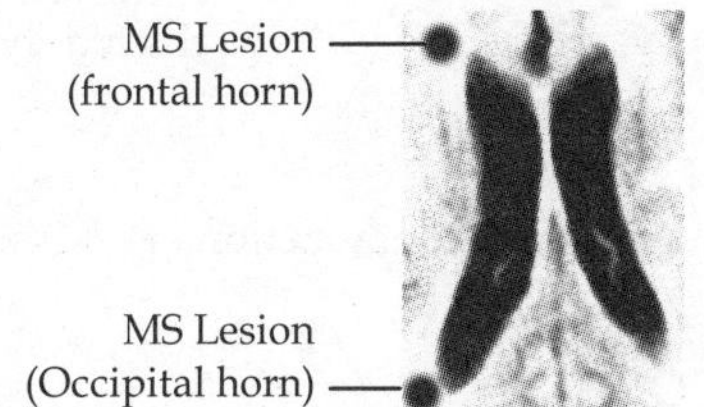

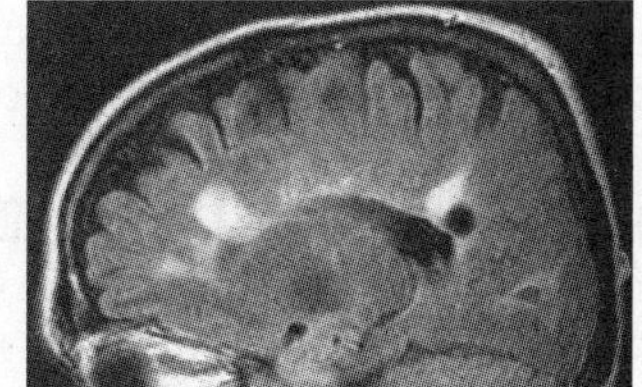

Periventricular MS Lesion

8. **B i.e., Krabbe's disease** *[Ref: Sutton 7/e p.1801–02; Grainger 5/e p. 1674-71, 1336-39; Haga 5/e p. 449-52]*

Krabbe's diseases (Globoid cell leukodystrophy) is characterized by:

- Focal ***bilateral thalamic, posterior internal capsule and basal ganglia lesion showing hyperdensity & calcification in CT scan***[Q] and hypointensity on T2 MRI.
- Extensive ***involvement of deep white matter***[Q], more severely posteriorly & centrally.
- Cerebellar white matter abnormality sparing the dentate nuclei; & involvement of pyramidal tracts within brain stem.
- MCT shows hypodensity of white matter. MRI- T2 image also detect abnormality in deep *periventricular white matter with cavitatory changes, adjacent to frontal horns.*

9. **C i.e. Blurring of Grey white matter junction of ipsilateral temporal lobe**
[Ref: Dahnert Wolfgang 7/e p. 312; Harrison 17th/ 2250; The Comprehensive evaluation and treatment of epilepsy by Schomer (1997)/55]

Atrophy of hippocampus, fornix and mamillary body are established MRI findings in Mesial Temporal Sclerosis. Blurring of grey white matter at junction of ipsilateral temporal lobe is not listed as a feature of mesial temporal sclerosis.

10. **D i.e. Vein of Galen malformation** *[Ref: Osborn p-150-151, 289, 320-24; Sutton 7/e p-1697; Neuroradiology AMP series 3/e p-141-42; Nelson 18/e p-2511, Danhert 6/e p-333]*

Midline hypoechoic mass with dilated lateral ventricles (on USG), bruit on auscultation, hydrocephalus and high output cardiac failure in neonates / infantsQ is diagnostic of **vein of galen malformation.**

11. **B i.e., Ballooning of dorsal sellae** *[Ref: Sutton 7/e p –1626- 27]*

- **Sutural diastasis** (1st sign in children), **increased convolutions (copper beating of skull vault)** *and* **thinning & erosion of dorsal sellae** (cardinal sign in adults) are features of **raised ICT**.
- ***Expansion & ballooning of sella is seen in pituitary adenoma***Q***. Expansion & erosion of internal auditory meatus (IAM) is seen in acoustic neuroma***Q.

12. **B i.e. Diffuse axonal injuries** *[Ref: Dahnert 6/e p. 281; Osborn p-202-212, Harrison 16/e p. 2448, Chapman 4/e p.417; Neuroradiology AMP series 3/e p. 538-42]*

Diffuse axonal injuries (DAI) – shearing injuries caused by sudden rotational or accelerating / decelerating forces. Patient ***typically lose consciousness at the time of impact***Q***. On CT small petechial hemorrhages are seen***Q

13. **D i.e. Video EEG with ictal 99m TcHMPAO Brain SPECT** *[Ref: Grainger 4/e P-2311, 2505, 2407-10]*

Any recurrent or resistant (to drugs) seizure activity may be due to non detectable underlying structural lesion **(cryptogenic epilepsy)**. ***Hippocampal Sclerosis***Q is the most common structural lesion, which is associated with ***temporal lobe epilepsy, the most common of the partial epilepsies***Q.

Pre operative Investigational Algorythm for Localizing Epileptogenic Lesion is

I. **Structural Imaging (MRI, CT)**
*MRI*Q is preffered over CT

Diagnose lesion in most (90%) cases | Undiagnosed

II. **Functional Imaging** (SPECT, PET, functional – MRI)
1. *Ictal SPECT with* ***HMPAO***Q, which shows hypermetabolic foci during ictal phase is the ***most practical & best method***Q
2. *Interictal PET with FDG,* which shows hypometabolic seizure foci is IInd preferred method.
3. **Addition of** ***Video EEG***Q further helps in localization of epileptic foci.

III. Once the epileptogenic focus has been identified preoperative lateralization of hemispheric dominance for language function may be necessary. It is done by:
1. Noninvasive activation studies with H_2 ^{15}O PET or f MRI.
2. Invasive WADA test with Catheter angiography.

Know these facts:
1. Ictal investigations are more sensitive than interictal.
2. SPET has poorer resolution than PET; But SPECT is cheap & good investigation with wider availability as compared to PET which is very expensive & available at selected places making it non practicle.

14. **B i.e. Lumber puncture** *[Ref: Harrison 15/e P-2331]*

Raised **ICT** (example in Brain Tumor) ***is an absolute contraindication for L.P. as there is risk of brain herniation & sudden death.***Q

INFECTION

15. **A i.e. Tuberculosis meningitis** *[Ref: Haga 5/e p 412-13, 159-79; Wolfgang 7/e p 311, 332-33, 287; Harrison 8/e p 3410-40; Osborn 3/e p 678-712]*

Subacute or chronic granulomatous tubercular meningitis has a characteristic proclivity to develop **basal cisternal** ***exudates ischemic infarcts of basal ganglia and internal capsule and communicating hydrocephalus***[Q] as a sequelae.

16. **A i.e. Toxoplasmosis** *[Ref: Chapman 3/e P-513, 414, 422; Osborn 3/e p. 691]*

Conditions causing ring-enhancement with CT (contrast)
- ***Toxoplasmosis***[Q]
- Cysticercosis
- ***Tuberculoma***[Q]
- Pyogenic abscess
- Glioma metastasis
- Craniopharyngeoma
- Gaint aneurysm

EPIDERMOID

17. **C i.e. Restricted diffusion** *[Ref: Osborn 3/e p 900-1, 639-42, 843; Wolfgan 7/e p 272-288; Haga 5/e p 550-45, 806, 700-1, 494]*

Epidermoids can be differentiated from arachnoid cyst characteristically by hyper-intense diffusion weighted images because of restricted diffusion of epidermoid cyst[Q]. FLAIR and proton images are less specific than DWI.

CALCIFICATION

18. **A i.e. Pineal gland; B i.e. Choroid plexus** *[Ref: P.J. Mehta 14/e P-328; Chapman 3/e P-407]*

Physiological calcification in skull X Ray is seen in
1. ***Choroid plexus***[Q]
2. ***Pineal gland***[Q] in old age.
3. Petroclinoid ligament
4. Falx cerebri
5. Lateral edges of diaphragm sellae

Intracranial Neoplasms showing Calcification

Mnemonic-DEar Ca^{++} PLease COME Home"
- **Dermoid (arcs of calcification similar** to those seen in walls of aneurysm and small central defect in occipital bone; mostly in posterior fossa & skull base), Epidermoid (multiple small arc calcifications) & **Teratoma.**
- **Craniopharyngeoma** (mainly in children, ***midline suprasellar calcification***[Q] in 75% cases)
- **Astrocytoma, Aneurysm**
- **Pinealoma, Papilloma, Lipoma** (lipoma of corpus callosum show ***marginal or bracket calcification***[Q])
- **Choroid plexus papilloma** (mainly in children, lateral or 4th ventricle calcification in 25% cases); **Chordoma** (irregular calcification usually originating from clivus)
- **Oligodendroglioma/gliomas** (commonest cerebral

19. **C i.e. Meningioma > A i.e. Ependymoma** *[Ref: Danhert 7/e p. 240-41, 288, 309; Sutton 7/e p. 1628-32]*

Calcification is seen in both meningioma & ependymoma; but is more common a feature of meningioma[Q].

Ependymoma	Meningioma
- Slow growing tumour - Arises either from ependymal surface of ventricular system or from ependymal cell rest within nervous tissue	- M.C. primary intracranial tumour of nonglial origin
On CT - Isodense to slightly hypodense with calcification	- Hyperdense as compared to brain on non contrast CT
- Mild to moderate inhomogenous enhancement	- Calcification present

Disease	Characteristic calcification
Pineal calcification	Most common intracranial calcification
Hypo, pseudohypo & hyper-**parathyroidism**, hypothyroidism, hypoxia, TORCH	Basal ganglia calcification
CMV (intrauterine)	*Peri/Circum-ventricular calcification*[Q]
Toxoplasmosis	*Intraparenchymal diffuse multiple foci of noduler calcification (multiple scattered flecks in cortex & linear streaks in basal ganglia)*[Q]
Craniopharyngoma	*Midline suprasellar calcification*[Q] (may be curvilinear)
Lipoma of corpus callosum	*Marginal (bracket) calcification*[Q]

tumor glioma calcify in 5% case & usually in slow growing & less malignant tumors; rare oligodendroglioma shows calcification in 50% and posterior fossa gliomas in 20% cases; oligodendroglioma can show *serpiginous calcification*).

- **Meningioma** (calcification may be **characteristically heavy, ball like & amorphous** or less typical speckled or noduler, in a **characteristic parasagittal** or other typical meningioma site like base of tumor lying *against the vault or sphenoid ridge*. The presence of *local hyperostosis* and increased/***prominent meningeal vascular markings leading upto the site of attachment***Q also help to confirm the diagnosis).
- Medulloblastoma, Metastases
- Ependymoma
- Hamartoma

★ Astrocytoma calcify less frequently but are most common tumor.

Oligodendroglioma	Serpiginous calcification; ribbon like/ dense nodular calcification
Meningioma	***Parasaggital, heavily ball like & amorphous calcification***Q ***against the vault or sphinoid with local hyperostosis & prominent meningeal vascular markings***Q
Pituitary adenoma	Figure of eight appearance
Acoustic schwannoma	Icecream cone appearance
Neuroparagonimiasis	***Soap bubble calcification***Q
Cysticercosis	***Rice grain calcification***Q

Hydatid cyst	***Not calcify in lung***Q
Pulmonary hemartoma	***Popcorn calcification***Q
Silicosis/Sarcoidosis	***Egg shell calcification***Q
Constrictive pericarditis	***Pericardial calcification***
Carcinoid synsrome	***Cardiac calcification***Q
Sturge Weber Syndrome	***Rail road (tram track) or gyriform calcification***Q
Pseudogout	***Meniscal cartilage calcification***Q

20. B i.e. Cytomegalovirus 21. C i.e. Craniopharyngioma 22. C i.e. Craniopharyngioma

23. B i.e. Lipoma of carpus callosum *[Ref: Sutton 7/e p 1630, 1752; Nelson 17/e p. 1707; Chapman 4/e p 455, 463]*

- *In* ***CMV*** *there is -* ***microcephaly***Q, B/L-Symmetrical stippled & ***periventricular calcification***Q
- In **Toxoplasma –** calcification consists of *multiple scattered flecks in cortex & linear streaks in the basal ganglia. Mnemonic-* CMV calcifications are Circum Ventricular and Toxoplasma calcifications are intraparenchymal.
- In congenital syphilis – ***hot cross bun skull***Q.
- **Lipomas of corpus callosum** may show highly characteristic ***margical calcification (i.e. bracket sign)***Q.
- Pituatory macroadenoma is also a suprasellar mass which typically has *cottage loaf or figure of eight appearance.*

Craniopharyngeomas are derived from ***Rathke's pouch***Q, near pituitary stalk. These are large, ***cystic***Q, locally invasive tumors, many are ***calcified***Q. It is ***most common suprasellar tumor in children***Q. Presentation is:

Clinical

- More than half **craniopharyngiomas** occur in ***children (8-14 years)***Q **presenting with** ***headache***Q, ***visual disturbance***Q and ***endocrinal abnormalities***Q. Second peak is in middle age. X Ray/CT demonstrates midline ***solid/cystic suprasellar mass with calcification***Q that extends superiorly & posteriorly. Occasionally, when the tumor is cystic, curvilinear calcification may be seen in the cyst wall.
- Signs of ↑ ICT – headache, vomiting, papilledema & hydrocephalus
- ***Anterior pituitary dysfunction***Q ***& Diabetes insipdus***Q, ***Growth retardation***Q
- Other – ***visual field defect***Q, personality change. Cognitive deterioration, cranial nerve damage, sleep difficulties & weight gain

Radiological

- On CT & X Ray – ***Suprasellar calcification with cystic lesion***Q
- ***On MRI- Mixed cystic and solid suprasellar mass***Q

★ **Medulloblastoma** mostly arise from cerebellar vermis & ***medulloblastoma of posterior fossa are the most common malignant brain tumor of children***Q.

★ **Pilocytic (spindle shaped) low grade astrocytoma** is the **most common** ***brain tumor***Q, ***most common posterior fossa tumor of children***Q.

24. D i.e. Wilson's disease 25. B i.e. Wilson's disease

26. A i.e. Hyperparathyroidism; C i.e. Hypoparathyroidism; D i.e. Hypothyroidism *[Ref: Chapman 4/e P-430] [Ref: Chapman 4/e P-430; Sutton 7/e p. 1798; Dahnert 5e/P 240]*

HypoparathyroidismQ, ***pseudo-hypoparathyroidism***Q, ***hyperparathyroidism***Q ***& hypothyroidism***Q cause basal ganglia calcification. Calcification usually occurs in globus pallidus.

Causes of Basal Ganglia Calcification

1. Endocrinal - ***Hypo & Pseudo hypo-parathyroidism***Q*,(Albright's syndrome),* ***Secondary hyperparathyroidism***Q ***Hypothyroidism***Q
2. Toxic - **Hypoxia *(Birth anoxia)***Q Co/Pb = Carbonmonoxide/Lead poisoning
3. Chemo/Radio - Therapy
4. Infection - ***TORCH***Q (toxoplasma, congenital rubella, cytomegalo virus, Herpes simplex) - HIV - ***Cysticercosis***Q - TB
5. Metabolic - ***Fahr's ds***Q, Cockayne's syndrome, mitochondrial disorder (Cytopathy)
6. ***Vascular malformation***Q - Mineralizing micro angiography
7. Tumor
8. Physiological with aging, idiopathic, familial

CRANIOPHARYNGIOMA

27. **D i.e. Craniopharyngeoma** **28.** **B i.e. Craniopharyngeoma**
29. **B i.e. Craniopharyngioma** **30.** **B i.e. Craniopharyngioma**
31. **C i.e. Craniopharyngioma** *[Ref: Nelson 17/e p. 1707, OP Ghai 6/e p. 526; Sutton 7/e p. 1752; Grainger 4/e p. 2344]*

- Most common cause of intra cranial calcification = ***Pineal body calcification***Q
- Most common calcifying brain tumor in child = ***Craniopharyngioma***Q > Oligodendroglioma
- Craniopharyngioma causes characteristic ***suprasellar calcification with cystic appearance***Q
- **Craniopharyngioma** arises from remnants of ***rathke's pouch***Q (mesodermal structure from which anterior pituitary gland is derived) near pituitary stalk. It presents as ***suprasellar cystic lesion with a tendency for calcification (80%). It is the most common suprasellar tumor in children***Q.
- **Medulloblastoma** mostly arises from cerebellar vermis & ***Medulloblastoma of posterior fossa are the M. C. malignant brain tumor of children***Q.
- **Pilocytic (spindle shaped) low grade Astrocytoma** is the **most common** ***brain tumor***Q, ***most common posterior fossa tumor of children***Q.

Craniopharyngioma

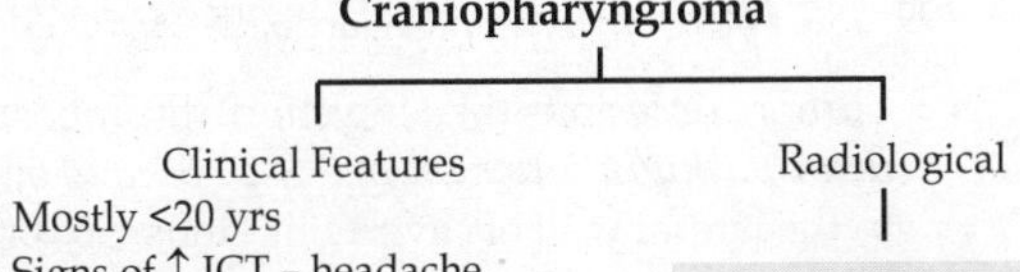

Clinical Features
- Mostly <20 yrs
- Signs of ↑ ICT – headache, vomiting, papilledema & hydrocephalus
- ***Anterior pituitary dysfunction***Q & ***Diabetes insipdus***Q, ***Growth retardation***Q
- Other – ***visual field defect***Q, personality change. Cognitive deterioration, cranial nerve damage, sleep difficulties & weight gain

Radiological
- ***Suprasellar cystic lesion with calcification***Q on CT scan
- ***Mixed solid-cystic suprasellar mass***Q on MRI

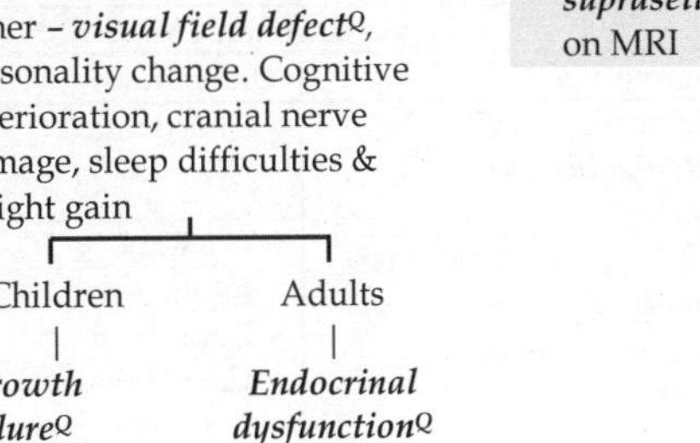

Signs of raised **ICT** & ***visual field defects***Q may be seen in either age group.

INTRACRANIAL VASCULAR MALFORMATIONS

32. **A i.e. Reticulated popcom like configuration** *[Ref:Haga 5/e p 265-66, Wolfgang 7/e p 276; Osborn 3/e p 285-321]*

T2 gradient echo MRI is the investigation of choice for identification of **cavernous angioma (cavernous hemangioma or cavernoma)**, which typically demonstrates a mass characterized as ***popcorn in appearance (mulberry shaped lesion)***Q.

INTRACRANIAL TUMORS

33. **A i.e. Meningioma** **34.** **B i.e. Meningioma** **35.** **B i.e. Meningioma**
36. **C i.e. Erosion** **37.** **A, C, D, E**
[Ref: Wolfgang 7/e p. 309-11; Haga 5/e p. 99-101; Osborn 3/e p. 584-601; Sutton 7/e p – 1629; Neuroradiology 3/e p. 268]

- **Meningioma** is the ***most common intracranial – extra axial (extra-parenchymal), dural based neoplasm***Q; 90% of which are *supratenotorial* mostly in *parasagital area or fronto-parietal convexity in close association with falx cerebri.*
- Meningioma is 2nd ***most common spinal tumor in the intradural-extra medullary location***Q (next only to nerve sheath tumor). ***Thoracic (dorsal) spine is most frequent site***Q followed by cervical > lumbar spine.
- Symptoms & sign depends on location eg *intracranial lesions l/t raised ICT features* like headache, nausea, vomiting etc and spinal lesions l/t sensory-motor weakness of limbs (lower limbs in dorsal spine & all four limbs in cervical spine lesion) *with bladder bowel involvement.* Classic patient is *middle to old aged (35-70yrs) female (F:M=4/2:1)*
- **Meningiomas** l/t ***hyperostosis (osteosclerosis), , enlarged meningeal grooves/vascular channels/foramen spinosum, tumor calcification (Psammoma/sand bodies), pneumosinus dilatans (enlarged blistering paranasal sinuses), invasion & interruption of sinus (eg mushrooming in superior saggital sinus) and rarely sutural diastasis and erosion (least common)***Q on plain x-ray.
- On **noncontrast imaging**, ***meningioma is chracteristically homogenous mass with a broad dural base***Q, which appears **hyperdense (on NECT), isointense to slightly hypointense (on T1WI) and isointense to mildly hyper intense (on T2WI).**
- **Meningiomas (almost** all />90%) ***characteristically display rapid, strikingly intense (pronounced) and homogenous contrast enhancement***Q on **CECT & CE-MRI (T1WI).**

38. **B i.e. Meningioma** *[Ref: Wolfgang 7/e p 253, 270-73, 309-11, 224, 323; Osborn 3/e p. 529-63, 429-32, 311-13, 288, 394, 499, 488; Harrison 18/e p-3384-86, 3298-99, 3365]*

- Tumors or lesions (like infection, thrombosis, aneurysm, fistula) of **cavernous sinus** can cause ***neuropathy/involvment of 3rd, 4th 6th and 5th (V_1 >>V_2) cranial nerves*** because of their anatomical proximity to the lateral wall of cavernous sinus. So for pin pointing the diagnosis we have to focus on other features like sex, age, incidence and MR findings.
- Now lets focus on **differential diagnosis of cavernous sinus masses** which indicates that Schwannoma & meningioma are common; cavernous sinus hemangioma is very rare and astrocytoma is almost not a cause cavernous sinus masses.

Unilateral Mass	
Common	**Uncommon**
- *Schwannoma*Q - *Meningioma*Q - Metastasis - Aneurysm (cavernous-internal carotid artery) - Carotid cavernous fistula	- Chordoma - Lymphoma **Very Rare** - Lipoma - Epidermoid - *Cavernous hemangioma*Q - Osteo cartilagenous tumors - Plexiform neurofibroma (NF_1)

Bilateral Mass	
Common	**Uncommon**
- Invasive pituitary adenoma - Meningioma - Metastases	- Lymphoma - Cavernous sinus thrombosis

- Lets focus on astrocytoma to see wheter it can be completely ruled out or not
  - Astrocytomas either **do not /mildly enhance** (*low grade astrocytoma*) or **strongly enhance** (anaplastic/malignant astrocytoma, glioblastoma multiformae, PA, PXA, SEGA) but when they enhance they characteristically enhance ***inhomogenously (heterogenously) mostly***Q (except in PXA >PA).
- Now we are left with cavernous hemangioma, meningioma and schwannoma
  - **Cavernous sinus hemangioma** is a *rare benign tumor seen in young or middle aged (4th & 5th decade) predominantly females (F:M = 9:1 to 3:1).* It presents as *homogenous hypointense on T1 and highly hyperintense on T2* weighted images. ***Contrast enhancement is homogenous***Q, which distinguish them from other lesions. So it seems a probable answer but lets rule out other options.
  - **Trigeminal Schwannoma** (neuroma) is a common cause of cavernous sinus mass. It presents ***predominantly in females (F:M=2:1) of 35 to 60 years age***Q. But it is characterized by high chances (30-40%) of ***heterogeniety of both density and contrast enhancement***Q (b/o tumor necrosis & cyst formation in larger > 1 mm tumors). So schwannoma can be easilyruled out.
  - **Meningiomas** are common cause of cavernous sinus mass. It presents ***predominantly in females (F:M=4:1 to 2:1) of 35 to 70 years and even in younger patients in a/w NF2***Q. Meningiomas are characteristically **homogenous hyperdense mass (with broad dural base)** on CT and ***characteristically show homogenous (uniform) intense contrast enhancement***Q. So this is the answer because it is far more common than CSH.

- Dont get confused that ----book mention, meningioma may be heterogenous without understanding the logic behind it. Brodly speaking any tumor may give any appearance but we are concerned about its typical / characteristic/ most common pattern of appearance. This and most of PGME question about CNS tumors are very broad concept based. Now let me rephrase this question to make it more clear : **What would be your first diagnosis of cavernous sinus mass which appears hyper intense on T2 WI and shows homogenous contrast enhancement** in a 20 yr old female.

Astrocytomas is rule out because it is characteristically (mostly) inhomogenous/heterogenous causing ***mixed intensity in T2WI and heterogenous contrast enhancement***Q

Schwannoma, CSH and meningioma all are **more common in females >30years** and **show hyperintensity on T2WI**

- **Schwannoma** is common, but very commonly shows **heterogenous contrast enhancment** (30-40%) so it is ruled out
- CSH is very **rare but mostly shows homogenous contrast enhancment,** so it can't be ruled out
- **Meningioma** is common and mostly (90%) shows **homogenous contrast enhancement**, so it is first diagnosis

39. **B i.e. Medulloblastoma**
40. **C i.e. Astrocytoma** *[Ref: Neuroradiology AMP series 3/e p-331]*

Posterior Fossa tumors in children

Features	Astrocytoma	Ependymoma	Medulloblastoma
Cyst Formation	*Very common*Q	Common	Rare
CT scan	*Hypodense*Q	Isodense	Hyperdense
CSF seeding	Rare	No	**Yes** (15-40%)
Transforaminal spread	No	**Yes**	No
Calcification	~10%	**40-50%**	10-15%
T2WI	**Hyper** (intense)	Hyper/Iso	Iso
T1WI	Iso/Hypo	Iso/Hypo	Iso/Hypo
Postgadolinium (contrast)	*Nodule enhance*Q	Mild	Moderate

41. **B i.e. Hemangioblastoma**

Well demarcated cystic lesion with a mural nodule in cerebellar hemisphere (l/t raised ICT = nausea, vomitting, headache, dizziness, vertigo and cerebellar features like ataxia or disequilibrium) may be caused by JPA and HB and is differentiated by

Juvenile Pilocytic Astrocytoma (JPA)	Hemangioblastoma (HB)
• Seen typically in **children & young adults (adoleseents)**, with most becoming symptomatic during **first two decades (<20 years) of life**. When associated with **NF-1**, it presents earlier in slightly *younger (2-3 years) children.*	• Present typically in **young adults to middle age** with a peak incidence in **3rd to 5th decade of life (20 to 50 years** age) and are rare in children. When a/w **von Hippel Lindau syndrome**, HB are multiple and become symptomatic at an *earlier age (29-39 yrs).*
• **Intratumoral calcification** is occasionally seen (5-25%), but despite prominent vascularity hemorrhage & necrosis are rare	• Vascularity is more but calcification is lesser than JPA
• On MRI, cystic portion more than mural nodule appears **hyperintense on T_2** and **hypointense** to isointense on **T1** images. Cystic portion is homogenous whereas mural nodule in some cases with calcification may l/t heterogenous appearance (although most are homogenous). • **Homogenous contrast enhancement** is **characteristic** but calcific focus does not enhance and *may l/t heterogenous or variable enhancement* (although uncommon but relatively more common than HB).	• On MRI, cystic portion is homogenously **hypointense on** T_1 and **hyperintense on T_2 images (like JPA). Mural nodule is more variable most are inhomogenously isointense**/hypointense **on T1 and slightly hyperintense on T_2 images** • **Prominent serpentine flow (signal)** voids are characteristic • **Contrast enhancement** of mural nodule is **characteristically homogenous and intense** on T_1 images.

42. **A i.e. Hemangioblastoma**
43. **C i.e. Tumors of Schwann cells are common** *[Ref: Harrison 18/e p 3078, 3384; Osborn 3/e p 605-07-104-106; Wolfgang 7/e p 337-39, 295-96, 274-352, 242, 278, 274, 352; Haga 5/e p 1662, 108-10, 59-62]*

Von Hippei-Lindau (VHL) syndrome is associated with ***multiple hemangioblastomas***Q ***of infratentorial craniospinal axis, retina and pancreas. Supratentorial HB are uncommon***Q.

44. **A i.e. (Subependymal giant cell astrocytoma (SGCA))** *[Ref:Osborn 3/e p 583-571, 562, 432;Wolfgang 7/e p 334; Haga 5/e p 86-82, 79, 63-65]*

Foramen of Monro (FM) is a *Y shaped structure* that connects the two lateral ventricles with the third ventricle. FM masses are uncommon in young children. **Subependymal giant cell astrocytoma (SGCA)** ***occurs in older children & young adults with tuberous sclerosis***[Q]. **Pilocytic astrocytoma** also occurs in this age group. **Subependymoma and central neurocytoma** occurs in adults. All FM masses can cause **obstructive hydrocephalous** and lead to **raised intracranial tension.**

Well delinated Intraventricular –Mass around foramen of Monro with Calcification & Obstructive Hydrocephalus.

- ***In older children & young adults (<20yrs)***[Q],
- *Lateral wall of lateral ventricle overlying head of caudate nucleus near foramen of monro* (almost always).
- Features of *tuberous sclerosis like cortical tubers & sub ependymal hamartomatous nodules*
- *Large, multinucleated giant cells* with *GFAP reactivity &/or neuron specific enolase* and swollen astrocytes with abundant glossy eosinophilic cytoplasm
- ***Heterogenous (cystic & heavilly calcified) vascular mass showing strong/intense but heterogenous contrast enhancement***[Q].

Subependymal Giant Cell Astrocytoma

- Occurs in *young adults (average 31-yrs, rang 17-53 yrs)*, rare in children & older adults.
- Exclusively in lateral ventricle near septum pellucidum & FM.
- *Indistinguishable from oligodendroglioma on light microscopy* but demonstrate *neuronal origin on electron microscopy* (synapse, process, granules & microtubules) and *immunohistochemistry (enolase & synaptophysin)*.
- **Heterogenous** (multiple small cyst & heavy calcification) mass with mild to moderate inhomogenous contrast enhancement

Central Neurocytoma

- More common (60%) **infratentoral/posterir fossa tumors (in 4th ventricle mostly) are plastic ependymomas** which occur predominantly in **1-6yr children**. Less common **infratentoral** (40%) tumors arise *near atrium of left ventricle or foramen monro, which occur predominantly* in 2nd through 4th decade.
- **Perivascular pseudorosette, peritumoral edema** and CSF seeding (mainly in infra tentorial).
- **Heterogenous** (mixed density / intensity; d/t heavy calcification & cyst) mass with *peritumoral edema* (hypodense halo on CT) and *mild to moderate but heterogenous contrast enhancement.*

Ependymoma

- In ***middle and elderly adults***[Q] (40/60yr average age of asymptomatic / symptomatic)
- **4th ventricle** (lower medulla) > frontal horn of **lateral ventricle near septum pellucidum & FM** (this mostly becomes symptomatic).
- **Avascular, homogenous,** grade I tumor; although large tumors may contain **calcification** & microcystic changes (**less common**).
- ***Homogenous, avascular/hypovascular mass with variable no or minimal contrast enhancement***[Q].

Subependymoma

★ Broadly NE-CT of all is hypo-isodense; T1WI is iso-hypo intense and T2 WI is iso-hyper intense (general not absolute rule)

45. **D i.e. Gd-MRI** *[Ref: Harrison 18/e p 3391; Wolfgang 7/e p 309, 221; Haga 5/e p 419-403-24]*

Investigation of choice for ***meningeal carcinomatosis is Gd enhanced MRI***[Q] (especially for detection of *focal spread, bulky disease and metastases from solid tumor). Demonstration of tumor cells / tumor markers in CSF is definitive & often considered gold standard*; but has suboptimal/moderate overall sensitivity, and is more sensitive in detecting *diffuse leptomeningeal involvement from hematological malignancy*.

46. **A i.e. CT** *[Ref: Osborn 3/e p 448-49; Haga 5/e p 100, 521-24]*

NE (non contrast enhanced) CT is the ***investigation of choice to see temporal bone lesions***[Q], *(bony lesions such as fractures & destruction)*, whereas **MRI** is better to see the ***soft tissue masses (such as lipoma, hemangioma, meningioma, lymphoma, schwannoma, and non neoplastic lesions like meningitis, fibrosis, sarcoidosis, hemorrhage, vascular loop, AVM or aneurysm) inside the internal auditory canal of temporal bone***[Q].

47. **A i.e. Neurofibromatosis** *[Ref: Wolfgang 7/e p 319-22, 337, 333, 329; Haga 5/ep 803-4, 98-99, 1007; Osborn 3/e p 790/98, 72-94]*

- **Neurofibromatosis type 1** is associated with ***widening (enlargement) of neural foramina***[Q] ***(mostly secondary to dumbbell neurofibroma along exiting spinal nerve root or less commonly d/t dural ectasia, arachnoid cyst or lateral menngocele)***[Q], scalloping of posterior vertebral bodies, enlargement of internal auditory canal (d/t dural dysplasia), enlargement of *optic foramen* (d/t optic glioma), enlargement of *orbital margins & superior orbital fissure* (d/t plexiform neurofibroma) and *sclerosis of optic foramen* (d/t optic nerve sheath meningioma).
- NF1 causes ***empty orbit***[Q], *Herlequin appearance of orbit and herniation of middle cranial fossa structures into orbit d/t sphenoid bone hypoplasia.*

- Both *neurofibromas (common in NF1) and Schwannomas (common in NF2)* are benign nerve sheath tumors mostly found in *intradural extramedullary location*. Both are derived from Schwann cells, however, neurofibromas also have colagen & fibroblasts. Vestibular or acoustic Schwannoma (or neurilemmoma or acoustic neuroma of 8th cranial nerve) seen in NF2 l/t *internal auditory canal (IAC) enlargement (erosion* d/t mass centered on long axis of IAC forming acute angles with dural surface of petrous bone) and *widening or obliteration of ipsilateral cerebello pontine angle cistern.*
- NF-**2** is located on chromosome **22** and NF**1** on chromosome **17**(Mn 1 for 1 & 2 for 2). NF2 have propensity for developing **MEN/MES** i.e. **m**eningioma, **e**pendymoma (gliomas) and **S**chwannoma (**n**euromas). Nerves without Schwann cells are *olfactory and optic nerve.*
- **Schwannomas** & **neurofibromas**, on CT, appear as *sharply marginated, unilateral, spherical, or lobular posterior mediastinal mass, with pressure erosion of adjacent rib or vertebral bodies or enlargment of neural foramen* with occasional *punctate intralesional calcifcation.* Owing to their high lipid content, interstitial fluid and areas of cystic degeneration – *Schwannomas* are often of *lower attenuation* than skeleton muscle. **Neurofibromas** are often more homogenous & of *higher attenuation* than schwannomas (owing to fewer of above histological features). These may *heterogenously enhance on contrast administration.* On MRI both show variable intensity on T1WI but typically have similar signal intensity to the spinal cord. On T2WI these characteristically have *high signal intensity peripherally and low signal intensity centrally* **(*target sign*)** owing to collagen deposition. *Both schwannoma & neurofibroma enhance on gadolinium* administration.

48. **C i.e. Widened neural foramen** *[Ref: Haga 5/e p 705, 1007-3; Wolfgang 7/e p 222, 320, 450; Osborn 3/e p 803-5, 82]*

- **Lateral meningocele** is ***non solid, CSF containing leptomeningeal outpouching through widened neural foramen usually into paraspinal, intrathoracic space***Q. And it is generally associated with spinal deformities like, posterior (dorsal) scalloping, erosion of pedicles, thinning of neural arch & ribs, widening of spinal canal & neural foramen and kyphoscoliosis.

49. **D i.e. Wyburn-Mason syndrome** *[Ref: Osborn 3/e p 106-7, 287; Wolfgang 7/e p 273]*

- **Wyburn-Mason syndrome** (or **Bonnet-Dechaume Blanc syndrome mesencephalo-oculo-facial or mesencephalo-optico retinal angiomatosis syndrome)** is characterized by *neuro (mesencephalo) – optico / oculo / retinal – facial angiomatosis* (vascular-malformations).
- Wyburn-Mason syndrome presents with ***telangiectasia of skin***Q (i.e cutaneous vascular nevi) on face + ***retinal cirsoid aneurysm***Q and arterio-venous malformation ***(AVM) involving the visual pathways and midbrain***Q (= *entire optic tract = optic nerve, thalamus, geniculate bodies and calcarine cortex).* The lesions are typically unilateral mostly. It may be a/w AVMs of postrior fossa, neck, mandible/maxilla presenting in childhood.
- **Rendu-Osler-Weber syndrome (hereditary hemorrhagic telangiectasia)** is AD neurocutaneous syndrome that result in a variety of systemic ***fibrovascular dysplasia (i.e. telangiectasia, AVM, AV hemangioma/fistula, and aneurysm) affecting mucous membrane, skin, lung, brain and GI tract***Q. Telangiectasi is primarily found in the skin & mucous membranes. AVM and fistula are found manly in liver > brain > lung > spine. Aneurysm can invovle any size vessel. Frequent bleeding into mucous membrane, skin, lungs, genitourinary and gestrointestinal system is d/t vascular weakness.
- **Klippel-Trenaunay syndrome (KTS)** is *angio-osteo-hypertrophy* i.e. hypertrophy of soft tissue & over growth of bone l/t abnormalitie of finger/toes /limb and venous varicosities d/t large angiomatous nevus (AVM). Several KTS patients exhibit CNS findings of Sturg-Weber syndrome and are called **Klippel-Trenaunay-Weber syndrome**. They exhibit cutaneous angiomata, soft tissue /bony hypertrophy and leptomeningeal vascular malformation.

50. **A i.e. Sturge Weber syndrome** *[Ref: Grainger 4/e P-2348; Wolfgang 7/e p. 329]*

Sturge Weber syndrome is a kind of ***phakomatoses***Q (better termed as ***neuroectodermal dysplasias***Q) characterized by (Mn = **"Progressive PAST"**)

Progressive	- **Progressive** hemiparesis, hemianopsia, mental retardation
P	- *Port Wine Stain*Q (d/t cutaneous angiomas)
A	- Angiomas (Leptomeningeal angiomas with primarily parieto-occipital distribution)
S	- Seizures
T	- *Tram line* ***Calcification***Q (of occipital & parietal lobes)

Other neuroectodermal dysplasias / phakomatoses are :

Neuro	= **Neuro**fibromatosis
Surgeon's	= **S**turge Weber Syndrome
T	= **T**uberous Sclerosis (Bourneville's disease)
V	= **V**on – Hippel – Lindau disease

5

RADIODIAGNOSIS

NEPHROLOGY

KIDNEY

51. **D i.e. Increased vascularity** *[Ref: AMPIS- GU Imaging 3/e p. 140-142]*

Hypoperfusion (not increased vascularity), focal/segmental hypoechogenecity, and perinephric fluid (pus) collection in grossly or focally enlarged kidney on biphasic/ triphasic CE-CT or USG (investigation of choice in pregnancy) is seen in **acute pyelonephritis**.

52. **B, C i.e. MRI, PET-Scan**
53. **C i.e., Non contract CT scan of the abdomen**
54. **C i.e. CT Scan**
55. **A i.e. Intravenous urography**
56. **D i.e. MCU**
57. **C i.e., Voiding cystogram**
58. **B i.e. Contract MCU**

[Ref: AMPIS 3/e p 1-6; Swartz 8/e p 1547; Sutton 7/e p 1017, 898-99, 920; Armstrong 5/e p 217-233, Nelson 17/e P-1802]

- Patients with **suspected urolithiasis (stone)** present with painful hematuria and /or recurrent UTI. **Ultrasound and KUB X-ray** are the ***initial screening modality***Q followed by **unenhanced (i.e. non contrast) helical or spinal CT** (imaging modality of choice) if screening is negative. However, **IVU (intravenous urography)** or **IVP** is still the best investigation if CT is not available.
- The ***test of choice at most centers for diagnosing an acute stone is a non contrast helical CT Scan***Q. Helical CT (Non contrast) *has the advantage of detecting uric acid stones in addition to the traditional radioopaques stones, and CT does not expose the patient to the risk of radio contrast agents.*
- ***Calcification is best detected by CTscan***Q. MRI and PET scan have no role in diagnosing renal stone.
- **Intravenous urography (IVP)** is the only method which can *detect early renal tuberculosis and papillary necrosis*. It is the **most sensitive** and **investigation modality of choice** for early renal TB. However in **advanced cases** it should be integrated with ***cross sectional CT images***Q.

Investigation of Renal tuberculosis

Early stage

- ***IVU*Q *is the most sensitive imaging method*** because of its ability to detect calcification to show detailed calyceal anatomy and to demonstrate multiple lesions that typically occur.
- It's D/D is Papillary necrosis but unlike it TB is ***usually unilateral. If B/L it is not symmetrical.***

<u>IVP</u> is investigation of choice

Advanced stage

- *CT* (is good in demonstrating the changes as calcification, pelvicaliceal dialation, parenchymal loss & extrarenal spread)
- CT>*IVP > USG* (sensitivity order)

<u>CT</u> is investigation of choice

Also Remember:

- **IVP** is still the *most valuable & most sensitive examination of the urinary tract* as it gives excellent anatomical images. **USG** is 2nd most useful examination of urinary tract, next to IVP in adults & ***investigation of first choice in children***Q.
- **CT** is employed when USG is inconclusive as in *obese* patient, mass in *upper pole of left kidney (hidden area), macroscopic heamaturia* (suspecting renal cell CA).
- **Voiding/Micturating cystourethrogram (MCU)** is most accurate method of demonstrating ***vesicoureteric reflux***Q and to ***evaluate posterior part of urethra***Q whereas **retrograde cystourethrography** is most appropriate to evaluate the **anterior part of urethra**.

- ***Micturating/Voiding cystourethrography is the best method to visualize posterior urethra, posterior urethral valve & vesico ureteric reflux*** Q. In post urethral valve,Voiding Cystourethrogram (VCU) shows dialation of prostatic urethra & filling defect corresponding to the valve.

Urethra can be imaged in two ways:

- Anterograde techniques (done along with voiding cystourethrography or with voiding following excretory urography)	Best for visualization of posterior urethra
- Retrograde techniques (Folder catheter is passed through the urethra & radiocontrast material is injected)	*Best for Anterior (Penile) Urethra*

- VU Reflux occurs when urinary bladder contracts so contrast studies of urinary bladder done during micturation is best way to see VU Reflux. Radionucleotide cystogram is Inv of 2nd choice. It's advantage is that it avoids the need for bladder catheterization. The disadvantage is its lack of anatomical detail. So it may be useful in follow up (not initial assessment).

5

RADIODIAGNOSIS

59. **C i.e. Bilateral nephrostogram** *[Ref:Haga 5/e p2576-78;Grainger 5/e p1537-38, 820, 910-11, 164, Sutton 7/e p898-99, 924-25, 946, 902; Genitourinary imaging –AMPIS 3/e p 3, 223; Pediatric urinary imaging 3/e p 241-43]*

- The **low dose CT (Liu) protocol for stone** detection still results in approximately double the effective dose equivalent in comparison with **IVU** (2.8m Sv for CT, 1.33 mSv for conventional IVU). However, normal CT abdomen l/t 10 mSv and IVP l/t 2.5 mSV exposure i.e. equivalent to 500 and 120 chest x-ray respectively.
- **Voiding (micturating) cystourethrography (VCUG)** is performed after the bladder is filled with contrast material via a transuretheral or suprapubic catheter. After catheter is withdrawn the patient voids *under fluoroscopic (=continuous running x-ray) observation and spot radiographs (oblique voiding image)* of bladder & urethra are obtained. VCUG is the most appropriate way to evaluate *posterior urethra & retrograde urethrography (RGU)* is most appropriate way to evaluate *anterior urethra.* **MCUG/VCUG** has a **high radiation dose, but it is the only technique that can visualize male urethra adequately** including its posterior part. However VCUG may not demonstrate few abnormalities of male anterior urethra because the normal anterior urethra is not fully distended to the degree seen at RGU. So VCUG is used for evaluation of *female urethra & male posterior urethra.* It is **indicated in all boys with suspected urethral pathology** and is often done in those.

1. Under 3 years of age with UTI who have an abnormal US or DMSA scintigram
2. When ureteric dilatation is found
3. For terminal hematuria- accompanied by lower urinary tract symptomalogy
4. Renal failure of undetermined cause with abnormal ultrasound
5. In certain voiding problems, particularly when a thick walled bladder is seen on US
6. For infant screening in thoe who have an older sibling with VUR

- **Radionuclide (radioisotope) cystogram** is a simple procedure with **lower radiation dose** and is *more sensitive than VCUG in detecting vesico-ureteric reflux*; however it provides poor anatomical details than conventional VCUG.
- Radionuclide cystography (RC) may be **direct** (i.e. similar to MCUG, ^{99m}Tc is instilled in bladder through catheter) or **indirect** (i.e. following IVinjection of ^{99m}Tc DTPA, ^{123}I-hippuran or commonly ^{99m}Tc MAG3; so catheter is not required but toilet training is necessary as it takes more time for tracer to reach bladder so only older/toilet trained children can tell the exact time of when to start indirect micturating radionuclide cystogram). So RC is indicated **whenever renal (vesico-ureteric) reflux must be excluded** (direct in younger & indirect in older toilet trained children). This group mainly includes *young girls with a history of UTI and boys who require followup cystography (having previously had an MCUG).* A direct radiosotope cystogram is adequate *for diagnosing VUR* in girls who are not toilet trained and have a UTI or abnormal ^{99m}Tc-DMSA findings. For *follow up of known VUR, a RC should be carried out. The last 2 conditions (i.e. follow up of known VUR in boys and diagnosing VUR in girls) are included in contraindication list of MCUG* in Grainger (1538)- why- because of high radiation.
- **Nephrostomy** is placement of pigtail catheter in a dilated renal pelvis or ureter usually under ultrasound guidance or during surgery (both a/w no radiation) and rarely under fluoroscopy or CT guidance (>3.5 MSv radiation exposure). However, the indication for CT guidance is limited and include renal transplants, unilateral kidney, high risk patients, unusual anatomic variation or a kidney with a urinoma a/w hydronephrosis (i.e. conditions in which higher margin of safety is needed and good anatomical detail is required to prevent damage).
- **Nephrostogram** is a very simple procedure in which contrast is pushed into nephrostomy tube positioned for therapeutic purposes. It is very *similar to antegrade pyelogram,* in which dye is injected in *pelvi calyceal system directly* to provide anatomical detail of renal pelvis & or ureter unavailable from US or IVP. Nephrostogram has a *low radiation exposure* because after infusion of contrast into collecting system (via already placed nephrostomy tube) only few spot films of ureter down to the level of obstruction are taken. Nephrostogram is indicated to assess the obstructing lesion, either to evaluate its status (continued presence of a calculus or response of malignancy to treatment) or obtain further information if the cause of obstruction has not yet been determined.
- **Retrograde pyelography** is visualization (opacification) of pelvicalyceal system & ureter by injecting dye through cystoscopically placed catheter in ureter
- You may get different radiation doses in different books/sites b/o varying protocols i.e. an IVP done to see pelvis only would expose to less radiation than IVP done to see whole excretory system.

60. **B i.e. Cysteine** *[Ref: Nelson 17/e P-403, 1613; Campbell's urology 5/e P-3270; Schwartz 7/e P-1776; Harrison 15/e P-2273; Shinde 5/e P-213; Harper 26/e P-301]*

Stone	Radiological appearance
- Calcium *phosphate*Q (apatite), - Ca – hydrogen – phosphate (Brushite) - Ca – mono - *oxalate*Q	**Densely radiopaque**
- Ca – di – oxalate - *Struvite*Q (Magnesium – ammonium - phosphate)	**Moderately radiopaque**
- *Cystine*Q	**Faint (slight) radiopaque** d/t sulfer content
- *Orotic acid*Q - *Uric acid*Q - *Xanthine*Q - Dihydroxyadenine - Indinavir - *Triamterene* - Matrix	**Radiolucent**

Orotic Acid Urea

- Hereditary orotic acidurea is AR disorder caused by deficiency of ***UMP Synthase***Q [Uridine Mono Phosphate synthase; a bifunctional enzyme having activity of Orotate – phosphor ibosyl – transferase & Ortidine – 5' –monophosphate decorboxylase, which converts orotic acid to UMP] resulting in excessive accumulation of orotic acid.
- Clinically presents as **Macrocytic Hypochromic Megaloblastic anemia**Q *not responsive to folic acid and B_{12}, with normal serum levels of B_{12} & folic acid,* **growth retardation,** neurological abnormalities and **orotic acid urea.**
- *Allopurinol*Q, 5 – *azauridine,* 5 – flurouracil produce **secondry (2°) orotic aciduria.**
- 2° Orotic acid urea also occurs in parentral nutrition, essential amino acid deficiency & Rye's syndrome.

★ Allopurinol treatment may lead to Xanthine & orotic acid stones, which are radiolucent.

61. **B i.e. Systemic hypertension**

62. **B i.e. Renal vein thrombosis**

- **Nonvisualization of kidney** (or **absence of nephrogram**) occurs in *complete renal ischemia secondary to occlusion of main renal artery,* (global absence) or ***focal renal infarction/ischemia*** secondary to focal arterial occlusion or ***renal vein thrombosis***Q or space occupying lesions (segmental absence).
- **Persistent dense nephrogram** (both increasingly or immediate) is seen in ***systemic hypotension, severe dehydration***Q, renal artery stenosis, renal vein thrombosis, ***tubular obstruction & damage and urinary tract obstruction (eg ureteral obstruction)***Q but not in systemic hypertension. Although hydronephrosis usually l/t ***scalloped/shell i.e. non smooth rim nephrogram***Q.

63. **C i.e. Rapid (Bolus) injection of dye** *[Ref: Smith's urology 16/e p-65; Grainger 5/e p-873; Cecil medicine 6/e p-291-99; Chapman 5/e p. 209-11; Wolfgang 7/e p. 901-11]*

Dense nephrogram or intensified renal images are obtained (iatrogenically) by –

- ***Rapid/bolus injection of same contrast dose concentration (preferred method)***Q.
- **Increased contrast concentration** is less preferred than rapid injection method. The quantity that can be used safely depends on weight & hydration of patient.
- **Abdominal (ureteric) compression** may be used to temporarily obstruct the upper urinary tract but is demanding.
- **Dehydration** method used in past is not used now b/o more chances of precipitation of proteins in renal tubules, obstruction, oliguria & anuria.

64. **B i.e. Hyperdense nephrogram** *[Ref: Wolfgang 7/e p. 961-62; Sutton 7/e p. 978; Armstrong 5/e p. 247-49; AMPIS 3/e p. 147, 317-18; Chapman 5/e p. 211-12]*

Characteritic IVP features of papillary necrosis include ***ball in cup or egg in cup configuration, signet ring sing or ring shadow of papilla, lobster clew sign, club shaped (saccular) calyx***Q, amputated calyces, multiple cavities, nonopaque filling defects and ***diminished density of contrast material in nephrogram***Q.

65. **B i.e. Presence of collaterals**

66. **C i.e. Spiral CT Scan (CTA)**

[Ref: Wolfgang 7/e p. 974/83; Sutton 7/e p. 432-33, 964-65; Harrison 18/e p. 2048-49; AMPIS 3/e p. 284-97; Grainger 5/e p. 841-46]

- ***The presence of arterial collaterals indicates that renal artery stenosis is hemodynamically significant***Q. The diameter of stenotic segment may also give an indication of hemodynamic significance, but is only reliable if the stenosis is either very severe or minimal.
- **Conventional contrast renal arteriography** (or **digital substraction angiography or intraarterial catheter angiography**) is the **gold standard** for ***diagnosis of renal artery stenosis***Q against which all other modalities are compared.
- On angiography, the ***presence of collateral vessels to the ischemic kidney***Q suggest a **functionally significant lesion** (i.e. a lesion that occludes >70% of *lumen of affected renal artery).*
- A **lateralizing renal vein renin ratio** (>1.5 of affected side/contralateral side) has a 90% predictive value for a lesion that would respond to vascular repair and result in BP control.

- **After percutaneous arteriography**, the ***next most sensitive and specific screening test for diagnosis of RAS is CT angiography***[Q] (using spiral and more recently **multidetector CT**) almost equvalent to DSA. However, it requires use of large amount of iodinated contrast medium (like IVP) precluding its use in renal insufficiency and also exposes to ionizing radiation.
- **Captopril enahanced radionuclide renal scintigraphy,** is *most widely performed screening test for diagnosis of renovascular hypertension,* (neither most sensitive nor most specific). ^{99m}Tc MAG 3 is slightly preferred over ^{99m}Tc-DTPA; ^{131}I OIH is not used now. It can be used as screening test to establish hemodynamic significance of RAS, to predict the outcome of revascularizaation and in the follow up after successful revascularization. Disadvantages include low sensitivity in patients with azotemia or underlying renal dysfunction & with bilateral RAS. Branch artery stenosis cannot be diagnosed and *provides functional not anatomical data.*
- Summary: The **decreasing order of sensitivity & specificity for diagnosis of renal artery stenosis (related renovascular hypertension)** is **conventional** contrast / intraarterial-catheter **angiography >CT angiography** (using spiral/MDCT) > **CE-MRA (dynamic) > SSFP** non contrast. enhanced MRA > **captopril enhanced radionuclide renal scintigraphy** (**^{99m}Tc MAG3 and ^{99m}Tc LLEC** preferred over ^{99m}Tc DTPA). All have their pros & cons.
- This question is ideal to emphesize the "phenomenon of contradiction (poc) in medical preperatory exams. After referring Harrison, it may seem to some students that best screening method is captopril enhanced RRS and 99mTc DTPA is the best radionuclide, but both are only relative truths. In last 12 years we have explained this question at least 4 times but the answer always remained same. It is not always possible to elaborate all answers to such a huge extent but research done to find a perfect answer is far more extensive and exhaustive.

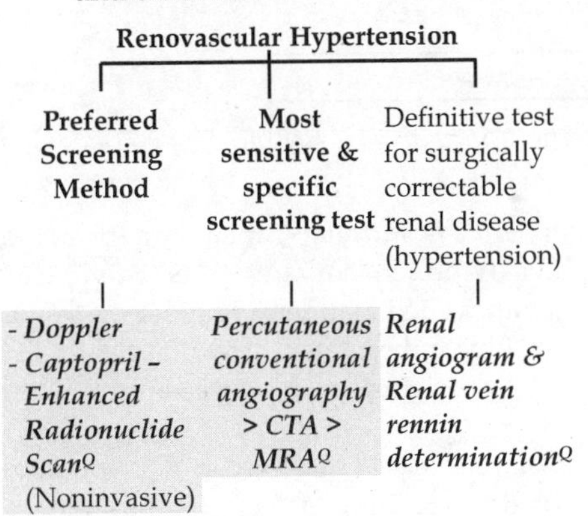

Investigational algorhythm of RAS

- IVP and non captoril RRS are no longer used. **USG** or **Doppler** is a logical first step
- Patient who are strongly suspected of RAS on clinical & USG grounds may be further investigated with **CTA, MRA or percutaneous angiography** for **anatomical detail** and **captopril enhanced RRS** for **functional detail**.
- **CT angiography** is an extremely useful investigation but exposes the patient to a considerable amount of radiation and should not therefore be used as a first line investigation.
- MR angiography has advantage that it avoids ionizing radiation. Its disadvantage has been image degradation by patient movements (especially respiration), inability to see distal renal arteries and poor resolution compared with CT.
- The **conventional gold standard** investigation for diagnosis of RAS has been ***percutaneous arteriography***[Q]. Its place as a diagnostic tool has been much reduced in view of the non invasive investigations considered above.

67. **A i.e. Wilm's tumor** *[Ref: Grainger 4/e p.1570, 1578; Wolfgang 5/e p. 933, 984, 927, 950; Pediatric USG –Hayden p331]*

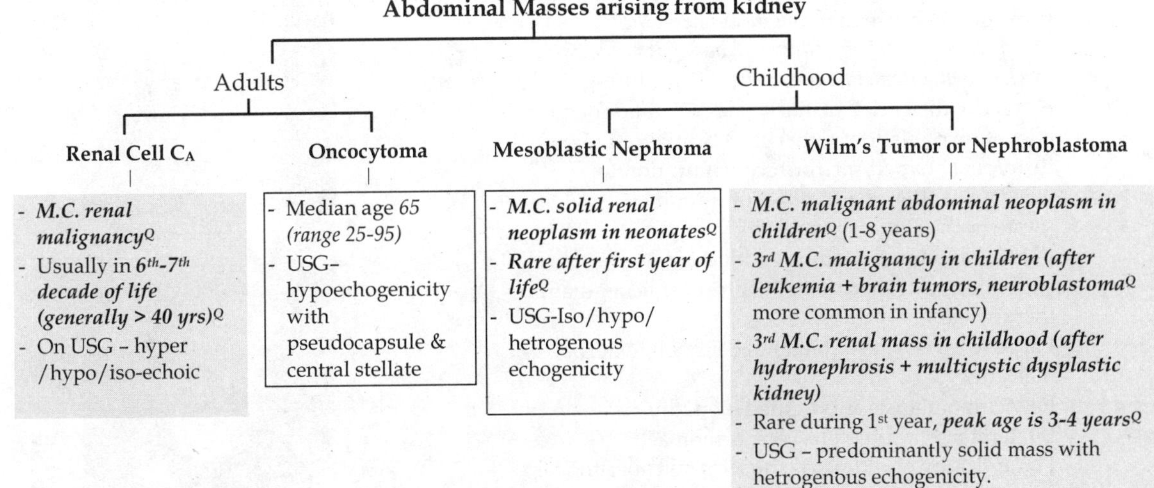

Abdominal Masses arising from kidney
Adults
Childhood
Renal Cell CA
Oncocytoma
Mesoblastic Nephroma
Wilm's Tumor or Nephroblastoma
- M.C. renal malignancy[Q]
- Usually in 6th-7th decade of life (generally > 40 yrs)[Q]
- On USG – hyper /hypo/iso-echoic
- Median age 65 (range 25-95)
- USG– hypoechogenicity with pseudocapsule & central stellate
- M.C. solid renal neoplasm in neonates[Q]
- Rare after first year of life[Q]
- USG-Iso/hypo/ hetrogenous echogenicity
- M.C. malignant abdominal neoplasm in children[Q] (1-8 years)
- 3rd M.C. malignancy in children (after leukemia + brain tumors, neuroblastoma[Q] more common in infancy)
- 3rd M.C. renal mass in childhood (after hydronephrosis + multicystic dysplastic kidney)
- Rare during 1st year, peak age is 3-4 years[Q]
- USG – predominantly solid mass with hetrogenous echogenicity.

Approach to this case – On the basis of age you can easily rule out RCC_Q & Oncocytoma (found in adult age group); Mesoblastoma (which is rare after 1 year of age). So anwer is Wilm's tumor.

At the age of 3 years (1-8 years) – *Wilm's tumor is most common malignant abdominal mass (2nd m.c. is neuroblastoma)*Q;
- **3rd m.c. renal mass (after hydronephrosis & multicystic dysplastic kidney)**
- ***3rd m.c. malignancy (after leukemia & brain tumor)*Q. Note *in infancy 3rd m.c. malignancy is neuroblastoma*Q.**

URETHRA

68. **A i.e. MRI** *[Ref: Nelson 17/e P-1803; Sabiston 16/e P-1669]*

Radiological Investigation for urethral stricture

1. **Retrograde *urethrography*Q**
   - It should not be done within *3-4 weeks* of significant urethral trauma (can cause extravasation of the dye into the spongy tissue, lymphatics & veins of pelvis).
   - Mainstay of investigation.
2. **Micturating Cysto Urethro*gram*Q**
3. **Endoscopy**
   - Is confirmatory
   - Is of two types (a) Retrograde urethroscopy (b) Antegrade cystourethroscopy.
4. **Sonographic – urethrogram**
5. **High frequency *ultrasound*Q**

BLADDER

69. **A, B i.e. Pelvic hematoma, Pelvic lipomatoma** *[Ref: Peter Armstrong 5/e p 256-57; AMPIS 3/e p 371-73; Grainger 5/e p 889-90; Wolfgang 7/e p 916, 999]*

- **Inverted pear shaped** or **inverted teardrop bladder** is seen in ***pelvic hematoma*Q**, aneurysm (bilateral common or external iliac artery), ***pelvic lipomatosis*Q** and pelvic lymphadenopathy. (Mn-"**Pelvic-HaLL**").
- **Neurogenic bladder** may present as either 1) large atonic smooth walled bladder with poor or absent contractions & large residual volume; or 2) very thick, hypertrophic trabeculated (irregular) walls showing marked sacculations, small volume with an elongated shape (k/a **christmas or pine tree appearance**) d/t bladder out flow obstruction.
- **Bladder tuberculosis** presents with *thickened calcified bladder wall, shrunken bladder* (scarred bladder with decreased capacity), **thimble bladder** (diminutive irregular bladder) & filling defect (d/t multiple granulomas)
- **Ureteral tuberculosis** presents with **saw toothed/beaded /Corck-screw/pipestem – ureter** with filling defects. Tuberculous prostatitis present with ***watermelon sign*** (on T_2WI MRI).

Tear-Drop/Pear shaped Urinary Bladder

Accumulated blood (eg perivesicle hematoma) or urine or any cause that *compresses upon the extraperitoneal part of bladder narrowing it at the base /neck into an attenuated (thin) stem*, while lifting markedly distended urinary bladder, out of pelvis (elevation of bladder floor) gives a **inverted tear drop/pear shaped/piriform configuration** to urinary bladder on excretory urography (cystogram). It may be caused by
- **Pelvic hematoma** (trauma eg **bladder contusion/ extraperitoneal rupture**, anticoagulant therapy etc.)
- Large **A**neursysms of bilateral common/ external iliac artery
- Pelvic **l**ipomatosis & **l**ymphadenopathy
- Bilateral pelvic mass (abscess, urinomas)
- Hypertrophy of ilio-psoas muscles, retroperitoneal fibrosis and thrombosis of IVC are other rare causes.

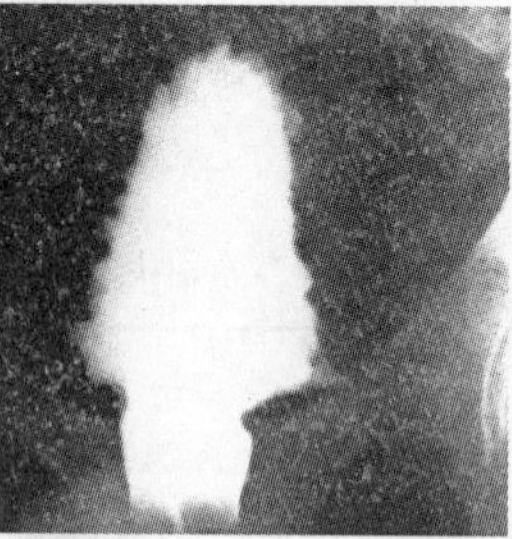

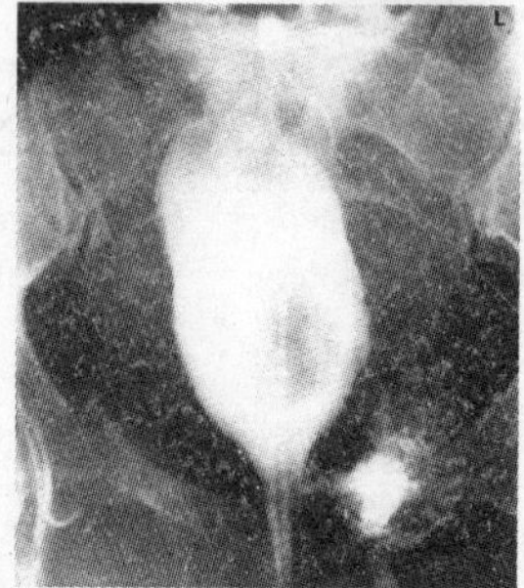

70. **A i.e. Schistosomiasis; C i.e. TB; D i.e. Carcinoma** *[Ref: Chapman*

Bladder Calcification

In the lumen

- Calculus
- Foreign body
- Encrusted foley catheteter

STC	*Squamous & Transitio* other primary neoplasm
S	*Schistosomiasis*[Q]
T	*Tuberculosis*[Q]
C	Cystitis: Cyclophosphamide/Cytox irradiation, alkaline incrusted, intersti

Mn- "STC"

PROSTATE

71. **A i.e. Guided prostatic biopsy** *[Ref: Sutton 7/e p – 637, 1005, 896- 97]*

The major role of transrectal USG is to guide prostatic biopsies[Q].

72. **A i.e. Adeno C_A; B i.e. Normal prostate tissue; E i.e. BPH** *[Ref: Sutton 7/e p. 1004-06; Grainger 5/e p. 900-05; Wolfganf 7/e p. 924]*

- **Hypoechoic lesions of prostate** (on USG) include: Mn-**"Normal ABCD of prostate"** i.e. **Normal** prostatic tissue (cluster of prostate retention cysts, prominent ejaculatory ducts); Atrophy; ***Adenocarcinoma (most common cause)***[Q]; Benign prostatic hypertrophy, BCG (Calmette Guerin bacillus) intravesicle therapy l/t granulomatous prostatitis; Chronic & acute prostatis; and Dysplasia of prostate.
- **Hypointense T2 signal** of prostate (on MRI) is seen in ***adenocarcinoma***[Q], post biopsy haemorrhage, inflammation/fibrosis/scarring, post-normal & radiation treatment and dystrophic changes.
- In normal USG, the central zone of prostate appears hypoechoic, while peripheral zone appears hyperechoic. In **BPH**, adenomatous nodules are seen predominantly ***hypoechoic***[Q]. **Prostatic carcinoma** most often demonstrates a ***hypoechoic echo texture***[Q].

USG of Benign prostatic hyperplasia (BPH)

- *Trans rectal* (better than trans abdominal) USG can measure *accurate prostate volume*. However, symptoms, complication & treatment are not closely related to volume (although occasionaly, decision to choose retropubic or transrectal approach may depend)
- Adenomatous nodules are seen as ***well defined echo – poor nodules, located centrally***[Q] (originating in transitional zone) *expanding the central gland and compressing peripheral* (hyperechoic) zone.
- *Cyst & foci of calcification with dense shadowing* are frequent
- Rarely nodule may be *hyperechoic.*
- Assessment of effects on rest of urinary system is routienly done.

USG of Carcinoma prostate

- 85% of C_A appear in peripheral hyperchoic zone & ***classically appear as focal hypoechoic nodule or ill defined area of reduced echogenocity***[Q].
- 50% of C_A are *multifocal or bilateral*
- Few carcinomas are of *similar echogenocity to normal peripheral zone* or may originate in central gland. Rarely may be *hyperechoic.*
- Doppler & contrast enhance sensitivity, but histopathology is still required & ***major use of transrectal USG is to guide prostatic biopsies***[Q].

...LOGY II: OTHERS

...rlequin Appearance of Orbit

...minate
...id bone)
...een in.
...plasia or
...(d/t

Innominate line representing greater wing of sphenoid

Empty Bare Orbit (NF1, Metastasis, Meningioma)

Plain Chest X-Ray

- PA and lateral views are routinely done to evaluate the ***lungs, 40% of which is obscured by other structures including ribs***Q.
- ***Exposure is made on full inspiration***Q for optimal visualization of lung bases, centering at T5. The breast should be compressed against the film to present them obscuring the lung bases.
- **High Kilovoltage (kVp)** is *preferred* and *widely used* technique because radiographic *visibility of bony thorax is reduced* with only slight change in over all visibility of lungs. Further more with high (120-170) kVp the mediastinum is better penetrated thereby *permitting visibility of hidden areas of lung* (such as behind the heart etc), mediastinal lines and interfaces. It also results in *lower radiation exposure* and *shorter exposure time* so that *movement blurr due to cardiac pulsation is minimized.* The only disadvantage of high kVp technique is diminished visibility of calcium. Using a **low kilovoltage (kVp)** produces a *high contrast film with miliary shadowing and calcification* being more clearly seen than on a high kVp film.
- *To reduce scatter and improve contrast* a **grid /filter** (at least 10:1 aluminum interspace with a minimum 103 lines/inch) or **air gap** (15-25 cm gap between patient & x-ray film) is necessary. An air gap of 15-25 cm necessitates an increased **Focal film distance (FFD)** of 8 feet (2.44 m) to reduce magnification and produce a sharper imge.
- ***In most patients the right hemidiaphragm is higher than the left. This is d/t heart depressing the left side and not to the liver pushing up the right hemidiaphragm***Q; in dextrocardia with normal abdominal situs the right hemidiaphragm is the lowest. In 3% left side is higher mostly when the *stomach or splenic flexure is distended with gas.* A difference > *3cm in height is considered significant.*

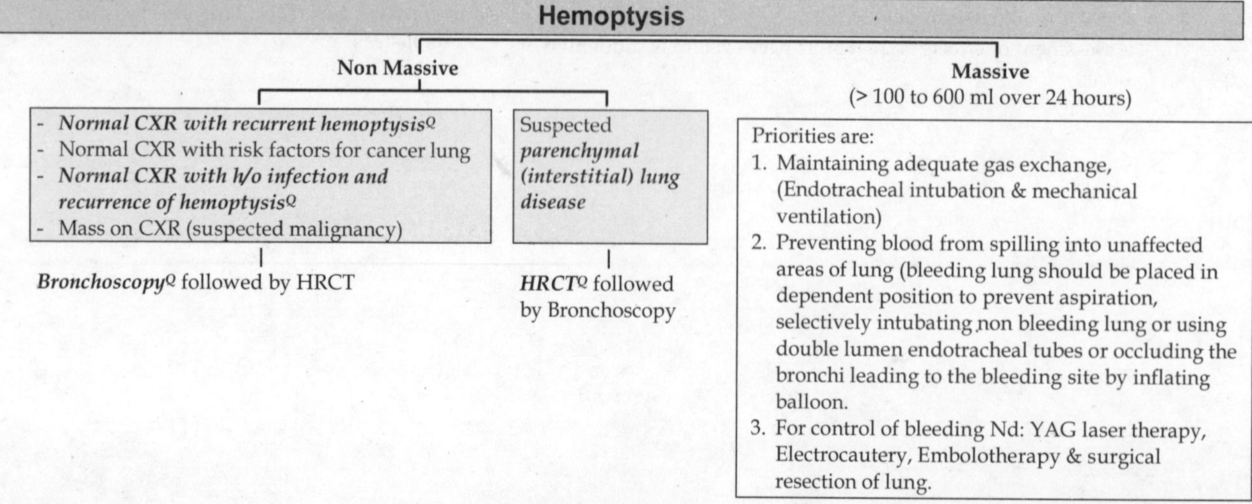

Hemoptysis
Non Massive
Massive
(> 100 to 600 ml over 24 hours)
- Normal CXR with recurrent hemoptysisQ
- Normal CXR with risk factors for cancer lung
- Normal CXR with h/o infection and recurrence of hemoptysisQ
- Mass on CXR (suspected malignancy)
Suspected parenchymal (interstitial) lung disease
BronchoscopyQ followed by HRCT
HRCTQ followed by Bronchoscopy
Priorities are:
1. Maintaining adequate gas exchange, (Endotracheal intubation & mechanical ventilation)
2. Preventing blood from spilling into unaffected areas of lung (bleeding lung should be placed in dependent position to prevent aspiration, selectively intubating non bleeding lung or using double lumen endotracheal tubes or occluding the bronchi leading to the bleeding site by inflating balloon.
3. For control of bleeding Nd: YAG laser therapy, Electrocautery, Embolotherapy & surgical resection of lung.

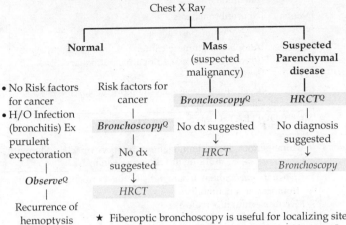

Algorithm for Evaluation of Non massive Hemoptysis

Chest X Ray

- **Normal**
  - No Risk factors for cancer
  - H/O Infection (bronchitis) Ex purulent expectoration
  - → *Observe*[Q] → Recurrence of hemoptysis → *Bronchoscopy*[Q] → No dx suggested → *HRCT*
  - Risk factors for cancer → *Bronchoscopy*[Q] → No dx suggested → *HRCT*
- **Mass (suspected malignancy)** → *Bronchoscopy*[Q] → No dx suggested → *HRCT*
- **Suspected Parenchymal disease** → *HRCT*[Q] → No diagnosis suggested → *Bronchoscopy*

★ Fiberoptic bronchoscopy is useful for localizing site of bleeding & visualizing endobronchial lesions. In massive hemoptysis, rigid bronchoscopy is preferrec over fiberoptic bronchoscopy b/o better airway control & suction capability.

Massive Reccurent Hemoptysis (MRH)

- **Systemic Artery (Bronchial Vessels)**[Q]: MRH originates from systemic (bronchial) artery in *Most of patients*[Q].
- **Pulmonary arteries**[Q] are culpable in **5-10%**[Q] of patients with *chronic disorders such as TB with Rasmussen aneurysm formation.*

↓

Bronchial Artery Embolization (*BAE*)[Q] is well accepted & effective form of treatment for MRH typically from 1) TB 2) Sarcoidosis 3) Fungal cavity 4) AVMal formation 5) In-operable ronchiectasis (espically cystic fibrosis) 6) Acute / chronic Abscess.

Diagnostic Algorithm of Solitary Pulmonary Nodule

- Some 40% of solitary pulmonary nodules are malignant with other common lesions being granulomas & benign tumors.
- CT scan is most sensitive imaging modality available for identification of pulmonary nodules of ≥ 3mm diameter but relatively insensitive to smaller nodules. The specificity for small nodules is also poor.
- Spiral scanning has improved detection rate for pulmonary nodule but has not improved specificity.
- The presence of calcification indicates benign lesion but 14% of carcinomas (malignant) show calcification.
- The cavitation not necessarily indicates malignant lesion.

CT scan is most sensitive for detecting large pulmonary nodules (≥ 3mm) but neither sensitive nor specific for smaller nodules the maximum CT scan can show is calcification & cavitation, which are not always diagnostic of benign & malignant lesions respectively. So the best investigation to come to a diagnosis (i.e. most specific) will be ***image guided (transthoracic needle aspiration) biopsy***[Q].

Solitary Nodule on X Ray
↓
CT Scan (*Next investigation* for getting more details, which are indicative of some diagnosis)
↓
Image guided Biopsy[Q], (*Best investigation to come to a diagnosis*)

Causes of Miliary Mottling (Diffuse fine=1-4mm nodules)

- **Inhalational diseases**
  - Silicosis + Coal workers *pneumoconiosis*[Q]
  - Siderosis
  - Berylliosis
  - Extrinsic allergic alveolitis (chronic phase)
- **Allergic (chronic)**
  - Simple pulmonary eosinophilia (**Loffler's syndrome**)
  - Tropical eosinophilia
- **Granulomatous diseases**
  - *Eosinophilic granuloma*[Q]
  - *Sarcoidosis*[Q]

Causes of Reticular Pattern (Honey comb Lung)

G	Gaucher disease
OO	**O**xygen toxicity, **O**ccupational lung disease (asbestosis, hard metal =C, Co, tun geston pneumoconiosis and paraquat poisoning)
D	**D**rugs = **B**leomycin, **B**usulfan, **C**yclophosphemide, Melphalan, Nitrofurantoin
B	**B**rit-Hogg – Dube syndrome, **B**one marrow transplantation
A	**A**rthritis (Rheumatoid), **A**myloidosis, **A**llergic alveolitis (extrinsic), **A**lveolar proteinosis
T	**T**.B, **T**uberous sclerosis
H	**H**istiocytosis X (Langerhan's cell histiocytosis)

- **Infectious diseases**
  - ***Tuberculosis*Q (most common)**
  - Bacterial: ***Salmonella, nocardiosis*Q**, brucellosis
  - **Fungus**: ***histoplasmosis*Q**, coccidioidomycosis, blastomycosis (all common), aspergillosis, cryptococcosis (both rare)
  - **Virus**: ***Varicella (most common in adults)*Q**, Mycoplasma pneumonia
- **Metastases (Secondaries)**
  - From thyroid carcinoma, melanoma, adenocarcinoma of breast, stomach, colon, pancreas
  - Lymphoma, leukemia, lymphangitis carcinomatosis, alveolar cell carcinoma (?)
- **Cardiac** causes of **pulmonary edema**, multiple **pulmonary infarcts.**
- Bronchiolitis obliterans, Gaucher disease, Alveolar microlithiasis (rare)
- ***Rheumatoid arthritis nodules*Q**, Wegner's granulomatosis, Caplan's syndrome, amyloidosis, hydatid, AVM, & abscess l/t multiple (>5mm mm) Larger nodules.

Leaves	**L**ymphangioleiomyomatosis, **L**ymphocytic intertitial pneumonia
Noone	**N**eurofibromatosis
S	**S**cleroderma, **S**arcoidosis
I	**I**diopathic, **I**diopathic interstial fibrosis (cryptogenic fibrosing alveolitis), **I**diopathic pulmonary hemosiderosis
C	**C**ystic lung disease, **C**ystic bronchiectasis, **C**ystic fibrosis

Mn: "**GOOD BATH Leaves Noone SIC**"

Homogenous or non homogenous air space opacification with Bulging of Fissure is seen in-

- ***Klebsiella pneumonia*Q** (characteristic, most imp. but unusual)
- Streptococcus pneumoniae
- Mycobacterium tuberculosis
- Yersinia pestis
- Lung abscess
- CA bronchus

★ Varicella pneumonia is ***most serious complication*Q**, developing ***more commonly in adults (≈20%)*Q** following chicken pox. CXR shows nodular infiltrates & interstitial pneumonitis (i.e. miliary shadows).

Causes of U/L Radiolucent Hemithorax

Due to U/L Air trapping

1. Pneumatocoal
2. ***Pneumothorax*Q**
3. ***Emphysema*Q**
4. Bullae
5. Mc Leod's Syndrome (there is air trapping on expiration as it is a late sequale of childhood bronchiolitis)

Due to U/L Decreased Soft tissue mass (not lung mass)

1. Mastectomy
2. Poland's Syndrome (Absent pectoralis muscle)
3. Polio (atrophy of pectoralis muscle)

Due to **Tilted Patient** (radiolucent is the side to which patient is turned)

1. Scoliosis
2. Poor technique

★ Always remember that ***decreased U/L lung mass as in pulmonary agenesis pulmonary hypoplasia, collapse & pneumonectomy are the causes of U/L radiodense hemithorax with I/L mediastinal displacement.***

Hypertransradiant (Radiolucent) Hyperinflated lung on CXR is seen in

- ***Emphysema*Q**
- Pulmonary embolism
- Pneumothorax
- Polland's syndrome
- Patient rotation
- Macleod syndrome

CXR in Emphysema

- ***Barrel shaped Kyphotic chest*Q**
- ***Hyper inflation*Q** of lung causes ***lower lying flat diaphragm*Q (tarrace pattern)Q, *increased intercostals space*Q**, increased sterno-diaphragmatic & costo-diaphragmatic angles & increased retrosternal air space

***Tubular Heart*Q**

Note – Hyperinflation l/t increased radiolucency.

Ground Glass Appearance

- It is radiological marker of *pathology in air space or* ***interstitium***[Q].
- Presents with increased lung density which on chest X Ray obscures broncho vesicular markings (but present on CT ; if bronchial & vascular markings are absent both in X Ray & CT then k/a consolidation)
- So any disease of alveoli & interstitium (described in Q 7 of AI – 2002) can give rise to this but important causes are –

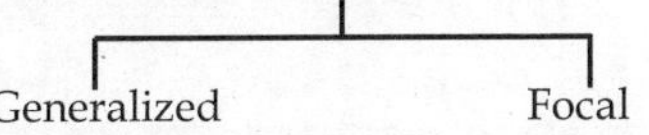

Generalized	Focal
- ***Interstitial Pneumonias***[Q] - Allergic alveolitis/Alveolar proteinosis - ***Hyline membrane disease***[Q] - ***Obstructive TAPVC***[Q] d/t Pulmonary edema caused by pulmonary hypertension.	- Broncho alveolar A - Lymphoma - Pulmonary infiltration with eosinophillia syndrome

Total Anomalous Pulmonary Venous Drainage (TAPVD)

Due to Interstial & alveolar edema caused by pulmonary venous hypertension Obstructed TAPVD usually presents in neonatal period with cynosis and severe respiratory distress and it is difficult to differentiate it from pulmonary hypertension & severe pulmonary disease. Radiological features of TAPVD are-

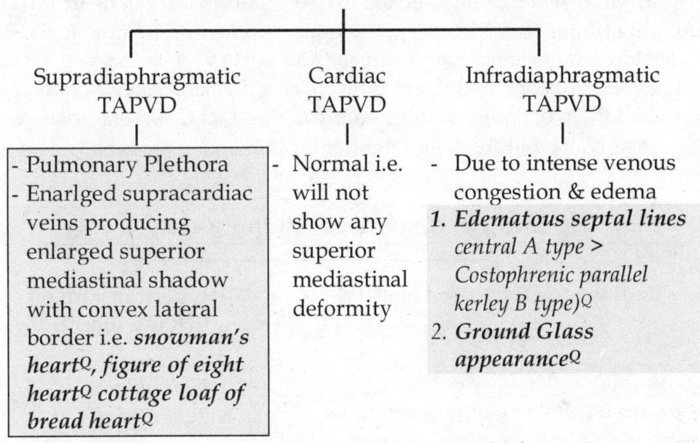

Supradiaphragmatic TAPVD
Cardiac TAPVD
Infradiaphragmatic TAPVD
- Pulmonary Plethora
- Enarlged supracardiac veins producing enlarged superior mediastinal shadow with convex lateral border i.e. snowman's heartQ, figure of eight heartQ cottage loaf of bread heartQ
- Normal i.e. will not show any superior mediastinal deformity
- Due to intense venous congestion & edema
1. Edematous septal lines central A type > Costophrenic parallel kerley B type)Q
2. Ground Glass appearanceQ

Note :

- Ground glass ap. of cardiac origin is differentiated from pulmonary origin by *presence of edematous septal lines & fissures.*
- **L→R shunts shows *hyperemic or plethoric lung field*[Q].**

Radiological Signs of Air Space (Acinar) disease

1. Nodular pattern (< 3 cm)
2. Acinar nodules (5-10 mm)
3. Ground glass opacification (increased lung density, obscures vessel markings)
4. ***Air Bronchogram***[Q]
5. ***Air Alveologram***[Q]

Air bronchogram within opacity is seen in

Infective	Inflamatory	Neoplastic
↓	↓	↓
Pneumonia	- Radiation Pneumonitis - Progressive Massive fibrosis	Alveolar cell C_A Lymphoma Lympho S_A

Air Bronchogram

- Normal intrapulmonary airways are not usually visible radiographically if however surrounding air spaces are opacified, the *airways are seen as linear branching structures.* **The resulting air bronchogram is a reliable sign of an intrapulmonary pathology**[Q] **for which *consolidation is the most common cause*[Q].**
- So presence of *air bronchogram or other signs of air space disease excludes any pleural or mediastinal pathology.*
- Causes: In any condition l/t parenchymal opacification which can be caused by replacement of air in distal air spaces by

- Tissue	=	Bronchoalveolar Cell C_A Lymphoma Metastasis Kaposi S_A Pseudo Lymphoma
- Blood	=	Contusion Infarction DIC, Hemophillia, Anticoagulants
- Exudate	=	Pneumonia
- Transudate	=	Oedema Fat embolism

Loculated (Encysted/Encapsulated) Pleural Effusion

- **Loculated (encysted/encapsulated) pleural effusion** are differentiated from free pleural fluid by **gravitational methods**. ***Loculated PE (true pleural pathology) can be differentiated from peripheral pleural based lung lesions by absence of airbron chogram***[Q]. Extrapleural opacities have much sharper outlilne, with tapered sometimes cancave edges where they meet the chest wall.

- Loculted effusion is often a/w free pleural fluid or other pleural shadowing and *may extend into fissures. Theyh have considerable width, but little depth and look like a biconvex lens.* The appearance of locuated PE varies with its location and radiographic projections used. It is **sharply marginated when the surface is parallel to Xray beam and is ill defined when viewed en face (end on)**[Q]. So a collection loculated in lateral pleural space will appear sharply marginated on frontal radiograph and ill defined on lateral film. For effusions loculated anteriorly or posteriorly, the converse is true.
- **Loculated PE may not be confined to any bronchopulmonary segment and may make an obtuse angel with the chest wall.**[Q]
- **Fissural interlober loculated effusions**, seen particularly in **heart failure** produces the **pseudo (phantom) tumor or vanishing tumor** as it may disappear rapidly following treatment and recur in the same place on repeated occasion. Viewed in *lateral view it is sharply marginated and biconvex, with a tail passing through the fissure* .The enface affearance depends on thickness of effusion (quantity of fluid). *Thin effusions produce a vague area of opacity and thick effusions appear clear edged and mass like.* LPE in oblique fissure is poorly defined on frontal radiograph, but a lateral film is diagnostic since the fissure is seen tangentially and the typical **lenticular (biconvex)** effusion is demonstrated.

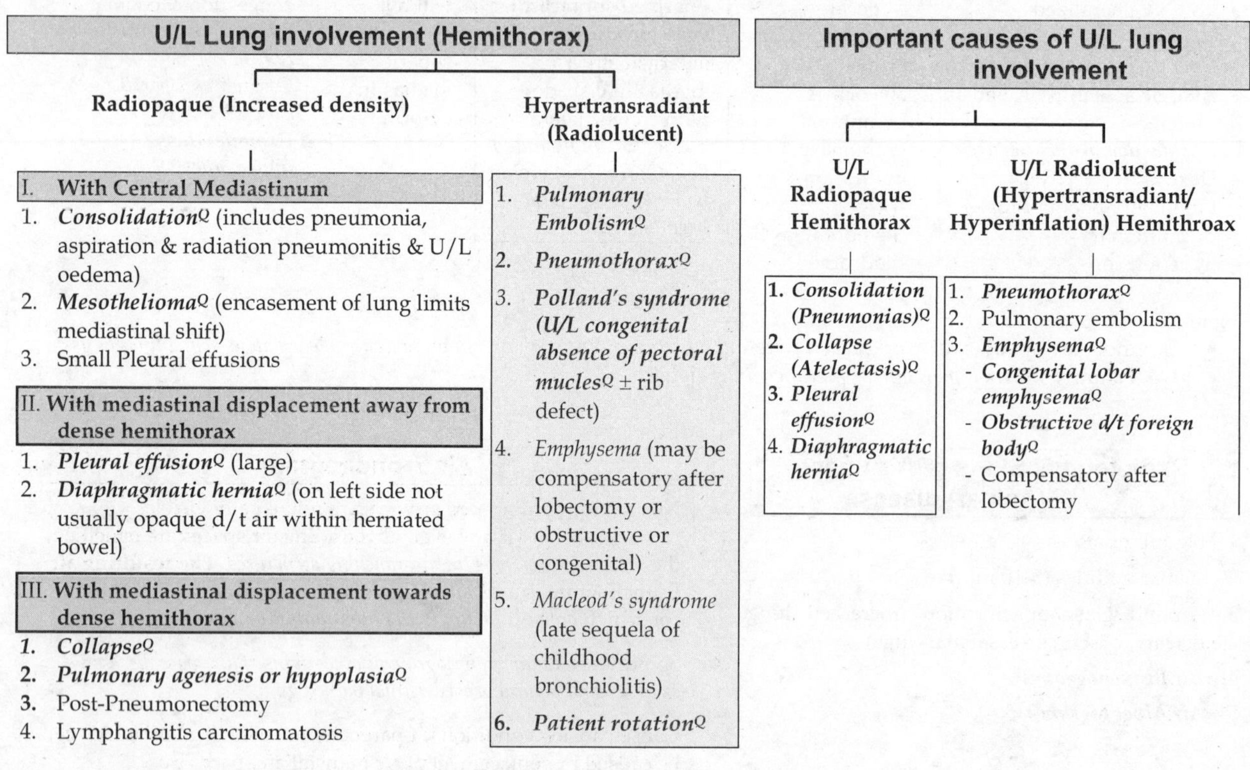

U/L Lung involvement (Hemithorax)
Radiopaque (Increased density)
Hypertransradiant (Radiolucent)
I. With Central Mediastinum
1. Consolidation[Q] (includes pneumonia, aspiration & radiation pneumonitis & U/L oedema)
2. Mesothelioma[Q] (encasement of lung limits mediastinal shift)
3. Small Pleural effusions
II. With mediastinal displacement away from dense hemithorax
1. Pleural effusion[Q] (large)
2. Diaphragmatic hernia[Q] (on left side not usually opaque d/t air within herniated bowel)
III. With mediastinal displacement towards dense hemithorax
1. Collapse[Q]
2. Pulmonary agenesis or hypoplasia[Q]
3. Post-Pneumonectomy
4. Lymphangitis carcinomatosis
1. Pulmonary Embolism[Q]
2. Pneumothorax[Q]
3. Polland's syndrome (U/L congenital absence of pectoral mucles[Q] ± rib defect)
4. Emphysema (may be compensatory after lobectomy or obstructive or congenital)
5. Macleod's syndrome (late sequela of childhood bronchiolitis)
6. Patient rotation[Q]
Important causes of U/L lung involvement
U/L Radiopaque Hemithorax
U/L Radiolucent (Hypertransradiant/ Hyperinflation) Hemithroax
1. Consolidation (Pneumonias)[Q]
2. Collapse (Atelectasis)[Q]
3. Pleural effusion[Q]
4. Diaphragmatic hernia[Q]
1. Pneumothorax[Q]
2. Pulmonary embolism
3. Emphysema[Q]
- Congenital lobar emphysema[Q]
- Obstructive d/t foreign body[Q]
- Compensatory after lobectomy

Foreign Body Inhalation

- *Foreign body* more commonly enters ***more vertically orientated right bronchus***[Q] leading to involvement of ***right lung***[Q]
- *Peanuts* are the most commonly inhaled foreign body.
- It is *most common cause of acute collapse* with peak age incidence in *1-2 years* of age. Symptoms are ***sudden onset***[Q] *of* ***wheezing***[Q]***, choking, & cough***[Q] ***with respiratory distress, stridor and decreased breath sounds on affected side***[Q]**.**
- Radiological findings of foreign body inhalation

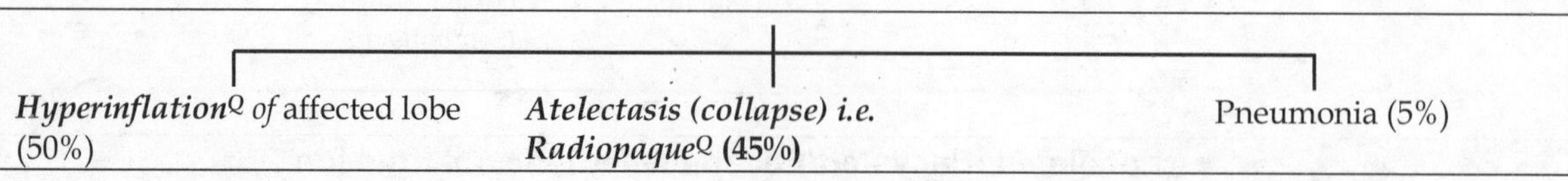

Pediatric Rspiratory Distress (Difficulty)

Multicystic Air Filled (Radioopaque) Intrathoracia (Chest) Lesions

Respiratory Distress with Contralateral Mediastinal Shift

Congenital Lobar Emphysema

- Due to dysplastic or deficient bronchial cartilage or/& bronchial compression d/t aberrant pulmonary artery l/t distal lobe go into emphysematous condition.
- Most commonly found in infants and presents with ***progressive respiratory distress + progressive cynosis within first 6 months of life***Q.
- Male: Female ratio is 3:1. Frequently associated with ***VSD, TOF, PDA***
- Immediately afer birth on CXR affected lobe is radiopaque which with in few days become hyperlucent d/t clearance of lung fluid, & over inflation of affected lobe
- Radiological
  - ***Left Upper lobe (40%>) Rt middle lobe(30%>) Rt upper lobe (20%) whole lung is not involved usually***Q) involvement. Hazy mass like opacity immediately after birth (d/t delayed clearance of lung fluid in affected lobe).
  - ***Air trapping and hyperlucent expanded lobe***Q (after clearing of fluid) which will later on cause compression collapse of adjacent lobe & opposite mediastinal shift.

Conginatal Cystic Adenostatoid Malformation (CCAM)

- *Rare*
- It is multicystic mass of pulmonary tissue; consisting of harartomatous proliferation of terminal bronchioles at expense of alveolar development; usually ***communicating with normal tracheobroncheal tree & receiving blood supply from narmal pulmonary artery & vein***Q. ***(difference from bronchopulmonary sequestration)***Q
- Slight predilection for *upper lobe* (whole lung is rarely involved)
- Associated with **Hydrops fetalis, maternal polyhydramnios**, & other congenital malformation.
- X Ray just after birth show –C/L mediastinal shift by radiopaque soft tissue mass. With progression fluid is absorbed and radiolucent areas representing air appear.

Congenital Diaphragmatic Hernia

- ***Commonest***Q
- ***70% are left sided***Q
- **Scaphoid *abdomen***Q due to migration of abdominal contents
- ***Malrotation & Malfixation of small bowel*** are associated problems
- Respiratory distress is most severe due to associated pulmonary hypoplasia, surfactant deficiency & persistent fetal circulation
- Immediate postnatal X Ray shows *radiopaque hemithorax* with C/L mediastinal shift. Once G.I. tract starts to fill with air *radioluciencies* appear & there will be progressive deviation of mediastinum.
- ***Absence of gas containing bowel in the abdomen***Q on X Ray
- *Intrathoracic multiple air filled loops usually* ***left sided*** *(70%) on X Ray*

Bochdalek Hernia Q	Morgagnian Hernia	Eventration of Diaphragm
• *Most common* diaphragmatic hernia in children • Through persistent posterior ***pleuro-peritoneal canal***Q • 75% ***left sided***Q • Presents with: - ***respiratory distress***Q - ***air filled loop in thorax***Q - ***scaphoid abdomen***Q - associated with dextro-cardiac & malrotation of bowel.	• *Rare* • *Anteriorly* placed hernia with the defect between sternal & costal attachments • of diaphragm • Mostly ***right sided***Q • Mostly asymptomatic, so may not be diagnosed until adulthood.	• An abnormally elevated position of one or both hemi diaphragm from paralysis or atrophy of the muscle fibers • ***Right sided***Q is more common • Most are minor, transitory, local diaphragmatic elevations, found incidently within the first few years of life & disappears with age • *Paradoxical respiration* is treated by plication of redundant diaphragm; to minimize paradoxical movements & mediastinal shift.

- All of the three conditions mentioned above may be cause of *loops of bowel in hemithorax on X-ray leading to mediastinal (heart shadow) shift* &
- Bochdalek hernia is mostly left sided (but not always).
- Morgagnian hernia & Eventration of diaphragm are mostly right sided (but not always).

No (Minimal) Respiratory Distress and No Mediastiral Shift

Oesophageol Duplication Cyst

- M. C. involve ***distal esophagus***Q, f/b cervical f/b mid esophagus
- Usually associated with ***vertebral anomalies***Q ***(spina bifida, hemivertebrae, fusion defects)***, esophageal atresia & small bowel duplication.
- CXR – Posterior mediastinal mass
  - ± Air fluid level
  - ***Thoracic vertebral anomalies***Q
  - Displacement of esophagus by paraesophageal mass

Bronchogenic (Lung) Cyst

- Mediastinal type is more common than intrapulmonary
- Carinal – mediastinal variety is mc.
- Usually ***do not communicate with tracheo bronchial tree***Q
- Mostly presents with symptoms of infection.
- ***M. C intrathoracic foregut*** *cyst*Q (from ventral segment), esophageal cyst is also foregut cyst (dorsal segment)
- Usually presents with symptoms of infection

Bronchopulmonary Sequestration

- Mass of aberrant non functioning pulmonary tissue that does ***not communicate with normal bronchial tree or pulmonary – arteries***Q
- Receives its blood supply from ***systemic circulation***Q
- Presents usually with recurrent infection & asymptomatic pulmonary mass at older age

Pneumatocele Formation

- Feature of childhood pneumonia mostly d/t ***staph aureus***Q
- May be seen in ***Pneumocystis carinii pneumonia (in AIDS)***
- Uncommon in neonates but may be seen with *E.Coli & H. influensae*
- Presents with C/F of Pneumonia

Pulmonary Thrombo-Embolism (PTE/PE)

Chest Xray

- ***Normal/Near-normal in dyspneic patient***[Q]
- Focal (localized peripheral) oligemia **(westermark sign)**
- Peripheral pleural based wedge shaped density above the diaphragm ***(Hampton's hump***[Q]*) d/t pulmonary infarct.*
- Enlarged right descending pulmonary artery **(Palla sign)**
- Long curvilinear densities reaching pleural surface (**Fleischner lines**)
- Pleural effusion on left > right (**Felson's sign**)
- Peripheral air space opacification, linear atelectasis, enlargement of central pulmonary arteries, consolidation & cavitation.

CECT (CT Pulmonary Angiography with IV Contrast)

- **Contrast enhanced CT pulmonary angiography (CT with intravenous contrast)** is the **principal imaging test for diagnosis of PE**[Q]**. It has virtually replaced invasive pulmonary angiography as the main stay investigation & a diagnostic test for PE**. Conventional pulmonary angiography, does however remains the **gold standard test.**
- **Spiral or helical chest CT scan with intravenous contrast (CT pulmonary angiography)** is the ***principal imaging test for the diagnosis of pulmonary embolsm***[Q]**.** It acquires image with < *1 m resolution* and visualizes *up to 6th order branches* and small peripheral emboli with a resolution *superior to conventional invasive contrast pulmonary angiography.* It obtains excellent images of right & left ventricle and can be used for diagnosis as well as *risk stratification.* In patients with pulmonary embolism, *RV enlargement indicates 5 times more likelihood of death within next 30 days.*
  Inadequate breath holding can impair the image quality b/o change in arterial flow rates and motion artefact during breathing. The advent of **multidetector CT** (*MDCT*) allows examination of whole lung during single breath –hold. It is noninvasive.

Lung (Ventilation- Perfusion =VP) Scan

- **Ventilation - perfusion lung scanning** is now ***second line diagnostic test***[Q] for PE, and mostly used in patients who *cannot tolerate intravenous contrast. Its utility is greatest when accompanied with a normal chest x-ray* implying that a ventilation – perfusion mismatch is not due to parenchymal disease. **High probability (>80%)** scan have ≥ 2 large segmental V-P mismatches (perfusion defects & normal ventilation) with a normal chest radiograph. And **very low probability scans** have <3 small perfusion defects with normal chest radiograph.
  Perfusion seen is done by injecting *microparticles (10 – 100μm) of Tc99 micro – aggregate albumin (MAA)* in patients lying supine. Ventilation scintigraphy is performed by inhaling Krypton – 81, (best), Xenon 133, Tc99 – diethylenetriamine penta acetic acid (DTPA), or technegas. Last two can't be administered during perfusion scan as both are labelled with Tc99. *Eight images* (anterior, posterior, obtique & lateral on both sides) are aquired.
- ***2nd most frequent used*** imaging investigation for suspected PTE is **V-P Scan**[Q]. It uses IV injection for Tc99 labelled albumin or inhalation of radioactive gas (Krypton-81, Xenon-133, Tc99 DTPA or Carbon particles known as Techegas) The cardinal sign is ***Mismatched Perfusion defect***[Q] (i.e. under perfused part of the lung on perfusion scan while the ventilation scan remains normal).

Pulmonary Angiography

- ***Most Specific test*** for establishing a diagnosis of pulmonary thromboembolism is ***pulmonary arteriogram***[Q]**.**
- **Conventional pulmonary angiography**: Non invasive CT with contrast have virtually replaced invasive pulmonary angiography as a diagnostic tool. However, it remains the ***gold standard test***[Q]**.**

Contrast Enhanced MRI

It is excellent for diagnosis of deep thrombosis (DVT) if USG is equivocal (MR venography), may detect large proximal PE but is **unreliable for smaller segmental PE.**

Diagnostic strategy in cases of suspected PTE

Chest X Ray / Quantitative Plasma-D-dimer-Elisa (reflects plasmin break down of fibrin & indicates endogenous thrombolysis, has ***high negative predictive value & can be used to exclude PTE***[Q])

High (> 500 mg/mL)

Chest CT with intravenous contrast (non invasive & **investigation of choice)**

Lung Ventilation Perfusion Scan (noninvasive, after CXR, a **V-P Scan is the 2nd *most commonly requested***[Q] imaging investigation for a suspected case of PTE)

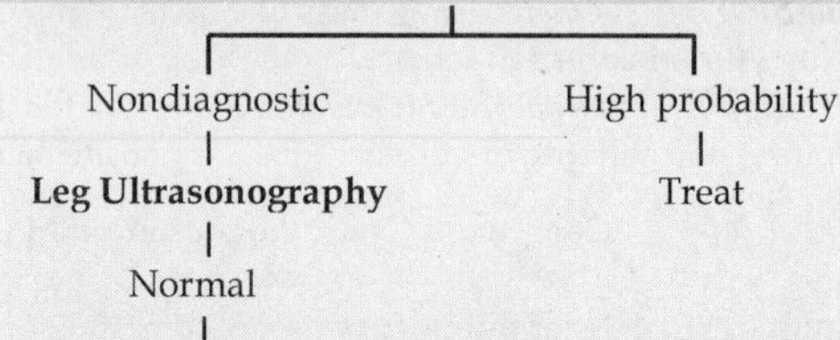

Pulmonary Arteriography[Q] *(**most definitive diagnostic method***[Q] but invasive & costly so done when dx can't be confirmed by other methods)

Advantages & Disadvantages

Dx Test	Advantages	Disadvantages
Plasm D-dimer ELISA	Normal results make PE highly unlikely	Level is elevated in various systemic illnesses
Lung (V-P) Scanning	***Standard initial imaging test for PE***[Q]**.** High probability scans are reliable for detecting PE normal/near normal scans are reliable for precluding PE	Most scans are neither high probability nor normal/near normal; most are equivocal
Pulmonary angiography	***Gold standard for diagnosis***[Q]	*Invasive, Costly & Uncomfortable* ; so not a first line investigation
CT angiography (helical)	- Noninvasive, widely available test that has replaced ***pulmonary angiography (conventional) as the main stay investigation for PE***[Q]. - Stratifies risk, obtains images of RV & LV	- Initially it was a sensitive method of detecting *central segmental, lobar & main pulmonary artery emboli upto 4th order vessel (~ 7mm* diameter) i.e., from aortic arch to inferior pulmonary vein. However, with advent of helical & multidetector CT (MDCT) has improved resolution of *peripheral arteries upto 6th order.*

Egg shell calcification of lymphnodes

Silly	-	***Silicosis (m.c.)***[Q]
Cool	-	Coal workers pneumoconiosis
Sardar	-	***Sarcoidosis***[Q]
Loves	-	***Lymphoma after radiotherapy***[Q]
His	-	Histoplasmosis
Progressive	-	Progressive massive fibrosis
Tubercular	-	***Tuberculosis***[Q]
Cox	-	Coccidiodomycosis

Approach to Respiratory involvement in AIDS

Pneumocystis carinii/ Jiroveci Pneumonia (PCP)

- It is a ***protozoa***[Q], previously thought to be fungi
- ***M.C. opportunistic infection in AIDS***[Q]
- C/P- ***Dry non productive cough***[Q], ***dyspnea***[Q], ***fever***[Q] with tachypnea, tachycardia & cynosis and few ausculatory findings.
- Radiological – Classical finding is ***B/L diffuse infiltrates beginning in the perihilar region***[Q], mid & lower zone (ground glass infiltrate).
  - Cavities & Pneumothorax are well recognized complications.
  - Less common complications are mediastinal lymphadenopathy: pleural effusion, miliary disease & discrete pulmonary nodules.
  - In patients receiving ***pentamidine aerosol,*** there is ***increased frequency of upper lobe infiltrates & pneumothorax***[Q]

Kaposi Sarcoma

- ***M.C. AIDS associated maligancy***[Q]
- Pulmonary involvement is mostly associated with ***cutaneous & visceral involvement.***
- Radiological
  - B/L pulmonary perihilar infiltrates associated with *thickening of interlobular septa & nodularity of fissure*
  - ***Pleural / Pericardial effusion & mediastinal lymphadenopathy are common features.***[Q]

Tuberculosis

- Early stage: appears similar to reactivation of TB with typical pattern of upper lobe infiltrates & cavitation
- Late stages: similar to primary T.B. like pattern with diffuse interstitial or miliary infiltrates, no/little cavitation and prominent ***intrathoracic lymphadenopathy***[Q].
- **TB infection in HIV** patients present with **productive cough, cavitatory apical disease** of upper lobes (high CD4 count), disseminated disesase, diffuse or lower lobe bilateral reticulonodular infiltrates consistent with **miliary spread, pleural effusions, hilar &/or mediastinal lymphadenopathy with extrapulmonary** (bone, brain, meninges, GI tract, lymph nodes esp cervical, genitourinary) involvement.

Lymphocytic Interstitial Pneumonitis

- Radiologically presents as mid or lower zone reticular or reticulonodular infiltrate
- Distinguished from opportunistic infection by *slow progression of radiological change & neither pleural nor lymph node enlargement.*

CMV

- Very rare cause of pneumonia in AIDS
- ***M.C. cause of pneumonia in renal transplant patients***[Q]
- ***M.C. cause of chorioretinitis in AIDS***[Q].

Tree in Bud appearance

Tree in bud appearance (or gloved finger appearance) is depiction of normally invisible branching course of intralobular bronchiole on HRCT. It indicates the *endobronchial spread* of disease l/t bronchiolar luminal impaction with mucus, pus or fluid, bronchiolar wall thickening, peribronchiolar inflammation and dilatation of distal bronchioles. On HRCT, it appears as **peripheral** (within 5mm of pleural surface) *small (2-4mm) centrilobular well defined nodules connected to linear branching opacities with more than one contiguous branching sites.* It is seen in-

- **Infections (most common)**
  1. ***Bacterial (most common): Mycobacterium tuberculosis (mc)***[Q], M.avium intracellular complex (Lady Windermere syndrome), Staph.aureus, H.influenzae
  2. Viral : ***CMV, Respiratory***
- **Idiopathic**
  1. Bronchiolitis obliterans (obliterative/ constrictive-bronchiolitis)
  2. Diffuse panbronchiolitis
- **Immunological disorder**
  1. Allergic bronchio-

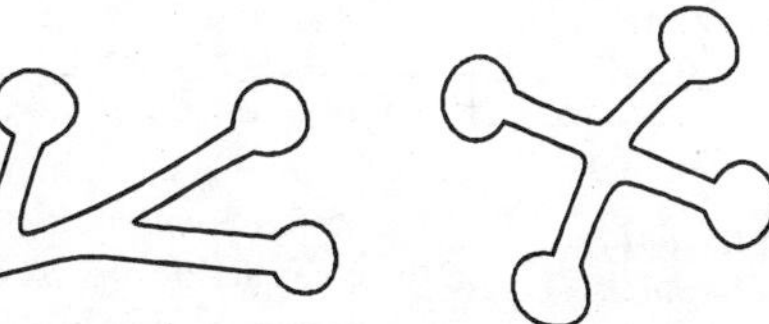
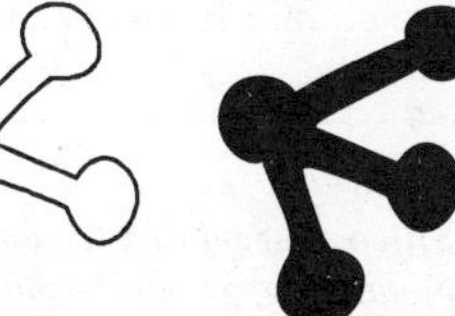

Tree in bud appearance

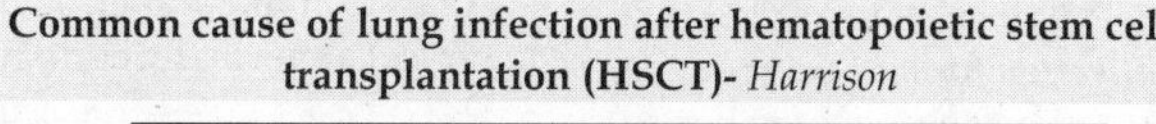

Common cause of lung infection after hematopoietic stem cell transplantation (HSCT)- *Harrison*

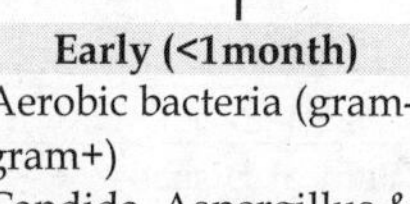

Early (<1month)	Middle (1-4 months)	Late (>6 Months)
Aerobic bacteria (gram-, gram+) Candida, Aspergillus & other molds HSV (rare cause of pneumonia reported almost exclusively in allogenic HSC transplant recepient patients)	CMV, Seasonal respiratory virus (**RSV** & para influenza viruses) Pneumocystis Toxoplasma	Pneumocystis S.pneumoniae

M.tuberculosis has been an uncommon cause of pneumonia among HSC transplant recipients in western countries (<0.1-0.2%) but is common (5.5%) in counties where prevelance of TB is high *(Harrison -1125).*

*syncytial virus (RSV)*Q
3. Fungal : ***Invasive aspergillosis, pneumocystis jiroveci (sometimes)***Q

- **Congenital**

1. Cystic fibrosis
2. Kartagener syndrome (dyskinetic cilia syndrome)
3. Yellow nail syndrome

pulmonary aspergillosis
2. Congenital immune-deficiencies

- **Connective tissue disorder**

1. Rheumatoid arthritis
2. Sjogren syndrome

- **Neoplasm**

1. Primary pulmonary lymphoma
2. Laryngotracheal papillomatosis

Tumor emboli (of gastric, breast, renal & Ewing's cancer)

Inhalation of toxic fumes and Aspiration pneumonitis

Common respiratory viruses include *rhinovirus, corona virus, RSV, Meta pneumoviruses, parainfluenza* viruses, adenoviruses, influenza (A, B) virus, HSV, enterovirus.

Human-RSV can cause severe lower respiratory tract disease with pneumonitis in elderly (often institutionalized) and in patients with immuno compromized disorders or treatment including **HSCT and solid organ transplant recipients** HRSV occurs in 18% HSCT patients.

Lung Complications

Not specific to HSCT

These infections tend to occur b/o TBI/ *chemotherapy associated neutropenia in early phase post HSCT* and include.

- Bacterial pneumonia (gram + staph.aureus >gram-ve)
- Pneumocystis jiroveci (carinni) pneumonia (classic bilateral perihilar or diffuse symmetric interstitial pattern which may be *finely granular, reticular or ground glass appearance*; occasionally *crazy paving appearance*; and sometimes *tree in but appearance*)
- Fungal infections (Aspergillus, Candida, Mucor, Cryptococcus): Invasive aspergillosis may be angioinvasive (more common) and airway invasive. Angioinvasive aspergillosis presents with *halo sign* (early sign representing necrotic center & rim of hemorrhagic infarction) and *hypodense & air crescent sign* (late sign indicating recovery & good prognosis). Airway invasive aspergillosis may cause tree in bud appearance.
- **Tuberculosis**

Specific to HSCT

An immunosuppressive state continues for about 1 year after allogenic HSCT; which can be divided into early (upto 100 days) and late phase. Neutropenic phase lasts upto 10-12 days with peripheral stem cells and upto 3 weeks with bone marrow. These include

- ***CMV pneumonia (most common)***Q
- Idiopathic pneumonia syndrome
- Bronchiolitis obliterans

Radiological Approach to Industrial Lung Disease

Predilection for Mid & Upper ZoneQ

(Whole lung may be involved with predominant mid & upper zone involvement)

I. Silicosis:

- **D/t *Silica dust related to coal & gold*Q *minning; granite, sandstone, slate*Q** quarrying; foundry, ceramic & pottery work.
- *Multiple, well defined, uniform in density, 2-5 mm nodular shadow* ***with a predilection for mid & upper zone*** *and* posterior aspect of lung but ***relatively sparing the bases***Q.
- Linear shadows & septal also appear
- *B/L hilar* ***lymphadenopahty***Q, nodes may calcify diffusely or in ***egg shell (peripheral) pattern***Q.

II. Coal workers PneumoconiosisQ:

- *D/t coal dust mainly* ***carbon***Q
- *Small indistinct, faint nodules of 1-5 mm appear in* ***mid zone***Q. Eventually involve whole lung.
- The development of Progressive massive fibrosis (PMF) is marked by

Predilection for Lower ZoneQ

(Whole lung may be involved with predominant lower zone involvement)

Asbestosis Related Lung Disease:

- Asbestos is the generic term used for *heat resistant fibrous silicates.* They are classified into 2 groups. 1) Straight, rigid, needle like ***Amphiboles*** (*eg commercial crocidolite* = blue/black asbestos & *amosite* = brown asbestos; and non- commercial contaminating amphiboles such as **actinolite, tremolite & anthophyllite**); 2) **Serpentines (nonamphiboles)** such as commercial **chrysolite = white asbestos.**
- **Aspect (length-to-diameter) ratio** decides carcinogenicity. *Amosite & crocidolite are* relatively malignant, whereas *anthophyllite, chrysotile and tremolite* are benign.
- Apart from **pleural effusion**, which may be present as early as **5 years** post exposure, the **typical abnormalities** do not appear **until 20 years** or more after initial exposure.
- D/t *asbestos, exposure may occur in* ***asbestos industry, ship building & textile manufacture industry***Q.

Pleural Disease

Pleural Effusion

- **Benign pleural effusion** are often *small (<500ml)*, sterile, serous or *typically hemorrhagic, may be persistent or recurrent and may be simultaneously or sequentially bilateral*
- **Small, hemorrhagic recurrent bilateral** exudates of mixed cellularity and usually donot contain asbestos bodies. Therefore, the diagnosis is

Parenchymal Disease

Asbestosis

- **Asbestosis** is *chronic progressive diffuse pulmonary parenchymal (interstitial) fibrosis* (i.e. term used for lung not pleural disease). It (interstitial fibrosis) **begins around respiratory bronchioles,** particularly in the **lower posterior lobes adjacent to visceral pleura.** With advancing disease, the fibrosis extend into the *adjacent alveolar septa of adjacent alveoli*, eventually involving the coalescence of small nodules or appearance of large opacities of 1cm mainly in mid & upper zone, bilaterally. It tends to migrate towards hila creating peripheral areas of emphysema & bullae. Fibrotic mass may calcify or cavitate.

- ***PMF & caplan's syndrome (in Rheumatoid arthritis)***[Q] is more common in coal workers Pneumoconiosis in comparison to silicosis.

Wide spread throughout lung

I. Siderosis:

- D/t *Iron oxide dust.*
- B/L widespread reticulo nodular shadows

II. Stannosis:

- D/t *tinoxide*
- Multiple very small, very dense (denser than calcium d/t high atomic no. of tin) discrete opacities of 0.5 – 1mm distributed through out lung
- Dense septal line

III. Barytosis:

- D/t *$BaSO_4$ dust*
- Very dense nodules through out lung.

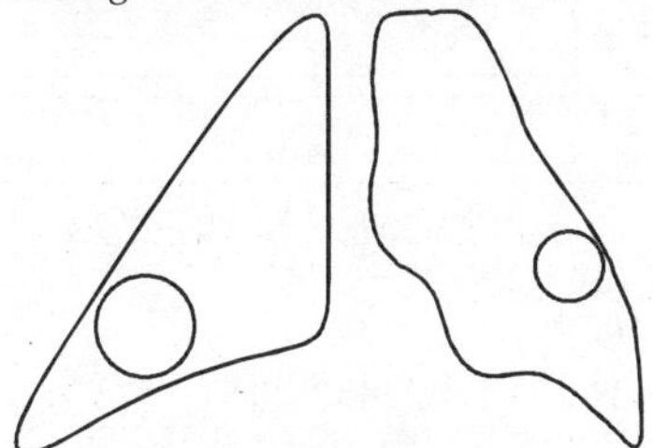

B/L Pleural thickening, plaque, calcification in peripheral, lower & posterior lobes: Asbestos related

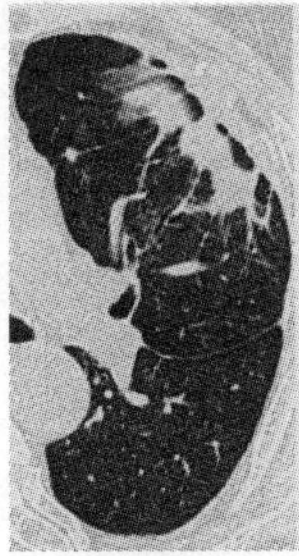

Comet Tail Sign

based largely on exclusion of other causes of effusion. Large effusion raises possibility of underlying CA or Mesothelioma

Pleural Plaques

- **Pleural plaques is most common** manifestation of asbestos exposure, which grossly are discrete foci of pearly white fibrous tissue, usually 2-5 mm thick. On histology, the plaques are relatively acellular, (hypocellular) with undulating collagen bundles arranged in **basket- weave appearance.** *Asbestos fibers (mostly chrysolite) are often seen but asbestos bodies are usually absent.*
- ***Pleural plaques almost exclusively involves parietal pleura***[Q] (visceral pleura typically spared) and are classically distributed along the **posterolateral chest wall between 7th and 10th ribs,** *lateral chest wall between 6th & 9th ribs & dome of diaphragm & mediastinal pleura.*
- Pleural plaques are usually **bilateral, multifocal plaques in mid & lower zones over diaphragm** with edges thicker than central portion. They typically **spare apices & costophrenic angles and viceral pleura.**
- Pleural plaques are *specific* to asbestos exposure and *cause no functional impairment* (i.e. are asympotmatic), *no hilar adenopathy* and mostly (90%) are *not calcified.*

Pleural Calcification

- **Pleural calcification** is **hallmark** of asbestos exposure. It may be seen as dense lines paralleling the chest wall, mediastinum, pericardium, diaphragm. **Bilateral diaphragmatic calcifications with clear costophrenic angles are pathognomic** and advanced calcifications are *leaf like with thick rolled edges.*

Diffuse Pleural Thickening

- **Diffuse pleaural thickening** (which is *not specific*) is differentiated by presence of **fusion of parietal & visceral pleura with subsequent impairment in lung function** *eg reduced FVC & gas transfer DLco.* By contrast pleural plaques involve parietal pleura only.

entire lobule and in most severe cases may l/t parenchymal remodelling & honey combng.

- **Asbestos bodies** are almost always identifiable microscopically in *fibrous tissue or macrophages (bronchoalveolar lavage fluid).*
- On plain radiography the ***earliest sign is fine reticular or nodular pattern in lower zone***[Q]. With progression, this *becomes coarse &* ***causes loss of clarity of diaphragm & cardiac shadow, so called shaggy heart***[Q].
- HRCT (in prone position to negate gravity related phenomenon) shows **subpleural pulmonary arcades** (i.e. *multiple subpleural curvilinear branching lines & dot* like reticulo nodularities), *pleural based nodular irregularities, parenchymal bands and septal lines* (of thickened, fibrotic inter lobular septa). The fine reticulation eventually progress to a coarse linear pattern with honey combing. The abnormalities are most severe in subpleural lower (posterior) lobes.

Atelectatic Asbestos Pseudotumor

- **Round atlectasis (folded lung)** is benign mass produced d/t infolding of redudant pleura accompanied by segmental/subsegmental parenchyma. It occurs most commonly in **peripheral lungs in the dorsal region of lower lobes** (i.e. *postero-media/postero-lateral basal region of lower lobes*) and is frequently *bilateral.*
- *Mostly round/lentiform= lens shaped/wedge shaped peripheral mass, always seen adjacent to the visceral pleura;* appearance suggest that retraction of collagen in pleura is the cause of collapse. It shows a relatively **stable appearance** i.e. shows little progression and occasionally decrease in size (difference from true tumor).
- **Comet tail or vaccum cleaner sign** is presence of crowded bronchi & blood vessels that extend from the border of collapsed lung mass to the hilum like tails of comet.
- **Crow's feet sign** is presence of linear bands radiating (emanating) from collapsed lung mass into lung parenchyma.
- **Swiss cheese air bronchogram**, volume loss of affected lobe (always) with hyperlucency of adjacent lung (±) are other features.

Asbestos related Malignancy

- **Lung cancer** (broncho-alveolar carcinoma = adeno + squamous), **Malignant Mesothelioma and gastrointestinal cancer** increase in asbestos exposure.

Heart Borders on Chest X-ray PA-view/Radiographic Anatomy of Heart

Right Heart Border (Formed by)

a. *Superior vena cava (SVC)*Q
b. Right lateral aspect of **ascending thoracic arota** (in old age especially d/t tendency of aorta to dilate and elongate) and ***right brochio cephalic vein***Q sometimes)
c. *Right atrium (RA)*Q
d. *Inferior vena cava (IVC)*Q

Left Heart Border (Formed by)

f/e. **Aortic Knuckle** or **knob** (i.e. posterior part of transverse **aortic arch**) ± left **subclavian vein** (its shadow is above aortic knuckle)
g. ***Pulmonary conus (trunk of main pulmonary artery)*** Q
h. **Left ventricle** (LV, lowest and largest segment and also forms inferior or diaphragmatic border)
i. *Left atrial appendage*Q

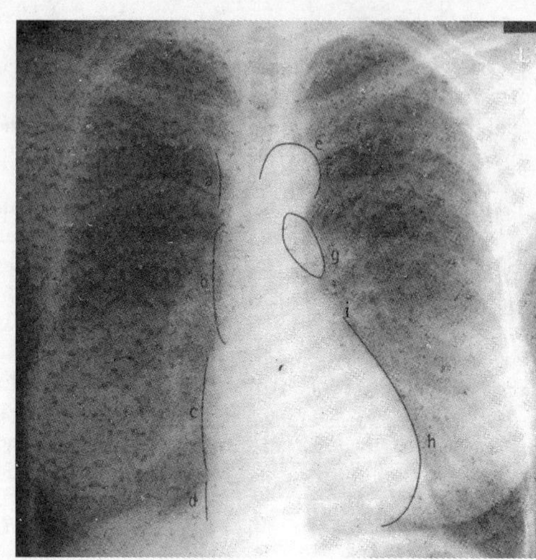

Cardiothoracic Ratio (CTR)

$$\text{CTR} = \frac{\text{Maximum transverse diameter of heart (right heart border to midline + left heart border to midline)}}{\text{Maximum width of thorax above costopheric angles, measured from the inner edge of ribs}}$$

CTR is maximally **0.5**; however, is usually greater in children.

Right heart border is formed by

Right Atrium (not right ventricle)Q
Superior Venacava (SVC)Q
Inferior Venacava (IVC) Q
Sometimes ***ascending thoracic arch of aorta, right innominate vessels or right brachiocephalic vein***Q

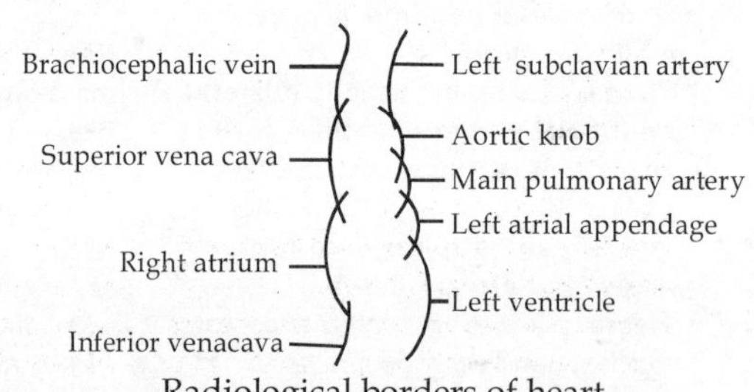

Radiological borders of heart

Left heart (mediastinal) border is formed by

- *Aortic knuckle (arch/knob)*
- ***Pulmonary trunk of left pulmonary artery/main pulmonary artery***Q.
- ***Left atrial appendage***Q
- *Left ventricle (outer border)*

Radiological Feature of

Left Atrial Enlargement

- *LA does not form any part of cardiac* border in normal subjects (on PA view) because it lies in midline & posteriorly. It usually, enlarges postriorly & to the right causing **indentation & displacement of oesophagus posteriorly** (on barium swallow) .
- ***Elevation of left main bronchus***Q is the **earliest *evidence (feature) of left atrial enlargment***Q. Subequently there is **splaying of carina (i.e. carinal angle widens** and become *right or obtused angled* as compared to normal 51-71 degree).
- The right border of an enlarged left atrium is visible as **double contour (shadow/density)** adjacent to the right heart border usually within the main cardiac shadow.
- ***Double right heart border** is formed* d/t bulging of left atrium into right lung & eventually forming right heart border. The borders of left & right atria are differentiated by the fact that left atrial border passes medially towards spine & border of right atrium is limited below by entry of IVC (inf. venacava). With massive enlargment LA can form the most part of right cardiac border
- Left border of LA is rarely visible, although **left atrial appendage**, when dilated, is seen as a bulge below the main pulmonary artery.
- On lateral view postero-superior part of cardiac shadow becomes prominent.

Right Atrium Enlargement

- In early stage, only RA appendage fills the space b/w front of heat & back of sternum (prominent anterosuperior part on lateral view).
- It causes an *increase in the curvature of right heart border, which becomes more convex, prominent and also protudes to the right* away from midline (>3cm beyond right lateral vertebral border). It is often accompanied by *enlargment of superior venacava* and **increase in RA height** (most reliable sign). In normal individuals, the distance b/w top of aortic arch and the junction of SVC & RA is more than the distance between the later & right cardiophrenic angle. When the reverse happens (i.e. SVC/RA to RCPA distance >AA to SVC/RA distance), the RA is said to be enlarged.

Left Ventricle Enlargment

- On PA view, there is *prominent left heart border with rounding*. Hypertrophy produces *rounding of cardiac apex* whereas dilatation causes elongation/displacement of cardiac apex to the left or to the left & downwards
- Lateral view shows prominent *postero-inferior* part of cardiac shadow

Right Ventricle Enlargement

- RV enlarges mainly to the left & anteriorly, so there is *prominence of left heart border on PA* view and prominence of *anterior part of cardiac shadow with encroachment of retrosternal space* in upper part on lateral view.
- **Pulmonary conus (outflow tract) becomes prominent.**
- It may form left cardiac border and can rotate LV to the left with **elevation of cardiac apex**. This rotation tends to swing the aorta to right, so that **aortic knukle becomes less prominent**.

Oesophageal markings on Barium column (Filled oesophagus)

Normal impressions

- **Aortic arch & left main bronchus** on *left antero lateral aspect* of thoracic oesophagus, best seen in *right anterior oblique view*
- Occasionally the **confluene of pulmonary veins**, as they enter the back of left atrium, produce an extrinsic impression on the **front of oesophagus**

Abnormal impressions

Right sided aortic arch & descending aorta

Oesophagus is **indented on its right by aortic knuckle** & usual left aortic arch impression is absent.

Coarctation of aorta

Reversed-'3' impression on left side of oesophagus by prestenotic & poststenotic dilatations

Aneurysms of aortic arch & descending aorta

- Localized displacement of oesophagus
- As aorta becomes atheromatous & assumes tortous course, it *displaces lower end of oesophagus anteriorly & to the side*
- *Transient intermittent obstruction* & transmitted pulsations (on fluroscopy)
- Distal oesophagus is *narrowed in one plane; & obstruction in erect & supine positions may be relieved by turning the patient prone.*

Aberrant right subclavian artery

Characteristic smooth, oblique indentation on posterior wall[Q]

Left atrium/ ventricle enlargement

- Anterior impression on lower oesophagus which is displaced posteriorly & to the right
- Enlargement of left ventricle produces a similar indentation to that of left atrium but at a lower level.

Others

- Enlargement of thyroid gland displaces & narrows the upper oesophagus & trachea
- Large parathyroid may indent lateral margin of oesophagus
- Mediastinum shift from whatever cause, displaces the oesophagus, so apical lung fibrosis will draw the mediastinum with the oesophagus to that side
- *Displacement of middle third of oesophagus is most often caused by mediastinal lymphadenopathy. Although usually indenting the anterior margin* of the mid oesophagus, disease extension may produce a *stricture* resembling a primary carcinoma.

Thymic Tumors

Normal Thymus Gland

- It is the *commonest cause of mediastinal abnormality in infants* and is usually seen as *triangular soft tissue mass projecting to one side* (usually right) of mediastinum.
- It may ***disappear during severe neonatal infections, or after major surgery corticosteroid treatment***[Q], but may reappear following recovery from illness.
- Thymus gland is completely absent in *Di-George's syndrome*, an immune deficiency disease involving T lymphocyes.
- It is seen as *a triangular arrow head or bilobed structure* in children and young adult patients on CT but undergoes fatty involution in adults & elderly.
- Enlargement of thymus gland can be d/t *thymoma, thymic hyperplasia, thymic carcinoma, lymphoma, thymo lipoma, carcinoids & germ cell tumors & thymic cysts.*

Thymic Hyperplasia

- Although uncommn & rare, it is the most common anterior mediastinal mass in paeditric age group.
- The most common association of thymic hyperplasia is **mysthenia gravis** (65%) and **thyrotoxicosis** (eg *Grave's disease*, treatment of hypothyroidism etc. Other associations include *Addison's disease, acromegaly, SLE, RA*, and after **stress atrophy,** where the thymus gland initially atrophies in patients on chemotherapy, or corticosteroid treament, irradiation, stress, severe illness (burns) or after treatment for Cushing's disorder and then becomes larger than its previous normal size (i.e. enlarges) once the treatment is stopped or stress is ended. The phenomenon is called **rebound thymic hyperplasia**. It is

Thymoma

- It is the ***most common tumor of thymus in adults and most common primary tumor of anterior mdidastinum in adults***[Q].
- Most (90%) thymomas arise in *upper anterior mediastinum* usually anterior to ascending aorta, lying on the right ventricle outflow tract and pulmonary artery.
- It is rare under 20, extremely unusual below 15 and usually presents at *50 year age* (earlier in those who present with mysthenia gravis)
- Thymoma is often asymptomatic 50% but can also present with **mysthenia; red cell aplasia, hypogammaglobulinemia**. About 10-25% mysthenics have thymoma and 25-50% of thymoma patients have mysthenia gravis.
- It may cause ***mediastinal widening***[Q] and displacement of heart and great vessels posteriorly (but not trachea)- in benign cases; and *can invade mediastinal fat & pleura* in invasive malignant variety.
- It may be undetectable on chest x-ray when small, indicating the need of **CT** (which is **investigation of choice & most sensitive**).
- Thymomas give rise to *asymmetrical focal swelling* which appear as well defined round or oval soft tissue mass projecting to one side of anterior mediastinum. It may contain punctate or curvilinear calcification and areas of low attenuation d/t cystic degenration. MRI is also useful for diagnosis.

differentiated from recurrent malignant disease on the basis of a *known reason for rebound and presence of normal shaped enlarged thymus*

- Rarely cause visible enlargement, but when it does, both lobes are enlarged, *usually uniformly with a diffuse symmetrical enlargment.* Radiological signs include.

1. **Wave sign** is a rippled thymic contour (border) d/t indentation by *anterior rib ends.*
2. **Notch sign** is indentation at the junction of thymus with *heart.*
3. **Sail sign** is a *triangular density projection* from superior mediastinum on one or both sides.
4. Shape change with respiration & position

Thymic Carcinoid

- It presents with *cushing's syndrome (d/t ACTH serection), hyperparathyroidism and inappropriate ADH secretion.*
- Radiographic & CT features resemble thymoma

Thymolipoma

- Can grow to a very large size before discovery and,being soft, mould themselves to the adjacent mediastinum and diaphragm, mimicing cardiomegaly or lobar collapse.
- Very large soft tissue mass with less radiographic density than expected for its size, which alters it shape on respiration indicates thymolipoma

5

RADIODIAGNOSIS

Causes of Expansile (Focal) Rib lesion

Neoplastic

Metastases (Secondary Malignant)

- From bronchus, kidney, prostate or breast
- ***Leukemia/lymhoma***Q
- ***Ewing's sarcoma (most common malignant tumor affecting ribs of children & adult)***Q, **Neuroblastoma** in children
- **Desmoid tumor, Osteosrcoma** (rare)

Primary Malignant

- **Multiple myeloma/Plasmacytoma** (common)
- **Chondrosrcoma** (calcified matrix; mc)
- **Askin tumor (PNET)** uncommon tumor of intercostal nerves
- Lymphoma, fibrosarcoma, ***osteosarcoma (rare)***Q

Primary Benign Tumor

- Fibrous dysplasia (most common; predomnantly posterior location)
- Osteochondroma (exostosis), Enchondroma (both at costo chondral/costovertebral junction)
- Eosinophilic granuloma (LCH), Xanthogranuloma
- Giant cell tumor, Aneurysmal bone cyst
- Osteoid osteoma, Osteoblastoma, Chondroblastoma
- Benign cortical defect, Hemangioma, Enostosis (bone island, lipoma, **chondroma, neurofibroma**)

Nonneoplastic

- Fibrous dysplasia, **Paget's disease**
- ***Brown's tumor of hyper parathyroidism***Q
- Osteomyelitis (tubercular, fungal, **actinomyces infection**)
- *Gaucher's disease, Hurler's syndrome* (generalized expansion sparing proximal ends), **Thalassemia** (trabecular pattern & expansion most marked proximally)

Mediastinal tumor

Anterior M

From sternum anteriorly to pericardium & brachiocephalic vessels posteriorly. It contains the **thymus gland**, anterior medinstinal lymphnodes and internal mammary arteries & veins

- ***Thymoma (m.c.)***Q
- ***Teratoma*** Q
- Ectopic thyroid
- **Lymphoma/Leukemia** (nodal) **mc** a/t Grainger.

Middle M.

Between ant & post mediastinum. It contains heart, ascending & *transverse arches of aorta, venacava, brachiocephalic arteries & veins,* ***phrenic nerve,*** trachea, main bronchi and their contiguous lymph nodes and *pulmonary artery & veins.*

- ***Congenital cyst***Q (pleuropericardial, & bronchogenic) – 2nd ***most common***Q
- **Vascular masses (most common)**
- Lymph node enlargement (from metastasis or granulomatous ds.)

Posterior M.

From pericardium & trachea to vertebral column. It contains descending thoracic aorta, esophagus, thoracic duct, azygous/hemizygous veins, posterior mediastinal lymph node & neurogenic structures

- ***Neurogenic tumor (m.c.)***Q
- Meningoceles / meningomyeloceles
- Esophageal diverticula
- Gastroenteric cyst

M. C. mediastinal mass (over all) = ***Thymoma***Q

CT scan is the imaging modality of choice for mediastinal masses.

Definite diagnosis can be obtained by percutaneous FNA biopsy or endoscopic trans-oesophageal or endobronchial ultrasound guided biopsy (preferred), video assisted thoracoscopy, mediatinoscopy and mediastinotomy.

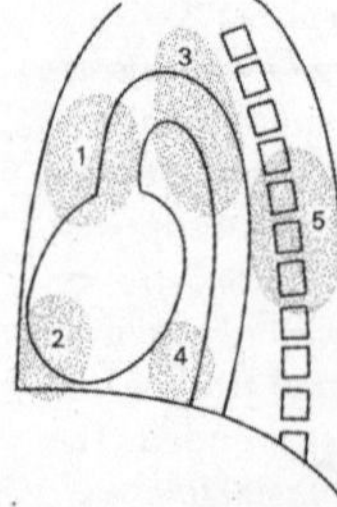

ANTERIOR
1. Thyroid tumour
Thymic tumour or cyst
Teratoma/Dermoid cyst
Lymphadenopathy
Aortic aneurysm
2. Pericardial cyst
Fat pad
Morgagni hernia

MIDDLE
3. Thyroid tumour
Lymphadenopathy
Bronchogenic cyst
Aortic aneurysm
4. Hiatus hernia

POSTERIOR
5. Neurogenic tumours
Soft tissue mass of v infection or neoplas
Lymphadenopathy
Aortic aneurysm

Atrial Septal Defect (ASD)

- In **atrial septal defect (ASD)**, there is a defect between both atrium leading to **left to right (L→R) shunt** from *left atrium to right atrium, to right ventricle* (RV), *pulmonary artery (PA) and then pulmonary circulation.* Increased blood flow through pulmonary circulation causes **hilar dance** (increased pulsations of central pulmonary artery), ***pulmonary plethora***Q, increased size of pulmonary veins & anteries with size larger than accompanying bronchus (**kissing cousin sign**), dimeter of right descending pulmonary artery > trachea just above aortic knob, enlarged hilar vessels and visualization of vessels below 10th posterior rib (all indicating prominent pulmonary vasculature d/t over circulation).
- **ASD** may show ***cardiomegaly, normal sized left atrium & left ventricle and enlarged right atrium, right ventricle and main pulmonary artery***Q. Due to RV hypertrophy, there is *clockwise rotation of heart l/t loss of visualization of superior venacava (SVC)* and small appearing aorta with normal aortic knob.
- *Pulmonary pressure remains normal for decades* and usually after 40 years of age onset of pulmonary hypertension causes increased R→L shunting **(Eisenmenger syndrome)**.

Heart	RA	RV	Main PA	Pulmonary vessels & blood flow	LA	LV	Aorta	PAH
↑	↑	↑	↑	↑	Normal	N	↓/N	No/ Late

Ventricular Septal Defect (VSD)

- In VSD, there is a defect between both ventricles leading to L→R shunt from left ventricle (LV) to right ventricle (RV) to pulmonary artery (PA) → pulmonary vein → left atrium (LA) →LV. So all these chambers enlarge with pulmonary vessels being affected last
- In nonrestrictive large shunts (>75% of aortic diameter) pulmonary artery hypertension & Eisenmenger syndrome develops early. *Calcification of PA is pathognomic of PAH.*

Heart	LV	RV	PA (main)	Pulmonary vessels & blood flow	LA	LV	RA	Aorta (thoracic)	PAH
↑	↑	↑	↑	↑	↑	↑	N	↓/N	Early

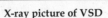

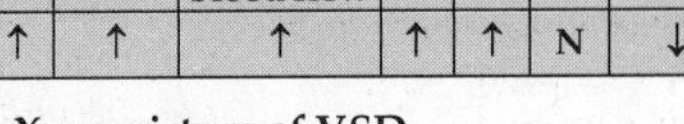

X-ray picture of VSD

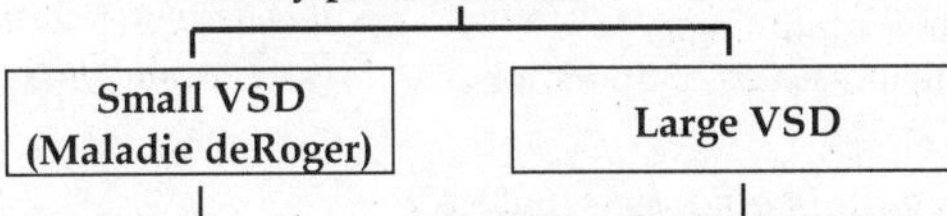

Small VSD (Maladie deRoger)
- Normal/Asymptomatic
- No/Minimal cardiomegaly
- No/Minimal increase in pulmonary vasculature

Large VSD
- Gross cardiomegaly
- **Dilation** of
  - ***Both ventricles (RV & LV)***Q
  - ***Left atrium (LA)***Q
  - ***Pulmonary artery (PA)***Q
- Increased pulmonary vascular marking, (PA & PV) pulmonary edema & pleural effusion.

★ In **PDA**, RA & RV are normal; LA, LV, PA and often/proxomal aorta are enlarged (↑).

Pulmonary Blood Flow (PBF)

Increased (Plethoric lungs d/t over circulation)

With left atrial (LA) enlargement

Indicates shunt distal to mitral valve=increased volume without escape defect
- *VSD*Q (small aorta in intracardiac shunt)
- **PDA** (aorta & pulmonary artery of equal size in extra cardiac shunt)
- *Ruptured sinus of Valsalva aneurysm*
- *Coronary arterio-venous fistula*
- Aortopulmonary window

Without LA enlargement

Indicates shunt proximal to mitral valve=volume increased with escape mechanism through defect.
- ASDQ
- **Partial anomalous pulmonary venous return (PAPVR)**+ sinus venosus (ASD)
- **Endocardial cushion defect (ECD)**

Increased PBF with Cynanosis

Mn-**"Double – ACT-5"**
- **Double** out let right ventricle (DORV type I) Taussig Bing anomaly (DORV type II)
- Aortic atresia
- Common atrium
- ***Truncus arteriosus***Q
- Total anomalous pulmonary venous connection (*TAPVR*Q; supracardiac, cardiac)
- Tingle = single ventricle
- Transposition of great vessels = **TGV± VSD**
- Tricuspid atresia ± transposition & VSD

Decreased (Oligemic lungs)
- ***Pulmonary stenosis/atresia***Q
- ***Ebsteins anomaly***Q
- ***Tetralogy of Fallot (TOF)***Q
- Tricuspid atresia with **pulmonary stenosis**
- TGA with pulmonary stenosis (PS)
- Single ventricle with PS

(Mn-"**PET** with **PA/PS**")

Ebstein's Anomaly

Downward displacement of abnormal septal & posterior leaflets of tricuspid value into right ventricle (towards the apex) producing atrialization of RV and complex TR.

↓

Large RA & small ineffective RV (right ventricle)

↓

Poor Right ventricular output → Patent foramen ovale or ASD

↓

*Pulmonary oligemia*Q ← R → L shunt

5

RADIODIAGNOSIS

Radiological Features of Left Ventricle Failure / Congestive Cardiac Failure (produced due to pulmonary venous hypertension).

Stage I

Equalization (at pulmonary capillary wedge pressure 13-15 mm Hg) f/b **cephalization of pulmonary vascularity** (at 16-18 mmHg PCWP). It is characterized by:

- ***Constriction & blurring of lower zone vessels*** Q
- Effacement of hilar angle
- ***Dilatation & prominence of upper lobe vessels*** Q. Exceptions to this pattern of redistribution are basal emphysema & pulmonary parenchymal diseases of upper lobe.

Stage 2

Interstial pulmonary edema (at PCWP-19-24 mm Hg) occurs d/t presence of fluid within peribroncho-vascular interstial tissue. It is seen as:

- *Peribronchial thickening /cuffing & indistinct vessel margins*
- **Kerley A lines** is 3-4 cm long lines of interlobular septal thickening radiating from hila to mid & upper long zones..
- **Kerley (septal) B lines** i.e. short horizontal reticulations within lateral subpleural lung bases.
- ***Perihilar haze*** Q d/t hilar interstitial edema
- *Pseudoeffusion* d/t thickened pleural fissures and ***back ground haze (ground glass appearance)*** Q.

Stage 3

Alveolar edema (at PCWP >25 mm Hg) occurs when the interstitial fluid accumulates at rates faster than it can be removed by the lymphatics. It is seen as

- *Bat's wing appearance* d/t bilateral perihilar & basilar air space opacification
- *B/L small pleural effusion* usually occurs when systemic venous pressure is also elevated as in right heart failure.

★ *Cardiomegaly is also seen in CHF* Q.

Normal Pulmonary Vasculature

- Visualization can only be achieved on good erect PA chest film. Under exposure may make vessels appear more prominent but this will not alter their size & distribution (that is of major importance).
- Pulmonary circulation begins with **main pulmonary artery**, which forms convexity on left mediastinal border b/w arch of aorta & straight left heart border. *Upper normal limit for MPA is 3cm (on CT)*. Main pulmonary trunk (artery) is straight/slightly concave/or even mild convex (in normal young females). It measures **<4.5 cm** (left ward distance from vertical line at carina to most lateral aspect of MPA contour) MPA divides into right & left pulmonary artery (left PA being its continuation).
- The *left pulmonary artery lies above the left main bronchus*, before passing posteriorly, whereas on *right side the artery is anterior to the bronchus, resulting in right hilum being the lower.*
- With in the lung the **arteries** can be identified as they ***divide in a constant manner, following the branching pattern of the airways, these branches tapering smoothly and can be seen as far as the outer third of lung (i.e. not normaly visible in outer third of lung)*** Q. However, they are visible *only in medial third of lung* in conditions a/w **pulmonary oligemia** (↓PBF). Whereas, in **pulmonary plethora**, they become visible in *the outer third of lung parenchyma* also.
- Pulmonary veins can be differentiated by position & course in some areas only. *Pulmonary veins* in right lower zone run in a *horizontal* direction entering left atrium, compared with the more vertical course taken by the arteries. Because of difficult differentiation, **pulmonary vessels** or **vascularity** is more practical term than PA or pulmonary veins.
- The peripheral lung markings are mainly vascular, veins & arteries having no distinguishing characteristics. Centrally they can be differentiated. The *arteries accompany the bronchi*, lying postero-superior, whereas veins do not follow the bronchi but *drain via the inter lobular septa* eventually forming superior & basal veins which converge on left atrium. This **confluence of veins** may be seen as a round structure to the right of midline superimposed on heart (sometimes *simulating an enlarged left atrium*). Pulmonary *veins have fewer branches, and are straighter, larger and less well defined.*
- The **descending branch of right pulmonary artery** usually does **not exceed 16 mm in men & 15 mm in women** (for **left,** size given in various books vary b/w **<15 & 14mm**).
- Normal pulmonary vasculature shows a marked difference between upper and lower zones. **At 1st intercostal space the normal vessels should not exceed 3mm in diameter**. The *lower lobe vessels are larger than the upper lobe vessels in erect position* (in supine vessels equalize). **Pulmonary vessels (distribution)** within lower prehilum approximates 2/3 of total vascularity, whereas for upper prehilum it is 1/3rd. The right paracardiac vessels are invariably prominent.
- **Pulmonary vessels taper** near transition of middle & outer 1/3rd with vessel size <1-2mm in extreme lung periphery.

Pulmonary (Arterial) Hypertension (PAH)

It is defined as an elevation in ***mean pulmonary arterial pressure*** **above 30mmHg during execise** and *above 25mmHg at rest in systole*. An increase in PAH most commonly occurs as a result of *intrinsic lung disease, which results in an increae in pulmonary vascular resistance* and subsequent *increase in PA pressure*. PAP can also increase as a result of an *increase in* *pulmonary venous pressure* (which may be d/t impaired left ventricle function or obstruction to left sided cardiac flow eg MS etc). So radiological features may be slightly different depending on cause i.e. pulmonary arterial or pulmonary venous hypertension. **Radiological features of PAH** include.

Vascular Signs

- **Enlargement of central pulmonary arteries** (***main pulmonary artery & its branches down to the segmental level***)Q and ***tapering of peripheral arterial branches*** (*vessels beyond segmental level*)-termed ***pripheral pruning***Q are seen
- Enlargement of central main pulmonary artery may be extremely large with *complete infilling of pulmonary artery/ventricular concavity of left heart border* on X-ray.
- Widest diameter of main pulmonary artery (MPA) ≥**29mm** measured on transverse section (CT) at level of PA bifurcation has 90% sensitivity & specificity
- Diameter **ratio of MPA to ascending aorta** (measured at same level) **>1 i.e. diameter of MPA>AA** has strong correlation in <50yrs age.
- Transverse diameter of right descending pulmonary artery at midpoint **>17mm** (Grainger); diamete of left and right pulmonary artery **>16mm** (Wolfgang); maximum diameter of descending branch of pulmonary artery (measured 1cm medial & 1 cm lateral to hilar points) **>16mm for males** & **>15mm for females** (Sutton)
- Pulmonary arteries with in lungs are enlarged but there is rapid tapering of vessels (beyond segmental level) as they run towards the periphery. The **important feature is discrepancy between central and peripheral vessel size**, central pulmonary arteries being large or near normal sometimes and **peripheral arteries disproportionately small (pruning or tapering)**.
- Vascular complications include *sub pleural pulmonary infarct,* dissection & **calcified plaques of central pulmonary arteries (pathognomic**, a feature not seen in nonhypertensive pulmonary arteries; is often *curvilinear & egg shape calcificaiton* mimicking enlarged lymph nodes, from which it is differentiated by *absence of lobulation and presence of smooth border*).
- **Pulmonary veins** are *small in pre capillary pulmonary hypertension whereas enlarged in post capillary causes.*

Mediastinal & Cardiac Signs

- ***Cardiac enlargement (right heart i.e. RA and RV enlargement & hypertrophy)***Q demonstrating a large, triangular heart.
- Mild *pericardial thickening & effusion.*
- Dilatation of IVC, coronary sinus & SVC (On MRI/CT)

Lung Parenchymal Signs

- *Mosaic perfusion without dilatation of bronchi* (increase in vessel diameter in areas of hyper attenuation & tapering of peripheral vessels in areas of hypo attenuation)

Pulmonary Venous Hypertension (PVH)

Causes

- By increased resistance in pulmonary vein secondary to **left- sided heart disease** eg. *left ventricle out flow obstruction* (coarctation of aorta, AS, hypoplastic left heart), ***LVF, mitral valve disease***, *left atrial myxoma* or less commonly **mediastional disease** eg. fibrosing mediastinitis, pulmonary venoocclusive disease.
- Severity of mitral stenosis is represented by degree of PVH but in AS it is more indicative of myocardial failure than severity of stenosis.

Radiological Features

- ***Reversal of normal gravity dependent pattern or upper lobe venous diversion is first radiological sign***Q. It is seen as:
  - *Upper lobe veins distend* initially reaching the size of, & then eventually becoming larger than lower lobe vein.
  - *Increased upper zone flow is also associated with reduction of flow in lower zone & attenuation of lower zone pulmonary artery.*
  - *Right descending pulmonary trunk (RDP)* is normally the most prominent vessel on frontal view. *Attenuation of mid or distal portion* of RDP is indicative of PVH & so is the *enlargement of superior pulmonary vein.*
- **Interstitial pulmonary oedema & kerley (septal / interstitial) B lines** appear if PV pressure continues to rise.
  - **Kerley B** lines are ***horizontal, subpleural lines 1-3 mm in thickness, ≤ 1cm in length***, found most frequently in *lower zones* peripherally at ***costophrenic angles and parallel to each other but perpendicular (at right angle) to pleural surface***Q**.** It is differentiated from **blood vessels** as later is seen with ***less clarity , branch uniformly & not visible in outer 1 cm of lung***Q
  - Septal lines disappear on t/t & persistant lines are seen in – long standing PVH, pneumoconiosis, lymphangitis carcinomatosis, interstitial fibroisis.
  - ***Perihilar haze***Q (i.e. loss of clarity of hilar & lower lobe vessels) & ***peribronchial cuffing***Q (thickening of proximal ilitary wall) are the features of interstial oedema.
- **Aleolar oedema** occurs when PV pressure increases > 25mmHg in acute phase or > 30 –35 mmHg in chronic cases.
  - Air space nodules, B/L symmetrical consolidation in mid & lower zone and *pleural effusion*

Long standing PVH

is associated with *hemosiderosis,* which appears radiologically as ***fine ilitary calcification or fine nodular pattern scattered throughout lung***Q

Severe long standing PVH

Pulmonary ossiclesQ (bone formation) never larger than 1cm in diameter can develop.

Certain opacification pattern

- **Perihilar batswing** pattern of air space consolidation is indicative of *LVF & renal failure*
- **Right upper zone alveolar oedema** is seen in *severe mitral regurgitation.*

Radiological features of Mitral Stenosis

Due to left atrial enlargment

- *Straightening of the left border of cardiac silhoute (earliest sign)*Q
- *Lifting of left bronchus and splaying of carina*Q
- *Posterior displacement of oesophagus on barium shallow*Q
- *Double atrial shadow (double density seen through right upper cardiac border)*Q

Due to Pulmonary venous *hypertension*Q

- **Pulmonary vascular cephalization** i.e. redistribution of pulmonary blood flow to upper lobes
- ***Dilation of upper lobe pulmonary veins & constriction of lower (inverted moustache sign) = 1st radiological feature of pulmonary venous hypertension***Q
- Interstitial edema seen as ***kerley's B septal costophrenic***Q & central A lines
- Alveolar edema
- ***Pulmonary hemosiderosis seen as ilitary shadows***Q
- Pulmonary ossified nodules

Due to elevated pulmonary vascular resistance & **Pulmonary arterial hypertension**

- *Cardiomegaly (rt atrial & ventricle enlargement)*Q
- Enlargement of main pulmonary artery & central pulmonary vessels (right & left pulmonary arteries & right inferior pulmonary artery) and its branches upto segmental level
- **Peripheral pruning** (i.e. tapering of peripheral vessels beyond segmental level)

Other features:

- Normal or slightly enlarged cardiothoracic ratio
- Normal or under sized LV
- Dilated left atrial appendage & enlarged LA
- Small aortic knob (d/t decreased cardiac output)
- **Calcification** of *mitral valve leaflets* (not annulus) and rarely *left atrial wall* (in long standing disease) and *pulmonary artery* (from PAH)

- In mitral stenosis, there is increase in PCW pressure which causes radiological changes

PCWP (mm hg)	Finding
5-12	*Normal*Q
12-17	***Cephalization of pulmonary vessels***Q (only in chronic conditions)
17-20	***Kerley lines***Q, subpleural effusion
>25	***Alveolar flooding edema***Q

- Radiographic changes of mitral valve ds (mainly rheumatic)

1. ***Left atrial enlargement is seen as straightening of left border which bulges immediately below left bronchus & elevating it***Q, f/b *double density to aneurysmal enlargement.* (when left atrium reaches to ≤ 1 inch of chest wall)
2. ***Upper lobe blood diversion*** seen as distension of upper lobe veins & constriction of lower lobe veins.
3. ***Interstial edema seen as Kerley's septal costophrenic B lines & central A lines.***Q
4. *Alveolar edema* seen as perihilar confluent shadows.
5. *Pulmonary hemosiderosis* seen as fine punctate densities throughout lung (miliary shadow) usually after years & in MS.
6. *Pulmonary ossified nodules* seen as discrete calcified densities at the lung base, is d/t PAH in long standing MS.
7. *Pulmonary arterial hypertension* seen as enlargement of main pulmonary artery & central pulmonary vessels with peripheral vessel pruning.

Causes of Gross Cardiac Enlargement (Increased Cardiac Silhouette Sign)

- ***Pericardial effusion***Q ***(globular/flask shaped heart, crisp cardiac outline)***
- ASD
- Cardiomyopathy & ischemic heart disease
- ***Multiple valvular disease (aortic and mitral valve disease particularly with regurgitation)*** Q
- Congenital heart disease eg **Ebstein anomaly**Q (i.e. atrialization of RV+ complex tricuspid regurgitation.)

Causes of Small heart

- Normal variant
- Emphysema
- Addison's disease
- Dehydration / malnutrition
- Constrictive pericarditi

Radiographic Mediastinal Signs

Silhouette's (Obscured Margin) Sign

- The **normal radio-opaque margins** of soft tissue mediastinal structures (such as *heart, aortic arch, hilum, azygoesophageal recesses) and diaphragm* are visible on chest x-ray because they are outlined by adjacent air containing radiolucent lung (i.e. b/o normal soft tissue air inteface/contrast).

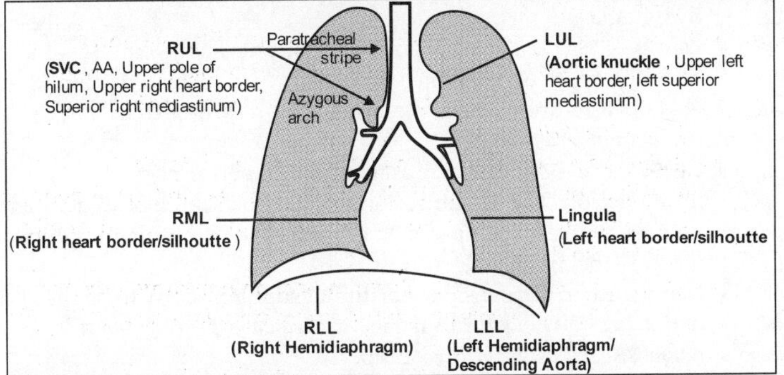

- **Silhouette (obscured margin) sign** is based on the principle, which says that **if two structures have approximately the same radiographic density, and are in intimate contact with each other, then the interface between them is obliterated".** However, if there is even a small gap between them, then they are seen with their borders as separate entities. An intrathoracic lesion touching a border of heart, aorta or diaphragm and having similar radiographic density (opacity) will obliterate that border on X-ray. And a lesion not anatomically contigious with a border of these structures or having markedly dissimilar density will not obliterate that border.
- **Silhouette's invisible or obscured border sign** is caused by any *intrathoracic opacity eg consolidation, pneumonia, mass, fluid, atelectasia* of same density as the adjacent normal structure. This sign is used to diagnose variety of lung/chest conditions and to localize it to a specific lobe /region of lung. Silhoutte sign is very useful in localizing lung lesions as all structures forming cardiac silhoutte (heart border, ascending descending aorta, aortic knob & hemidiaphragm) are in contact with a specific portion of lung.

Silhoutte structure (which may be **obscured** by pathology)	**Lung lobe/portion** in contact
Upper right heart border (Superior vena cava), Ascending aorta & Upper pole of hilum = Superior right mediastinum or Right Aortic border	**RUL** (Right upper lobe, anterior segment) & anterior segment of RML
Right heart border/Right cardiac sithoutte	**RML** (Right middle lobe, medial) >>> Right medial lower lobe
Aortic knudcle/knob/arch	**LUL** (Left upper lobe apico-posterior segment)
Upper left heart border (left superior mediastinum)	**LUL** (Left upper lobe anterior segment)
Left heart border (Left cardiac silhoutte)	**Lingula** (anterior) segment of LUL
Anterior hemidiaphragm Position of oblique fissure is best index of lower lobe volume.	Lower lobe (anterior- basal segments)
Left hemidiaphragm, Descending aorta	Left lower lobe (LL)
Right hemidiaphragm	Right lower lobe (RLL)

- ***Obscuration of right heart border (right cardiac silhoutte) on PA view***[Q] and movement of horizontal fissure and lower half of oblique fissure toward one another on lateral projection is diagnostic of ***right middle lobe collapse.***
- With the exception of absence of horizontal fissure on left, radiological features of lingual collapse are similar to right middle lobe collapse.
- In right upper lobe collapse, *lateral end of horizontal fissure moves upward & medially* (towards superior mediastinum) & its *anterior end moves upward* towards apex. And the upper half of oblique fissure moves anteriorly. Both fissures become concave superiorly.

Cervico-Thoracic Sign

- It is based on the fact that upper most border anterior mediastinum ends at the level of clavicle while middle (higher) & posterior (highest) mediastinum projects above clavicle.
- Therefore, *a well defined mass* (which is *sharply outlined* by apical lung) above the clavicles is always **posterior**, whereas an **anterior mass** being in contact with soft tissues (of same density) rather than aerated lung, is *ill defined (have unsharp borders)*

Hilar-Overlay Sign

- It allows differentiation of true cardiomegaly from large anterior mediastinal masses. In **cardiomegaly** the *hilum is displaced laterally* whereas in the presence of **anterior mediastinal mass** the *hilum* is seen projecting *medial to the lateral border of mass.*
- With the mediastinal mass, the hilium is seen through the mass whereas with cardiomegaly the hilum is displaced so that only its lateral border is visible.

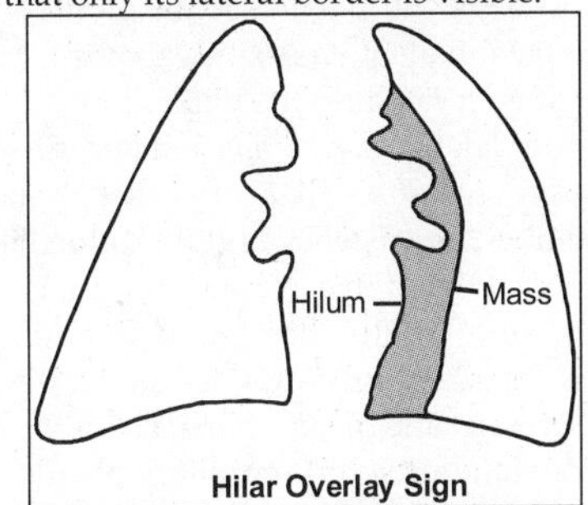

Hilar Overlay Sign

Hilar Bifurcation (Convergence) Sign

- It differentiates hilar masses from vascular structures in cases of hilar enlargment.
- If the vessels (eg pulmonary arteries) are seen to arise directly from the hilar shadow (i.e. *vessels converge into lateral border of cardiac silhoutte) then the enlargement is vascular,* but if they appear to arise medial to the lateral aspect of the hilar shadow, the enlargment is caused by an extravascular mass.

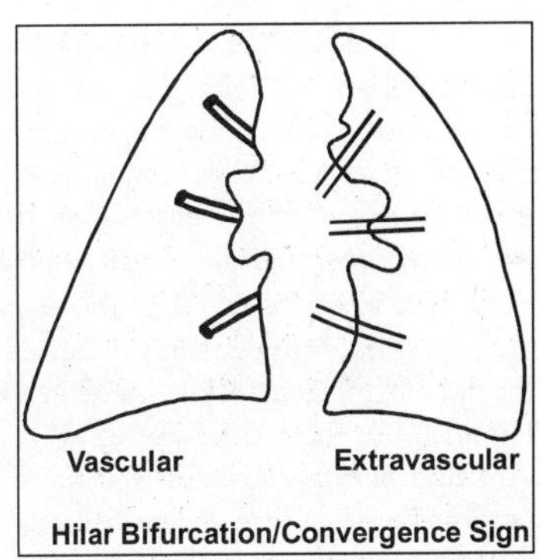

Hilar Bifurcation/Convergence Sign

Agatston Coronary Artery Calcification Scoring

- **Coronary calcium** is used as a *surrogate marker to detect the presence and quantify the amount of atherosclerosis*. Both **electron beam (EB) CT and MD-CT** permit accurate detection and quantification of coronary artery calcium. With the *exception of renal failure* patients, calcification occurs almost exclusively in the context of *atherosclerosis*.
- **Agatston** developed a scoring system, which takes into account the *area (in pixels)* and the *CT density of calcified lesion (defining calcification as densities ≥130 Hounsfield units)* for *quantifying coronary artery calcification* in patients evaluated with *EB-CT scans using 3mm slice thickness*. Each lesion in each slice is scored based on maximum density with a particular scale i.e. **1 = 130 to 199 HU; 2 = 200-299 HU; 3 = 300-399HU; 4 = 400HU or greater**. Then a total score is obtained by summing the scores from all slices, broadly indicating grade of coronary artery disease (& risk of cardiovascular events ±. **0 = No; 1 to 10 = Minimal; 11 to 100 = Mild; 101 to 400 = Moderate; >400 = Severe.**
- Currently, **MDCT calcium scoring** is widely used to calculate coronary clacium load, using 2.5 to 3 mm nonenhanced axial CT images obtained with a prospective ECG gated acquisition. Modified Agatston score equivalent, takes into account the area of each calcified lesion and the maximum CT value within the lesion. The *volumetric and absolute mass quantfication scoring algorithms* are also available, showing increased accuracy, consistency and reproducibility (however, not been validated in clinical setting).
- It is important to understand that the amount of coronary calcium correlates moderately to overall atherosclerotic plaque burden. On the other hand, not every atherosclerotic coronary plaque is calcified and calcification is a sign of neither stability nor instability of an specific plaque. *The absence of coronary calcium rules out the presence of coronary artery stenoses with high predictive value. However, even pronounced coronary calcification is not necessarily a/w hemodynamically relevant luminal narrowing.* ***So even the detection of large amounts of calcium does not indicate the presence of significant stenosis & it should not prompt invasive coronary angiography in otherwise asymptomatic individuals.***

Vascular Rings

- **Vascular rings** is a condition in which an anomalous configuration of the arch and / or its associated vessels completely or incompletely surrounds the trachea & oesophagus causing compression of these structures. Neonates present with respiratory distress and older children present with stridor or dysphagia.
- *Fourth developmental arch* is most important. The two most common types of complete vascular rings, which account for 85-95% of cases are *double aortic arch and right aortic arch with left ligamentum arteriosum*
- Chest x-ray is the first & most commonly performed investigation. The identification of right aortic arch or ill defined arch location and compression of trachea in symptomatic child indicate the diagnosis.
- Many authorities consider **barium oesophagoscopy** to be the *most important study in patients with suspected vascular ring and it is diagnostic in vast majority of cases.*
  - A double aortic arch produce *bilateral & posterior compression of oesophagus, which remain constant regardless of peristalsis.* The right indentation is usually slightly higher than left and posterior one is usually wide & course in a downward direction from right to left.
  - Right subclavian artery takes a retrooesophageal course, there is a posterior defect slanting upward from left to right. The posterior defect is less broad than in double aortic arch.
- Echocardiography can be used but structures without lumen such as ligamentum arteriosum or an atretic arch are difficult to be identified.
- Plain x-ray & barium swallow can not reliably distinguish among the types of vascular rings. Cross section images by **CT, MRI and digital substraction angiography (DSA)** can be useful diagnostic tool in delineating the anatomy and aiding in presurgical planning & post surgical assessment. MR angiography (MRA) is an excellent substitute for DSA but young patients may require general anesthesia & where there is already airway compromise, this should be avoided.
- ***MRI is preferred as it is non invasive and avoids radiation risk***[Q]. Multidetector CT is rarely used b/o radiation implication. Angiography (an invasive method) is rarely required unless cardiac catheterization is necessary for investigation of associated cardiac anomalies and if MRI is equivocal (same protocol applies for coarctation of aorta i.e. MRI > CT > Angiography).

Radiological Evaluation of Ischemic Heart Disease

Cascade of ischemia & Viability

- Stenoses of epicardial artery l/t reduced perfusion & diminished myocardial oxygen delivery. However, *even moderate to severe stenosis can be asymptomatic at rest and cannot be detected using various imaging & perfusion studies at rest.* ***Pharmacolgical or physical stress increases*** the contractile function, O_2 demand & perfusion (3-4 folds) and precipitate myocardial ischemia – because the flow in normal coronary artery is increased by vasodilation (a/t demand) but the moderate & severe stenoses become flow limiting *resulting in perfusion deficits* (seen in radionuclide imaging), *wall motion abnormalities* (seen in ECHO or CMR) and *symptomatic angina* (on ECG).

Investigations

- Although MDCT or catheter angiography can detect coronary artery luminal obstruction but cannot assess the functional /hemodynamic relevance of the lesion. Therefore, beyond establishment of clinical diagnosis, **stress perfusion imaging** can also risk stratify patients.
- **Perfusion scanning** not only enables a diagnosis of ischemia to be made but it can also help distinguish ischemic muscle from scar d/t infarction. **Ischemic areas** seen on **exercise (stress) scan** as region of reduced uptake show normal activity on resting scans. Whereas, **infarcted area (scars)** in which there is little, if any, remaining viable myocardium will **show a persisting defect on the resting scan**.

- Cascade of ischemia l/t initial *hypoperfusion in subendocardial layer of myocardium* f/b *transmural perfusion deficits* (with more severe stenoses). Progression of ischemia *l/t diastolic f/b systolic wall motion abnormalities*. Finally ECG changes can be detected and symptomatic angina may occur. As perfusion abnormalities are the first step in this cascade of ischemia, **direct visualization of perfusion defects** seems to be the **diagnostic test of first choice** in patients with suspected coronary artery disease (CAD). Both CMR & nuclear imaging can measure myocardial perfusion.
- Viable means alive and nonviable is dead cell. By this definition, histology is the only & ultimate method for detection of viability. So a number of indirect methods have been used to detect the presence of living (viable) myocytes for in vivo assessment and include

1) *Recovery of contractile* function following revascularization.
2) *Response to inotropic stimulation* (eg dobutamine MRI or ECHO).
3) Presence of *glucose metabolism* eg FDG, PET.
4) Presence of *active cellular transport mechanisms* eg ^{201}Tl SPECT; and
5) ***Absence of scarred myocardium on delayed enhanced (or DE) MRI***[Q].

- Myocytes may be viable in the setting of severly reduced or even absent contractile function (=akinetic areas) resulting from either acute or chronic reduction in perfusion. It is crucial to identify the myocardium that is viable and not infarcted.

- **Ischemic myocardium** that is **viable and can restore (recover) function after reperfusion** usually demonstrate **stress induced reversible (left ventricle) wall motion impairment** i.e. *hypokinesia* (reduced wall motion), *akinesia* (absent wall movement) & *dyskinesia* (paradoxical wall movement) which improves on rest.	**Infarcted, noviable myocardium (i.e. Scarring or Fibrosis)** can be identified as it - fails to recover systolic function on extended pharmacological stress - ***retains contrast on DE MRI***[Q] **(gold standard)** - ***does not recover function after reperfusion***[Q] - ***irreversible wall motion changes*** i.e. localized contraction abnormalities even in resting state.

- **Ventricular function** i.e. **wall motion and ejection fraction** (>66%=normal; <50%=significant; <30%=sever; and <10%=very severe impairment) can be demonstrated by **ECHO, radionuclide imaging** (first pass or gated blood pool), EBCT, MDCT, conventional left ventriculography & **multilevel cine-MRA** with short axis breath hold tagging sequences to highlight abnormal regional wall movement and reduced myocardial thickening in systole (probably **most accurate method** for assessing ventricular function).
- *Ventricular dysfunction may persist* in spite of there being patent coronary arteries *even at rest* in two condition of IHD which are

Radionuclide Studies

- **Nuclear cardiac imaging** is a first line technique for evaluating myocardial perfusion, viability & function. **Myocardial perfusion imaging (MPI)** or **SPECT** (single photon emission CT) using **^{201}Tl or ^{99m}Tc labelled agents** is the most common procedure.
- **PET** (along with **CMR**) **using metabolic tracers such as 18F-FDG** (glucose analog) is regarded as **gold standard for tissue viability** (fatty acids are used as substrate in normoxic heart but glucose becomes major substrate in ischemic conditions). It can be combined with flow tracers such as **13 N ammonia** or **Rubidium 82** to assess myocardial perfusion.
- Radionuclide studies are non-invasive & simpler to perform than angiocardiography. They provide information on myocardial blood flow & cardiac function but provide little anatomical detail. In cardiology it can be of 2 types

1. **Myocardial perfusion scintigraphy**, using *thallium-201 (^{201}Tl)* traditionally or ^{99m}Tc labelled agents such as *sesta MIBI teboroxime*, tetrofosmin. These agents are taken up in proportion to blood flow, so *regions of reduced myocardial perfusion appear as areas of reduced uptake*. The site & sizes of ischemic areas can be assessed & distinction between ischemic & infarcted regions can made by *comparing peak stress (physical or pharmacological) and resting images*
2. **Radionuclide angiography** or multiple gated **(MUGA)** equilibrium blood pool imaging uses ^{99M}Tc attached to RBC to image the blood pool (^{99M}Tc is injected IV, 15 min after reducting agent stannous pyrophosphate). Because insufficient radioactive counts are collected from each cardiac cycle, images from successive cardiac cycles are combined with the use of electronic gating. Each cardiac cycle of ECG is divided into a number of equal intervals. Data from each interval in each successive cycle (from~400-500 cycles) are summed to give a representative cycle which is then displayed as a moving image on TV monitor or **cine** (from cinema) **loop**. RA are used to calculate the ventricular ejection fraction in patients with valvular disease & myocardial disorder and for wall motion analysis in patients with ischemia heart disease (IHD).

- Radionuclide perfusion imaging can be of 4 types: (1) **Exercise (stress) image or distribution image** (initial phase or first pass extraction images) performed within minutes (max 30) of stress to accentuate temporary ischemic defects; and 3 late images to assess viability are : (2) **Reditribution image** obtained at rest after 2-3-4-6 hours; (3) **Delayed image** (optional) at 24 hours; (4) **Booster reinjection image/Very delayed redistribution image** after 18-24-72 hours. In redistribution images, there is washout in normal areas but slow continued accumulation of tracer in areas of greatly reduced perfusion and increased uptake in viable ischemic zone (in comparison to stress images). **Permanent defect on redistribution (rest) image is indicative of nonviable myocardium** as in myocardial infarction/fibrosis. 50% of irreversible persistent defects improve significantly after booster reinjection.

Echocardiography (ECHO)

- **While echocardiography** usually is the *most appropriate method for assessing cardiac (ventricular) function and structural complicaton of IHD* such as VSD, papillary muscle dysfunction

5

RADIODIAGNOSIS

Stunned Myocardium

- It is slow recovery of previously ischemic & nonfunctioning myocardium in form of prolonged but temporary ventricular dysfunction that **follows a period (episole) of transient but profound ischemia**. It can be seen after relief of ischemia by thrombolysis, PCI, coronary bypass grafting, reversal of vasospasm, or a after exercise.
- In other words, it is a prolonged contractile dysfunction after a **transient profound acute ischemic insult & coronary reperfusion**. i.e. despite a prompt & complete return of blood flow, it may take usually days and (sometimes) even weeks for injured myocardium to recover fully to achieve its normal contractile abilities.
- In stunning, there is abnormal ventricular function but the myocardium is viable, has contractile reserve and can regain normal functon with revascularization.
- Stunning can be identified by recovery of LV function **during extended pharmacological stress testing with echocardiography, radionuclide imaging or cine-MRA**.

Hibernating Myocardium

- It is a more **chronic** condition *resulting from months or years of ischemia* causing ventricular dysfunction that persists until normal blood flow is restored.
- In other words, it is a result of repetitive periods of stunning usually seen in clinical situations like *chronic stable/unstable angina*, silent ischemia & after MI.
- Like stunning, hibernating myocardium shows contractile reserve, is viable, can regain function with revascularization and can be identified with pharmacological stress testing with ECHO, cine-MRA & radionuclide imaging.

(causing MR), ventricular thrombus, aneurysm, false aneurysm or valve function and wall motion abnormalities. In those patients where ECHO is difficult, **breath hold CMR** (cardiac magnetic resonance) is the *next best* alternative. Although this information can be obtained by CTA but at cost of high radiation exposure.

- **Strees echocardiography** also can differentiate infarcted viable but **lethargic myocardial muscle**. The resting regional left ventricular function is compared with any changes induced when the heart rate is increased eg by exercise or *IV agents such as adenosine dipyridamole, dobutemine, arbutamine.* This may allow the identification of dyskinetic areas of ventricular muscle from underlying coronary artery disease.

CMR

- **Stress CMR** to assess myocardial ischemia may be of 2 types: 1) **dobutamine stress MR (DSMR)** less preferred b/o concerns relating to patient safety & monitoring inside MR machine; 2) **perfusion CMR** (using Gd contrast and adenosine for vasodilator stress) show *hypoperfused (ischemic) areas as decreased signal intensity on T1* (first pass) images. The standard CMR technique for detection of myocardial viability is **delayed contrast enhancement (DE)- MRI**. It is regarded as **gold standard** for detection of **irreversibly damaged (nonviable) myocardium**. The underlying concept is that infarcted tissue accumulates Gd and can be visualized as bright/hyper enhanced regions on T1WI acquired at least 10 min after Gd injection. Actually viable myocytes actively exclude extracellular contrast Gd by intact sarcolemma. Therefore the hyperenhancement effect of nonviable myocardium may be regarded as being d/t absence of any viable myocyte rather than any inherent properties of nonviable /necrotic tissue. So recent MI shows poor perfusion with first pass contrast medium imaging but delayed enhancement with Gd based perfusion agents. DE-MRI or high T1 signal is not specific and can be seen in other conditions causing myocardial damage such as *sarcoidosis or myocarditis*.
- **Breath hold DE-MRI** using patient specific inversion times (T1) to null signals in normal myocardium is widely used for *assessing viability* when planning revascularization and may be as accurate as PET. In acute phase following MI, DEMRI is *the best method for determining the size of infarct*.
- SSPF cine MRA and tagging sequences can assess myocardial mass, and consequences of MI such as LV dysfunction or aneurysm.
- MRI can show areas of myocrdial thinning following infarction & even altered signals in subacute infarction, but there is little clinical utility for MRI as yet in ischemic heart disease (used mainly for research purposes).

Radiological Evaluation of Pneumoperitoneum & Abdominal trauma

CT Scan Abdomen

- CTscan-abdomen is the **most sensitive** investigation for detection of **free peritoneal air** (i.e. **pneumoperitoneum**), *intra abdominal or pelvic hemorrhage (hemoperitoneum), spleen injury* (commonest injured organ following blunt trauma abdomen), *liver injury* (2nd most common), *adrenal*

Plain Radiography

- ***Erect chest radiograph***Q is **superior to erect abdominal view** for demonstration of ***pneumoperitoneum***Q (i.e. ***free intra abdominal gas)***Q since, in the later view, the divergent x-ray beam penetrates the gas between diaphragm and liver obliquely and this area is usually overexposed for detecting small amount of gases.

injury (most common retroperitoneal injury) *bowel and mesenteric injuries*. Whereas, CT is relatively insensitive to acute pancreatic injuries.

- In order not to miss small (minimal) pneumoperitoneum, **abdominal CT images** *should be viewed in the* ***lung window settings***. Bubbles of free air may be detected *over the liver*, anteriorly *in mid abdomen*, trapped *between* the leaves of *mesentery or in the peritoneal recesses*.
- **Sentineal clot sign** (i.e. clotted blood of higher attenuation 45-75HU) near the site of bleeding with lower attenuation and unclotted blood elsewhere in peritoneal cavity indicate hemoperitoneum.
- CT scan is the **imaging modality of choice for diagnostic evaluation of abdominal trauma**. CT is as accurate as DPL in detecting blunt abdominal injury with extra advantages of detailed anatomical evaluation of injuries, quantification of hemorrhage, detection of active arterial extravascation and better detection of retroperitoneal injuries. Wit these advantages diagnostic peritoneal lavage (DPL) has now almost become obsolete (to be used only in few hemodynamically unstable patients).
- **Helical CT** is preferred over conventional CT as it is fast, better (less artifacts & respiratory misregistration) and offers optimal IV contrast enhancement. **Contrast enhanced CT** is imaging modality of choice for ***spleenic & liver injuries***[Q]. **MDCT** provides excellent quality coronal, saggital reconstructions and is ***diagnostic modality of choice for detection of bowel & mesentric injuries***[Q]. Administration of IV **iodinated contrast** is mandatory as it makes detection & location of parenchymal contusions & hematoma more clear and identifies great vessels and provides information regarding integrity of organs or extent of the injury.
- **Erect chest film is best view for showing small pneumoperitoneum**, particularly on right side with gas under diaphragm because the **X-ray beam is passing almost tangentially (horizontally)** to the free gas and the exposure of diaphragm is optimal to show small amounts of gas. On the left it can be difficult to distinguish free gas from stomach & colonic gas.
- Number of conditions can simulate pneumoperitoneum on erect X-ray (**k/a pseudo-pneumoperitoneum**) such as *Chilaiditi's syndrome* (i.e. distended bowel b/w liver & diaphragm), *subdiaphragmatic fat/abscess*,diaphragmatic irregularity, *curvilinear lung collapse*, intramural gas cysts in *pneumatosis intestinalis*, omental fat, distended viscus, subpulmonary pneumothorax, and apposition of gas distended loops mimicking the double wall sign. CT or lateral decubitus x-ray can differentiate by demonstrating gas b/w liver and abdominal wall.
- Pneumoperitoneum can be detected in 76% of cases using an erect film only and in 90% cases if left lateral decubitus projection is also included. So in a suspected case a **horizontal ray radiograph either an erect chest or left lateral decubitus (with right side up) abdomen X-ray**, is mandatory. The patient should ideally remain in position for **10 min** before the **horizontal ray film** is taken, because it takes this time for gas to rise to the highest point in the abdomen.
- In patients who are unfit to sit or stand for an erect film **left lateral decubitus abdomenal radiograph is the projection of choice** (i.e. **2nd best view**) to show a small pneumoperitoneum. In this view free gas is seen b/w the edge of liver & lateral abdominal wall or sometimes over pelvis (in females, this may be the highest point). This is the *best view to show a gas filled dialated duodenal loop*, one of the commonest sign of acute pancreatitis. As little as **1ml** of free gas can be demonstrated radiographically, on either an erect chest or a left lateral decubitus abdominal radiograph.
- A **supine abdomen and an erect chest** are regarded as **basic standard radiographs in the acute abdomen.** In many patients particularly who are *old, unconscious or critically ill, have suffered trauma*, perforation (l/t pneumoperitoneum) may be clinically silent or is over shadowed by another serious medical or surgical condition, and the supine abdominal radiograph may be the only view that can be obtained. So it is important to be able to recognize the signs of pneumoperitoneum on supine view which are

Signs of right upper quadrant gas (best place to look for small collection)

1. **Doge's cap's sign** is triangular collection of gas in Morrison's pouch (posterior hepatorenal fossa)
2. *Perihepatic* (over the liver), *subhepatic* (postero inferior margin) and *parahepatic* (lateral to right edge) hyperlucency d/t gas
3. **Cupola/Mustache/Saddlebag sign** is large amount of gas trapped below central tendon of diaphragm.
4. Free gas may outline **falciform ligament** (most common), **fissure of ligamentum teres** (which is posterior free edge of falciform ligament k/a ligamentum teres sign) and **ligamentum teres notch** (inverted V shaped hyperlucent area along under surface of liver)

Signs of large collection of gas

- **Football or air done sign** is large amount of gas in center of abdomen over a fluid collection/or large pneumoperitoneum outlining entire abdominal cavity.
- **Rigler's double wall sign or bas-relief sign** is visualization of both inner and outer walls of a bowel loop d/t air out lining both (luminal & serosal surface) is k/a Rigler's sign and the bowel loops then take on **a ghost like appearance**.
- **Tell tale triangular sign** is small triangular collection of gas b/w 3 loops of bowel.
- Free gas may outline & visualize *diaphragmatic muscle slips, both lateral umblical ligaments* (**inverted V sign**), medial umblical ligaments (containing obliterated umblical arteries) and *middle umblical ligament* (**urachus sign**).
- Scrotal air through open processus vagnalis (in children)

Zenker (Pharygo-Esophageal) Diverticulum

- **Zenker (pharygo-esophageal) diverticulum** is an acquired ***pulsion diverticulum herniating through Kilian dehiscence***Q, an area of congenital weakness between the horizontal & oblique fibers of **cricopharyngeus muscle**. It is *outpouching of posterior hypopharyngeal wall (mucosa & sub mucosa)* through oblique & transverse muscle bundles (*pseudo-diverticulum*) of cricopharyngeal muscle at pharyngoesophageal junction in the midline of Killian dehiscence (**triangle of Laimer**), at level of $C_{5\text{-}6}$.

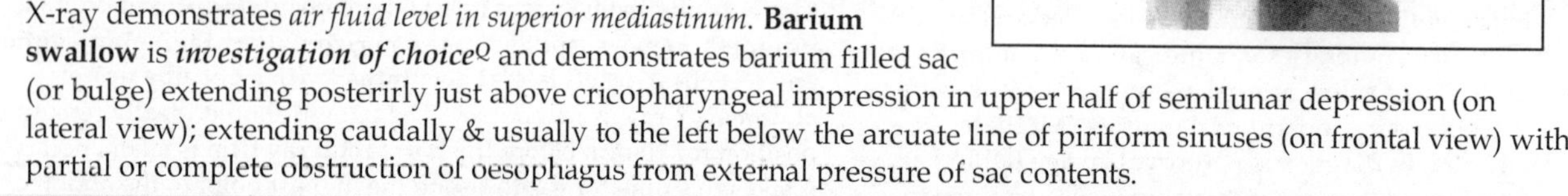

- It may present with upper *oesophageal dysphagia* (as diverticulum fills preferentially Zeinker diverticulum (Posterior) with food & obstructs the lumen of oesophagus), *compressible neck mass, regurgitation (± aspiration) of undigested pouch content (food), noisy deglutition and halitosis (foul breath).* Aspiration (30%), perforation & carcinoma (0.5%) are possible complications.
- X-ray demonstrates *air fluid level in superior mediastinum.* **Barium swallow** is ***investigation of choice***Q and demonstrates barium filled sac (or bulge) extending posterirly just above cricopharyngeal impression in upper half of semilunar depression (on lateral view); extending caudally & usually to the left below the arcuate line of piriform sinuses (on frontal view) with partial or complete obstruction of oesophagus from external pressure of sac contents.
- Once suspected, clinically & radiologically, ***the diagnosis of Zenker's diverticulum is estabilished by barrium swallow***Q. No other study is often required. ***Endoscopy is usually difficult & potentially dangerous***Q, owing to obstruction of true oesophageal lumen by the diverticulum l/t increased risk of diverticular perforation.

★ **Killian-Jamieson Pouch (diverticula)** are protrusion arising on anterolateral wall of proximal cervical oesophagus just below the level of cricopharyngeus, in region of anatomic *weakness caused by passage of inferior laryngeal nerve.*

Hypertrophic Pyloric Stenosis (HPS)

- It is *idiopathic hypertrophy & hyperplasia of pyloric circular muscle fibers and redundancy of pyloric mucosa.* The hypertrophied muscle project into gastric antrum. There is a constant assocaition with ***hyperplasia of antral mucosa.***
- It is a common developmental condition (3 in 1000 live births), ***affecting boys more than girls (M:F = 4/5 :1)***Q. There is a *familial predisposition.*
- Affected infant usually presents **between 2-6 weeks of age**, with *projectile non bilious vomiting* (D/D include pylorospasm, hiatus hernia & preampullary duodenal stenosis). HPS is **never seen beyond 3 months of age** except in premature infants in

Barium Study

Performed if USG is inconclusive or *gastroesophageal reflux is suspected. Combination of narrowing & elongation of pylorus is the hallmark* of HPS on barium study.

Pyloric signs include

1. **String sign**, is passing of thin barium streak through narrowed & elongated pyloric canal. It is **most specific sign**.
2. Pyloric canal is almost always *curved upward posteriorly*
3. **Double/triple track sign or double string sign** is produced by barium caught between crowded mucosal folds in pyloric canal overlying the hypertrophied muscle & parallel lines may be seen.
4. **Diamond sign or twining recess is transient triangular tent** like cleft/niche in midportion of pyloric canal *with apex pointing inferiorly* secondary to mucosl bulging between two seperated hypertrophied muscles *on the greater curvature side* of pyloric canal.
5. **Apple core lesion**, pyloric segment looks like apple core with under cutting of distal antral & proximal duodenal bulb.

Antral signs include

1. **Pyloric teat sign** is *out pouching along lesser curvature* b/o disruption of antral peristalsis.
2. **Shoulder sign** is impression of hypertrophied muscle on distended gastric antrum.
3. **Antral beaking** is noted as thick *muscle narrows the barium column as it enters the pyloric canal.*
4. **Olive pit sign** is impression of pyloric muscle upon antrum seen as tiny amount of barium at orifice.
5. **Caterpillar sign** is gastric hyperperistaltic waves.
6. **Kirklin mushroom sign** is indentation of base of duodenal bulb.

whom enteral feeding has been started late.

- Despite the recurrent vomiting, child has a voracious appetite that leads to *cycle of feeding & vomiting* that invariably results in ***severe dehydration, hypochloremic-hypokalemic metabolic alkalosis*** with eventual decrease in urine PH
- Diagnosis can be made clinically on the basis of **history** and **palpation of an olive mass** in the **subhepatic region** (right upper quadrant) and ***presence of visible gastric (antral peristaltic) waves***Q.
- Diagnosis of the HPS can be established (confirmed) by either *USG (method of choice)*Q or barium study.

Ultrasonography (USG)

It is the **method of choice** to directly visualize the HPS. The examination is typically performed *with a high frequency linear transducer (>5MH$_2$)* (as the pylorus & duodenum are very superficial in an infant) with infant in *right posterior oblique position* (to move any fluid present in fundus into antral & pylorus region. The *stomach should not be emptied prior to examination* as this makes identification of antropyloric area difficult. If fluid is administered to make visualization better, it should be removed at the end of examination to prevent vomiting/aspiration. Features include)

1. **Doughnut appearance/Bull's eye or target sign** is hypoechoic (black) ring of hypertrophied pyloric muscle around echogenic (reflective) mucosa & submucosa on cross /transverse section images.
2. **Shoulder/cervix-sign** is indentation of hypertrophied muscle on fluid filled gastric antrum on longitudinal section.
3. **Antral nipple sign** is protrusion (evagination) of redundant pyloric mucosa into distended antrum.
4. **Double tract sign** refers to fluid trapped in center of elongated pyloric canal is seen as two sonolucent streaks in center.
5. Exaggerated peristattic waves & delayed gastric emptying of fluid into duodenum
6. **Elongated pylorus with thickened muscles (most specific)** is indicated by
   - **Length > 15mm, muscle thickness >3mm and transverse serosa to serosa diameter >15mm** is consistent with HPS. At least 2 values should be positive. A thickness <2mm is unequivocally normal and between 2 & 2.9mm is abnormal but non specific & can be seen in pylorospasm & gastritis also. Though *pylorospasm is transient & mostly resolve in 30 minutes and* there is considerable variation in measurement or image appearance with time during thickness. (GI imaging)
   - **Pyloric canal length ≥ *16-17mm, muscle wall thickness ≥ 3-3.2mm*Q**, pyloric volume > 1.4cm3, pyloric transverse diameter ≥13mm with pyloric canal closed and length (mm) + 3.64x + 3.64 x thickness (mm) >25 (Wolfgang)
   - Pyloric length >16mm & muscle thickness > 4mm (Swartz)

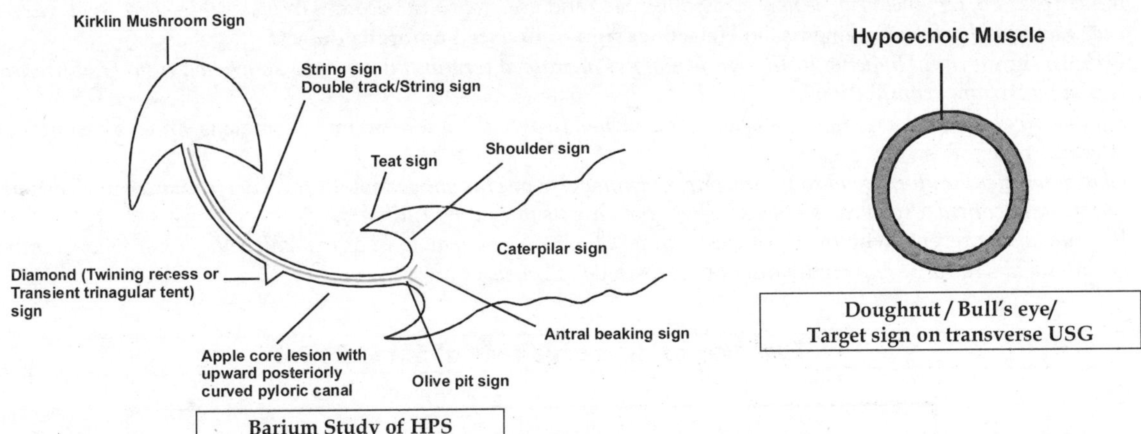

Barium Study of HPS

Doughnut / Bull's eye/ Target sign on transverse USG

Benign Ulcer	Malignant Ulcer
- Young age	- Old age
- Commonly seen on *lesser curvature*Q	- Commonly seen on *greater curvature*Q
- Margins of ulcer are **not** elevated, beaded & heaped up	- ***Heaped up*Q *& Beaded (nodular)*Q *margins***
- Sharply *punched out defect*Q with relatively straight walls	- Overt neoplastic tissue extending into the surrounding mucosa & wall
- *Base* of ulcer is ***smooth & clean***Q d/t peptic digestion & may show patent or thrombosed blood vessel	- Shaggy & ***necrotic base***Q
- Mucosal folds *radiate from crater in sponge like manner*Q	- Gastric folds are amputated or clubbed & ***do not reach the edge of the ulcer crater***Q
- **Ulcer mound** d/t mucosal edema - **Ulcer collar** – a lucent ring that separates the ulcer crater from gastric mucosa - **Hampton's line** - **Penetrating Sign** – i.e. the ulcer crater should project into stomach wall rather than into a mass in stomach wall.	- ***Carman's meniscus sign***Q – the barium which is trapped in ulcer bed gives meniscoid appearance (inner margin is concave towards lumen) - **Kirkland complex** – heaped margins touching bed, cause lucent rim around ulcer on barium meal - **Intraluminal crater** – the crater erodes into the mass within the gastric cavity.

RADIODIAGNOSIS 5

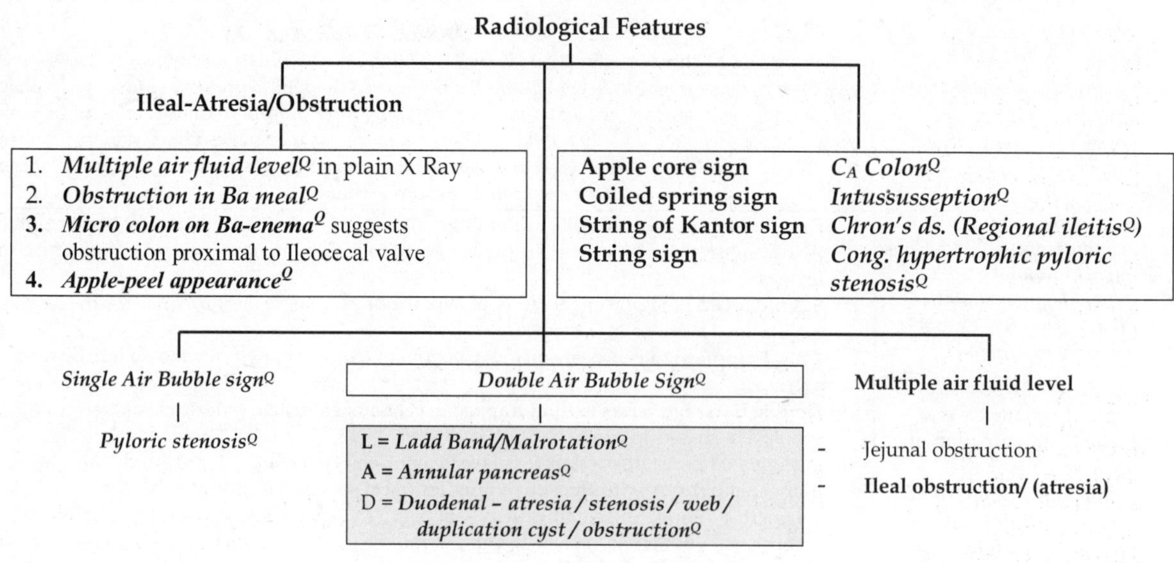

Ileocecal Tuberculosis

- It is the most common site of gastrointestinal tuberculosis (80 –90%). The *ileum particularly terminal part and ileocecal valve* are most commonly affected. The main radiological features are – ***mucosal fold thickening, discrete (usually transverse or star shaped & circum ferential) ulcers and stricture formation involving terminal ileum associated with funneled contracted caecum***Q.
- In ileocecal TB, *terminal ileum is narrowed & thickened* and *ileocecal valve* becomes *irregular thickened, rigid, incompetent, wide gaping and patulous* giving rise to **Fleischner sign or inverted umbrella defect**.
- **Steirlin sign** is ***rapid hyper motality (emptying) of narrowed terminal ileum into shortened rigid & obliterated cecum on barium examination***Q.
- ***Symmetrical annular napkin ring stenosis & widened ileocecal angle***Q (normal IC angle is 90° & it becomes obtuse in ileocecal tuberculosis).
- ***Characterstically ulcers tend to be descrete, & transverse or star shaped (stellate) + deep fissures with elevated margins, in contrast to chron's disease where they are usually longitudinal***Q.

★ Rt colonic TB presents with *rigid shortened contracted cone shaped amputated cecum with hourglass stricture*. Amputated cecum means retraction of cecum out of ileal fossa d/t fibrosis of mesocolon.

Radiological Investigations of Small Bowel

- **Plain Xray**
- **Barium studies such as**
1. Barium follow through
2. ***Enteroclysis (=small bowel enema)***Q
3. Double contrast & air contrast enteroclysis
4. Ileostomy emema, small bowel meal, peroral penumocolon examination

Enteroclysis = Small bowel enema

Preparation	Same as Barium meal follow through with or without laxatives
Procedure	Jejunal intubation by catheter through nasal route under fluoroscopy Dye is given and films are taken
Dye	Dilute barium/barium suspension followed by methylcellulose solution for double contrast view.

Barium meal follow through proved superior to enteroclysis, because of better muscosal detail.

- **Angiography**
- **Nuclear imaging** such as **FDG-PET, leukocyte scan** (for assessing inflammation), **^{99m}Tc scan** for meckel's diverticulum
- **Ultrasonography**

- **CT scan** (NE,CE), **CT** ***enteroclysis & CT enterography***Q
- **MRI and MRE (MR enteroclysis** using small bowel intubation, administration of biphasic contrast agent, heavily T2W single shot turbo spin echo **(SSTSE)** image for MR fluoroscopy & for monitoring the infusion process, T2W images imploying half-fourier acquisition single shot turbo spin echo **(HASTE)** and true **FISP** sequences, and dynamic T1W images using a post godolinium **FLASH sequence with fat suppression,**

Causes of radiopaque material in bowel

- Chloral hydrate
- Heavy metals
- Iron
- Phenothiazine
- Salicylate

Mnemonic – **"CHIPS"**

Calcification in right hypochondrium

- ***Gall stone, calcified (porcelain) gall bladder***Q
- Calcified lymph node/vessel/costal cartilage
- Hepatic adenoma, ***hemangioma***Q, metastases
- ***Calcification in substance of kidney***Q
- Phlebolith

Gasless Abdomen (Adult)

- High obstruction eg gastric outflow obstruction, congenital atresia
- Excessive vomiting eg ***acute pancreatitis***Q
- Fluid filled bowel eg closed loop obstruction, total active colitis, mesenteric infarction (early), bowel wash-out
- Large bowel mass (pushing bowel laterally)
- Ascites
- Normal

In children other causes of high obstruction & vomiting include

- Oesophageal atresia without fistula distally
- Hypertrophic pyloric stenosis
- Duodenal atresia, Annular pancreas, Choledochel cyst, volvulus (2° to malrotation)
- **Congenital diaphragmatic hernia**Q

Stepwise diagnostic approch to a patients with suspected chronic pancreatitis.

I. **CT scan** (calcification, atrophy &/or dilated duct seen for diagnosis)

↓

II. **MRI/MRCP with secretin-enhancement (sMRCP)**(Diagnostic criteria=Cambridge class III, dilated duct, atrophy of gland, filling defect in duct suggestive of stone)

↓

III. **Endoscopic ultrasound (EUS)** with quantification (≥5) of parenchymal & ductal criteria

↓

IV. **Pancreatic function test (with secretin)**- gastroduodenal (SST) or endoscopic (ePFT) collection method. Diagnostic criteria: peak $[HCO_3]$<80meq/L

↓

V. **Endoscopic Retrograde Cholangio pancreaticography (ERCP)**
DC: Cambridge III, dilated main pancreatic duct & >3 dilated side branch

Acute Pancreatitis

- Any severe acute pain in abdomen or back should suggest the possibility of acute pancreatitis. ***Abdominal pain,***is the major symptom of acute pancreatitis characteristically, the pain which is steady & boring in character, is located in ***epigastrium & periumbilical region***Q and often ***radiates to the back***Q as well as to the chest, flank & lower abdomen. The patient often obtains ***relief by sitting with the trunk flexed and knees drawn up***Q.
- When a patient with *possible predisposition to pancreatitis* (such as **gall stone, alcoholism**, *ERCP, hypertrigyceridemia, trauma, surgery and drugs like azathioprine, sulfonamides, estrogen, tetracycline, valproic acid, 6-merceptopurine & anti HIV drugs)* presents with severe & constant abdominal pain frequently a/w *nausea, fever, emesis, tachycardia, leukocytosis, hypocalcemia and hyperglycemia*, the diagnosis of **acute pancreatitis** is usually entertained.
- **Diagnosis of acute pancreatitis requires** 2 of the following: typical **abdominal pain, 3 fold or greater increase in serum amylase &/or lipase** (which usually establishes/clinch the diagnosis if gut perforation, ischemia or infraction are excluded, however, levels does not indicate the severity) and **confirmatory findings on cross sectional abdominal imaging.** ***A CTscan can confirm the diagnosis of acute pancreatitis***Q even with less than a 3 fold increase in serum amylase and lipase levels. It also indicates *severity of disease, risk of morbidity and mortality and evaluates complication* of acute pancreatitis. However, a CTscan within 3-5 days of symptom onset may *underestimate the extent of tissue injury* (hence repeated again). Sonography is useful to evaluate gallbladder if gall stone disease is suspected as etiology.

Liver Scan

Liver Colloid Scan

- **Liver Colloid Scintigraphy** (also k/a **Liver-Spleen-Bone marrow Scan**) uses **^{99m}Tc Sulfur Colloid** to localize *functional reticulo endothelial system (RES)* cells eg Kupffer cells. RES function and so radionucleide accumulation lies with in **liver (85%)**, *spleen (10%) and bone marrow (5%) and even abscess*. So it can be used for RES localization, bone marrow (hematopoietic system) localization or distribution and abscess localization. However bone marrow localization cannot be used to *determine sites of erythropoiesis*.
- **Colloid shift** (away from liver to bonemarrow & spleen) is seen in *diffuse hepatic dysfuncton/decreased hepatic perfusion* (such as cirrhosis, hepatitis, chronic

Hepato-Biliary Scintigraphy (IDA-Imaging)

- **^{99m}Tc acetanilide iminodiacetic acid analogs (IDA)** like *HIDA, BIDA, PIPIDA, DIDA, DISIDA & TMB-IDA* are used which are taken up by **hepatocytes** (dependent on substance's lipophilicity there is a trade off between hepatic uptake & renal excretion; BIDA most & HIDA least lipophilic)
- Albumin binding of tracer prevents it from renal excretion and so it is *taken up by functioning normal hepatocytes* (5-15 min post injection). Delayed liver uptake implies hepatocyte dysfunction or CHF (less likely). *Hepatocytesw secrete tracer without conjugation* **visualizing CBD** in 10-30 min **and gall bladder** in 20-60min. Tracer is excreted into duodenum within 1hr; no enterohepatic recirculation (no reabsorption).
- So, IDA compounds are taken up by functioning hepatocytes,

progressive congestion), *increased bone marrow activity* (eg hemolytic anemias, hematopoietic disorders), and increased spleenic activity/perfusion (eg hypersplenism) and long term corticosteroid.

- **Focal hot liver scan** is seen in ***Focal nodulr hyperplasia (d/t Kupffer cells)***Q, Budd Chiari syndrome (increased perfusion of caudate lobe wit decreased activity elsewhere), IVC/SVC obstruction (increased perfusion of quadrate lobe) and regenerating nodules of cirrhosis. (Mn "**Hot FBI is regenerating**")

Summary: Colloid scan demonstrates functioning tissue by targeting RES cells (eg Kupffer cells) of liver. So lesions containing functioning RES cells (like **focal nodular hyperplasia**) form **hot spots**. Whereas mass lesions without RES cells l/t nonfunctioning areas.

excreted unchanged in bile & not resorbed from the gut. It will allow imaging of liver parenchyma, trace the flow of bile, in the ducts, gall bladder & bowel. Its uses are: a) Assessment of liver function b) Biliary obstruction c) In liver trauma to see bile leaks d) Choledocal cyst e) Demonstration of G.B. function.

[18F] FDG-PET

- Highly sensitive in detecting **hepatic metastasis** from various primaries like colon, pancreas, parotid, oesophagus & sarcomas. It is more sensitive than CT for early detection of hepatic metastases **from recurrent colorectal cancer**
- Its sensitivity for *hepatocellular carcinomas* & their metastases is only 50% and can not detect poorly differentiated HCC. It is *also not suitable for benign primary liver lesions like hemangiomas, hepatocellular adenomas and FNH.*

Magnetic Resonance Cholangio Pancreatography (MRCP)

Magnetic Resonance Cholangio-Pancreatography (MRCP)

- **Magnetic reasonance cholangio pancreatography (MRCP)** is **non invasive** technique, which **uses heavilly T_2 weighted images of MRI (not CT) without contrast (mostly) to create 2D or 3 dimensional image of biliary (pancreatic) tree using maximum intensity projection (MIP) algorithm**Q.
- **Heavilly T_2 weighted biliary & pancreatic system images** of excellent diagnostic quality are obtained with high sensitivity & specificity for evaluation of *biliary duct dilation, strictures and intraductal anomalies* and benign & malignant disorders of biliary and pancreatic system. **In (heavily) T_2 weighted images, stationary or slowly moving fluid such as bile (even wihtout contrast)** is high in signal intensity, whereas all the surrounding tissues including retroperitoneal fat & solid visceral organs, are lower in signal (ie look darker).
- The ***'high signal bright bile technique'*** is preferred & performed using either CE- FAST (contrast enhanced Fourier aquired steady state) or *FSE (fast spin echo) pulse sequences in coronal plane without intravenous contrast agent.*

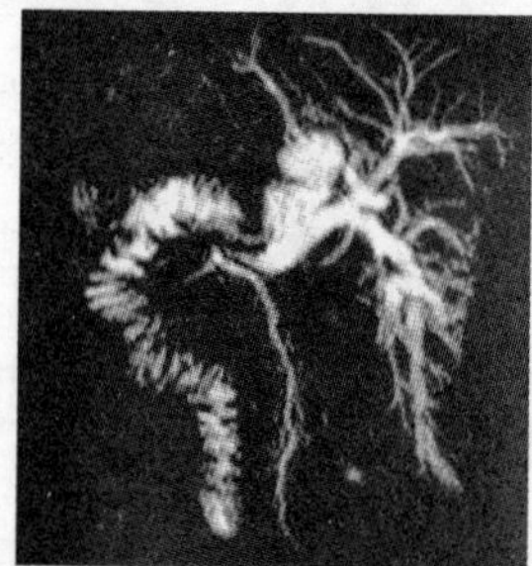

Single shot breath hold, **heavily T_2 weighted FSE/TSE MRCP** images demonstrating **high contrast fluid signals from biliary and pancreatic system**.

- *CE-FAST* is a variant of *gradient echo imaging* & utilize T_2-w breath hold sequences. It is more accurate in demonstrating *choledocholithiasis*. Whereas, FSE is *spin echo imaging* and more accurate in imaging *cause of obstruction in malignant biliary or pancreatic disease.*
- **Both hold T_2 weighted sequences** are obtained by refinement of **fast /turbo spin echo (FSE/TSE)** sequences to permit **single shot acquisitions** (single shot FSE/TSE sequence). Long echo train lenghts of 128 (180°) spin echos, often linked with **half Fourier K space filling (HASTE),** produce heavilly T_2 weighted images from a single excitation pulse (90%). The visulization of **static, long T_2 pancreaticobiliary fluids** resulting from long effective echo times **gives perfect contrast for MRCP (even without contrast injection).**
- MRCP images can be breath hold, non breath hold, respiratory gated, single thick slab acquisition (in 2-3s), multiple 2D slices (in 10-15s) even **3 dimensional (3D)** images in single breath hold. **Maximum intensity projection (MIP) algorithm** allows rotation of summed images, removes overlying high signal from stomach & small bowel and displays cholangiogram to best advantage.
- It is a ***non – invasive alternative to evaluate biliary tree***Q, **eliminating the morbidity associated with ERCP & PTC**. MRCP can visualize *common bile duct, common hepatic duct, & main right and left ducts.* It has replaced PTC (percutaneous transhepatic cholangiography) & ERCP in significant proportion. Since conventional MRCP does not rely on contrast excretion, it is *suitable for jaundiced patient, a major advantage over CT- intravenous cholangiography (CT – IVC).* **Surgical clips** may create **susceptibility artifact mimicing a stone**, which may obscure the region of interest by producing *areas of signal void.* So in postoperative patients cautions must be used to avoid false postive (stone) diagnosis.
- **Contrast enhanced MRCP** uses **intravenous hepatobilary contrast** eg. ***Mangafodipir trisodium, gadobenate dimeglumine & gadoxetic acid disodium***. Images are taken *30 min* after IV infusion to allow hepatocyte uptake and biliary excretion, therefore depends on near normal hepatocyte function (as with CT – IVC) and uses T_1 weighted images (allowing more manipulation). It is used for liver donor transplant workup, assessments of bile leak & biliary communication with cysts, detecting segmental obstruction. However, it is not as sensitive as MRCP for detecting choledocholithiasis.

Acute Pancreatitis	Chronic Pancreatitis	CA – Pancreas
- Renal Halo Sign - Gasless abdomen[Q] - ***Colon cut off sign***[Q] - Sentineal loop[Q]	- **Beaded** appearance - **String** of pearls appearance - Chain of **lakes** appearance - **Rat** Tail stricture / **Nipping** or narrowing of origins of side branches ± CBD.	- **Double** duct Sign - **S**crambled egg app. - **I**nverted 3 sign - **R**ose thorning of 2nd part of duodenum
Mnemonic- **"Read GCS"**	Mn: **"Be a strong Lovely Rat"**	Mnemonic- **"Double SIR"**

Causes of Air in Biliary tract

Air coming from GI tract through fistulas caused by
- Trauma
- Surgery
- *Malignancy*[Q]
- Duodenal Ulcer
- *Gall stone ileus*[Q]

Air Produced within Biliary tract
- *Emphysematous cholecystitis*[Q]

Air coming from GI tract d/t failure of closure of sphincter of oddi l/t reflux of duodenal gas
- Passage of Stone
- Passage of Ascaris (Biliary ascariasis)
- Surgery (endoscopic sphinct –erotomy, sphinctero plasty, papillotomy)

Adenomyomatosis of Gall bladder

- Adenomyomatosis is a special case of Gall Bladder cholesteatosis and belongs to the group of Hyperplastic Cholecystoses.
- It appears as a hyperechoic tumerous thickening of the gall bladder wall (generalized or focal) originating from hypertrophied Rokitanski-Aschoff Sinuses (Intramural Diverticulae).
- This disorder is ***charachterized by coexistant cholesterol deposits with their typical comet tail artifacts and cystic intramural inclusions. Types include***

Generalised form
- Generalised (diffuse) or segmental thickening of GB wall
- ***Pearl necklace gall bladder*** is tiny extraluminal extension of contrast on OCG/MR Cholangiography (T2WI)
- ***Comet tail***[Q] *is sound reverberating* ***artifact*** *between cholesterol crystals in RA sinus* ***(Pathognomonic).***
- ***String of Beads sign (bright high signal intensity areas in thickened gall bladder wall*** on T2WI of MRI (92% specific).

Localised form in fundus

Fundal nodular filling defect

Annular form

'Hourglass configuration of GB with transverse congenital septum.

- *Adenomyomatosis should also be differentiated from diffuse infiltrating gall bladder carcinoma. Gall bladder carcinoma lacks the Rokitanski-Aschoff sinuses and intramural comet-tail like artifacts.*

Xanthogranulomatous cholecytitis

It is inflammatory disease characterized by intramural extravasation of inspissated bile due to rupture of occluded Rokitansky – Aschoff sinus. On USG, it shows Intramural hypoechoic nodule.

Gall bladder carcinoma has 4 patterns

a. Gall bladder replaced by ill defined mass
b. Immobile intraluminal well defined oval mass
c. Focal or diffuse wall thickening with gall stone
d. Tumour inseperable from liver.

Comet-tail-like artifacts in gallbladder ultrasound:

Differential Diagnosis

	Emphyse-matous cholecystitis	Cholestea-tosis	Adenomyo-matosis	Microliths	Pneumonia
Size	Large	Normal	Normal or Smaller	Normal	Normal
Shape	Round	Normal	Hourglass furrows	Normal	Normal
Lumen	Sludge	Normal	Constricted	Floating (calculi < 5mm)	Normal
Wall	Hypoechoic wall thickening	Often normal or slightly thickened	***Hyperechoic, thickened,*** cystic inclusions	Normal	Normal
Comet-tail- like artifacts	Intramural or intraluminal gas collections	Intramural, partly few, partly diffuse	***Localized, intramural or diffuse***	Floating in the lumen	Position-dependent gas collections at the anterior wall

USG Features of Thyroid Lesion

Features	Benign	Malignant
Margins	Well marginated	- Ill marginated - Poorly defined
Echogenicity	Iso/hypo/hyperechoic	- ***Mostly hypoechoic***[Q]
Internal contents	- Purely cystic - Internal debris	- Cystic with mural nodules - Papillary excrescence
Halo	Sonoleucent peripheral halo d/t - Fibrous capsule & - Compressed blood vessels	Incomplete halo
Calcification	- Peripheral - Egg shell - Scattered echogenic large & coarse	- Fine & punctuate - Internal microcalcification
Vascularity	Peripheral vascularity	Internal vascularity

★ In general on USG lesions may be **cystic (anechoic**=dark black) and **solid (hypoechoic**=grey/light black or **hyper echoic** =seen white on USG). **Calcification** in any solid/cystic lesion l/t production of *hyper reflective/hyperechoic zones with acoustic shadowing*.

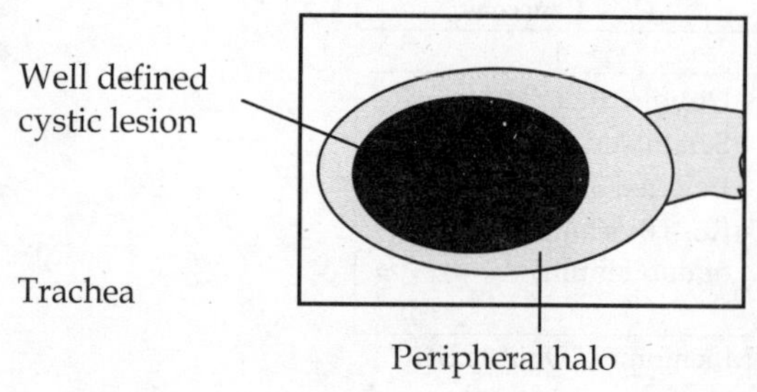

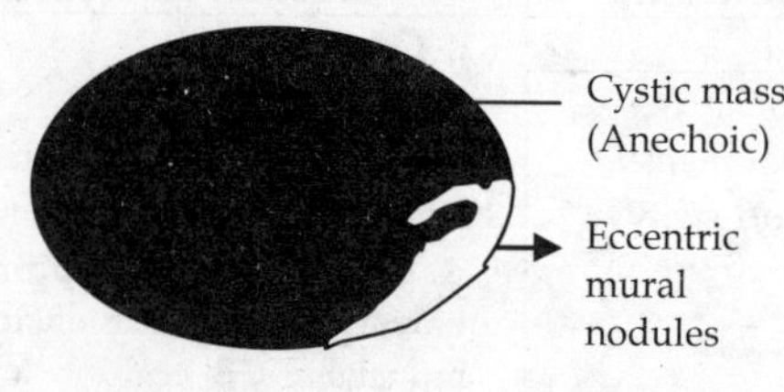

X Ray Hand

- Markedly ***Short 4th metacarpel bone*** → **Pseudo-hypoparathyroidism**
- ***Arrow head distal phalynx***Q → **Acromegaly** (characteristic feature is increased thickness of heel pad)
- ***Subperiosteal erosion***Q of radial aspect of middle phalynx of middle & index finger & Erosion of tuft → **Hyperparathyroidism** (other features are Brown's tumor, salt-pepper skull, Basket work app.)
- 1. Gull's wing appearance
  2. Licked-candy-stick appearance
  3. ***Tufting of distal phalynx***Q *(d/t new bone formation)*
  4. *Sausage digits*

  → **Psoriasis**

  Mnemonic- **"Girls Licking Tomato Sause"**

Mnemonic	Causes of Intervertebral Disc Calcification
All	= ***Alkaptonuria***Q ***(Ochronosis***Q***)***
Ankylosed	= ***Ankylosing Spondylitis***Q (i.e. non rheumatic ankylosis)
Degenerated	= Degenerative spondylosis
D	= DISH (Diffuse idopathic skeletal hyperostosis)
C	= ***CPPD(Ca-Pyrophosphate Dihydrate Deposition/Pseudogout)***Q
H	= Hemochromatosis
Girls	= Gout

Disease	Radiological features
Hyper PTH Mnemonic- **"Brown Erosed Salt Basket"**	- ***Brown's tumor (m.c. mandible)***Q - ***Subperiosteal*** Erosion ***(Hallmark)***Q - ***Salt pepper (pepper pot) appearance***Q - Basket work app.
Gaucher's ds	- ***Bone in Bone appearance***Q
Achondroplasia	- ***Trident Hand***Q - Tomb stone iliac bone - Cheuron sign (V shaped long bone epiphysis)
Pseudogout	- ***Calcification of menisical cartilage***Q

Radiological approach of Inflamatory Arthritis

- Periarticular soft tissue swelling
- Periarticular osteopenia (osteoporosis)
- Joint space narrowing
- Periostitis
- ***Erosions***Q
- Syndesmophytes
- Malalignment

Rheumatoid & its variants

- Symmetrical
- Small joints esp MCP & PIP joints
- Osteoporosis
- ***Erosions***Q
- ***Examples***
  - Rheumatoid arthritis
  - SLE
  - Scleroderma
  - Dermatomyositis

Seronegative Arthritis

- Asymmetrical
- Large joints – SI, spine & DIP joints of hand
- Osteoporosis less marked
- ***Periostitis***Q
- ***Syndesmophytes***Q
- ***Examples***
  - Ankylosing spondylitis
  - Psoriatic arthropathy
  - Reiter's Syndrome
  - Enteropathic arthritis

Characteristic Joint Involvement & Radiological Features (specific in arthritis)

Osteoarthritis
- *DIP (Heberden's node) = M.C.*Q*, PIP (Bouchard's node)*Q *& CM joint of thumb (CMI = 2nd M.C.)*Q along with hip, knee & spine are involved
- *Wrist & MCP joints are spared*Q
- Radiologically : **LOSS**
  1. *Loose bodies*Q — L
  2. *Osteophytosis*Q — O
  3. *Subchondral Cyst*Q — S
  4. *Subchondral bone sclerosis*Q — S

Gout
- *1st MTP joint*Q is M.C. involved
- Radiologically :
  - *Tophi*Q-eccentric soft tissue swelling which may *calcify*.
  - ***Strongly bierfringent needle shaped MSU (Sodium biurate) crystals***Q

Rheumatoid Arthritis
- Involve *MCP joint*Q *(M.C.) and PIP joint*Q
- ***Does not involve DIP joint***Q. Axial skeletal involvement is limited to cervical spine
- *Swan Neck Deformity*Q (Hyperextension at proximal interphalyngeal joint & hyper flexion at the distal interphalyngeal joint.
- *Boutonniere deformity*Q (Hyperflexion at proximal interphalyngeal joint, hyper extension at distal interphalyngeal joint
- *Hitch Hiker Thumb*Q (Ist metacarpophalyngeal joint flexion with interphalyngeal joint extension).
- *Hammer Toes*Q (Lateral deviation and or hyperextension at the metatarsophalyngeal joint and flexion of proximal or distal interphalyngeal joint)
- Ulnar deviation at M-P joint
- Ulnar translocation of carpus & erosin of ulnar stytoid

Pseudogout
- Knee is M.C. involved
- Radiologically:
  - *Chondrocalcinosis*Q is diagnostic (articular cartilage calcification)
  - ***Weakly positive bierfringent Rhomboid crystal***Q

Ankylosing Spondylitis
- *Sacroiliac joint*Q involvement is essential; spine & hip joints are usually involved.
- Radiologically : **BASSS**
  1. ***Bamboo/Rugger Jersy spine***Q — B
  2. *Anthesitis*Q — A
  3. *Sacroiliatis*Q — S
  4. *Syndesmophytes*Q, (delicate, vertically oriented) — S
  5. *Squarring of vertebrae*Q

Psoriatic Arthritis
- *DIP & MCP*Q joints are involved
- ***1st CM joint is not involved***Q
- Radiologically : **FOG-C**
  - **F**loating, nonmarginal, vertical syndesmophytes
  - **O**pera glass deformity
  - **Gull's wing appearance** (due to erosion of articular rather than Periarticular surface)
  - ***Cup and Pencil deformity***Q

Systemic Sclerosis (Scleroderma)

It is multisystem connective tissue disorder characterized by overproduction of collagen causing exuberant interstitial fibrosis and sclerosis of many organs. It is associated with ***CREST***Q -

C	=	Calcinosis of skin
R	=	Raynaud's phenomenon
E	=	Esophageal dysmotality
S	=	Sclerodactyly
T	=	Telangiectasia

Radiological features of Systemic Sclerosis

Musculoskeletal
1. Sausage digit
2. Sclerodactyly = Tapered finger i.e. atrophy & resorption of soft tissue and soft tissue calcifications.
3. ***Auto amputation = Pencilling = Acrosteolysis i.e. erosion of tip of distal phalynx***Q beginning at volar aspect
4. Calcinosis i.e. punctate soft tissue calcification.
5. Erosion of superior aspect of ribs.
6. Widening of periodontal membrane.

Pulmonary
1. B/L peripheral & bibasilar involvement
2. Ground glass appearance
3. Honey combing
4. ***Subpleural nodules***Q
5. Aspiration pneumonia

GI tract
1. Barrett oesophagus
2. Stricture
3. Dialation of esophageal sphincter

Radiological Features of Scurvy

Mnemonic-

Mnemonic	Features
True	*Trummer field zone*Q (metaphyseal lucency)
Pearly	*Pelkan spur*Q (Metaphyseal fracture)
Whiteness from	*Frankel white line*Q (radio dense metaphyseal end towards growth plate)
Wimbar	*Wimberger Sign*Q (small epiphysis marginated by sclerotic radiodense rim)

Adult

OsteoporosisQ

✶ Other radiological features are d/t increased bleeding tendancy l/t sub periosteal hematoma, periosteal elevation & ***cornor's sign*** (periosteal infarct)

- Metaphysis: Frankel's while line, trumerfeld lucent zone, Pelikan's spur due to fracture.
- Wimberger's sign (small epiphysis surrounded by sclerotic rim)
- Subperiosteal hemorrhage with periosteal elevation

Rickets (Children)

- ***Metaphysis: indistinct, frayed, splaying, and cupping of margin***Q. Patchy sclerosis in case of intermittent dietary deficiency
- Widened epiphysis with hazed cortical margin
- Generalized reduction in bone density
- Looser's zone (less common)
- Severe cases show Genu valgum, bow legs, thoracic kyphosis, pigeon chest, ***ricketic rosary***Q, skull bossing, cox vera.

1. ***Widening of physis (growth plate)***Q
2. ***Splaying & cupping of metaphysis***Q
3. Irregular metaphyseal margins
4. Rachitic Rosary ***(flaring of anterior ends of ribs)***Q
5. Bowing of extremity eg. genu valgum
6. ***Triradiate pelvis***Q

Also remember:
- Most obvious changes occur at metaphysis in rickets
- Initial abnormality in rickets is loss of normal 'zone of provisional calcification'.

RADIODIAGNOSIS 5

- Ground glass appearance of bone with pencil thin cortex.

Osteomalacia: Mn- **"Losse Pencilin Fish"**	- ***Looser's zone***[Q] *or* ***Pseudofracture***[Q] (Hallmark) - Pencilling-in- of vertebral bodies - ***Cod – fish (marked biconvex) vertebrae***[Q]
Renal Osteodystrophy (d/t CRF):	- It combines findings of ostemalacia, hyperparathyroidism and bone sclerosis - Osteomalacia l/t Looser's zone - Hyper PTH l/t Subperiosteal Erosion of bone - *Osteosclerosis l/t Rugger Jersey* ***spine***[Q] (End plate sclerosis with alternating bands of radiolucency)
Hyperparathyroidism **Mn:** O.P. = Lost = Brown = Erosed = Salt = Basket =	 **O**steo**p**enia **Loss** of lamina dura **Brown**'s tumor ***Subperiosteal Erosion (pathognomic)***[Q], Subchondral erosion & intracortical erosions l/t cigar shaped lucencies ***Salt & Pepper/Pepper-pot skull***[Q] Basket work appearance of cortex

Hypothyroidism

- Thyroid is important in growth regulation. Its deficiency l/t marked decrease in cartilage cell proliferation of growth plate & osseous tissue abutting growth zone. Radiological manifestation of these pathological process include:
  - ***Delayed appearance & closure of epiphysis***[Q]
  - ***Retarded skeletal growth & maturation***[Q]
  - ***Epiphyseal dysgenesis***[Q] ***(Fragmented epiphysis)***[Q]
  - Decrease longitudinal growth l/t short thick bones
- Other features are :
  - Osteoporosis (osteopenia)
  - Delayed dentition

Causes of Cupping & Fraying of Metaphysic

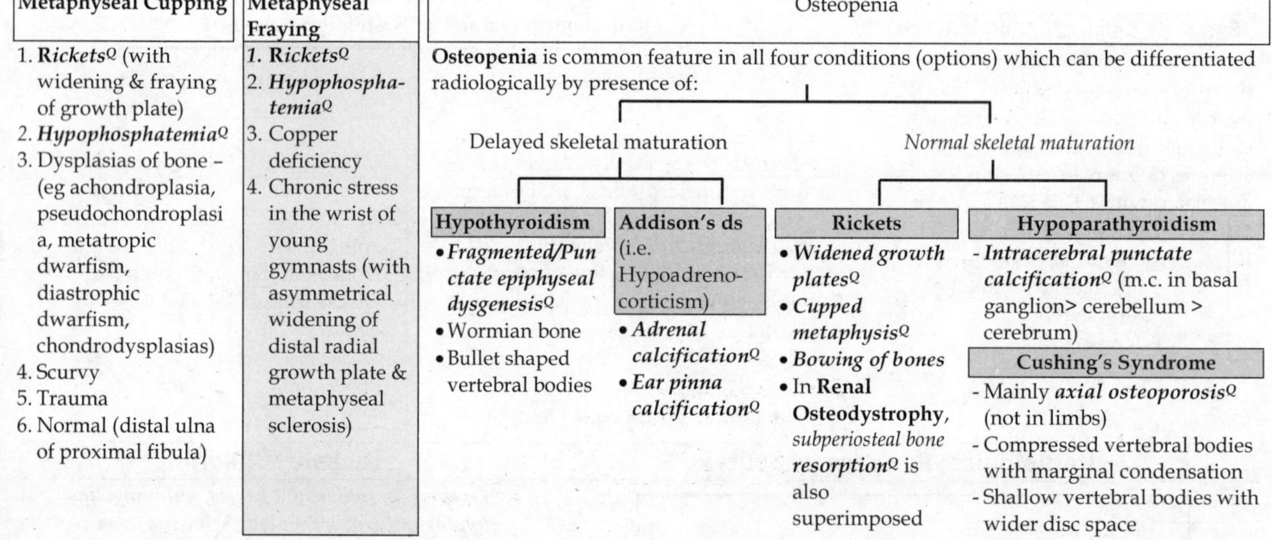

Metaphyseal Cupping

1. ***Rickets***[Q] (with widening & fraying of growth plate)
2. ***Hypophosphatemia***[Q]
3. Dysplasias of bone – (eg achondroplasia, pseudochondroplasia, metatropic dwarfism, diastrophic dwarfism, chondrodysplasias)
4. Scurvy
5. Trauma
6. Normal (distal ulna of proximal fibula)

Metaphyseal Fraying

1. ***Rickets***[Q]
2. ***Hypophosphatemia***[Q]
3. Copper deficiency
4. Chronic stress in the wrist of young gymnasts (with asymmetrical widening of distal radial growth plate & metaphyseal sclerosis)

Osteopenia

Osteopenia is common feature in all four conditions (options) which can be differentiated radiologically by presence of:

Delayed skeletal maturation

Hypothyroidism
- ***Fragmented/Punctate epiphyseal dysgenesis***[Q]
- Wormian bone
- Bullet shaped vertebral bodies

Addison's ds (i.e. Hypoadreno-corticism)
- ***Adrenal calcification***[Q]
- ***Ear pinna calcification***[Q]

Normal skeletal maturation

Rickets
- ***Widened growth plates***[Q]
- ***Cupped metaphysis***[Q]
- ***Bowing of bones***
- In **Renal Osteodystrophy**, *subperiosteal bone* ***resorption***[Q] is also superimposed

Hypoparathyroidism
- ***Intracerebral punctate calcification***[Q] (m.c. in basal ganglion> cerebellum > cerebrum)

Cushing's Syndrome
- Mainly ***axial osteoporosis***[Q] (not in limbs)
- Compressed vertebral bodies with marginal condensation
- Shallow vertebral bodies with wider disc space

Easy way to remember causes of Metaphyseal cupping is

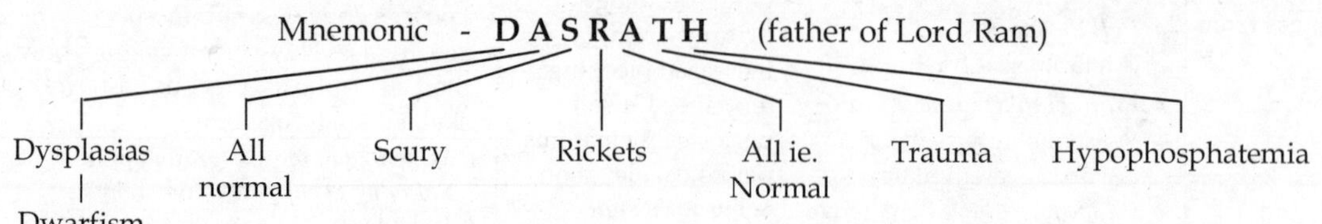

Radiological Approach of Radiolucent Lesion

Simple Bone Cyst (Centric)
- **< 20 years age**
- ***Proximal Humerus***[Q] (50%), Proximal femur (25%)
- ***Metaphyseal***[Q]
- ***Centric Expansile radiolucent lesion***[Q] (i.e. centrally located)
- Fallen fragment sign (it is a single chamber cavity ,so any fractured cortex settles in the most dependent portion)

Aneurysmal Bone Cyst = ABC (Eccentric)
- **< 20 years age**
- Femur, tibia, spine
- Metaphyseal
- ***Eccentric*** (not in centre) ***Blow out/ Ballooned-out radiolucent lesion***[Q]
- Trabeculated/Bubbly appearance due to pseudoloculation

Osteochondroma (M.C. bone tumor)
- **< 20 years**
- Distal femur, Proximal tibia, Proximal humerus
- **Metaphyseal/ Diaphyseal**
- ***Sessile or pedunculated bony stalk***[Q]
- **The cortex & cancellous bone of O.C. blends with cortex & cancellous bone of host.**

Osteoclastoma
- ***20-40 years***[Q]
- Proximal tibia, distal femur, lower end radius, proximal humerus
- ***Metaphysis /Epiphysis***[Q]
- ***Soap Bubble appearance***[Q]

In Summary

S.B.C., ABC & OC all occur in < 20 years age and metaphyseal region (OC may become diaphyseal with gradual growth of bone) and these are differentiated by presence of fallen fragment sign & centric location in S.B.C.; presence of trabeculated/Bubbly/Pseudoloculated appearance & eccentric location in ABC; and presence of sessile or pedunculated bony stalk whose cortical & cancellous bones are in continuation with normal bone and direction away from epiphysis in O.C.

Feature	ABC	Osteoblastoma
Number	Involvement of contigous vertebrae may occur	Usually solitary
Calcification or ossification	Not present	***Calcification or ossification***[Q] of osteoid tissue with in the tumor may cause punctate or amorphous ***increase in density (i.e. more radiodense)***[Q]
Margins & Reactive Sclerosis	Absence of bone reaction (sclerosis) & poorly defined margins	Margins are more defined and reactive sclerosis is present
Fluid-fluid level	Present	Absent
Trabeculation	Present	Absent
Location	Eccentric	Uniform fusiform

Disease	Radiological Feature
Osteosarcoma	• *Variable mixture of radiopacities & radiolucency* ***(hallmark)***[Q] • ***Sun burst/ sun ray appearance***[Q] (IInd) • ***Codman's triangle***[Q] (non specific)
Osteoclastoma	***Soap Bubble appearance***[Q]
Ewing's Sarcoma	***Onion peel appearance***[Q]
Paget's disease	• In Osteolytic Hot phase - **A**dvancing wedge/**B**lade of Grass/**C**andle flame appearance (Mn = **ABC**) • In Mixed phase - ***Cotton Ball Skull***[Q] - ***Picture Frame Vertebrae***[Q] • In Cool Phase - Bowing - Bone density increased

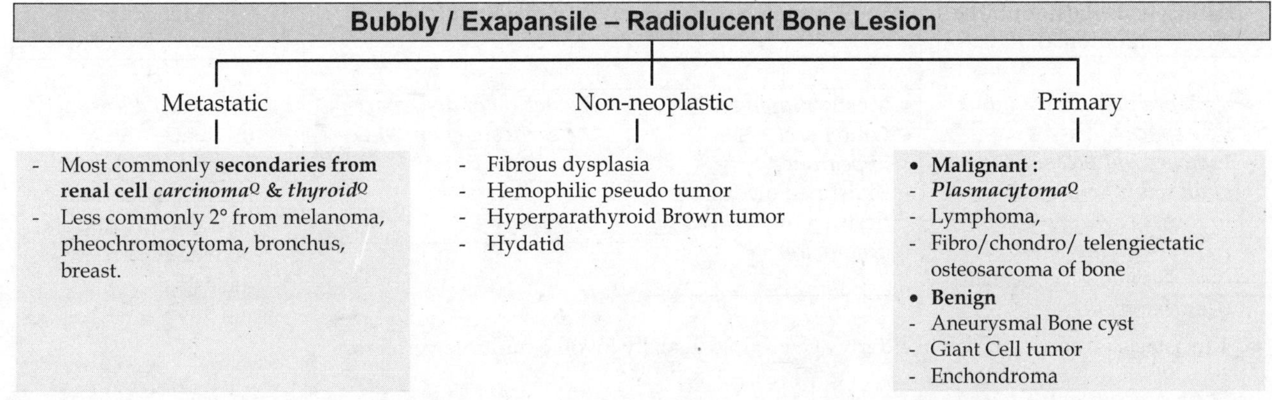

Bubbly / Exapansile – Radiolucent Bone Lesion
Metastatic
- Most commonly secondaries from renal cell carcinoma[Q] & thyroid[Q]
- Less commonly 2° from melanoma, pheochromocytoma, bronchus, breast.
Non-neoplastic
- Fibrous dysplasia
- Hemophilic pseudo tumor
- Hyperparathyroid Brown tumor
- Hydatid
Primary
• Malignant :
- Plasmacytoma[Q]
- Lymphoma,
- Fibro/chondro/ telengiectatic osteosarcoma of bone
• Benign
- Aneurysmal Bone cyst
- Giant Cell tumor
- Enchondroma

Bone-Metastases / Secondaries

A/t Devitta onchology

Mostly Blastic
- *Prostate*Q
- *Carcinoid*Q (Abdominal & bronchial)

Usually lytic but frequently blastic
- *Breast*Q

Invariably lytic
- *Kidney*Q
- *Thyroid*Q

✶ **Large expansile secondaries** are also from *thyroid & hypernephroma*Q.

A/t Radiology

Calcifying Bone Metastases
- Breast
- **Osteosarcoma**Q
- Thyroid
- Testis
- Ovary
- Mucinous adenocarcinoma of GI tract
(Mn-**"BOTTOM or BROOM-2t"**)

With Sunburst Periosteal Reaction

Prostate carcinoma, Neuroblastoma (skull), Retinoblastoma, GI tract cancer (**Mn-"PNR-tract"**; is infrequent)

Bone Metastase with Soft tissue Mass

Kidney, Thyroid (Mn "**KiT** is soft")

Permeative Bone Lesions

Mycosis fungoides, Burkitt lymphoma (Mn "**My Burr Permeates Well**")

Osteolytic Bone Metastases

Sign of destruction; may begin in *spongy bone (a/w soft tissue mass in ribs)* and often involve *vertebral pedicles* (not invoved in multiple myeloma) eg include Neuroblastoma (in children), Kidney, Thyroid, Colon, Lung & Breast.
(Mn:**New ki Te Col**ors **B**lue = New kite's colour is blue")

Osteoblastic Bone Metastases

Indicates slow growing neoplasm
- ProstateQ
- LymphomaQ
- Brain (Medulloblastoma)
- Bowel (Malignant carcinoid & mucinous adenocarcinoma)
- Bladder (TCC)
- Breast
- Bronchus

Mn-"**Problem lies in 5Bs**")
However, **BPL** i.e. *breast, prostato & lymphoma* cause *mixed bone metastases.*

Sonographic findings of Spina bifida

Spina bifida is most common in **lumbosacral region** (90%).

1. ***Ventriculomegaly***Q with hydrocephalus
2. **Banana sign** – ***Cerebellum is stretched***Q around the brain stem with ***effacement of cisterna magna***Q.
3. **Lemon sign** – Flattening of frontal bones on transverse image.
4. Bony decept in spine
5. V shaped profile d/t outward flaring of two posterior ossification centres.
6. Presence of intact sac on posterior aspect of spine
7. Sac filled with fluid or solid tissue in meningocele or myelomeningocele.

	Cord Edema	Myelomalacia /Cord atrophy
Etiology	Reflects focal accumulation of intracellular & interstitial fluid in response to injury	In end stage of cord trauma and result of trauma, ischemia and release of vasoactive substances & cellular enzyme.
MRI *T1WI*Q *T2WI*Q	• Ill defined *hypointense area* • Focus of *hyperintensity*	• Poorly marginated *hypointense area* • ***Hyperintense***Q cord parenchyma

Radiological Peculiarities

Histiocytosis (Eosinophillic granuloma)
- *Vertebra plana with intact disc space*Q
- *Punched out lucencies in skull vault*Q may coalesce to form ***geographical skull***Q
- *Destructive lesion in skull base, mastoid, sell or mandible (floating teeth*Q*)*

Ewing's SA
- Mostly *diaphyseal*Q
- ***Onion peel appearance***Q
- Ill defined medullary destruction *(moth eaten appearance)*

Tuberculosis
- ***Reduction of disc space is the earliest sign in M.C. paradiscal type.***Q
- ***Cold abscess***Q
- Deformity

Metastasis
- ***Preserved disc space***Q until late
- Paravertebral soft tissue mass is more common in multiple myeloma than metastasis

✶ Metastasis is more common in elderly age group & usually involve multiple vertebra.

Ossification of Posterior Longitudinal Ligament [OPLL]

- OPLL is a dense, ossified strip of variable thickness along the posterior margin of vertebral bodies resulting in spinal cord compression
- Often called 'Japanese disease'
- ***Most common in mid and lower cervical spine***Q.
- Multilevel involvement is characteristic.
- On **CT scan,** Involved portion of the ligament is replaced by high density of calcium.
- **MRI scan** is the ***investigation of choice***Q for spinal stenosis
  Ossification is represented by ***low signal on all pulse sequences***Q
  On gradient echo sequences owing to magnetic susceptibility (blooming effect,) ***osteophytes size may be exaggerated resulting in overestimation of canal stenosis***Q.

BI-RADS (Breast Imaging Reporting & Data System) Categories (Americal College of Radiology)

Category	Description (For mamography, USG MRI)	Malignancy Likelihood
0	**Need additional imaging evaluation** (or prior mamogram for comparion) because of incomplete or technically unsatisfactory information	--
1	**Negative** (Mammography, USG, MR) finding. Routine mamogram in 1 year is recommended.	0%
2	**Benign findings** on mammography, USG, MR. Routine mamogram in 1 year is recommended.	0%
3	**Probably benign findings**. Initial short interval follow up suggested (in 6 months)	2%
4	**Suspicious abnormality. Biopsy should be considered.** 4a=low (3-50%): 4b= intermediate (50-80%) and 4c= moderate(80-90%) probability of malignancy	3-90%
5	**Highly suggestive of malignancy** (≥95%)- appropriate action should be taken eg surgical treatment, however, biopsy (image guided core needle biopsy) usually required	>90%
6	**Biopsy proven malignancy**	100%

Breast

Mammogram	Benign	Malignant
Opacity	- ***Smooth margin***Q - ***Low density***Q - Homogenous - Thin halo	- ***Ill defined margin***Q ***(speculated,***Q **comet tail, stellate)** - ***High density***Q - **Inhomogenous** - Wide halo
Calcification	- ***Macrocalcification***Q (>0.5 mm diameter) - *Egg shell curvilinear* (in fat necrosis & cyst) - *Popcorn* (in fibroadenoma) - *Floating calcification* (in milk of calcium cyst) - Tramline / tortous calcification - Rod like wide spread calcification (some with radiolucent centre) - Lobular calcification	- **Microcalcification** (<0.5 mm dia) - **Granular (amorphous, dot like elongated)** calcification - **Casting calcification** (fragmented cast of calcification within ducts).

Indications: Standard Techniques used for Screening Early Stage Ca Breast

Mammography
- **50 years – asymptomatic women**
- **≥35 years – asymptomatic women with risk factor** (Ist degree relative has breast C_A, has ductal hyperplasia)
- **35 years – symptomatic women (evidence of early stage C_A breast)**Q
- Breast lump in man
- Follow up after excision

Breast (Real time) USG
- **< 35 years – symptomatic women**
- Breast lump during pregnancy or lactation
- Second look procedure after mammography, scintimammography, MRI
- Breast mass with negative mammogram
- Guidance of needle biopsy
- Breast inflammation
- Follow up after chemotherapy

Skin	Normal	Thickened
Nipple / Areola	± Retracted	± Retracted
Cooper ligament	Normal	Thickened
Ducts	Normal	Focal dialation
Subcutaneous retromammary space	Normal	Obliterated
Surrounding parenchyma	Normal	Disrupted

Mammographic Appearance of Breast

- The mammographic appearance of breast depends on the relative amount of fat and glandular tissue which are present. ***Young woman's breast contains a large proportion of glandular tissue which appears as a soft tissue density***[Q] and lowers the sensitivity of mammogram.
- **Mammographic appearance of breast (Based on the relative amount of fat and glandular tissue)**

- **Glandular breast** (dense breast): In young woman, where breast contains large amount of glandular tissue
- **Adipose breast:** (Fatty breast) In older women where most of the glandular tissue has involuted
- **Involuting breast:** When mixture of soft tissue and fat density present.

Fat Containing Breast Lesions

Fat- Containing breast lesion[Q] *(Fat contained within a lesion proves benignity i.e. the lesion is benign)*

- Lipoma
- Galactocele
- Traumatic lipid cyst = fat necrosis
- Oil cyst
- Hamartoma

- *Mammography is the screening modality of choice* for breast cancer because it can detect micro calcification which is often the only manifestation of DCIS.
- The sensitivity of ultrasound for detecting DCIS is significantly lower than mammography that is why USG is not a useful screening test for breast cancer.
- ***MRI can not detect calcification***[Q]

Breast MRI

- Lobular carcinoma which is difficult to detect and measure by conventional method because of multifocal and infiltrating growth pattern.
- Staging of primary breast cancer
- Occult primary tumour with malignant axillary lymphadenopathy and normal mammogram and breast USG.
- Screen younger women with high familial risk of breast cancer.
- Assessing the integrity of breast implant

Triple Assessment

In any patient who presents with a breast lump or other symptoms suspicious of carcinoma, the triple diagnostic approach is used to confirm the diagnosis. ***Triple assessment***[Q] comprises of :-

- Clinical examination
- Radiological imaging – mammography or ultrasound
- Pathological assessment – cytology or biopsy.

Pheochromocytoma & Paraganglioma

- Pheochromocytomas & paragangliomas are catecholamine producing tumors that arise from **paraganglion (chromaffin) cells anywhere in autonomic nervous system.** These well vascularized tumors arise from **cells of sympathetic (adrenal medulla) or parasympathetic (eg glomus vagale, carotid body) paraganglia.** Term pheochromocytoma is used for *symptomatic catecholamine producing tumors, including those in extraadrenal, retroperitoneal, pelvic and thoracic site*. Whereas, paraganglioma term is used for catecholamine producing tumors in head and neck (Harrison)/ extraadrenal region (Haga). These may secrete little or no catecholamines.
- Pheochromocytoma originate in **adrenal medulla** mostly (90%); whereas, most common site for extraadrenal pheochromocytoma is **paravertebral sympathetic ganglia in organ of Zuckerkandl** (near aortic bifurcation) or rarely in bladder.
- **Rule of tens:** pheochromocytomas are **extraadrenal/ multicentric/ in children/bilateral/malignant/familial or syndromic/ nonfunctioning** in 10% of cases (each). Syndromic cases are a/w MEN type IIA & IIB, von Hippel Lindau disease, neurofibromatosis, Sturge-Weber syndrome, Carney's triad, tuberous sclerosis and isolated
- Plasma – catecholamines, free metanephrins; & chromogranin A and urinary (24 hour) vanillyl mandelic acid, catecholamines, fractioned & total metanephrines are elevated on biochemical testing. The diagnosis is based on *demonstration of catecholamine excess by biochemical tests and localization of tumor by imaging (CT, Gadolinium MRI, I^{131} or I^{123} MIBG, In^{111}Somatostatin analogues scintigraphy or F^{18} dopamine PET).*
- **CT and MRI are similar in sensitivity for localization of adrenal pheochromocytoma**. CT should be performed with contrast and T_2 WI MRI with gadolinium contrast is optimal. **Contrast enchanced CT is currently the investigation of choice in detecting, evaluating& confirmaing adrenal lesions including adrenal pheochromocytoma** (Grainger, AMPIS) because of cost and availability.
- **MRI** is also excellent for evaluating & confirming adrenal masses including pheochromocytoma and is (if available) or will become **investigation of choice** (Sutton, Wolfgang). On MRI pheochromocytomes are hypointense on T1 WI and usually **markedly hyperintense (light bulb appearance) on T_2 weighted images** d/t lung T_2 relaxation times. Although this typical T_2 WI is neither sensitive (as they are more often heterogenous with intermediate or high T_2 signal intensity) nor specific (as may be seen in adrenal metastases).

familial pheochromocytoma.

- Characteristic clinical findings include **episodes of palpitations, headache, profuse sweating (classic triad),** tremor; anxiety, tachycardia, **sustained or paroxysmal hypertension,** panic attacks, pallor, nausea, abdominal pain, weakness, weight loss, paradoxical response to antihypertensive drugs, orthostatic hypotension, polyuria, polydypsia, constipation, dialated cardiomyopathy, erythrocytosis, elevated blood sugar and hypercalcemia. **The episodes lasts <1 hour and may be precipitated by biopsy, surgery,** positional changes, exercise, pregnancy, urination (especially bladder pheochromocytoma).
- ***Due to risk of catastrophic hypertensive crisis and fatal cardiac arrhythmia, fine needle aspiration cytology (FNAC) of pheochromocytoma is contraindicated***[Q]. Injection of intravenous contrast dye or glucagon, anesthesia and surgical procedure can also trigger the catestrophic crisis.
- However, **MRI is slightly better than CT for imaging extradrenal pheochromocytomas & paragangliomas and in detecting recurrence after surgery.**
- Investigation of choice for **locally recurrent, metastatic, Ectopic & Extra – adrenal pheochromocytoma** is ***metaiodobenzylaguanidine (MIBG) Scan***[Q] **(using I^{123} or I^{131}). Sensitivity of imaging modalities for extraadrenal pheochromocytomas: MIBG > MRI (contrast enhanced T_2 WI) > CT (CE) > USG.**
- Both CT, MRI can suggest the diagnosis of pheochromocytome but it must be confirmed clinically & biochemically. MIBG is the only definitive imaging test, but a positive MIBG scan (sensitivity 80-90% specificity 90-100%) should always be correlated with CT or MRI
- **Sensitivity of imaging modalties** for **adrenal pheochromocytoma.**

CT=MRI > MIBG >USG

Features of Hyperparathyroidism

O.P.	=	Osteopenia
Lost	=	Loss of lamina dura
Brown	=	Brown's tumor
Erosed	=	*Subperiosteal Erosion (pathognomic)*[Q], Subchondral erosion & intracortical erosions l/t cigar shaped lucencies
Salt	=	*Salt & Pepper/Pepper-pot skull*[Q]
Basket	=	Basket work appearance of cortex

Thyroid Cancer

Papillary CA
- **Most common**
- **Best Prognosis**
- **Lymph node** metastasis is most common in this type
- Occurs d/t **Radiation Thyroglossal Cyst Hashimoto ds**

Follicular CA
- **No use of FNAC** as benign and malignant types can't be differentiated
- **Occurs in Endemic goiter**
- **Bone secondaries** is m.c. in the type
- **Hurthle cells** are seen
- **Takes up I_2 ,so radio iodine is used in treatment**
- **Hurthle cells** seen in –
  - **Follicular CA**
  - **Hashimoto ds**

Medullary CA
- Occurs with **MEN***
- **Calcitonin** is marker
- **Amyloid pattern** is seen
- ↑ S. Ca^{++}

Mnemonic - **"Multiple Endocrine Neoplasia"**

Anaplastic

External Radiation + CT is used in treatment

Echogenicity of Thyroid nodules
- *The echogenecity of thyroid nodule refers to its brightness compared to the normal thyroid parenchyma*
- *A nodule is charachterized as hypoechoic,isoechoic,hyperechoic or anechoic*
- *Hypoechogenecity is associated with thyroid malignancy.* ***'Malignancies always have a Hypoechoic or nonhomogeneous hypoechoic structure'***

Differentiation of thyroid nodules according to ecgo-genicity

Echogenecity of the Nodule	Most likely diagnosis
Hyperechoic, isoechoic	Adenomatous (colloid) noodule
Hypoechoic	Follicular adenoma Malignoma Metastasis
Mixed echogenicity	Large nodules (follicular adenomas as well as colloid nodules) with regressive changes
Anechoic	Cyst

Ultrasound features of carcinoma in a Thyroid Nodule

Feature	Carcinoma/Malignancy
Structure	***Hypoechoic/ Nonhomogeneous/*** Solid
Regressive changes	Rare
Microcalcifications	***Common***
Peripheral rim	Variable
Internal vascularity	Common(70-100 percent)
Lymph nodes	Relatively common

Note : *A hypoechoic lesion may be benign or malignant,* however a ***hyperechoic lesion is most often benign***

Characteristics	Benign Adrenal adenoma	Malignan Adrenal carcinoma
Size	Smaller (<4-5 cm)	Larger
Appearance	Well circumscribed, sharply defined ***Smooth regular margins***^{Q} *Homogenous*	Not Irregular margins Heterogenous
Calcification, Necrosis, Haemorrhage	*Rare*^{Q} (may be seen in larger masses l/t heterogenous appearace)	Common
Non contrast CT scan	*Low attenuation*^{Q} (<10HU) d/t lipid content	High attenuation (>10HU)
Contrast enhanced CT scan	- ***Relatively rapid washout of contrast material (due to lack of large interstitial spaces)*** - *Mild homogenous enhancement* - ***< 37 HU on delayed CECT (> 5-15 minutes after contrast injection) due to relatively rapid washout*** is charachteristic (diagnostic) of adenoma.	***Delayed (slow) washout***^{Q} May invade adjacent organs extending into IVC, and involve lymph nodes and metastases to the liver, lung and bone. Functional imaging using **(F-18) FDG-PET/CT** can be used to map the full extent of spread.

Radiological picture of **Leukemia** & **Metastatic Neuroblastoma** in **Childhood.**

1. ***Metaphyseal translucencies***^{Q} –most characterstic sign, is presence of *translucent dark band running across the metaphysis below growth plate.*
2. **Metaphyseal cortical erosion**
3. ***Metaphyseal osteosclerosis***^{Q}
4. ***Periosteal reaction & new bone formation***^{Q}
5. ***Osteolytic lesions***^{Q} – any bone may be involved, commenest are shaft of long bones

✶ **Osteoporosis,** translucent areas with bone destruction & collapse are found in adults

✶ Metastatic neuroblastoma is differentiated from leukemia by seperation of suture of skull in former condition.

Causes of 'Hair on End' Skull Vault

1. **Hemolytic anemias**
   - ***Thalassemia major / Cooley's anemia (most common)*** ^{Q}
   - ***Sickel cell anemia***^{Q}
   - Others ex spherocytosis, elliptocytosis, G6PD deficiency, pyruvate kinase deficiency.
2. Neoplastic
   - Hemangioma, Meningioma, Metasasis
3. Others
   - Cynotic heart disease
   - Iron deficiency anemia
   - Ewing's sarcoma, Syphilis, Infantile Cortical hyperostosis (caffey's ds)

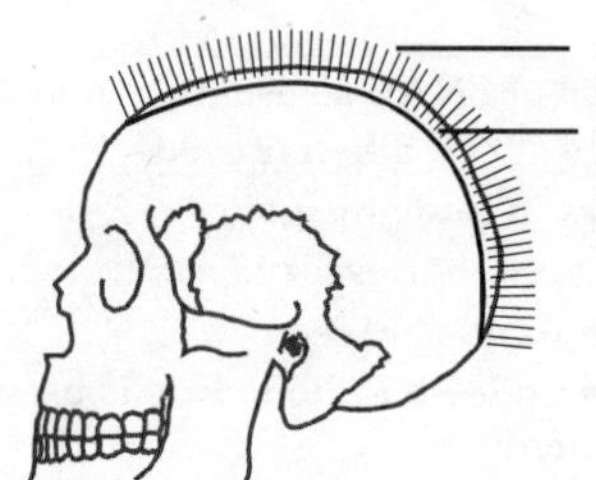

Floating teeth^{Q} i.e. No obvious supporting bone for the teeth is seen in.

- ***Langerhans cell histiocytosis***^{Q}
- Hyperparathyroidism
- Metastases
- Multiple myeloma
- Lymphoma, Leukemia

Sickle Cell Disease

- Caused by substitution of ***glutamic acid by valine at 6th position***^{Q} in β-chain of Hb
- Radiological changes

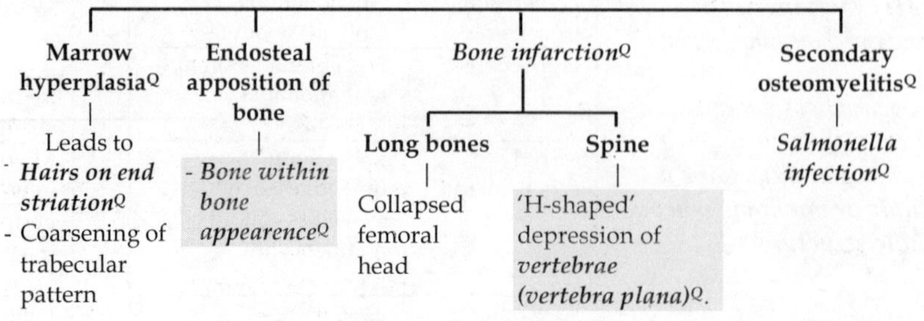

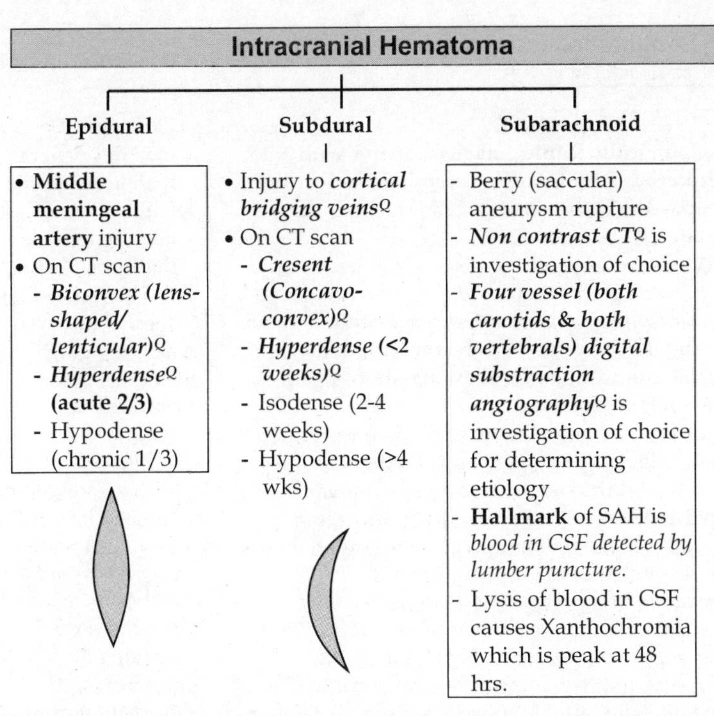

EDH	SDH
• Across dural attachment not sutures • CT *Biconvex*Q - 2/3 *Hyperdense*Q - 1/3 Mixed appearance i.e. Hyperdense & Hypodense	• Across sutures but not dural attachments • CT-*cresentic* ***(Concave-convex)***Q - Acute SDH (< 2 weeks) – Hyperdense - Subacute SDH (2-4 weeks) – Isodense - Chronic SDH (> 4 weeks) - Hypodense

It is difficult to diagnose isodense hematomas then it becomes necessary to rely on indirect signs:
- Contralateral displacement of ventricle or pineal (absent in B/L cases)
- Absence of visible sulci on affected side
- Squeezing of frontal horns to give a *rabbits ear's appearance* & effacement of basal cisterns suggesting B/L isodense lesion.

Sub Arachnoid Haemorrhage (SAH)

- Most common intracranial lesion after head injury is ***subdural hematoma***Q. Most common cause of SAH is ***Head trauma***Q. M.C. cause of spontaneous SAH is ***ruptured saccular aneurysm***Q. Other causes include bleeding from a vascular malformation (AV mal formation or dural AV fistula) and extension into the subarachnoid space from a primary intracerebral hemorrhage.
- Sudden rise in ICP accounting for **sudden transient loss of consciousness** which may be preceded or followed by (a brief moment of) **excruciating headache (worst headache of life)**. Although sudden headache **in the absence of focal neurological symptoms** is the hallmark of aneurysmal rupture, *focal neurological deficit may occur*.

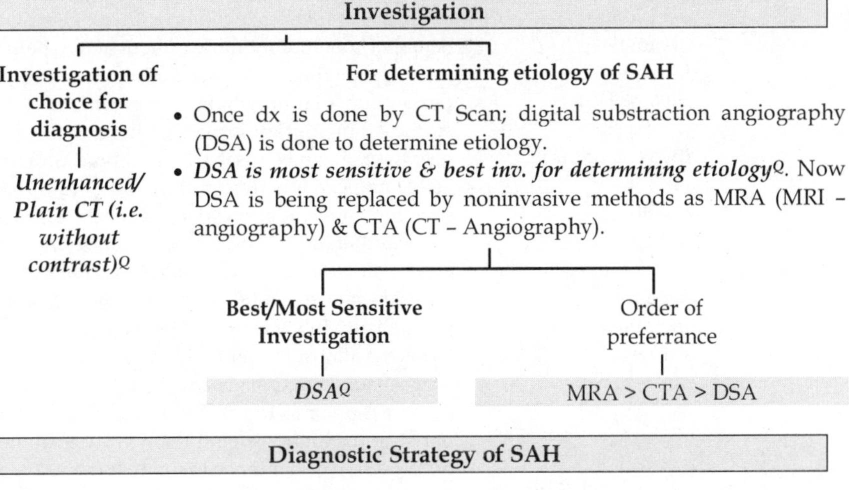

Investigation
Investigation of choice for diagnosis
Unenhanced/ Plain CT (i.e. without contrast)Q
For determining etiology of SAH
• Once dx is done by CT Scan; digital substraction angiography (DSA) is done to determine etiology.
• DSA is most sensitive & best inv. for determining etiologyQ. Now DSA is being replaced by noninvasive methods as MRA (MRI – angiography) & CTA (CT – Angiography).
Best/Most Sensitive Investigation
DSAQ
Order of preferrance
MRA > CTA > DSA

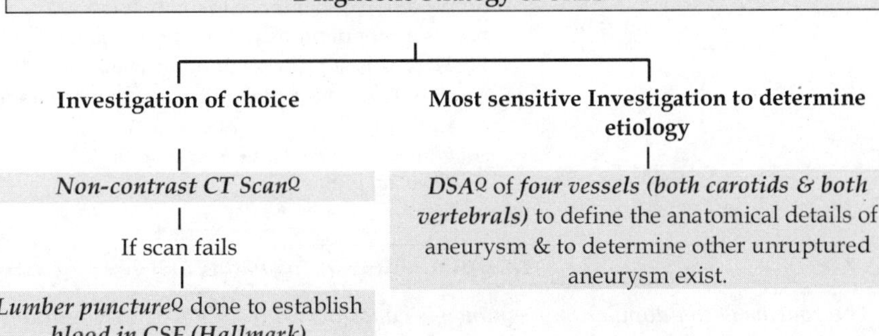

Diagnostic Strategy of SAH
Investigation of choice
Non-contrast CT ScanQ
If scan fails
Lumber punctureQ done to establish blood in CSF (Hallmark)
Most sensitive Investigation to determine etiology
DSAQ of four vessels (both carotids & both vertebrals) to define the anatomical details of aneurysm & to determine other unruptured aneurysm exist.

ASR Guideline for Imaging in Abdominal Trauma

Category A

Includes **hemodynamically unstable** patients following clinically obvious abdominal trauma & with unresponsive profound hypotension need *rapid clinical evaluation & immediate resuscitation with volume replacement.*

- If does not respond and remain hemodyn-mically unstable → Immediate **Diagnostic peritoneal lavage (DPL)** without imaging.
- If time & circumstances permit during resuscitation → **Conventional x-rays of chest & abdomen** to identify pneumothorax /peritoneum or bone injury **USG** for intraperitoneal free fluid can support a decision to operate immediately *Routine DPL is obsolute* b/o invasive nature, lack of specificity & inability to predict the need for therapeutic surgery.

Category B

- Include **hemodynamically stable** patients, patients with mild to moderate responsive hypotension presenting after blunt abdominal trauma, & unstable patients who stabilize after initial resusciatation.
- In patient with clinical evaluation suggesting a *lesser index of suspicion for significant intra abdominal injury, plain x-rays, (chest, abdomen), hematocrit with blood* chemesteries & urinalysis should be performed. And if these tests are unremarkable in the setting of a reliable clinical abdominal examination, a period of clinical observation is only needed.
  - However, if a reliable abdominal exam can not be performed (in **unconscious patient** or prolonged non abdominal surgery is anticipated) or **if a clinical evaluation suggests organ injury, hemo peritoneum or peritonitis,** further imaging is needed. The need for initial radiograph is also obviated if the clinical condition at initial evaluation merits a CT.
  - ***USG is not a good modality for further imaging***[Q] as it is *relatively much sensitive than CT for liver & spleen injuries & highly insensitive for renal, pancreatic, mesenteric, gut, bladder and retroperitoneal injuries.* If d/t circumstance, a negative USG is the sole imaging modality used to triage a patient, for safety reasons it must be followed by a 12-24 hrs of in hospital observation. However, any positive USG finding would warrant a CT.
  - In contrast **CT is an excellent modality** for detecting solid organ & gut injuries together with even small amount of hemoperitoneum. Identification of active hemorrhage, parenchymal blush, or pseudoaneurysm in spleen, gut perforation, diaphragmatic / pancreatic injury indicates surgical /angiographic management. Stable patients with negative CT can be discharged without observation.
- Stable patients who respond to initial fluid therapy should undergo **x-rays of cervical spine, chest & pelvis** b/o high chances of injury to these areas. ***Erect x-ray chest is superior to erect abdominal view for demonstration of free intrabdominal gas***[Q], since in erect abdomen view the x-ray beam is passing through any free gas under the diaphragm at an oblique angle (whereas almost tangentially in chest x-ray) and this part of film is usually overexposed. Upright chest x-rays may demonstrate upto 1cc of free air but it may take 10 min for air to rise to the highest point. Plain x-ray abdomen are insensitive for detection of hemoperitoneum and >800 cc volume is necessary for demonstration of *classical dog/bladder ear sign*
- **FAST (Focussed Assessment with sonography in Trauma)** is commonly used for the initil assessment of abdominal trauma, to detect free fluid and visceral organ injury. *Radionucleotide scanning & MRI do not play a role in initial evaluation & screening of abdominal trauma.*

Category C

- Includes patients with **hematuria**
- Patients with microscopic *hematuria (<35 RBC/hpF)* need no specific urinary tract imaging.
- Patients with *microscopic hematuria (>35RBC/hpF),* with macroscopic hematuria *or with fracture/diastasis of symphysis pubis & its rami plus any hematuria* need imaging of urinary tract.
  - If urethral meatus has gross blood, if there is a floating prostate, or if a foley catheter can not be passed, a **retrograde urethrogram** should first be performed to rule out urethral injury.
  - If clinical evaluation or urethrogram indicates no urethral injury, a computed tomography **(CT) cystogram should be added to abdominal CT.**

Doppler Ultrasound Analysis in Pregnancy

- The ***routine use of doppler in pregnancy is constroversial***[Q]. **TVS** (transvaginal sonography) is *method of choice for monitoring infertility disorders, diagnosis of ectopic pregnancy & differentiating abnormal & normal 1st trimester pregnancy.* The advantages of TVS is that it can be performed in empty bladder and its ability to use higher frequency trandsducer nearer the organs of interst thus providing higher resolution of uterus, ovaries, cul de sac & adnexa.

- Doppler may prove ***valuable in assessment of pregnancy complications & at risk factus***[Q]. Both *fetoplacental & uteroplacental circulations* can be assessed. ***As normal pregnancy progresses, placental blood flow increases d/t reduction in placental vascular resistance***[Q].
- *Increased placental resistance* results in reduced blood flow, manifesting as *decreased or absent end diastolic flow. Systolic diastolic (S/D) ratio, resistive & pulsatility indices* are used to quantify these changes. ***Increased values of S/D ratio & R-P indices and reduction in end diastolic flow are associated with IUGR & poor fetal outcome***[Q]. (d/t fetoplacental insufficiency). Other associations include *pregnancy induced hypertension, oligohydramnios, & cesarian section for fetal distress.*
- Doppler USG is either continuous wave or duplex (pulsed) wave. The duplex wave from uterine & umblical arteries is useful in assessment of IUGR whereas colour & power doppler are invaluable in assessment of fetal heart & outflow tracts and other fetal vessels such as intracerebral & renal arteries.
- Although, predictive value of continuous wave doppler for IUGR is relatively low, *reversed diastolic flow* indicates severely hypoxic fetus. In head spared IUGR, diastolic flow to brain (cerebra artery obtained by colour doppler) is increased, an indication that the head is spared from the diminished flow to the body.

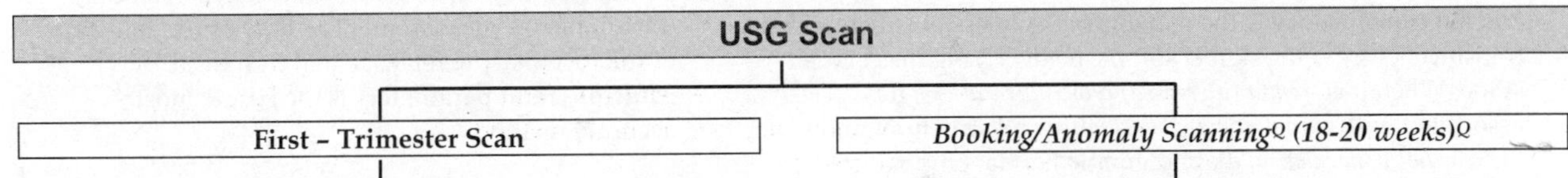

First – Trimester Scan

Either trans abdominal (TAS) or trans vaginal (TVS) helps to detect

1. Pregnancy confirmation
2. Accurate dating
3. Number of fetus
4. Uterine/Adnexal pathology
5. *Gross anomalies*

Booking/Anomaly Scanning[Q] (18-20 weeks)[Q]

In addition to 1st trim. Scan

1. ***Detailed fetal anatomical survey to detect any structural abnormality***[Q] including cardiac
2. *Placental localization.*

Dx of Ectopic Pregnancy

Transvaginal USG (*most accurate method*[Q])

1. ***Absence of intrauterine pregnancy***[Q] gestational sac in uterus with positive pregnancy test
2. ***Free Fluid in peritoneal cavity & pouch of douglas***[Q]
3. ***Adnexal mass***[Q] clearly separated from ovary
4. Rarely cardiac motion in mass
5. Mass can be located in one of the lateral fornix.

- ***Transvaginal sonography (TVS) is the first line investigation in hemodynamically stable female, presenting with suspected ectopic pregnancy***[Q]. *Absence of intrauterine gestational sac* on TVS and *β -hCG level higher than 1000 mIU/ml* has sensitivity of 93% & positive predective value of 86%.
- On TVS signs of unruptured ectopic pregnancy are:
  - ***Complex adenexal mass***, which is mostly separate form uterus & ovary.
  - Mass may contain embryo (only true sign) or yolk sac.
  - **Doughnut** or **bagel sign** i.e. ***hyperechoic ring surrounding gestational sac***[Q].
  - **Pseudo sac** i.e., endometrial cavity may contain hyperechogenic areas & fluid.
- *Intraperitoneal fluid in pouch of Douglas* on TVS is indicative of fallopian tube rupture or tubal abortion.
- The ultrasound appearance of **gestational trophoblastic disease** (i.e., hydatiform mole, invasive mole = choriocarcinoma destruens & choriocarcinoma) is most commonly ***large for gestational age uterus with echogenic soft tissue mass, distending the endometrial canal, and having multiple small cystic spaces***[Q]. In complete hydatiform mole, the small spaces corresponds to hydropic villi.

B-HCG

1. Lowest level of BHCG at which gestational sac is visible on –
   - TVS – 2000 IU/L
   - TAS – 6500 IU/L
2. B-HCG > 2000 IU/L, with empty uterine cavity on TVS
3. ***Failure to double the value of B HCG by 48 hours***[Q] with empty uterus.
4. Lower level of B-HCG compared to gestational age
5. ***β - HCG levels < 6500 IU/L***[Q], is seen in Ectopic pregnancy & missed abortion
6. ***Failure to double β HCG level by 48 hours (2 days)***[Q]

Ultrasound Assessment of Gestational Age

1st trimester

- **Gestational sac** is visualized by *TVS at 4 weeks* & by *TAS at 5 weeks*. During early 1st trimester mean sac diameter, (MSD) correlates well with menstrual age, with similar confidence limits to crown rump length.
- **Embryo** is consistently visualized from *6 weeks by TVS and 7 weeks by TAS* (trans abdominal sonography). ***Crown rump length is the most accurate method of pregnancy dating b/w 6 & 10 weeks***Q.
- Spinal flexion, in later 1st trimester onwards , may produce a false low value. Hence, the ***biparietal diameter should be measured once the fetal head is apparent***Q.
- **Nuchal translucency** is the maximum thickness of subcutaneous translucency b/ w the skin & soft tissue overlying the cervical spine. When it is *>3mm (increased) b/w 10&14 weeks*, it is associated with *chromosomal abnormality* and structural anomalies like *cardiac abnormality*, diaphragmatic hernia, omphalocele, & body stalk abnormalities.

2nd & 3rd trimester

- **Biparietal diameter** can be measured from around 9 weeks onwards and is the *most accurate single parameter of pregnancy dating.*
- **Head circumference** is more accurate predictor of gestational age *when the skull shape is abnormal.*
- **Abdominal circumference** is less accurate than BPD as abdomen suffers first in asymmetrical growth retardation. So *ration of head to abdominal circumference is useful indicator of asymmetircal growth retardation*
- **Femur length** is used when head is in a position unsuitable for measurement of BPD or for detection of microcephaly & fetal skeletal dysplasia.
- **Multiple fetal parameters** is the best & most accurate method.

QUESTIONS

Eye

1. Bare orbit is/are seen in: *(PGI Nov 2010)*
A. Metastasis
B. Neuroblastoma
C. Optic nerve glioma
D. NF -1
E. Pseudotumorcerebri

2. All are X-ray findings of retinoblastoma except :
A. Widening of optic canal *(AIIMS 1999)*
B. Intra cerebral calcification
C. Intraocular calcification
D. Secondaries in cranial bones

Respiratory System

General

3. True about chest X-ray: *(PGI Nov 2009)*
A. 40% lung tissue seen obscured by bony structure & mdiastinum
B. 60% lung tissue seen obscured by bony structure & mediastinum
C. Right dome higher than left dome
D. Right dome pushed up by liver
E. Should be taken in expiration

4. Normal hilar shadow in X-ray chest is produced by all except *(AIIMS 97, DNB 01)*
A. Pulmonary artery
B. Bronchus
C. Lower lobe viens
D. Upper lobe veins

5. True about chest X-ray is all except:
A. Left hilum is higher *(PGI 97, DNB 99)*
B. Left dome is higher
C. All fissures are clearly seen on lateral film
D. None

Hemoptysis

6. A young man with pulmonary tuberculosis presents with massive recurrent hemoptysis. For angiographic treatment, which vascular structure should be evaluated first: *(AI 2004)*
A. Pulmonary artery
B. Bronchial artery
C. Pulmonary vein
D. Superior vena cava

7. A young man with tuberculosis presents with massive recurrent hemoptysis. Most probable cause would be.
A. Pulmonary artery *(AIIMS 02, 03, DNB 04)*
B. Bronchial artery
C. Pulomary vein
D. Superior vena cava

8. A young patient of 30 yrs male presents with recurrent hemoptysis. On X-Ray no abnormality is seen. Next investigation is.
A. HRCT *(AIIMS 2001)*
B. Spiral CT
C. Helical CT
D. Bronchoscopy

9. A 40 years old man presents with a recurrent hemoptysis and purulent cough. X-ray was found to be normal. To next investigation done to aid in diagnosis is :
A. MRI *(AIIMS 2002)*
B. Bronchoscopy
C. HRCT
D. CT guided biopsy

Pulmonary Nodule

10. All of the following produce cavitating nodules in the lung except *(AIIMS 93, DNB 96)*
A. Sqamous cell CA
B. Caplan's syndrome
C. Hamartoma
D. Silicosis

11. What does not make diagnosis of solitary pulmonary nodule *(AIIMS 91, DNB 94)*
A. Tuberculoma
B. Bronchial adenoma
C. Hamartoma
D. Neurofibroma

12. A patient presents with a solitary pulmonary nodule (SPN) on x-ray. The best investigation to come to a diagnosis would be : *(AIIMS 2002)*
A. MRI
B. CT Scan
C. USG
D. Image guided biopsy

Miliary Shadow

13. "Millary shadow" on chest X-ray is seen in *(PGI 2003)*
A. Tuberculosis
B. Rheumatoid Arthritis
C. Pneumoconiosis
D. COPD
E. Metastasis

14. Miliary mottling seen in *(PGI Dec 06)*
A. T.B.
B. Sarcoidosis
C. Silicosis
D. P. carinii pneumonia

15. Miliary mottling found in: *(PGI June 06)*
A. Rheumatoid arthritis
B. TB
C. Pneumucystis carinii pneumonia
D. Congestive heart failure
E. Pulmonary edema

16. Millary mottling on X-ray chest is seen in:
A. Histoplasmosis *(PGI 2000)*
B. Sarcoidosis
C. Secondaries from Ca. colon
D. Gonococal pneumonia

17. All show miliary shadow on chest X-Ray except *(AI 1991)*
A. Pneumoconiasis
B. Sarcoidosis
C. MS
D. Staphylococcal Pneumonia

18. Miliary shadow in chest X-ray is seen in A/E: *(PGI 1999)*
A. TB
B. Loeffler's pneumonia
C. Klebsiella
D. Varicella pneumonia

19. **Bulging fissures in lungs is seen in :**
A. Klebsiella pneumonia (*PGI 1999*) ☐
B. Staph pneumonia ☐
C. Pulmonary oedema ☐
D. Pneumoconiosis ☐

20. **Honeycombimg of lung in C.X.R. is seen in** (*PGI 2003*)
A. R.A. ☐
B. T.B. ☐
C. Scleroderma ☐
D. Carcinoma ☐
E. Interstitial lung disease ☐

21. **Radiological finding(s) of eosinophilic granuloma is/are:**
A. Hilar involvement (*PGI May 12*)
B. Miliary shadowing
C. Honey comb appearance
D. Whiteout lung
E. Splitting of pleura

Hyperinflated Lung

22. **Increased radiolucency of one sided hemithorax may be caused by all except**
A. Obstructive Emphysema (*AI 91, DNB 95*) ☐
B. Pneumothorax ☐
C. Expiratory film ☐
D. Patient rotation ☐

23. **Hyperinflation of lung in CXR is seen in-**
A. CCF (*PGI Dec 2004*) ☐
B. Congenital lobar emphysema ☐
C. Diaphragmatic hernia ☐
D. Foreign body ☐
E. Mucoviscidosis ☐

24. **Hypertranslucency of lung unilaterally is seen on all except :** (*PGI 2000*)
A. Pneumothorax ☐
B. Resection of mammary gland ☐
C. Pulm art. obstruction ☐
D. Pneumonectomy ☐

25. **In rt. sided hemithorax on chest X-ray PA view what can be excluded:**
A. CCF (*PGI 97, DNB 98*) ☐
B. TB ☐
C. Pulmonary infarct ☐
D. None of the above ☐

26. **All are true regarding emphysema finding in X-Ray except:** (*AIIMS 92, DNB 02*)
A. Low flat diaphragm - Tarrace pattern ☐
B. Tubular heart ☐
C. Decreased inter costal space ☐
D. Increased radiolucence ☐

Interstial & Pleural Pathology

27. **Ground glass appearance is not seen in**
A. Hyline membrane disease (*AI 2001*) ☐
B. Left to right shunts ☐
C. Pneumonia ☐
D. Obstructive TAPVC ☐

28. **Uremic lung most often results due to :**
A. Pulmonary edema (*PGI 1998*) ☐
B. Fibrosis ☐
C. Alveolar injury ☐
D. CVC liver ☐

29. **All of the following are true about loculated pleural effusion except-** (*AI 2002*)
A. It makes an obtuse angle with the chest wall ☐
B. The margins are diffuse when viewed end on ☐
C. Not confined to any bronchopulmonary segment ☐
D. Air bronchograms are seen within the opacity ☐

30. **A patient presented with minimal Rt. sided pleural effusion. The best method to detect this would be**
A. Rt. lateral (*AIIMS 2001*) ☐
B. Left Lateral ☐
C. Left lateral decubitus ☐
D. Right lateral decubitus ☐

Pediatric Respiratory Distress

31. **The most likley diagnosis in a newbron who had a radiopaque shadow with an air fluid level in the chest along with hemivertebrae of the 6th thoracic vertebra on plain X-ray is:** (*AIIMS 2002*)
A. Congenital diaphragmatic hernia ☐
B. Oesophageal duplication cyst ☐
C. Bronchogenic cyst ☐
D. Staphylococcal pneumonia ☐

32. **A child has respiratory distress, chest X-Ray shows multiple air filled space, the differential diagnosis is all except.**
A. Congenital lung cyst (*AIIMS 1998*) ☐
B. Congenital Diaphragmatic hernia ☐
C. Congenital lobar aplasia of lung ☐
D. Congenital adenomatous malformation ☐

33. **Pappu 2 yrs old boy presents in the causality with H/O sudden onset of respiratory difficulty & strider on ausculation ↓ed breath sound & wheeze on the RT side. The X-Ray shows RT opaque hamithorex what will be diagnosis-** (*AI 2002*)
A. Pnumothorax ☐
B. Acute epiglottitis ☐
C. Massive plural effusion ☐
D. Foreign body aspiration ☐

34. **A child with acute respiratory distress showing hyperinflation of unilateral lung in X-ray is due to-**
A. Staphylococcal bronchopneumonia (*AI 2002*) ☐
B. Aspiration pneumonia ☐
C. Congenital lobar emphysema ☐
D. Foreign body aspiration ☐

35. **A new born baby with acute respiratory distress on day 1. X Ray chest PA view showed neumerous gas luscencies in entire left hemithorax, most likely diagnosis is** (*AIIMS 1992*)
A. Congenital lobar Emphysema ☐
B. Pneumatocoel hernia ☐
C. Congenital diaphragmatic hernia ☐
D. Congenital lung cyst ☐

36. **A neonate presents with respiratory distress, contralateral mediastinal shift and multiple cystic air filled lesions in the chest. Most likely diagnosis is-**
A. Pneumonia (*AI 2001*) ☐
B. Congenital Lung Cyst ☐
C. Congenital diaphragmatic hernia ☐
D. Congenital lobar Emphysema ☐

37. **Apgar scores were 3, and 6 at 1 and 5 minutes. At 10 minutes child shows features of breathlessness on CXR - mediastinal shift was there, possible causes:** (*PGI 2000*)
A. Bilateral choanal atresia ☐
B. Pneumothorax ☐
C. Congenital diaphragmatic hernia ☐
D. Hyaline Membrane disease. ☐

38. **In X-ray, loops of bowel on left side of hemithorax and shift of heart shadow:**
A. Eventration of diaphragm *(PGI 1998)* □
B. Foraman of bochdalek hernia □
C. Morganian hernia □
D. Any of the above □

39. **A 3 year old female child developed fever, cough and respiratory distress. On chest x-ray consolidation is seen in right lower lobe. She improved with antibiotics but on follow up at 8 weeks was again found to have increasing consolidation in right lower lobe. Your next investigation would be:** *(AIIMS Nov 07)*
A. Bronchoscopy □
B. Bacterial culture of the nasopharynx □
C. CT scan of the chest □
D. Allergen sensitivity test □

Pulmonary Embolism

40. **A 55 year old man who has been on bed rest for the past 10 days, complain of breathlessness and chest pain. The chest x-ray is normal (or shows Hampton's hump). The next step in investigation should be:** *(AI 2004)*
A. Lung ventilation – perfusion scan □
B. Pulmonary arteriography □
C. Pulmonary venous wedge angiography □
D. Echocardiography □

41. **In pulmonary embolism, findings in perfusion scan is :**
A. Perfusion segmental defect *(PGI 2K)* □
B. Perfusion defect with normal lung scan & radiography □
C. Tenting of diaphragm □
D. Normal chest scan □

42. **Hampton hump is feature of?** *(AIIMS 07, DNB 08)*
A. Pulmonary tuberculosis □
B. Pulmonary embolism □
C. Pulmonary hemorrhage □
D. Bronchogenic carcinoma □

43. **Best method to diagnose pulmonary embolism:**
A. Pulmonary angiography *(PGI 97, DNB 99)* □
B. Scintillation perfusion scan □
C. CT scan □
D. X-ray chest □

44. **Gold standard for diagnosing pulmonary embolism:**
A. X-ray chest *(PGI 97, DNB 99)* □
B. Ventilation perfusion scan □
C. Blood gas analysis □
D. Doppler □

Infectious Disease

45. **A 25 year old man presented with fever, cough, expectoration and breathlessness of 2 months duration. Contrast enchanced computed tomography of the chest showed bilateral upper lobe fibrotic lesions and mediastinum had enlarged necrotic nodes with peripheral rim enhancement. Which one of the following is the most probable diagnosis?** *(AI 2003)*
A. Sarcoidosis □
B. Tuberculosis □
C. Lymphoma □
D. Silicosis □

46. **A patient suffering from AIDS presents with history of dyspnea and non- productive cough x-ray shows bilateral perihilar opacitics without pleural effusion and lymphaden-opathy. Most probable etiological agent is :**
A. Tuberculosis *(AIIMS 2002)* □
B. CMV □
C. Kaposis sarcoma □
D. Pneumocystis carinii □

47. **A Bone marrow transplant receipient patient, developed chest infection. ON chest Xray Tree in Bud appearance is present. The cause of this is:** *(AIIMS Nov 2010)*
A. Klebsiella □
B. Pneumocystis □
C. TB □
D. RSV □

Industrial Lung Disease

48. **Extensive pleural thickening and calcification especially involving the diaphragmatic pleura are classical features of:** *(AI 2003)*
A. Coal worker's pneumoconiosis □
B. Asbestosis □
C. Silicosis □
D. Siderosis □

49. **A 48 years old man, resident of Baroda outskirts near a textile mill presents to his family physician with respiratory symptoms. Doctor advices X Ray chest which showed – fine reticular & nodular pattern in lower zone with loss of clarity of diaphragm & cardiac shadows. He also doubts about the presence of small pleural effusion. The probable diagnosis is?** *(AI 93, DNB 96)*
A. Stannosis □
B. Asbestosis □
C. Silicosis □
D. Coal worker's pneumoconiosis □

50. **A 35 yrs old with a history of asbestos exposure presents with chest pain. X-ray shows a solitary pulmonary nodule in the right lower zone. CECT reveals an enhancing nodule adjoining the right lower costal pleura with comet tail sign and adjacent pleura with comet tail sign and adjacent pleural thickening. The most likely diagnosis is:** *(AI 2012)*
A. Mesothelioma □
B. Round atelectasis □
C. Pulmonary sequestration
D. Adenocarcinoma

Malignancy

51. **Which of the following organs should always be imaged in a suspected case of broncogenic carcinoma.**
A. Adrenals *(AIIMS Nov 2004)* □
B. Spleen □
C. Kidney □
D. Pancreas □

52. **In lung X-ray, heterogenous shadow is due to:** *(PGI 97, DNB 99)*
A. Haemangiorma □
B. Pulmonary infarction □
C. Metastatic lesion □
D. TB □

Mediastinum

53. **Lt border of the heart in C.X.R. is formed by:** *(PGI 04)*
A. Pulmonary artery □
B. Pulmonary vein □
C. Abdominal aorta □
D. Arch of aorta □
E. Rt ventricles □

54. Left border of heart on chest X-ray is formed by:
A. Aortic arch *(PGI Nov 2010)* □
B. Left Pulmonary artery □
C. Right atrium □
D. Left ventricle □
E. Right ventricle □

55. Left sided cardiac bulge seen on chest X-ray is/are d/t: *(PGI May 10, DNB 08)*
A. Enlargement of left atrial appendage □
B. Azygous vein enlargement □
C. Coronary artery aneurysm □
D. Pulmonary edema □
E. Right atrial hypertrophy □

56. Which does not form right border of heart on X-ray:
A. Superior vena cava *(PGI May 13)* □
B. Inferior vena cava □
C. Right Atrium appendages □
D. Main Pulmonary trunk □
E. Aortic arch □

57. All are seen on right side of cardiac shadow in X-Ray chest PA view except
A. Superior venacava *(AIIMS 91, DNB 94)* □
B. Rt. atrium □
C. Ascending Aorta □
D. Inferior venacava □

58. Structure forming right border of heart
A. SVC *(PGI June 2006)* □
B. IVC □
C. Rt. atrium □
D. Lt. atrium appendage □
E. Pulmonary vessels □

59. Right side of mediastinum shadow is not formed by:
A. Superior venacava *(AI 95, DNB 96)* □
B. Right innominates □
C. Right atrium □
D. Right ventricle □

60. Right border of the heart in CXR is formed by
A. Pulmonary artery. *(PGI June 07)* □
B. Superior vena cava □
C. Rt atrium. □
D. Rt ventricle □

61. In X-Ray right border of mediastinum is formed by all except: *(AI 1998)*
A. SVC □
B. Right Atrium □
C. Right Ventricle □
D. Right Brachiocephalic Vein □

62. Earliest CXR feature of left atrial enlargement is *(AI 08)*
A. Elevation of the left main bronchus □
B. Double cardiac shadow □
C. Widening of carina □
D. Pericardial effusion □

63. Posterior marking on Ba column in Ba swallow study is caused by? *(AIIMS Nov 09)*
A. Aortic knuckle □
B. Left atrium □
C. Aberrant right subclavian artery □
D. Pulmonary artery sling □

64. Base of heart is formed by
A. Rt. ventricle *(PGI 06, DNB 07)* □
B. LV □
C. LV + RV □
D. RA + RV □
E. RA + LA □

65. All are true about thymus swelling except: *(AIIMS 1999)*
A. Widening of mediastinum on X-Ray □
B. Sharp border with shail like appearance □
C. Steroid administration reduces size of swelling □
D. Shift of trachea on X-ray □

66. Soft tissue mass in chest with rib erosion in X-Ray is seen in all except: *(AIIMS 1996)*
A. Leukemia □
B. Ewing's sarcoma □
C. Multiple myeloma □
D. Osteosarcoma □

67. The following is not the differential diagnosis of an anterior mediastinal mass.
A. Teratoma *(AIIMS 2002)* □
B. Neurogenic tumor □
C. Thymoma □
D. Lymphoma □

Cardio Vascular System

Septal Defect

68. Characterstic X Ray finding in ASD is:
A. Enlarged left ventricle *(AIIMS 93, DNB 95)* □
B. Enlarged left atria □
C. Pulmonary pletheora □
D. PAH □

69. X-ray picture of VSD: *(PGI June 2004)*
A. Small Lt. ventricle □
B. Small Rt. Ventricle □
C. Dilated Lt. atrium □
D. Dilated pulmonary veins □
E. Dilated pulmonary arteries □

70. How to differentiate ASD from VSD in X-ray: *(AI 2011)*
A. Enalrged LA □
B. Normal LA □
C. Pulmonary Congestion □
D. Aortic shadow □

71. Plethoric lung fields are seen in all of the following conditions, except: *(AIIMS 06, DNB 07)*
A. Atrial septal defect (ASD) □
B. TAPVC (Total Anomalous Pulmonary venou connection) □
C. Ebsteins' anomaly □
D. Ventricular septal defect □

72. Left heart failure findings are all except:
A. Kerley B lines *(AIIMS May 11, 10, 09)* □
B. Redistribution of blood vessels to apex (increased flow in upper lobe veins) □
C. Oligemic lung field (pulmonary oligemia) □
D. Cardiomegaly □

73. Chest X-ray picture in CCF- *(PGI Dec 2004)*
A. Cardiomegaly □
B. Thick interlobar septum □
C. Superior mediastinal widening □
D. Multinodular parenchymal lesion □

74. All are seen in congestive cardiac failure except: *(AI 2000)*
A. Kerly B lines □
B. Prominent lower lobe vessel □
C. Pleural Effusions □
D. Cardiomegaly □

75. Which is the objective sign of identifying pulmonary plethora in a chest radiograph? *(AI 11, 06)*
A. Diameter of the main pulmonary artery > 16 mm □
B. Diameter of the left pulmonary artery > 16 mm □
C. Diameter of the descending right pulmonary artery > 16 mm □
D. Diameter of the descending left pulmonary artery > 16 mm □

76. Prunning of Pulmonary arteries is seen in: *(AI 2009)*
A. Pulmonary hypertension ☐
B. Chronic Bronchitis ☐
C. Pulmonary infections ☐
D. Pulmonary transplant ☐

77. Features of pulmonary venous hyper tension are A/E
A. Perihilar haze *(PGI 06, JIPMER 05, DNB 07)* ☐
B. Peribroncheal cuffing ☐
C. Upper lobar diversion ☐
D. Uniformly branching lines parallel to pleura ☐
E. Pulmonary ossicles & fine nodular pattern ☐

78. Earliest feature of pulmonary venous hypertension
A. Kerley B lines *(AI 08, DNB 10)* ☐
B. Upper lobar diversion of vessels ☐
C. Left atrial enlargement ☐
D. Pleural effusion ☐

79. Radiological feature of Mitral stenosis is are
A. Double contour of right heart border ☐
B. Straightening of left heart border ☐
C. Splaying of carinal angle *(PGI May 12, June 09)* ☐
D. Prominent aortic knuckle ☐
E. Kerley lines ☐

80. A patient is having Mitral stenosis. His x-ray will show all of the following finding *except* *(AIIMS 2002)*
A. Lifting up of left bronchus ☐
B. Double atrial shadow ☐
C. Obliteration of retrosternal shadow on lateral x-rays ☐
D. Posterior displacement of esophagus on barium swallow. ☐

81. All are radiological features of Mitral stenosis except
A. Straight left border of heart *(AIIMS 2000)* ☐
B. Oligemia of upper lung fields ☐
C. Pulmonary hemosiderosis ☐
D. Lifting of left bronchus ☐

82. Left cardiac border bulge can be sen in all, except
A. Enlarged azygous vein *(AI 2000)* ☐
B. Left appendicular overgrowth ☐
C. Coronary artery aneurysm ☐
D. Pericardial defect ☐

83. In all of the following increased cardiac silhouette sign is seen except:
A. Tetralogy of Fallot's *(AIIMS 04, DNB 02)* ☐
B. Pericardial effusion ☐
C. Aortic regurgitation ☐
D. Ebstein anomaly ☐

84. Which of the following is virtually diagnostic of aortitis on chest X-Ray? *(AI 08)*
A. Calcification in descending aorta ☐
B. Calcification of ascending aorta ☐
C. Calcification of pulmonary artery ☐
D. Focal oligemia ☐

85. Oblitration of left cardiac shadow on PA view is due to:
A. Lingular lesion *(AIIMS 91, DNB 98)* ☐
B. Left hilar lymphadenopathy ☐
C. Left lower lobe lesion ☐
D. Left upper apical lobe lesion ☐

86. If the right cardiac silhouette is obliterated, it means the pathology involves: *(AIIMS May 08)*
A. Right lower lobe ☐
B. Right atrium ☐
C. Right middle lobe ☐
D. Right ventricle ☐

87. A young patient presented with 3 days cough, fever and difficultly in breathing. On X-ray, homogeneous paracardiac opacity was found in right lung near right cardiac silhouette and lateral border is ill defined. What is the diagnosis? *(AIIMS May 13)*
A. Pneumonia affecting medial zone of right middle lobe
B. Pneumonia affecting superior zone of right lower lobe
C. Loculated pleural effusion
D. Pneumonia of anterior zone of right middle lobe

88. Consolidation of which portion of the lung is likely to obliterate the Aortic knuckle on X-ray chest: *(AI 2011)*
A. Left Lingula ☐
B. Right Upper lobe ☐
C. Apex of lower lobe ☐
D. Left upper lobe (posterior part) ☐

89. The patho-physiological phenomenon that occurs during atheromatous plaque formation and is used for screening of 'asymptomatic coronary plaques' on CT scan is: *(AI 2012)*
A. Increased outer diameter of coronary artery ☐
B. Decreased inner diameter of coronary artery ☐
C. Calcium deposition in the atheromatous plaque ☐
D. Lipoid degeneration in the plaque. ☐

90. To visualize vascular sling causing tracheal /external airway compression which of the following would you best prefer? *(AIIMS Nov 09)*
A. Catheter angiography of aorta and pulmonary artery ☐
B. MRI ☐
C. CT ☐
D. PET-CT ☐

91. Which of the following is not true: *(AIIMS Nov 2011)*
A. Hibernating myocardium can be detected by Low dose butamine scar ☐
B. Rest reinjection thallium scan is used in hibernating myocardium ☐
C. Akinetic areas does not benefit from revascularization. ☐
D. Late Gd MRI enhancement is suggestive of scar but Gd scan is not used for hibernating myocardium detection. ☐

92. Drug used to perform stress ECHO:
A. Thallium *(AIIMS May 08, DNB 09)* ☐
B. Dobutamine ☐
C. Adrenaline ☐
D. Adenosine ☐

93. The most recent advance in noninvasive cardiac output monitoring is use of:
A. PA catheter *(AIIMS 2002)* ☐
B. Thermodilution technique ☐
C. Echocardiography ☐
D. Electrical impedance cardiography technology ☐

94. About diagnosing air embolism with transesophageal echocardiography, which of the following is false:
A. It can quantify the volume of air embolised ☐
B. It is a very sensitive investigation *(AIIMS 2002)* ☐
C. Continuous monitoring is needed to detect venous embolism ☐
D. Interferes with doppler when used together ☐

95. Best investigation for cardiac temponade is *(AI 1994)*
A. 2-D Echocardiography ☐
B. M-Mode Echocardiography ☐
C. Real time echocardiography ☐
D. USG ☐

5

RADIODIAGNOSIS

Gastrointestinal System

Abdominal Trauma

96. Which of the following is the best view for detecting minimal pneumoperitoneum? *(AI 2012)*
A. Erect view of abdomen ☐
B. AP view of abdomen ☐
C. Right lateral decubitis abdominal x-ray with horizontal beam ☐
D. Left lateral decubitus abdominal x-ray with horizontal beam ☐

GI Tract

97. Investigation of choice for Zenker's divertculum is:
A. Barium swallow *(AIIMS Nov 2011)* ☐
B. Endoscopy ☐
C. Esophageal Menometry ☐
D. CT ☐

98. What is least useful as diagnostic procedure in case of acute haemetemesis
A. Barium meal *(AIIMS 91, DNB 94)* ☐
B. Endoscopy ☐
C. Gastric content aspiration ☐
D. Angiography ☐

99. Diffuse esophageal dilatation on barium swallow is seen in:
A. Achlasia *(PGI June 05)* ☐
B. Trypanosomiasis ☐
C. Etidronate therapy ☐
D. Scleroderma ☐

100. All correlates with USG findings of congenital pyloric stenosis except: *(AIIMS Nov 2011)*
A. > 95% accuracy ☐
B. Segment length >16mm ☐
C. Thickness >4mm ☐
D. High gastric residues ☐

101. Following are common features of malignant gastric ulcer on Barium meal, EXCEPT: *(AIIMS May 2004)*
A. Location on the greater curvature ☐
B. Carman's meniscus sign ☐
C. Radiating folds which do not reach the edge of the ulcer ☐
D. Lesser curvature ulcer with a nodular rim ☐

102. Radiological finding in ileal atresia :
A. Microcolon on Ba enema *(PGI 2000)* ☐
B. Double bubble sign ☐
C. Coil spring appearance in Ba-Enema ☐
D. Obstruction in Ba meal ☐

103. All of the following are diagnostic barium follow through features of ileocecal tuberculosis EXCEPT *(AI 08)*
A. Apple – core appearance ☐
B. Pulled up contracted cecum ☐
C. Widening of ileocecal angle ☐
D. Strictures involving terminal ileum ☐

104. Ileocecal tuberculosis presents with all except
A. Rapid emptying of narrowed terminal ileum ☐
B. Inverted umbrella sign *(PGI –06, JIPMER-07)* ☐
C. Stellate ulcer with elevated margins ☐
D. Longitudinal ulcers are more common ☐
E. Napkin ring stenosis ☐

105. Investigation for small intestine includes all except:
A. Enteroclysis *(PGI Dec 2005)* ☐
B. Radionucleide scan ☐
C. MRI enteroclysis ☐
D. CT enteroclysis ☐
E. USG enteroclysis ☐

106. After taking a drug a patient developed some abdominal problem for which he consulted a physician, who adviced X-ray. X ray findings was radiopacity in bowel. Probably he might have taken A/E:
A. Salicylate *(AIIMS 95, DNB 97)* ☐
B. Iron ☐
C. Phenothiazine ☐
D. Corticosteroid ☐

107. Gasless abdomen is a feature of: *(MP 01, DNB 09)*
A. High obstruction ☐
B. Acute pancreatitis ☐
C. Congenital diaphragmatic hernia ☐
D. All ☐

108. DD for Rt. upper quadrant calcification:
A. Gallstone *(PGI June 06)* ☐
B. Renal stone ☐
C. Calcification in vessels ☐
D. Hepatic hemangioma ☐

Pancreas

109. A patient complains of epigastric pain, radiating to back off and on. The investigation of choice is: *(AIIMS 99)*
A. MRI ☐
B. CT Scan ☐
C. USG ☐
D. Radio nucleotide scan ☐

110. Widening of C loop of duodenum is a feature of:
A. Pancreatic head growth *(AIIMS 1991)* ☐
B. Carcinoma stomach ☐
C. Splenic involvement ☐
D. Involvement of upper rt renal pole ☐

111. ERCP in pancreatitis is done to know about : *(PGI 2001)*
E. Gall stones ☐
A. Associated cholangitis ☐
B. Ascites ☐
C. Pancreatic divisum ☐
D. Annular pancreas ☐

Hepatobiliary System

112. According Couinaud's classification of functional segments of liver, which of the following is Segment IV of liver?
A. Left lobe *(AIIMS Nov 07)* ☐
B. Right lobe ☐
C. Caudate lobe ☐
D. Quadrate lobe ☐

113. Solitary hypoechoic lesion of the liver without septate or debris is most likely to be- *(AIIMS Nov 2005)*
A. Hydatid cyst ☐
B. Caroli's disease ☐
C. Liver abscess ☐
D. Simple cyst ☐

114. Hyperchoice hepatic metastases on USG are seen in which of the following malignancies: *(AI 2012)*
A. CA ovary ☐
B. CA colon (Mucinous adenocarcinoma) ☐
C. Urinary bladder ☐
D. Mucinous cystadenoma ☐

115. Which one of the following hepatic lesions can be diagnosed with high accuracy by using nuclear imaging?
A. Hepatocellular carcinoma ☐
B. Hepatic adenoma *(AIIMS Nov 2004)* ☐
C. Focal nodular hyperplacia ☐
D. Cholangiocarcinoma ☐

116. A 22 year old man presents with a solitary 2 cm space occupying lesion of mixed echogenicity in the right lobe of liver on ultrasound examination. The rest of the liver is normal. Which of the following tests should be done next: *(AIIMS Nov 02)*
A. Ultrasound guided biopsy of the lesion ☐
B. Hepatic Scintigraphy ☐
C. Hepatic angiography ☐
D. Contrast enhanced CT scan of the liver ☐

117. Which of the following is true regarding the principle of use of MRCP? *(AIIMS Nov 12)*
A. Intraluminal dye is used to create the three dimension view of the structures
B. Dye is instilled percutaneously first then MRI is used
C. Use of heavily T2-weighted image without contrast to create the three dimensional image of the billary tree using MIP algorithm
D. Use of systemic gadolinium as a contrast agent to create the three dimensional image of the billary tree

118. True about are MRCP: *(PGI Dec 07)*
A. MRI is used to obtain the image ☐
B. CT is used for the images ☐
C. It shows the biliary tree ☐
D. Dye has to be injected endoscoically ☐
E. It is an invasive procedure ☐

119. All of the following modalities can be used for in-situ ablation of liver secondaries, except *(AI 2006)*
A. Ultrasonic waves ☐
B. Cryotherapy ☐
C. Alcohol ☐
D. Radio frequency ☐

120. X-Ray appearance of CBD stone on cholangiography is:
A. Meniscus appearance *(AIIMS 1998)* ☐
B. Sudden cut off ☐
C. Smooth tapering ☐
D. Eccentric occlusion ☐

121. Air in biliary tract is seen in all except:
A. Gall stone ileus *(AIIMS 1995)* ☐
B. Sclerosing cholangitis ☐
C. Carcinoma gall bladder ☐
D. Endoscopic papillotomy ☐

122. Thickened gall bladder wall in USG seen in-
A. Acute cholecystitis *(PGI Dec 2004)* ☐
B. Mucosal thickening ☐
C. Cholesterosis ☐
D. Ascites ☐
E. AIDS cholangitis ☐

123. True about features of cholecystitis on USG : *(PGI 2001)*
A. Thick fibrosed gallbladder wall ☐
B. Stone impacted at neck of gall bladder ☐
C. Perigallbladder halo ☐
D. Increased vascularity ☐

124. Computed Tomography (CT scan) is least accurate for diagnosts of: *(AI 2011)*
A. 1cm size Aneurysm in the Hepatic Artery ☐
B. 1cm size Lymph node inthe para-aortic region ☐
C. 1cm size Mass in the tail of pancreas ☐
D. 1cm size Gall stones ☐

125. Focal and diffuse thickening of gall bladder wall with high amplitude reflections and 'comet tail' artifacts on USG suggest the diagnosis of: *(AI 09)*
A. Xanthogranulomatous cholecysitis ☐
B. Carcinoma of gall bladder ☐
C. Adenomyomatosis ☐
D. Cholesterolosis ☐

Pediartric Abdomen

126. A newborn baby not passed meconium for 48 hours since birth, presents with vomiting and distension of abdomen. The most appropriate investigation for evaluation would be? *(AIIMS Nov 07)*
A. Barium enema study ☐
B. Manometry ☐
C. Rectal biopsy ☐
D. Fecal fat estimation ☐

127. A newborn baby has not passed meconium for 48 hours since birth. She has vomiting and distension of abdomen. The most appropriate investigation for evaluation would be *(AI 08)*
A. Anorectal manometry ☐
B. Rectal biopsy ☐
C. Lower G1 contrast study ☐
D. Trypsin estimation ☐

MUSCULOSKELETAL SYSTEM

Arthritis

128. A 40 year old male female patient on long term steroid therapy presents with recent onset of severe pain in the right hip. Imaginf modality of choice for this problem is:
A. CT scan *(AIIMS May 05, DNB 06)* ☐
B. Bone scan ☐
C. MRI ☐
D. Plain X-ray ☐

129. Heberden's nodes are found in: *(AIIMS May 2005)*
A. PIP joints in osteoarthritis ☐
B. DIP joints in osteoarthritis ☐
C. PIP joints in rheumatoid arthritis ☐
D. DIP joints in rheumatoid arthritis ☐

130. Tufting of distal phalanx is characteristically seen in
A. Gout *(AIIMS 91, DNB 01)* ☐
B. Psoriatic arthropathy ☐
C. Hypoparathyroidism ☐
D. Hyperparathyroidism ☐

131. Chondrocalcinosis is seen with
A. Gout *(AIIMS 91, DNB 94)* ☐
B. Osteoarthritis ☐
C. Pseudogout ☐
D. Septic arthritis ☐

132. Calcification of intervertebral disc is seen in
A. T.B. spine *(AIIMS 90, DNB 95)* ☐
B. Prolapse of intervertebral disc (PID) ☐
C. Non rheumatic ankylosis ☐
D. Rheumatic ankylosis ☐

133. Calcification of Intervertebral Disc is seen in *(AI 2000)*
A. Gout ☐
B. Rheumatoid ☐
C. Alkaptonuria ☐
D. Psoriasis ☐

134. Calcification of meniscal cartilage is feature of:
A. Achondroplasia *(AI 91, DNB 96)* ☐
B. Hyperparathyroidism ☐
C. Gaucher's ds. ☐
D. Pseudogout ☐

135. Calcification around the joint is seen in:
A. Pseudogout *(PGI 99)* ☐
B. Hyperparathyroidism ☐
C. Rh. arthritis ☐
D. Gout ☐

136. Which one of the following is a recognized X-Ray feature of rheumatoid arthritis?

A. Juxta-articular osteosclerosis ☐
B. Sacroilitis (AI 2003) ☐
C. Bone erosions ☐
D. Peri-articular calcification ☐

137. Radiological features of scleroderma are A/E:
A. Diffuse periosteal reaction (AI 93, DNB 94) ☐
B. Esophageal dysmotality ☐
C. Erosion of tip of phalynx ☐
D. Lung nodules ☐

Deficiency Diseases

138. All are radiological sign of Vit C defeciency except
A. White line of Frenkel (AIIMS 95, DNB 99) ☐
B. Wimberger line ☐
C. Osteoporosis of bone ☐
D. Widening of epiphysis ☐

139. In scurvy all the following radiological signs are seen except: (AI 2004)
A. Pelican spur ☐
B. Soap bubble appearance ☐
C. Zone of demarcation near epiphysis ☐
D. Frenkel's line ☐

140. Radiological findings of scurvy are A/E:
A. Epiphyseal widening (PGI 1999) ☐
B. Metaphyseal porosis ☐
C. Metapyseal infarction ☐
D. Pelkan spur ☐

141. Earliest evidence of healing in rickets is provided by
A. S. Ca^{++} (AI 95, DNB 97) ☐
B. S. PO_4^{3-} ☐
C. Radiological examination of growing bone ends ☐
D. S. Alkaline Phosphate level ☐

142. Radiological features of rickets include:
A. Narrowing of epiphysis ☐
B. Cupping of metaphysis (PGI Dec 05) ☐
C. Ricketic rosary ☐
D. Pelikan's spur ☐

143. Splaying and cupping of the'metaphysis is seen in :
A. Rickets (PGI 1999) ☐
B. Scurvy ☐
C. Paget's disease ☐
D. Lead poisoning ☐

144. Fraying and cupping of metaphyses of long bones in a child does not occur in:
A. Rickets (AI 2003) ☐
B. Lead poisoning ☐
C. Metaphyseal dysplasia ☐
D. Hypophosphatasia ☐

145. Looser's zones is seen in : (PGI 2002)
A. Osteoporosis ☐
B. Hyperparathyrodism ☐
C. Osteomalacia ☐
D. Multiple myelorna ☐
E. Paget's disease ☐

146. Flaring of anterior ends of the ribs is characteristically seen in (AI 08)
A. Neurofibromatosis ☐
B. Scurvy ☐
C. Rickets ☐
D. Hypothyroidism ☐

147. Which endocrine disorder is associated with epiphyseal dysgenesis? (AI 2003)
A. Hypothyroidism ☐
B. Cushings syndrome ☐
C. Addison's disease ☐
D. Hypoparathyroidism ☐

Malignancy

148. 76 year old man presents with lytic lesion in the vertbrae. X-Ray skull showed multiple punched out lesions. The diagnosis is (AIIMS 2000)
A. Metastasis ☐
B. Multiple myeloma ☐
C. Osteomalacia ☐
D. Hyperparathyroidism ☐

149. A lady Dimple has a lytic lesion in X-Ray of upper end of humerus. The diagnosis is, (AIIMS 1999)
A. Osteosarcoma ☐
B. Osteochondroma ☐
C. Unicarmel bone cyst ☐
D. Osteoclastoma ☐

150. A classical expansive lytic lesion in the transverse process of a vertebra is seen in:
A. Osteosarcoma (AI 2003) ☐
B. Aneurysmal bone cyst ☐
C. Osteoblastoma ☐
D. Metastasis ☐

151. X-ray shows soap bubble appearance at lower end of radius, treatment of choice is
A. Local excision (AIIMS 98, DNB 02) ☐
B. Excision & Bone grafting ☐
C. Amputation ☐
D. RT ☐

152. Radiological feature of osteosarcoma is:
A. New bone formation (AIIMS 99, DNB 2K) ☐
B. Sunray appearance ☐
C. Cotton wool app. ☐
D. Osteoid formation ☐

153. Dense calcification is seen in (AIIMS 96, DNB 97)
A. Chondroblatoma ☐
B. Chondrosarcoma ☐
C. Osteosarcoma ☐
D. Fibrosarcoma ☐

154. Expansible pulsating secondary metastasis is a feature of
A. Basal cell carcinoma (AIIMS 90, DNB 91) ☐
B. Renal cell carcinoma ☐
C. Osteogenic sarcoma ☐
D. Carcinoma prostate ☐

155. Lytic lesion in skull are seen in following except:
A. Multiple myeloma (PGI 97) ☐
B. Metastasis ca bronchus ☐
C. Thalassemia ☐
D. Ca prostate ☐

Infection

156. X-ray finding of ostemyelitis within 8 day is: (PGI 99, DNB 99)
A. Cystic swelling ☐
B. Soft tissue swelling ☐
C. New bone formation ☐
D. Seyuestrum formation ☐

Spine

157. Sonographic finding of Spina bifida
A. Ventriculomegaly (PGI June 2004) ☐

B. Obliteration of cisterna magna ☐
C. Small BPD ☐
D. Abnormal curvature of cerebellum ☐
E. Club foot ☐

158. An eight year old boy presents with back pain and mild fever. His plain X-ray of the dorsolumbar spine reveals a solitary collap-sed dorsal vertebra with preserved disc spaces. There was no associated soft tissue shadow. The most likely diagnosis is:
A. Ewing's sarcoma *(AI 2003)* ☐
B. Tuberculosis ☐
C. Histiocytosis ☐
D. Metastasis ☐

159. On MRI the differential diagnosis of spinal cord edema is: *(AIIMS May 06)*
A. Myelodysplasia ☐
B. Myelomalacia ☐
C. Myeloschisis ☐
D. Cord tumors ☐

160. Which of the following is not true regarding Ossified Posterior Longitudinal Ligament (OPLL)? *(AI 2009)*
A. Most commonly involves thoracic spine ☐
B. Gradient echo MR sequence may overestimate the canal stenosis ☐
C. MRI is best for diagnosis ☐
D. Low signal intensity on all MR sequences ☐

Breast

161. Mamographic abnormality seen in CA breast is-
A. Change in density *(PGI June 2005)* ☐
B. Microcalcification ☐
C. Change in architecture ☐
D. All ☐

162. On mammogram all of the following are the features of a malignant tumor except: *(AIIMS 2003)*
A. Spiculation ☐
B. Microcalcification ☐
C. Macrocalcification ☐
D. Irregular mass ☐

163. Which of the following features on mammogram would suggest malignancy *(AIIMS May 06)*
A. Well defined lesion ☐
B. A mass of decreased density ☐
C. Areas of speculated microcalcifications ☐
D. Smooth borders ☐

164. Investigation to diagnose stage-I carcinoma breast:
A. B/L mammogram *(PGI 2000)* ☐
B. X-ray chest ☐
C. Bone scan ☐
D. Liver scan ☐

165. The sensitivity of Mammography is low in young females because? *(AI 2009)*
A. Less glandular tissue and more fat ☐
B. Young females are less cooperative ☐
C. Young breast have dense tissue ☐
D. Because of less fat content ☐

166. Triple assessment for carcinoma breast includes:
A. History, clinical examination, biopsy/cytology ☐
B. Clinical examination, Mammography, biopsy/cytology *(AI 2009)* ☐
C. History, clinical examination, Ultrasonography ☐
D. Observation, Ultrasonography, biopsy/cytology ☐

167. Which of the following does not contain Fat on mammography? *(AI 2009)*
A. Post-traumatic cyst ☐
B. Hamartoma ☐
C. Seborrhic keratosis ☐
D. Galactocele ☐

168. The most sensitive investigation for DCIS (Ductal carcinoma in-situ) of breast? *(AIIMS Nov 10, AI 09)*
A. Mammography ☐
B. Ultrasound ☐
C. MRI ☐
D. PET Scan ☐

169. Birads stands for: *(AIIMS Nov 12)*
A. Breast Imaging reporting and data system
B. Best Imaging reporting and data system
C. Best Imaging Reporting and data system
D. Best imaging reporting and data system

Endocrine System

170. X-ray of which bone (s) would be diagnostic in hyperparathyroidism :
A. Skull *(PGI 2000)* ☐
B. Phalanges ☐
C. Long bones ☐
D. Scapula ☐
E. Spine ☐

171. Pathognomic feature of hyperparathyroidism:
A. Osteopenia *(AIIMS 92, 98, DNB 96)* ☐
B. Loss of Lamina dura ☐
C. Brown's tumor ☐
D. Sub periosteal resoption of phalynges ☐

172. The diagnostic procedure not done in case of pheochromocytoma. *(AIIMS May 07)*
A. CT scan ☐
B. MRI ☐
C. FNAC ☐
D. MIBG scan ☐

173. Which one of the following imaging modalities is most sensitive for evaluation of extra- adrenal phaeochromocytoma. *(AIIMS 03)*
A. Ultrasound ☐
B. CT ☐
C. MRI ☐
D. MIBG scan ☐

174. Light bulb appearance in MRI scan is/are seen in:
A. Pheochromocytoma *(PGI May 12)* ☐
B. Adrenal adenoma ☐
C. Adrenal cortical tumor ☐
D. Adrenal calcification ☐
E. Adrenocortical carcinoma ☐

175. Post irradiation thyroid tumor is: *(AIIMS 92, DNB 94)*
A. Follicular CA ☐
B. Papillary CA ☐
C. Lymphoma ☐
D. Hurthle cell tumor ☐

176. Radio iodine is used in treatment of
A. Papillary CA thyroid *(AI 92, DNB 95)* ☐
B. Medullary CA thyroid ☐
C. Follicular CA thyroid ☐
D. Anaplastic CA thyroid ☐

177. Which of the following feature of thyroid nodule on Ultrasongram is not suggestive of malignancy?
A. Hyperechogenisity *(AIIMS May 10, AI 09)* ☐
B. Hypoechogenisity ☐
C. Nonhomogenous ☐
D. Microcalcification ☐

178. Which of the following is not a CT feature of Adrenal adenoma? *(AI 10, 09)*
A. Low attenuation ☐

5

RADIODIAGNOSIS

B. Homogenous density and well defined borders (regular margins) □
C. Contrast is taken up early (enhances rapidly), contrast stays in it for a relatively longer time and washes out late (slowly) □
D. Calcification is rare □

Hematology

179. Which one of the following is the earliest radiographic manifestation of childhood leukemia? *(AIIMS Nov 04)*
A. Radioleucent transverse metaphyseal band □
B. Diffuse demineralization of bones □
C. Osteoblastic lesions in skull □
D. Parenchymal pulmonary lesions on chest films □

180. A 2 yr old boy suffering from leukaemia following are the x-ray finding *(PGI 2003)*
A. Osteolytic lesion in flat bones □
B. Metaphysial osteoporosis □
C. Periostial new bone formation □
D. Osteosclerosis of long bone □
E. Transverse line of dark band below the growth plate □

181. "Hair –on end" appearance is seen in:
A. Thalassaemia *(AIIMS May 08)* □
B. Sickle cell anemia □
C. Hemochromatosis □
D. Megaloblastic anemia □

182. Wide diploic space of skull with brush border (hair on end) appearance is characteristic of *(AI 91, DNB 96)*
A. Congenital haemolytic anaemia □
B. Multiple myeloma □
C. Raised intracranial tension □
D. Meningioma □

183. All are radiological features of sickle cell anemia except:
A. Vertebra plana *(PGI June 08)* □
B. Floating teeth □
C. Bone infarct □
D. Marrow hyperplasia □
E. Secondary ostcomyelitis □

Trauma

184. Investigation of choice for temporal bone injury:
A. CT scan *(AIIMS May 2010)* □
B. MRI □
C. Angiography □
D. Plain x-ray a □

185. Subdural haematoma most commonly results from
A. Rupture of intracranial aneurysm *(AIIMS 2004)* □
B. Rupture of cerebral AVM □
C. Injury to cortical bridging veins □
D. Hemophilia □

186. Characteristic of subdural hematoma is
A. Convex Hyperdensity *(AIIMS 98, DNB 95)* □
B. Concavo convex Hyperdense □
C. Biconvex hyperdense □
D. Concavo convex hypodense □

187. Which of the following is classic CT appear-ance of an acute Subdural hematoma: *(AI 04)*
A. Lentiform-shaped hyperdense lesion □
B. Cresent-shaped hypodense lesion □
C. Cresent-shaped hyperdense lesion □
D. Lentiform-shaped hypodense lesion □

188. Investigation of choice for acute subarachnoid haemorrage *(AI 98, DNB 99)*
A. Angiography □
B. CT-Scan □
C. MRI □
D. Enhanced MRI □

189. CT scan of a patient with history of head injury shows a biconvex hyperdense lesion displacing the grey-white matter interface. The most likely diagnosis is:
A. Subdural hematoma *(AI 2003)* □
B. Diffuse axonal injury □
C. Extradural hematoma □
D. Hemorrhagic contusion □

190. Hard dense biconvex appearance on cranial CT scan is seen in: *(PGI May 12)*
A. Subdural hemorrhage □
B. Extradural hemorrhage □
C. Foreign body □
D. Intracerebral hemorrhage □
E. Hypertensive hemorrhage □

191. The first investigation of choice in a patient with suspected subarachnoid haemorrhage should be :
A. Non-contrast computed tomography *(AI 2004)* □
B. CSF examination □
C. Magnetic resonance imaging (MRI) □
D. Contrast-enhanced computed tomography □

192. Best test to determine etiology of SAH
A. Enhanced CT *(AIIMS 95, DNB 97)* □
B. Unenhanced CT □
C. Intra arterial digital Substraction Angiography □
D. MRI □

193. Splenic injury is diagnosed on X-ray by:
A. Half stomach shadow *(PGI 1997)* □
B. Obliteration of splenic shadow □
C. Rib fracture □
D. Gas under diaphragm □

194. In a patient with abdominal trauma who is hemodynamically stable, what would be the investigation of choice? *(AIIMS Nov 09)*
A. FAST □
B. DPL □
C. Barium meal □
D. Erect x- ray abdomen □

195. Investigation of choice for diagnosis of spleenic rupture
A. Peritoneal lavage *(AIIMS 93, DNB 98)* □
B. Ultrasound □
C. CT scan □
D. MRI □

196. For the evaluation of blunt abdominal trauma, which of the following imaging modalities is ideal? *(AIIMS 2004)*
A. Ultrasonography □
B. Computed tomography □
C. Nuclear scintigraphy □
D. Magnetic resonance imaging □

OBSTETRICS

Pregnancy

197. True about antenatal doppler analysis is all except
A. Reduction in end diastolic flow is associated with poor out come *(JIPMER – 2006, PGI –06)* □
B. Reduction in EDF is associated with IUGR □
C. In normal gestation placental resistance is high □
D. S/D ratio is high in IUGR □
E. Investigation of choice in pregnancy □

198. Which one of the following regarding antenatal assessment of umbilical arteries by Color Doppler study is TRUE? *(AI 08)*
A. There is decreased S/D ratio in smoker and nicotine abusing pregnant females □
B. The reduced diastolic flow at term indicates good prognosis □

C. The flow velocities and the S/D ratio are useful to evaluate high risk pregnancies ☐
D. In otherwise normal pregnancies the increased S/D ratio is normal in smoking females ☐

199. USG can detect gestation sac earliest at: *(DNB 95, 98)*
A. 5-6 weeks of gestation ☐
B. 7-8 weeks of gestation ☐
C. 10 weeks of gestation ☐
D. 12 weeks of gestation ☐

200. Earliest sign of fetal life is best detected by
A. X-Ray *(AI 2004)* ☐
B. Feto scopy ☐
C. Real time USG ☐
D. Doppler ☐

201. Ultrasonogrsphy of umbilical artery is done to know about: *(PGI 1997)*
A. Heart beat ☐
B. Gastational age ☐
C. Fetalweight ☐
D. Fetal maturity ☐

202. Parameters used to estimate gestational age in last trimester: *(PGI 1997)*
A. CR length ☐
B. Abdominal circumference ☐
C. BPD ☐
D. Femurlength ☐

203. USG done at 18-20 weeks mainly to: *(DNB 99, 02)*
A. Detect fetal abnormality ☐
B. Determine sex ☐
C. Estimate liquor ☐
D. Determine maturity ☐

204. Which one of the following congenital malformation of the fetus can be diagnosed in first trimester by ultrasound? *(AI 2006)*
A. Anencephaly ☐
B. Inencephaly ☐
C. Microcephaly ☐
D. Holoprosencephaly ☐

205. Anencephaly can be diagnosed by USG at
A. 10-12 weeks of gestation *(AIIMS 96, DNB 03)* ☐
B. 14-18 weeks of gestation ☐
C. 20-24 weeks of gestation ☐
D. 24-28 weeks of gestation ☐

206. Best for unruptured ectopic pregnancy is:
A. Per abdominal US *(PGI 1997)* ☐
B. HCG ☐
C. Trans vaginal US ☐
D. Amniocentesis ☐

207. The investigation of choice for an ectopic pregnancy is:
A. CT scan *(AIIMS Nov 09, May 08)* ☐
B. Transvaginal USG ☐
C. Serum HCG levels ☐
D. MRI ☐

208. All are signs /features of ectopic pregnancy on USG except *(PGI – 2003)*
A. Pseudo sac ☐
B. Hyprechoic ring ☐
C. Adenexal mass ☐
D. Echogenic mass with multicystic spaces within endometrial cavity ☐
E. Doughnut sign ☐

209. Ectopic pregnacny, characteristic finding in USG is:
A. Absence of gestational sac in uterus *(AIIMS 1998)* ☐
B. Complex adenexal mass ☐
C. Resistance in coloured Doppler ☐
D. Free fluid in peritoneal cavity ☐

210. Most accurate assessment of gestational age by USG is done by *(Jipmer 04, DNB 06)*
A. Femur length ☐
B. Gestational sac size
C. Menstrual history ☐
D. Crown rump length ☐

211. USG can diagnose all except: *(PGI 98, DNB 2K)*
A. Anencephaly ☐
B. Neural tube defect ☐
C. Placenta previa ☐
D. Down's syndrome ☐

212. On USG finding of cystic hygroma in fetus is suggestive of *(AIIMS 1997)*
A. Down's syndrome ☐
B. Marphan's syndrome ☐
C. Turner's syndrome ☐
D. Klinfelter's syndrome ☐

Gynecology

213. Missed IUD (IUCD) is recognized by
A. X-Ray *(AIIMS 91, DNB 92)* ☐
B. USG ☐
C. Barium meal ☐
D. CT Scan ☐

214. The method to diagnosis misplaced intra uterine device is *(AIIMS 91, DNB 92)*
A. Ultrasound ☐
B. X-Ray abdomen (Erect view) ☐
C. Uterine sound & Hysteroscopy ☐
D. All of the above ☐

215. Radiological investigation of female of reproductive age group is restricted to *(AI 1993)*
A. Menstrual Period ☐
B. First 10 days of Menstrual Cycle ☐
C. 10-20 days of M.C. ☐
D. Last 10 days of M.C. ☐

216. Maximum radio opaque shadow in ovary is seen in
A. Teratoma *(AIIMS 1997)* ☐
B. Dysgerminoma ☐
C. Mucinous cystadenoma ☐
D. Granulosa cell tumor ☐

Pediatrics

217. Invertogram to be done in a new born :
A. Immediately *(PGI 1998)* ☐
B. After 2 hours ☐
C. After 4 hours ☐
D. After 6 hours ☐

218. First sign of hydrocephalus in children is :
A. Post clinoid erosion *(PGI 1998)* ☐
B. Large fhead ☐
C. Sutural diastasis ☐
D. Thinned out vault ☐

219. William's syndrome is associated with *(AIIMS 1998)*
A. Congenital Supravalvular Aortic stenosis ☐
B. Congenital Subvalvular Aortic stenosis ☐
C. VSD ☐
D. ASD ☐

220. Radiological findings of battered baby syndrome is :
A. Multiple Inuries not explained by one cause ☐
B. Multiple fractures in different stage of healing ☐
C. Excessive callus formation *(AIIMS 1994)* ☐
D. All ☐

Answers and Explanations:

EYE

1. **A i.e. Metastasis; D i.e. NF -1** *[Ref: Chapman 5/e p 254: Osborn 1/e p – 82-83; Wolfgan's 7/e p 320; Grainger 5/e p 1664-65]*

Bare orbit is seen in **metastases (lytic type), neurofibromatosis (NF) type 1, and meningioma**Q.

2. **B i.e. Intracerebral calcification** *[Ref: Wofgang 7/e p. 355-56]*

- Retinoblastoma is the malignant congenital intraocular tumor arising from primitive *photoreceptor cells of retina* (included in primitive neuroectodermal tumor).
- Histologically, it shows ***Flexner-Wintersteiner rosettes***Q **(50%)** ***Home-Wright rosettes***Q ***& fleurettes***Q.
- Clinically presents with ***cat's eye reflex/leukokoria***Q.
- ***Retinoblastoma is the most common cause orbital calcification***Q (nodular or punctate calcification & is favourable prognostic sign.)
- ***Enlargement of orbit & orbital canal***Q occurs d/t involvement of optic nerve & intracranial extension.
- ***Metastasize to meninges, cranial bones***Q, bone marrow, lung, liver, lymph node.

RESPIRATORY SYSTEM

GENERAL

3. **A, C i.e. 40% lung tissue seen obscured by bony structure & mdiastinum; Right dome higher than left dome**
4. **C i.e. Lower lobe veins** 5. **B i.e. Left dome is higher**

[Ref: Chest & CVS imaging: AMP series 3/e p-7-11; Sutton 7/e p-2-14; Felson (2202 ed) P-185; Snells 7/e P-137-39; Grainger 4/e P-289]

- PA and lateral views are routinely done to evaluate the *lungs, 40% of which is obscured by other structures including ribs*Q. *In most patients the right hemidiaphragm is higher than the left. This is d/t heart depressing the left side and not to the liver pushing up the right hemidiaphragm*Q
- The *lower lobe pulmonary veins* do not cross the hila in their course to the left atrium and therefore do not contribute to the hilar shadow.
- ***Left hilum is higher than right***Q. Pulmonary arteries & upper lobe veins mainly contribute to hilar shadows. ***All fissures are seen clearly on lateral film***Q.

HEMOPTYSIS

6. **B i.e. Bronchial artery** *[Ref: Grainger 4/e P-609]*

In 95% of cases of **massive recurrent hemoptysis,** the source of blood are ***systemic bronchial artery***Q rather than pulmonary artery; So these are the vascular structures which should be evaluated first.

Type of Bleeding	Source
- Hemoptysis	- ***Bronchial artery***Q
- Epidural hemorrhage	- ***Middle meningeal artery***Q
- Subdural hemorrhage	- ***Bridging veins***Q
- Sub arachnoid hemorrhage	- ***Berry saccular aneurysm***Q
- Intracerebral hemorrhage	- Intra parenchymal vessels
- Menstruation	- ***Spiral arteries***Q
- Epitaxis	- Plexus of vein (M.C.) & sphenopalatine artery

7. **B i.e. Broncheal artery** *[Ref: Grainger 4/e P-609; Crofton & Douglas – respiratory diseases 5/e P-516]*

- In great majority of patients hemoptysis originates from **systemic rather than pulmonary arteries** and the **bronchial vessels are almost universally involved.** (Grainger)
- Massive hemoptysis in a patient of T.B. is usually d/t erosion of bronchial artery which bleeds at systemic pressure. (Crofton)

8. **D i.e. Bronchoscopy** *[Ref: Harrison 18/e p. 282-86]* 9. **B i.e. Bronchoscopy**

As a rule, you can remember, for almost all cases of hemoptysis the investigation of choice is Bronchoscopy followed by HRCT;
Except for hemoptysis associated with ***parenchymal (interstitial) lung disease*** where investigatim of choice is HRCT> Bronchoscopy, and in suspected bronchitis where you observe and wait for recurrence for performing Bronchoscopy.

PULMONARY NODULE

10. **C i.e. Hamartoma** *[Ref: Sutton 7/e P-138, 140; Harrison 15/e P-1448]*

- **Hamartoma** produces ***noncavitating popcorn calcification***[Q].
- Various infections, neoplasms, granulomatous lesions (wegner's rheumatoid-caplan's, pneumoconiosis, traumatic & vascular infarcts) produce **cavitatory lesions.**

11. **D i.e. Neurofibroma** *[Ref: Grainger 4/e P-485; Sutton 7/e P-21]*

- Primary complex in TB, produce solitary pulmonary nodule.
- Bronchial adenoma & Pulmonary hamartoma mostly produce solitary nodules d/t their benign nature.
- Neurofibroma is almost always present at multiple foci.
- It is important to note that **Hamartoma** produces **non cavitatory lesions.**

12. **D i.e. Image guided biopsy** *[Ref: Sutton 7/e P-19-22/35-37, Wolfgang 7/e p. 432-35]*

CT scan is most sensitive for detecting large pulmonary nodules (≥ 3mm) but neither sensitive nor specific for smaller nodules the maximum CT scan can show is calcification & cavitation, which are not always diagnostic of benign & malignant lesions respectively.
So the best investigation to come to a diagnosis (i.e. most specific) will be ***image guided (transthoracic needle aspiration) biopsy***[Q].

MILIARY SHADOW

13. **A i.e. T.B; B i.e. R.A; C i.e. Pneumoconiosis; E i.e. Metastasis** 14. **A i.e. T.B.; B i.e. Sarcoidosis**
15. **A i.e. Rhematoid arthritis; B i.e. TB; E i.e. Pulmonary edema**
16. **A i.e. Histoplasmosis; B i.e. Sarcoidosis; C i.e. Secondaries from C_A colon**
17. **D i.e. Staphylococcal pneumonia** 18. **C i.e. Klebsiella** 19. **A i.e. Klebsiella pneumonia**
20. **A i.e. Rheumatoid arthritis; C i.e. Scleroderma; E i.e. Interstitial disease**
[Ref: Wolfgang 7/e p. 514, 428; Chapman 5/e p. 73-85; Sutton 7/e p. 132; P.J. Mehta 14/e p. 309; Harrison 15/e p. 1107, 957]

- **Miliary nodules (mottling)** is seen in ***tuberculosis, fungal infections (eg histoplasmosis), varicella virus, brucellosis, salmonell, nocardiosis (bacteria)***[Q], ***sarcoidosis, secondaries, pneumoconiosis, pulmonary edema & Loffler's syndrome but not in klebsiella & staphylococeal pneumonia***[Q].
- **Klebsiella pneumonia** is most common cause of ***bulging of fissure***[Q] and **Staphylococcus pneumonia** commonly l/t ***pneumatocele formation***[Q]

21. **A i.e. Hilar involvement; B i.e. Miliary shadowing; C i.e. Honey comb appearance**
[Ref: Wolfgang 7/e p. 428-27, 501-502; Grainger 5/e p. 322, 1783-85]

- **Split pleura sign** (ie pleural fluid between enhancing thickened parietal & visceral pleura) in CT is seen in **empyema.**
- **Entire (whole) lung collapse** results in ***complete opacification or white out of the affected hemithorax***[Q].
- **Eosinophilic granuloma** may radiologically present with ***diffuse fine milliary nodules (miliary mottling), reticulo-nodular lung disease, honey comb appearance and hilar involvement.***[Q]

HYPERINFLATED LUNG

22. **C i.e. Expiratory film** *[Ref: Chapman 4/e P-114]*

How can a normal expiratory film leads to increased radiolucency of hemithorax? So the answer is very obvious. ↑ed Radiolucency of one side means there is U/L lung pathology. Obst. Emphysema & U/L Pneumothorax may lead to U/L lung collapse & radiolucency. Patient rotation may also lead to false impression of U/L radiolucency. But expiration film in normal conditions may never be a cause of this.

23. **B i.e. Congenital lobar emphysema** *[Ref: Chapman 4/e p. 114]*

Congenital lobar emphysema cause hyperinflation of lungQ.

24. **D i.e. Pneumonectomy**
[Ref: Grainger 4/e P-651, 1227; Sutton 7/e P-260; Chapman 4/e P-118 & 115]

- ***Pulmonary agenesis***Q & ***Pneumonectomy***Q are the causes of ***radiopaque lung with I/L mediastinal shift***Q.
- **Pulmonary artery obstruction (i.e. Pulmonary embolism)** l/t ***radiolucent lung***Q.

25. **A i.e. CCF** *[Ref: Sutton 6/e P-327]*

Congestive cardiac failure is a condition which ***presents with B/L changes in chest X Ray***Q – so it can be excluded by seeing U/L hemithorax on chest X Ray, if it is normal.;

26. **C i.e. Decreased intercostals space** *[Ref: Sutton 7/e P-168; Grainger 4/e P-453]*

In **emphysema**, ***intercostals space is increased (not decreased)***Q

INTERSTIAL & PLEURAL PATHOLOGY

27. **B i.e. Left to Right Shunt**
[Ref: Nelson's 16/e P-1399; Grainger 4/e P-820, 640, 641, 311, 591; Wofgang 5/e P-421; Chapman 4/e P-124, 142]

Ground glass appearance is seen **in interstitial pneumonias, hyline membrane disease and obstructive TAPVC**Q **but not in left to right shunts** which show hyperemic **(plethoric) lung field.**

28. **A i.e. Pulmonary edema** *[Ref: Harrison's 15/e P-1556]*

Salt & water retention in uremia

↓

Pulmonary congestion & edemaQ in the absence of volume overload (due to increased permeability of alveolar capillary membrane)

↓

Butterfly wing distribution of Pulmonary edema = Uremic lungQ

29. **D i.e. Air bronchogram are seen within the opacity**
[Ref: Felson P-69; Lee Stanley P-465; Grainger 4/e P-311, 591; Wolfgang 5/e P-421; Chapman 4/e P-124, 142; (Ref: AMPIS: Chest Imaging 3/e p 379-80; Sutton 7/e p 91; Wolfgng 7/e p 446-47]

- **Loculated (encysted or encapsulated)pleural effusions can be differential from peripheral pleural based llung lesions by absences of air bronchogram.**
- Loculated PE are sharply mrginated on profile, obique, tangential views and **ill defined on enface (end on) view**Q.
- **Loculated PE may not be confined to any bronchopulmonary segment and may make an obtuse angel with the chest wall.**Q

30. **D i.e. Right lateral decubitus** *[Ref: Wofgang 5/e P-428/30; Sutton 7/e P-380]*

Ipsilateral decubitus is investigation of choice for minimal pleural effusionQ

PEDIATRIC RESPIRATORY DISTRESS

31. **B i.e. Oesophageal duplication cyst** *[Ref: Pediatric Imaging 3/ep 155; Wolfgang 7/ep 840]*

Most likely diagnosis is a **asymptomatic or mildly symptomatic** (ie dysphagic/dyspneic) newborn **who had posterior mediastinal mass with airfluid level in chest X ray[Q] associated with vertebral anomalies (hemivertebra, spina bifida, fusion defects) on plain Xray[Q]** is – **Oesophageal duplication cyst.**

32. **C i.e. Congenital lobar aplasia of lung** *[Ref: Wofgang 5/e P-482, 996; Grainger 4/e P- 252, 254]*

- **D/D of Multiple air filled (cystic appearing) intrathoracic mass in new born are**
  1. *Congenital diaphragmatic hernia[Q]*
  2. Congential lobar emphysema
  3. Broncho-pulmonary malformations
     - ***Bronchogenic (Lung) Cyst[Q]***
     - Broncho-pulmonary sequestration
     - ***Congenital Cystic adenomatoid malformation[Q] (CCAM)***
  4. Pneumatocoel formation.

- ***In congenital lobar aplasia, there is hyperlucency not multiple air filled spaces (which are seen in congenital lobar emphysema.)[Q]***

33. **D i.e. Foreign body aspiration** **34.** **D i.e. Foreign body aspiration**
[Ref: Grainger 4/e P-651, 1227; Sutton 7/e P-260; Chapman 4/e P-118 & 115; Wolfgang 5/e P-405]

Child (not new born) presently with acute/ sudden onset respiratory distress (difficulty) & strider ; and decreased breath sound and wheeze unilaterally (esp on right side) along with hyperinflation (50%) or radiopacity (45%) of unilateral lung on chest X ray indicate the diagnosis of foreign body aspiration.

Now approach to this case: In *pneumothorax* there will be *no wheeze & stridor* and it will present with *radiolucent hemithorax. Acute epiglottitis* may present with *wheeze & stridor* but there will be *B/L lung involvement* and the symptoms are *acute but not sudden. Massive pleural effusion* presents with U/L radiopaque hemithorax but *without wheeze & stridor* and the onset is *not sudden.* Childish age, h/o ***sudden onset[Q]*** of symptoms of respiratory difficulty and *airway obstruction* ***(wheeze & stridor)[Q]***, involvement of ***right lung[Q]*** and U/L radiopaque hemithorax all indicate towards diagnosis of foreign body aspiration.

35. **C i.e. Congenital diaphragmatic hernia** **36.** **C i.e. Congenital diaphragmatic hernia**
[Ref: Sutton 7/e P-252-54; Nelson's 16/e P-1232; Grainger 4/e P-387,402, 639-40; Wolfgang 7/ep 498-99; Pediatric Imaging 3/ep 64-65]

- **Neonate presenting with acute respiratory distress on day 1 with chest X ray showing multiple air filled (cystic) lesions and contralateral mediastinal shift** is most likely suffering from **congenital diaphragmatic hernia.** Bag & mask therapy during resusciatation may worsen the respiratory distress.
- It is very easy to understand that intestinal coils migrating from abdomen (making it scaphoid) to chest, causing mediastinum to shift contralateraly. The swallowed air in the loops, is cause of multiple cystic air filled lesions in chest. So diagnosis is congenital diaphragmatic hernia. Bronchogenic cyst usually presents with minimal symptomps & no mediastinal shift.
- **Congenital diaphragmatic hernia may be Bochdalek hernia, Morgagni hernia, eventration[Q]**, septum transversum defect or hiatal hernia.

37. **B i.e. Pneumothorax; C i.e. Cong. diaphragmatic hernia**

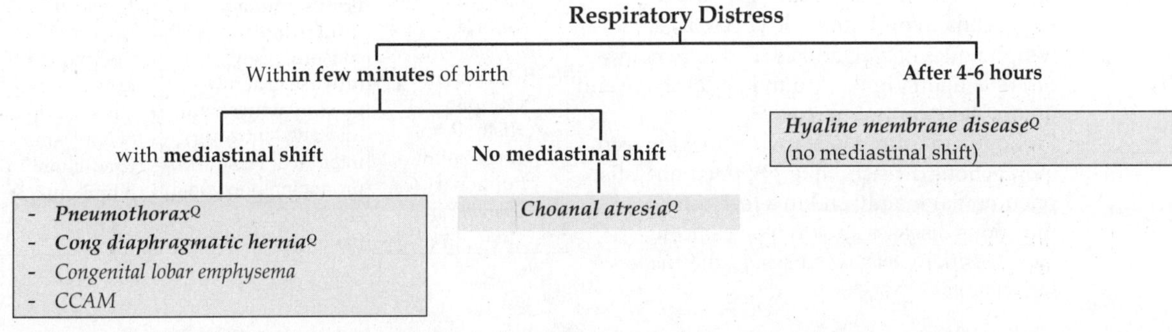

38. **D i.e. Any of above** *[Ref: B & L 24/e P-873; Sutton 6/e P-254-55, 560]*
39. **C i.e., CT scan of chest** *[Ref: Grainger 5/e p- 401- 5, 301, 391, 326- 28, 411- 12; Harrison 17/e p. 1593 – 94, 1609]*

- Consolidation is an increase in parenchymal density obscuring margins of airways & vessles. It is a radiological sign of air space disease. (eg. pneumonia etc). CT scan is frequently requested in patients with air space disease and the CT features are occasionally diagnostic.
- In this child to rule out underlying predisposing lung pathology eg. pulmonary sequestration ect, CT scan would be the investigation of choice.
- Even in hypersensitivity pneumonitis (HP), high resolution CT has become the imaging procedure of choice. Lung biopsy (through flexible bronchoscope) may be diagnostic but not pathognomic. Traid of mononuclear bronchiolitis, interstitial infiltrates of plasma cells & lymphocytes and single non necrotizing randomly scattered parenchymal granuloma without mural vascular invasion is consistent with but specific for HP.

PULMONARY THROMBOEMBOLISM (PTE)

40. **A i.e. Lung Ventilation Perfusion Scan**
41. **A i.e. Perfusion segmental defect; B i.e. Perfusion defect with normal lung scan & radiography**
42. **B i.e., Pulmonary embolism** 43. **A i.e. Pulmonary angiography**
44. **B i.e. V-P Scan** *[Ref: Grainger 5/e p. 536-43; Braunwald- Heart disease P-1896; Harrison 18/e P-2170-77; 15/e p. 1510-11]*

- **An elderly (55 yr old) man on prolonged bed rest (>3 days)** predispose him to deep vein thrombosis **(DVT)**. And if he ***complains of dyspnea (mc symptom), tachypnea (mc sign), breathlessness and chest pain with a normal or near normal chest Xray*** or CXR showing ***Hampton's hump***[Q], **Pella sign, Westermark sign, Felson's sign or Fleischner lines** the probable diagnosis is **pulmonary thromboembolism (PTE).**
- **Contrast enhanced CT pulmonary angiography (CT with intravenous contrast)** is the **principal imaging test for diagnosis of PE[Q]. It has virtually replaced invasive pulmonary angiography as the main stay investigation & a diagnostic test for PE**. Conventional pulmonary angiography, does however remains the **gold standard test.**
- **Lung scan = ventilation - perfusion (VP) scan** has become the **2nd line diagnostic test for PE**, used mostly for patients who cannot tolerate intravenous contrast (of CECT). A **high probability scan for PE** is defined as one that indicates **≥2 segmental perfusion defects in the presence of normal ventilation**[Q]. Abnormal ventilation scans (indication abnormal non ventilated lung) exclude PE as a possible cause of perfusion defect and provide lung diseases as asthma, COPD etc as possible explanation for perfusion defect.

INFECTIOUS DISEASE

45. **B i.e. Tuberculosis** *[Ref: Wolfganf 7/e p. 549-51; Harrison18/e p.2124-25, 2806-8; Chapman 5/e P-92; AMPIS: Chest Imaging 3/e p. 119, 60-6]*

- **B/L Upper lobe fibrosis** makes lymphoma unlikely. It may be seen in other conditions and m.c. in tuberculosis. Diagnosis of silicosis is based on relevant *occupational history* (10-12 years exposure is usually necessary). Expectoration is common in T.B. & usually not found in silicosis, sarcoidosis & lymphoma.
- ***Tuberculosis is most common cause of necrotic lymphnode with peripheral rim enhancement***[Q] ***on CT.*** In contrast to enhanced enlarged mediastinal lymphnodes of TB, enlarged lymph nodes of **sarcoidosis** tend to remain discrete, maintain their round nodal shape and **do not have central nercosis**[Q]
- Predominant upper lobe involvement is seen in infectious diseases (like **TB**, pneumocystis pneumonia) mainly and in a few non infectious diseases eg *sarcoidosis, silicosis, hypersensitivity pneumonitis and Langerhans cell histocytosis.*

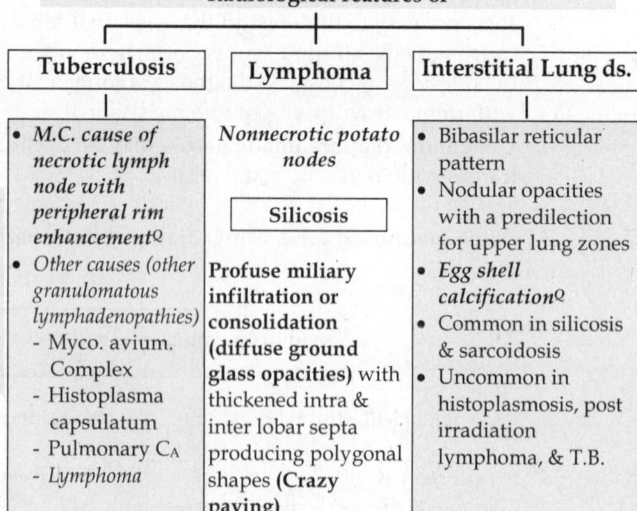

46. **D i.e. Pneumocystic carinii** *[Ref: Harrison 18//e P-1547-49; Sutton 7/e p. 154-58; AMPIS Chest Imaging 3/e p. 134-139]*

- **Non productive or minimal productive cough** (white sputum) **with a normal chest X ray or faint to dense bilateral perihilar infiltrates (opacity) without pleural effusion & lymphadenopathy in AIDS^Q patient** indicate diagnosis of **pneumocystis (P. jiroveci, P. Cavini) pneumonia.** Patients with PCP may complain of a characteristic retrosternal chest pain that is worse on inspiration and is described as sharp or burning. HIV associated PCP may have an indolent course.
- **TB infection in HIV** patients present with **productive cough, cavitatory apical disease** of upper lobes (high CD4 count), disseminated disesase, diffuse or lower lobe bilateral reticulonodular infiltrates consistent with **miliary spread, pleural effusions, hilar &/or mediastinal lymphadenopathy with extrapulmonary** (bone, brain, meninges, GI tract, lymph nodes esp cervical, genitourinary) involvement.

47. **D i.e. (RSV)** *[Ref:Wiliams 7/e p 433; Wolfgang 7/e p 430/482; 529, 815; Chest Imging 3/e p 153-35; Harrison 18/e p 1120-25, 1486-88]*

- Most common cause of **tree in bud (bronchiectasis) appearance** is Mycobacterium tuberculosis (endobronchial).
- Most common specific cause of tree in bud appearance in **HSL (bone marrow) transplant patients** is **CMV (30-70%) > RSV (18%) > M. tuberculosis (5-6%) > Pneumocystis > Invasive aspergillosis.**

INDUSTRIAL LUNG DISEASE

48. **B i.e. Asbestosis** 49. **B i.e. Asbestosis**

[Ref: Wolfgang 7/e p 472-73; Grainger 5/e p 372-73; Armstrong 5/e p 77/79; Haga 5/e p 372-73; Sutton 7/e p 189-95; Robbins 6/e p 732; Fraser-Muller p-2424]

- **Asbestos related lung disease** presents with **pleural effusion** (*small, blood stained, persistent, recurrent, bilateral*), **pleural plaques** (bilateral, multifocal, exclusively involving parietal pleura along posterolateral & lateral chest wall b/w 6-10th ribs and sparing visceral pleura, apices & costophrenic angles), **pleural calcification** (bilateral diaphragmatic calcification with clear CP angles is pathognomic), **diffuse pleural thickening** (involves visceral pleura & l/t impaired lung function), **asbestosis, pseudotumor (round atlectasis) & malignancy**.
- **Asbetosis** may present with *fine to coarse reticulonodular pattern* causing loss of clarity of diaphragm & cardiac shadow (**Shaggy heart**) *on* x ray. HRCT (investigation of choice) shows *subpleural pulmonary arcade, pleural based nodular irragularities, parenchymal bands & septal lines*
- **Round atelectasis** occurs mostly in ***peripheral, lower, dorsal (posterior) lobes adjacent to visceral pleura***^Q and presents with ***Comet tail/Vaccum cleaner/ Crow's feet sign and Swiss cheese air bronchogram***^Q

- ***Pulmonary fibrosis in asbestosis is bilateral and maximal at bases whereas in coal workers pneumoconiosis and Silicosis upper half of the lung is mainly involved.***^Q
  Radiological features of Asbestosis:
  - ***Pleural thickening and calcification primarily localized along lateral chest wall and diaphragm***^Q.
  - Differentiated from postinflamatory and post-traumatic pleural thickening & calcification by it's ***Bilateral involvement and sharp costophrenic angles in asbestosis***^Q.
  - Pleural thickening & calcification may be seen following minor exposure whereas pulmonary fibrosis only follows significant exposure

Approach to Industrial lung disease

Predominant Mid & Upper zone involvement^Q	**Predominant Lower zone involvement**^Q	**Wide spread whole lung involvement**
1. Silicosis^Q - Related to coal, gold, granite, slate, sandstone & ceramic industry - *Multiple, well defined, 2-5 mm nodules relatively* ***sparing bases*** - ***BIL Hilar lymphadenopathy with peripheral (egg-shell) calcification***^Q **2. Coal Worker's Pneumoconiosis** - Due to coal dust mainly carbon small, indistinct, - Faint nodules of 1-5 mm mainly in midzone - Progressive massive fibrosis (PMF) & Caplan's syndrome (in RA) is more common in CWP as compared to in silicosis	**Asbestosis**^Q - Due to asbestos exposure in ***asbestos, ship building & textile manufacture industry***^Q - Radiologically ***earliest sign is fine reticular or nodular pattern in lower zone***^Q. With progression becomes coarse & causes ***loss of clarity of diaphragm & cardiac shadow (shaggy heart)***^Q - ***B/L pleural plaques in mid & lower zone over diaphragm***^Q are specific to asbestosis. - ***Small (<500 ml) blood stained pleural effusion.***^Q	1. Siderosis (iron oxide dust) 2. Stannosis (tin oxide dust) 3. Barytosis ($BaSO_4$ dust)

50. **B i.e. Round atelectasis** *[Ref: Haga 5/e p 887]*

Round atelectasis (folded lung or **atelectatic asbestos pseudotumor)** characteristically presents with *comet tail sign*Q i.e. the presence of crowding of bronchi & blood vessels that extend from the border of the mass of collapsed lung to the hilum like a tail of comet.

MALIGNANCY

51. **A i.e. Adrenals** *[Ref: Sutton's Radiology 7th/e p-108; Lee & Seagel 3/e p. 1191]*

Adrenal gland is m.c. site of endocrinal gland involvement in bronchial carcinomaQ.
Because Adrenal metastases are so common in lung cancer, the adrenal glands should be included in the CT examination of all patients presenting with a lung cancer. Q

- Metastasis may occur any where in the body but nodal involvement is most common in bronchogenic carcinoma– Hilar, Mediastinal, Supraclavicular
- Nodal involvement is followed by liver, bones, brain, adrenal gland and skin.

52. **C i.e. Metastasis** *[Ref: Sutton 6/e P-409]*

Pulmonary metastasis is ***radiologically hetrogenous***Q due to occurance of ***cavitation (more common in squamous cell carcinoma) & calcification (most often in osteogenic S_A***Q & rarely in chondrosarcoma.)

MEDIASTINUM

53. **A i.e. Pulmonary artery; D i.e. Arch of aorta**
54. **A i.e. Aortic arch; D i.e. Left ventricle; B i.e. Left Pulmonary artery**
55. **A i.e. Enlargement of left atrial appendage** *[Ref: Grainger 5/e p 467-74; Sutton 7/e p 265-66/240; Peter Armstong 5/e p 108/117; Clark's 12/e p 215; Chapman 5/e p 114-18; Wolfgang 7/e p 609; AMPIS 3/e p 342; Chest X Ray made Easy by J. Corne, M. Caroll, I. Brown/20]*

Left heart border on chest X-ray PA view is formed by- <u>A</u>ortic <u>K</u>nuckle, <u>P</u>ulmonary <u>C</u>onus, <u>L</u>eft <u>a</u>trial <u>A</u>ppendage and <u>L</u>eft <u>V</u>entricle. So **left sided cardiac bulge** is seen in ***enlargement of left atrial appendage***Q.

Mn- "**AK PC LAAV** = एक Personal computer LoVe" forms left heart border.

56. **D i.e. Main Pulmonary trunk; E i.e. Aortic arch**
57. **C i.e. Ascending aorta**
58. **A i.e. SVC; B i.e. IVC; C i.e. Rt atrium**
59. **D i.e. Right ventricle**
60. **B i.e., Superior vena cava; C i.e. Right atrium**
61. **C i.e. Right Ventricle**
[Ref: Dahnert Radiology Review Manual 5th/636-637, 458; Harrison 17th /1467; P.J. Mehta 15th/160-61]

Right heart border on chest x-ray PA view is formed by ***right atrium with its draining tributaries SVC & IVC***Q. Right aspect of ***ascending thoracic aorta and right innominate/brachiocephalic vessels***Q are also involved sometimes in forming right border. But ***right ventricle does not form the right border of the heart or mediastinum. It forms the anterior border of heart visible on lateral film.***

62. **A i.e. Elevation of the left main bronchus**

Left atrial enlargment presents radiologically with ***elevation of left main bronchus (earliest feature)***Q, ***splaying or widening of carina***Q (to right or obtused angle), indentation & displacement of oesophagus posteriorly, ***double contour/shadow/density or double right heart border***Q, and prominent left atrial appendage.

63. **C i.e. Aberrant right subclavian artery** *[Ref: Sutton 7/e p-572-73; Haga 5/e p-1025]*

An **aberrant right subclavian artery** arises from the aortic arch distal to the origin of left subclavian artery, and passes upwards & to the right behind the oesophagus. This gives rise to a ***classical smooth, oblique indentation on posterior wall of barium filled oesophagus***Q.

64. **E i.e. RA + LA** *[Ref: BDC vol. 1 pg 217]*

The **base of heart** forms its posterior surface. It is formed mainly ***by the left atrium***Q and ***by small part of right atrium***Q.

65. **D i.e. Shift of trachea on X Ray** *[Ref: Sutton 7/e P-64-66; Wolfgang 7/e p. 547-46, 454, 449; Pediatric Imaging AMPIs 3/e p. 93; Grainger 5/e p. 209-12, 245-248, 256-57]*

Prominent but normal thymus is the *most common pseudotumor of anterior mediastinum*. On imaging anterior mediastinal tumors displace the trachea and oesophagus posteriorly and laterlly in a contradistinction to a ***normal enlarged thymus which does not displace adjacent structures***Q. – *Paediatric imaging 93*

66. **D i.e. Osteosarcoma** *[Ref: Chapman 5/e P-27-28; Wolfgang 7/e p. 18, 79, 119; Sutton 7/e p. 49, 113, 125; Grainger 5/e p. 1777-79, 1696, 1482, 1646, 342, 254]*

- **Soft tissue mass with rib erosion** can be seen in **leukemia** (osteolytic expanding geographical lesion caused by collection of leukaemic cells/chloroma-Grainger 1777), **lymphoma** (rib involvement is common with multiple lytic occasionally expanding lesions with soft tissue masses-Grainger 1779), **Ewing's sarcoma** (osteolytic destructive rib lesions d/t primary Ewing's or secondaries from it b/o large soft tissue component; *while sclerosis when present should not be interpreted as tumor bone production, as seen in osteosarcoma*, but is a secondary reactive phenomenon- Grainger 1646) and even **Osteosarcoma**, (but it is rarest and is more commonly a/w *sclerosis and calcification*).
- General rule: **Rib erosion /destruction** is caused by many *infective*, (granulomatous infections like TB & fungal are more common), metabolic (Pagets & Brown tumor) and **neoplastic lesions**. (*secondary more common than primary*; and **malignant primary more common than benign primary**). *Chondrosarcoma & osteosarcoma* have tendency to calcify.

67. **B i.e. Neurogenic tumor** *[Ref: Armstrong 5/e p. 55; Harrison 18/e p. 2095-96, 2181/e-20/21; Grainger 5/e p. 1479]*

Neurogenic tumors (arising in posterior nerve structues) ***are the most common posterior mediastinal tumor but these do not occur in anterior mediastinum***Q. And posterior mediastinum is the most common location for neurogenic tumors.

68. **C i.e. Pulmonary plethora**

69. **C, D & E i.e. Dilated left atrium; Dilated pulmonary veins & Dilated pulmonary artery**

70. **B i.e. Normal LA** *[Ref: Wolfgang 7/e p. 592-93, 633-34, 676; Chapman 5/e p. 115-18; Felson 2002 – 216; Braunwald 6/e P-1526; Nelson's 17/e p. 1509-10]*

- Characteristic findings of **ASD** include ***enlarged heart, RA, RV, PA and PV with normal LA & LV and decreased aorta and SVC***Q
- Characteristic findings of **VSD** include ***enlarged heart, RA, RV, PA, PV and LA***Q. So ***pulmonary overcirculation/congestion occurs both in ASD & VSD but LA remains normal in ASD & enlarges in VSD***Q.

71. **'C' i.e. Ebstein's anomaly** *[Ref: Wolfgang 7/e p. 593-90; Sutton 7/e p. 290; Grainger 5/e P 533-34; OP Ghai 6/e P 399, 410]*

Pulmonary plethora (hypercirculation) occurs in *ASD, VSD & TAPVC*Q whereas **oligemic lungs** occur in *Ebstein anomaly*Q. L→R shunts increse and R→L shunts decrease pulmonary blood flow.

72. **C. i.e. Oligenic lung field** **73.** **A i.e. Cardiomegaly; B i.e. Thick interlobar septum**

74. **B i.e. Prominent lower lobe vessels** *[Ref: Wofgang 7/e P-597-98; AMP series 3/e p. 347]*

In **CCF/ Left heart failure** there is ***cephalization of pulmonary vascularity (i.e. dilatation of upper lobe & constriction of lower zone vessels)***Q, ***Kerley A lines (interlobular septal thickening)***Q, ***Kerley (septal) B lines, perihilar haze and pseudoeffusion***Q.

75. **C i.e. Diameter of descending right pulmonary artery > 16mm**
[Ref: Grainger 5/e p 532-33; Wolfgang 7/e p 594-96; Sutton 7/e p 8, 286-88; Vidyasagar 2007 p-138]

- The **maximum normal diameter** of the **descending branch of right pulmonary artery** is ***16 mm for males and 15 mm for females***Q. It forms the *lower border of right hilium (on PA view)*. ***Diameter of descending right pulmonary artery > 16mm***Q ***for males & > 15mm for females denotes pulmonary hypertension.*** *(Sutton)*
- A recognized method of *assessing pulmonary artery size (to find out pulmonary plethora = overcirculation &/or pulmonary artery hypertension)* is by measuring the size of right descending pulmonary artery. **Enlargement indicating plethora/PAH** is diagnosed if the transvere diameter of RDP artery at its midpoint is **greater than 17mm**Q (Grainger).

76. A i.e. Pulmonary hypertension

Pulmonary arterial hypertension is characterized by ***pruning of peripheral pulmonary arteries***^Q (i.e. *disproportionate increase in caliber of fibrous central arteries* from sustained increase in PBF with a *decrease in caliber of small muscular/peripheral arteries*).

77. D i.e. Uniformly branching lines parallel to pleura

78. B i.e., Upper lobar diversion of vessels *[Ref: Grainger 5/e p-530-32; Danhert 7/e p. 586; Sutton 7/e p – 288-89]*

Upper lobe venous diversion is the first radiological sign of pulmonary venous hypertenson^Q **(PVH).** *Other features of PVH include* ***Kerley B lines (parallel to each other but perpendicular to pleura), perihilar haze, peribroncheal cuffing, pulmonary ossicles, fine punctuate (nodular) calcification***^Q ***and perihilar bats wing pattern.***

79. A, B, C, E i.e. Double contour of right heart border, Straightening of left heart border, Splaying of carinal angle, Kerley lines *[Ref: Grainger 4/e P-833, 877; Denhert 5.e p. 644-645; Harrison 15/e P-1345]*

80. C i.e. Obliteration of retrosternal shadow on lateral X Ray

81. B i.e. Oligemia of upper lung field *[Ref: Grainger 5/e p-471-472; Harrison 15/e P-1345]*

There is ***dialation of upper lobe pulmonary veins and constriction (l/t olegemia) of lower lobe veins causing inverted moustache sign***^Q***, in mitral stenosis.***

Radiological features of mitral stenosis include ***straightening of left heart border, lifting of left bronchus, splaying of carina, double contour of right heart border (double atrial shadow), posterior displacement of oesophagus (on barium swallow), Kerely B lines, pulmonary hemosiderosis and small aortic knob (knuckle)***^Q.

82. A i.e. Enlarged Azygous Vein *[Ref: Snell's anatomy 7/e P-57 & 128; Sutton 7/e p. 5]*

Azygous vein is a right sided structure^Q and all others are left sided. Azygous vein lies *in the angle between the right main bronchus & trachea* and size is < 10mm diameter on erect X-ray. Its size **decreases** on valsalva, in spiration; and **increases** in supine position, pregnancy, portal hypertension, IVC & SVC obstruction, right heart failure, constrictive pericarditis and enlarged subcranial nodes. So Azygous vein can't give rise to left cardiac bulge.

83. A i.e. Tetralogy of Fallot's *[Ref: Nelson 16/e, p 1386; Chapman 5/e, p 115]*

In **tetralogy of fallot's** ***heart size is normal***. Roentgenographically, the typical configuration as seen in anteroposterior view consist of a narrow base, concavity of the left heart border in the area usually occupied by the pulmonary artery and normal heart".

84. B i.e. Calcification of ascending aorta *[Ref: Sutton 7/e p – 312 –14]*

- ***Saccular aneurysm with pencil – thin (linear) dystrophic calcification most commonly in ascending aorta commencing near the aortic root***^Q is charcteristic feature of **syphilitic aortitis.**
- Aortic aneurysm in Marfan's syndrome often involves *sinuses of valsalva, & ascending aorta.* It can also affect aortic ring resulting in AR. The aneurysm is classically *flask shaped with loss of usual indentation at sino – tubular junction.*
- Takayasu's aortitis affects segments of aorta including main aortic branches & pulmonary arteries.

85. A i.e. Lingular lesion

86. C i.e. Right middle lobe

87. A i.e. Pneumonia affecting medial zone of right middle lobe

88. D i.e. Left upper lobe (posterior part) *[Ref: Juhl's 7/e p 302; Sutton 7/e p 175- 79, 14; AMPIS 3/e p 39-41; Webb & Higgin's 2/e p 40-41; Wolfgang 7/e p 448]*

- Consolidation of **apical portion of left upper lobe (LUL)** will obliterate or obscure the **aortic knuckle (knob)** portion of cardiac shadow on chest x-ray (Mnemonic-**LUL** sounds like **Knuckle**")
- Consolidation of **lingula** (anterior) obscures **left heart border (i.e. left cardiac silhouette)** and consolidation of **righ middle lobe (RML)** obliterates **right heart border (right cardiac silhoutte)**. Mn= ***"Lingula is left and RML is right".***
- **Homogenous paracardiac opacity in right lung, near right cardiac silhouette (or right heart border)** with ill defined lateral border (of opacity) in a patient with fever, cough and difficulty in breathing is indicative of **pneumonia involving** medial zone of **right middle lobe**.

89. **C i.e. Calcium deposition in the atheromatous plaque** *[Ref: Haga 5/e p. 1186-90; CVS Imaging 3/e p. 358-60]*

- **Screening** of asymptomatic **coronary plaques on CT scan** (EBCT & MDCT) uses ***calcium deposition***Q as a *surrogate marker for detecting the presence & amout of atherosclerosis.*
- CT attenuation within non calcified fibrous plque (91-116) is greater than within noncalcified lipid-rich plaques (47-71 HU). However, large variability currently *prevents accurate classification of non calcified plaques by CT.*

90. **B i.e. MRI** *[Ref: Granger 5/e p-1475, 550, 557-47; Sutton 7/e p-407-10, 866; Dahnert 6/e p-592-93; Pediatric imaging AMP series 3/e p-106-7]*

To visualize vascular sling causing tracheal (external airway) compression, MRI is investigation of choiceQ.

91. **C i.e. Akinetic areas does not benefit from revascularization**
[Ref: Wolfgang 7/e p 1130-22; Grainger 5/e p 520, 152; Sutton 7/e p 319; CVS Imaging 3/e p 360-50, Armstrong 5/e p 124-22; 105, 110]

- **Akinetic areas** in myocardial wall ***may also be d/t hibernating & stunned myocardium, which can restore function (recover) after reperfusion (revascularization)***Q.
- Stunned & hibernating myocardium can be identified by recovery of LV function (such as wall movement) during ***extended stress (like pharmacologically dobutamine induced stress) testing with radionuclide*** (*^{201}Th / ^{99m}Tc) imaging, ECHO or Cine-MRA*Q.
- **Delayed contrast enhancement (DE)-MRI using gadolinium is the** ***gold standard for detection of irreversibly damaged (nonviable) myocardium (i.e. scar, fibrosis, infarcted)***Q.

92. **B i.e. Dobutamine** *[Ref: Grainger 5/e p- 432; Sutton 7/e p – 277; Harrison 17/e p.1399 – 1400]*

- **Stress echocardigraphy** has same technique used to access the heart function at rest eg. cardiac output, ejection fraction, shortening fraction & segmental wall motion analysis) but ***with a stressor as exercise or dobutamine infusion***Q. It can cause emergence of regions of akinesis or dyskinesis not present at rest.
- Stress echocardiography is primarily indicated to confirm the suspicion of ischemic heart disease & to estimate its severity. **Regional wall motion abnormality** i.e., decreased systolic contraction of an ischemic area of myocardium, *occurs before symptoms or ECG changes. New regional wall motion abnormalities, decrease in ejection fraction* and increase in end systolic volume with stress, are all indicators of myocardial ischemia.
- Response of gradient to dobutamine stimulation is of diagnostic & theraputic value in patients with *low – gradient, low output aortic stenosis (AS).* It's also used to assess myocardial viability in patients with *poor systolic function of concomitant coronary artery disease (CAD).*
- In selected situations (eg men, multivessel disease, LAD disease when imaging single vessel diseae), it is very sensitive in detecting myocardial ischemia. The same is true for stress ECG and radionuclide perfusion scan.

93. **D i.e. Electrical impedance cardiograph technology** *[Ref: Journal of Medicine & Braunwald]*
- PA catheter & thermodilution technique are invasive procedure.
- Echo is noninvasive old technique to measure cardiac output
- Recent noninvasive advance to measure C.O. is electrical impedance Cardiographs technology.

94. **D i.e. Interferes with Doppler when used together**
[Ref: Sutton 7/e P-276, 318-19; Grainger 4/e P-697, 706-7; Lee 12/e P-274, 450]

- ***Doppler modalities are generally available on modern trans esophageal echo systems to increase its effectiveness***Q.
- **Trans Esophageal Echocardiography** is the ***most sensitive investigation for diagnosing air embolism***Q.
- Continuous monitoring is required for detecting venous embolism.
- It can quantify volume of embolism.
- It is used in wide range of abnormalities including heart valve malfunction, endocarditis, evaluation of thrombus in left atrium, & congenital heart defects.

95. **A i.e. 2 D Echocardiography** *[Ref: Grainger 4/e P-716]*

- M- Mode Echo is also k/a One dimensional echo, it uses stationary beam so informations are updated very rapidly. It is often more conventient for assessing distance & motion of selected cardiac structure. 2-Dimensional echo has replaced it for most diagnostic purposes. It is expected that 3D imaging will replace most 2D imaging in future.
- 2-D-Echocardiography is investigation of choice for:
  - ***Pericardial effusion***Q
  - ***Cardiac Temponade***Q
  - *Valvular heart ds*
  - *Cardiomyopathy*

GASTROINTESTINAL SYSTEM

96. **D i.e. Left lateral decubitus abdominal x-ray with horizontal beam** *[Ref: AMPIS-chest imaging 3/e p 5; Abdominal trauma imaging 3/e p. 34-37; Wolfgang 7/e p 771-72; Sutton 7/e p-663-68; Grainger 5/e p 239-589-90-599]*

Abdominal CT in lung window setting is the ***most sensitive investigation for detection of free peritoneal air*** *(i.e. pneumoperitoneum)*Q followed by ***erect radiograph (i.e. erect x-ray chest PA view)***Q f/b ***left lateral decubitus (with right side up) abdominal x-ray with horizontal beem***Q f/b ***erect abdomen view***Q ***f/b supine abdomen view***Q.

97. **A i.e. Barium swallow:** *[Ref. Swartz 9/e p 848; Armstrong 5/e p 151, 154; Wolfgang 7/e p 892; GI Imaging 3/e p 57]*

Investigation of choice to confirm Zenker's diverticulum is barium swallowQ.

98. **C i.e. Gastric content aspiration** *[Ref: Harrison 15/e P-254; CMDT – 2003 P-540]*

- Patient is already having frank haematemesis (upper GI bleed coming through mouth). So there is no diagnostic role of gastric aspiration. It may be of some value, when there is doubt of upper GI bleed.
- ***Endoscopy is the investigation of choice for upper GI bleed***Q. Endoscopy is helpful in dx of Oesophagitis, gastritis, ulcer, reflux, carcinoma, varicose veins. **Barium meal** is helpful in diagnosing ulcer & gastritis. **Angiography** tells about bleeding vessel.

99. **A i.e. Achlasia; B i.e. Trypanosomiasis** *[Ref: Sutton 7/e p. 552,554]*

- In **Achlasia & Trypanosomiasis**, there is ***diffuse dilatation of oesophagus***Q.
- In **scleroderma** only ***lower esophagus dialates***Q.
- Oral biphosphonates like etidronate are poorly absorbed & have a potential to produce ulceration and reflux.

100. **D i.e. High gastric residues** *[Ref: Schwartz 9/e p 1425-26; Wolfgang 7/e p 858-59; Armstrong 5/e p158-60; Pediatric imaging 3/e p 126-28]*

Ultrasonography is the ***investigation of choice to confirm diagnose of hypertrophic pyloric stenosis with accuracy > 95% (approching almost 100%)***Q. USG visualizes ***thickened and elongated pyloric canal***Q. USG criteria for diagnosis include ***>16 mm pyloric length and >4mm pyloric muscle wall thickness***Q. ***Gastric residues are low b/o recurrent emesis***Q.

101. **D i.e. Lesser curvature ulcer with nodular ring**
[Ref: Robbins Basic Pathology 6/e P-800; Harsh Mohan 4/e P-536; Maingot 10/e P-16]

Malignancy in gastric ulcer is indicated by **greater (not lesser) curvature location, Carman's meniscus sign and amputated/clubbed radiating gastric folds which donot reach the edge of ulcer crater**Q.

102. **A i.e. Microcolon on Ba enema; D i.e. Obstruction in Ba meal**
103. **A i.e. Apple core sign**
104. **D i.e., Longitudinal ulcers are more common.**
[Ref: Grainger 5/e p- 670, 658, 630, 698- 99, 1484; Sutton 7/e p. 627- 28; Wolfgang 5/e p- 862]

- ***Apple core sign is seen in carcinoma of colon***Q whereas *ileocecal tuberculosis* presents with ***stricture of terminal ileum, widening of ileocecal angle and pulled up contracted cecum***Q on barium study.
- **Iliocecal TB** presents with ***discrete (transverse, stellate, circumferential) not longitudinal ulcers with elevated margins, inverted umberella (Fleischner) sign, symmetrical annular napkin ring stenosis and Steirlin sign (rapid emptying of narrowed terminal ileum)***Q.

105. **E i.e. USG enteroclysis** *[Ref: Sutton 7/e p. 616-617; Grainger 5/e p. 660-62]*

Investigation of small intestine include CT/MR- enteroclysis, enteroclysis (small bowel enema) and radionuclide scan but not USG enteroclysis.

106. **D i.e. Corticosteroid** **107.** **D i.e. All**

108. **All [A, B, C, D]** *[Ref: Wofgang 7/e p. 773; Chapman 5/e p. 128; S. Das 6/e p. 418]*

- **High obstruction, acute pancreatitis & congenital diaphragmatic hernia** can cause **gasless abdomen.**
- Calcified gall stone/hepatic hemangioma/renal stone and vessel may cause right upper quadrant calcification. Whereas, iron, salicylates & phenothiazine can cause radio paque material in bowel.

PANCREAS

109. **B i.e. CT Scan** *[Ref: Harrison 18/e p. 2631-41]*

In patients complaining epigastric pain radiating to back off and on the diagnosis of **acute pancreatitis** can be confirmed by **CT scan.**

110. **A i.e. Pancreatic Head Growth** *[Ref: Das manual on Clinical Surgery 5/e P-368]*

On barium meal, the ***loop of duodenum is widened***Q also k/a **Pad Sign** in cases of **carcinoma head of pancreas.**

111. **A i.e. Gall stone, D i.e. Pancreatic divisum, E i.e. Annular Pancreas**
[Ref: Sutton 7/e P-806-10; B&L 24/e P-1127; Harrison 18/e P-2630]

Uses of ERCP

1. For **diagnosing acute & chronic pancreatitis**
   The hallmark of acute pancreatitis are:
   a. *Calculi*
   b. *Block of main pancreatic duct*
   c. *Dialation & beading of the main pancreatic duct*
   d. *Cavities*
2. For evaluating conditions which might have predisposed to pancreatitis like:
   a. ***Pancreas divisum***Q
   b. ***Annular pancreas***Q
3. Assessment of complications of acute pancreatitis like:
   a. Abscess
   b. Pseudocyst
4. Interventional – ***gall stone disimpaction in acute pancreatitis***Q, pancreatic duct stone extraction, balloon dialation of minor papilla in pancreas divisum.

HEPATOBILIARY SYSTEM

112. **D i.e., Quadrate lobe** *[Ref: Rumac's diagnostic USG 2/e P 89- 91; Grainger 5/e p- 726, 763- 64]*

Functional segmental liver anatomy according to Couinaud & Bismuth classifications

It divides liver into *8 segments* based on distribution of 3 *major hepatic veins.*

- **Middle hepatic vein**
  - *Divides liver into right & left lobe*
  - Also seperated by main portal vein incisura, cantile line passing through IVC & long axis of gall bladder.
- **Left hepatic vein** divides left lobe into *medial & lateral sectors.*
- **Right hepatic vein** divides right lobe into *anterior & posterior sectors.*

Segment	Liver lobe
I	**Caudate lobe**Q
II	Left lateral – superior
III	Left lateral – inferior
IV	***Quadrate lobe***Q
a	Left medial – superior
b	Left medial - inferior
V	Right inferior – anterior
VI	Right inferior – posterior
VII	Right superior – posterior
VIII	Right superior – anterior

113. **D i.e. Simple cyst** *[Ref: Rumack's Diagnostic Ultrasound 3/e p 86, 89, 94]*

***A solitary hypoechoic lesion without any septae or debris* is most likely to be a simple cyst.**

Ultrasound appearances of

Hydatid cyst	Caroli's disease	Liver abscess
- Simple cyst with hydatid sand - Daughter cyst - Calcification - Floating endocyst	- Type V choledocal cyst - Multiple intrahepatic biliary cyst - Sludges and stones within cysts	- Cystic lesion with irregular margins & floating internal echos - Septation, debris & Fluid-Fluid interface may be seen

5

RADIODIAGNOSIS

114. **B i.e. CA colon (Mucinous adenocarcinoma)** *[Ref: Chapman 5/e p 169-72; AMPIS 3/e p 164-67, 256-57, 515; Wolfgang 7/e p 745-46; Sutton 7/e p 740, 757, 772-74; Grainger 5/e p 750-51, 1236, 1564]*

- **Hepatic metastasis** may be *hypoechoic (most common), hyperechoic and cystic or mixed echogenicity.* **Hypoechoic or hyporeflective** lesions *with no distal shadowing or enhancement* is produced by *highly cellular and hypovascular lesions.* Hypoechoic metastases are seen in *lymphoma, sarcoma and most adenocarcinoma such as breast, lung and pancreas (Sutton).* **Echopenic liver metastasis** include lymphoma, pancreas, cervical cancer, lung (adenocarcinoma) and nasopharyngeal cancer (Wolfgang).
- **Hyper-reflective** or **hyper-choic** (or **echogenic**) lesions with *distal shadowing or enhancement* is produced by ***vascular metastases due to many blood-tissue interfaces from the tortous abnormal vessels. They are often seen in metastases from colorectal cancer and other gastrointestinal primaries and with vascular metastases from islet cell tumors, carcinoid, choriocarcinoma and renal cell carcinoma***Q. **Calcification** which may be recognized by *marked reflectivity and acoustic shadowing* (i.e. hyperechogenecity), is most often seen in metastases from *mucinous adenocarcinoma of colon* (Sutton) / mucin secreting *metastases from GI tract (Grainger)/mucinous metastases from colon* & ovary (Berry). **Echogenic liver metastases** include ***colonic carcinoma (mucinous-adenocarcinoma)***Q-54%, hepatoma (25%) and treated breast carcinoma (21%)-Wolfgang.
- Presence of ill defined hypoechoic halo (indicating an aggressive tumor) around the hyperchoic lesion produces a **bull's eye** or **target appearance**. It is seen in ***metastases from bronchogenic carcinoma & gastrinoma***Q (Sutton/Berry)
- Metastases of increased reflectivity can mimic hemangiomas and predominantly cystic metastases (eg ovary) can mimic simple cyst. (Grainger). **Cystic metastases** usually develop in patients who have a primary lesion with a cystic component for example **ovarian cancer** or **cystadenocarcinoma of pancreas** (Sutton). Cystic metatases are seen with *adenocarcinoma of pancreas, ovary and colon* (Berry).
- **Hypervascular liver metastases** include *primary neuroendocrine tumor (eg pancreatic islet cell tumor, neuroendocrine carcinoma = carcinoid, pheochromocytoma), renal cell carcinoma (hypernephroma), thyroid cancer, choriocarcinoma, melanoma,* and also sarcomas, breast cancer, *ovarian cystadenocarcinoma* (Wolfgang).

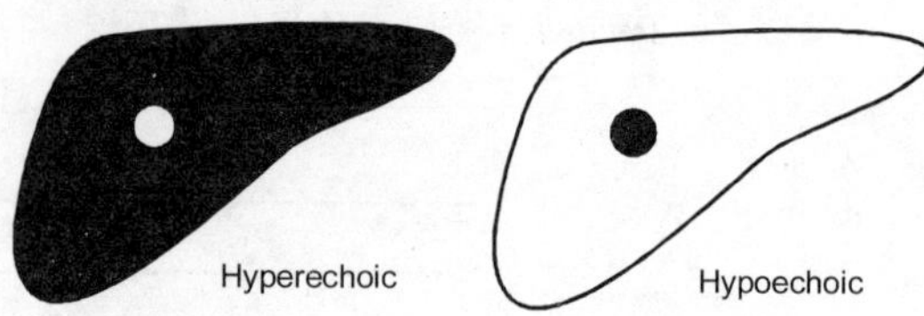

- **Cystadenomas** (both **serous and mucinous**) are benign cystic tumors (eg of ovary). On USG serous cystadenoma presents with large (>10cm), thin walled, usually unilocular, **anechoic** (smooth black; darker than hypoechoic) masses which may be bilateral. Sonographically **mucinous cystadenomas** are larger (15-30cm), multilocular (thin septal), usually unilateral, showing **variegated echogenicity sign** in cystic mass (anechoic empty space, hypoechoic/low level echos d/t mucoid material in the dependent portion of mass and difference in chemical composition of fluid, protein content & hemorrhage l/t different echogenocity). On MRI (T2WI) *stained glass appearance* is seen.
- **Sumary: Cystadenoma** is never hyperechoic, although it may be *anechoic, hypoechoic or show variegated echogenicity.* (Anechoic means more hypoechoic, hypoechoic lesions are seen as black and hyper echoic lesions are seen as white on USG). **Colorectal carcinoma (mucinous adenocarcinoma)** gives rise to ***hypervascular metastasis and produce hyperechoic (echogenic) lesion on USG***Q.
- It is important to understand that cystic lesions are an-echoic mostly but all hypoechoic lesions are not cystic. Similary calcified lesions are hyperechoic and produce shadowing but all hyperechoic lesions are not calcified and produce shadowing.

115. **C i.e., Focal Nodular Hyperplasia** *[Ref: Wolfgang 7/e p. 1133-35; Hepatobiliary Imaging 3/e p. 227, 216; Sabiston 16/e p. 1015--1016; Bailey & Love 24/e 1068]*

TIBIDA hepatobiliary scanning has 92% sensitivity for diagnosing **focal nodular hyperplasia**. And 60% FNH lesions show **sulphur colloid uptake**.

Focal nodular hyperplasia - Only liver tumour which consistently contains functioning RE cells & shows uptake of labeled colloids. FNH also contains functioning hepatocytes and takes up IDA compound. Histology typically shows presence of bile ductules within FNH but ducts do not communicate with biliary tree, so there is no excretory pathway. This explains why FNH lesions characteristically show prolonged retention of IDA on delayed images.

Hepatic Adenoma: *This benign tumour contains little functioning RE cells, so colloid scan will show non functioning area.* IDA scan will show normal Hepatocytes.

Hepatic carcinoma: Contain little or no functioning liver tissue. Both the colloid and IDA uptake is very low.

Liver parenchyma is primarily made up of two types of cells:

(1) Hepatocytes → Perform excretory & synthetic function

(2) Kuppfer cells → They have Reticuloendothelial function

116. **B i.e. Hepatic scintigrahy** *[Ref: Rumack vol. 2nd - 126]*

MC benign liver tumor in young adult is cavernous Hemangioma[Q] which is typically < 3cm, well defined, at posterio-superior segment of (Rt.) lobe of liver. It is homogenous – hyperchoic in 80% and mixed density in rest. Cavrnous Hemangioma suspected on U/S examination; dx confirmed by.

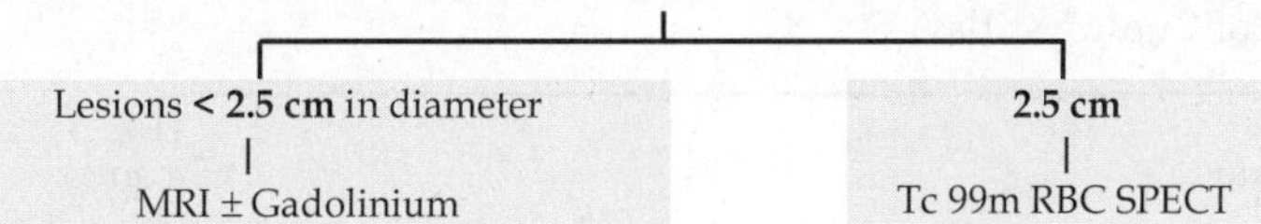

- MRI has added advantage of being more specific than SPECT (or Hepatic scintigraphy or RBC scintigraphy) in diagnosing other hepatic lesions.
- Dynamic CECT is less specific than MRI and scintigraphy.
- Therefore, in this context, ***best answer is MRI followed by hepatic scintigraphy f/b Dynamic contrast in enhanced CT Scan***[Q].

117. **C i.e. Use of heavily T2-weighted image without contrast to create the three dimensional image of the billary tree using MIP algorithm**

118. **A i.e. MRI is used to obtain the image C i.e., It shows the biliary tree** *[Ref: Grainger 5/e p 777, 766; Blumgart Surgery of Liver, Billiary tract and pancreas 5th/315; Sutton 7/e p 1822, 716-18; AMPIS 3/e p. 273]*

- **Magnetic reasonance cholangio pancreatography (MRCP)** is **non invasive** technique, which **uses heavilly T_2 weighted images of MRI (not CT) without contrast (mostly) to create 2D or 3 dimensional image of biliary (pancreatic) tree using maximum intensity projection (MIP) algorithm**[Q].
- Contrast enhanced MRCP uses intravenous hepato biliary contrasts **eg mangafodipir trisodium, gadobenate dimeglumine & gadoxetic acid disodium**[Q].

119. **A i.e. Ultrasonic waves** *[Ref. Rath & Mohanti p.376-377; Gunderson 3/e p. 435]*

Ultrasonic waves (i.e. USG) have ***been used to improve placement of probe delivering intralesional ethanol injection, radiofrequency ablation and cryotherapy***[Q]. It is not used for insitu abalation of liver tumor (primary & secoandary).

Treatment modalities for liver secondaries

- Liver transplant (in patients with single lesion < 5 cm or three or fewer, lesions < 3 cm) but usually not recommended
- Hepatic artery embolization & chemotherapy ***(chemoembolization)***[Q]
- Intralesional insitu abalation via ultrasound guided
  - -Percutaneous ethanaol (alcohol) injection
  - -***Cryotherapy***[Q]
  - -***Radiofrequency ablation***[Q]
  - -*Microwave coagulation therapy.*

120. **A i.e. Meniscus appearance** *[Ref: Sutton 7/e P-726; Wolfgang 7/e p. 688, 751, 718; AMPIS 3/e p. 285, 275]*

Impacted stone in CBD gives **cresentic shadow** or ***Meniscus Sign***[Q]. **Rat tail/ Nipple like occlusion of CBD (with irregular shouldered tapering)** is seen in **pancreatic ductal adenocarcinoma** &/or chronic pancreatic (±). **Smooth tapering** is seen in ***benign strictures of CBD***[Q].

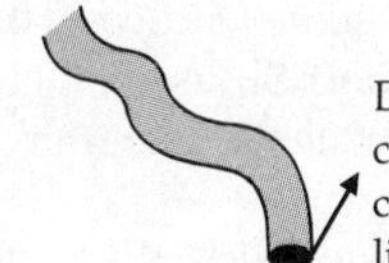

121. **B i.e. Sclerosing Cholangitis** *[Ref: Sutton 7/e P-714; Grainger 4/e P-984; CSDT 2003-600]*

Air in biliary tract can be seen in gall stone ileus, carcinoma GB, and endoscopic papillotomy but not in sclerosing cholangitis[Q].

122. **A i.e. Acute cholecystitis; B i.e. Mucosal thickening; C i.e. Cholesterosis; D i.e. Ascites** *[Ref: Sutton 7th/ 715,717]*

On USG, gall bladder thickening is seen in following conditions

A) Biliary	- *Acute & chronic cholecystitis*[Q] - *Cholesterosis*[Q]	B) Non-biliary	- Liver cirrhosis - CCF - Hypoalbunemia - Portal hypertension
			- Viral hepatitis - CRF - *Ascites*[Q]

123. **A i.e. Thick fibrosed gall bladdar wall; B i.e. Stone impacted at neck of gall bladder**
C i.e. Perigall bladdar halo *[Ref: Sutton 7/e P-714-15; B&L 24/e P-1097; Harrison 15/e P-1782-83]*

USG is the *standard initial imaging technique* for the investigation of patient with ***gall stone, jaundice & cholecystitis***[Q]. USG features of **Cholecystitis:**

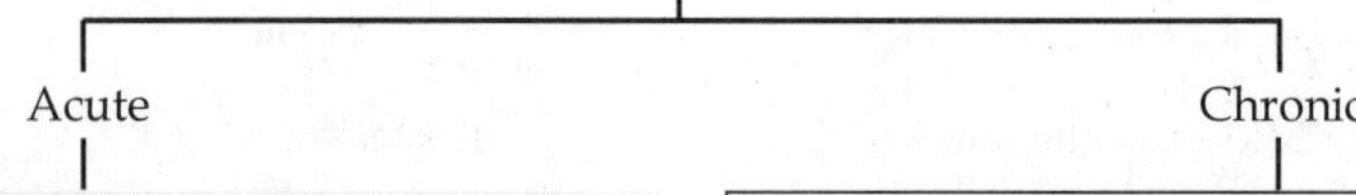

Acute	Chronic
1. *Circumferential halo of low echogenicity around g.b.*[Q] 2. *Mural thickening of > 3mm*[Q] in fasting state 3. *Calculi*[Q] may be present in Biliary tree 4. Echogenic bile	**1.** *Contracted gall bladder*[Q] **2.** Obliteration of lumen, so that acoustic shadowing at the porta may be all that is visible

124. **D i.e. 1 cm size Gall stones** *[Ref: Grainger 5/e p 767-68, 1427; Schiff 10/e p 652; AMPIS 3/e p 306, 334, 223,209; Wolfgang 7/e p 716-17]*

- **CT scan** has a very ***limited role in diagnosis of gall stone (Cholelithiasis) as only a minority (20-60%) of gall bladder stones are visible***[Q] which show calcification. Most (70%) stones are cholesterol stones and 93% of them are radiolucent). CT scan, however, can evaluate complications such as pancreatitis, pericholecystic fluid, abscess or perforation.
- **Ultrasound** is the ***most accurate modality for the diagnosis of gall bladder stones***[Q], which appear as *echogenic foci producing acoustic shadows*. Stone mobility is also identified (although not essential for making diagnosis). Small stones are differentiated from small polyps by the demonstration of mobility or the presence of an acoustic shadow. Non visualization of gall bladder on US may be d/t previous cholecystectomy, nonfasting, abnormal gall bladder position, *emphysematous cholecystitis* or *because the gall bladder' is filled with stones*. The latter can be identified by **double-arc shadow sign = hypoechoic line between two echogenic lines in** gall bladder fossa (i.e. 2 parallel curved echogenic lines seperated by a thin anechoic space with dense acoustic shadowing distal to the deeper echogenic line).

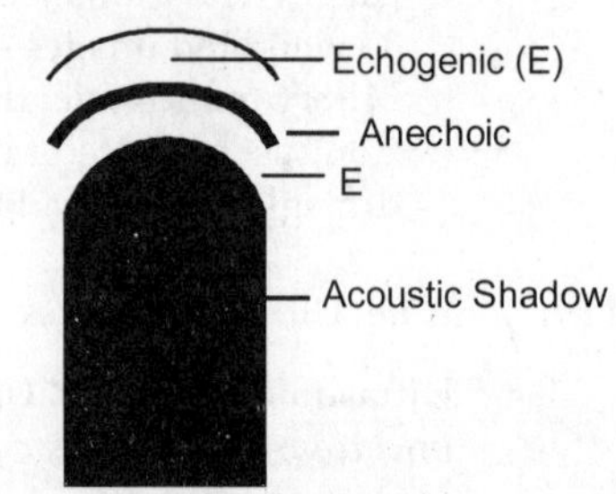

Double Arc Shadow Sign

- **CT scan** is one of the most accurate procedure in detection of lesions in **pancreas** (including tail), **retroperitoneum (eg paraaortic lymph nodes)** and **liver** (focal lesions like aneurysm, hemangioma etc).

125. **C i.e. Adenomyomatosis** *[Ref: Wolfang 7/e p 741, 715; AMPIS-Gall blader Imaging 3/e p 286; Sutton 7/e p 723-24; Schmidt (2005) p 130; Head-neck Imaging 2/e p 555; Haga 5/e p 1434-37]*

- **Adenomyomatosis** of **gall bladder** is chracterized by ***diffuse (generalized), segmental (annular) or localized hyperplastic muscular wall thickening***[Q], mucosal overgrowth and **intramural diverticula /crypts/or sinus tracts** (so called **Rokitansky-Aschoff Sinuses)**. It characteristically pesents with **comet tail artifacts/sign** (on USG), **pearl necklace sign** (on oral cholecystogram or MR cholangiogram) and **string of beads sign** (on MRCP T_2WI).
- ***Most thyroid carcinomas are hypoechoic***[Q]. Whereas *most thyroid adenomas are hyperechoic or isoechoic at ultrasound.*

PEDIATRIC ABDOMEN

126. A i.e., Barium enema study *[Ref: Sutton 7/e p – 850; Swartz 8/e 1497- 99; Baily & Love 24/e P- 1246-47, 1154 –56]*

- Main **indications for water soluble contrast barium enema** are ***neonatal low gastrointestinal obstruction***Q, suspected post –necrotizing enterocolitis strictures, ***Hirschsprung's disease***Q and after colonic surgery. Colonoscopy has replaced barium enema in inflammatory bowel disease allowing concurrent biopsy & avoiding ionizing radiation.
- For **anorectal malformation**, infant is held upside down for 3 – 4 minutes , with a metallic object or coin strapped to the site of anus or metal bougie inserted into the blind anus and *a radiograph is taken in inverted position.*

  The distance between the top end of rectal gas and metal indicator indicates the length of malformed rectum. Sufficient gas may have collected in large intestine, *6 hours after birth*, to cast radiographic shadow. But sometimes 24 hours wait is required.
- *Neonates with delayed passage of meconium beyond first 24 hours of life with abdominal distension & bilious vomiting* are indicative of **Hirschsprung's disease**. However, it can also present with *chronic constipation starting from 1st few weeks of life without fecal soiling* in children & adults, in whom per-rectal examination reflects contracted rectal wall and may provide temporary relief from constipation.

Barium- enema	Erect & supine abdominal X- ray	Anorectal manometry	Rectal Biopsy
- ***Confirms the diagnosis and indicate the length and site of involved bowel***Q. - PR should not be done before radiological examination.	- Distended loops of small & large intestine with fluid levels consistent with low intestinal obstruction - Intramural gas indicates enterocolitis & free peritoneal gas perforation.	- Useful screening test in ***constipated young child or adult who is otherwise fit*** - ***Should not be done in ill neonates***Q because of poor anal tone & a normal absence of rectosphenteric inhibitory reflex in some.	- ***Confirms diagnosis of Hirshsprung's disease***Q

127. C i.e. Lower GI contrast study *[Ref: Sutton 7/e p – 859]*

Lower GI contrast study confirms the diagnosis & indicate the type of involvement, in cases of lower intestinal obstruction causing failure to pass meconium timelyQ.

MUSCULOSKELETAL SYSTEM

ARTHRITIS

128. C i.e., MRI *[Ref. Sutton 7/e p. 1181]*

A known complication of *long term steroid uptake and chronic alcoholism* is ***avascular necrosis of hip.***
MR scanning is the most sensitive and specific means of detecting changes in avascular necrosisQ. Sensitivity & Specificity approach 100%.

129. B i.e., DIP joints in osteoarthritis *[Ref: Peter Armstrong –353; Sutlon 7/e P-1204; Chapman 4/e P-95; Ref: Harrison 16/e 2040]*

Heberden's nodes ***(bony enlargement of distal interphalageal joints)***Q ***are the most common form of idiopathic osteoarthritis***Q. A similar process at ***proximal interphalangeal joint***Q leads to **Bouchard's nodes.** (Mnemonic – **"DH & PuB"** ie dissection half & pub or **HaD BP**).

★ In **osteoarthritis,** the *most commonly* involved joint is *DIP (Herberden's node)* followed by *CM joint of thumb (2nd m.c.), Wrist and MCP joints* are *spared* in O.A.

130. B i.e. Psoariatic arthropathy *[Ref: Grainger 4/e P-2009; Sutton 7/e P-1217, 1362]*

Tufting of distal phalynx is characteristic of **psoriatic arthropathy.**

131. **C i.e. Pseudogout** *[Ref: Grainger 4/e P-2014]*

Chondrocalcinosis term is used for finding of radiopaque crystals in hyaline or fibrocartilage. It is seen in ***calcium pyrophosphate dihydrate crystal deposition disease (CPPD)***Q, of which ***pseudogout***Q is a manifestation.

132. **C i.e. Nonrheumatic ankylosis** *[Ref: Chapman 4/e P-84]*

Calcification of intervertebral disc is seen in nonrheumatic ankylosing spondylitisQ

133. **C i.e. Alkaptonuria** *[Ref: Chapman 4/e P-84]*

Features	Disease
Fish Mouth Vertebrae	- ***Sickel Cell Anemia***Q ***Homocystinuria***Q
Cod Fish Vertebra (Biconcave vertebra)	- Osteomalacia, Osteoporosis, Hyperparathyroid
Rugger jersey spine (sclerosis of upper & lower spine borders)	- ***CRF induced osteomalacia***Q - Osteopterosis (marbel bone disease)
Calcification of Intervertebral disc	- ***Alkaptonuria (m.c.)***
Picture Frame vertebrae	- Paget's disease
Vertebrae plana	- ***Eosinophilic granuloma***Q

134. **D i.e. Pseudogout** *[Ref: Wofgang 5/e P-53]*

Pseudogout also k/a ***familial chondrocalcinosis / CPPD*** presents with deposition of ***calcium pyrophospate dihydrate crystals*** in synovial fluid & within leucocytes (characterstic ***weakly positive birefringent diffraction***Q pattern) leading to calcification esp. of ***meniscus***Q *& outer fibers of annulus fibrosus.*

135. **A i.e. Pseudogout** *[Ref: Harrison 15/e P-1997]*

In **pseudogout (CPPD)**, there is ***intra & peri-articular calcification***Q due to radio dense deposits are deposited in menisci & articular hyaline cartilage.

136. **C i.e. Bone Erosion** *[Ref: Peter Armstrong –353; Sutlon 7/e P-1204; Chapman 4/e P-95; Harrison 16/e p. 2040]*

All inflamatory arthritis share a lot of radiological features in common. **Rheumatoid arthritis** is differentiated from other inflammatory seronegative arthropathies by ***symmetrical***Q***, small joint (esp MCP & PIP joints) involvement***Q***, more osteoporosis & bony erosions***Q. In seronegative arthritis, there is asymmetrical, large joint (esp SI, spine & DIP joint of hand) involvement, more periostitis & less osteoporosis.

137. **A i.e. Diffuse periosteal reaction** *[Ref: Wolfgang 5/e P-854-55; Chapman 4/e p. 129, 229, 611; Sutton 7/e p. 34, 199, 200]*

Scleroderma presents with ***oesophageal dysmotality, subpleural (lung) nodules, acrosteolylsis (erosion of tip of phalanx)***Q *but not with* **diffuse periosteal reaction.**Q

DEFICIENCY DISEASES

138. **D i.e. Widening of Epiphysis**
139. **B i.e. Soap Bubble appearance** *[Ref: Sutlon 7/e P-1356, 1212]2*
140. **A i.e. Epiphyseal widening**

- **Widening of physis (growth plate below epiphysis)** also known as Epiphyseal growth plate (not epiphysis) is character stick feature of ***rickets***Q
- **Enlargement or Widening of Ephphysis** (bone ends) is seen in ***Juvenile chronic Arthritis***Q
- ***Soap bubble appearance***Q is characteristic of **giant cell tumor**

141. **C i.e. Radiological Examination of growing bone ends** *[Ref: Ghai 5/e P-84; Grainger 5/e p- 1104-05, 4/e p. 1933]*

Response to treatment in rickets following administration of vit D_3 orally or parentrally is ***monitored on repeated X Ray plates of growing bone ends.***Q

142. **B, C i.e. Cupping of metaphysis, Ricketic rosary** *[Ref: Sutton 7/e p. 1353, 1356]*

143. **A i.e. Rickets** **144.** **B i.e. Lead poisoning** *[Ref. Chapman 4/e P. 48]*

- *Splaying and cupping of metaphysis and recketic rosary*Q is seen in **rickets.**
- Remember : *Lead poisoning*Q (Bismuth, Arsenic, P, mercury fluride, radium also), Radiation & Hypervitaminosis D leads to **solitary dense metaphyseal band** not cupping & fraying.

145. **C i.e. Osteomalacia** *[Ref: Sutton 7/e P-1339, 1355, 1365]*
146. **C i.e. Rickets** *[Ref: Wofgang 5/e P-19, 133]*

- *Flaring of anterior ends of rib is charcteristically seen in rickets*Q and **beaded ribs** are found in *osteogenesis imperfecta*Q.
- Other causes of **multiple anterior rib flaring** are – *achondroplasia, scurvy, thanatophoric dysplasia* & normal variants.

147. **A i.e. Hypothyroidism** *[Ref: Ghai 5/e P-447; Grainger 4/e P-1950-1952; Wofgang 5/e P-105]*

MALIGNANCY

148. **B i.e. Multiple Myeloma** *[Ref: Sutton 7/e p.1339, 1355, 1365]*

- Old age, male sex & vertebral involvement (lytic lesion) indicate towards diagnosis of Metastasis & Multiple myeloma. But *Absence of primary and characterestic* ***multiple punched out lesions on X-Ray skull is diagnostic of Multiple myeloma***Q.
- **Multiple Myeloma** has two cardinal features: (1) Generalized reduction of bone density (Osteopenia); (2) Localized areas of radiolucency **(Punched out**Q**/Rain drop lesions**Q**) in red marrow areas i.e. axial skeletal – spine & skull.** In multiple Myeloma lytic lesions of spine are usually associated with some collapse & soft tissue extension i.e. paravertebral soft tissue shadows (differentiation from Metastasis). Differentiation from inflamatory lesions can be made as the intervertebral disc space & articular surfaces are not affected.
- In children with CRF, the combination of rickets & hyperparathyroidism leads to **R*otting Fence Post appearance.***Q

149. **C i.e. Unicameral bone cyst** *[Ref: Tachdjian's Pediatric orthopaedics 3/e P-1901-7]*

Simple/Solitary/Unicameral Bone cyst nearly always occurs during first two decades of life, mostly in metaphysis of proximal humerus (50%) or femur with a male predominance (Male-female ratio = 2:1).

150. **B i.e. Aneurysmal Bone Cyst** *[Ref: Sutlon 4/e p.1261; Chapman 4/e p.52; Osborn Pasricha-Treatment of skin disease 4/e p.882; Turek 638, 639; Tachdjian's orthopaedics 3/e p.1936]*

- Both aneurismal bone cyst & osteoblastoma can present as expansile lytic lesion of posterior element of spine in young age group.
- **Osteobastoma** is differentiated by presence of ***more radiodense mottled*** *(calcification/ossification)* ***appearance***Q with ***more defined margins due to reactive sclerosis***Q. Whereas **ABC** presents as ***purely lytic lesion with trabeculated appearance***Q. **Metastasis** presents as ***multiple predominantly osteolytic***Q non expansible lesions.

151. **B i.e. Excision & Bone grafting** *[Ref: Turek's orthopedics 4/e P-617]*

- The diagnosis of patient is Osteoclastoma
- Osteoclastoma also known as Giant cell tumor, is mostly a ***locally malignant***Q tumor occurring usually ***between 15 and 40 years***Q of age in the ***epiphyseal***Q **&** ***metaphyseal region.*** **The** ***lower end of femur***Q, the ***distal radius***Q and upper tibia are common sites.
  Radiologically, it presents with characterstic loculated ***Soap bubble appearance***Q.
- GCT is treated by:
  - ***Currettage and Bone grafting***Q/Acrylic cement for tumors of long bones without articular collapse
  - ***Excision & Autograft replacement*** – By I/L upper end fibula in lower end radius tumors
  - ***Resection*** – for tumors of distal ulna, proximal fibula, small bones of hand & feet, scapula (i.e. bones which can be resected without undue effects)
  - ***Amputation*** – for wide spread aggressive tumors with sof tissue invasion.

152. **B i.e. Sunray appearance** *[Ref: Green span-orthopaedic radiology 3/e P-658; Turek Orthopaedics 4/e P-630]*

The X Ray findings of osteosarcomas are characterized by:

- *Variable mixture of radiopacities* (due to osteogenesis) & *radiolucencies* (due to destructive change & replacement by radiolucent osteoid)
- ***Sun Burst / Sun ray appearance***Q
- ***Codman's triangle***Q (also found in infection & Ewing's S_A so not specific)

153. **B i.e. Chondrosarcoma** *[Ref: Turek – Orthopedics 4/e P-603; Wolfgang 7/e p. 125-26]*

- **Most common** bone tumor = ***Osteochondroma***
- Bone tumor with **Dense calcification** = ***Chondro Sarcoma***
- Bone tumor with **Calcified secondaries** = ***Osteosarcoma***

154. **B i.e. Renal Cell carcinoma** *[Ref: Chapman 4/e p. 25]*

155. **D i.e. Ca Prostate** *[Ref: Wolfgang 7/e p. 125; Harrison 15/e P-628; Devitta P-2228]*

Expansile pulsating secondary metastasis is seen in renal cell carcinomaQ.
Ca prostate produces ***mainly osteoblastic secondaries***Q.

INFECTION

156. **B i.e. Soft tissue swelling** *[Ref: Harrison 15/e P-826]*

Radiological features of **Acute osteomyelitis:**

< 7 days	***Soft tissue swelling***Q
> 10 days	***Periosteal reaction***Q
After 2-6 weeks	***Lytic changes***Q when 50-75% of bone density has been lost

SPINE

157. **A, B & D i.e. (Ventriculomegaly), (Obliteration of cisterna magna) & (Abnormal curvature of cerebellum)** *[Ref: Sutton 7/e p. 1052, 1121]*

USG findings of spin bifida are ventriculomegaly, hydrocephalus, increased biparietal diameter (BPD), obliteration (effacement) of cisterna magna, stretching (abnormal curvature) of cerebellumQ**.**

158. **C i.e. Histiocytosis** *[Ref: Sutlon 7/e P-1340; Chapman 4/e P-565 &75; Simon 2/e P-14]*

Most common cause of single vertebral body collapse in child with maintained disc space is **Eosinophilic Granuloma**Q

159. **B i.e. Myelomalacia** *[Ref: MRI of Brain & Spine by Scott W. Atlas, 3e/P 1802, 1810]*

Both ***cord edema***Q and ***myelomalacia***Q appear as:
On T1 – Ill defined hypointense area
On T2 – Hyperintense area

160. **A i.e. Most commonly involves thoracic spine**: *[Ref: Grainger Radiology 4th/1376; John R. Haaga 5th/786-87, Anne G. Osborn/848]*

Ossification of the Posterior longitudinal ligament most commonly involves the cervical spine and not the thoracic spine.

BREAST

161. D i.e. All

162. C i.e. Macrocalcification

163. C i.e. Areas of spiculated microcalcification

164. A i.e. B/L mammogram

165. C i.e. Young breast have dense tissue

166. B i.e. Clinical examination, Mammography, biopsy/cytology

167. **C i.e. Seborrhic Keratosis** *[Ref: Chapman 5/e p. 237-47; Sutton 7/e p. 1451-86; Wolfgang 7/e p. 555-62; Grainger 5th/1190, 1188; AIIMS-MAMC-PGI Series; Diagnostic Radiology – Breast imaging 2/e p. 530; Silverstein 2/e p. 123-24]*

- ***Most sensitive investigation (i.e. investigation of choice) to diagnose early (stage I) carcinoma breast and ductal carcinoma in situ (DICS) is bilateral mammography*Q.**
- The **sensitivity of mammography is low in young females** because ***young breast contains large proportion of dense glandular tissue***Q which appears as soft tissue density.
- **Mammographic abnormalities** seen in **(malignant) carcinoma breast** include **spiculate (stellate), ill-defined, irregular, inhomogenous, high (or asymmetric) density mass** with associated **architectural (parenshymal) distortion** of surrounding breast tissue (resulting in **V shape or tent sign**). Malignant calcifications are **usually <0.5 mm (i.e. microcalcification); however, microcalcification** is not specific to carcinoma. And **macro calcifications are mostly (not all) benign**Q.
- **Galactocele, hamartoma & traumatic cysts** are **fat containing breast lesions** but ***seborrhic keratosis is not a fat containing breast lesion.***
- **Triple assessment for carcinoma breast** include, **clinical examination, mammography and ultrasound guided needle biopsy (FNAC & core biopsy)**Q.

168. **A i.e. Mammography**

- This answer is also an example of POC. You are free to believe that MRI is correct answer. But the latest (2012) book by authors of AIIMS-MAMC & PGI for Breast Imaging says this - Currently, nearly 90% of **ductal carcinoma in situ (DCIS)** are diagnosed while they are clinically occult because of mamographic detection of microcalcification (in 76%), soft tissue densities (11%) or both (13% cases). ***For diagnosis of DCIS, mammography is far superior (to MRI) because of its ability to pick up microcalcification*Q. *MRI cannot detect this characterirstic finding*Q**. Only 40-50% of DCIS display an enhancement pattern typical of malignancy. These can be diagnosed on MRI alone. Remaining **50-60% can not be diagnosed on MR alone or not at all on MR**.
- This question is based on some basic concepts of DCIS & breast imaging which are
- ***Earliest finding of DCIS is microcalcification. Mammography is most sensitive and MRI is least sensitive in detecting microcalcification*Q**. (Another Q about the inability of MRI to detect calcification has already been asked many time and you have answered it but never tried to apply, that concept here.)
- **Mammography** is most sensitive for **detecting early DCIS** and therefore is the ***screeining modality of choice*Q**. And MRI can't detect 50-60% early DCIS. However, because of discontinuous spread of DCIS through the ductal system, **mammography may underestimate the extent of lesion**.
- MRI is superior to mammography in *determination of disease extent, size, infiltration, microinvasion and staging of DCIS (this all is done for invasive and relatively* **late DCIS**).
- *Screening with MRI is superior to mammography in detecting invasive breast cancer* ***in younger women where the sensitivity of mammography is low due to presence of mammographically dense breast parenchyma*Q.**
- *Although* ***mammography remains more sensitive for detecting Ductal carcinoma in sits [DCIS]*Q.**
- But if you still want to believe that some latest British American research is behind this question. Then my advice is, stop reding books & go for journals as you would get many of them to contradict most of the lines written in your reference text books.

169. **A i.e. Breast Imaging reporting and data system** *[Ref: Sabiston 19th/834; Wolfgang 7/e p 562, 553]*

"BIRADS" stands for "Breast Imaging Reporting and Data System".

ENDOCRINE SYSTEM

170. **A i.e. Skull; B i.e. Phalanges** *[Ref: Sutton 7/e P-1339,1362]*

171. **D i.e. Subperiosteal resorption of bone (phalynges)**

Hallmark or characteristic feature of hyperparathyroidism is–**subperiosteal Erosion of bone, particularly radial aspect of middle phalynx of middle & index finger.**Q

172. **C i.e. FNAC** **173.** **D i.e. MIBI Scan**

174. **A i.e. Pheochromocytoma**

[Ref: Sutton 7/e p 832-46; Wolfgang 7/e p 937-38,962-63; Harrison 18/e p 2952-67: AMPIS: GU Imaging 3/ep 387-92; Haga 5/ep 1823-29, 2523; Grainger 5/ep 1723-27]

- *MIBG sean is most sentiive for evaluation of extra-adrenal (et pic) pheochromocytomakQ*, and for identification of metastatic or locally o whole body image technique.
- **Light bulb appearance** (brigh high signal intensity close to that of fluid), is sometimes seen in pheochromocytomas on moderately T2 weighted images. It is neither sensitive nor specific and not frequently seen in practice.
- ***Due to risk of catastrophic hypertensive crisis and fatal cardiac arrhythmia, fine needle aspiration cytology (FNAc) of pheochromocytoma is contraindicated***Q.
- **Sensitivity of imaging** modalities

*MIBG*Q > *MRI*Q ≥ CT Scan > USG

175. **B i.e. Papillary CA** *[Ref: Schwarts 7/e P-1681]*

Radiation is an etiological agent **for papillary carcinoma** thyroid & **external radiation is used in treatment of anaplastic cancer thyroid.**Q

176. **C i.e. Follicular Cell CA** **177.** **A i.e. Hyperechogenesity**

[Ref: Biley & Love 24/e P-797-804; Differential Diagnosis in Ultrasound :a teaching atlas' bySchmidt (2005)/436; Grainger 4th/1375 ; 'Surgical Ultrasound' by Mantke,Peitz (2007)/199

Hyperechoic structure on Ultrasonaography suggests a benign lesion. Malignancies always have a Hypoechoic or nonhomogeneous hypoechoic structure.

178. **C i.e. Enhances rapidly, contrast stays in it for a relatively longer time and washes out late:**

[Ref: Grainger 5/e p. 1724; 4/e p. 1388; Adrenal imaging: Blake & Boland 1/e p. 54; GI imaging: AMP series 3/e p. 396-397; Wolfgang 6th/919]

Adrenal adenoma on contrast enhanced CT/MRI show rapid uptake and relatively rapid washout of contrast material than do non adenomasQ.

HEMATOLOGY

179. **A i.e. Radioleucent transverse metaphyseal bands**

180. **A i.e. Osteolytic lesion in flat bones; C i.e. Perioteal new bone formation; D i.e. Osteosclerosis of long bones; E i.e. Transverse line of dark band below the growth plate.**

[Ref. Sutton Radiology 7/e pg 1327; Grainger & Allison's 4/e P-1327]

- ***Metaphyseal translucencies are the earliest and most characteristic features of childhood leukemia***Q.
- ***Childhood leukemias present with metaphyseal translucencies, cortical erosion, & osteosclerosis, periostead new bone formation and osteolytic lesions in bones***Q.

181. **A i.e. Thalassemia**

182. **A i.e. Congenital hemolytic anemia** *[Ref: Chapman 4/e P-489]*

Congenital hemolytic anemias eg thalassemia present with ***wide diploic space of skull with brush border (hair on end, appearance)***Q.

183. **B. i.e. Floating teeth** *Ref: David Sutton Textbook of radiology & imaging 7th/ed p- 1323-24 ; Grainger 12/e p.1904-1905; Radiological differential diagnosis Chapman 4th/ed p-391*

Sickel cell anemia presents with vertebrae plane, bone infarct, marrow hyperplasia and secondary osteomylitis but not with floating teethQ.

Trauma

184. **A i.e. CT scan** *[Ref: Diagnostic Radiology; Neuroradiology imaging AMP series 3rd/e pg-339; Haga 5/e p-521; Cumming otorhinology 5/e p-11.5]*

- ***CT is undoubtedly superior to demonstrate bony abnormalities including fractures and inflammatory diseases in temporal bone[Q].***
- ***Diagnosis of temporal bone fracture is primarily done by CT scan[Q].*** CT scan evaluation of temporal bone consists of routine surveys of temporal bone by *5 mm thick sections* followed by *high resolution scan* (HRCT) for assessing *petromastoid complex.* It is superior to demonstrate bony abnormalities along with detection and localization of soft tissue masses in inflammatory conditions of temporal bone.
- **MRI is supplementary** and is used to evaluate associated intracranial pathologies eg hemorrhage & contusion in adjacent brain, *to determine the site of CSF leak* and for improved visualization of soft tissue lesions. MRI is the imaging standard *for detection of facial nerve canal, internal auditory canal (IAC) and jugular foramen lesions.*
- X-ray is inadequate & detects only 17-30% of fractures of temporal bone.

185. **C i.e. Rupture of cortical bridging veins**

186. **B i.e. Concave Convex hyperdense**

187. **C i.e. Crescent shaped hyperdense lesion**

188. **B i.e. CT Scan**

189. **C i.e. Extradural Hematoma**

190. **B i.e. Extradural hemmorhage**

[Ref: Harrison 18/e p. 3379-80; Sutton 7/e p. 1779; Osborn p. 205; Love & Bailey 23/e p. 550; Sabiston 15/e p. 1359]

- **Acute subdural hematoma** most commonly results from ***rupture of cortical bridging veins[Q]*** in elderly d/t minor direct cranial trauma or acceleration force (whiplash). ***Investigation of choice is CT[Q]*** which shows ***crescentric (concavo-convex) shaped hyperdense lesions[Q].***
- **Epidural hematoma** (d/t middle meningeal artery injury) are characteristically a/w **lucid interval** and appear on CT as ***lenticular (bi convex) hyperdense lesion[Q].***

191. **A i.e. Non Contrast CT** *[Ref: Harrison 18/e P-2261-63; CMDT-2003 P-965]*

192. **C i.e. Intra arterial digital Substraction angiography** *[Ref: Grainger 4/e P-2368, 1442; CMDT 2003- 965]*

- ***First investigation of choice for suspected subarachaoid hemorrhage (SAH) is non contrast CT followed by lumbar puncture[Q].***
- **Angiography of 4 vessels (2 carotid + 2 vertebral)** is the investigation of choice to determine **the etiology of SAH**. (MRA> CTA> Intra arterial DSA)

193. **B i.e. Obliteration of splenic shadow; C i.e. Rib fracture** *[Ref: Sutton 7/e P-692]*

On X Ray, factors suggestive of **splenic injury** are:

- *fracture of left lower ribs[Q]*
- *obliteration of splenic & psoas shadows[Q]*
- elevation of left diaphragm
- indentation of stomach & presence of free fluid between coils of investine are suggestive of spleenic rupture.

194. **A i.e. FAST** *[Ref: Grainger 5/e p-589-93; Diagnostic Radiology, Genitominary imaging 3rd/e pg-359-60, 33-36]*

Investigation of choice for abdominal trauma in hemodynamically stable patient is FAST (focussed assessment with sonography in trauma)[Q].

195. **C i.e. CT Scan** *[Ref:Sutton 7/e p. 692; Grainger 4/e p.1442]*

196. **B i.e. Computed tomography**

- ***CT Scan[Q]*** is the imaging modality of choice in all blunt abdominal trauma (both in children as well as adults).
- ***Spleen is the most commonly injured organ in blunt injury abdomen.[Q]***
- ***Contrast – enhanced CT[Q]*** is the investigation of choice for detecting splenic injuries
- ***Kehr sign[Q]*** (after elevating foot end referred pain over left shoulder d/t irritation of under surface of diaphragm by blood) is seen in splenic ruptures.
- On X-ray fracture of left lower ribs, obliteration of splenic & psoas shadows, elevation of left diaphragm, indentation of stomach & presence of free fluid between coils of intestine are suggestive of splenic repute.

OBSTETRICS

PREGNANCY

197. **C i.e. In normal gestation placental resistance is high; E i.e. Investigation of choice in pregnancy** *[Ref: Sutton text book of radiology and imaging 7/e p. 1046, 1039]*

In antenatal doppler (not routinely done) high S/D ratio & RP indices and reduced end diastolic flow are a/w IUGR and poor fetal out come[Q]. In normal gestation placental resistance is low[Q].

198. **C i.e. The flow velocities & S/D ratio are useful to evaluate high risk pregnancies** *[Ref: Grainger & Allison's diagnostic radiology 5/e p- 1212]*

Colour doppler analysis of umbilical arteries play an important role in assessment of high risk fetus (pregnancy)[Q].

199. **A i.e. 5-6 weeks of gestation** *[Ref: Sutton 7/e P-1041; Grainger 4/e P-2178]*

Gestation sac is visible at

- ***4-5 weeks by Trans vaginal USG[Q]***
- 5 weeks by Transabdomina USG

200. **D i.e. Doppler**

Doppler is an interpretation of audible signals of USG
By listening fetal heart sounds and seeing blood flow, we can detect fetal life at earliest.

201. **A i.e. Heart beat** *[Ref: William's obs 21/e P–234/1106]*

USG of umbilical artery is done to know about ***heart beat[Q]***.

202. **B i.e. Abdominal circumference; C i.e. BPD; D i.e. Femur length (FL)** *[Ref: Dutta obs. 5/e P-71, 77/340]*

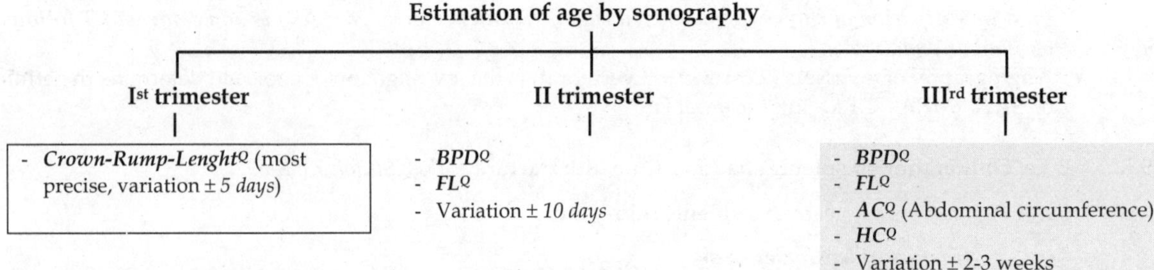

✶ BPD > 9.2 Cm indicates fetal pulmonary maturity corroborated by L:S ratio.

203. **A i.e. Detect fetal abnormality** *[Ref: Dutta obs. 5/e P-104]*

USG done at 18-20 weeks is to detect fetal anomaly[Q].

204. **A i.e. Anencephaly**

205. **A i.e. 10-12 weeks of gestation**

- Earliest detectable congenital anomaly on USG is ***Anencephaly.[Q]***
- **Anencephaly** can be diagnosed
  - ***Earliest at 10 weeks[Q]***
  - ***Best at 12 weeks[Q] (100% accuracy)***

206. **C i.e. Tranvaginal US** *[Ref: Dutta obs. 5/e P-197-99; Grainger 5/e p. 1206-5, 1230]*
207. **B i.e., Transvaginal USG**
208. **D i.e. Echogenic mass with multicystic spaces within endometrial cavity**
209. **A i.e. Absence of gestational sac in uterus** *[Ref: Shaws 13/e P-270]*

Best method of diagnosing unruptured ectopic pregnancy is ***combination of transvaginal sonography & quantitative B-HCG values[Q].***

210. **D i.e. Crown rump length**
[Ref: Grainger & Allison's diagnostic radiology 5/e p- 1206 Sutton : textbook of radiology & imaging 7/e p – 1040-43]

***Most accurate estimation of gestational age by USG is done** by **crown rump length**[Q].*

211. **D i.e. Down's Syndrome** *[Ref: Dutta 4/e P-259, 439; Ghai 5/e P-406, 479]*

- In anencephaly, absece of vault.
  In NTD, presence of meningo-myelocoel &
  In placenta previa location of placenta seen by USG confirms the diagnosis.
- Although on prenatal U/S increased nuchal fold thickness, and reduced length of femur & humerus are suggestive of Down's syndrome but the diagnosis is confirmed by chromosomal study (trisomy of 21st autosome) either by amniocentesis or chronic villous sampling.

212. **C i.e. Turner's Syndrome** *[Ref: Nelson essentials of pediatrics 3/e P-139 (not text book)]*

Turner's syndrome (XO) may have
- **Cystic hygroma**
- Widely spaced nipples
- Webbed neck
- Infertility
- Normal I. Q.

GYNECOLOGY

213. **B i.e. USG**

214. **D i.e. All of above** *[Ref: Grainger 4/e P-2221; Dutta 5/e P-579]*

Investigation of choice in displaced IUD is ***Ultrasound,*** but we can also diagnose this by X-Ray abdomen (metal in IUD produces radioopaque shadow) & Hysteroscopy (Endoscopic visualization of uterus).

215. **B i.e. First ten days of M.C.** *[Ref: Grainger 4/e P-233]*

- **Ten day Rule** : Radiological investigation in a reproductive age gp. female should be carried out ***within 10 days of last Menstrual Period i.e. Ist 10 days of M.C.***[Q] **(i.e. *within in 10 days of onset of menstruation).***
- This was stated in the belief that there was then least likelihood of conception taking place (but if it did, the embryo would be most sensitive to radiation) it is now believed that fetus is relatively insensitive to radiation in early stages of pregnancy, any adverse effect leads to spontaneous abortion.
- The fetus is most sensitive to radiation, at ***8-15 weeks*** gestation for increased incidence of ***Down's Syndrome*** and slight reduction in IQ.

216. **A i.e. Teratoma** *[Ref: Shaws 13/e P-350-52]*

In teratoma, there may be presence of tooth & other calcified bodies giving rise to radio-opaque shadows.

PEDIATRICS

217. **D i.e. After 6 hours** *[Ref: B & L 24/e P-1247]*

- **Invertogram** is done to detect ***imperforate anus***[Q].
- It is done ***after six hours of birth***[Q] in infant as sufficient air may have collected in large intestine to cast a x Ray Shadow.
- If the distance between highest level of ***gas in rectum & metal bougie inserted into the blind anal canal is > 2.5 cm***[Q]; the abnormality is **high.**
- In high lesion, the ***presence of proteus or pseudomonas in urine***[Q] is indicative of fistula. I.V. Urogram & gas in bladder also indicate, fistula, but with definite radiation risk.

218. **C i.e. Sutural diastasis**
[Ref: Sutton 7/e P-1728, 1809; Love & Baiely 24/e P-613; Nelson text book of pediatrics 17/e P-1990]

In infants, the diagnosis of ***hydrocephalus is confirmed by USG (as the fontanel are open)***Q and in most cases, it tells about the level of obstruction & cause (like Dandywalker & arachnoid cyst.) *[Sutton 7/e P-1728]*

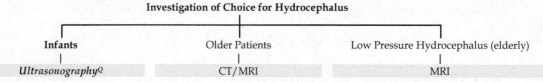

Investigation of Choice for Hydrocephalus

Infants	Older Patients	Low Pressure Hydrocephalus (elderly)
*Ultrasonography*Q	CT/MRI	MRI

- Also Remember
  - ***Aqueductal Stenosis***Q is m.c. of obstructive / non-communicating hydrocephalus.
  - ***Subarachnoid hemorrhage***Q (which is usually a result of intraventricular hemorrhage in premature infant) is m.c. of nonobstructive / communicating hydrocephalus.
  - In an infant *accelerated rate of enlargement of head* is the most prominent sign.
  - Clinical presention is: ***open anterior fontanel***Q, ***setting sun eye sign***Q, UMN signs & ***cracked pot / macewen sign***Q on percussion.
  - Skull X Ray shows ***copper beaten sign, indicative of chronic raised intra cranial pressure (ICP)***Q.
  - In ***adults, erosion of dorsum sellae***Q occurs earliest in hydrocephalus.

219. **A i.e. Congenital Supravalvular Aortic stenosis** *[Ref: Harrison 15/e P-2216; Nelson text book of pediatrics 17/e P-388]*

William's Syndrome or Idiopathic Hypercalcemia of Infancy

It is characterized by:
1. Hypercalcemia d/t abnormal sensitivity to vitamin D
2. ***Supravalvular aortic stenosis***Q & other congenital defects
3. Mental retardation
4. Elfin facies (Round face with full cheeks & lips)

220. **D i.e. All** *[Ref: Sutton 7/e P-1384-85]*

- **Battered Baby / Caffey Syndrome** is a term used to define a clinical condition in young children, who have received nonaccidental injury on one or more occasions at the hands of adults responsible for child's welfare.
- I think this definition is self explanatory - as the child is beaten regularly there are multiple injuries & fractures in different stages of healing.
- Due to lack of proper splintage, fracture either does not unite or unite with excess callus formation.

4 DIAGNOSTIC FEATURES & SPECIFIC SIGNS

QUESTIONS

SKULL & SPINE

1. **Geographic lytic lesions in vault of skull with bevelled edges are seen with**
   A. Multiple myeloma (AIIMS 97, DNB 98) ☐
   B. Eosinophilic granuloma ☐
   C. Hyperparathyroidism ☐
   D. Reticular cell CA ☐
2. **Multiple Punched out lesions on skull X-Ray is found in:**
   A. Down's (AIIMS 1994) ☐
   B. HyperParathyroidism ☐
   C. Multiple Myeloma ☐
   D. All ☐
3. **Vertebra plana is seen in-** *(PGI June 05, AIIMS 98, DNB 99)*
   A. Eosinophilic granuloma ☐
   B. Trauma ☐
   C. Paget's disease ☐
   D. Malignancy ☐
4. **Schober's sign is for :** *(PGI 1998)*
   A. Flexion of lumbar spine ☐
   B. Chest expansion ☐
   C. Pain with motion of hip ☐
   D. Neck pain and stiffness ☐

MUSCULOSKELETAL SYSTEM

5. **Epiphyseal enlargement is seen in**
   A. Rickets (AIIMS 97, DNB 95) ☐
   B. Scurvy ☐
   C. Spondo-epiphyseal dysgenesis ☐
   D. Juvenile Rheumatoid Arthritis ☐
6. **Fraying and cupping of metaphyses of long bones in a child does not occur in:**
   A. Rickets (AI 2003) ☐
   B. Lead poisoning ☐
   C. Metaphyseal dysplasia ☐
   D. Hypophosphatasia ☐
7. **Dense metaphyseal band is seen on:** *(PGI June 08)*
   A. Hypervitamininosis A ☐
   B. Hypervitaminosis B ☐
   C. Scurvy ☐
   D. Hypervitaminosis D ☐
8. **Wind Swept deformity is seen in:**
   A. Ankylosing spondylitis (AIIMS 1998) ☐
   B. Scurvy ☐
   C. Rheumatoid arthritis ☐
   D. Rickets ☐
9. **Trident hand is seen in:** *(AIIMS 98, DNB 01)*
   A. Achondroplasia ☐
   B. Mucopolysacchoroidosis ☐
   C. Diphyseal achlasia ☐
   D. Cleidocranial dystosis ☐
10. **Champagne glass pelvis is seen in**
    A. CDH (Jipmer 02, DNB 04) ☐
    B. Down's syndrome ☐
    C. Cetinism ☐
    D. Achondroplasia ☐
11. **Bone within bone appearance is seen in-**
    A. CML (AIIMS 93, Jipmer 2K, DNB 97) ☐
    B. Osteoporosis ☐
    C. Osteopetrosis ☐
    D. Bone infarct ☐
12. **X-ray view of choice for lumbar spondylosis is/are:** *(PGI May 12)*
    A. AP view
    B. PA view
    C. Lateral view
    D. Lt oblique view
    E. Rt oblique view
13. **Scottish terrier sign is seen in-** *(AI 95)*
    A. AP view ☐
    B. PA view ☐
    C. Lateral view ☐
    D. Oblique view ☐
14. **Beheaded Scottish terrier sign is-**
    A. Spondylosis (AIIMS 92, Jipmer 90, 99, DNB 98) ☐
    B. Spondylolisthesis ☐
    C. Lumbar canal stenosis ☐
    D. Slipped Disc ☐
15. **In spondolysthesis following radiological features seen:**
    A. Scotty dog (PGI Dec 06) ☐
    B. Scotty dog wearing a collar ☐
    C. Beheaded Scotty dog terrier sign ☐
    D. Nepolean sign ☐
16. **Least useful for diagnosing spondylolisthesis**
    A. MRI (AIIMS Nov 11) ☐
    B. CT ☐
    C. X ray spine lateral view ☐
    D. X ray spine AP view ☐
17. **Pesudo fracture of looser's zone is seen in** *(AIIMS 1997)*
    A. Osteoporosis ☐
    B. Osteopetrosis ☐
    C. Osteomalacia ☐
    D. Scurvy ☐
18. **Looser's zones is seen in:** *(PGI 2002)*
    A. Osteoporosis ☐
    B. Hyperparathyrodism ☐
    C. Osteomalacia ☐
    D. Renal osteodystrophy ☐
    E. Paget's disease ☐
19. **Radiographic appearance of Pindborg's tumor is:** *(AI 2002)*
    A. Onion - peel appearance ☐
    B. Sun burst appearance ☐
    C. Cherry - blosom appearance ☐
    D. Driven - snow appearance ☐
20. **"Sunray appearance" on X-rays is suggestive of:**
    A. A Chondrosarcoma (AIIMS 95, 04, DNB 05) ☐
    B. A metastatic tumour in the bone ☐
    C. An Osteogenic sarcoma ☐

5 RADIODIAGNOSIS

D. An Ewing's sarcoma

21. Sun ray appearance is seen in:
A. Osteosarcoma *(PGI Dec 05)*
B. Ewing sarcoma
C. Osteoclastoma
D. Multiple myeloma

RESPIRATORY SYSTEM

22. All are true about Kerley B line except: *(AIIMS 1997)*
A. Horizontal
B. Runs from hilar area to peripheral area
C. Due to thickening of septa
D. Due to pulmonary venous hypertension

23. Kerley B lines seen in: *(PGI Nov 2009)*
A. Pleural effusion
B. Mitral stenosis
C. Pericardial effusion
D. Interstitial edema
E. Lymphangitis carcinomatosis

24. Kerley's 'B' lines are found in: *(PGI 03)*
A. Interstitial edema
B. Pulmonary venous congestion
C. Pericardial effusion
D. Mitral stenosis

25. Floating water-lily sign is feature of:
A. Lung Hydatid *(AIIMS Nov 07)*
B. Bronchial adenoma
C. Lung abscess
D. Aspergilloma

26. Water lilly sign is seen in chest X-ray of :
A. Pulmonary hypoplasia *(AIIMS 91, DNB 93)*
B. Echinococcus
C. Pneumonia
D. Sarcoidosis

27. Popcorn calcification is characteristically seen in *(AI 1997)*
A. TB
B. Metastasis
C. Pulmonary hamartoma
D. Fungal invagination

28. Egg shell calcification is seen in all except
A. Sarcoidosis *(AIIMS 1998)*
B. Silicosis
C. Post irradiation lymphoma
D. Bronchogenic CA

29. Egg shell calcification is seen in *(PGI June 09)*
A. Sarcoidosis
B. Silicosis
C. Lung Ca & bronchiolitis
D. Pneumoconiosis
E. Lymphoma following radiation treatment

30. Egg shell calcification are seen: *(PGI 03, 06, 01)*
A. Sillicosis
B. T.B.
C. Carcinoma metastatic to Lymphonode
D. Lymphoma
E. Sarcoidosis

31. Egg-shell calcification in hilar lymph nodes is seen in :
A. Sarcoidosis *(PGI 2001)*
B. Histoplasmosis
C. Tuberculosis
D. Carcinoma lung
E. Silicosis

Cardiovascular System

32. Spring water cyst is another name for:
A. Hydatid cyst of lung *(PGI 97, DNB 01)*
B. Lung amoebic cyst
C. Pleuro pericardial cyst
D. Enterogenous cyst

33. Following can cause rib notching except: *(AIIMS Nov 09)*
A. Blalock Taussig shunt
B. Waterston Cooley's shunt
C. Pulmonary atresia with large VSD
D. Aorta disruption

34. Superior rib notching is /are caused by: *(PGI June 09)*
A. Hyperparathyroidism
B. Poliomyelitis
C. Blalock-Tausig shunt
D. Marfan syndrome.
E. Coarctation of aorta

35. Rib notching is found in : *(PGI 2001)*
A. Neurofibromatosis
B. Lymphangiomyomatosis
C. Aortic aneurysm
D. Taussig-Bing operation
E. Aortic obstruction

36. Which of the following causes rib-notching on the chest radiograph? *(AI 2006)*
A. Bidirectional Glem shunt
B. Modified Blalock-Taussing shunt
C. IVC occlusion
D. Coarctation of aorta

37. True regarding radiological picture of coaritation of aorta A/E *(PGI 04, WB 05, DNB 06)*
A. Involvement of upper two ribs
B. Bilateral
C. Inferior rib notching
D. Usually before 5 years of age
E. '3' sign

38. Inferior rib notching is seen in *(AI 08)*
A. Coarctation of aorta
B. Rickets
C. ASD
D. Multiple myeloma

39. In which of the following a 'Coeur en Sabot' shape of the heart is seen: *(AI 2K, 04)*
A. Tricuspid atresia
B. Ventricular septal defect
C. Transportation of great arteries
D. Tetralogy of fallot

40. Snowmann appearance is seen in: *(PGI Nov 2009)*
A. Total anomalous pulmonary venous Connection
B. Ebstein anomaly
C. Tetralogy of fallot
D. VSD
E. Transposition of great vessel

41. "Snowman" sign is seen in: *(AIIMS May 08)*
A. TGV
B. TOF
C. TAPVC
D. Aortic dissection

42. Figure of 8 in chest X Ray is seen in
A. Ebstein Anomaly *(AI 2K, PGI 10)*
B. Total Anomalous pulmonary venous connection (TAPVC)
C. Tetrology of fallot (TOF)
D. Transposition of great vessels (TGA)

43. Flask shaped heart is seen in following except: *(PGI 1997)*
A. Ebstein anomaly
B. Pericardial effusion
C. TOF
D. TAPVC

44. Egg on side appearance is seen in: *(PGI 09, DNB 07)*

A. TAPVC
B. Ebstein anomaly
C. TGA
D. TOF
E. VSD

45. "Egg-on-side" appearance is seen in:
A. TOF *(AI 10, AIIMS May 08)*
B. Uncorrected TGV
C. TAPVC
D. Constricted pericarditis /TA

ENT

46. 'Thumb print' sign seen in: *(PGI June 08)*
A. Candida
B. Aspergillus
C. Thrrmomyces
D. Epiglotis

Gastrointestinal System

47. Double bubble sign is seen in A/E
A. Lad's band *(PGI June 09, Dec 04)*
B. Annular pancreas
C. Pancreatic pseudocyst
D. Duodenal atresia
E. Diaphragmatic hernia

48. Double bubble sign seen in: *(PGI Dec 07)*
A. Duodenal atresia
B. Ileal atresia
C. Pyloric stenosis
D. Pancreatic divisum
E. Volvulus

49. Double bubble sign on X-Ray is seen in:
A. Duodenal atresia *(AIIMS May 09, 99)*
B. Oesophageal atresia
C. Colonic atresia/Hirschprung's disease
D. Pyloric stenosis

50. X-Ray feature of pyloric stenosis is
A. Single bubble appearance *(AIIMS 97, DNB 99)*
B. Double bubble appearance
C. Triple bubble apperance
D. Multiple air fluid levels

51. Radiological signs of crohn's disease: *(PGI June 08)*
A. String sign of Kantor
B. Pipestem appearance
C. Pseudo polyp
D. Backwash ileitis

52. Radiological feature of ischemic colitis is
A. Saw toothing *(PGI 96, UP 99, Karnataka 01)*
B. Craggy popcorn appearance
C. Thumb printing
D. Cobble stone appearance

53. Lead pipe appearance is seen in
A. Chron's disease *(PGI 94, UP 02, DNB 03)*
B. Ulcerative colitis
C. Schistosomiasis
D. Carcinoma colon

54. String of Kantor is seen in
A. Chron's disease *(UP 03, Kerala 2000, AIIMS 96)*
B. Ulcerative colitis
C. TB
D. Carcinoma

55. Soap Bubble appearance in X-ray is seen in
A. Multiple cystic Kidney *(AIIMS 1999)*
B. Neuroblastoma
C. Cystic lymphagiectasis
D. Meconium ileus

56. Radiological sign of ischemic colitis is
A. Popcorn appearance *(AIIMS 94, DNB 95)*
B. Thumb print apperance
C. Cobrahead app.
D. Inverted 3 sign

57. String sign is suggestive of: *(AIIMS 93, DNB 97)*
A. Toxic Megacolon
B. Hypertrophic Pyloric stenosis (HPS)
C. Ulcerative Colitis
D. IBS

58. A newborn presenting with intestinal obstruction showed on abdominal X-ray, multiple air fluid levels. The diagnosis is not likely to be- *(AI 2002)*
A. Pyloric obstruction
B. Duodenal atresia
C. Illeal atresia
D. Ladd\s bands

59. Feathery appearance in jejunum is due to:
A. Valvulae conniventes *(PGI 99, DNB 2K)*
B. Haustrations
C. Luminal gas
D. Vascular network

60. X-Ray appearance of CBD stone on cholangiography is:
A. Meniscus appearance *(AIIMS 98, DNB 03)*
B. Sudden cut off
C. Smooth tapering
D. Eccentric occlusion

61. Chain of lakes appearance in ERCP is seen is *(AI 1996)*
A. Acute Pancreatitis
B. Chronic Pancreatitis
C. Carcinoma Pancreas
D. Ductal Adenoma

62. Central dot sign is seen in: *(AIIMS May 11, Nov 08)*
A. Caroli's disease
B. Primary sclerosing cholangitis
C. Polycystic liver disease
D. Liver hamartoma

63. "Spongy appearance" with central sunburst calcification is seen in
A. Pancreatic adenocarcinoma
B. Mucinous cyst adenocarcinoma
C. Somato statinoma *(AIIMS May 07)*
D. Serous cyst adenoma

64. A 45 yrs female presents with recurrent epigastric abdominal pain and jaundice. USG shows clausters of cysts, cysts are having lobulated margins, in the head of pancreas. MR reveals a multicystic mass with a bunch of grapes appearance and a grossly dialated pancreatic duct. The most probable diagnosis is: *(AI 2012)*
A. Serous cystadenoma
B. Mucinous cystadenoma
C. Intraductal papillary mucinous neoplasm (IPMN)
D. Solid pseudopapillary epithelil neoplasm

Urology

65. Rim sign in IVP is seen in *(AIIMS 98)*
A. Polycystic Kidney
B. Hydronephrosis
C. Chronic pyelonephritis
D. Hypernephroma

66. Cobra head deformity is characterstic of
A. Posterior urethral valve *(AIIMS 97, DNB 09)*

B. Ureterocoel ☐
C. Bladder tumor ☐
D. Cytitis ☐

67. IVP of polycystic kidney disease shows: *(PGI Nov 2009)*
A. Cobra head ☐
B. Dropping lilly ☐
C. Flower base appearance ☐
D. Spider leg deformity ☐
E. Fish hook appearance ☐

68. B/L spider leg sign on IVP suggests *(DNB 08)*
A. Renal stone ☐
B. Polycystic kidney ☐
C. Hypernephroma ☐
D. Hydronephrosis ☐

69. Spider leg appearance is found in :
A. Polycystic kidney *(PGI 1999)* ☐
B. Pyelonephritis ☐
C. Hydronephrosis ☐
D. Renal artery stenosis ☐

5

RADIODIAGNOSIS

Answers and Explanations:

SKULL & SPINE

1. **B i.e. Eosinophillic Granuloma** *[Ref: Turek's orthopedics 4/e P-753]*

Features	Disorder
*Geographic lytic skull*Q *Vertebrae plana*Q	**Eosinophillic granuloma**/Hand-Schuller Christian ds/ Histocytosis

2. **C i.e. Multiple myeloma** *[Ref: Grainger 4/e P-1914]*

Features	Disease
Multiple punched out lesions	Multiple *myeloma*Q
Hair on end skull vault	*Thalessemia*Q, Sickel cell Anemia
Erosion of dorsum sella	Raised ICT (earliest & most common)
Silver Beaten app. of vault	Raised ICT
Sunray calcification with spicules	Meningioma

3. **A, D i.e. Eosinophilic granuloma; Malignancy** *[Ref: Sottun 7th/ 1187]*

Vertebra Plana

Vertebra plana is a condition manifested by increased density & collapse of a vertebral body, with normal adjacent disc spaces or increase in width. **Vertebra plana** is marked flattening and increased density of vertebrae with the contour appearing like the edge of a coin or disc and not being wedge shaped. The causes are-

1. Osteochondritis of vertebral body (Calve's disease)
2. ***Histiocytosis, Eosinophilic granuloma***Q
3. Leukemia
4. Ewing's sarcoma
5. ***Metastasis***Q
6. TB

Increased density and collapse of vertebrae with normal disc space

Feature	Found in
• *Vertebrae plana*Q • *Picture frame vertebra*Q • *Calcification of Intervertebral disc*Q	*Eosinophilic granuloma*Q Paget's ds Alkaptonuria
• *Fish mouth vertebrae*Q	Sickle cell anemia Homocystinuria
• *Cod Fish Vertebrae*Q	Osteomalacia Osteoporosis Hyperparathyroidism
• *Rugger jursy spine*Q	CRF induced Renal osteodystrophy Osteopetrosis

4. **A i.e. Flexion of lumber spine** *[Ref: Harrison 15/e P-1950]*

Schober's test is measure of ***flexion on lumber spine***Q. This test is done in ***ankylosing spondylitis***Q

MUSCULOSKELETAL SYSTEM

5. **D i.e. Juvenile Rheumatoid** *[Ref: Sutton 7/e P-1356/1215; Chapman 5/e p. 479]*

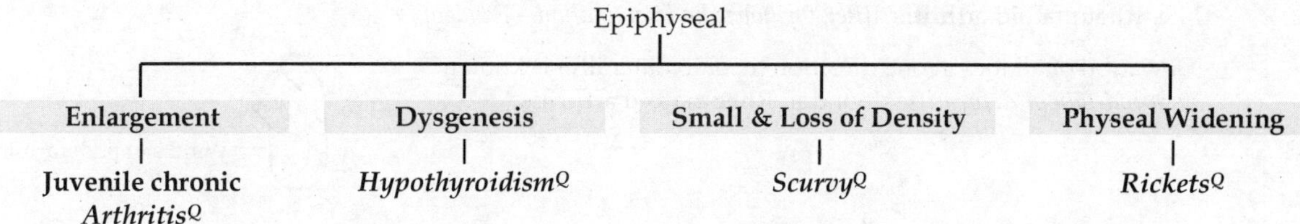

Disease	Radiological feature
Hypothyroidism	*Fragmented / Punctate Epiphysis*[Q] *Epiphyseal dysgenesis*[Q]
Rickets	*Widened physis (growth plate)*[Q] *Cupped & Frayed metaphysis*[Q]
Juvenile chronic arthritis	*Overgrowth/enlargement of epiphysis*[Q] with squaring & angulation
Scurvy C, W, P, F, T, S	- **Wimberger sign** (W) is ***loss of epiphyseal density with a pencil thin cortex or small epiphysis***[Q] marginated by sclerotic rim - **Frankel' line** (F) is ***radiodense zone of provisional calcification***[Q] – due to excessive calcification of osteoid –at growing metaphyseal end - ***Trummerfeld zone*** (T) is *metaphyseal radiolucent zone* – due to lack of mineralization of osteoid seen beneath Frenkel's line. - **Metaphyseal corner fractures** through the weakened lucent metaphysis (**Pelkan spurs**) resulting in **cupping of metaphysis** (C) - **Periosteal reaction & new bone formation** due to **subperiosteal hematoma (S)**

6. **B i.e. Lead poisoning** *[Ref. Chapman 4/e P. 48]*

- Remember : ***Lead poisoning***[Q] (Bismuth, Arsenic, P, mercury fluride, radium also), Radiation & Hypervitaminosis D leads to **solitary dense metaphyseal band** not cupping & fraying.
- Causes of **Cupping & Fraying of metaphysis**

Metaphyseal Cupping	Metaphyseal Fraying
1. R*ickets*[Q] (with widening & fraying of growth plate) 2. ***Hypophosphatamia***[Q] 3. Dysplasias of bone – (eg achondroplasia, pseudochondroplasia, metatropic dwarfism, diastrophic dwarfism, chondrodysplasias) 4. Scurvy 5. Trauma 6. Normal (distal ulna of proximal fibula)	1. ***Rickets***[Q] 2. ***Hypophosphatamia***[Q] 3. Copper deficiency 4. Chronic stress in the wrist of young gymnasts (with asymmetrical widening of distal radial growth plate & metaphyseal sclerosis)

Easy way to remember causes of Metaphyseal cupping is

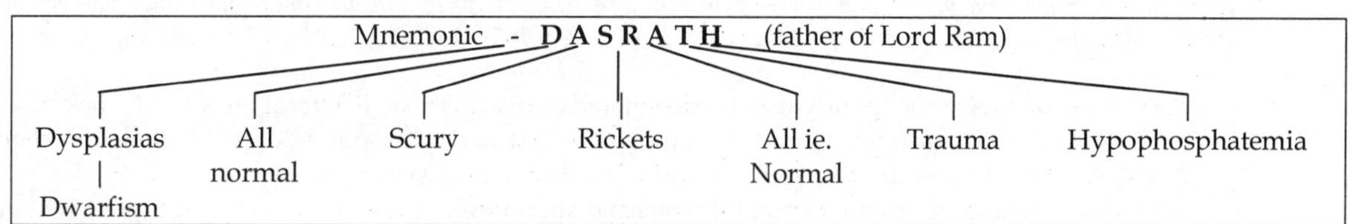

7. **D. i.e. Hypervitaminosis D** *[Ref: Aids to differential diagnosis – Chapman 4/e p.47]*

Metaphyseal bands

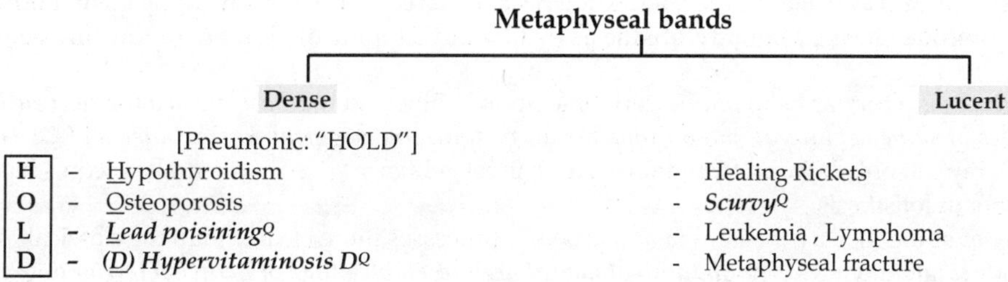

Dense
Lucent
[Pneumonic: "HOLD"]
H - Hypothyroidism
O - Osteoporosis
L - Lead poisining[Q]
D - (D) Hypervitaminosis D[Q]
- Healing Rickets
- Scurvy[Q]
- Leukemia , Lymphoma
- Metaphyseal fracture

8. **C i.e. Rheumatoid arthritis** *[Ref: Orthopaedic Examination – Pandey]*

Deviation of all toes in one direction (usually laterally) is known as ***wind-swept deformity***[Q] found in **Rheumatoid arthritis.**

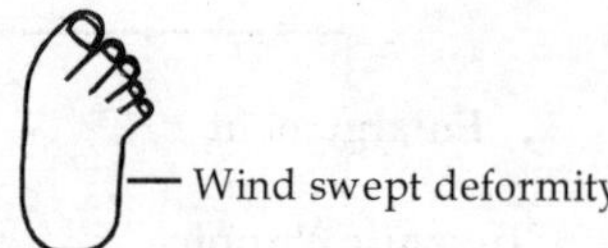

9. **A i.e. Achondroplasia**

10. **D i.e. Achondroplasia** *[Ref: Wolfgang 5/e p. 217; Adams 13/e P-49; Maheswari 3/e P-268]*

In **achondroplasia,** due to squaring of iliac bones, broad and flat acetabular roofs and a small sciatic notch the pelvis look radiologically as- ***champagne glass***[Q].

Anchondroplasia is a *AD (autosomal dominant)* condition which presents as

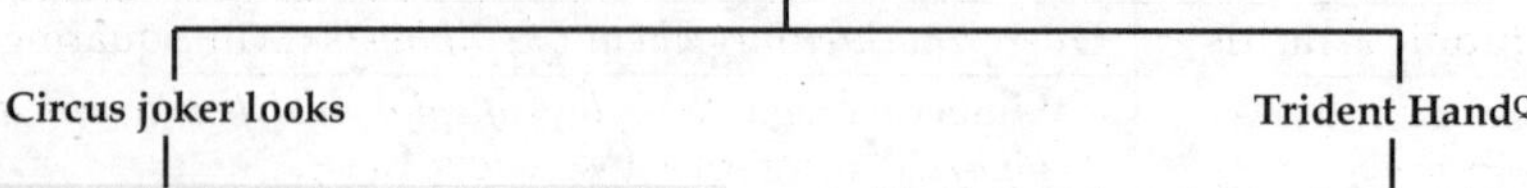

Circus joker looks

- ***Disproportionate Dwarfism***[Q] as the growth of *trunk is normal* and shortening is mainly present in *proximal segments of limbs*
- Normal intelligence
- Large skull
- Increased lumber lordosis
- Near normal life except who develop spinal canal stenosis

Trident Hand[Q]

Hands are short & broad, central 3 digits being divergent & almost equal length.

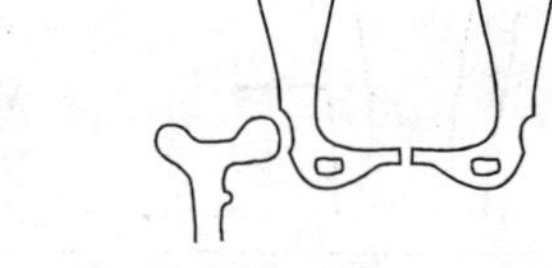

Champagne glass pelvis in achondroplasia

11. **C i.e. Osteopetrosis** *[Ref: Robbin's Pathological basis of disease 7/e p. 1281]*

In **osteopetrosis,** there is reduced osteoclastic bone resorption resulting in diffuse symmetrical skeleton sclerosis. Also k/a **marble bone disease** d/t its stone like quality of bones; however the bones are abnormally brittle & fracture like a piece of chalk. It can present radiologically as-

- Sclerosis of all bones ***more prominent at base of skull***[Q].
- Sclerosis of vertebral end plate l/t characteristic ***sandwitch or broad stripped (rugby jersey spine)*** [Q]
- ***Bone in bone appearance***[Q] d/t sclerotic foci within the bone.

12. **C i.e. Lateral >> A i.e. AP view**

13. **D i.e. Oblique view** **14.** **B i.e. Spondylolisthesis**

15. **C i.e. Beheaded Scotty dog terrier sign; D i.e. Napolean hat sign** **16.** **D i.e. X ray spine AP view**

[Ref: Watson & Jones 6/e p. 268; Turek's 6/e p. 503; Gray's Anatomy p. 18; Greenspan Orthopaedic Radiology 4/e p 397; Maheshwari 3e/p 237; Wolfgang 7/e p 228-29, 206; Sutton 7/e p 1658, 1662-63; Clark's 12/e p 182-86]

- **X ray view of choice for spondylosis (ie degenerative disc disease) is lateral view > AP view >>>** oblique view. Radiological features of spondylosis (not to be confused with spondylolysis) include *reduction in disc height, Schmorl's node, endplate osteophytes* and other degenerative changes.
- Xray view of choice for **lumbar spondylolysis** and **spondylolisthesis** (minimal) is **oblique (right or left posterior oblique) > lateral >>> AP view**. The degree of obliquity in PO views should be such that posterior elements of vertebrae show the classic **"Socttie Dog appearance". A defect in pars interarticularis appears as collar** on the Socttie dog neck. **If defect is bilateral (ie appears on both right & left posterior oblique views), a spondylolisthesis** (ie forward slipping of **vertebra on the one below it) is more likely.**
- **Spondylolisthesis** is a forward slip of one vertebrae upon another; so it is ***best viewed (or seen earliest) in sagittal images of spine i.e. lateral and oblique X rays of spine and saggital & axial views of CT & MRI***[Q]. AP views of X ray can only be used to demonstrate indirect evidences (eg. inverted Napoleon's hat sign) of late/severe spondylolisthesis.
- **Oblique view of spine** display the lamina and articular processes more clearly than the classical anteroposterior & lateral views. The ***shadow of neural arch resembles that of Scottish terrier dog***[Q].

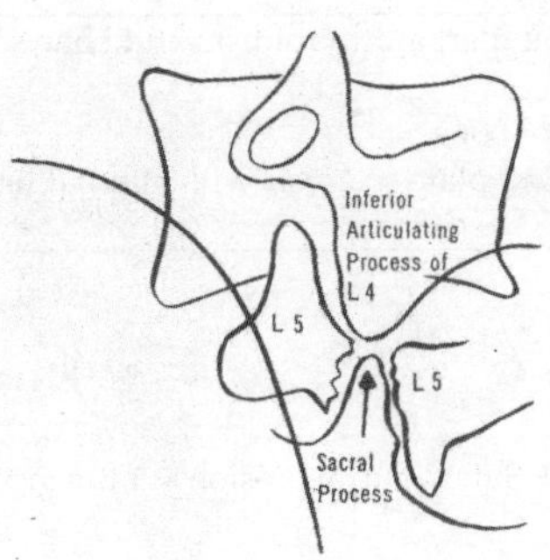

- Ear is superior articular process
- Nose is transverse process
- Eye is pedicle
- Neck is ***pars inter articularis***[Q].
- Front paw is inferior articular process

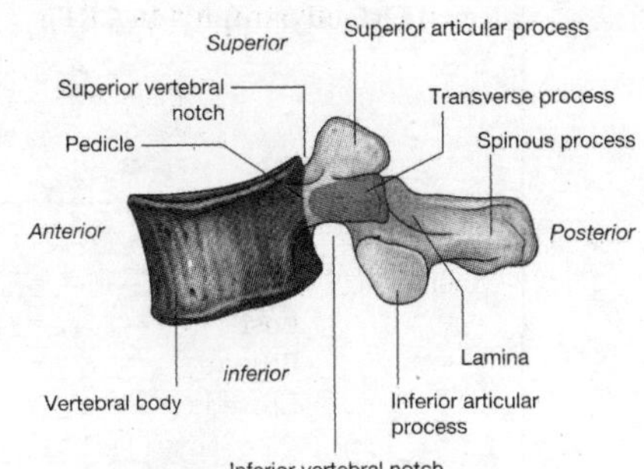

- **Spondylothesis** is forward slip of one vertebrae upon another. Majority of cases are due to *stress fracture of pars interarticularis* leading to ***broken neck or presence of collar on the Scottie dog***[Q]. More displacement will lead to ***Beheaded (without head) Scottie terrier sign***[Q].
- **Spondylolisthesis :** ventral slipping or gliding of all or part of one vertebrae on a stationary vertebra beneath it. Most common is between $L_5 - S_1$ and between $L_4 - L_5$.
- ***"Inverted Napoleon's Hat***[Q]***"*** sign: A severe degree of spondylolisthesis at $L_5 - S_1$ can be identified on A-P view by ventrocaudal displacement of L5 over sacrum and creates curvilinear densities.
- **Lumbor spondylolysis is traumatic, degeneration or deficient** congenital development of the articulating portion of vertebra. Pars inter articularis prevents vertebra slipping (spondylolisthesis) and a defect in it can be congenital or treaumatic.

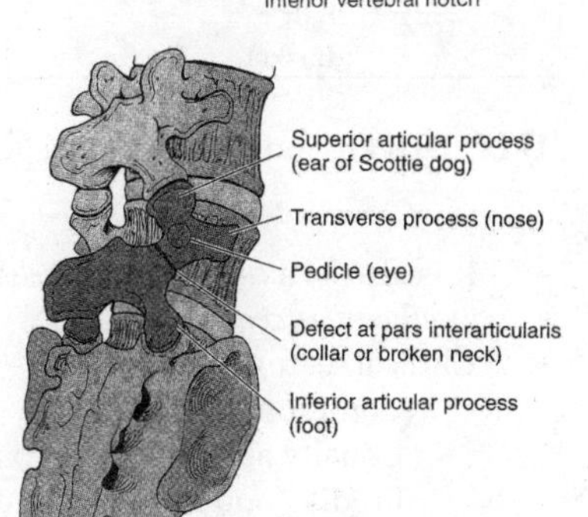

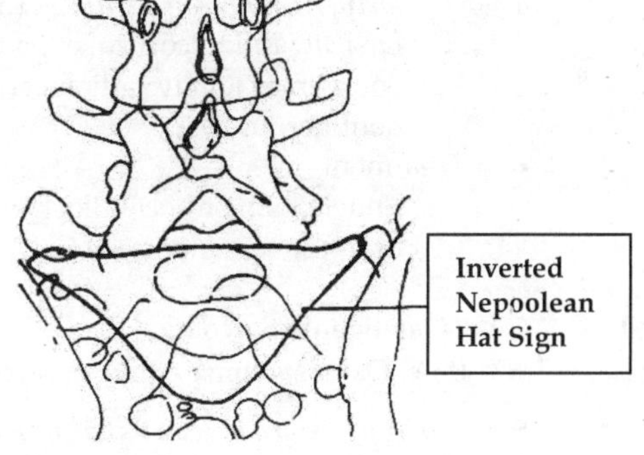

Scotty dog appearance

(In oblique view of spine, in a normal vertebra; the pars interarlicularis looks like a 'Scotty dog')

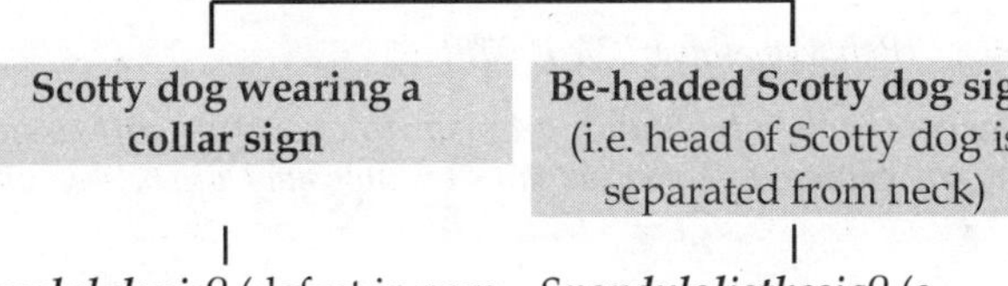

Scotty dog wearing a collar sign	**Be-headed Scotty dog sign** (i.e. head of Scotty dog is separated from neck)
Spondylolysis[Q] (defect in pars interarticularis without slipping of vertebrae)	***Spondylolisthesia***[Q] (a defect with slip of vertebrae)

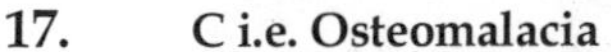

17. **C i.e. Osteomalacia**
18. **C i.e. Osteomalacia** *[Ref: Sutton 7/e P-1339, 1355, 1362-65]*

The most **specific feature of Osteomalacia** is presence of ***looser transformation zones***[Q] also k/a **Milkman's pseudofractures** or **umbau zone**.

Disease	Radiological feature
Osteoporosis Mn – **"Fish In Pan"**	- Cod **fish** vertebrae - **Pencilling-in**-vertebrae (loss of density of vertebral body with radiodense end plates)
Osteomalacia Mn – **"Lost Fish In Pan"**	- ***Looser's zone***[Q]***/ Pseudo fracture***[Q] ***(Hallmark)*** (B/L radiolucent band of uncalcified osteoid due to pressure of pulsating artery) - ***Cod Fish***[Q] **(marked biconcave) vertebrae** - Pencilling in vertebrae
Osteopetrosis/Marbel Bone disease /Alberg Schowenberg disease	- ***Bone within Bone appearance***[Q] - Erlenmeyer flask deformity of long bone ends (flask shaped metaphysis) - ***Rugger jersey spine***[Q] - ***Increased density of bones***[Q]

Renal Osteodystrophy(d/t CRF):	- It combines findings of ostemalacia, hyperparathyroidism and bone sclerosis - Osteomalacia l/t Looser's zone - Hyper PTH l/t Subperiosteal Erosion of bone - *Osteosclerosis l/t Rugger Jersey* ***spine***[Q] (End plate sclerosis with alternating bands of radiolucency)
Hyperparathyroidism Mnemonic: O.P. = Lost = Brown = Erosed = Salt = Basket =	 - **Osteopenia** - **Loss** of lamina dura - **Brown**'s tumor - ***Subperiosteal Erosion (pathognomic)***[Q], Subchondral erosion & intracortical erosions l/t cigar shaped lucencies - ***Salt & Pepper/Pepper-pot skull***[Q] - Basket work appearance of cortex

19. D i.e. Driven Snow appearance *[Ref: Oral pathology by Shafer Hine Levy 4/e P-286-7; Burket's Oral Medicine 9/e p. 163-4]*

Pindborg Tumor

- It is also k/a *calcifying Epithelial Odontogenic Tumor (CEOT).* It resembles an ameloblastoma in that it is *locally invasive.*
- Clinical features:
  - Commonly in *middle age.*
  - Usually asymptomatic, patients are aware of *painless swelling.*
  - Predilection for *mandible* over maxilla (2:1).
  - Prevalence in *molar* region is three times more than premolar (bicuspid) region.
- Radiological feature:
  - ***Driven Snow Appearance***[Q] (it is scattered flecks of calcification throughout the radiolucency)
  - *Liesgang Rings* (cortical expansion with areas of spotty calcification)
  - Sometimes totally radiolucent with an impacted tooth, leading to mistaken clinical diagnosis of dentigerous cyst.
- Treatment :
  - Enucleation or Local Block excision without exploration of regional nodes & follow up radiation (as used for squamous cell C_A).

20. C i.e. Osteogenic Sarcoma

21. A > B i.e. Osteosarcoma > Ewing sarcoma *[Ref: Maheshwari 3/e p. 218]*

Sun ray appearance is seen usually in osteosarcoma when the tumor grows into overlying soft tissue and new bone is laid down along the blood vessels. *Sunray appearance and Codman's triangle may also be seen in Ewing's sarcoma.*

Classical radiological features	*Found In*
Sun ray appearance, Codman's triangle	*Osteosarcoma*[Q]
Onion peel appearance	*Ewing*[Q]
Soap bubble appearance	*Osteoclastoma*[Q]
Spickeled/Mottled/Patchy calcification	*Chondrosarcoma*[Q]
Wormian bones	*Osteogenesis imperfecta*[Q]
Trethowan's sign	*Stipped capital femoral epiphysis*[Q]
Aneurysmal sign	TB spine.
Honey comb appearance	*Admantinoma*[Q]
Driven Snow appearance	*Pindborg Tumor*[Q]

X-ray features of Osteosarcoma

- Area of irregular destruction of metaphyses
- Erosion of the overlying cortex
- New bone formation in the matrix of the tumor
- Irregular periosteal reaction (periosteal reaction in osteomyelitis is smooth)
- Codman's triangle
- Sun-ray appearance.

RESPIRATORY SYSTEM

22. B i.e. Runs from hilar area to peripheral area

Kerley A lines radiate from hilum not kerley B lines which are best seen in costophrenic angles[Q]**.**

Kerley lines

Kerley B lines

- ***Horizontal (transverse)***[Q], non branching 1-2 mm thick, 1-3 cm long lines at **lung base** (best seen at ***costophrenic angles***[Q]) & are ***perpendicular to pleural surface***[Q]
- Seen at PCWP = ***17-20 mmHg***[Q]
- Due to ***thickening of interlobular septa***[Q] caused by:
  1. ***Pulomonary venous hypertension***[Q] (MS, LVF)
  2. Lymphatic obstruction (pneumoconiosis, Lymphangitis carcinomatosis, sarcoidosis)
  3. Interstial pneumonitis

Kerley A lines

- 1-2 mm thick, 2-6 cm long non branching lines ***radiating from the hilum***[Q]
- D/t thickened deep interlobular septa

Kerley C lines

- Fine interlacing lines throughout the lung producing spider web appearance

23. **B, D, E i.e. Mitral stenosis, Interstitial edema, lymphangitis carcinomatosis**

24. **A i.e. Interstitial edema; B i.e. Pulmonary venous congestion; D i.e. Mitral Stenosis**
[Ref: Sutton 7/e P-12, 289; Chapman 4/e P-128]

Costopherenic/Kerley B / Septal lines

These are 1-2 mm thick and 1-3 cm long, ***horizontal***[Q] transverse, nonbranching, lines at *lung bases* which are *perpendicular to the pleural surface* and best seen at ***costophrenic angles***, formed due to ***visible interlobular lymphatics***, (which may be d/t ***pulmonary venous hypertension***[Q] or lymphatic obstruction). Causes of Kerley B Line

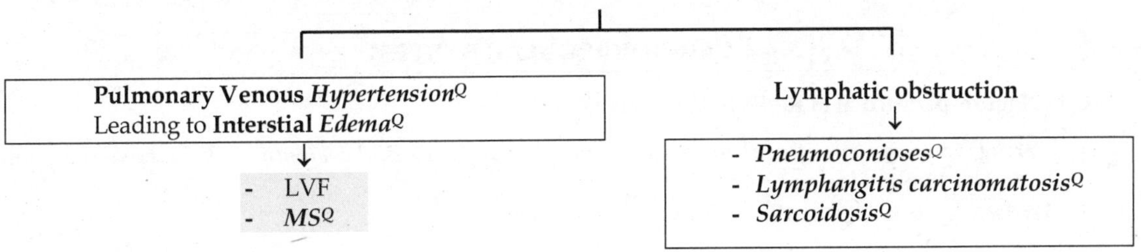

25. **A i.e. Lung hydatic**

26. **B i.e. Echinococcus** *[Ref: Wofgang 5/e P-494; Grainger & Allison's diagnostic radiology 5/e p- 284,1762]*

- Chest- X Ray of **Echinococcus** (hydatid disease) shows: (as fluid decreases and air increases due to rupture of membrane in bronchi)

1. *Oval mass that is easily deformable, l/t lobulation or eccentricity, but* ***almost never calcify***[Q].
2. ***Meniscus /Moon/Air crescent of mycetoma/ Double arch sign***[Q]
3. Cumbo sign/ Air fluid level
4. ***Water lilly / Camalotte Sign***[Q]
5. ***Serpent Sign/Rising sun sign***[Q]
6. Mass in cavity
7. Empty cyst sign

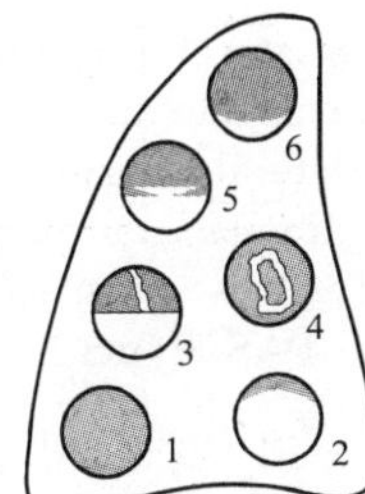

- Cyst has three layers in the wall, two in the cyst itself (ecto & endo cyst) and third derived from surrounding lung (pericyst). The **unruptured cyst** presents as *homogenous spherical or oval mass* (1). If the *inner two layers are intact* airway communication results in ring opacity containing a rounded homogenous density i.e. *air crescent of mycetoma* (2). **Disruption of inner layers** result in – air fluid level (3), a ***floating membrane (camolote / water lilly sign)***[Q], dry cyst with crumpled membrane lying at its bottom (*double wall, rising sun / serpent sign*) and a cyst with all its content expectorated (empty cyst sign).
- *CT scan is highly specific for diagnosis of perforated pulmonary hydatid cyst (air bubble sign).*

27. **C i.e. Pulmonary Hamartoma** *[Ref: Wofgang 5/e P-490, 541; Bhadury P-48]*

Calcification type	Condition associated
Pop corn calcification	*Pulmonary hamartoma*[Q], mediastinal lymph nodes of acute histoplasmosis.
Egg shell (peripheral) calcification Rice grain calcification Tram track (Rail road) calcification **Basal ganglion calcification**	***Silicosis*[Q], *Sarcoidosis*[Q]** ***Cysticercosis*[Q]** ***Struge Weber syndrome*[Q]** Hyper parathyroidism
Cardiac calcification Pericardial calcification	Carcinoid syndrome Constructive pericarditis
Not calcify	***Hydatid cyst in lung*[Q]**

28. **D i.e. Bronchogenic carcinoma**

29. **A, B, D, E i.e. Sarcoidosis, Silicosis, Pneumoconiosis, Lymphoma following radiation treatment**

30. **A i.e. Silicosis; B i.e. T.B.; E i.e. Sarcoidosis** *[Ref: Chapman 4/e P-148; Wofgang 5/e P-434]*

31. **A i.e. Sarcoidosis; B Histoplasmosis; C i.e. Tuberculosis; E i.e. Silicosis**

Egg shell calcification means peripheral rim calcification of lymph nodes. It is found in:

Silly	- *Silicosis (M.C. cause)*[Q]
Cool	- *Coal worker's pneumoconiosis*[Q]
Sardar	- *Sarcoidosis*[Q]
Likes	- *Lymphoma following radiotherapy*[Q]
His	- *Histoplasmosis*[Q]
Progressive	- Progressive massive fibrosis (Fibrosing Mediastinitis)
Tubercular	- *Tuberculosis*[Q]
Cox	- Coccidiodomycosis

Common causes of Egg shell calcification of nodes

- **Pneumoconiosis** (M.C.)
  1. ***Silicosis*[Q]** *(M.C.)*
  2. ***Coal Workers Pneumoconiosis*[Q]**

  not seen in Asbestosis, berylliosis, baritosis, talcosis
- *Sarcoidosis*[Q]
- **Lymphoma following Radiotherapy**[Q]

★ **Rare causes are:**

1. Fibrosing mediastinitis
2. Fungal + Baterial infection
   - a- ***Histoplasmosis*[Q]**
   - b- Coccidiodomycosis
   - c- Blastomycosis
   - d- ***Tuberculosis*[Q]**
3. Amyloidosis

CARDIOVASCULAR SYSTEM

32. **C i.e. Pleuro-pericardial cyst** *[Ref: Wofgang 5/e P-494]*

- **Spring water cyst** also k/a ***Pleuro-pericardial cyst*[Q]** or ***pericardial coelomic cyst*[Q]** is most commonly found in pericardiophrenic angle more often on right side.
- **Hydatid cyst** is also k/a ***Water-lilly/Camalotte cyst*[Q]**

33. **B i.e. Waterston Cooley's shunt** **34.** **A, B, D, i.e. Hyperparathyroidism, Poliomyelitis, Marfan syndome**

35. **A i.e. Neurofibromatosis; C i.e. Aortic aneurysm; D i.e. Taussig-Bing operation; E i.e. Aortic obstruction**

36. **D i.e. Coarctation of aorta.** *[Ref. Chapman 4/e p. 53-54; Grainger & Allison's 5/e p- 221, 454, 551; Sutton 7/e p. 48]*

Unilateral inferior rib notching is seen in <u>B</u>lalock- Taussig operation, <u>A</u>ortic coarctation (involving left subclavian artery or anomalous right subclavin artery) and <u>S</u>ubclavian artery occlusion (Mn **"BAS"**) whereas, **bilateral inferior rib notching** is seen in <u>V</u>enous (svc, ivc) obstruction, <u>P</u>ulmonary oligaemia (Fallot's tetralogy, pulmonary atresia/stenosis, truncus type IV), <u>A</u>orta coarcation /occlusion /aortitis, <u>S</u>ubclavian atheroma (Takayasus disease), **<u>hyper</u>**parathyroidism, **<u>neuro</u>**genic, and intercostal pulmonary arterio-venous **<u>fistula</u>** (Mn- **"V-PAS-Hyper Nerve Fistulas"**)

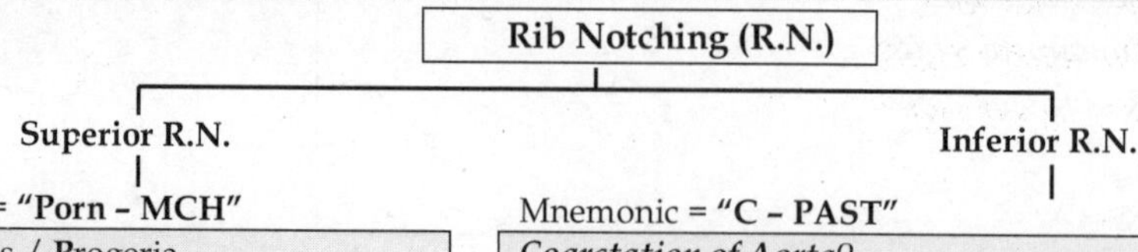

Superior R.N. — Mnemonic = **"Porn - MCH"**	Inferior R.N. — Mnemonic = **"C - PAST"**
Poliomyelitis / Progeria **O**steogenesis imperfecta **R**estrictive lung disease ***N*eurofibromatosis**[Q] **M**arfan's syndrome **C**onnective tissue disease - RA, SLE, Scleroderma, sjogren's syndrome **H**yperparathyroidism	***Coarctation of Aorta*[Q]** **P**ulmonary-oligemia / A-V malformation/atresia/stenosis ***Aortic thrombosis*[Q]*/obstruction/aortitis/disruption*** **S**ubclavian artery obstruction - Takayasu disease, atheroma ***Taussig Blalock operation*[Q]** (subclavian to pulmonary artery anastomosis for TOF) Chest wall A-V malformation - intercostals - pulmonary AV fistula Superior venacava obstruction, IVC obstruction Neurofibromatosis, Hyperparathyroidism

37. **A i.e., Involvement of upper two ribs D i.e., Usually before 5 yrs age** *[Ref: Grainger 5/e p- 550-51]*

Coarctation of aorta (CA)

- *Mostly (95%) involving aortic isthmus*
- *Most (80%) patients are male.*
- *Turner's syndrome* is associated with CA in females.
- *Infantile* type is usually *proximal* to ductus arteriosus, whereas *adult type* is *distal to ductus arteriosus & left subclavian artery.*
- Consequently, whitest adults present with hypertension & signs of collateral vessels on chest x-ray, infants present with hypertension, CHF & failure to thrive.
- Prominent ascending aorta, small descending aorta with intervening notch &, left ventricle enlargement.

Rib –signs

- ***Inferior rib notching***[Q] takes several years to develop and is d/t *pressure erosion by intercostal arteries.*
- *'3' sign*[Q] is d/t enlargement of *left subclavian artery* above the coarctation
- ***Rib signs are unusal before 10 years of age***[Q] & mostly affect $4-8^{th}$ ribs.
- ***Usually bilateral but asymmetrical & mostly spares fist two ribs***[Q] where intercostal arteries arise from costocervical trunk which is proximal to the usual site of CA. But

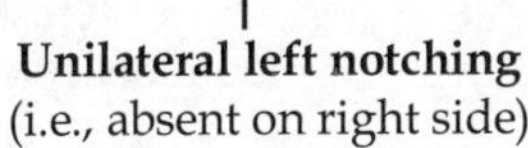

Unilateral left notching
(i.e., absent on right side)

Anomalous origin of right subclavian artery distal to coarctation

U/L right notching
(i.e., absent on left side)

- Stenosed / occluded left subclavian artery
- Coarctation is proximal to left subclavian.

38. **A i.e. Coarctation of aorta**
[Ref: Grainger & Allison's diagnostic radiology 5/e p- 551]

Inferior rib notching in coarctation of aorta is d/t pressure erosion of intercostal arteries[Q] It usually takes several years to develop, so is unusual before 10 years of age.

39. **D i.e. Tetralogy of fallot**

Radiological feature	Disorder
Dock's sign (inferior notching of 3-8 ribs but does not involve 1st & 2nd ribs), E-sign, reverse figure of 3 sign	**Coarctation of aorta**
Jug handle appearance	**Primary pulmonary hypertension**
Maladie de roger defect	**Small VSD (< 0.5 cm diameter)**
Great Hilar dance (pulmonary plethora) on fluoroscopy	**ASD**
Great Box shaped heart	**Tricuspid atresia**
Moneybag/Water bottle/Flask or pear shaped heart	**Pericardial effusion**
Coeur en Sabot[Q] i.e. ***Boot Shaped heart***[Q] (normal sized)	**TOF (Fallot's tetrology)**
Square root sign, Egg in cup appearance[Q]	**Constrictive pericarditis**
Egg on side appearance[Q] Egg shaped heart	**D-Transposition of great arteries (D-TGA)** **Uncorrected TGA**
Convex Left heart border	**L-TGA**
Straight left upper cardiac border	**Ebstein Anomaly**
Sitting duck heart Concave main pulmonary segment & right aortic arch	**Persistent Trunkus arteriosus**
Snowman sign[Q] ***Figure of 8 sign***[Q] ***Cottage loaf sign***[Q]	**Total Anomalous Pulmonary Venous Connection (TAPVC) supracardiac variety**
Tubular heart	**Emphysema**
Ground glass appearance	Infra cardiac TAPVC
Pulmonary plethora, narrow pedicle & globular heart	D-TGA (uncorrected)
Globular heart with oligemic lung field	Tricuspid atresia
"Stag-antler" or "Hands – UP" Sign	CCF
Double aortic knuckle	Dissection of aorta
Double cardiac shadow / density (Buttressing)	Left atrial enlargement

Scimitar sign/vein / syndrome or Turkish Sword appearance	Partial APVC > TAPVC (congenital venolobar syndrome)
Cardiac wall calcification	Endomyocardial fibrosis
Pop –corn calcification in centre of cardiac silhouette	Calcified aortic valve
Glassy heart (speckled appearance) on Echo	Amyloidosis
Ground glass ventricular septum	HOCM
Spade like deformity on echo	Atypical hypertrophic cardiomyopthy (HOCM)
Four bump heart	MS/MR d/t left atrial appendage enlargement
Goose neck deformity on LV angiography	Primum ASD

40. **A i.e. Total anomalous pulmonary venous Connection** **41.** **C i.e., TAPVC**

42. **B i.e. Total Anomalous Pulmonary Venous Connection (TAPVC)**

43. **D i.e. TAPVC** *[Ref: Sutton 7/e p. 395-97; Grainger 4/e P-820; Nelson's 16/e P-1399; Wofgang 5/e P-604-03]*

Due to dilation of SVC (superior vena cava) & left vertical vein, **TAPVC (total anomalous pulmonary venous connection** / return) of supra diaphragmatic variety shows ***double contour / "Figger of 8" / Snowman configuration of cardiac silhouette***[Q].

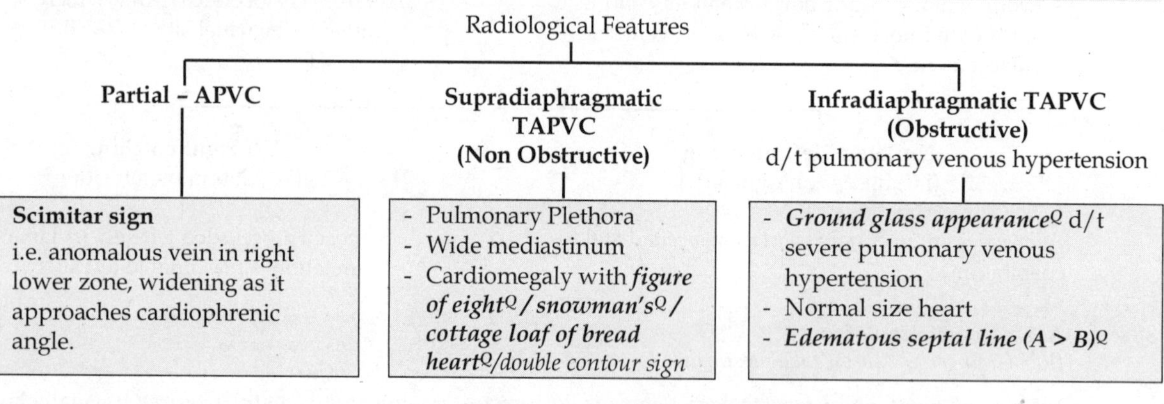

44. **C i.e. TGA** **45.** **B i.e. Uncorrected TGV**

[Ref: Grainger 5/e p. 451, 454; Sutton 7/e p – 385- 86]

Transposition of great arteries (TGA)

D- loop transposition / Uncorrected TGA

- Heart is *slightly enlarged & rounded (cardiomegaly)* with dilated right atrium projecting into right side and prominent right ventricle bulging into left hemithorax; thus producing contour k/a ***egg on side (egg on string) appearance***[Q].
- ***Pulmonary plethora***[Q]
- ***Narrow pedicle***[Q] because main pulmonary artery is behind aorta.

L-loop transpositon / Physiologically corrected transposition[Q]

- ***Long smooth curve to left heart border***[Q] because of abnormal leftward origin of aorta.

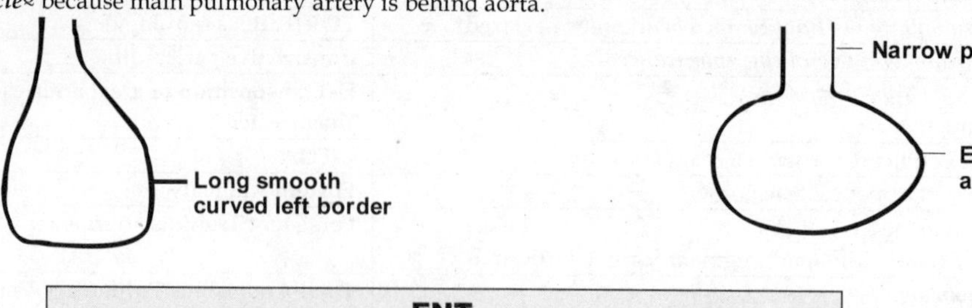

ENT

46. **D. i.e. Epiglottitis:** *[Ref: Berry Neuroradiology 2nd/ed p-575; Chapman 4th/ed 262]*

Thumbprint sign[Q] is a finding on *lateral cervical spine radiograph that suggests dignosis of epiglottitis*[Q]. This appearance is due to thickening of aryepiglottic folds, which causes it to appear more radiopaque, resembling the distal thumb.

Differential Diagnosis of Thumb print sign in colon[Q]
- ***Ulcerative colitis***[Q]
- ***Ischaemic colitis***[Q]
- *Crohn's colitis*
- *Pseudomembranous colitis.*

GASTROINTESTINAL SYSTEM

47. **E i.e. Diaphragmatic hernia** **48.** **A i.e. Duodenal atresia**

49. **A i.e. Duodenal atresia** *[Ref: Wofgang 5/e P-998; Sutton 7/e p. 1362]*

50. **A i.e. Single bubble appearance**

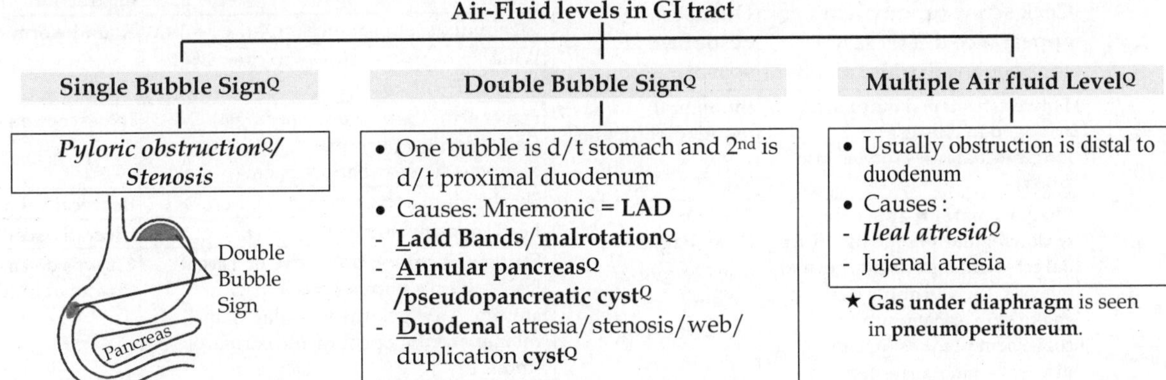

Air-Fluid levels in GI tract
Single Bubble Sign[Q]
Pyloric obstruction[Q]/ Stenosis
Double Bubble Sign
Pancreas
Double Bubble Sign[Q]
• One bubble is d/t stomach and 2nd is d/t proximal duodenum
• Causes: Mnemonic = LAD
- Ladd Bands/malrotation[Q]
- Annular pancreas[Q] /pseudopancreatic cyst[Q]
- Duodenal atresia/stenosis/web/ duplication cyst[Q]
Multiple Air fluid Level[Q]
• Usually obstruction is distal to duodenum
• Causes :
- Ileal atresia[Q]
- Jujenal atresia
★ Gas under diaphragm is seen in pneumoperitoneum.

It is easy to understand that if there is obstruction at pylorus there will be only single air bubble of stomach and 2nd air bubble of duodenum will not be present (nor the multiple air bubbles in intestine) whereas in **duodenal** atresia, one bubble will be of stomach & other of 1st part of normal duodenum.

51. **A. i.e. String sign of Kantor** **52.** **C i.e. Thumb printing**

53. **B i.e. Ulcerative colitis** **54.** **A i.e. Chron's disease**

[Ref: Sutton 7/e p. 1300-1370; Wolfgang 5/e p. 772-998]

Radiological features

Chron's Disease

- **Bull's eye** or **Target lesions**[Q] are small collection of barium surrounded by radiolucent halo
- **String sign of Kantor**[Q] is greatly narrowed terminal ileum
- ***Comb sign***[Q] is prominent vasa recta of mesenteric vessels

Ulcerative Colitis

- **Lead-pipe appearance**[Q] d/t fibrosis causing loss of normal haustral pattern
- **Collor button ulcer**
- ***Pseudopolyp***[Q] are mounds of inflamed tissue between ulcerate mucosa
- ***Backwash ileitis***[Q]

Ischemic Colitis

- **Thumb printing**[Q] is focal indentation of endematous bowel wall into the air filled colonic lumen.

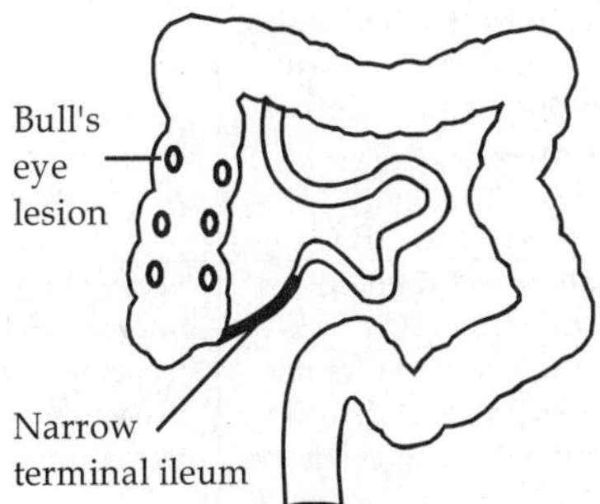

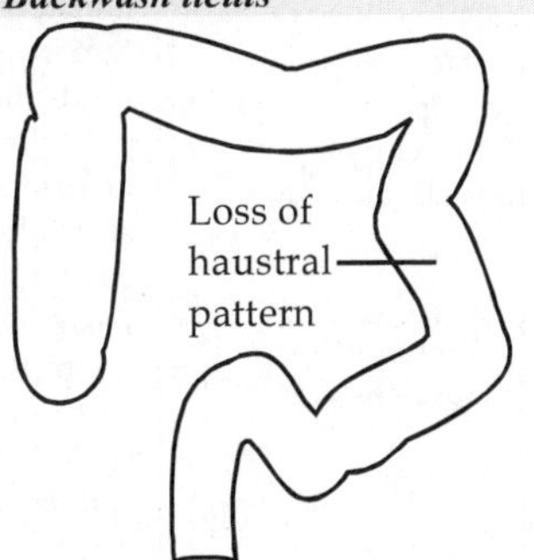

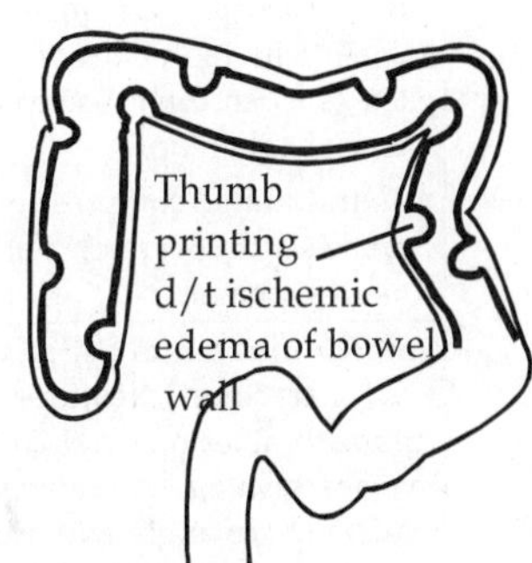

55. **D i.e. Meconium ileus** **56.** **B i.e. Thumb printing** **57.** **B i.e. Hypertrophic Pyloric Stenosis**

[Ref: Wofgang 5/e P-846/748]

Meconium ileus is small bowel obstruction secondary to sticky tenacious meconium d/t deficiency of pancreatic secretions. It is the *earliest clinical manifestation of cystic fibrosis.* It usually presents with *abdominal distension, bilious vomiting and failure to pass meconium within 48 hours.* It has ***Bubbly/Froathy/Soap Bubble***[Q]***/Apple sauce appearance***[Q] d/t admixture of gas with meconium.

Barium meal (swallow) appearance of Oesophageal Disorders	
Bird's beak appearance (very dilated oesophagus with smooth narrowing at its lower end) (barium meal)	**Oesophageal achlasia**
Cock screw (undulated) appearance d/t tertiary contractions (barium meal)	**Diffuse oesophageal spasm**
Tiny flash shaped outpouchig arranged in clusters or longitudinal rows (on barium study).	**Intramural pseudodiverticulosis**
Shaggy (contour) appearance with irregular plaque like filling defects with intervening normal mucosa (early), **cobble stone** or **snake skin appearance or coalescent plaques** (in late disease) which correspond to **white plaques seen in endoscopy; Foamy oesophagus** (tiny 1-3 mm bubble like lucencies producing foamy appearance).	**Candida Oesophagitis (double contrast barium)**
Shelf like indentation from anterior wall or well localized circumferential narrowing (at C5/C6) with **minimal proximal dilatation** and **jet effect** (on barium swallow)	**Cricopharyngeal/ oesophageal web** (when a/w Fe deficiency anemia, glossits & pharyngeal atrophy it is k/a **Plummer Vinson Syndrome**)
Lucent, tortuous, worm like filling defectss which distort the mucosal pattern (on barium swallow); *thickened longitudinal esophageal folds with fusiform seperation* (on mucosal spot films); **beaded or serpiginous longitudinal filling defects** (best seen on *mucosal relief views of collapsed oesophagus in prone RAO position* with high density barium paste/suspension to increase mucosal adherence). ★ Extraluminal compression makes a shllow angle with wall of oesophagus.	**Esophageal varices** (dilated subepithelial veins d/t increased collaterals). **Uphill varices** (d/t *portal hypertension*) are confined to *distal half* **& down hill varices** (d/t *SVC obstruction*) involve *upper & middle part of oesophagus* Endoscopy is investigation of choice
Smooth intramural filling defect with characteristic features of submucosal lesion i.e. *smooth, rounded, semilunar indentation that makes* a **sharp angle with the wall of oesophagus with intact mucosa, splitting/narrowng the barium column, & widening the oesophageal** diameter and splaying longitudinal esophageal folds.	**Leiomyoma of esophagus**
Annular apple core lesion with overhanging margins (or **irregular stricture with**	**Carcinoma Oesophagus**

Radiological features	Disorders
Beak sign; Double track or Tram track sign, Shoulder sign; **String sign**	**Hypertrophic pyloric stenosis**
Seagull /Mercedez Benz/ Crow Feet Sign	**Radiolucent gall stone with gas**
Multiple gas fluid level (step ladder pattern)	**Intestinal obstruction**
Cigar bundle appearance on X-ray Winding highway railway tract on USG ***Medusa Head colonies***[Q] on CT scan	**Round worm**
Pincer sign, ***Claw appearance sign***[Q], ***Coiled spring appearance***[Q], Target sign, Meniscus sign (on barium enema)	**Intussception**
Shark mouth appearance	**Ileocecal valve**
Lead pipe appearance[Q]	**Ulcerative colitis**
String of *Kantor*[Q], Bull's eye or Target lesion, Ram's horn stomach (narrow antrum, wide pylorus with flared up tubular antrum opening into corpus of stomach)	**Chron's disease (Regional ileitis)**
Thumb printing sign[Q]	**Ischemic colitis** (*hallmark*[Q]) also in Amoebic & Ulcerative colitis
Saw tooth *appearance*[Q] (on barium enema)	**Diverticula of colon (Diverticulosis)**

Apple core lesion, Napkin's sign (on barium enema)	**Carcinoma colon**
Bilious vomiting in 1st month (hallmark), current jelly stools/ malena with *double bubble sign* (x-ray); clockwise **whirlpool sign** (USG), **apple-peel/twisted ribbon/Corckscrew & spiral appearance** (barium study); **whirl like pattern** (CT); **barber pole sign** (angio)	**Midgut volvulus** (torsion of gut around SMA)
Whirl sign (CT); **bird of prey sign** (tapered beak like distal aspect of twist on barium enema); **white stripe sign & three line sign** (respectively d/t obliquely oriented center line/ outerwall & center-line of U shaped loop), **northern exposure/bent tyre tube sign** (greatly distended paralyzed loop with fluid-fluid level arising from pelvis & extending towards diaphragm), **Coffee bean sign** (midline crease corresponding to mesentry of largely gas distended loop)- on plain X-ray.	**Sigmoid volvulus**
Distension of small bowel & colon (loops wider than L1 vertebral body ± air fluid level in right lower quadrant is (1st & most common sign), *loss of mosaic multifaceted bowel gaa pattern, large bowels may be impossible to differentiate from small bowel*, ***fixed bowel or persistent loop sign, bowel wall thickening, thumb printing***[Q], ***pneumatosis intestinalis***[Q] (black lines of intramural gas a/b white lines of intestinal wall), **bubbly appearance** of bowel wall, **gas in portal venous system** (plain horizontal beam cross table x-ray); **zebra pattern**; **Y pattern & ring pattern** (on USG)	**Necrotizing enterocolitis** (ischemic bowel disease of premature infants)

shouldering) on barium oesophagogram; other features may be *irregular narrowed segment of lumen, diffuse nodular filling defects*, irregular /smooth tapering strictue, bulky endophytic mass and fixed **varicoid appearance** (i.e. b/o submucosal spread of tumor, the appearance may mimic that of varices, however, unlike varices it is fixed & does not change in size & shape at fluoroscopy)	

Adynamic ileus pattern, nodular haustral pattern (thumb printing – transverse banding = markedly thickened & distorted haustral folds most prominent in transvere colon) –on plain x-ray; **accordion sign** (oral contrast traps between distorted thickened closely spaced transvere edematous folds of low atenuation; is typical but seen only in severe cases), **target sign** and rarely pneumatosis coli ± portal vein gas – on CT; barium enema is contraindicated	**Pseudomembranous colitis** (Clostridium difficile diseas)
Bowler's hat sign, lace like/reticular surface pattern (characteristic of villous adenoma >> tubular adenoma)	**Colonic polyp**

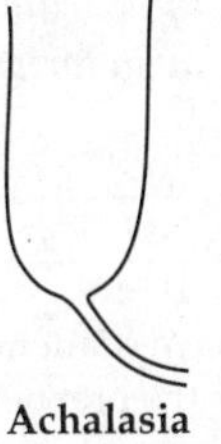
Achalasia

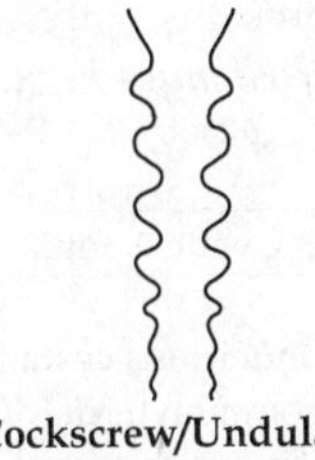
Cockscrew/Undulated appearance

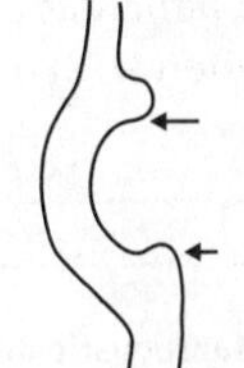
Leiomyoma of Oesophagus (sharp angle)

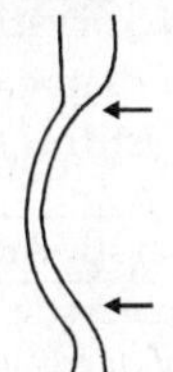
Extraluminal Compression (shallow angle)

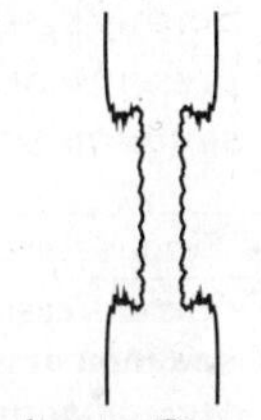
Carcinoma Oesophagus (Apple core with over hanging shoulders)

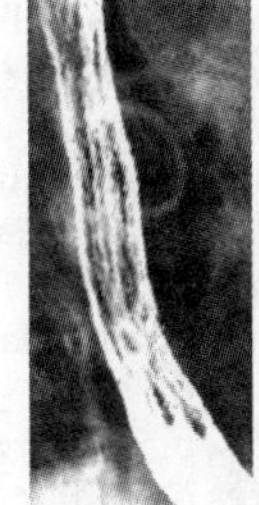
Oesophageal Candidiasis

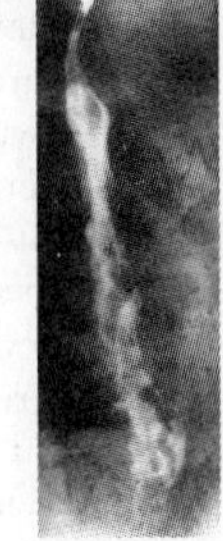
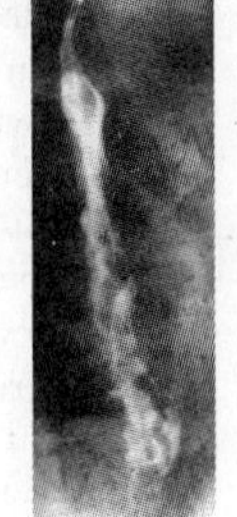
Oesophageal Varices

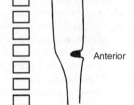

Oesophageal Web (Shelf like identation)

58. **A i.e. Pyloric obstruction**
59. **A i.e. Valvulae conniventes**
60. **A i.e. Meniscus appearance**
61. **B i.e. Chronic Pancreatitis**

[Ref: Bailey & Love 24/e P-1199; Nelson 17/e P-1234; Sutton 7/e P-726; 6/e p. 924-25; Wolfgang 5/e P-998]

- Impacted stone in CBD gives cresentic shadow or ***Meniscus Sign***[Q].
- In chronic pancreatitis ***cholangiopancreatography (ERCP)***[Q] is *most sensitive* imaging modality. It shows ***Chain of lakes appearance***[Q], String of pearls appearance and Beading appearance.
- On X Ray, ***numerous irregular calcification*** are pathognomic of chronic pancreatitis.

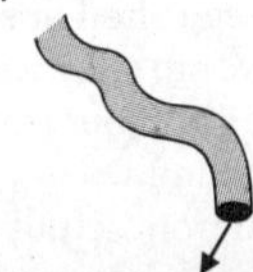
Due to impacted stone, dye can't flow down giving **cresentic/ C-shaped/meniscus like shadow**

★ ***String of beads sign is seen in small bowel obstruction***[Q]

Radiological pictures of

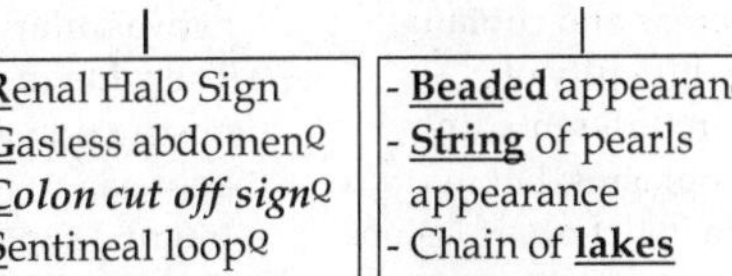
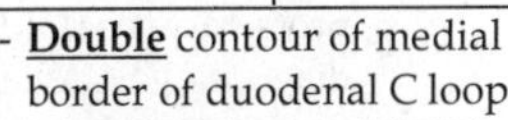

Acute Pancreatitis

- <u>R</u>enal Halo Sign
- <u>G</u>asless abdomen[Q]
- ***<u>C</u>olon cut off sign***[Q]
- <u>S</u>entineal loop[Q]

Mn - "Read GCS" on abdominal X-ray

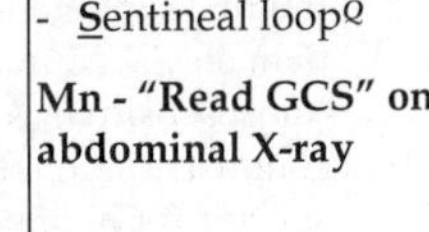

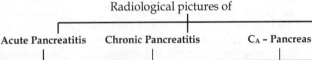

Chronic Pancreatitis

- **<u>Beaded</u>** appearance
- **<u>String</u>** of pearls appearance
- Chain of **<u>lakes</u>** appearance
- **<u>Rat Tail</u>** stricture of CBD

Mn - "Be a strong Lovely Rat" or "Be a String of Rat tail lakes" on ERCP

CA – Pancreas

- **<u>Double</u>** contour of medial border of duodenal C loop
- **<u>Double</u>** duct sign (ERCP)
- ***<u>Dialated/Widened</u> Duodenal-C loop***[Q]
- ***<u>Mucosal irregularity</u>***[Q]
- <u>S</u>crambled Egg appearance
- <u>I</u>nverted/Reverse – 3 sign of frost berg
- <u>R</u>ose thorning of medial wall of 2nd part of duodenum

Mn–"Double SIR" or "Double Decker Music SIR"

62. **A. i.e. Caroli's disease** *[Ref: Haga 4th/e p.1364; Manorama Berry Diagnostic Radiology Manorama Berry 2nd/e p-150]*

Central dot sign is ***considered pathognomonic of carolis disease***Q. This sign consists of cystically dilated intra hepatic biliary radicles with a "dot" of increased density represented by portal radicle with the lumen of duct.

Caroli's disease

- *Communicating cavernous ectasia of* the *intrahepatic bile ducts.* (IHBD).
- *AR* congenital disorder
- Segmental, saccular dilatation of the IHBD.
- A/W: - *Choledochal cyst* and
  - AR polycystic kidney disease (*ARPKD*)

Signs	Disease
*Central dot sign*Q	**Caroli's disease**
Pruned- Tree appearance / ***Beaded appearence***Q*/ Skip lesions*	**Primary sclerosing cholangitis**
Light bulb appearance	**Liver Hemangioma (on T2W MRI)**
Water lily sign /HoneycombingQ	**Liver hydatid**

63. **D i.e. Serous Cystadenoma** *[Ref: Sutton 7/e p – 792- 94; Grainger 5/e p- 804]*

Serous cystadenoma or microcystic adenoma of pancreas classically presents with ***spongy appearance***Q d/t presence of multiple < 2cm diameter microcyst often with ***a large calcified mass having a characteristic sunburnt pattern within a central fibrotic scar***Q.

Serous Cystadenoma (Microcystic Adenoma)

- **Serous cystodenoma (or microcystic adenoma)** is a *benign tumor of elderly women (grandmother lesion)*. It occurs more commonly in ***females (M:F = 1:2 to 4) of 35-85 years (mean 65yrs)***Q.
- There is ***slight predilection for pancreatic head & neck***Q, although any part of pancreas may be affected.
- SCA are typically large (average size 11cm), well demarcated, **lobulated, multicystic tumor** with at **least ≥6 cysts, each measuring 0. 2-2.0cm**. The cysts are usually too small to be resolved (identified) individually at CT or USG, and the mass may appear solid – with a classical **cluster of grapes appearance**.
- The multiple cysts are seperated by **fibrous septa that radiate from center forming a central stellate scar**, that can calcificy giving it a ***characteristic (virtually pathognomic) sunburst or stellate pattern of calcification***Q within a central fibrotic scar.
- Grossly, SCA is well circumscribed with lobulated margins with **honeycomb or sponge like appearance** on cross section. Histologically the cysts are lined by glycogen rich cuboidal/flat epithelial cells derived from centroacinar cells of pancreas and contain proteinaceous fluid. The difficulty of diagnosing SCA lies not in differentiating them from othe cystic neoplasms, but in appreciating that they are infact cystic lesions because of the solid appearance of tumors with high stromal content and multiple tiny cysts seperated by thin septa lined by epithelial cells – i.e. **cluster of grape appearance.**
- The tumor is **hypervascular (highly vascular)** and contrast *enhancement of internal septa* results in typical **honey-comb or Swiss-cheese** appearance.
- SCA may ***displace, encase or obstruct (from out side) pancreatic duct & CBD, l/t dilation of duct but with no communication of lesion with the main pancreatic duct***Q

Mucinous Cystic Neoplasm (MCNs)

- **Macrocystic adenomas** or **mucinous cystadenoma /cystadenocarcinoma** are best referred to under common term MCNs as the preoperative distinction between cystadenoma & cystadenocarcinomas is difficult in the absence of metastases.
- ***Often located in tail (90%)/ body, infraquent in head***Q.
- They have a **strong female predilection** (>95% M:F=1:9) with mean age of occurance is *50 years* (range 20-95) are referred to as ***mother lesions***.
- It is a well demrcated (encapsulated), well circumscribed, thick fibrous walled mass with **smooth external surface (smooth contour)**. MCNs are *typically large (mean 10-12 cm dia), solitary and multilocular* cysts with *few large compartments (<6 cysts of >2cm diameter with thin <2mm septa)* and micro cystic in most cases but they can be unilocular with single compartment.
- Internal articeture of cyst may contain septa (**hypovascular internal septation**), **solid papillary excrescences** protuding into the interior (sign of malignancy) and **a very vascular solid component or mural nodule.**
- Dystrophic calcification (**amorphous discontinuous peripheral mural** or curvilinear) can be seen in **thick fibrotic wall (capsule)or septa**.
- All MCNs should be considered as low grade malignant neoplasm with great propensity for invasion of adjacent organs. It may cause vascular encesement and spleenic vein occlusion. *Disruption or distortion of adjacent organs with obliteration of adjacent fat planes* suggests local invasion. *Irregularity of septal wall* suggest malignant change.
- It is predominantly avascular mass with solid components (mural nodule) and cyst wall demonstrating small areas of vascular blush & neovascularity (on angio).
- They ***do not communicate with pancreatic duct***Q, but can cause ductal obstruction. Clinically present with abdominal pain, palpable mass, anorexia.
- Internal septation & papillary excrescences are often better seen on USG than on CT. Mural nodule is best appreciated on high resolution EUS (most sensitive) & MRI > MRCP > MDCT. Mural nodule enhances on contrast administration. **Peripheral egg shell or septal calcification** are specific for mucinous cystic lesions & are *predictive of malignancy*. Internal septation may not be visulized on CT without contrast enhancement (mild). Septa & wall enhance late and mild.
- Multilocular MCN are differentiated from serous cystadenoma by ***younger age group (mother/grandmother), lesser & larger cyst (<6 of >2 cm dia), location of calcification (peripheral/central) and pattern of lesion enhancment (particularly of tumor nodule in MCN and typically in septa in SCA).***
- Unilocular MCN are differentiated from pseudocyst by absence of radiographic signs of acute/chronic pancreatitis, **presence of solid**

5

RADIODIAGNOSIS

- When symptomatic, patients present with ***abdomminal pain, weightloss, abdominal mass and rarely jundice***Q. It may be a/w **Von-Hippel Lindau disease.**
- On USG it appears as solid echogenic (not cystic anechoic) mass b/o multiple interfaces produced by numerous microscopic cysts or may appear as multilocular cyst or mixed solid & cystic lesions
- On unenhanced CT, SCA appear as hypodense (near water) attenuation masses that frequently show **central stellate scar (fibrous central scar)** with or without **characteristic central stellate calcification**. The arrangement of cyst around a central fibrous scar in a sunburst pattern with coarse calcification is characteristic. Contrast enhancement of septa results in typical **swiss-cheese or honey combing appearance**.
- On MRI, it appears as well defined, lobulated hypointense (on T1) and hyperintense (on T2) with a **cluster of grapes appearance**. Tumor septa are seen as dark thin strands on T2 which enhance minimally with delayed enhancement of central scar (on CE-FLASH); calcification l/t signal voids in central scar.
- On ERCP, CBD & pancreatic duct may be displaced, encased or obstructed by tumor **but with no communication of lesion with the main pancreatic duct.**
- Serous cystadenoma is a **well circumscribed, lobulated (externally & internally = septa)**, multicystic (≥6 cyst of <2cm) tumor which produces almost solid-multicystic **cluster of grapes appearance**. The multiple cysts are seperated by **fibrous septa that radiates from center** forming a **central stellate scar** that can calcify giving it a characteristic (virtually) **pathognomic sunburst or stellate pattern of calcification**. The tumor is hypervascular and contrast enhancement of internal septa results in typical **honey comb** or **swiss cheese appearance**. It can obstruct pancreatic duct (l/t dilatation) but **with no communication of lesion with the main pancreatic duct.**

component in cystic mass, normal pancreatic tissue adjacent to cyst, and lack of communication of cyst with main pancreatic duct (on ERCP) favors the diagnosis of MNCs.

Intraductal Papillary Mucinous Neoplasm (IPMN=IPMT)

- IPMN is mucin producing tumor which develops from *proliferation of epithelial lining of main pancreatic duct or its side branches l/t variable ductal dilation.*
- It presents in *6th to 7th decade with a slight male predominace*. Intermittent ductal obstruction occurs & recurrent abdominal pain is most common. Other features may be backpain, jaundice, weight loss, endocrine & exocrine insufficiency l/t DM, steratorrhea (in chronic obstruction).
- **Main duct IPMT** does **not** present as **a cystic lesion**. It occurs *predominantly in head* and only occasionally in tail. Owing to mucin production, there is partial or diffuse dilation of main duct; the **ductal dilation is disproportionate to the degree of parenchymal atrophy**. Excessive mucin secretion may l/t **bulging of major papillas into the duodenal lumen**; a **pathognomic sign** on ERCP & cross sectimal imaging (CT/MRI) and is seen more often in malignant tumors. Prolonged obstruction may l/t *chronic pancreatitis*, in which case the pancreas is markedly fibrotic. ERCP may demonstrate *thick jelly like mucus protuding from a bulging patulous duodenal papilla*, plugging of papilla of vater, amorphous ***intraluminal filling defects in main pancreatic duct, dilated main + branch PD without obstructive ductal stricture and intraductal mural nodule***Q (also on CT,MR).
- The occurance of malignancy is significantly higher in main duct and mixed IPMNs than in side branch IPMNs. The presence of **solid mural nodule, thick septa/wall, wall** calcification, segmental or diffuse dilation of main pancreatic duct >10mm in diameter (Haga)/> 15 mm (AMPIS), intraductal filling defect size >3mm, bulging duoenal papilla, cysts larger than 3 cm, indicates an **increased likelihood of malignancy.**
- **Side branch/branch duct IPMT** and **mixed IPMTs** (in which side branch tumors extends into the main duct or vise versa) present as ***unilocular or multilocular cystic lesions that mostly communicate with the main pancreatic duct***Q with narrow neck at cyst duct junction.
- Presence of vascular encasement, peripancreatic lymphadenopathy & metastases confirm malignancy. Side branch lesions >30 mm are considered malignant. On endoscopic US (EUS) main duct type tumors with >10 mm dilated MPD, branch duct type tumor (>40mm)with irregular septa, and large mural nodules (>10mm) strongly suggest malignancy. Malignant lesions may form fistulas (with duodenum, CBD=lesions of head; colon, stomach = body tail lesions).
- Branch duct IPMT occurs mainly in *uncinate process* >> tail > body and presents with dilatation of multiple side branches (mc) ± dilated MPD.

64. **C i.e. (Intraductal papillary mucinous neoplasm (IPMN): (without any doubt)** *[Ref: Grainger 5/e p. 804-805; Wolfang 7/e p 705-6, 747-50, 765-66, 742; AMPIS 3/e p 342-48; Haga 5/e p 1665-50; Sutton 7/e p 794-93]*

- **Bunch of grapes appearance with lobulated margins** is highly suggestive (and **characteristic) of serous cystadenoma**. It is actually a cystic tumor with multiple tiny cyst (>6 in number))measuring < 2cm in size with a *high stromal content* seperated by thin septa lined by epithelial cell. Therefore *these lesions appear solid owing to the compact arrangement of multiple small cyst forming* myriad of (many) interfaces and produce **finely lobulated microcystic lesion with internal septation** producing classic **cluster of grapes appearance.**
- In **mucinous cystadema** the cysts are mostly large (average 10cm) unilocular or multilocular (<6) with a less prominent lobulation. **Intraductal papillary mucinous tumor (IPMT)** produce cystic appearance b/o dilated pancreatic ductal system distal to IPMT, so it is more like a distended ductal system covered by normal pancreatic parenchyma. So in mucinous cystadenoma cysts are much larger & lesser, whereas in IPMT there is no true microcystic pattern to produce almost solid bunch of grape appearance.
- Now lets focus on *grossly dilated ductal system which indicates total or near total ductal obstruction*. All of them can l/t ductal obstruction & gross dilatation the only difference is that it is *almost always early, intraluminal*

*with out obstructive ductal stricture, **intense and communicating*** (i.e. cyst communicates with pancreatic duct) in IPMT, whereas it is b/o compression of duct from outside, in mucinous & serous cystadenoma (in which case it is gradual & non communicating).

- Serous cystodenoma occurs in females over age of 60 years (range 35-85yrs; F:M = 2/4 : 1) whereas IPMN mainly occurs in males between 60 & 80 years.
- All of these can cause jaundice, abdominal pain when present in head of pancreas.

UROLOGY

65. **B i.e. Hydronephrosis**
66. **B i.e. Ureterocoel**
67. **D i.e. Spider leg deformity**
68. **B i.e. Polycystic Kidney**
69. **A i.e. Ploycystic Kidney** *[Ref: Sutton 7/e P-970; Wofgang 5/e P-922; Bailey 24/e p. 1308]*

Chronic hydronephrosis is most common ***cause of abdominal mass in first 6 months of life.***[Q] On IVP it shows:
- Early = ***Rim Sign***[Q] (thin band of radiodensity surrounding clyces)
- Delayed = Opacification & dialation collecting system

Polycystic or Congenital cystic kidney presents with abdominal mass, loin pain, heamaturia, infection, hypertension & uremia; but usually not before age of 30 years.
On excretory urography it has ***B/L spiders' leg apearance***[Q].
Decapping surgery *(Rovsing's operation)* is rarely indicated, as it only relives pain (no prognostic change)

Egg in cup appearance
Ball in cup/ Signet ring appearance

Ureteric orifice looks like **Cobra Head or Adder Head** in
- ***Ureterocoel***[Q]
- Impaction of stone at ureteric orifice
- Tumor, partially obstructing ureteric orifice
- Following retrograde catheterization

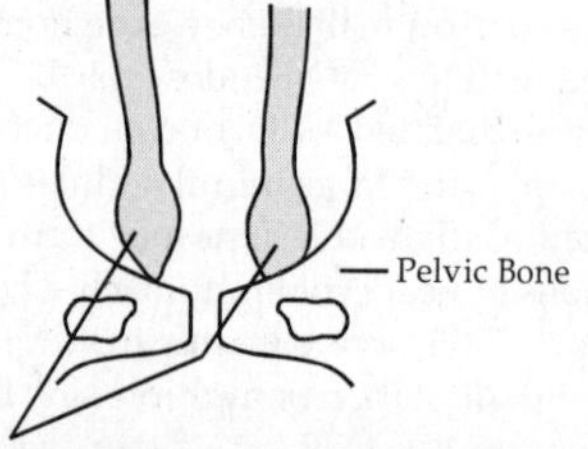

Urographic - Cobra/Adder (i.e. snake) Head Appearance
Spring Onion appearance

Radiological Feature	Disease
Rim / Cresent Sign[Q] d/t ureteric & pelvic dialatation l/t cortex compression	**Hydronephrosis**
Soap Bubble ***appearance***[Q]	**Hydronephrosis**
Flower vase appearance of ***ureter***[Q]	**Horse shoe kidney**
Drooping flower appearance[Q]	**Ectopic ureter**
Cobra (Adder) head appearance[Q]	**Ureterocoel**
Thimble ***bladder***[Q]	**Tubercular cystic (chronic)**
Sandy ***patches***[Q]	**Schistosomiasis of bladder**
Fish hook bladder[Q]	**BPH**
B/L Spider leg appearance[Q] Swiss-cheese nephrogram Sub burst nephrogram	Polycystic kidney
Egg in cup appearance, ***ring shadows/ ring sign, lobster claw sign or calyceal horns and diminished density of contrast in nephrogram***[Q]	Papillary necrosis (analgesic nephropathy)
Tree barking or **Corduroy appearance** (in IVU or RGU) i.e. multiple linear radiolucencies in ureter	**Squamous metaplasia** of ureter l/t mucosal thickening

5

INVESTIGATION OF CHOICE

QUESTIONS

Central Nervous System

1. **Investigation of choice for juvenile nasoangiofibroma**
   A. X-Ray *(AIIMS 1997)* ☐
   B. Angiography ☐
   C. USG ☐
   D. CT Scan - contrast enhanced ☐
2. **The procedure of choice for the evaluation of an aneurysm is:**
   A. Ultrasonography *(AI 2006)* ☐
   B. Computed tomography ☐
   C. Magnetic resonance imaging ☐
   D. Arteriography ☐
3. **The best investigation to diagnose a case of acoustic neuroma is:** *(AIIMS May 08)*
   A. Gadolinium enhanced MRI ☐
   B. CT scan ☐
   C. Audimetric analysis ☐
   D. PET scan ☐
4. **A patient is suspected to have vestibular Shwanomma. The investigation of choice for its diagnosis is:** *(AI 2004)*
   A. Contrast enhanced CT scan ☐
   B. Gadolinum enhanced MRI ☐
   C. SPECT ☐
   D. PET scan ☐
5. **Which of the following is the best choice to evaluate radiologically a posterior fossa tumor?** *(AI 2003)*
   A. CT scan ☐
   B. MRI ☐
   C. Angiography ☐
   D. Myelography ☐
6. **Ideal imaging method for diagnosis of hydrocephalous in infant is** *(AI 1991)*
   A. X-Ray ☐
   B. CT Scan ☐
   C. USG ☐
   D. MRI ☐
7. **Parameningeal Rhabdomyosarcoma is best diagnosed by-** *(AIIMS 2001)*
   A. MRI ☐
   B. CT Scan ☐
   C. SPECT ☐
   D. PET ☐
8. **The best X Ray view for minimal pleural effusion**
   A. A – P *(AI 1992)* ☐
   B. PA ☐
   C. Lateral ☐
   D. Lateral decubitus ☐
9. **Decubitus view is useful in diagnosisng:**
   A. Pleural effusion *(PGI 2001)* ☐
   B. Pleural effusion with dependent hemithorax ☐
   C. Pericardial effusion ☐
   D. Middle lobe consolidation ☐
10. **Best view for right pleural effusion in X-Ray chest**
    A. Supine *(AI 1993)* ☐
    B. Prone ☐
    C. Right lateral decubitus ☐
    D. Left lateral decubitus ☐
11. **The following will be most helpful radiological investigation in a patient suspected of left pleural effusion**
    A. Right lateral decubitus *(AIIMS 1992)* ☐
    B. Left lateral decubitus ☐
    C. Left lateral erect ☐
    D. Right lateral erect ☐
12. **Inter lobar pleural effusion can be detected in best way in**
    A. Lateral decubitus *(AIIMS 1993)* ☐
    B. Reverse lardotic ☐
    C. Lateral oblique ☐
    D. Posterior oblique ☐
13. **Right anterior oblique view of chest X-ray true is/are:**
    A. Cassette near right shoulder *(PGI June 08)* ☐
    B. Cassette near left shoulder ☐
    C. Arch of Aorta best seen ☐
    D. Left atrial enlargement can be diagnosed ☐
    E. Mitral & Tricuspid valves better seen ☐
14. **X-Ray view for supra orbital fissure**
    A. Towne's *(AIIMS 1997)* ☐
    B. AP ☐
    C. Cald well ☐
    D. Basal ☐
15. **Tracheal bifurcation on X-ray corresponds to**
    A. T_5T_6 *(PGI 2001)* ☐
    B. T_4T_5 ☐
    C. Sternal angle ☐
    D. Thoracic inlet ☐
16. **Best view for visualizing sella turcica on X-Ray:** *(AI 1994)*
    A. A P View ☐
    B. Town's view ☐
    C. Lateral view ☐
    D. Open mouth view ☐
17. **Caldwell lac view (occipito - frontal) can visualise:**
    A. Sphenoid sinus *(PGI 2002)* ☐
    B. Nasal bone ☐
    C. Maxilary bone ☐
    D. Ethmoid ☐
    E. Frontal sinus ☐
18. **Basal skull view (submentovertical view) X-ray is best to visualize :** *(PGI 2000)*
    A. Ethmoid sinus ☐
    B. Frontal sinus ☐
    C. Sphenoid sinus ☐
    D. Maxillary sinus ☐
    E. Nasopharynx ☐

ENT

19. **A 30 year old man presents with 6 month history of nasal discharge, facial pain and fever. On antibiotic therapy, fever**

subsided. After 1 month again had symptoms of mucopurulent discharge from the middle meatus and the mucosa of the meatus appeared congested and oedematous. Next best investigation would be: *(AIIMS Nov 07)*
A. MRI of the sinuses.
B. Non-Contrast CT of the nose and para-nasal sinuses
C. Plain x-ray of the para-nasal sinuses
D. Inferior meatus puncture

Cardiovascular System

20. Test of choice for Reversible Myocardial Ischemia?
A. Thallium scan *(AI 2009)*
B. MUGA scan
C. Resting ECHO
D. Coronary angiography

21. In a Down's syndrome patient posted for surgery, the necessary pre-operative investigation to be done is –
A. CT Brain *(AI 2009)*
B. Echocardiography
C. Ultrasound Abdomen
D. X-Ray cervical spine

22. Investigation of choice for Aortic Dissection is
A. Aortography *(AIIMS 1997)*
B. CT scan
C. MRI
D. X-Ray chest

23. Investigation of choice in aortic dissection is
A. USG *(AI 1996)*
B. CT Scan
C. MRI
D. Digital substraction Angiography

24. Investigation of choice for pericardial effusion is
A. CT Scan *(AIIMS 93, 97)*
B. MRI
C. Echocardiography
D. X Ray Chest

25. The most accurate investigation for assessing ventricular function is:
A. Multislice CT *(AI 2006)*
B. Echocardiography
C. Nuclear scan
D. MRI

26. Cardiotoxicity caused by radiotherapy & chemotherapy is best detected by *(AI 1999)*
A. ECHO
B. ECG
C. Radionucletide Scan
D. Endomyocardial Biopsy

Respiratory Ststem

27. Investigation of choice for detection & char-acterization of interstitial lung disease is
A. MRI *(AI 08, AIIMS 05, DNB 09)*
B. Chest X-ray
C. High Resolution CT scan
D. Ventilation perfusion scan

28. Investigation of choice in Bronchiectasis is
A. X-Ray *(AIIMS 1994)*
B. Bronchoscopy
C. Bronchography
D. USG

29. Best diagnostic aid for broncheitasis is:
A. Bronchoscopy *(AIIMS 1992)*
B. X- Ray
C. Bronchography
D. CT Scan

30. High resolution computed tomography of the chest is the ideal modality for evaluating
A. Pleural effusion *(AI 2003)*
B. Interstitial lung disease
C. Lung mass
D. Mediastinal adenopathy

31. Most sensitive investigation for air embolism is *(AI 1999)*
A. Decreased tidal volume of CO_2
B. Decreased tidal volume of NO_2
C. Doppler ultrasound
D. Central Venous Presure

32. In patient with high clinical suspicion of pulmonary thromboembolism, best investigation would be?
A. D-dimer *(AIIMS Nov 07)*
B. CT angiography
C. Catheter angiography
D. Color Doppler

33. Investigation of choice for pulmonary embolism *(AI 1998)*
A. CT scan
B. Contrast CT
C. Ventillation - Perfusion Scan
D. MRI

34. Pulmonary embolism is best diagnosed by *(AI 1996)*
A. USG
B. X Ray Chest
C. Ventilation - Perfusion Scan
D. CT Scan

35. Best method for detecting minimal Bronchiectasis
A. Bronchogram *(AI 1992)*
B. CT Scan
C. Radio nucleotide scan
D. Chest X Ray

36. Best view to diagnose pneumothorax :
A. Lateral oblique *(PGI 1998)*
B. PA view in full expiration
C. PA view in full inspiration
D. AP view in full expiration

Excretory System

37. In Renal cell carcinoma investigation of choice to evaluate inferior venacava & renal vein for thrombus
A. IVP *(AIIMS 1999)*
B. Coloured Doppler
C. USG
D. CT scan

38. Functional analysis of kidney is best done by
A. Radionuclide scanning *(PGI 1997)*
B. IVP
C. Ultrasound
D. MRI

39. Investigation of choice for studying Renal Cortical mass
A. 99 Tc DTPA *(AIIMS 1993)*
B. 53 Cr Study
C. 99 Tc DMSA
D. 99 Tc Pyrophosphate

Gastrointestinal System

40. Investigation of choice in diffuse esophageal spasm is
A. Manometry *(AI 08)*
B. Esophagoscopy
C. Barium examination showing tertiary contractions
D. CT thorax

41. Gastro-oesophageal reflux is best detected by
A. Endoscopy *(AIIMS 1992)*
B. USG

C. Barium study ☐
D. Isotope scan ☐

42. **Investigation of choice for gall stone** *(DNB 04)*
A. X-Ray ☐
B. USG ☐
C. Cholecystography ☐
D. CAT Scan ☐

43. **Investigation of choice in obstructive jaundice is**
A. ERCP *(AI 1997)* ☐
B. USG ☐
C. Cholecystography ☐
D. Laproscopy ☐

44. **Most common investigation done for obstructive jaundice** *(AIIMS 1999)*
A. CT scan ☐
B. USG ☐
C. X-Ray ☐
D. ERCP ☐

45. **Minimal Ascites can be best detected by:**
A. USG *(AIIMS 98, 92)* ☐
B. Plain X-ray abdomen ☐
C. MRI ☐
D. CT scan ☐

46. **The investigation of choice for acute cholecystitis is:**
A. USG *(PGI 2002)* ☐
B. HIDA-Scan ☐
C. CT-Scan ☐
D. OCG ☐
E. X-Ray ☐

47. **Best investigation for acute cholecystitis is** *(DNB 07)*
A. ERCP ☐
B. Oral cholecystography (OCG) ☐
C. HIDA scan ☐
D. IV cholangiography ☐

48. **Investigation of choice for recurrent GIST:**
A. MIBG *(AIIMS Nov 08)* ☐
B. PET ☐
C. MRI ☐
D. CECT ☐

Musculoskeleton System

49. **Best radiographic view for fracture of C_1, C_2 vertebrae is**
A. AP view *(AI 08, AIIMS 09)* ☐
B. Odontoid view ☐
C. Lateral view ☐
D. Oblique view ☐

50. **Best investigation for Traumatic paraplegia**
A. CT Scan *(AIIMS 1992)* ☐
B. Routine Tomography (MRI) ☐
C. X Ray spine ☐
D. Myelography ☐

51. **The gold standard for assessing bone mineral density (BMD) & diagnosis of osteoporosis is:** *(AIIMS 04, AI 12, 05)*
A. Dual energy X-ray absorptiometry ☐
B. Single energy X-ray absorptiometry. ☐
C. Ultrasound. ☐
D. Quantitative computed tomography. ☐

Obstetrics

52. **Neural tube defect is best detected by**
A. USG *(AI 1995)* ☐
B. Chromosomal analysis ☐
C. Amniocentesis ☐
D. Placentography ☐

53. **Earliest congenital malformation that may be detected on USG is** *(AI 1994)*
A. Down's syndrome ☐
B. Hydrocephalous ☐
C. Anencephaly ☐
D. Sacral Agenesis ☐

Answers and Explanations:

CENTRAL NERVOUS SYSTEM

1. **D i.e. CT Scan-Contrast inhanced** *[Ref: P.L. Dhingra ENT 3/e P-300]*

Angiofibroma is very vascular tumor of ***teenage boys***Q. ***CT scan***Q is the investigation of choice to see the extent of invasion.

Juvenile Nasopharyngeal Angiofibroma/Nasopharyngeal fibroma

CT Scan with contrast *inhancement*Q
- ***Investigation of choice***Q
- Anterior bowing of posterior wall of maxillary sinus ***(antral sign)***Q is pathognomic

MRI

When soft tissue extension is present intracranially/infratemporal fossa or into the orbit

2. **D i.e. Arteriography** *[Ref: Wolfgang Dan hert 5/e p-604-605; Grainger & Allison's 4/e p. 841-843, 956-958, 2379]*

Arteriography is considered the gold standard in evaluation of ***arteriovenous fistula, aneurysm and aortic dissection***Q.

- Aneurysm is a sac filled with blood in direct communication with the interior of an artery. A true aneurysm is due to local dilatation of the artery, whereas a false aneurysm is a sac with walls formed of condensed connective tissue which communicates with the lumen of the artery through its apparatus in its wall. Aneurysm may be classified into congenital, infective, degenerative, dissecting, post stenotic, post inflammatory (arteritic; necrotic), traumatic and cirsoid.
- *Arteriography is the gold standard for all types of aneurysms; but in dissecting aneurysm* (aortic dissection) the investigation of choice is *MRI in stable* patients and *TOE (trans oesophageal echocardiography) in unstable patients.*
- For detecting aortic dissection, MRI has a **sensitivity** of 98.3%, TOE 97.7%, CT 93.8% & TTE 60% *(MRI > TOE > CT > TTE)*. MRI had **specificity** of 97.8%, CT of 87%, TTE 83% and TOE 77% *(MRI > CT > TTE > TOE)*. MRI and CT were more sensitive than TTE in **detecting thrombus formation** but not superior to TOE *(TOE > MRI > CT> TTE)*. CT was not effective in detecting the entrance site or regurgitation but MRI and TOE accurately identified both.
- ***Aortography (Arteriography)***Q is considered the ***gold standard*** in evaluation of aortic dissection. The diagnosis can be made by recognizing an initial flap or a *double lumen*, findings which are *pathognomic.* The indirect findings are - compression of true lumen, thickening of aortic valve, branch vessel abnormalities, aortic insufficiency or an ulcer like projection beyond the aortic intima wall.

3. **A i.e., Gadolinium enhanced MRI** 4. **B i.e. Gadolinium enhanced MRI**
[Ref: Sutton : textbook of radiology & imaging 7/e p -1598- 99, 1610-11; Ballenger's manual of otorhino- laryngology 4/e p- 1050]

Contrast enhancement using paramagnetic agent ***gadolinium DTPA in MRI*** leads to better visualization of acoustic neuroma (shwanomma). So ***Gadolinium enhanced MRI***Q became definitive investigation for **acoustic neuroma (vestibular shwanomma).**

- **Neuromas / Neurinomas / Neurolemmomas** *arise from Schwann cells* which invest the cranial nerves; therefore they are more correctly called Schwannomas. They can *arise from any cranial or spinal root except the optic and olfactory nerves,* which are myelinated by *oligodendroglia* rather than Schwann cells.
- *Schwannomas most frequently arise in eighth (VIII) cranial nerve* and are known as *vestibular or acoustic Schwannoma / Neuroma.* 8th nerve tumor are the most common tumors affecting the petrous pyramid – *as 80% arise within the internal auditory meatus (IAM),* usually from vestibular nerve. *Fifth* (V) cranial nerve is the *second most common site.*
- Tumors arising from Vth (5), VIIth (7), XIth (11) or XII (12) cranial nerves may affect temporal bone. These are all very rare except in cases of *neurofibromatosis (NF) type 2.*
- **Thin section T2 MRI** is the *standard investigation to demonstrate or exclude the presence of an acoustic neuroma.* Vestibular Schwannomas are iso to hypo intense globular mass centered over IAC on T_2 images and the *enlargement of internal auditory canal* is distinguishing feature that differentiates them from other cerebello pontine angle masses. However, ***gadolinium enhancement on T_1 weighted images is usually used to confirm diagnosis***Q.

- Gadolinium enhancement is also required in NF2, for follow UPS after partial or total removal of acoustic neuroma.
- Now, latest MRI scanners using either **gradient-echo or spin- echo 3DFT constructive interference in steady state (CISS)** can produce thin section T_2 images.
- **Meningiomas** are 2nd most common tumors arising in cerebello pontine angle. Unlike Schwannomas, meningiomas *usually calcify* & tend to have *broad attachment* to the petrous ridge, which may show characteristic *hyperostosis*. Meningiomas show intense contrast enhancement with gadolinium MRI (Gd-MR).

5. **B i.e. MRI**

- MRI is best choice for all space occupying lesions of brain (Either in anterior, middle or posterior fossa).
- MRI is specially useful in diagnosis of *infratentorial (posterior fossa)* ***neoplasm***[Q] because it is free of beam hardening artifact & has higher contrast to noise ratio causing excellent identification of neoplasm. In CT scan beam hardening artifact causes difficulties in interpreting posterior fossa tumors.
- MRI (± Contrast & angiography) is I^{st} recommended (better) investigation of almost all conditions of spine & brain except :

  Noncontrast CT[Q]=Acute Head injury (non shear) ,Headache, Migraine.
  Acute parenchymal hemorrhage
  Subarachnoid hemorrage (SAH)[Q]
  Hemorrhagic infarct
  Angiography (?MRA) = Aneurysm
  Doppler USG, MRA, CTA = Carotid stenosis

6. **C i.e. USG** *[Ref: Sutton 7/e P-1728, 1809; Love & Baiely 24/e P-613; Nelson text book of pediatrics 17/e P-1990]*

Investigation of Choice for Hydrocephalus

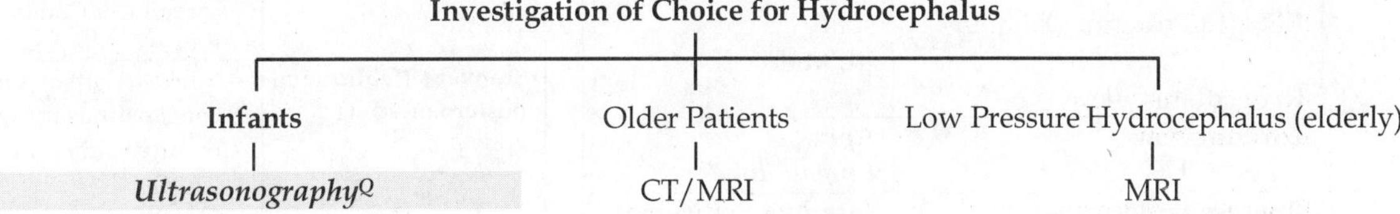

7. **A i.e. MRI** *[Ref: Harrison 15/e P-2337; Grainger 4/e P-2309, 2337]*

- PET & SPECT are functional brain imaging modalities so these cannot be used for dx of parameningeal Rhabdomyosarcoma.
- Other informations indicating towards answer are

- Investigation of choice for primary or metastatic brain tumor = **MRI + Contrast** *(Harrison)*
- Inv. of choice for meningeal tumors = **MRI + Contrast** *(Ganong-2337)*
- Inv. of choice for meningeal disease = **MRI + Contrast** *(Harrison)*
- MRI is excellent for soft tissue imaging & CT is best for bone imaging.

8. **D i.e. Lateral decubitus** 9. **A i.e. Pleural effusion; B i.e. Pleural effusion with dependent hemithorax**
10. **C i.e. Right lateral decubitus** 11. **B i.e. Left lateral decubitus** 12. **B i.e. Reverse lardotic**
13. **A i.e. Cassette near right shouldes; C i.e. Arch of aorta best seen; D i.e. Left atrial enlargement can be seen**
14. **C i.e. Cald well** 15. **A i.e. T_5T_6; B i.e. T_4 T_5; C i.e. Sternal angle**
16. **C i.e. Lateral view** 17. **B i.e. Nasal bone; C i.e. Maxillary bone; D i.e. Ethmoid; E i.e. Frontal sinus**
18. **C i.e. Sphenoid Sinus** *[Ref: Hutchison's 20/e p. 43; AMPIS 3/e p. 7; Clarks 12/e p. 204, 219; Wofgang 5/e P-428-30; P.L. Dhingra ENT 3/e P-496; CSDT 10th -1256; Sutton 7/e p. 1597, 5]*

- **Pleural effusion** is best visualized by X Ray in **decubitus posture (on same side of pleural effusion). Ipsilateral lateral decubitus** ***is investigation of choice for minimal pleural effusion***[Q]
- **Ipsilateral (Same sided) lateral decubitus view** leads to collection of even minimal fluid in the lateral pleural recess; making diagnosis of minimal pleural effusion easy.
- *In pleural effusion, best view is –* ***ipsilateral lateral decubitus***[Q]
  - Right pleural effusion = Right lateral decubitus view.
  - Left pleural effusion = Left lateral decubitus view.

- First 300 ml is not visualized on PA view (collect in subpulmonic region first, then spill into posterior costophrenic sinus). *Lateral decubitus* views may detect as little as **25 *ml*[Q]**.
- ***Meig Salmon Syndrome*[Q]*: primary pelvic neoplasm* (ovarian thecoma, granulosa cell tumor, Brenner tumor, cystadenoma, adeno CA, fibromyoma of uterus) *cause pleural effusion, ascites + hydrothorax.*** These resolves with tumor removal.

Disorders	View
Supraorbital Fissure	*Cald well view*[Q]
Recurrent Shoulder Dislocation	*Striker's view*[Q]
Sella Turica Scaphoid Patella	Lateral skull view *Oblique view*[Q] *Skyline view*[Q]
Minimal Pleural Effusion	*Lateral decubitus (Ipsilateral)*[Q]
Pneumothorax	*PA view in full expiration*[Q]
Minimal Pneumoperitoneum	*Chest X-ray view > left lateral decubitus with horizontal beam*[Q] > standing/ erect abdomen

View (Chest X-Ray)	Structure seen
RAO (Rt Anterior Oblique)	Rt lung Lt. atrium Gall Bladder Mitral Valve
LAO (Lt. Ant. Oblique) RPO (Rt Posterior Oblique) Rt decubitus View	Tracheal Bifurcation Rt. Retrocardiac space Rt. Middle lobe
Lardotic view	*Apex*[Q] *Lingual lobe*[Q]
Reverse lardotic view	*Interlobar effusion*[Q]

★ In **lingual lobe** pathology there **is obliteration of left cardiac shadow.**

★ **Golden S Sign** seen in **Rt upper lobe collapse.**

Right Anterior Oblique View

Oblique views are mainly used for cardiovascular abnormality

Position of patient & Cassette	Centring of X-Ray beam	Useful for
- ***Right side of the patient's trunk is in contact with cassette*[Q].** - Patient is rotated so that left , side is away from cassette.	At the level of 6th thoracic vertebrae	- To separate heart, aorta & vertebral column - ***Ascending, arch & desending aorta*[Q]** - ***Enlargement of the heart or aorta with barium studius.***

Veiw	Structure Seen
Cald well (Occipito-Frontal) View Mn- **Fishing Lovely Front For M E**	- *Superior orbital Fissure*[Q] - Lamina papyracea & superior margin of orbit - *Frontal sinus (Best seen)*[Q] - Foramen rotundum - Maxillary sinus - Ethmoid sinus
Waters (O-M/Occipito Mental) View Mn - **Maximum Spherical Front In the Zym**	- *Maxillary sinus (Best seen)*[Q] - *Sphenoid sinus (if film is taken with open mouth)*[Q] - *Frontal sinus* - Intratemporal fossa - Zygoma & Zygomatic arch
Basal (submentovertical) View Mn - **"SPM"**	- *Sphenoid, Posterior ethmoid, maxillary sinus (in that order)*[Q] - Zygoma & Zygomatic arch - Mandible along with coronoid & Condyloid process
Stenver's (Oblique posteroanterior) view	- Whole length of petrous bone, petrous tip - Internal auditory meatus (IAM) - Semicircular canals (superior & lateral) - Middle ear cleft - Mastoid antrum & mastoid process.
Perobital view	- *Best view of IAM* if tomography is unavailable - Petrous pyramid & apex - Vestibuli

- **Clinically bifurcation of trachea corresponds to:** ***angle of louis*[Q] *(lower border of manubrium sterni) in*** *front* and ***disc between T_4 T_5 vertebrae*[Q] *behind.***
- Trachea is seen as a central radiolucent air filled structure in the upper thorax which divides **at the level of 4th thoracic vertebra** (T_4 a/t Clark's / usually at **D_5 or D_6 level in adults** (a/t AIMPS) into the right & left main bronchus.

ENT

19. B i.e., Non contrast CT for nose & paranasal sinuses

[Ref: Harrison 17/e p. 205 – 07]

- **Bacterial sinusitis** is uncommon in patients whose symptoms have lasted for > 7days. This diagnosis is reserved for patients with *purulent nasal discharge and persistent symptoms (i.e. symptoms lasting > 7 days in adults or > 10-14 days in children).*

- CT or sinus radiography *is not recommended in routine cases,* particularly *early in course of disease* (< *7 days*) d/t high prevalence of acute viral rhinosinusitis.
- However, **CT (noncontrast) of sinuses** is the ***radiological investigation of choice in evaluation of persistent, recurrent, or chronic (lasting > 12 weeks) sinusitis***Q.

★ **Pott's puffy tumor** is advanced frontal sinusitis with soft tissue swelling & pitting edema over frontal bone d/t communicating subperiosteal abscess.

CARDIOVASCULAR SYSTEM

5

RADIODIAGNOSIS

20. A i.e. Thallium Scan: *[Ref: Grainger Radiology 5th/513- 515; Harrison 17th/1519]*

Nuclear cardiac imaging using radiotracers like thallium is the first line technique for evaluating reversible myocardial ischemia

Nuclear cardiac imaging

- **Nuclear cardiac imaging** is a first line technique for evaluating ***myocardial perfusion, viability (reversible MI) and function***Q. Technique involves IV administration of perfusion agents (radiotracers)
  - ***Thallium 201***Q
  - *Tc*[99] *labelled agents* i.e. Sesta MIBI, Tetrofosmin, Teboroxime
- Myocardial perfusion & dense tracer distribution depends upon difference in blood flow to normal and ischemic myocardium.
- Done in both rest and stress

Resting perfusion abnormalities seen in
- Reduced perfusion in viable myocardium (***reversible ischemia)***Q
- Myocardial infarction
- Fibrosis
- Area supplied by severe (> 85%) stenosis.

Stress technique
- Increases the difference between flow in normal & abnormally perfused myocardium
- Useful in coronary artery disease because *resting ischemia only occurs when artery is 85-90% occluded.*

MUGA : (multiple-gated blood pool imaging)
- Equilibrium radionuclide angiography
- Involves the imaging of Tc99 labeled albumin or red cells
- Used when : Echocardiography is technically difficult
  Poor LV function requires accurate quantification.

ECHO

Main value of echocardiography in ischemic heart disease (IHD) is in demonstrating
- Effect of IHD on ventricular function
- Detecting structural complications such as VSD, Papillary muscle dysfunction, Ventricular thrombus

21. B i.e. Echocardiography *[Ref: Sutton Radiology 7th/1150; Dahnert Wolfgang Radiology Review Manual 6th/70-71]*

Congenital heart disease (especially endocardial cuchion defects) is frequently found in Down's syndrome children.Echocardiography is therefore considered a necessary pre-operative investigation.

Down's Syndrome (Trisomy 21)

Skull	**Axial Skeletoss**	***Congenital heart disease (40%)***Q	**Ribs**	**GIT**
- Brachycephaly - Delayed closure of sutures & fontanelle - Hypoplasia of sinuses	*Atlanto-axial subluxation* (25%)	- Endocardial cushion defect - VSD - TOF	11 pairs	- Umbilical hernia - ***Double bubble sign***Q (duodenal atresia) - Hirschprung's disease

22. C i.e. MRI *[Ref: Grainger 4/e P-841, 956-58; Cardiovascular imaging 3/e p. 451]* **23. C i.e. MRI**

MRI followed by CT Scan is imaging modality (investigation) of choice for aortic dissection.Q

Investigation of choice for aortic dissection

- Stable patient → *MRI*Q
- **Unstable patient** → **Trans-esophageal Echocardiography followed by CT Scan**

Aortic dissection

- Most patients are in *50-70 years* age group present with *very sudden onset pain,* often accompanied by *tearing sensation.* It is usually felt in the *precordium & substernal* region but may be in back *between scapula.* These patients are usually misdiagnosed as having cardiac ischemia, which increases risk of complications.
- Dialation & dissection in ***Morphan Syndrome***Q are probably caused by a failure to resist shearing stress in media. In ***Ehlers-Danlos***Q collagen molecule abnormalities predispose to dialation & saccular aneurysms but not to dissection these patients have normal resistance to shearing stress.
- Stanford classifies it into two types as **Type A** (*involving ascending aorta*) – which is *more common* & carry high probability of complications & mortality; and **Type B** (*not involving ascending aorta*).

★ ***Aortography is the gold standard***Q

24. **C i.e. Echocardiography** *[Ref: Braunwald – heart disease 6/e P-1839; Ref: Wofgang 5/e P-585; Bhadury P-104; Grainger 4/e p. 716; Sutton 7/e P-332]*

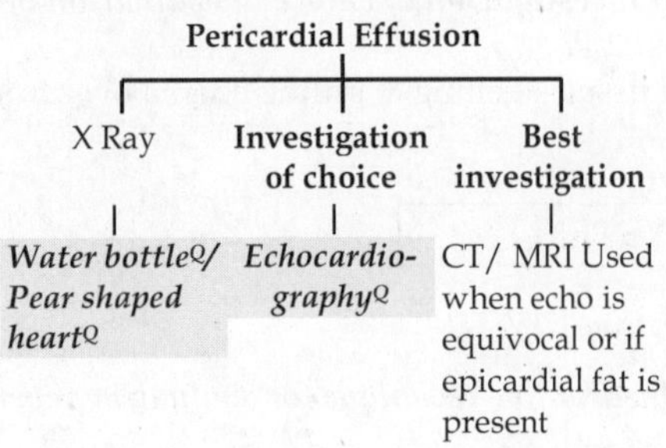

Pericardial Effusion

- P.E. is pericardial fluid > *50 ml*
- ***Best diagnosed by Echocardiography –M Mode***[Q] – there is seperation of epi & pericardial echoes extending into diastole.

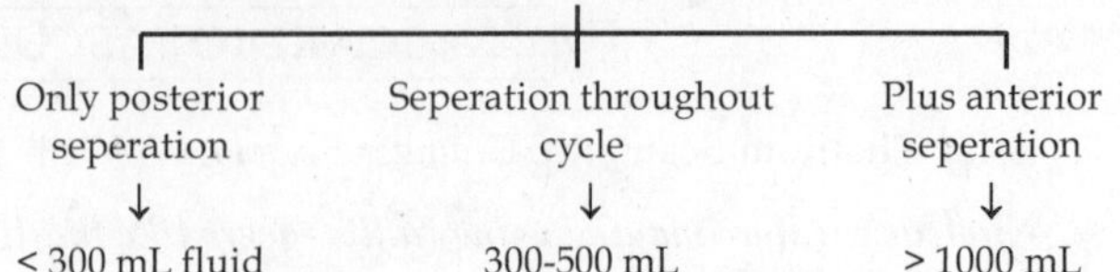

- CXR – signs are seen for >250 mL fluid, these are:
  1. ***Watter Bottle configuration***[Q] – Symmetrical enlargement of cardiac silhouette.
  2. *Fat Pad Sign* – Seperation of retrosternal from epicardial fat line > 2 mm.
  3. *Differential density sign* – Increased lucency at heart margins d/t difference in contrast between pericardial fluid & heart muscle.

25. **B i.e. Echocardiography** *[Ref: Sutton 7/e p. 318-319]*

Transthoracic echocardiography is the most commonly used cardiac imaging examination after the chest X-ray and probably approaches the electrocardiogram in its clinical utility. It is harmless and relatively comfortable for the patient and is the first-line technique for evaluating most abnormalities of the cardiac chambers, valves and great vessels.

Diagnotic utility	Chest X-ray	Transthoracic echocardiogram	Transesophageal echocardiogram	Nuclear medicine technique	Multislice CT	MRI	Angiography
Anatomy							
Myocardium	+	++	+++	+	++	+++	++
Valves	+	++	+++	0	+	++	++
Coronaries	0	0	+	0	++	++	+++
Pericardium	+	+	+	0	++	+++	+
Pulmonary vessels	+++	0	0	0	+++	++	++
Calcification	+++	+	+	0	+++	+	+++
Function							
Myocardium	++	++	+++	++	+	+++	++
Valves	+	++	+++	0	+	+	++
Coronaries	0	0	+	++	++	+	+++
Limitations							
Radiation hazard	-	0	0	- -	- - -	0	- - -
Risk/discomfort	0	0	- -	-	-	-	- - -
Spatial resolution	- -	- -	-	- - -	-	-	0
Temporal resolution	- -	-	-	- - -	- -	- -	0
Operator skill	-	- - -	- - -	- -	-	- - -	- - -
Cost	-	-	- -	- -	- -	- - -	- - -

+++ = Major utility; ++ = moderate utility, + = minor utility; 0 = no utility/no limitations; - = minor limitation; - - = moderate limitation; - - - major limitation

26. **D i.e. Endomyocardial Biopsy** *[Ref: Harrison 15/e P-2588]*

- RT and CT cause fibrosis; which can be **best diagnosed** by seeing the tissue under microscope – **Endomyocardial** ***Biopsy.***[Q]
- IInd best answer is **Radionucleotide** ***scan***[Q].

RESPIRATORY STSTEM

27. **C i.e. HRCT** *[Ref. Grainger 4/e p. 278, 279; Sutton 7/e p. 33; Hanga CT & MRI of whole body 4/e p. 838]*

High Resolution CT (HRCT) is *investigation of choice for* ***interstitial lung disease (parenchymal lung disease)*** and ***bronchiectasis***Q as it can delineate the lung parenchyma upto the level of secondary pulmonary lobule.

Principles of HRCT are:

1. Narrow beam collimation leading to thin section (≈ 1.5 mm) .
2. Small field view l/t increased resolution.
3. ***High spatial reconstruction algorythm (edge enhancing or sharp algorythm)***Q ***eg. Bone algorythm,*** that makes structure visible sharper & reduce smoothing, but it makes image noise more obvious.

28. **C i.e. Bronchography** *[Ref: Wofgang 5/e P-464; Harrison 15/e P-1486]*

- For diagnosing bronchiectasis **investigation of choice is *HRCT (highresolution CT) > Bronchography*Q (not scopy).**
- Bronchiectasis CXR Shows:

G	- Grape cluster *pattern*Q	
H	- Honey comb *pattern*Q	
O	- TOOth paste pattern	Mnemonic- **"Ghost**
S	- Signet ring pattern	
T	- Train /Tram - track *pattern*Q	

29. **D i.e. CT Scan** **30.** **B i.e. Interstitial Lung disease**

[Ref: Harrison 15/e P-1454, 1501; Consise Text Book of Radiology – Peter Armstrong -538]

- **Routine chest CT** examinations consists of adjacent *8-10 mm sections* through the area of interest.
- Intravenous contrast medium may be injected when the primary purpose of examination is to show the mediastinum or hilar structures.
- **High resolution CT (HRCT)** uses very thin *1-2 mm* ***thick.***Q HRCT of lung is *designed primarly to diagnose* :
  - ***Bronchiectasis***Q
  - ***Interstial Lung disease***Q as fibrosing alveolitis, asbestosis etc.
  - When lung biopsy is required, HRCT is useful for determining *most appropriate area from which biopsy sample should be taken.*

31. **C i.e. Doppler Ultrasound** *[Ref: Lee 12/e P-274, 450]*

Diagnosis of Air Embolism

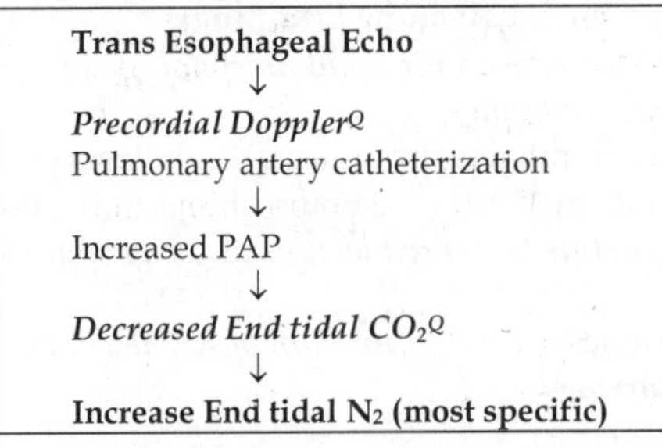

Trans Esophageal Echo
↓
Precordial DopplerQ
Pulmonary artery catheterization
↓
Increased PAP
↓
Decreased End tidal CO2Q
↓
Increase End tidal N2 (most specific)

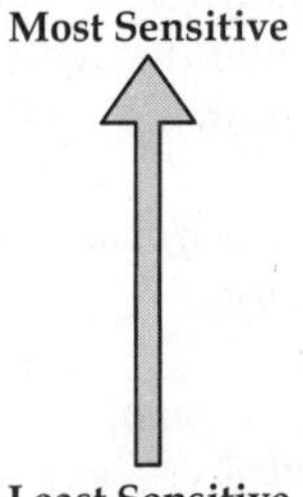

- On precordial / oesophageal stethoscope – ***Mill Wheel Murmur***Q is diagnostic of air embolism.

32. **B i.e. CT angiography** *[Ref: Harrison 17/e p. 1653 – 55; Grainger & Allison's diagnostic radiology 5/e p- 536- 43]*

33. **B i.e. Contrast CT** **34.** **D i.e. CT Scan**

[Ref: Grainger & Allison's diagnostic radiology 5/e p-536-43; Braunwald- Heart disease p1896l; Harrison 17/e p.1653-55]

Investigation of choice (IOC) is ***CT angiography (contrast CT) followed by pulmonary arteriography followed by a ventilation – perfusion scan***Q.

35. **B i.e. CT Scan** *[Ref: Wofgang 5/e P-464-65; Sutton 7/e P-45]*

Bronchiectasis

- **High Resolution CT** ***Scan***Q with sensitivity 97% & specificity almost 100% has become the ***investigation of choice***Q.
- Investigation of **IInd choice is** ***Bronchography***Q which is now occasionally *used in recurrent hemoptysis when all other investigations are* ***negative***Q, to demonstrate bronchopleural fistulas and congenital lesions such as sequestration & agenesis. It is ***C/I in massive hemoptysis***Q, active infections (TB, pneumonia) & impaired pulmonary function.

36. **B i.e. PA view in full expiration**

Disorders	View
Supraorbital Fissure	***Cald well view***Q
Recurrent Shoulder Dislocation	***Striker's view***Q
Sella Turica	Lateral skull view
Scaphoid	***Oblique view***Q
Patella	***Skyline view***Q
Minimal Pleural Effusion	***Lateral decubitus (Ipsilateral)***Q
Pneumothorax	***PA view in full expiration***Q

EXCRETORY SYSTEM

37. **B i.e. Coloured Doppler** *[Ref: Grainger 4/e P-1570]*

Renal Cell CA

- Best investigation for defining extent of **venous invasion and the proximal extent of thrombus in the inferior vena cava** → *MRI*Q *> Colour Doppler USG*Q
- Investigation of choice for **diagnosis and staging** → *Contrast-CT Scan*Q > MRI
- When contrast – CT is C/I or frequent followup is required in high risk patient → MRI

Condition	Investigation of choice
- **Small intestine tumor**	CT Scan with contrast
- **Cardiotoxicity** by CT & RT	Endomyocardial Biopsy
- **Dental pathology** & TM Joint pathology	Pantomography
- **Pregnant lady with upper abdominal mass**	MRI
- **Renal T.B. (Early)**	*IVP*Q
- **Renal T.B. (advanced stage)**	CT > IVP > USG

38. **A i.e. Radionuclide scanning** 39. **C i.e. 99 – Tc – DMSA**
[Ref: Love & Bailey 23/e P-1168-1170; O. P. Gahi 5/e P-364, Bhaduri 4/e P-343; Sutton 7/e p. 912]

DTPA (Renogram)	DMSA (Isotope Scanning)
- DTPA is freely filtered at glomerulus with no tubular reabsorption or excretion (i.e. GFR = Excretory function) - DTPA is useful for ***evaluating perfusion and excretory function of each kidney***Q - Indications: 1. Measurement of ***relative renal function***Q ***in each kidney.*** **2.** ***Urinary tract obstruction***Q 3. Diagnosis of ***Renovascular cause of hypertension***Q 4. Investigation of ***Renal transplant***Q	- T_C.99 DMSA is used for ***renal morphological (anatomic) imaging***Q - This compound gets fixed in renal tubules & images may be obtained after 1-2 hours of injection. Lesions such as ***tumors & benign lesions as cysts show filling defect***Q - Used to assess ***cortical function of Kidney***Q and ***detect renal scarring***Q.

GASTROINTESTINAL SYSTEM

40. **A i.e., Manometry** *[Ref: Harrison 17/e p. 1850; Bailey & Love 24/e p – 1020 –21]*

- *Prolonged ambulatory oesophageal manometry is the best investigation to* ***diagnose diffuse oesophageal spasm***Q. Solid bolus & edrophonium may induce both chest pain & motor abnormalities on manometric studies, whereas cold sollows only produce chest pain. Pressure on manometry may be 400-500 mmHg.

- **Barium swallow** shows that normal sequential peristalsis is replaced by uncoordinated simultaneous contraction producing ***Corkscrew appearance***[Q] i.e., multiple ripples, curling, sacculation & pseudo diverticula in the walls.

41. **A i.e. Endoscopy** *[Ref: Love & Bailey 24/e P-1001]*

- **G-O-Reflux is best diagnoses by *24 hours Acid study*[Q]** & the next best investigation is ***Endoscopy***[Q].
- *24 hours PH recording (Acid Study[Q])* is the ***gold standerd for GOR diagnosis.***

42. **B i.e. USG** **43.** **B i.e. USG** **44.** **B i.e. Ultrasonography**
[Ref: Sabiston 16/e P-1081; Pretest Schwartz 7/e Q-551; Wofgang 5/e P-665; Grainger 4/e P-1310]

- **USG** is most sensitive in detecting gall stone & is the **first screening** method and ***investigation of choice for gall stone (obstructive jaundice)***[Q].
- Most common cause of obstructive jaundice is stone in gall bladder or CBD. And the stones are best visualized by USG. Other advantage of USG is that it's a noninvasive & cheap procedure, easily available every where.
- If asked **obstructive jaundice d/t tumours** condition, then investigation of choice will be **CT Scan.**
- *Though **CT Scan** may yield similar information, is more expensive and is not good as ultrasound when the stones are concerned.*

USG

No ductal dilatation	*Extrahepatic ductal dilatation with or without intrahepatic dilatation*	*With only intrahepatic ductal dilatation*
ERCP	*ERCP*	*PTC*

45. **A i.e. USG** *[Ref: Harrison 15/e P-1763]*

Earliest detection	Investigation
Ascites	*USG*[Q]
Pericardial effusion	***Echocardiography***[Q]
Bronchiectasis	***CT-Scan***[Q]
Fetal life	*Doppler*[Q]
Pleural effusion	*I/L lateral decubitus view*[Q]
Pneumoperitonum	*Erect chest X-ray or left lateral decubitus abdominal X-ray*[Q]

46. **A i.e. USG** **47.** **C i.e. HIDA Scan**
[Ref: Schwartz 7/e P-1452; Bailey & Love 24/e p. 1097; Maingot 10/e P-75]

HIDA Scan & PIPIDA are ***best test to rule out acute cholecystitis***[Q] with.≈100% negative predictive value. It can be pseudo positive in chronic malnutrition, & Parenteral nutrition & alcoholic liver disease.

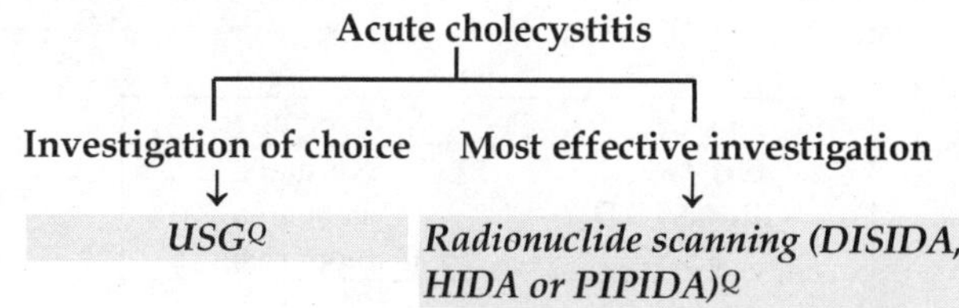

48. **B. i.e. PET > D. i.e. CECT** *[Ref: Maingot's Abdominal operation by Rechiry Maingots; The Onchologist 2008; 13 (suppl 2): 8-13 www. The Oncologist.com]*

- ***Tumour response to therapy in sarcomas, including GISTs is best moinitored by using both PET & CT***[Q], by combined PET/CT scanners for both anatomic & functional tumour evaluation.
- *Because sarcomas often show high metabolic activity* related to intense glycolysis, *PET using 18FDG is best for staging, restaging & tumour evaluation after treatment.*

GIST (Gastrointestinal Stromal Tumour)

- Mesenchymal tumour of GIT with either smooth muscle or neural differentiation.
- Immunohistochemically *C-KIT (CD-117) & CD 34 positive.*
- Most common site is *small bowel > stomach.*
- **Investigations** for tumour evaluation:

CECT

- *Method of choice in the initial diagnosis &* staging of GISTs.
- Is limited for evaluating tumour response to treatment & thus recurrence because sarcomas, including GISTs may not change size in response to therapy.

18 FDG-PET

- Is ***best for evaluation of tumour response to treatment & recurrence***[Q] by virture of its functional characteristic
- When *combined with CT, provides greater specificity and accuracy* in predicting the outcome.

5

RADIODIAGNOSIS

MUSCULOSKELETON SYSTEM

49. **B i.e. Odontoid View** *[Ref: Turek 5/e p – 806]*

Open mouth odontoid (peg) view is the best radiographic view to visualize upper cerical C1, C2 vertebraeQ***. Atlanto-axial (C1-C2) articulation and integrity of dens & body of C2 are best seen on the odontoid view***Q***.***

50. **B i.e. MRI** *[Ref: Maheshwari 3/e P-154; Grainger 4/e P-2451]*

MRIQ is the ***investigation of choice for imaging traumatic spine*** **(ex paraplegia)**. CT is second best investigation

51. **A i.e. Dual energy X Ray absorptiometry**
[Ref: Harrison 18/e 2602, 3125, 3102; Orthoteers.com; Bone Density & osteoporosis: An update of physicians]

Dual Energy X-ray Absorptiometry (DEXA) is the gold standard and investigation of choice for diagnosis of osteoporosis and assessing bone mineral density (BMD)Q***.***

DXA/DEXA/Dual Energy X-ray Absorptiometry

- It is a highly accurate X-ray technique that has become the *standard for measuring bone density* in most centers.
- Standard X-rays cannot detect bone loss until 30% of bone has been lost; where as DXA can detect as little as *1% of bone loss.*
- However DXA is a *two dimensional* scanning technique and *cannot estimate the depths or posteroanterior length* of the bone. Thus small people tend to have lower then average bone minerals density (BMD). Bone spurs, which are frequent in osteoporosis, tend to falsely increase bone density of the spine.
- Though it can be used for measurement of any skeletal site, clinical determinations are usually made of the *lumbar spine and hip.* Portable DXA machines have been developed that measures the heel (Calcaneus), forearm (radius & ulna) and finger (phalanges)
- In DXA, two scores are used

1) **T – score:** is *more important* and compares individual results with to those in *young population* (of same race & gender)

t-score	Interpretation
Upto – 1 S.D.	Normal
- 1 to -2.5 S.D.	Osteopenia
< - 2.5 S.D.	**Osteoporosis**

S.D. = Standard deviation

2) **Z – Score**: Compares individual with *same age* population (same race & gender) .

- FDA approved **indications for BMD tests** are:
  1. Estrogen deficient women at risk of osteoporosis
  2. Glucocorticoid treatment equivalent to ≥ 7.5 mg of prednisole, or duration of therapy > 3 months
  3. ***Primary hyper parathyroidism***Q
  4. Vertebral abnormalities on X-ray suggestive of osteoporosis (osteopenia, vertebral fracture)
  5. Monitoring response to an FDA-approved medication for osteoporosis
  6. Repeat BMD evaluation at > 23 month intervals, or more frequently if medically justified.
- Biochemical markers of bone metabolism in clinical use are

Bone Formation	Bone Resorption
- *Serum bone specific alkaline phosphatase*Q - *Serum osteocalcin*Q - *Serum peptide of type I procollagen*Q	Urine & serum cross linked **N – telopeptide** Urine & serum cross linked **C – telopeptide** Urine total free **deoxypyridinoline** Urine hydroxyproline Urine hydroxylysine glycosides Serum tartrate – resistant acid phosphatase Serum bone sialoprotein

- Noninvasive techniques for measurement of Bone mass in osteoporosis

1. ***Dual Energy X Ray Absorptiometry (DEXA)***Q **= Gold standard & investigation of choice**
2. Single Energy X Ray absorptiometry (SEXA)
3. USG
4. CT Scan – provides a true density but expensive & has greater radiation exposure.

OBSTETRICS

52. **C i.e. Amniocentesis** **53.** **C i.e. Anencephaly** *[Ref: Harrison's 18/e p. 508-18, 58, 865]*

- **Neural tube defects (NTDs)** i.e. ***anencephaly, meningomyelocele, encephalocele and spina bifida***Q can be caused by *antifolate & antiepileptic drugs, maternal diabetes, lower maternal folate status, reduced activity of 5, 10, methylene – THF reductase (MTHFR) enzyme* (d/t C677 T-polymorphism in MTHFR gene) and possibly by mutation of other enzymes eg. methionine synthase and serine-glycine hydroxymethylase. Folate supplementation at the time of conception and in first 12 weeks of pregnancy reduce 70% incidence of NTDs (and also hare lip and cleft palate).
- ***Neural tube defects are best detected by amniocentesis***Q. Earliest detectable congenital anomaly on USG is ***anencephaly***Q**.** It can be diagnosed as early as at ***10 weeks***Q**.** It is best diagnosed (100% accuracy) ***at 12 week.***Q
- Karyotypic analysis (for chromosomal abnormalities), biochemical & molecular analysis of DNA obtained from cells can be done in either chronic villi of 1st trimester or amniotic fluid of 2nd trimester fetus.

Test	Done at	Comment
Amniocentesis (removal of small amount of amniotic fluid)	***14-16 weeks***Q (early 2nd trimester)	- M.C. used procedure; M.C. reason to perform this is **advanced maternal age (>35 yrs),** the best known correlate of trisomy - Other reasons are - 1. **Abnormal (maternal serum) triple marker assay**Q *(HCG*Q*, α-Fetoprotein*Q and ***unconjugated estriol***Q in ***maternal***Q serum) and **inhibin** also (in **quad marker assay**) predict risk of *trisomy 21 or 18* 2. **Mid trimester USG abnormalities**Q – estimated risk of chromosomal abnormality is dependent on USG finding & is ***maximum in cystic hygroma***Q *>Omphalocele > congenital heart ds > nonspecific > choroid plexus cyst* 3. More recently, 1st trimester screening involving measurement of **nuchal translucency** (on USG) and *levels of PAAP-A and HCG* are used to identify women at increased risk.
Early Amniocentesis	12-14 weeks	Has greater risk of spontaneous abortion or fetal injury but provides results at an earlier stage of pregnancy
Chrionic Villus Sampleing (CVS) (Transcervical/ abdominal biopsy of fetal trophoblastic tissue/chorion)	Earlier *(8-12 wks)*Q preferably 10-12 wks.	- 2nd m.c. procedure. It allows for an *earlier* ***detection***Q of abnormalities & a safer pregnancy termination (d/t early diagnosis), if desired - Spontaneous abortions are more common in comparison to amniocentesis but is overall a safe procedure (spontaneous abortions <0.5 to 1%) - ***Risk of limb defects***Q increases if CVS is done **<10 *weeks***. So it is applicable during very narrow window of time
Percutaneous Umbilical Blood Sampling (PUBS) (fetal blood for lymphocytic culture)	2nd – 3rd trimester of pregnancy (> 18 wks)	- Done under USG control. Usually performed when USG abnormalities are detected late in 2nd trimester. - Also done to clarify cytogenetic results of amniocentesis as detection of *mosaicism.*
Pre implantation molecular diagnostic testing (eg- PCR)	***Before implantation invitro fertilization***Q **at 8-10 cell stage**	To detect single gene disorder such as –Mn : "**SC ST**" S - Sickle Cell Anemia C - Cystic fibrosis ST - Sachs-Tay disease (Tay-Sachs ds)

★ **Endometrial biopsy** is done ***at Premenstrual period***Q **to** avoid risk *of* ***endometriosis.*** **Chordocentesis** is done at *18 week*Q. Amniocentesis is not useful in cleft lip detection. ***Golden*** **Amniotic fluid** is diagnostic of ***Rh incompatibility***Q. **Saffron coloured meconium** is seen in ***post maturity***Q.

5

RADIODIAGNOSIS

NOTES